NEOPLASMS—
COMPARATIVE PATHOLOGY OF GROWTH IN ANIMALS, PLANTS, AND MAN

NEOPLASMS—
COMPARATIVE PATHOLOGY OF GROWTH IN ANIMALS, PLANTS, AND MAN

HANS E. KAISER, D.Sc., Editor

Department of Pathology
University of Maryland
School of Medicine
Baltimore, Maryland

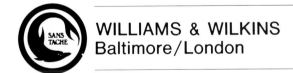

WILLIAMS & WILKINS
Baltimore/London

Copyright © 1981
The Williams & Wilkins Company
428 E. Preston Street
Baltimore, MD 21202, U.S.A.

Made in the United States of America

Library of Congress Cataloging in Publication Data

Main entry under title:

Neoplasms—comparative pathology of growth in animals, plants, and man.

Includes index.
1. Tumors. 2. Growth disorders. 3. Pathology, Comparative. 4. Tumors, Plant. I. Kaiser, Hans Elmar, 1928–xxxx [DNLM: 1. Neoplasms—Pathology. 2. Histology, Comparative. 3. Cell transformation, Neoplastic. QZ200 N439]
RC255.N46   616.99′2′071   80-12316
ISBN 0-683-04503-2

Composed and printed at the
Waverly Press, Inc.
Mt. Royal and Guilford Aves.
Baltimore, MD 21202, U.S.A.

In Memoriam

Martin Nordmann   1895–1980

Eminent researcher, teacher and physician, Professor Nordmann, through his distinguished contributions to medical science in his chosen field of clinical pathology, has constructed his own enduring monument. The present volume is greatly indebted to him, not only for his invaluable co-authorship, but also for his early interest in, and continuing strong support for, the objectives of the entire undertaking. Fortunate indeed are those who, as in my own case, could benefit from his warm and perceptive encouragement and profit from the fruits of a lifetime of such high professional achievement. It must remain, however, a source of deep regret for all those who labored on this work that he who made so vital a contribution to its initiation, concept and aims did not live to see its completion.

Hans E. Kaiser

The search for truth is sometimes easy and often hard.
It is difficult to master it fully yet impossible to miss it wholly.
Each scholar adds a little of his essence to
our knowledge and from all the facts there
assembled arises a certain grandeur.

Aristotle

Through knowledge of the vital processes in plants, the pathologist, too, gains most valuable insights toward an understanding of disease—on the basis of such an understanding, he, above all others, must become increasingly persuaded of the validity of the cellular theory.

Rudolf Virchow

Preface

This book, the first of its kind, is designed to illuminate the topic of neoplasms, the "cancer problem," from a broad comparative viewpoint using as its basis the normal growth patterns of the organisms involved. Neoplastic growth in animals and plants, and in man, is seen within the framework of abnormal growth. The neoplasms are viewed from the different aspects of comparative oncology, such as immunology and epidemiology, with selected examples to illustrate species-specific diversification.

The phenomenon of growth, one of the characteristics of life, can be looked at from many points of view as a part of normal biology. For this reason, abnormal growth should be seen within the framework of comparative pathology, and we should investigate it from all possible angles to gain a better understanding.

Because abnormal growth is a common pathological phenomenon of living matter, it cannot be understood in all its diversity unless we have a thorough knowledge of what constitutes normal growth in the various organisms.

The known types of neoplasms found in both the animal and plant kingdoms are examined in the sense of the two-kingdom approach, within the framework of the various types of pathological growth, such as granulomas, hyperplasias, cysts, and other forms.

It would be impossible in this book to elucidate comparative oncology in all its different aspects. Therefore, the following course has been adopted: (a) the authors of the various chapters have been invited to contribute only from their own fields of specialization; (b) only selected subtopics of the particular fields have been chosen to illustrate important aspects in these areas.

It is hoped that the comparisons presented here will facilitate a better understanding of the characteristics common to all neoplasms, as opposed to the particular characteristics typical only of certain groups or special types of neoplasms. It is also hoped that the present volume will clarify the phylogenetic stages that lead to the picture as we see it today, including not only the characteristics of the neoplasms of man but also those of higher animals and of plants.

An additional purpose of this book is to suggest a key according to which future research findings can be arranged on the basis of histological characteristics. Comparative functional histology and histopathology, knowledge of the distribution of chemical compounds in normal organisms and in pathologically modified organisms, and an understanding of the different types of ontogenetic development in living organisms will provide a foundation for comprehending the biological phenomenon of neoplastic growth, based on a broader and deeper understanding of comparative pathology.

The theoretical background for the present work involves the conviction that a comparison of larger numbers of phenomena than any attempt made previously, offers the possibility of a more penetrating perception and deeper understanding. It is for this reason that, through the co-authors, an effort has been made to shed light from the most varied angles on the problem of neoplastic growth.

H. E. KAISER
M. NORDMANN

Contributors

Andrew Ahlgren University of Minnesota, Minneapolis, Minn.

Ira H. Ames Department of Anatomy, State University of New York, Upstate Medical Center, Syracuse, N.Y.

A. Anders Genetisches Institut der Justus Liebig Universitaet Giessen, Giessen, FRG

A. V. Arstila Department of Cell Biology, University of Jyväskylä, Jyväskylä, Finland

Jose Barbosa University of Minnesota, Minneapolis, Minn.

Irene K. Berezesky Department of Pathology, University of Maryland, School of Medicine, Baltimore, Md.

Harriet Berg St. Paul-Ramsey Medical Center, St. Paul, Minn.

Umberto Binda Istituto di Anatomia e Istologia Patologica della Universitá, Milan, Italy

S. Boonyanit Department of Obstetrics and Gynaecology, Siriraj Hospital Medical Faculty, Mahidol University, Bangkok, Thailand

Joseph Buckley University of Minnesota, Minneapolis, Minn.

Walter J. Burdette College of Pharmacy, The University of Houston and The University of Texas, Health Science Center at Houston, Houston, Texas

Mario Cagnoni Department of Medicine, University of Florence, Florence, Italy

A. Camagna Ospedale Civile di Urbino, Urbino, Italy

James W. Carpenter U.S. Department of the Interior, Fish & Wildlife Service, Patuxent Wildlife Research Center, Laurel, Md.

Bruce Chesebro National Institute of Allergy and Infectious Diseases, Rocky Mountain Laboratory, Hamilton, Mont.

Emil Y. Chi Department of Pathology, University of Washington, Seattle, Wash.

Germaine Cornélissen University of Minnesota, Minneapolis, Minn.

Luciano Donati Ospedale Civile di Urbino, Urbino, Italy

Werner Düchting Department of Electrical Engineering, University of Siegen, FRG

Leland N. Edmunds, Jr. Department of Cellular and Comparative Biology, State University of New York at Stony Brook, Stony Brook, N. Y.

Peter J. Fischinger Laboratory of Viral Carcinogenesis, National Cancer Institute, NIH, Bethesda, Md.

Arthur E. Frankel Laboratory of Viral Carcinogenesis, National Cancer Institute, NIH, Bethesda, Md.

Constantine J. Gillespie Library, National Institutes of Health, Bethesda, Md.

Alfonso Giordano Istituto di Anatomia e Istologia Patologica della Universitá, Milan, Italy

Frederick Goetz University of Minnesota, Minneapolis, Minn.

Keith Griffiths Tenovus Institute for Cancer Research, Welsh National School of Medicine, Cardiff, Wales, United Kingdom

Piergiovanni Grigolato Istituto di Anatomia e Istologia Patologica della Universitá, Milan, Italy

Erna Halberg Chronobiology Laboratories, Department of Laboratory Medicine and Pathology, University of Minnesota, Minneapolis, Minn.

Franz Halberg Chronobiology Laboratories, Department of Laboratory Medicine and Pathology, University of Minnesota, Minneapolis, Minn.

Erhard Haus University of Minnesota, Minneapolis, Minn.

Howard M. Hayes, Jr. Environmental Epidemiology Branch, National Cancer Institute, NIH, Bethesda, Md.

Ronald B. Herberman Laboratory of Immunodiagnosis, National Cancer Institute, NIH, Bethesda, Md.

A. C. Hildebrandt Department of Plant Pathology, University of Wisconsin, Madison, Wis.

Raymond T. Jones Department of Pathology, University of Maryland, School of Medicine,

Baltimore, Md.

Millicent Kalil Department of Botany, University of Wisconsin Center-Waukesha County, Waukesha, Wisc.

Terukazu Kawasaki Second Department of Internal Medicine, Faculty of Medicine, Kyushu University, Fukuoka, Japan

Willard L. Koukkari Department of Botany, Biological Sciences Center, University of Minnesota, St. Paul, Minn.

Ernst Krokowski Zentral-Roentgeninstitut mit Strahlenklinik, Stadtkrankenhaus, Kassel, FRG

Marilyn Kuzel University of Minnesota, Minneapolis, Minn.

David Lakatua St. Paul-Ramsey Medical Center, St. Paul, Minn.

Renato Lauro II Clinica Medica, University of Rome, Rome, Italy

Francis Levi Chronobiology Laboratories, Department of Laboratory Medicine and Pathology, University of Minnesota, Minneapolis, Minn.

Howard Levine Department of Pediatrics, University of Minnesota, Minneapolis, Minn.

James B. Lewis Cold Spring Harbor Laboratories, Cold Spring Harbor, N.Y.

A. Lima-de-Faria Institute of Molecular Cytogenetics, University of Lund, Lund, Sweden

Barbara B. Lippincott Department of Biological Sciences, Northwestern University, Evanston, Ill.

James A. Lippincott Department of Biological Sciences, Northwestern University, Evanston, Ill.

I. Locatelli Ospedale Civile di Urbino, Urbino, Italy

Jack Mandel University of Minnesota, Minneapolis, Minn.

Midori Matsuoka Second Department of Internal Medicine, Faculty of Medicine, Kyushu University, Fukuoka, Japan

Mark Nesbit University of Minnesota, Minneapolis, Minn.

Eugene W. Nester Department of Microbiology, University of Washington, Seattle, Wash.

Martin Nordmann Formerly Institut für Klinische Pathologie, Hanover, FRG and Eberhard-Karls Universitaet, Tuebingen, FRG

Meliton N. Novilla Department of Pathology, Lilly Research Laboratory, Eli Lilly Co., Greenfield, Ind.

Teruo Omae Second Department of Internal Medicine, Faculty of Medicine, Kyushu University, Fukuoka, Japan

Donald J. Ortner Department of Physical Anthropology, Museum of Natural History, Smithsonian Institution, Washington, D.C.

Henry C. Pitot McArdle Laboratory for Cancer Research, The Medical School, University of Wisconsin, Madison, Wisc.

Alan Radke University of Minnesota, Minneapolis, Minn.

D. V. R. Reddy International Crops Research Institute for the Semi-Arid Tropics, Begumpet, Hyderabad, India

J. A. Romberger U.S. Department of Agriculture, Forest Service, Beltsville, Md.

Linda Sackett St. Paul-Ramsey Medical Center, St. Paul, Minn.

Mauricio Garcia Sainz Instituto Mexicano del Seguro Social, Mexico City, Mexico

L. E. Scheving Department of Anatomy, University of Arkansas for Medical Sciences, Little Rock, Ark.

Leonard Schuman University of Minnesota, Minneapolis, Minn.

M. Schwab Genetisches Institut der Justus Liebig Universitaet Giessen, Giessen, FRG

Mary W. Smith Department of Pathology, University of Maryland, School of Medicine, Baltimore, Md.

Edward A. Smuckler Department of Pathology, University of California, San Francisco, Calif.

Robert B. Sothern University of Minnesota, Minneapolis, Minn.

Thomas K. Soulen Department of Botany, Biological Sciences Center, University of Minnesota, St. Paul, Minn.

Thomas Spelsberg Department of Molecular Medicine, Mayo Medical School, Rochester, Minn.

John J. Stegeman Woods Hole Oceanographic Institution, Woods Hole, Mass.

Leroy C. Stevens Jackson Memorial Laboratory, Bar Harbor, Me.

Brunetto Tarquini Department of Medicine, University of Florence, Florence, Italy

Patrizio Tatti Ospedale Civile di Urbino, Urbino, Italy

George Tritsch Roswell Park Memorial Institute, Buffalo, N. Y.

Benjamin F. Trump Department of Pathology, University of Maryland, School of Medicine, Baltimore, Md.

Michio Ueno Second Department of Internal Medicine, Faculty of Medicine, Kyushu University, Fukuoka, Japan

Keiko Uezono Second Department of Internal Medicine, Faculty of Medicine, Kyushu University, Fukuoka, Japan

M. Vasta Ospedale Civile di Urbino, Urbino, Italy

Edmee Perez Vega Instituto Mexicano del Seguro Social, Mexico City, Mexico

E. Wagner Biologisches Institut II, Universitaet Freiburg, Lehrstuhl für Botanik, Freiburg, FRG

Donald F. H. Wallach Therapeutic Radiology Department, Radiobiology Division, Tufts University, New England Medical Center, Boston, Mass.

Lee Anne Wallach University of Minnesota, Minneapolis, Minn.

Elizabeth K. Weisburger Carcinogen Metabolism and Toxicology Branch, National Cancer Institute, NIH, Bethesda, Md.

Hans W. Wendt Department of Psychology, Macalester College, St. Paul, Minn.

L. Wetterberg Department of Psychiatry, St. Göreans Hospital, Karolinska Institute, Stockholm, Sweden

Douglas Wilson Tenovus Institute for Cancer Research, Welsh National School of Medicine, Cardiff, Wales, United Kingdom

E. B. Wittlake Arkansas State University, Museum, State University, Ark.

Acknowledgments

I am grateful to many persons without whose assistance this book would not have been completed. The greatest burden was borne, of course, by the contributors whose names are listed separately.

Special thanks are owed to the reviewers who have spent much time and effort in the improvement of the manuscript. The most significant contribution in this effort was made by Hans Falk. Among those reviewers who were most helpful are M. Ariel, L. M. Black, F. M. Hueber, H. H. Smith, W. A. Priester, M. Meeker, H. B. Tepper, R. Borchert, L. C. Vander Beek, J. C. Sutherland, K. Maramarosch, and S. E. Nawab. Additional reviewers have been approached by the contributors. I add my appreciation in their own behalf and thank them.

The following served as editors: B. Berz, J. P. Dickson, A. J. Feulner, D. P. Hammond, C. P. Lalire, J. Paradiso and N. Powers; for the artwork I am indebted to R. Rochkind. Of great assistance in computer retrieval and reference work were W. Sewell, C. Beebe, H. Gilbert, H. Listfeld, M. Listfeld, V. Hahn, J. Marquardt, C. Mc.Kissick, J. Miles, Jr., D. Mills, J. Ostrow and N. Petry.

Substantial help was provided by K. Baker, H. W. Casey, J. M. Dennis, C. C. H. Feng, G. Handlier, D. Hoffmann, I. Theloe and P. Zanibelli. A. Ally, D. Benton, B. Greer, C. McDonnell, P. Nikodem, and C. Wood-Robinson aided in the preparation of the manuscript. At Williams & Wilkins, Carol Eckhart, Production Coordinator, has provided attention to both detail and the author's wishes, with unfailing patience and courtesy. The assistance and patience of my wife Charlotte Kaiser were invaluable for the completion of this undertaking.

Hans E. Kaiser

Contents

I. FORMS OF ABNORMAL GROWTH AND HISTOGENESIS OF NEOPLASM

II. DISTRIBUTION AND FUNCTION OF NORMAL TISSUES

III. GENERAL REVIEW OF NORMAL GROWTH

IV. PATHOLOGIC (NEOPLASTIC) GROWTH

CLINICAL AND COMPLEMENTARY ASPECTS OF
NEOPLASTIC GROWTH

V. COMPARATIVE ASPECTS OF NEOPLASTIC GROWTH

Introduction

This treatise considers the problem of neoplastic growth, cancer and allied diseases, from a broad comparative aspect within the framework of abnormal growth. We intend to compare the processes involved in the transformation of normal to neoplastic cells as these take place in the different species. The different neoplasms will be examined from various aspects of comparative oncology such as pathohistology, biochemistry, virology, immunology, epidemiology, and genetic susceptibility. Species specific diversification will be illustrated by selected examples.

In the industrialized world, neoplastic diseases are a prime cause of death, ranking just after the cardiovascular disorders. In countries of the third world, these diseases rank third to parasitic and/or infectious and cardiovascular diseases. In contrast to the other disorders cited above, neoplastic growth, as a facet of abnormal growth, constitutes a basic phenomenon of life. Its spectrum is much broader than that of cardiovascular diseases and it is much more closely associated with the diseased organism through the processes of growth and transformation of normal body cells of the species involved. There is a partial remodeling, as it were, of the living matter of the organism concerned. This development occurs with respect to morphology (ultrastructure at the cellular level, and macroscopic tumor growth) and also to function (biochemical pathways, immunologic response).

The phenomenon of growth, as one of the basic characteristics of life, can be regarded from many points of view as a part of normal biology. It is for this reason that abnormal growth can best be examined within the framework of a comparative pathology. The field of comparative oncology is enormous. As we seek to present this discipline in all its various aspects, two basic criteria have been applied: the contributions of participating authors must be directed toward their own fields of specialization, and only selected subtopics of the particular fields were chosen to illustrate the most advanced aspects in these areas.

The investigations reported in these pages will demonstrate that progress in oncological research has been very uneven. This is particularly true of the morphological, biochemical and biophysical aspects of comparative oncology, as well as of studies of plant and invertebrate neoplasms.

In this book, we shall review the known types of neoplasms found in both the animal and plant kingdoms from the standpoint of the two-kingdom approach and within the framework of other types of pathological growth, such as granulomas, hyperplasias, cysts, and others.

A comparative review of the neoplasms reported to be present in the different groups of organisms is needed for two reasons: that we may conduct a comparative evaluation and that we may detect and identify hitherto unknown neoplasms. Two important conclusions can be drawn from the above:

1. In pathology, a phylogenetically regressive development to earlier phylogenetic stages may occur, but never an evolutionary forward development beyond the normal condition already achieved phylogenetically. The phylogenetic-systematical, or taxonomic, appearance of pathological changes must always be preceded by normal phylogenetic development, never the other way around.

2. If compared with the normal cells or tissues from which they are derived, neoplastic cells and tissues show only a modification toward the negative; morphologically and functionally, they are always of lesser value.

The comparison of the neoplasms already described and the assumption that hitherto undetected neoplasms still exist in the organisms rest upon these two facts.

Neoplastic tissues usually exhibit some characteristics of the tissues from which they derive, although highly undifferentiated neoplasms, such as a spindle-cell sarcoma, may constitute a partial exception. Neoplasms are tagged with the name of the normal tissue from which they derive; consequently, a thorough understanding of the normal tissues must form the basis for comparison of the neoplasms from the different phyla, which differ from each other because of the presence or absence of certain tissues. Thus, it is the principle of histogenesis that is the determining factor in such comparisons; all other parameters are not applicable. This statement becomes perhaps more readily acceptable if it is recalled that, even in the phyla and subgroups of a single kingdom, certain organs are not always found everywhere. The animal phyla of Tardigrada and Pentastomida, among others, for example, lack respiratory and excretory organs; their functions are performed by other structures, such as the integument. These facts indicate a special systematic distribution pattern of neoplasms in those organisms with true tissues, the metazoan animals, and the vascular plants (the histonia animalia and histonia plantae). The phylogenetic age of tissues varies, as evidenced by fossil remains. Hence neoplasms, too, are not all of the same phylogenetic age. True plant tissues are millions of years younger than true animal tissues.

It is important to bear in mind that the biologic value of the same type of tissue in different phyla may also vary, as, for example, in the case of the ontogenetic potential of a mesenchymatic stem cell which is able to produce cartilage and bone in a mammal, but not in a *Hydra* or flatworm.

Just as a coin has different sides, so does pathologic growth. The normal distribution of chemical compounds can partially explain these modifications. If the problem of neoplastic growth is viewed not only morphologically but also biochemically and biophysically, then we may approach a functional explanation of the general aspects and species-specific diversities of abnormal growth. Biochemical pathways of carcinogens in the cells and their reaction with cellular enzymes vary in different species. This variation explains the positive or negative neoplastic developments of the same initiator in different species. A comparison of closely and distantly related species, and their reaction to a particular carcinogen, can provide an insight into the processes that may lead to carcinogen-

esis. By the comparative approach, the pathways of carcinogenesis can be evaluated more meaningfully.

The mammal exhibits the highest tissue diversification in vertebrates, e.g. stratified epithelia, bone, etc. This can be better understood, once we realize that medicine itself has undergone a radical change. From being organ oriented, it has developed into a science based on biochemistry and the research in ultrastructures, and it is along these lines that we try to recognize, understand, and cure the diseases of man. In the foreground of these investigations are the processes taking place in the various types of cells, without which there would be no functions. Thus medicine has expanded the subjective, restricted point of view based on one species, man, leaving veterinary medicine aside, for a comparative treatment of diseases. From a practical viewpoint, such a comparison can be effected in two ways: first, through the incorporation of as many species as possible and second, through a treatment of the problem of neoplastic growth from the standpoint of various scientific aspects. In both cases we are faced with a multidisciplinary approach. The clinical sciences, especially pathology, provide the fundamental material for such a comparison, namely the most frequently, and from a special diagnostic standpoint, most carefully examined cases of human neoplasms. This, of course, is a tremendous change.

The philosophical background of the present work derives from the conviction that a comparison of a larger number of phenomena than hitherto undertaken offers the chance for a more penetrating perception which will result in a better understanding. A comparison of species, tissues and tumors on the one hand and of the multiplicity of tumors in a single species, specifically, those of man, on the other offers the statistical probability of a greater comprehension of the neoplastic event. This comparison is arranged in a five-step sequence: (1) species, tissues and tumors, (2) multiplicity of tumors in a single species: man, (3) multilateral illumination of the tumor problem, (4) species-specificity of neoplastic growth, and (5) the cellular reaction to neoplastic stimuli as the common denominator. It is hoped that the comparisons presented here will enable us to understand better the characteristics common to all neoplasms, as opposed to particular characteristics typical only of certain groups or special types of neoplasms. It is also hoped that the present volume will clarify the phylogenetic stages that comprise the picture as we see it today, including not only the characteristics of the neoplasms of man, but also those of other higher animals and of plants. These neoplasms have developed in convergent lines over a time span of two billion years, beginning with the Pre-cambrian period (see Chapter 1).

The spontaneous neoplasms of man are the best known. In this book these human neoplasms represent a focal point for comparison with those of other organisms. Experimental neoplasms induced in various species, especially rodents, may serve as supplements and are needed, of course, for the clarification of special aspects of the problem. It is important to use several species because direct comparison with a single species and the extension of these results to man seem to leave room for doubt. This has been demonstrated clearly by the screening studies of chemical carcinogens. However, the application of knowledge gained on a comparative basis will doubtlessly contribute to an understanding of human neoplasms. Immediate autopsy and human biopsy material may also help to clarify certain aspects of experimental oncology.

The final objective of every oncological treatise, including comparative oncology, must be a better comprehension of the process leading to neoplastic growth, with an eye to the possibility of combating it, especially in man.

At this stage we must return from our experiences with many species and aspects to man. We have to continue our investigations, but, at the same time not lose sight of the question, from which partial aspects can we expect, at the present time, the most important progress in cancer treatment? These expectations will continue to open up new questions as oncological research progresses; they will bring about constant changes which will give up a better chance for the continuous improvement of our therapy. The possibilities can be summarized as follows.

Our basic understanding is derived from the seven fundamental causes of cancer which can be grouped into two categories: chemical and physical. These two causes in turn may act in different ways on the structures and components forming the building blocks of the cells, thus causing a transformation of the cells from normal to malignant. For a basic understanding of these processes we cannot overlook the chemical pathways because they form the nucleus of our knowledge as far as malignant transformation is concerned. But since we need to know

which parts of the cells are subject to transformation, a study of the ultrastructure of neoplastic cells and tissues is of decisive importance. Next to its increased growth potential and its inferiority with respect to normal cells, the neoplastic cell does not possess a definite characteristic of its own. But this cannot be expected since we are faced here with a change in metabolism, that is, an aberrant biochemical process. This, again, is a reason why the problem of neoplastic growth must not only be considered from the standpoint of different species but also under the aspect of the various subfields of science and the most differentiated life stages. For a clinical treatment, today the following sciences are especially in need of extended research:

Psychology plays a part in preventive, diagnostic and prophylactic treatment that cannot be underestimated. Of greatest practical importance are the application of oncological results as, for example, during surgery, treatment of metastases, chemotherapy, radiation therapy etc. Another area which promises good results is the field of immunology, the defense mechanism of the body, strongly influenced by comparative oncology and further by the experiences gained during the regression of malignant tumors. Prophylaxis of metastatic growth should, in the future, become the center of clinical interest, and connected with it, organ transplantation. Since tumors and metastases can be regarded as the final stage of a broken-down metabolism, prevention of neoplastic cachexia assumes a considerable importance.

Finally, we can say that the multidisciplinary science of comparative oncology is one of the most interesting biological topics. On the other hand, cancer is one of the things most feared by man. But the species-specific and multidisciplinary approach is a fundamental science to a possible practical treatment of human tumors because a comparative oncology will open the doors for an applied solution of the cancer problem.

The contents of this volume reflect the ideas outlined above. The first part deals with forms of abnormal growth and the histogenesis of neoplasms. Chapter 1 defines neoplastic growth within the framework of abnormal growth, whereas the second chapter offers a comprehensive analysis of the principle of histogenesis. A discussion of the distribution of true tissues among organisms and the comparability of animal and plant tissues in Chapters 3 and 4 in Part

II provide the reader with a general review of normal growth in the various organisms.

Since we are dealing here with abnormal growth, we require a basic clarification of the boundaries and limitations of our topic. Growth as a basic phenomenon of life is a tremendously large topic. Therefore we have to establish on the one hand the boundaries between normal and abnormal growth, and on the other, where the border lines between abnormal and neoplastic growth lie. Furthermore, since we are able to distinguish between benign and malignant growth, we must evaluate the relationship between the different variations of growth from the point of view of pathology.

Each science has its own special, basic method. Actualism, which compares the timeless physical and other events of the present time with those of the past, is for geology while histogenesis is for oncology. The principle of histogenesis states that each neoplastic cell develops by transformation from a normal body cell. Such a change of the primary neoplastic cells is continued through the multiplication of these transformed neoplastic cells, resulting in a buildup of the primary tumor and its metastases. Such a neoplastic transformation is always accompanied by an inferiority of the resulting pathologic cells. With the exception of highly undifferentiated neoplasms such as certain spindle, round, or giant cell sarcomas, the parent tissue from which the neoplastic cells derived can be recognized.

The distribution of true tissues among the organisms as a precondition of neoplastic growth is reviewed in Chapter 3, and the comparability of tissues, best undertaken by a functional approach, in Chapter 4. This is logical because the purpose of each tissue is the fulfillment of one or more general and particular functions within the framework of the body.

Part III is devoted to the general review of normal growth and deals with a number of topics which, when combined, present the species-specificity of normal growth as a platform for abnormal growth.

Abnormal growth as we are confronted by it has been with us for millions of years and its different characteristics exhibit varying phylogenetic ages. The earliest beginning of cellular changes leading to today's characteristics of neoplastic growth may have started at the phylogenetic level of prokaryotic cells. A discussion of the time structure of a unicell, *Euglena*, by Edmunds and Halberg (Chapter 5), introduces the temporal aspects of growth problems encountered in human beings, other animals and plants. Rhythmic activity, as studied extensively in *Euglena*, is one of the cellular growth characteristics present in unicells, in organisms with pseudo-tissues and in organisms with true tissues. This phenomenon is revealed by the comparison of the rhythmic activities of *Euglena* and different tissues of mouse and hamster. Unicellular organisms can be used very appropriately in cases where a model is needed to investigate a characteristic of abnormal growth which is phylogenetically established in unicells. It would be unrealistic to use such a model to study factors of abnormal growth which can only occur in organisms with true tissues.

In Chapter 6 we examine fundamental aspects of normal organismal growth in animals. Special emphasis is given to the problems of indirect development in animals, because neoplasms are able to develop at each stage of ontogeny, with the exception of certain stages of cell invariable or highly regenerative structures. The time structure of vascular flowering plants, which make up the majority of plant species, is considered in Chapter 7 by Koukkari and Soulen and organismic time and metabolic control of development by Wagner in Chapter 8. Characteristic of vascular plants are tissues which retain an embryonal potential, at least theoretically, throughout the life of the plant. An example are the apical or lateral meristems which are the reason for the ability of continued growth, also for species-specific variations in the vascular plants. Similar tissues do not exist in animals but comparable ones are present in structures such as imaginal disks in holometabolic insects. Cohnheim, in his theory about the development of neoplasms from embryonal cell rests, referred to comparable structures such as the meristematic tissues in plants. The inclusion of these aspects of growth in plants enlarges our understanding. Fundamental aspects of normal growth in plants are discussed by Romberger in Chapter 9. Chapter 10 compares the development of man to that of other organisms and deals with such questions as the continuous character of man's ontogeny, regeneration, cell invariability in the human body, and the different potential of similar tissues in various phyla. Chapter 11, the last of Part III, by Spelsberg and Halberg offers new aspects of molecular chrono-oncology describing circadian rhythms found in the activity of RNA-polymerase of rat liver.

Part IV, devoted to pathologic neoplastic

growth, is the most diversified part of the book and is divided into general and selected species-specific aspects. The subgroup concerned with general aspects deals with two topics: In the first, Chapter 12, Trump et al. investigate the problems of cell injury as the basic initial cause. The second chapter of this group, Chapter 13, by Kaiser, describes and evaluates on a comparative basis such questions as the development of neoplasms from ontogenetic stages or tissues with embryonal potential and related topics such as embryonal tumors in man, Wilms' tumor, tumors of larvae as known from the fruit fly, *Drosophila*, and neoplasms of plants involving meristematic tissues. In addition, tumors found in the young and related questions, such as regeneration and cell invariability, are discussed. The second subgroup of this part of the book dealing with selected species-specific aspects of neoplastic (malignant) growth is organized according to special fields within the framework of comparative oncology. The first area of interest is concerned with the chronobiology of neoplastic growth. Thus, Chapter 14 by Halberg and co-workers deals with the newly evolving discipline of chrono-oncology. Chapter 15, by Scheving, is devoted more to the applied implications of this field by illuminating the chronobiological aspects of comparative experimental chemotherapy. The next segment of this mosaic is a discussion of the biochemical aspects of neoplastic growth. Species-specificity of normal biochemical pathways is dealt with in Chapter 16. These are seen against a background of histological and normal growth problems. Species-specific differences of normal biochemical pathways are seen as the precondition of a varying susceptibility of species to carcinogenic agents, such as chemicals or viruses. Species-specific biochemical pathways of malignant growth are the subject of Weisburger's discussion in Chapter 17. Aflatoxin and N-nitrosaminemethylurea were selected as the compounds under investigation. The activities of cytostatic compounds are also described in this chapter, with melphalan as representative. A third topic is experimental carcinogenesis from the species-specific point of view. A review of the various theories of the biochemical processes in the neoplastic cell is given in Chapter 18 by Pitot. Chapter 19, by Stegeman, deals with the interaction between the environment and the cell. An example are the hydrocarbons found in oceanic sediments and their interaction with benzo(a)pyrene hydroxylase in benthic fishes.

The third group of investigations is devoted to ultrastructure and biophysics of neoplastic growth. The ultrastructural characteristics of neoplastic cells in connection with the biochemical and biophysical, therefore functional, processes are the topic of Chapter 20, by Trump and Jones. It summarizes our knowledge of the ultrastructure and involvement of the different cell organelles in the cancer cell of animals and man. The aspects of neoplastic growth from a biophysical viewpoint are highlighted by Wallach in Chapter 21. The last chapter of this group, Chapter 22, by Düchting, examines the role of the control theory as the mathematical regulatory method for a better understanding of normal and malignant cellular growth. By borrowing from the field of mathematics such aspects as geometric progression, we can obtain a much more far-reaching understanding of the topic of neoplastic growth. This method results in a widening of the spectrum of our knowledge when we proceed from the various aspects of normal growth in animal and plant species.

The next stone in our mosaic is represented by the virology of neoplastic growth. This section of the book is of necessity interwoven with other sections, such as biochemistry, genetics, etc. Viruses can be regarded as macromolecular proteins and they share certain characteristics with genes. From experience we know that as initiating agents they are able to interact with other initiators and promoters as additive toxins. Chapter 23 deals with selected aspects of species-specific viral action, especially in relation to the characteristics they have in common with genes. We have identified several viruses which do or may play a role in the development of neoplasms and related disorders in invertebrates. For several of those viruses, their actions have not yet been fully ascertained. This field is briefly reviewed in Chapter 24. In vertebrates, DNA- and RNA-viruses play a role as tumor initiators or promoters. The latter are known as oncornaviruses; they are discussed as far as their origin, interaction, and oncogenesis are concerned in Chapter 25 by Fischinger and Frankel. Special emphasis is placed on the phylogenetic aspects of host-virus interactions and the recently established distribution of these viruses in certain host groups. A number of plant neoplasms are also known to be caused by viruses. The best known neoplasm initiated by a plant virus is the so-called wound tumor virus disease discussed by Reddy in Chapter 26. A fast-developing discipline during the recent years was the molecular biology of tumor viruses; their relations to different hosts are described by Lewis in Chapter 27. Because of their close relationship, the fields of virology and genetics of neoplastic growth are treated together. The durability of species, at least as far as we have been able to observe on the basis of recent discoveries in biology, is due to heredity. The science dealing with this phenomenon in all organisms, including plants and animals, is genetics. The comparability of animal and plant tissues was discussed in Chapter 4. As we continue these thoughts, it is very important that we now review the chromosomal similarities of plant and animal species. It can be considered a breakthrough in the comparability of plants and animals that Lima-de-Faria and other researchers succeeded in fusing components of plant and animal cells. In Chapter 28, Lima-de-Faria reports on his work. There is no doubt that genetic processes play a role of more or less importance in neoplasms generally and in particular types of neoplasms specifically. It seems to be necessary to distinguish between neoplasms that are produced by hybridization and therefore genetic factors alone, and the role genetic processes play in providing for a susceptibility to neoplastic transformation. Basic information on this topic is available from the fish, *Xiphophorus*, as pointed out in Chapter 29 by Schwab and Anders. These investigations particularly show how different organisms contribute to the whole neoplastic picture in comparative oncology. There exist only a few species of invertebrates of which pure-bred strains have been obtained. One of the best known animals in this respect is the fruit fly, *Drosophila*, of which genetic tumors in different aberrant tissues have become known; these are described by Burdette in Chapter 30. In vertebrates, the mouse is the animal of which the most pure-bred strains are available. The genetic influence on the development of gonadal tumors has been selected as one example for the study of the development of teratomas in this species by Stevens, as reported in Chapter 31. The interaction between genetic and viral influences during tumor development in experimental neoplasia are discussed by Chesebro in Chapter 32. With regard to plants, one of the most widely cultivated, and economically very important, is the tobacco plant. Hybrids have been studied extensively with respect to tumor development due to genetic crossing. These findings are evaluated and explained by Ames in Chapter 33 on the basis of his own investigations. The author also refers to the idea of cell fusion between animals and plants as performed by Lima-de-Faria and H. H. Smith, cited above.

One field of interest for future research, especially with respect to therapy is that of immunology against neoplastic growth. This field also can profit from a new impetus by comparative oncology. Species-specific aspects of this field are reviewed by Herberman (Chapter 34).

The remaining portion of Part IV deals with further applications: first, the epidemiology of neoplastic growth and second, clinical and complementary aspects of neoplastic growth. Cancer prevention is just as important as cancer cure. To make cancer prevention useful, animal models are needed which are more short lived than man, live in a closely related environment, and are taxonomically closely related to man *i.e.*, a mammal. Dog and cat are definitely such species. Generally they are not slaughtered in contrast to most other domesticated mammals. Development of spontaneous neoplasms in these two species with their many different breeds increases their value. Use of these species will enable us to shed light on human epidemiology in future decades and suggest preventive measures. The knowledge we can gain from these species is dealt with by Hayes in Chapter 35. In Chapter 36, Boonyanit and Kaiser review our knowledge of the geographical occurrence of neoplasms in the various human races. It shows that geographical and race differences are related to religious, ethnic, and professional habits as they are practiced in different regions of the world. But these factors are not the only ones of importance. They are called exogenic in contrast to the endogenic factors dealt with in Chapter 37 by Halberg *et al.* on international geographical studies of oncological interest. Studies of this type have shown that variations exist in the time intervals of hormone levels, for example, in the breast glands of women from different places such as Minneapolis, Milano and cities in Japan. These findings helped establish a convincing relationship between the appearance of breast cancer and geographical locations.

The melanomas are a very interesting group of neoplasms. In their precursor stages they may rest for years but then are able to metastasize very rapidly once their developmental stage is approached. The cells of these tumors can develop from different germ layers found in the animal kingdom. Cells with the major characteristic, the melanin pigment, occur also in plants, fungi and other lower organisms. The binding characteristic of these pigment cells is provided by that group of pigments which bridges the boundary between eumetazoan and vascular plants. It also occurs in pseudo-tissues, such as the plectenchymata of fungi, as well as intracellularly and extracellularly in the exoskeleton of insects.

This tumor type, described here from a clinical and comparative viewpoint by Giordano, Grigolato, and Binda, is a rewarding topic in comparative oncology (see also Chapters 29 and 43). Another topic with clinical implications which is not yet well understood is the regression of malignant neoplasms known from man and other species. It is reviewed in Chapter 39. A comparison of regressive processes in different species should lead to a better understanding of the circumstances which result in regressions of malignant growth.

In general, cancer patients do not die of the effects of the primary tumor but because of metastatic growth and cachexia which often occur simultaneously. Both of these processes are intimately related to the general body metabolism. Thus, prevention and treatment of metastasis must be regarded as one of the central problems of future cancer control. This is evaluated statistically by Krokowski in Chapter 40 on the basis of a large amount of patient data. New insights into this problem can be expected from studies of experimental comparative pathology on metastases as indicated in Chapter 41. This field, concerned with clinical and complementary aspects of neoplastic growth, closes with the review of the applicability of comparative oncology to therapy in Chapter 42.

Comparative aspects of neoplastic growth as discussed in Part II must be based on the principle of histogenesis, *i.e.*, the transformation of normal cells into neoplastic cells and tissues. To gain a realistic species-specific spectrum of neoplasms, the tumors and related disorders have to be seen according to their appearance and deviation from the normal tissues as they occur in the different organisms.

In contrast to human medicine, where neoplasms are classified according to the organs in which they appear and then secondarily according to the tissues from which they derive, in comparative pathology the neoplasms can be classified only on the basis of the tissues from which they derive (Chapter 43). This is the case because the different animal and plant phyla, in addition to the vertebrates, do not necessarily have the same organs as man. On the other hand, the neoplasms of man are those which are most often and with most difficulty diagnosed and histologically categorized.

Part VI of the book provides a systematic review of neoplasms beginning with the phylogenetic approach and ending with the detailed investigation of the crown gall, the most intensively studied malignant plant neoplasm. To gain an insight into the phylogeny of neoplastic growth, it is necesary to use the theoretical approach based on the geological principle of actualism, as noted above. These problems are outlined in Chapter 44 which is devoted to the phylogeny and paleopathology of neoplasms. Fossilized cases of neoplastic growth are very rare. Fossil plant galls are known from younger geological periods and are described in Chapter 45 by Wittlake, whereas bone tumors from archeological human skeletons were investigated and reported by Ortner in Chapter 46.

The large-scale disappearances of the faunas of the paleozoic and mesozoic eras were worldwide and could not have been caused by orogenetic[1] or transgressive[2] phenomena, or diseases which did not occur worldwide. But in cases where a species or another small taxonomic unit is already weakened, where it is affected by an increase of one or more diseases, species may be destroyed by such a factor or at least the time leading to extinction may be shortened. Several environmental factors can play such a destructive role. The chapter on neoplasms and other diseases in *Mustela nigripes*, the black-footed ferret, which is one of the rarest mammals of North America, by Carpenter, Novilla and Kaiser, deals with this topic and shows that in rare cases diseases may lead to the extinction of a species.

Chapter 48 provides in tabular form a systematic review of animal neoplasms, while Chapter 49 by Kalil and Hildebrandt discusses general aspects of pathology, the distribution of plant tumors and related disorders. Cellular transformation and ultrastructure of the crown gall are dealt with by Chi and Smuckler in Chapter 50, whereas the characteristics and particularities of crown gall as a malignant plant tumor are reviewed in Chapter 51 by Lippincott and Lippincott.

Molecular events, such as the incorporation of nucleic acids from the crown gall causing *Agrobacterium tumefaciens* into the crown gall cells,

---

[1] Processes of mountain formation.

[2] Spreading of the sea of land areas followed by sedimentation.

are described and evaluated by Nester, Chapter 52. These processes offer an interesting extension to the genetic and biologic chapters.

The VIIth and final part of the book summarizes the conclusions which can be drawn from the bird's eye view of comparative oncology as presented in this book. The interactions of the many fields and subfields enable us to understand the complexities of neoplastic growth.

Chapter 53 by Kaiser evaluates prospects for the future and Appendix I (Chapter 54) by Arstila and Kaiser addresses the use of model microcosms for simulating the role of the environment in comparative experimental oncology. Appendix II (Chapter 55), also a practical advice, reviews cancer information sources as compiled by Gillespie.

A glossary of human tumors with various synonyms used today and the indexes comprise the final sections.

Note in proof: As this volume was being typeset, J. C. Harshbarger's 1979 supplement of the activities report, *Registry of Tumors in Lower Animals* (National Museum of Natural History, Smithsonian Institution, Washington, D.C.), was published. Information found therein negates the statement made in this volume on page 150, the final sentence in the fourth paragraph, regarding the absence of a prostate gland in cetaceans.)

I

Forms of Abnormal Growth and Histogenesis of Neoplasms

1

Neoplastic Growth

Hans E. Kaiser and Martin Nordmann

Growth is the one characteristic common to all living matter. The process is of species-specific duration and, as a rule, it continues from the parent cell or cells to the fully developed organism. The embryonal potential of this growth process varies, and significant variations can be distinguished in different organisms. For example, the meristematic tissues of plants have, at least theoretically, unlimited embryonal potential through the whole life of a vascular plant. In the case of invertebrates, more or less extended embryonal processes of larval stages may be introduced, and it is possible that in single stages extensive autolytic processes of whole organ systems may occur. The renewed buildup of replacement systems in the next larval stage derives again from cells with embryonal potential (Table 1.1). Individual components of the normal growth process are always synchronized and regulated (for example, by hormonal action). Innumerable ontogenies constitute the phylogenetic process. Hologeny comprises both processes, the ontogenetic and the phylogenetic process.

Pathological processes can interrupt the normal growth of an organism at any developmental stage. This pathological growth may fit into the regulatory framework of the organism, where it does not necessarily escape such regulation; or it may become autonomous, as in neoplastic growth and especially malignant growth. Based on the histological derivations of human neoplasms, it may be concluded that within the basic principle of histogenesis lies the sole fundamentally applicable basis for a comparative classification of neoplastic growth.

Distinctions can then be made among different types of abnormal growth in various organisms. Based on the cellular makeup and the tissue compositions of the organisms involved,

it is possible to distinguish the following anomalies and abnormalities:

I. Growth anomalies of unicellular organisms
   A. Cellular abnormalities at the prokaryotic stage
   B. Cellular abnormalities at the eukaryotic stage
      1. Nuclear anomalies
      2. Cytoplasmic anomalies
II. Anomaly of cell accumulations. This phenomenon is nearly unknown in animal phyla. The term applies only to the mesozoans and the majority of sponges, and is widely distributed in such organisms as the fungi and algae; it may also occur as plant galls in certain algae, fungi, lichens, and mosses
III. Growth disturbances in organisms with true tissues, eumetazoan animals (including man), vascular plants, and certain of the higher nonvascular plants, in the sense of the two-kingdom approach
   A. Phylogenetic growth disturbances: organ disharmonies, decentralizations
   B. Nonneoplastic ontogenetic growth disturbances
      1. Malformations
      2. Diminished growth
         a. Congenital failure of development
            (1) Agenesis
            (2) Aplasia
            (3) Hypoplasia
         b. Acquired: atrophy
      3. Excessive growth
         a. Hyperplasia
         b. Hypertrophy
      4. Disturbances of cellular differentiation: metaplasia
      5. Appearance of tumor-like masses during ontogeny
      6. Repair: granulation tissues
   C. Neoplastic growth
      1. Epithelial animal neoplasms
      2. Mixed animal neoplasms
      3. Mesenchymal or nonepithelial animal neoplasms
      4. True neoplasms of vascular plants
      5. Certain hypertrophic plant neoplasms
   D. Abnormal growth: a comparative view

Definition of the relationships among the different types of abnormal growth as seen from a

3

Table 1.1
Tissues with Embryonal Potential

Group of Organisms	Tissues with Embryonal Potential	Percent Occurrence
Invertebrates	Larval tissues	
Nemertinea	Certain types of complicated metamorphosis	
Arthropoda		
Crustacea	Embryonal larval cells of "Kentrogon"	Up to approximately 95% by time and potential
Cirripedia	Cells of imaginal buds of holometabolic insects	in certain exceptional cases, i.e., 17-year lo-
Insecta		cust (*Magicicada septendecin* and *Magicicada cassini*)
Vertebrates	Blastemas	Embryonal potential of 100% generally ceased after less than 0.5% of life span (75 yr) in man
	Embryonal connective tissue shows the embryonic potential but is very limited in appearance	
	Embryonal cell nests under pathologic circumstances (Cohnheim's Embryonal Cell Theory of Cancer)	
Vascular plants	Meristematic tissues	100% or less, dependent on type and location
	Apical and lateral meristems	
	Primary and secondary meristems	
	Intercalary meristems	

phylogenetic and comparative point of view may justifiably precede discussion of the relationships of neoplastic growth, that type of pathological development most important to man. The following types of abnormal growth may be distinguished, with certain added characteristics.

ABNORMAL GROWTH OF UNICELLULAR ORGANISMS

At the level of unicellular organisms, some forms of abnormal growth may be considered as preneoplastic conditions.

Ontogenetic Abnormalities

Cellular Abnormalities at the Prokaryotic Stage. We are dealing here with a nearly unknown pathology, especially that of the bacteria and blue-green algae.

Cellular Abnormalities at the Eukaryotic Stage. Of the cellular abnormalities at the eukaryotic stage, the most interesting are the pathological conditions of protozoans, where a distinction may be made between nuclear anomalies, for example, and cytoplasmic anomalies.

Phylogenetic Abnormalities

Phylogenetic abnormalities at the level of unicellular organisms are manifested by development of phylogenetic variations of unicellular organisms, e.g., of giant size, that soon become extinct. Characteristic examples are the foraminifera and the *Bolivionoides* species from the Senon of northwest Germany (6). These conditions must be considered as phylogenetically abnormal, but they are not pathological.

ABNORMAL GROWTH OF CELL ACCUMULATIONS

Ontogenetic Abnormalities

In this category belong certain plant galls of green and other algae, as well as growth abnormalities in fungi. Nothing is known from the animal kingdom. Galls on the green alga *Urospora mirabilis* have been described, as have deformations on *Boletus grannulatus* (Chapter 49).

Phylogenetic Abnormalities

Phylogenetic anomalies are unknown at the level of cell accumulations.

ABNORMAL GROWTH IN ORGANISMS WITH TRUE TISSUES

Abnormalities of Phylogenetic Growth

There have been disturbances of organ topography appearing in a number of different genera, as in ammonites, dinosaurs, etc., that have led at least partially to their extinction. They are all genus-specific. Our diagnosis of fossil remains has shown that so-called organ disharmonies, in which no vital functions have been affected during phylogeny, and that alone could not lead to extinction, can be distinguished from anomalies like the so-called decentralizations, e.g., the relationship among brainstem, vagus nerve, and the periphery of the body, which can be considered as reasons for extinction of the particular developmental lines affected. Decentralizations, which are always genus-specific, may also have occurred in those types of organisms exhibiting organ disharmonies, but their remains have been lost because of incomplete fossilization of internal organs and other soft portions of the body. The sauropod dinosaurs are a typical example; despite their occurrence in a different hierarchical order, they remind us somewhat of malformations. In the phylogenetic process, whole genera are involved, in contrast to the situation with malformations, in which only individuals or, at the most, families of individuals are affected.

Nonneoplastic Ontogenetic Growth Disturbances

Excessive Growth. Excessive growth may be manifest as hypertrophy or hyperplasia. Hypertrophy is an overgrowth resulting from an abnormal increase in the size of an organ or of cells. This condition is known in animals and plants, as well as man. The cells of the tissue under hypertrophy increase in size but not in number; it is therefore only an increase in unit size, an increase that ceases after the stimulus is gone. Thus, hypertrophy may occur, for example, through increased use of a muscle or because of hormonal stimulation in the breast; it regresses after the stimulus ceases to act. Circulation and food supply increase with the heightened demand. The different types of tissues in the bodies of organisms display varying capacities in this regard. This increase in unit number results in demands similar to those in hypertrophy.

It does not appear that hypertrophy exists in cell-invariable species. From experience with ontogenetic development during which proliferation is lost, as in the case with human neurons or cardiac musculature, it may be assumed that hypertrophy can exist in certain stages of ontogenetic development of cell-invariable species.

Disturbances of Cellular Differentiation: Metaplasia. If one type of cell changes into another, the process is called metaplasia. Metaplasia is always a change into cells of a related kind. Thus, proliferating fibroblasts and vascular endothelial cells may produce not only fibrous tissue and new vessels, but also other differentiated mesenchymal tissues, namely cartilage, bone, mucoid connective tissue, adipose tissue, and even hematopoietic cells, but they never produce epithelium or nervous tissue. Conversely, epithelium of one kind may change into epithelium of another kind, e.g., epithelia of the respiratory, alimentary, or urinary passages may become stratified and squamous; but epithelium never becomes converted into connective tissues (15).

Causes for this phenomenon, which occurs in animals and man, are chronic inflammation, impairment of nutrition, change of function, etc. Metaplasia is common during neoplastic development. It may be a precondition for neoplastic change, e.g., the change from columnar to squamous cell epithelium in the bronchial epithelium. It is also known from cells of the connective tissue, because of the omnipotency of the mesenchymal cell. In plant pathology it is considered a "changed condition of a structure or organ; hyperplastic class of symptoms characterized by overdevelopment other than that due to hypertrophy or hyperplasia. Examples: abnormal starch accumulation, virescence" (11).

The previously cited limitations of metaplasia are important for an understanding of neoplastic growth. These limitations may be expected to exist among the same tissues of convergent lines in relation to the growth potential in these particular groups. For example, a smooth-muscle cell in a lower aschelminth will have a more limited growth potential than in a highly developed mollusc. The mesenchymal cell of the aschelminth is incapable of changing into cartilage by way of metaplasia, but the mesenchymal cell in the squid or the horseshoe crab, for example, has this capability. Today, the aschelminths and the annelids exist side by side; they exhibit mesenchymal cells as well as smooth musculature, but the potentials of these mesenchymal cells and of the smooth musculature are not alike with respect to metaplasia, because of differences in the course of phylogenetic development as reflected by their present taxonomic positions.

These limitations of metaplasia demonstrate the following:

1. Variations in cellular metaplasia can occur because of the age of an organism, animal or plant. Plant meristematic or animal cells with high embryonal potential, such as cells during larval or early embryogenic development, may be capable of giving rise to a wide variation of abnormal cells, such as the mesenchymal cell, as can be observed in teratomas or in the tissue family of epithelia. Therefore, plant or animal cells may be capable of causing different metaplastic changes in different life periods.

2. In the completed adult organism, variation of metaplastic change may be increasingly restricted with advanced age, a condition that will, of course, be associated with increased loss of embryonal potential, as seen in the cardiac muscle cells, or, with respect to cell relations, in the incapability of nerve fibers to regenerate, as in the brains of mammals. The latter condition may perhaps result from the absence of Schwann cells, which clear the way for nerve regeneration. For different species of various phyla with varying regeneration potentials, this comparative pathological picture will become even more complicated.

3. On the basis of our present understanding of the problem, changes from embryonal potential cells of one tissue family to another are unlikely to occur. However, in certain cases this may indeed happen; our experience is simply too limited. For example, connective tissue of a given phylogenetic stage that under normal conditions has failed to construct the next higher type may not build such a tissue under either pathological conditions or in a neoplastic caricature; e.g., bone neoplasms cannot occur in an invertebrate. It is important to bear this in mind in the expectation that the phylogenetic taxonomic levels of the same tissue in different phyla or subunits may not be totally equal but may vary to a considerable extent.

4. In retrospect, it is possible to discriminate between direct and indirect neoplastic transformation with interpolated metaplasia. Direct neoplastic development leads to the production of a neoplasm that still shows its origin from the original tissue. Direct development, for example, is an origin or development of a squamous cell carcinoma from squamous cell epithelium. Indirect development, on the other hand, is development via the interpolated stage of metaplasia; it is also indicated when the origin of a squamous cell epithelium occurs via metaplasia of squamous epithelium developing as metaplastic epithelium from columnar cell epithelium. The pathological ontogenetic relationship of both conditions forms the basis for their differentiation (Table 1.2). Direct derivable neoplastic origin without metaplastic change, and such origin with metaplastic change, may constitute the most common types of neoplastic origin in the organisms of the various groups. Basic experience with metaplastic processes during phylogenetic development leads us to expect that particular tissues of the organisms are comparable with regard to neoplastic processes, on the basis of the principle of histogenesis. A smooth musculature, for example, will at least theoretically be able to produce a leiomyoma or leiomyosarcoma where the normal smooth musculature occurs.

However, four limitations apply to these general theoretical possibilities:

1. The metaplastic potential of a given tissue type (e.g., the mesenchyme) must be considered as being variable because of the phylogenetic-taxonomic position of the organism involved. As pointed out earlier, a mesenchymal cell in an aschelminth is incapable of changing into a bone cell during metaplastic transformation, but the mesenchymal cell of the vertebrate does have this capability.

Along the indirect course of histogenesis (via metaplasia), the potential spectrum of development from the normal stem cell to the preneoplastic transfer cell and, finally, the neoplastic cell must have increased with taxonomic progression during the earth's history. The stem cell of a particular tissue type in lower animals may not have been able to produce the variety of metaplastic precursors to neoplastic cells as occurred with the stem cell in taxonomically higher animals and plants with a broader normal tissue spectrum. This conclusion receives indirect support from the fact that lower animals may not at all produce true neoplasms e.g., interference of regenerative capacity, or may only produce such preneoplastic conditions as regenerative or hyperplastic effects. The resulting neoplasms of the tissues of lower animals can be compared with human neoplasms because of the fact that man has the largest and best known tumor spectrum. There are, of course, exceptions. This does not hold true for certain tissues not common in man, such as the oblique striated musculature. Certain other limitations of com-

Table 1.2
Metaplasia, A Particular Type of Cellular Change, Which May Lead to Neoplastic Growth.[a,b]

Direct Transformation	From Normal Cell	Exhibiting Cell Inferiority	To Malignant, Neoplastic Cell
+	Squamous cell epithelium	+	Squamous cell cancer
+	Pulmonary epithelium	+	Oat cell carcinoma
+	Connective tissue	+	Round or spindle cell sarcoma

Indirect Transformation (Metaplasia)	From Normal Cell	Via Change of Tissue Character and Cell Inferiority	To Malignant, Different Neoplastic Cell
++	Bronchiolar columnar epithelium	++	To squamous cell (bronchiogenic, epidermoid cancer of lung)
++	Columnar epithelium of endocervix	++	Squamous cell cancer of cervix
++	Columnar epithelium of gallbladder	++	Squamous cell cancer of gallbladder

[a] The most cases of malignant, neoplastic transformation produces inferior cells of the same tissue type. The origin may be undetectable in the case of highly malignant tumors, exhibiting only a nucleus and a narrow rim of cytoplasm.
[b] Connective tissue metaplasia, leading in nonneoplastic cases from connective tissue in scars, arteriosclerotic blood vessels and degenerated areas to cartilage and bone where these tissues do not belong.

parative potential must also be applied to a comparison with such plant tissues as meristems or functionally nonliving plant tissues.

2. Furthermore, a phylogenetic normal change must always precede a neoplastic change. As known from conditions in man, not only will we find limitations of the tissue family (epithelium will never change metaplastically to connective tissue), but also it is not possible that a phylogenetically higher state than the normal tissue condition can be reached in the pathological sequence. A ganoid fish, for example, will not be able to develop an osteoma or an osteosarcoma.

3. Cell-invariable tissues or organisms, at least theoretically, are able to produce only neoplasms in a pre-cell-invariable youth stage, as we know from the neuroblasts in man. This is well known with respect to the neuroblastomas. It can occur that an invertebrate will produce a bonelike calcifying metaplastic or neoplastic tissue, but never a real bone tumor, even via metaplastic development. Such a transformation cannot occur because, on the one hand, neoplastic tissues are always of lesser value than the normal tissues from which they derive and, on the other hand, a phylogenetically higher development is always attained by normal development.

4. Impairments of the general picture of cellular differentiation are also complicated by the presence of different types of sequences of ontogenetic stages in the organism, such as in the case of normal autolysis of whole tissues or even organs, primary or secondary embryogeny, and continuing and catastrophic development.

Appearance of Tumor-like Masses during Ontogeny. These are found in animals, including man, and plants. Hamartomas are congenital defects in development of tumor-like character, composed of a mixture of tissues normally found in the particular area concerned. In special cases they also can be considered as neoplasms, and neoplasms may derive from them. Pigmented nevi or moles are well-known examples.

Heteropias are usually congenital, but they may also originate through tissue displacement, as in the case of injuries. They indicate the presence of a tissue in an area to which it is foreign.

Repair. Distinction can be made between repair of first or of second intention. Repair is proliferation of tissues to fill a breach caused by injury or disease. It can be considered as a pathological as well as physiological process, for wounds are common incidents in the lives of all classes of animals and plants, and the capacity to repair them is clearly a necessary self-preservative function without which none but the most sheltered individuals would ever attain adulthood. If no wound ever stopped bleeding or ever healed, man and most other vertebrate species would become extinct in a single generation.

Different classes and species of living things differ greatly in their capacity to repair injuries and lost parts. In many plants and many of the lower invertebrates, a small fragment can regenerate a whole organism, for example, cuttings or slips from small terminal branches or twigs are the horticulturist's usual means of propagating many kinds of trees and shrubs, *Hydra* and many other coelenterates may be cut up in many fragments, and each fragment will grow into a complete organism. Earthworms may be cut in half, and each half will regenerate a new tail or head as required. Structurally more complex creatures do not show this total or nearly total power of regeneration; nevertheless, some species have retained the ability to grow complete new parts. Thus, crabs can regenerate complete claws when these have been lost; snails can regenerate eyes; even among vertebrates, newts and allied amphibia can regenerate lost limbs or tails, and some lizards can grow new tails. Mammals do not regenerate complex parts such as eyes or limbs, but they possess great power of regeneration of many individual tissues, especially vascular, connective, bony, hematopoietic, and most epithelial tissues. It is convenient to distinguish two types of regeneration following injuries in mammals, namely (a) repair, which is the proliferation of tissues at the site of injury to fill the gap, and (b) compensatory regeneration, which is the proliferation of tissues with specialized functions, e.g., liver epithelium or hematopoietic cells, to compensate for those destroyed. The local repair of physical injuries is effected by the proliferation of vascular and connective tissue (or, in bone, bony tissue) to fill the breach, as well as proliferation of the overlaying epithelium if a surface is broken. Two types of wound healing may be distinguished: (a) Healing by first intention occurs in the case of the clean incised wound, where only a few cells are destroyed. Some vascular endothelial cells follow the fibroblasts and the fibrin coagulum that escape from the body fluids and cement the incision together. The few destroyed cells are removed, and if this happens to the epithelium, a new layer of the epithelium grows over. If both sides of the incision are not closed in this way, a larger blood clot will form, and we approach the condition of healing with second intention, characterized by granulation tissue that later becomes a scar. (b) In the case of severe injury, unification of the surrounding tissue will be undertaken by granulation tissue, which will change into scar tissue later. Both tissues are composed of fibroblasts that continue to develop more and more collagen. Vessels, macrophages for tissue destruction, lymphocytes, granulocytes, and plasma cells are also present. The remaining scar tissue is similar in makeup to the tissues of tendons or fasciae. In certain cases, scar tissue can also be considered as a preliminary stage of neoplastic tissue. There is some variation in the repair of different tissues. Tendons with closed cut ends will be repaired by new, properly oriented tendinous tissue. A fractured bone first shows the stage of granulation and periosteal proliferation, then the formation of young bone or callus and medullation of the newly formed bone. Young cartilage is repaired through the formation of new cartilage from perichondrial granulation tissue. Repair of blood vessels occurs by sealing, the clotting of blood; this involves either occlusion of a whole vessel by internal thrombosis with collateral circulation or, sometimes, recanalization. The two types of repair of epithelia have already been mentioned. Blood is regenerated by hemorrhage. Repair of adult muscle tissue usually takes place by granulation and formation of fibrous scar tissue. The repair of nervous tissues varies. In the case of peripheral nerves, perhaps because of the presence of Schwann cells, the fiber is able to regenerate; this does not take place in the central nervous system, where cell body and fiber are incapable of regeneration. Regeneration of a peripheral nerve fiber includes the following steps: regeneration proximal to the injury; degeneration distal to the injury; proliferation of Schwann cells ("*Bahnung*"); regeneration of the nerve fiber. The regeneration of autonomous nerves is similar to that of the peripheral nerves. At the proximal end of an amputation stump, a so-called amputation neuroma may develop. It can also develop because of local injury.

Repair in plants depends on the meristematic potential. In addition to the primary meristems, such as the apical or lateral meristems, the so-called succeeding meristems (*Folgemeristeme*) are of utmost importance. Two main types of reparative growth are distinguishable in plants, namely reparation and regeneration. Reparation normally occurs after wounding. A wound, depending on its size, results in transformation of similar or dissimilar cells in response to physiologically new conditions. Meristematic, mitotically active, and fully differentiated mitotically inactive cells may be involved, depending on the size of the wound. One portion of the cells will be repairable, another portion will be totally destroyed, and some may be uninjured. It is possible to distinguish, according to theoretical embryonal potential, between (a) meristematic cells that still have active potential before the injury and (b) cells of fully differentiated tissues that regain their dividing ability after the stimulation of wounding and respond with differential activation, often including synthesis of genetic material and cell division. Not all cells of the wound margin exhibit similar reactions, but a topographic pattern of reaction may be observed instead (1).

Regeneration is a more demanding process than reparation in that under the influence of the old damaged organism a whole new part will develop (Table 1.3). Regeneration in animals is very highly developed in holothurians, where whole organ systems can be replaced, such as the intestinal tract. If regeneration supersedes whole parts and leads to the development of a new plant, the problem moves from repair of an organism to one of asexual reproduction. It is very well known, for example, that a cut leaf from the plant *Begonia* can develop a whole new plant by regeneration.

Neoplastic Growth

On the basis of clinical observations and experience with human tumors, a definition of spontaneously occurring tumors has been developed. This procedure should now be applied to the tumors of other organisms, specifically to include animals and plants. But we must consider not only definite tumors but also pathological growth in human beings, animals, and plants as primary stages of tumors, as well as the kind of growth that can be traced only to lower animals and plants, if we want to consider the comparative aspects of neoplastic growth and its phylogenetic development with respect to the convergent lines of abnormal growth in the different phyla.

Table 1.3
Species-Specific Grading of Regeneration

Grade	Appearance with Characteristics
1	Types of asexual reproduction: regeneration of *Hydra* sp.; fission of polychaetes, regeneration in lower plants, offshoots in vascular plants
2	Primary meristematic capacity in vascular plants
3	Primary high regenerative capacity as in planarians
4	Secondary meristematic capacity as in succeeding meristems ("Folgemeristeme" in German literature)
5	Secondary high regenerative capacity as replacement of whole organ systems or body portions: intestinal tract in holothurians, regeneration of an arm in starfish, regeneration of a limb in amphibians
6	Regenerative capacity of smaller structural units: regeneration of tube feet in sea urchins, regeneration of a portion of the liver in mammals
7	Continued cell replacement in normal and common tissue regeneration: cells of body fluids, integuments and others
8	Cell consistence in particular systems, as in neurons of mammals
9	Cell invariability in whole organisms as in rotatorians or tardigrades (?)
10	Cellular inflexibility of functional nonliving tissues, as in sclerenchymas and others in vascular plants

The following definition of neoplastic growth is proposed:

1. A neoplasm is an excessive uncontrolled new growth of tissue originating from the tissues of a particular host; it is a growth that does not cease after removal of the stimulus. The growth is uncoordinated with that of normal tissues; it is worthless to the host. It continues to multiply indefinitely, irrespective of any functional requirements.

2. Generally, a neoplasm is an uncoordinated irreversible mass of cells, with a continuing tendency toward growth.

3. The cells of the tumor are permanently altered cells of the body.

4. The neoplastic tissue exhibits nestlike cellular multiplication with cell units; these cells diverge somewhat from the mother tissue and are generally useless in relation to the primary tissue from which they originated. The increase of cell multiplication in the form of increased mitoses or amitoses and the increase in the substance of the nuclei are characteristic of such neoplastic growth.

5. Differentiation is decreased. The cells of neoplastic tissues are characterized by a loss of substance and structure of the cytoplasm and a diminishing cellular and tissue differentiation.

6. There is an increase in the density of the nuclei, indicating a change in the nuclear cytoplasmic relationship.

7. There is a decrease in the functional performance of neoplastic cells, resulting in total disfunction at the extreme.

8. Benign tumors are characterized by slowly increasing swelling; they are often surrounded by a capsule, and they do not infiltrate the surrounding tissue.

9. Malignant tumors have the following attributes: (a) They are anaplastic; the cells are less well differentiated than those from which they are derived. (b) They infiltrate and destroy the adjacent tissues. (c) They grow more rapidly than benign tumors. (d) They metastasize.

10. Subpoints a, b, and c of point 9 above apply to all malignant tumors, but not subpoint d, because malignant plant tumors do not metastasize. This is because the body fluids of plants normally do not contain free floating cells and because of the presence of rigid cell walls. Certain human and animal tumors generally do not metastasize, such as the squamous cell cancer of the skin in man.

11. The metastasizing potential for malignant spreading must be evaluated according to the different groups of organisms affected. Beginning with conditions in man, we can distinguish,

according to von Albertini (14), the following metastases:

Lymphogenic Metastasis. Peripheral lymphatic vessels, afferent lymphatic tissues and the lymph nodes, border sinus, intermediary sinus, and lymphatic tissues can lead to metastases. With respect to the different animal phyla, we can distinguish among (a) animals of the acoelomate type *e.g.*, flat worms; (b) animals with an open circulatory system, such as the insects; (c) animals with a closed circulatory system, where lymphatic capillaries are present *e.g.*, mammals; and (d) animals with a mixed circulatory system, such as the cephalopods and pulmonates.

Hematogenic Metastasis. Hematogenic metastasis occurs in humans when the cells of the loosely built neoplasm invade and penetrate the walls of small venules. In man, this type of metastasis is most often perceived in sarcomas, carcinomas, and mesotheliomas.

Theoretically, hematogenic metastasis is impossible in those animal phyla that lack a circulatory system.

With respect to metastasis, special conditions that are not yet known may occur in pulmonate snails and cephalopods, depending on the presence of a mixed circulatory system (15). Presently, these organisms are included among the animal phyla with an open circulatory system.

In the case of those phyla having a closed circulatory system, conditions most closely resemble those in the mammals, including the human being. Von Albertini also considered three other characteristic pictures of metastasis (lymphangiosis of the lung, pleuracarcinosis of an ovarial cancer, and hematogen metastasis of a hypernephroma) that will not be considered in detail.

Neoplasm without Stroma. We know of neoplasms without stroma, and this category includes the group of leukemias. They maintain the characteristics of free pathological cells without tissue character, but we must bear in mind that this is a condition derived from the normal tissue. The free-floating cells of blood are without stroma also, as are blood-forming tissue such as the red bone marrow, normal blood with normal cells and corpuscles in man, and leukemic blood with characteristic leukemic cells. Therefore, we are not dealing with a pathological reduction of cell accumulation. This could hold true only with regard to the experimental ascites tumor of the mouse, but the matter may be open to question. In the following chapter, the principle of histogenesis will be discussed again from the aspect of comparative pathology. The chorioepithelioma is perhaps the only malignant epithelial neoplasm (cancer) that proliferates without stroma (14).

References

1. Beiderbeck, R. (1977): *Pflanzentumoren*, p. 35. Eugen Ulmer Verlag, Stuttgart.
2. Berry, R. J. (1974): Modification of neutron effects upon cells by repair, and by physical and chemical means broadbeans. In: *Proceedings of the Symposium on the Effects of Neutron Irradiation upon Cell Function*, Vol. 2D, pp. 257–271.
3. Faivre, M. (1975): Étude du comportement et de la régeneration du jeune gametophyte du *Gymnogramme calomelanos* (Leptosporangiees, Filicinees) en fonction de divers facteurs. (Study of the behavior and regeneration of the young gametophyte of *Gymnogramme calomelanos* (Leptosporangiae, Filicineae) in function of various factors.) *Rev. Gen. Bot.*, 82:5–91.
4. Giles, K. L. (1971): Dedifferentiation and regeneration in bryophytes; selective review. *N.Z. J. Bot.*, 9:689–694.
5. Hoffmann, G. M., Nienhaus, F., Schönbeck, F., Weltzien, H. C., and Wilbert, H. (1976): *Lehrbuch der Phytomedizin*. Paul Parey Verlag, Berlin.
6. Kaiser, H. E. (1970): *Das Abnorme in der Evolution*, p. 166. Brill, Leyden/Netherlands.
7. Kaiser, H. E. (1970): Arteriosclerosis in the point of view of comparative pathology. In: *VIIth International Congress on Pathology*. Academia Nazionale dei Lincei, Rome.
8. Kohlenbach, H. W. (1977): Basic aspects of differentiation and plant regeneration from cell and tissue cultures. In: *Plant Tissue Culture and Its Bio-Technological Application: Proc. Int. Congr. Med. Plant. Res.*, 1(Sec. B):355–366.
9. Lee, E. C. M., and De Fossard, R. A. (1975): Regeneration of strawberry plants from tissue cultures. *Comb. Proc. Int. Plant Propag. Soc.*, 25:277–285.
10. Riedacker, A. (1976): Rythmes de croissance et de regeneration des racines des vegetaux ligneux. (Growth and regeneration rhythms of roots of woody plants.) *Ann. Sci. For.*, 33:109–138.
11. Roberts, D. A., and Boothroyd, C. W. (1972): *Fundamentals of Plant Pathology*. Freeman, San Francisco, Calif.
12. Shalnov, M. I. (1977): DNA enzymatic repair and evolution of the genome in yeast, *Drosophila* and other organisms. *Radiobiologiia*, 17:652–671.
13. Tarr, S. A. J. (1972): *Principles of Plant Pathology*. Macmillan, London.
14. Von Albertini, A. (1974): *Histologische Geschwulstdiagnostik*, Ed. 2. Georg Thieme Verlag, Stuttgart, FRG.
15. Willis, R. A. (1961): *Principles of Pathology*, Ed. 2. Butterworth, Washington, D.C.

2

Transformation to Malignancy

Hans E. Kaiser

GENERAL ASPECTS OF HISTOGENESIS[1]

The development of a neoplasm always involves a transformation of normal tissue or tissues into neoplastic tissue or tissues. In order to classify a neoplasm, first the tissue from which it arose must be identified by its histogenetic origin. Histogenesis is the most important working principle for the evaluation of a neoplasm. It is also important in the field of comparative pathology (pathohistology). Histogenesis is concerned with several facets of neoplastic development, namely: (1) cytogenesis, or what is the origin of the single neoplastic cell? and (2) histogenesis *per se*, or what is the histologic origin of neoplastic tissues? In certain stages where the condition of true neoplasms is phylogenetically not reached, it may not be possible to define a histogenesis. This is the case in abnormal growth in galls of vascular plants, or algae, fungi, lichens, or perhaps to a certain degree also in bryophyta. (3) Dysontogenesis is known as the origin of certain neoplasms deriving from pathological tissues.

These points need some more detailed explanation:

1. *Cytogenesis.* It is inadvisable to assess the derivation of a neoplastic cell from a normal cell only on the basis of its form. The difficulties inherent in such a diagnosis can be seen from the hematology, especially when considering different phyla whose body fluids may or may not be concerned with gaseous exchange. Even less valid are theories concerning the derivation of neoplastic cells from embryonal cells in human neoplasms alone. Such a viewpoint is wholly incomparable of different phyla and varying ontogenetic stages as in continued and catastrophic development. A comparison of neoplastic cells of benign tumors is much more permissible than for those in malignant growths, because the benign cells resemble the normal cells of the parent tissue much more closely than do the malignant ones; this is especially true of the highly malignant neoplasms, some of which can be diagnosed only on the basis of the form of the cells such as oat cell carcinomas, spindle- or round-cell sarcomas, etc. Neoplastic cells may resemble normal cells, but they are not equal; neoplastic cells in plants and animals are generally inferior in function as well as structure. The increase in cellular dissimilarity as a function of malignancy can be shown to a certain degree (Table 2.1). Variations in the differentiation of plant galls similarly range from simple structures of unspecific cells to complex structures, comparable to neoplasms in animals.

2. *Histogenesis per se.* Each tumor exhibits some more or less characteristic signs which are similar to those found in a normal tissue. Thus, we can establish some relationship between a particular neoplasm and the normal tissue from which it may have derived, but this observation does not permit the assumption of identicality. In principle, all neoplasms in animals and plants develop from tissues in the body of the tumor host. But the variation found in neoplastic tis-

---

[1] In this chapter dealing with transformation of neoplasms, some simplifications have been undertaken in the case of tissues not present in man or in such cases where the neoplasms of two tissues bear the same name (e.g., rhabdomyoma or rhabdomyosarcoma, possible in skeletal musculature as well as cardiac musculature). Concerning the neoplasms of nervous tissues, the most common classification of topics known from the clinical experience has been used, in contrast to Chapters 3 and 43, where the comparative pathologic approach, which is broader in scope, has been applied. These are the reasons of slight differences in the classification used in these chapters.

Table 2.1
Selected Changes during Transformation to Malignancy

NORMAL   CELLS

1. Pleomorphism
2. Theory of nuclear/ plasma relation
3. Increased rate of growth
4. Invasive growth
5. Increase of cellular inferiority
6. Loss of cell specific function including differentiation
7. Metastic growth in most malignant and human neoplasms (lack of metastasis in plant neoplasms)

MALIGNANT   CELLS

sues is much greater than that of normal tissues, owing to the tremendous variability (also autonomy) of neoplastic tissues. General characteristics may serve as a guide for a group diagnosis of neoplasms, but particular characteristics must be identified so that we can arrive at a specific diagnosis. For example, a metastasis of a malignant neoplasm may be traced to a cancer if the epithelial-like arrangement of the cells can be spotted. It can be diagnosed as a metastasis from a thyroid cancer if it can be determined that the metastasis produces thyroxine.

3. *Dysontogenesis.* This phenomenon cannot be considered here in detail. However, it should be noted that a stomach cancer may develop from the old scar tissue of an ulcer.

SPECIAL AND COMPARATIVE ASPECTS OF HISTOGENESIS

As stated above, based on the principle of histogenesis, the various neoplasms can be considered from the viewpoint of the structure of the parent tissue from which they derive. An evaluation can commence with the tumors of man, because our most extensive knowledge lies in the field of human spontaneous tumors. The normal human tissues are known; so are the tumors. Therefore, it is from the human neoplasms that currently the best understanding of these tumors on a histologic basis can be acquired. The histologic makeup of the tissues of other organisms has also been studied extensively, but in many species, tumors have not been observed to date. We know of tissues in other organisms that are not present in our own body; this is not only the case with plant tissues, but also with certain animal tissues; for example, the oblique striated musculature.

The comparative histology (Chapter 3) of normal tissues must form the basis for a comparative pathohistology of neoplasms, a conclusion that perhaps has not been sufficiently recognized in the literature to date. Four major groups of parent tissues can be distinguished in man: (a) epithelial tissues, (b) connective tissues, (c) muscle tissues, and (d) nervous tissues.

Epithelial Tissues

The main function of epithelial tissues is to serve as cover; other higher and important functions are absorption and secretion. Epithelia cover both outer and inner surfaces of the body. Characteristic of the mosaic-like arrangement of epithelial cells is the close mutual adherence of the cells. All glands can be considered as being recessed epithelial membranes for the purpose of surface enlargement. Normally, intercellular substances are not present between epithelial cells. Another characteristic of such cells is polarization; a base, a medial portion, and an apical portion can be distinguished. This arrangement is particularly characteristic of the glandular cells, but is also seen in the shift from a simple to a multilayered epithelium. In the human skin and, for example, in the esophagus, the epithelium is no longer simple—it is multilayered. Other, more complicated epithelial types are well known, such as the transitional epithelium in the urinary passages in vertebrates, and the ciliated epithelium, as observed in the respiratory tract, where movement of particulate matter is needed. Secreting ducts, in certain glands, display cuboidal or cylindrical epithelium.

Neoplasms of Epithelial Tissues. *Benign Forms.* Papillomas develop as a thickening of the lining epithelium growing out from the surface. If the areas of enlargement are composed only of epithelial tissue components, then they are known as pseudopapillae, but if they are composed of both primarily involved epithelium and the supporting connective tissue, we speak of true papillae. A papilloma is composed of several papillae. If the papillae are enhanced and a very great increase in thickness occurs, a proliferating papilloma is present. In man, many papillomas develop not only from squamous cell, cylindrical and transitional epithelium, but also from the cuboidal epithelium of glandular ducts and from such lining membranes as those associated with the ovaries and the mammary glands.

The proliferating papilloma is a transitional stage leading to the malignant condition. In general, although infiltrative growth is absent, this neoplasm has the ability to expand at the surface and to implant certain metastases ("Implantationsmetastasen"). These tumors are most common from the skin, the mucosa of the bladder, and the vocal cord.

In contrast to the papilloma which exhibits primary epithelial growth and subsequent secondary stromatic reaction, there are fibromatous pseudopapillomas, which result from a primary stromatic growth and a secondary or passive epithelial growth.

At this point, consideration should be given to the situation found in the non-human organisms of both kingdoms. As stated elsewhere (6), the epithelial lining membranes and the glands derived therefrom display in principle a similar arrangement throughout the world of organisms.

The glandular epithelia comprise the next group of epithelia. Two types can be distinguished, namely, the exocrine and the endocrine glands. Exocrine glands are tubular, alveolar, or tubuloalveolar. Endocrine glands occur either in a cordlike epithelial pattern with sparse connective tissue which carries vessels, or as the follicular type, as in the case of the thyroid gland.

The third type of epithelia is that of the reproductive epithelia. The fourth type is represented by the epithelia of joints, tendon sheaths and bursae, also known as desmal epithelium. In this category the epithelia of serous cavities may also be included and, with some reservation, those of the blood vessels which are also known as endothelia. The similarities, as found in the animal and plant kingdoms, consist of the following: (a) A lining layer of "epidermal" or covering cells is always present. (b) A connective or interstitial cell layer underlays this basic layer. (c) The lining layer is simple in vascular plants and invertebrates, with a few exceptions (e.g., in xerophyta the body covering is multilayered as well as certain regions of the integument in the highest chaetognatha), but multilayered in vertebrates. (d) Glands in both kingdoms are composed of secretory and supporting cells. The comparison between animal and plant neoplasms can be complicated in the case of inner lining membranes of plants (14).

This basic comparability of lining membranes and glandular structures forms the basis for a comparative histogenesis of epithelial neoplasms, in animals and plants in the broadest sense of the words.

Malignant Variations. The malignant variations are the carcinomas in the case of man and vertebrates.

Comparable to the situation among the papillomas, two main tumor types can be distinguished: the papillary carcinomas which are constructed like the papillomas and the infiltrative carcinomas.

Malignant papillomas and papillary cancers display the same features described above for the benign papillomas with transformation to malignancy: malignant signs of cellular morphology, in the tumors with fast growth the epithelium dominates and the stroma is scarce. In addition to the destructive growth, the proof of infiltrative growth at the base of the tumor is especially important.

Infiltrative carcinomas, which constitute the majority of surface carcinomas, show a solid composition (solid cell cones and filaments grow infiltratively downward). The basal cells of the normal epithelium are located at the periphery of the infiltrative growth; the superficial cells occur in the center. Cornification, if present, occurs in the center, e.g., horn pearls in squamous cell cancer.

On the basis of the histogenetic principle, we can shed some light on the possible distribution of neoplasms. Cellularly undifferentiated and cellularly differentiated squamous cell carcinomas can be distinguished. The undifferentiated types in man are rather rare, whereas the differentiated ones are more common. Different types of ripeness occur: the nonepidermoid type, the epidermoid type or the mucoid type in the case of pronounced differentiation.

Most cancers are fully differentiated but mixed types occur also.

A theoretical question of importance is whether we can expect metaplastic neoplasms in those organisms which have not reached the grade of the normal tissue type the tumor is imitating. The comparative material leaves this question open. It can be assumed that the phylogenetic and taxonomic relationship of species compared may exhibit a variation due to the affinity of the host species. In the case of a lower organism taxonomically more distant from another species with a higher new type of tissue, metaplasia may be more simple. But in a species taxonomically closer related to the host species of a new tissue type, a more diversified metaplastic caricature of this new tissue type may perhaps occur. As we know from tumors which originate at locations which show no squamous cell epithelium, as in the case of the transitional epithelium, e.g., in the bladder or the ciliated epithelium in the bronchi, metaplastic squamous cell cancers do occur; but they do not do so as primary cancers without metaplastic change of the transitional or ciliated epithelium.

If the principle of histogenesis is applied, neoplasms of a tissue type not normally present, are, in turn, not to be anticipated in a particular organism. However, metaplastic changes may mimic nonpresent tissue types within certain limits.

Special forms of malignant neoplasms of lining membranes are the lymphoepitheliomas and the transitional carcinoma (Quick-Cutler) (Chapter 43). (See also (15).

Neoplasms of Glandular Epithelia. Glands are secretory structures composed of epithelial cells and, depending on the size of the gland, of a more or less well developed stroma as supporting portion. Two components can therefore be distinguished: secretory epithelial cells and supporting connective tissue. This holds true for animals and plants alike. In both, unicellular and multicellular glandular structures can be observed. Goblet cells in mammals and mucous cells in other groups exemplify unicellular glands in animals; in plants, the secretory cells of nectaries serve as an example. The next step in glandular development beyond the single secretory cell is the epithelial secretory sheet. In mammals, for example, the epithelia of the choroid plexus and the gastric epithelium are composed of such sheets. In plants, these external or internal sheets can be considered the final stage of this development, because in the plant, glandular structures do not form such characteristic organs as are found in the animal. Glandular epidermal cells and hairs on the outer surface are examples of the external structures; cavities or ducts surrounded by inner secretory components such as the oil cavities, oil ducts, and resin ducts may serve as examples of the internal structure.

The remaining multicellular glands occur as invaginations of the epithelial lining membrane penetrating the underlying connective tissue. In plant glands, the upper cells are secretory, the lower ones, supporting. The invaginated glands

are the subject of the secretion on histogenesis of glandular neoplasms.

Neoplasms of Exocrine Glands: Exocrine Neoplasms. The benign neoplasms are usually adenomas; some papillomas are of lesser importance. Distinguishable by these glandular variations, alveolar, tubular or mixed adenomas occur. Those of the endocrine thyroid (15) are also comparable to the exocrine adenomas. The lack of glandular ducts results in storage and accumulation of secretory products.

The tubular adenomas are composed of simple tubuli lined with cubic or cylindrical cells. A subtype of the tubular adenomas, the so-called trabecular adenomas, are cords without lumina. Certain of these structures are considered to be intermediate stages in malignant growth. The cords are enlarged and may be infiltrating, as in the case of the "proliferating struma Langhans" of the thyroid. Cystic conversion constitutes another complication. The cause can be secretory retention or epithelial growth inside the cavity. Pseudopapillae and even papillae may occur. This kind of tumor is known as *cystadenoma papilliferum.* This type of growth, too, can be viewed as a transitional phase leading to a cancerous growth. The stroma is less well developed than in carcinomas. The cellular picture resembles more or less that of the normal tissue from which the adenoma derives.

Cancers of the glandular epithelium, the adenocarcinomas, are the most common type of cancer in man. They are malignant neoplasms. Phylogenetically as well as ontogenetically the glands are the culmination of the epithelial tissues. These neoplasms are mostly of the tubular or trabecular type. The diameter of the cords remains about the same, but different subtypes can be distinguished: (a) with taut cords—carcinoma adenomatosum—with more regular cylindrical cells, and (b) with coiled cords, resembling a corkscrew—carcinoma adenomatoides—with more atypical, fully differentiated cells. The trabecular carcinomas, the less well differentiated neoplasms, are solid in structure.

In the solid carcinomas, subtypes are as shown in Table 2.2. The cells of the solid carcinomas, without a lumen, are often uncharacteristic due to lack of differentiation.

Neoplasms of Endocrine Glands: Endocrine Neoplasms. With the exception of the adenoma of the thyroid cited above, the adenomas of endocrine glands exhibit the characteristics of the epithelia from which they derive. The number of cells, however, is increased. The endo-

Table 2.2
Subtypes of the Solid Carcinoma (15)

Type	Cross Section of Cord	Stroma
Simple	3 cell rows	Strong
Scirrhous	7 cell rows	Abundant
Medullary	More than 7 cell rows	Almost entirely absent

Table 2.3
Histogenetic Classification of Ovarian Tumors

A. Ovarian tumors of paramesonephric, celomic (germinal, Müllerian) epithelium
B. Ovarian tumors of nonspecialized, sex-undifferentiated mesenchyme or gonadal stroma
C. Ovarian tumors of specialized, sex-differentiated mesenchyme or sex cords (potentially steroid-producing ovarian tumors)
D. Ovarian tumors of germ cell origin
E. Ovarian tumors of mesonephric rests
F. Ovarian tumors arising from heterotopic (accessory tissue in the ovary)
G. Secondary or metastatic tumors of the ovary

crine adenomas are solid, often of the trabecular type. Furthermore, the adenomas often exhibit only one cell type in contrast to the gland from which they originate. The following malignant variations are found: (a) metastasizing adenomas of the thyroid gland, (b) metastisizing adenomas of the parathyroid glands, (c) carcinoma of the cortex of the adrenal gland, and (d) carcinoma of the islands of Langerhans.

Neoplasms of the Reproductive Epithelia. The neoplasms of the reproductive epithelia open up a large field of great interest to comparative pathology. The epithelial or meristematic elements of reproduction occur throughout the animal and plant kingdoms; the germinative cells are also more or less comparable (not on an ontogenetic basis—but on a morphologic and functional one). New research in this area is essential, especially since the classification of human neoplasms is not yet firmly established. A brief review of the neoplasms of the germinative epithelia of the ovary and testes in man is provided in Chapter 43.

Reproductive cells are found, of course, in all animals and plants, but in the case of those organisms of particular interest to us—those with true tissues—additional cells are present which serve such functions as, for example, the nourishment of the reproductive cells. These additional cells may also be present in various benign or malignant tumors dominated by the reproductive cells. Hence it is necessary to consider variations in these supernumerary cells under normal conditions, as they occur in the various phyla. It can be assumed that a wide pathological variability of germ cell tumors exists in the different types of organisms. Table 2.3, a histogenetic classification of human ovarian tumors (7), reveals a distinction between ovarian tumors of germ cell origin (the group of immediate interest to this review) and six other groups of tissues that contribute to the ovarian tumors, such as those of the paramesonephric or celomic epithelium. The benign tumors of germ cell origin comprise the benign cystic teratoma, the benign solid adult teratomas, the fetiform

teratoma, and the struma ovarii. Benign tumors of germ cell origin may undergo a secondary tumefaction leading to the development of secondary tumors in teratomas or in benign cystic teratomas. It is not yet known whether these secondary malignant changes, which can be mono-, bi-, or tri-dermal, result from failure to mature or whether the tissues have become mature and have again resumed active growth of an embryonic character. These malignant changes—often with a very poor prognosis—suggest that a controlled embryonic potential characterizes the meristematic tissue of plants which in turn give rise to the germ cells in the plant. Such comparisons between animals and plants may shed new light on certain aspects of malignant growth. There are also, secondary tumors in the struma ovarii and also the so-called carcinoid changes in ovarian tumors. The malignant tumors of germ cell origin in man comprise the dysgerminoma, the teilum tumor with its variation of the polyvesicular vitelline tumor, polyembryoma, choriocarcinoma, teratocarcinoma, and gonadoblastoma. In 1960, Teter classified the latter tumor, due to the predominance of germ cells, into four subgroups (See (7). Up to 90% of the tumors of the testis derive from germ cells. A distinction must be made between teratomas which may be benign or malignant, and the seminoma.

Neoplasms of Desmal Epithelium Type (Mesothelium of Joints, Tendon Sheaths and Bursae). Tumors of this kind comprise the benign giant cell synovioma and the malignant synovioma (see Chapter 43).

Primary Neoplasms of Desmal Epithelium of Coelomic Surfaces. No benign neoplasms of the desmal epithelium are known in man. The principal malignant neoplasm of this type is the mesothelioma or endothelioma. Von Albertini (15) has assigned this tumor to the cancers.

Melanogenic System

The next group of tissues and neoplasms, those of the melanogenic system, exhibits a diversified histogenesis on one hand but a unifying characterization due to the storage of melanin on the other hand (12). The normal and neoplastic tissues of the melanogenic system are not a morphological similar group such as epithelia but a heterogeneous one combined for clinical and biochemical reasons. The system differs therefore from all other tissue types. These specialized neoplasms of man derive from different categories and precursors of the four main tissue types but especially from those of the epithelial and connective tissues. (This is the reason why this section is placed between those of epithelia and connective tissues.) Beside the storage of melanin these cells do not constitute a special type of tissue in other respects. It is useful to discuss it in one group because of the very important, highly malignant tumors, deriving from them, known as melanomas. Melanin storing cells occur also in fungi, vascular plants, invertebrates, and other vertebrates than humans, making them a very significant model for comparative pathology.

Normal Histology of Melanogenic System. The melanogenic system is considered here as a special system because of the wide distribution of the cells with respect to species and body region, which complement the importance of the tumors concerned. The cells are characterized by the brown pigment, melanin, which occurs in plants and animals. In animals it is found in serous membranes of body cavity and in connective tissues of many organs of invertebrates, and in vertebrates such as mammals in the skin especially at the nipple, pigmentation of the external sex organs, anal pigmentation, hairs, eyes, and certain nuclei of the brain, for example, the nucleus ruber. The pigment is also responsible for the varying colors in the different races.

The melanin-producing cells, the melanocytes (melanophores) originate in the neural crest. Before they migrate to the epidermal/dermal junction the cells developed in the neural crest are called melanoblasts; once they are located beneath or between the basal cells of the skin, they are called melanocytes.

The pigment comes about in the Golgi apparatus in the form of elipsoid, electron dense granules known as melanosomes. Characteristic of early formation are surrounding membrane and longitudinal lamellae. In vertebrates, the pigment can be transferred to other epidermal cells. The synthesis takes place in the rough endoplasmic reticulum. Melanophores of epidermis and subepidermis differ in appearance. They are also found in larval creatures, for example, in amphibians. This helps explain the fact that normal cells, in addition to the exceptions mentioned in the Chapter 1, can become neoplastic in each stage of life. The wide distribution of the pigment is comparable to the wide distribution of other plant pigments. In fishes and amphibians the hormone stimulating the synthesis of melanocytes is produced by the pars intermedia of the pituitary, which is more strongly developed in these animals than in man. The compound is also known as melanotropin and it influences the cellular distribution of the pigment. The melanocytes with the many extending processes are responsible for color changes, as, for example, those taking place in fishes through the transfer of the granules either closer toward the nucleus of the cell (dark coloration) or further away from it (light coloration). The different melanins range in color from yellow via brown to black.

Neoplasms of Melanogenic System. In man the neoplasms of the system include: the benign cutaneous melanoma (pigmented nevus) with the epidermodermal or junctional nevus, the compound nevus, the juvenile melanoma (Spitz), intradermal nevus or common mole, further the blue nevus and the malignant cutaneous melanoma (melanosarcoma). These are cutaneous tumors. Melanotic tumors of extracutaneous origin have been found in the conjunctiva, external auditory meatus, hard palate, oral mucosa, tonsillar region, nasal cavity, larynx, esophagus, intestine, adrenal cortex, penis, vulva, and vagina.

Connective Tissue in a Broad Sense

These tissues are composed of cells and a matrix, the intercellular substance. Hence they are clearly distinguishable from epithelial tissues. Accordingly, connective tissues with an abundance of cells can be separated from those with abundant fibers.

A wide variety of connective tissues occurs in man (see Table 2.8). It can thus be assumed that, similarly, a wide variety may occur in all organisms. But there are broadly applicable principles governing the function of connective-parenchymatic tissues which transgress the dividing line between the metazoans and the vascular plants. For example, the respiratory pigments in man and animals, as well as in plants, are contained in these tissues, either in their cells or, in certain animals, in their intercellular substances.

Connective Tissues Rich in Cells. Mesenchyme. Mesenchyme is the embryonal connective tissue from which all other types of the group of connective tissues develop during ontogeny. The asteroid cells which produce a loose network, are connected by their cytoplasmic processes, exhibit a large polymorphous nucleus, multiple nucleoli, and are dispersed in a fluid containing proteins and minute amounts of polysaccharides. This fluid constitutes the intercellular substance. The cells readily become detached and can easily be observed.

Spinocellular Connective Tissue. This type of tissue, which may be regarded as a variation (subdivision) of the mesenchyme, occurs only in the stroma of the ovaries and the lamina propria of the uterus; the constituent cells perform delicate processes that connect them. This type of tissue produces the theca cells in the ovary whose function is hormone production. Argyrophilic fibrils and collagenous fibers occur in the muscles. In the uterus, this tissue is involved in the regeneration of the mucosa during menstruation. This tissue is also responsible for the pathological condition of endometriosis, in which spinocellular tissue components are transported to other locations in the body where they can produce benign lesions.

Reticular Connective Tissues. This tissue type is also closely related to the mesenchyme and is composed of a cellular network comparable to that of the spinocellular variety. The nuclei are smaller than those of the mesenchyme; the cells are characterized by their capacity for phagocytosis. Free cells occur in the meshes of the network. Characteristic of these connective tissues, as the name indicates, is the presence of reticulin fibers. This type of tissue occurs in the hematopoietic organs, lymph nodes, bone marrow, spleen, and the so-called reticuloendothelial system. This concept and its defensive role was elucidated by K. A. L. Aschoff (1866–1942).

The other cells of the reticuloendothelial system—the endothelia of the venous sinus of the spleen, of liver, of the adrenal gland, and the anterior lobe of the pituitary, the endothelia of the vessels and the epithelia of the lung alveoli, the membrane synovialis of the joints, as well as the pleural and peritoneal epithelium have been considered earlier; the micro-(meso)glia—will be discussed later.

The reticular connective tissues can be subdivided into the lymphoreticular connective tissue occurring in the lymphatic organs (spleen, lymph nodes, tonsils, and lamina propria of the intestinal mucosa) and the hematopoietic-reticular connective tissues, of which the myeloic or red bone marrow is composed. Bone marrow is found in all marrow cavities of the embryonal or juvenile skeleton; in the adult, it has remained only in the diploe, vertebrae, sternum, sacrum, hip bone, and the phalanges.

Connective Tissues with Abundant Fibers. Fibers (argyrophylic, collagenous, elastic) predominate in the structure and enhance the mechanical functioning of these connective tissues. This group of tissues comprises the following types:

Gelatinous Connective Tissue. This tissue can also be traced directly to the mesenchyme, whose cells it resembles. Between the cells the collagenous fibrils are surrounded by a mucoid substance. This tissue type occurs in the umbilical cord (Wharton's jelly), the villi of the placenta, and, with a subtype, in the pulp of the teeth. The normal tissue is unimportant in the adult human body, but very important for the histogenesis of neoplasms which develops from it.

Loose Interstitial Connective Tissue. This type of connective tissues is related to the reticular connective tissue and fulfills particular mechanical functions. Its rich content in collagenous and elastic fibers enables this tissue, as in the case of the connective tissues of the mucous membranes, to provide the structures of which it is a component with mobility. The interwoven collagenous fibers permit temporary deformation. The elastic fibers then return the structures involved to their initial position. The mobility of the tissue which surrounds all organs is only one important function for which the fibers are responsible; a second function, that of repair and defense, is dependent upon the cell content which can be divided into fixed cells, such as the fibroblasts and fibrocytes, the adipose cells, the pigmented cells, and the free cells, such as the histocytes, the mast cells, and the leukocytes. Other subdivisions of loose interstitial connective tissue comprise the lamellar connective tissue, membranous connective tissue, and areolar connective tissue.

Pigmented Connective Tissue. Pigmented cells can be present in connective tissue. The endogenous nonhematogenic pigment cells have been discussed earlier in the section on the melanogenic system. This type of connective tissue is of reticular makeup and is characterized by the melanin production and content of the cells. It occurs, for example, in the choroidea, iris, and skin.

Fibrillar Connective Tissue. The primary characteristic of this tissue type is the presence of the collagenous fibers produced by the only cell type in which that occurs, the fibrocytes. The fibrils of this tissue have the task of producing and maintaining tension. Based upon these functional demands, the following subtypes of this tissue can be distinguished: reticulose, fibrillar connective tissue, taut fibrillar connective tissue, fibrillar connective tissue in parallel strands (e.g., peritoneum), fibrillar connective tissue with flattened, cross-over pattern (e.g., fasciae, aponeuroses), and interwoven fibrillar connective tissue (e.g., membrana fibrosa of joints).

Supporting tissues. As their name implies, these tissues provide for fixation of the position of an organ or support of the whole body. This objective can be achieved either by the cells themselves or by the matrix; this suggests the following classification.

Supporting Tissues Rich in Cells. The tissues belonging to this group are the adipose, the chordoid, and the chondroid tissues.

Adipose Tissue. The adipose tissue cells, which are large and round, are encased in a network of reticular fibers. These tissues are derived from the reticular connective tissue. The nucleus of the cells is located at the margin of the cell (signet ring cells). Capillary networks may be abundant. According to the specific functions involved, supporting or constructive connective tissue (e.g., in the sole of the foot and the palm of the hand) and storing or subcutaneous adipose tissue may be distinguished. According to the ontogenetic development the multivacuolated cells, with high cytochrome and lipochrome content are known as brown adipose tissue, which is replaced by the univacuolated adipose tissue, also known as white adipose tissue. The brown adipose tissue remains in the human body only in a few locations; in contrast to its range of distribution in small hibernating rodents. Adipose tissue is a derivative of the mesenchyme.

Chordoid Tissue. This tissue occurs during embryonal life, as inductor of the axial skeleton, where it composes the notochord; as the precursor of the axial skeleton it remains in the postembryonal life in the human body only in the nuclei

pulposi of the vertebral column. The cells are bladder-like and filled with a watery, glycogen-containing fluid. These cells tighten the fibrous sheath (coat, "Schlauch"-tube) of the notochord. The tissue type is restricted to the phylum-group of chordates, the hemichordates, the urochordates, the cephalochordates and the vertebrates.

Chondroid Tissue. This tissue type, also of very limited distribution occurs at the junctions of tendons and bone, and in the menisci. The small, roundish cells are separated by a narrow matrix of fibrous consistency (16). The tissue plays a role also during bone reparation.

Supporting Tissues, Rich in Matrix. Cartilage. From an ontogenetic point of view two developmental types may be distinguished: the perichondrium and the cartilage *per se.* The cells for the perichondrium, a tissue rich in cells, are those which contain the branched fibrocytes, from which the chondrocytes, the cells of cartilage develop. The cartilaginous tissues derive directly from the mesenchyme. The chondrocytes are large, roundish, and pale staining cells, encapsulated by the matrix they produce. This matrix contains collagenic and elastic fibers which are normally masked. In the vertebrate hyaline, elastic and fibrocartilage may be distinguished which are more or less comparable to invertebrate cartilage occurring in mollusca, annelida, and arthropoda. (About invertebrate cartilages, see Chapter 3.)

Bone. In the human body, bone normally occurs exclusively in the skeletal system. Bone is important as protection for such organs as the brain in the skull, the spinal cord in the vertebral column, and the thoracic organs in the thorax; even in the extremities, as in the human thigh, the important vessels and nerves, especially the arteries, are located in such a way that they are protected by the long bones (in this case, the femur). Bone undergoes a continuous remodeling. In the ontogenetic development of bone there is a clear distinction between tissue development and organ development, between histogenesis and organogenesis. The different nature of development and growth can be easily distinguished. The histogenesis of bone is always the same, no matter, whether it takes place during embryonal, fetal, or adult life. This is important for the understanding of neoplastic development. In organogenesis, on the other hand, discrimination is possible between direct desmal or indirect chondral ossification. The bone cells develop directly from the mesenchyme but they also arise from the cells of the reticulum, or from fibroblasts. These cells then differentiate to form osteoblasts which in turn excrete the bone matrix. When these cells are imprisoned, as it were, by this matrix production, they change to osteocytes, the major cells of bone. The osteoclasts, which also develop from the mesenchyme are the cells which initiate and remain responsible for the destruction of bone during the process of remodeling. These mesenchymal cells develop especially from the endothelia of the vessels. The bone matrix is composed of fibers, which are collagenic and usually masked in normal bone slides, and cement substance (27% organic material and 56% inorganic material, with 17% water). Most of the inorganic matter consists of calcium phosphates. During the embryonal and first fetal periods, textural bone is found, and in the adult both lamellar bone or bone cortex, and spongy bone or spongiosa occur. As an organ, the individual bone is surrounded by the periosteum.

Neoplasms of Connective Tissues. *Neoplasms of Connective Tissues Rich in Cells.* Neoplasms of the Mesenchymal Type. Disregarding certain mixed tumors, it may be stated that neoplasms which completely resemble the structure of the mesenchyme are unknown. No benign mesenchymal tumors appear to exist. Due to the small degree of mesenchymal differentiation, highly undifferentiated malignant neoplasms, such as certain round cell, spindle cell, or polymorphic cell sarcomas (the Ewing sarcoma) may be considered as belonging to this group. But these tumors must fulfill certain preconditions: for example, connection of the cells in the form of a network; the shape of the cells; and the lack of such fiber products as reticular fibers and other cellular derivatives in the open spaces of the cellular network (15).

Neoplasms of the Spinocellular Connective Tissue Type. Benign as well as malignant neoplasms may develop from this tissue. If endometriosis occurs, remnants of spinocellular neoplasms may be transported to other regions of the body where they are able to produce benign, but also metastasizing, neoplasms. Spinocellular tissue of the ovary, responsible for hormone production, can produce a neoplasm known as thecoma, which may be benign or malignant.

Neoplasms of the Reticular Connective Tissue Type. The hematopoietic capacity of this tissue reveals that the neoplasms developing from it are those of the hematopoietic cell group on the one hand and those of the lymphoreticular group on the other. The cause of benign tumors is not wholly clear, but can be summarized under the term of reticuloma which may occur in the form of reticuloma simplex (simple reticuloma) without cellular differentiation and differentiated forms according to the heterogenous cell types such as lymphocytes. The malignant neoplasms are the simple reticulosarcoma without cellular differentiation (polymorphism, giant cells and other signs of malignancy such as mitoses are present) and those with cellular differentiation such as the lymphosarcoma or the myelosarcoma.

Neoplasms of the Pigmented Connective Tissue Type. The benign neoplasm of this group is the blue nevus (naevus bleu). This fibroma is composed of reticular cells that may also assume spindle form. The cytoplasm contains abundant melanin granules. The malignant variation is the melanosarcoma, which in turn is a form of a malignant melanoma. The melanogenic system has been discussed earlier, but the fact is that the malignant tumor of the pigmented version of the connective tissue can be separated as melanosarcoma from the malignant melanoma as the epithelial version. This separation is based on tissue origin.

Neoplasms of Connective Tissues with Abundant Fibers. Neoplasms of Gelatinous Connective Tissue. The benign neoplasms are the myxofibromas which are composed of loosely connected starlike and anastomosing cells embedded in a gelatinous matrix in which collagenous fibers are present. The malignant neoplasm is the myxosarcoma, richer in cells than the benign form and characterized by atypical and polymorphic cells.

Neoplasms of Loose Interstitial Connective Tissue. Neoplasms analogous to the normal type of tissue occurring in mucous membranes, subcutis, etc., exhibit a few cells similar to fibrocytes, rich collagenous fibers and occasionally adipose cells or mucinous degeneration. These forms are known as lipofibroma molle and lipofibroma myxomatodes, respectively. The malignant forms are varying sarcomas especially the undifferentiated round cell sarcoma without matrix as well as spindle cell sarcomas and polymorph-cellular sarcomas.

Neoplasms of the Fibrillar Connective Tissue Type. In this group, the benign tumors are the very common fibromas. These neoplasms are composed of spindle cells with elongated nuclei comparable to the fibrocytes; the fibers are collagenic. The fibromas may be divided into cell-rich or fiber-rich fibromas, according to the predominance of either component. The so-called fibrosarcoma assumes an intermediate position between the benign and the malignant. This semimalignant tumor type exhibits locally destructive growth but does not metastasize. The true malignant form is the spindle cell sarcoma, rich in atypical polymorphic cells exhibiting increased and abnormal mitoses.

Neoplasms of Supporting Tissue Type. *Supporting Tissue Type Neoplasms Rich in Cells.* Adipose Tissues. The benign tumors of adipose tissue, the lipomas, are composed of enlarged adipose cells. The tumor tissue does not contain collagenic fibrils and there is no lobulation as in normal adipose tissue. In conformity with the normal course of ontogenetic development, the tumor may exhibit a combined pattern of connective tissues as such and of adipose tissue, resulting in a variation known as fibrolipoma. Benign forms are often encapsulated.

Another parallel to normal ontogenetic development is found in a combination of neoplastic adipose tissue with blood vessels resulting in the angiolipoma. The malignant variation, the liposarcoma, displays a cell-rich, polymorph to reticular pattern with the inclusion of small adipose cells—a pathological return to an earlier developmental stage. Here, the adipose cells reveal a honeycomb structure, indicating return to a phylogenetically early pattern somewhat similar to brown adipose tissue. The alveoli of the adipose cells, of course, contain fatty substances.

Neoplasms of the Chordoid Tissue Type. The neoplasms of remnants of chordoid tissue are the chordomas, which appear in benign to malignant variations. The large, bladder-like cells of the benign forms exhibit small, peripherally located nuclei. Younger cells are smaller. Masses of a mucous matrix often appear among the neoplastic cells. The cells of the malignant variation are smaller and the vacuoles more restricted. Developmentally, the same trend can be perceived as described in the above with respect to the benign and malignant neoplasms of adipose tissue.

Neoplasms of Chondroid Tissue Type. Owing to the fact that this type of tissue may replace cartilage during histogenesis it is suggested that these tumors be considered a variation of neoplasms developing from cartilage. Such tumors do indeed exist in both benign and malignant variations, but they are often described as chondromas or chondrosarcomas; the term of "chondroidoma" and chondroid sarcoma would consequently be more appropriate.

Neoplasms of the Supporting Tissue Type, Rich in Cells. Neoplasms of Cartilage Type. The benign neoplasms of this type are known as chordomas. The more commonly occurring forms are neoplasms exhibiting an unripe structure resembling somewhat the perichondrium, with starlike cells. Variations of such neoplasms are the myxochondromas (a misnomer) or reticular chondromas.

Neoplasms with a ripe cellular structure are the hyaline chondromas and the fibrillar or elastic chondromas, respectively (13).

The malignant chondromas, or chondrosarcomas, develop in a manner similar to the benign neoplasms, but the cells may be more of the chondroblastic type. Ripe tissue cells also occur in the same type of neoplasm. The malignant forms vary from the highly differentiated to the anaplastic. Chondromas and chondrosarcomas are often combined with neoplasms of the bone, a fact readily explained by the ontogenetic development of this type of connective tissue, which will not occur in the neoplasms of the cartilage type in the invertebrates.

Neoplasms of Bone Tissue Type. Bone is the most complex of all connective tissues. Hence, the neoplasms of this tissue type also exhibit a highly complicated picture. All of the steps of osseous histogenesis may be reflected in the particular neoplasm under study. The histogenetic approach, however, consists in achieving an understanding of the variable components of bone neoplasms and in overcoming difficulties in their histologic diagnosis. The common point of bone development progress (histogenesis) offers multiple potential for tumorigenesis. Neoplasms that form bone display a complex picture, but those that destroy bone are relatively uncomplicated. In its development, a given neoplasm never takes advantage of all possible types of growth. The result is that in bone neoplasms, one type of tissue dominates the others, a condition reflected in such designations as fibro-, myxo-, chondro-osteoblastic sarcoma, among others.

Functionally, two separate areas of bone may be distinguished. Each represents a functional tissue unit. These units are characterized by an osteogenic and a myelogenic matrix. The benign neoplasms of the bone are the osteomas, a group in which many facts and/or interpretations are still open to question. The malignant forms are generally known as osteosarcomas.

Osteogenic neoplasms are benign tumors of the osteogenic matrix. They include the chondroblastic forms and the osteoblastic forms, such as fibroma ossificans, osteoma eburneum, osteoid osteoma, and giant osteoid osteoma.

The next group comprises those tumors which are neither specifically chondro- nor osteoblastic, such as the nonossifying osteofibroma, the desmoblastic osteofibroma, and the primary giant cell tumors.

The malignant forms are the spindle cell sarcoma, the myxosarcoma, and the osteogenic sarcoma *per se*. The osteoblastic sarcoma, the osteolytic sarcoma, and the chondroblastic sarcoma are neoplasms originating from the developmental stages of bone. The second group, the myelogenic neoplasms of the hematogenic matrix derive from the hematogenic tissues. The benign forms are the fibromas and reticulomas. Malignant types include the spindle cell sarcoma and the reticulosarcoma. The latter occurs either as an undifferentiated reticulosarcoma or Ewing sarcoma, or as the differentiated reticulosarcoma. These forms differ from each other by their fiber content (reticulin fibers) or exhibit a characteristic cellular differentiation, as seen in the lymphoblastic reticulosarcoma or the myeloblastic reticulosarcoma.

Less complex connective tissues are characteristic of many phases of bone development. Their designations are usually self-explanatory, hence, no detailed histologic description has been deemed necessary.

Muscular Tissues

Normal Subtypes of Muscular Tissue. In the human body there are three types of muscular tissue (Table 2.4): (a) smooth musculature, as in the tube of the intestinal tract or in the uterus; (b) skeletal or transverse striated musculature, of which individual muscles are composed; and (c) cardiac musculature, which can be subdivided into the cardiac musculature *per se*, and the so-called system for the conduction of stimuli, composed of the sinus node (Keith-Flack) and the atrioventricular node (Aschoff-Tawara).

These types of musculature derive from the mesoderm, with exception of the dilatator muscles and sphincter pupillae. The myoepithelial elements are also nonmesodermal. They are the basket cells and are found in the mammae and salivary glands. The other animal phyla present a much more complicated, but not necessarily confusing picture. In the animal kingdom five types of musculature can be distinguished. These, in turn, can be divided into subtypes.

1. Myoepithelial musculature: subtype A = in coelenterates and entoprocta, subtype B = in ectoprocta, and subtype C = in mammals, and, as noted above, in the human mammae and salivary glands, as well as in the skin.

Table 2.4
Neoplasms of Muscular Tissues (a Comparative, Theoretical Review)

Normal Tissue Type	Benign Neoplasms	Malignant Neoplasms
Myoepithelial musculature:		
Subtype A	Myoepithelioma A	Myoepitheliosarcoma A
Subtype B	Myoepithelioma B	Myoepitheliosarcoma B
Subtype C	Myoepithelioma C	Myoepitheliosarcoma C
Smooth musculature	Leiomyoma	Leiomyosarcoma
Oblique striated musculature	Rhabdomyoma obliquae	Rhabdomyosarcoma obliquae
Transverse striated musculature	Rhabdomyoma	Rhabdomyosarcoma
Cardiac musculature:		
Subtype A	Rhabdomyoma cardiaci A	Rhabdomyosarcoma cardiaci A
Subtype a	Rhabdomyoma cardiaci A, a	Rhabdomyosarcoma cardiaci A, a
Subtype b	Rhabdomyoma cardiaci A, b	Rhabdomyosarcoma cardiaci A, b
Subtype B	Rhabdomyoma cardiaci B	Rhabdomyosarcoma cardiaci B

2. Smooth musculature occurring in many phyla. Its exact distribution cannot be estimated. Many organisms now believed to be characterized by this type of musculature may reveal Type 3 under the electron microscope.

3. Oblique striated musculature, occurring in certain nematodes, such as *Ascaris*.

4. Transverse striated or skeletal musculature. The most widely distributed of the muscle tissues, it is also characteristic of the class of insects with an estimated species number of approximately 7 million. Several subtypes can already be distinguished; more will be determined in the future.

5. Transverse striated cardiac musculature: subtype A: transverse cardiac musculature *per se*; subtype a: characteristic of invertebrates, such as the crustacean *Homarus*; subtype b: characteristic of vertebrates, especially mammals; subtype B: the stimulus-conducting system in mammals, with the nodes of Keith-Flack and Aschoff-Tawara. Other subtypes, probably occurring in the invertebrates, await identification.

Characteristics of Normal Muscular Tissues in Man. Myoepithelial musculature (type C)—basket cells in the breasts, salivary and sweat glands and known as myoepithelial musculature develop from ectoderm. They are characterized by a central cell body, long cell processes, and myofibrils. Smooth muscle cells = spindle form, 40–200 μm in length and 4–20 μm thick, exhibit a central nucleus and myofilaments which are not united to myofibrils (hence, their smooth appearance).

The cells of the skeletal musculature consist of a plasmodium, up to several centimeters in length and 10–100 μm thick. The nuclei occur in larger numbers in each fiber and assume a marginal position. The myofibrils, formed from two types of myofilaments, permit rapid contractility. The cardiac musculature is composed of anastomosing and ramifying fibers. Oval nuclei occur in the centers of these fibers. Intercalated discs are another characteristic of this type of musculature. The transverse striation is poorly defined and due to many mitochondria the cells are cloudy in appearance. (For other muscular tissue types of the animal kingdom, see Chapter 3.)

Neoplasms of Muscular Tissue. *Smooth Musculature.* The benign tumor is the leiomyoma; an unmistakable characteristic is found in the increased number of nuclei. The young neoplasms, especially, resemble the normal tissue; the connective tissue stroma increases in older neoplasms; in some cases, even leading to the picture of a fibroma.

The malignant tumor is the leiomyosarcoma. Its structure presents a similarly characteristic polymorph-cellular picture, with giant cells. The stroma is sparse; many vessels are necrotic.

Transverse Striated Skeletal and Cardiac Musculature. In this kind of musculature, the benign neoplasm is the rhabdomyoma, characterized by highly atypical cells. The cells are larger than normal; the nuclei are polymorphic and rich in chromatin. The cytoplasm appears granulated and vacuolated; transverse striation is nearly always lacking. The malignant variation rhabdomyosarcoma, is very rare. The Birsch-Hirschfeld or Wilms' tumor is a dysontogenetic mixed tumor, a rhabdomyosarcoma of the kidney. Positive recognition of the presence of transverse striation appears to be a prerequisite of diagnosis of a rhabdomyosarcoma.

Benign neoplasms of the basket cells are known to occur in the ducts and secretory structures of the mammae. Malignant tumors of this type have not been found. Myoepithelioma of the skin has not been properly and clearly defined.

Nervous Tissues

The nervous system is designed to correlate impulses by the transmission of signals. Through nerve endings and sense organs, it also acquires information about the environment and the different parts of the body. In the conscious state, the mind is aware of some, but not of all, of this information.

The nervous system develops from the ectodermal epithelium. In the first stages of development, the ectodermal epithelium of the skin and the neuroectoderm can be distinguished. The swellings of the neural crests and the neural furrow are discernible. The neural furrow becomes the neural tube; the neural crests submerge. Both entities are composed of the neural epithelium.

From a topographic-histogenetic viewpoint the neuroepithelium of the neural tube, which produces the neurons and the glia of the central nervous system on one hand, and the neural epithelium of the neural crest, which produces the neurons and the glia of the peripheral nervous system on the other, can be observed. From a systemic-histogenetic viewpoint, however, the following image emerges: the cells of the neuroepithelium differentiate in two ways, either via the neuroblast to form the different neurites, or via the spongio- or glioblast to make up the different types of the glial cells. The microglia, which derive from the mesenchyme and invaginate the central nervous system with the vessels, are an exception. Other cells deriving from the neural epithelium are the oligodendroglia, the epithelia of the plexus choroidei, the pinealocytes and the pituicytes.

Thus, the nervous tissue is composed of two cell types: those accomplishing the conduction of stimuli, such as the neurons and a cellular periblem, with more functions than just support, the glia or neuroglia.

Finally, the cells developing from the paraganglia (theoretically end of the neural crest in the vertebrate) produce cells with endocrine functions, such as those of the adrenal medulla.

Adult Neurons are Main Cells in Human Body Characterized by Cell Invariability. It is assumed that such a property is essential to the effective functioning within the complex interconnections of the nervous system. Immature neurons and the ontogenetic stages of cell development leading to the formation of neurons do not show cell invariability. The same holds true for resting stages as understood through the Cohnheim theory (embryonal cell theory).

In order that the occurrence of neoplasms in the nervous system of the human body may be understood, four groups of the tissue components concerned should be cited.

1. (a) The cell-invariable, adult neurons, which

are unable to produce neoplasms; and (b) the ontogenetic stages of neurons during development, or their resting stages, which are able to produce neoplasms.

2. The cells of the glia or neuroglia, which, with their ontogenetic precursors, are able to develop neoplasms.

3. The paraganglia and endocrine structures, such as the adrenal medulla, the precursors of which are neurons. This group of cells could also be added as type c in group 1 above. Neoplasms of this group are listed in Chapter 43.

4. Neoplasms deriving from the pituicytes of the neurohypophysis have been described as another example; but these cells can be considered as modified astrocytes.

In tumors, aging of the structures involved also takes place. This can be observed, for example, in the change of an astroblastoma to an astrocytoma. Both types can appear in the same tumor. The comparative aspects of endocrine structures in relation to the epithelia and the nervous system will be discussed in another chapter. In any event, exocrine, endocrine or neurosecretory secretion develops from lining membranes.

Table 43.3 provides a review of the development of the cells of the nervous system after

Starck (13), modified by von Mayersbach (16), and adapted here to meet the requirements of comparative oncology.

Table 2.5 shows the original phylogenetic and ontogenetic dependence of animal secretion on the epithelia, occurring either in a direct or an indirect course of development, suggesting unicellular precursors. Secretion takes place either in the direct course of development (exocrine or endocrine secretion) or in the indirect through the development of the neural epithelium and the precursors of neurons. In the plant organism, secretion, which is much more restricted, develops through meristems, epithelial linings or even parenchymata. In this connection, the formation of the matrix in the connective tissues of animals may be viewed as a type of secretion, because the plant parenchymata are comparable to the connective tissues in animals as a whole. It is easy to understand that this function is partially dependent on meristems, as the nervous tissue does not exist in plants. But all cells including the plant react to stimuli.

The relationship between hormone production and histogenesis, from a comparative standpoint, is shown in Table 2.5.

Normal Histology of Nervous System. The neuron or ganglion cell is a morphological and

Table 2.5
Hormone Production and Histogenesis

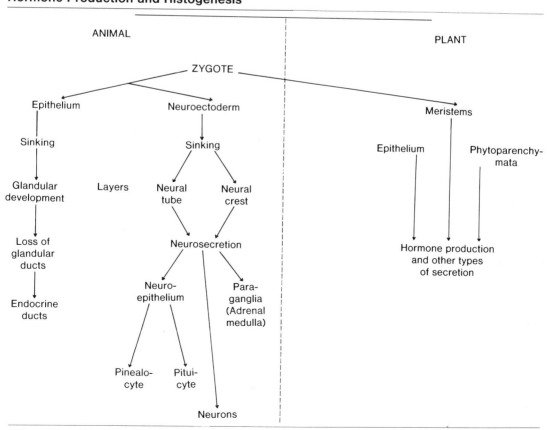

functional unit composed of the nerve cell with its processes and special structures. The cytoplasm of the nerve cell which surrounds the nucleus is the perikaryon. The processes which are usually involved in conducting stimuli to the perikaryon are the dendrites. Those processes conducting stimuli away from the perikaryon are the neurites or axons. Synapses connect processes of neurons with each other or with cells of other tissues such as muscles and glands. The nerve endings are generally branched, forming the so-called telodendria. If well developed they usually form the nerve end organs with the help of connective tissue support.

The nerve cells or neurons include the structure types: these are unipolar, bipolar, pseudounipolar, multipolar (Golgi II type with short neurites—multipolar, Golgi I type with long neurites—multipolar with adjusted dendrites, cell of Purkinje—multipolar without neurite) nerve cells or neurons. The perikaryon, 6–150 μm in size, is surrounded by the plasmolemma and houses the large nucleus; the latter usually contains only one large nucleolus. The cytoplasm contains the neurofibrils, a pronounced Golgi apparatus, and the Nissl bodies, with exception of the axon hill. Dendrites and axon-neurites occur as processes.

With respect to the cell connections, interneuronal synapses, myoneuronal synapses, and neuroglandular connections can be distinguished. These are the effectoric nerve endings. Concerning the receptoric nerve endings, free nerve endings, the nerve end bodies (lamellar bodies: corpuscles of Vater-Pacini, genital nerve bodies, Krause's end bulbs, Meissner's tactile cells and spindle bodies (muscle spindles and tendon spindles) can be distinguished.

The glial cells can be grouped into two categories; those of the central nervous system and those of the peripheral nervous system. The first group of macroglia comprises the protoplasmatic or fibrillar astrocytes, the oligodendroglia and the microglia. The peripheral glia is composed of the cells of Schwann and the so-called mantle cells. The Schwann cells, in turn, are the source of the medullation of the peripheral fibers, which is produced in the central nervous system by the oligodendroglia. In the periphery, we find medullated and unmedullated nerve fibers, some with, some without Schwann's sheaths in each instance.

Neoplasms of Nervous Tissues. The first group of tumors of the nervous tissues comprises the neural epithelium which exhibits the most pronounced embryonic potential.

The second group consists of the neoplasms deriving from the ontogenetic stages of the neurons of the central as well as peripheral distribution of nervous tissue, i.e., the neural axes and neural crests. This group also contains those cell types which cannot be considered specifically as nerve cells, but which derive from the neuroepithelium. Along with the pineal cells or the epithelial cells of the choroid plexus, these cells are offshoots of a development leading to one or another type of secretion, since it also occurs in the epithelium of the choroid plexus.

The third group comprises the neoplasms of glial elements, again divided into central and peripheral glia following the basic division of the nervous system. The microglia, for example, derive from mesenchymal origin, but it is still a controversial question whether all tumors of the peripheral nerve (say of the nerve sheath) derive from Schwann cells or from certain portions of the connective tissue components, as non-neuron elements of the peripheral nerve beside the Schwann cells.

It is suggested that the tumors of the peripheral nerves derive from both the Schwann cells and connective tissue cells. The high potential of the mesenchyme is well known. From this point of view it is perhaps justifiable to add here the rhabdomyomas of the nerves. (A detailed histologic description of human neoplasms and comparable structures in other organisms including the nervous system are given in Chapter 43.)

Neoplasms of Neural Epithelium. The full neuronal and glial potential of the neuroepithelium characterize the rare medulloepitheliomas. (Synonyms of the neoplasms are listed in the Glossary.)

Neoplasms of Conducting Tissue Components, Neoplasms of Embryonic Stages of Neurons, and Neoplasms of Neuraxis Originating from Derivatives. Medulloblastomas are neoplasms deriving from undifferentiated precursors of cells, which could have developed into cells of the neuronal or glial lines. They are solid tumors. No vesicles or tubes with cylindrical or cuboidal lining are observed (12). Variations include neuroblastomas, ganglioneuromas, and glioneuroblastomas. On the basis of the histogenetic principle, the neoplasms of the retina, the optic nerve, and the olfactory placode can be included in this group. They comprise the retinoblastomas and the retinogliablastomas, respectively, with or without stephanocytes, and the gliomas of the optic nerve.

Neoplasms of the Neural Crests Originating from Derivatives. Tumors of the Cranial and

Spinal Ganglia. A few rare tumors are included for these structures; they are composed of neuroblasts (see above) or of particular differentiated stages of the precursors of ganglion cells.

Neoplasms of the Sympathetic System and the Chromaffin Tissues. First among these tumors are the neuroblastomas. Their prognosis is poor. If these tumors are classified as sympathomas, they may be grouped as embryonal sympathomas, almost all of which are malignant, with such variations as sympathogonias and sympathoblastomas. Another variant is the ganglioneuroma. If, as Evans (6) suggests, the ganglioneuromas are diagnosed as a group, a distinction can be made between young and adult ganglioneuromas, corresponding to the age group of the patient when the tumors appear, not to the cell age of the neoplasm. The chromocytoma is a constituent group of tumors which develop from the caudal end of the spinal cord (?) and acquire the ability of producing pronounced endocrine or other types of secretion. As a result of their functional comparability they are grouped together here, one after the other. It is also possible to add these neoplasms to the group containing the tumors of the retina and of the optic nerve.

Paragangliomas are always composed of paraganglionic cells. The suprarenal paraganglioma and the carotid paraganglioma, the latter with benign and malignant forms, are variations. The meningiomas derive from meningocytic cells. The organ of origin is the arachnoid or subarachnoid. According to Masson's classification, these tumors comprise (a) pure arachnoid meningiomas (meningothelial); (b) mixed arachnoid and subarachnoid meningiomas, with a wet, lacunar, and a dry compact variation; and (c) subarachnoid meningiomas with a wet, lacunar, and a dry lamellar variation.

Another group of tumors deriving from the medulloepithelia are those of the choroid plexus, the benign choroid papillomas, and the more malignant chorioepitheliomas. Cells of the developing pineal are sooner or later capable of giving rise to neoplasms, namely, the pinealomas and the pineal embryomas. The latter bring about the development of different tissue types, comparable to the embryomas in the reproductive glands (ovary). This characteristic behavior demonstrates once again that all the neoplasms cited here are derivatives of undeveloped cells from the neuronal development of the nervous system.

The third group comprises the neoplasms of the second development of nervous tissues, the tumors which derive from glial cells:

Neoplasms of Glial Origin. Spongioblastomas. The spongioblastoma, also known as primary spongioblastoma (12), is a tumor originating from the neuroepithelium (medullar epithelium) but lacking any elements of neuron development. Hence, they are composed solely of elements of the glial development. Several subtypes, such as the cavitary, the solid and other varieties can be distinguished.

Neoplasms Deriving from Cells of the Central Glia. The following subgroup of neoplasms derives from the central glia. They are designated according to the glial cell types from which they arise. The astroblastomas are neoplasms of cells which simulate the characteristic patterns of astroblasts. The astrocytomas, in turn, are tumors made up of cells which simulate the differentiated astrocytes. Embryonal stages of this cell type, such as the astroblasts, are never found in this type of neoplasm. Fasciculated, reticulated, and intermediate types of this neoplasm correspond to the specific features of the cells involved. Malignancy varies in accordance with the subtype concerned. In the case of the ependymoglioma an ependymal lining consisting of tubules and vesicles on one hand and of a glial element on the other composes the tumor, of which the cell components develop from each other. The oligodendrogliomas are composed of the cell type after which they are named, the oligodendrocytes. The glioblastomas exhibit glial cells comparable to normal glioblasts. The glioblastoma multiforme is a tumor defined by its glial cells, which display sarcomatous and pleomorphic characteristics.

Neoplasms Deriving from Cells of the Peripheral Glia. These neoplasms constitute the last group of neoplasms of the nervous system. The neurofibromatosis of Recklinghausen, several subtypes of which can be distinguished, belongs to this category. A second group comprises the schwannogliomas, neoplasms deriving from the cells of Schwann. Finally, the rhabdomyomas of nerves that should be included here, for the following reasons: In the nerve structure, the different nerve bundles and units are separated from each other by connective tissues other than the glia. (For a comparison to invertebrates see Chapter 3, section on connective tissues.) The nerve also has vessels which nourish it; large nerves are often ensheathed together with a large artery and vein, e.g., the femoral nerve, femoral artery, and femoral vein. The mesenchymatic cell is multipotential and produces not only the different connective tissue elements, but can also produce muscle cells. If an abnormal production process occurs in the connective tissue structures of a nerve, the resulting condition constitutes a rhabdomyoma of the nerve. Similar to the individual muscle in which the covering connective tissue sheets can be considered part of this individual organ, the connective tissue sheet of the nerve covering it can be regarded as a portion of this organ.

General Comparative Aspects and Conclusions of Animal and Human Neoplasms (Zooneoplasms)

The neoplasms of man can serve as a starting point for the understanding of the histogenesis of animal neoplasms in general, vertebrates and invertebrates alike. Apart from a few exceptions, such as the oblique striated musculature and its possible tumors this holds true for most animal tissues. Human neoplasms deriving from normal tissues are the one fundament of histogenesis and plant neoplasms deriving from meristematic or fully differentiated plant tissues (succeeding meristems/"Folgemeristeme"; meristemoids) the other in a truly comparative oncology.

During the course of this study it becomes evident that the human being is an organism where the development of neoplastic growth reaches its highest peak and widest diversification. The reasons for this are the wide range of tissues in the human body and the additional often unnatural action of environmental and other influences acting upon them.

1. The human body as a representative of the mammalian body displays a high tissue differentiation, which we may regard as a peak in phylogenetic development. The tissues missing in comparison to other animals can be neglected, because of their low number.

2. The vertebrate body displays bone with all of its variations of neoplastic development, but also, with a few exceptions with invertebrates, the striated or multilayered epithelia. In this regard invertebrate hormone producing structures cannot be neglected, but they are of minor importance due to their being of another tissue type (glandular epithelia) and the fact that neoplasms of those endocrine glands in invertebrates had not been detected until now.

3. Due to the effects of technology and the exposure of our body to certain habits such as smoking, eating hot or reheated meals, wearing constraining or synthetic clothing, and exposure to pollutants as well as professional hazards, the number of neoplasms developing in man has increased tremendously. This can be seen from a comparison of industrialized and nonindustrialized nations (2) (Chapter 36). Thus, the neoplastic potential of human tissues has been enhanced tremendously, presenting us with a broad array of tumors as shown in Figure 2.1. (It is the number of cases which increased.)

In plants the transformation from normal to malignant cells proceeds always via meristematic potential which is either of primary or secondary origin.

The few special tissue groups, not present in the human body, can be considered as splinter groups as far as the principle of histogenesis in man is concerned.

In regard to this statement we now have to investigate the principle of histogenesis with respect to plant neoplasms of which more than 14,000 types are known to exist in different species. In plants we also can find the phylogenetic steps leading to true neoplasms if we look, for example, at galls of algae, etc. In the plant, the topic of neoplastic growth is also seen as a subunit of abnormal growth. The fact that some plant tumors are composed not only of the altered host tissue but also of the tissue of the causing organism is remarkable. This condition may be compared to a certain degree to tumor parenchyma and stroma in human tumors.

Histogenesis of Plant Neoplasms (Phytoneoplasms)

Introduction

Two extensive sources of spontaneous neoplasms are known: the human neoplasms, the histogenesis of which has been reviewed above, and the spontaneous tumors of the plants. The human neoplasms may serve as a central focal point for grouping the neoplasms of other animal species around them. Although the tumors of plants have often been described, owing to tissue differences and variations in the approaches of botanists and plant pathologists, their histogenesis has been discussed, yet not well established.

There is the problem in this section, because it appears to be necessary that the working principle of histogenesis be applied here as a basis for further comparisons and that similarities within the broad framework of a comparative oncology be indicated.

The histogenesis of the neoplasms of the remaining groups of eumetazoans can be readily

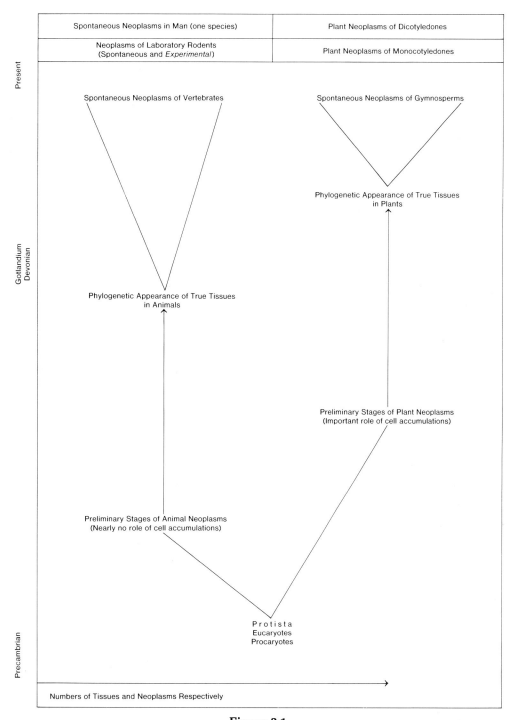

Spontaneous Neoplasms in Man (one species)	Plant Neoplasms of Dicotyledones
Neoplasms of Laboratory Rodents (Spontaneous and *Experimental*)	Plant Neoplasms of Monocotyledones

Spontaneous Neoplasms of Vertebrates

Spontaneous Neoplasms of Gymnosperms

Phylogenetic Appearance of True Tissues in Plants

Phylogenetic Appearance of True Tissues in Animals

Preliminary Stages of Plant Neoplasms (Important role of cell accumulations)

Preliminary Stages of Animal Neoplasms (Nearly no role of cell accumulations)

P r o t i s t a
Eucaryotes
Procaryotes

Numbers of Tissues and Neoplasms Respectively

Present

Gotlandium Devonian

Precambrian

Figure 2.1

approached from relevant aspects of human neoplasmic histogenesis. There are, of course, a few exceptions, such as neoplasms known from birds, which derive from the normal histogenesis of feathers. A full understanding of the histogenesis of neoplasms occurring in invertebrates must still be founded upon thorough knowledge of the histogenesis of human neoplasms, through which the character of the tissues of invertebrates can best be appreciated. Such a compar-

ison is presented in Figure 2.1. Nonetheless, the entire matter becomes complicated due to differences in the normal histogenesis of invertebrate and even vertebrate tissues.

Growth and malignancy of the same tumor may be different as shown in the case of the nephroblastoma:

> ...consider the nephroblastomas. In man, these tumors (sometimes designated Wilms' tumors, embryonal nephromas, or renal adenosarcomas) frequently metasta-

size and are often quickly lethal, particularly if untreated. In swine, nephroblastomas are common, but only rarely metastasize. In rabbits, nephroblastomas are relatively rare, histologically are practically identical with the counterpart in man, but have never been observed to metastasize. In fishes, nephroblastomas biologically seem to resemble the homologue in swine and in rabbits more than that in man. The fish nephroblastomas with which we are familiar, at least, have not metastasized.

C. J. Dawe and J. C. Harshbarger (3)

Other examples are known.

Nevertheless the principle of histogenesis remains the working principle of comparative oncology. Even identical tissues may vary to a certain degree in different phyla (see above and Chapter 43). Comparison of tumor development in the various phyla, taking into consideration cells, which have not achieved full maturity, presents further difficulties; including complications resulting from aging of the host and tumor itself. Hence, the histogenic differentiation of tumor tissues derived from immature cells may also vary. The dysontonogenetic appearance of tumors in different phyla has not been investigated to date from a comparative aspect. New insights may be gained from studies concerning this topic.

Tissues, normal and neoplastic, are composed of cells; cells, normal and neoplastic, are composed of organelles, which can be also considered subcellular structures. In turn, the latter are composed of molecules. For the histogenetic comparison between animal and plant tissues, more specifically, tissues of porifera and eumetazoan animals, higher algae, mosses and vascular plants, as a fundament we have adapted the histogenetic principle as outlined in the books by von Albertini (15), Evans (6), and Masson (12): (a) the comparability of the histogenesis of tissues, (b) the comparability of the cells during the histogenetic events, and (c) the biochemical, including genetic changes. Due to the topic of this chapter, problems a and b will be discussed in relation to the plants. The third problem, using selected examples, is discussed in Chapters 16–18, 28, 29, 31.

Following the discussion of the histogenesis of plant tumors, the various tissues serving the nine main life functions and the comparability of tissues occurring in the different phyla of organisms will be considered (Chapters 3, 4 and 6). This is an essential prerequisite to an understanding of the comparability of pathological growth.

Basic Principles. In a fully comparative approach to the histogenetic principle of neoplastic development, the plants, for which more than 1000 tumor types have been identified in the various families, cannot be excluded. Is it possible to relate these to each other on the basis of the histogenetic principle of plant neoplasms? The analysis of the extensive material suggests that such a relationship can be established, and that, therefore, the principle of histogenesis is also applicable to plant neoplasms.

Further, is it possible to relate the histogenesis of spontaneous human neoplasms to the histogenesis of spontaneous plant neoplasms? Again, this seems possible, and the same holds true, of course, for experimental neoplasms.

During the development of each organism, animal and plant alike, cells with embryonal potential can be distinguished. This embryonal potential in varying tissues and species ceases at different intervals of the particular life span (Chapter 13). Members have a different life span, according to the different tissues involved. In man, the cells with embryonal potential disappear normally during certain periods of embryonic development. But as stated by Cohnheim in his embryonal cell theory approximately 100 years ago, certain cells with embryonal potential may remain in a dormant stage for varying lengths of time. In addition, differentiated cells, even neurons of the cell-invariable nervous tissue (neuron elements—not to be confused with the glia) without a functional field may retain this potential:

Direct and Indirect Ontogeny

The main stages of ontogenetic development	The roundabouts of ontogenetic development
Development of germ cells	
Cleavage	Embryonal metamorphosis
Formation of germ layers	
Organ differentiation	Placentae
Development of germ cells	
Body form/metamerism	Larval metamorphosis (for details, see Chapter 6)

In principle, then, there is a true parallelism here, but only qualitatively, not quantitatively. This parallelism becomes more marked, when the opinion of several botanists is taken into consideration, namely, that the meristems should not be viewed as tissues, but as cell groups with embryonal potential. The collective embryonal cells of the plant meristems constitute the basic reason, at least theoretically, why an understanding of the growth of plant neoplasms is so important for a comparative viewpoint. The bulk of plant tissues, of course, as are those of the animal world, are fully differentiated tissues which will be discussed later.

General Histogenesis of Plant Neoplasms

1. The question of the meristematic, or continued embryologic tissues, to be discussed in one of the following chapters, lends special emphasis to the histogenesis of plant neoplasms. Theoretically, neoplasms can develop from such meristematic tissues as the apical and lateral meristems (lateral meristems are also known as cambium).

In the animal kingdom, cells which are precursors of fully differentiated cells are "blasts" and neoplasms deriving from them are blastomas, e.g., glioblast and neuroblast, and the equivalent tumors, glioblastoma and neuroblastoma. Plant neoplasms of meristematic origin (the meristem as a transitory form leading to fully differentiated cells) would in parallel manner be termed meristemoblastomas. It would furthermore follow that in accordance with the location of their occurrence, apical meristemoblastomas and lateral meristemoblastomas would succeed apical meristems and lateral meristems, respectively.

2. The fully differentiated plant tissues, also known as permanent plant tissues (a possibly misleading term owing to the ability of these tissues to regain meristematic potential under certain conditions) are also capable of reacting to carcinogenic stimuli, and hence are capable of tumor formation.

Topographically, from the standpoint of tissue location on one hand, and from that of tumor formation on the other (see Chapter 33 by Ames), the so-called meristemoids (as around the stomata in the epidermis of leaves) but mostly the so-called succeeding meristems ("Folgemeristeme" in the German literature), composed of cells of fully differentiated tissue regaining embryonal potential, are to be held responsible for the histogenetic change of normal to neoplastic plant tissues.

3. Those functional stages of fully differentiated plant tissues which are nonliving, lack the ability to form neoplasms. With respect to their potential for tumor formation the stages of abnormal plant growth can be subdivided into three groups: (1) hyperreactions, associated with the presence of stimuli, as in certain galls; (b) benign neoplasms; and (c) malignant neoplasms.

The most thoroughly investigated plant neoplasm, one that may be designated as truly malignant in a comparative sense, is the crown gall.

Review of the Plant Tissues of Tracheophyta (Vascular Plants)

Tissue Types of Plants Particularly in Relation to Special Histogenesis of Plant Neoplasms. It is possible to distinguish either between meristematic tissues with at least a theoretically unceasing embryonal potential and the fully differentiated tissues with absence of an embryonal potential which may be regained; but it is also possible to view fully differentiated tissues of the adult plant only, which contain meristematic units as part of their topographic makeup. It must be realized that plant tumors, such as the genetic ones, develop at a special stage (age) of plant development (see Chapter 33). To adopt these units to the requirements for the principle of histogenesis the following arrangement was chosen.

Meristems. Primary meristems are those tissues which derive directly from the meristem of the plant embryo without an intermediate stage of a fully differentiated tissue. They are also known as promeristems.

Secondary meristems are those which resume meristematic character after having given it up for a period of time, during which they existed as fully differentiated tissue. The name for this type is succeeding meristems.

1. Apical meristems as cell units producing first the whole plant embryo and then later remaining as cell cones (shoot and root apices) in the adult plant.

2. Lateral meristems remaining as cell sheets in the adult plant.

3. Intercalary meristems in special regions, e.g., internodes in grasses.

Fully Differentiated Tissue Units in a Topographical Sense.

1. Fully differentiated tissues with included meristemoids.

2. Fully differentiated tissues with the capability of partially retrogressive change into succeeding meristems.

3. Fully differentiated tissues with intercalary meristems.

4. Fully differentiated nonliving plant tissues.

The comparison of animal and plant neoplasms on the basis of a comparative histogenesis has never been attempted before. This bold new undertaking will remain preliminary at this time; but the approach has to be tried. It will have to be supported by experiments directed at unravelling the comparative histogenesis of neoplasms including those of the plants. The only way for a proper comparison with animal neoplasms is by such an approach. It will be seen that such a comparison will not depend only on just morphologic characteristics but also on certain principles, such as the regaining of embryonal potential during injury.

With the exception of genetic plant tumors, the first preliminary condition in the wound tumor or the crown gall disease is an injury to the plant. The same principle occurs to some varying degree in the animal (see Chapter 12, "Cell Injury as a Basic Initial Phenomenon"). The difference is provided by the occurrence of nonliving fully differentiated tissues in plants. Only the precursors of these are able to develop neoplasms as is the case for cell-invariable tissues in the eumetazoans including man. Other comparable factors are of biochemical or biophysical nature as stated above. The following conclusions can be reached: (a) Possible neoplastic development may derive from primary meristems, as cellular cones or sheets with embryonal potential. (b) Neoplasms possibly originating from succeeding meristems shall be discussed with the fully differentiated plant tissues from which the succeeding meristems derive as secondary structures. (c) The review of fully differentiated (permanent) plant tissues with special consideration of the meristemoids and succeeding meristems, which they include topographically or from which they derive secondarily. (d) Neoplasms to be considered as being derivatives of meristematic components of fully differentiated tissues.

Review of the fully differentiated plant tissues grouped in a comparison with the eumetazoans in general and the histogenetic distinction of the malignant neoplasms in the animal kingdom shows that cancers or carcinomas originating from epithelial tissues and the nonepithelial or mesenchymal malignant neoplasms derive from the connective tissue group and are known as sarcomas. Muscle and nerve tissue have no equivalent in the plant and neither do the neoplasms (tumors) emerging from them; they are also known as sarcomas if malignant.

Plant tissues having the same functional principles and similar makeup as types of animal epithelia, are reviewed in Table 2.6.

Significance of Nonmetazoan and Nontracheophytic Structures in Phylogeny and Framework of Neoplastic Growth

Abnormal growth of plants in a wider sense, and neoplastic growth in a more restricted sense exhibits a successive change from foreign matter reaction of the tissues to unlimited growth; just as in the animals, but in a somewhat different pattern. This may be easily assumed if we realize, that so-called galls have been found in algae, fungi, lichens, bryophyta, pteridophyta, gymnosperms, and angiosperms. The majority occurs in dicotyledons. Cell accumulations, pseudotissues, are much more widely distributed in plants, in the old sense of taxonomy, than in animals. Two types of structures have to be distinguished, plectenchymata and pseudoparenchymata, which simulate the character of true tissues by the swelling of the cell membranes. In the case of highest rhodophyceae and the basidiomycetes (fruit body of higher fungi), two types of arrangement occur in the rhodophyceae.

The next step is given by the tissues of the bryophyta, which lack true roots. In the following we should concentrate on the true tissues of the vascular plants. The facts of abnormal growth of pseudotissues are reviewed in Chapter 43.

Plectenchymata. Plectenchymata are pseudotissues composed of fiber systems which simulate true tissues of high algae and cormophytes. The cell connection is given by swelling of the cell membranes to form water-insoluble colloid matter surrounding the whole arrangement. In the red algae two types of plectenchymata can be distinguished.

Pseudoparenchymata. The pseudoparenchymata are tissues which arise by postgenital fusion of previously separated cells. Characteristic for this type of tissue are the sporophores of the mushrooms.

During the earth's history the true tissues of plants appeared phylogenetically millions of years later than the animal tissues. It is a fact that plant neoplasms generally contain cells

Table 2.6
Plant Tissue Comparison with Animal Epithelia

Types of Animal Epithelia	Comparable Plant Tissues
A. Lining epithelia B. Glandular epithelia 　a. Exocrine glands 　b. Endocrine glands	A. Lining membranes 　a. Covering and protective tissues—epidermis and periderm 　b. Absorptive tissues 　c. Secretory tissues 　d. Certain meristems, topographically included in non-hormone-producing cells or structures
C. Reproductive epithelia D. Desmal epithelia	C. Reproductive structures D. Comparable to a certain degree: 　a. Periderm 　b. Xylem, phloem

comparable to animal epithelia and connective tissues of animals. They can, therefore, be considered as being mixed tumors. The following review gives the two components found in the plant neoplasms most studied and a comparison with malignant animal neoplasms.

Review of the Meristematic Tissues. For general information consult Esau (4, 5).

Our main interest for the sake of this comparison should be devoted to fully differentiated tissues with the capability of at least partially retrogressive change into succeeding meristems. This change is a necessity for the different development of plant tumors.

The plant galls, as abnormal growth in plants, can be classified according to the part of the plant body they effect. A short review in tabular form of the tissue components of the root, shoot axis, bud, leaf, flower and fruit is given below.

Characteristics of Normal Apical Meristems. "Apical meristem" is practically a synonym for the shoot or apex above the youngest leaf primordium or the root apex. Initial and derivatives are distinguished by a more pronounced growth potential. The cells are relatively small and isodiometrical. The cell walls are tender and poor in cellulose; the cells are closely united, the nucleus is relatively large, the protoplasms are dense with small or no vacuoles. The whole structure appears conelike or flattened. Therefore it is also called a vegetative point.

Characteristics of the Normal Lateral Meristem or Cambium. This tissue is located between xylem and phloem. It is a cylinder surrounding certain portions of stem and root. It may also be separated in stripes. Two cell types are distinguished; the elongated cells with tapered ends, known as the fusiform initially and the relatively small ray initials. Secondary xylem and phloem are successors of these tissues: e.g., tracheids, fibers and xylem-parenchyma cells in the xylem, sieve cells, fibers and phloem, parenchyma cells in the phloem (4, 5).

The resting meristems are also characterized by intercalary growth zones on the fascicular cambia in the vascular bundles of the dicotyledons from which the secondary growth towards thickness in the shoot begins.

Characteristics of the Normal Succeeding Meristems. In contrast to the primary "Urmeristemie" deriving directly from the embryo, succeeding meristems develop as tissues with newly gained embryonal potential from the cells of fully differentiated tissues which have regained their embryonal powers.

The cells are elongated prismata and, in contrast to the apical meristems, contain large vacuoles. Examples of this type of tissue are the "Korkkambien" or phellogens and the interfascicular cambia.

Characteristics of the Normal Meristemoids. The meristemoids are also secondary in character. They are restricted to a limited region, where, for example, they produce such structures as stomata or trichomes, but also to the leaf or the accumulations of medullary rays. On the one hand they may stimulate cell division in their surrounding area, but on the other they prevent dividing activity by producing so-called sealing zones which may be important for the differentiation pattern of plants.

Phellogen as a Selected Secondary Meristem. The phellogen is the meristem which gives rise to the development of the periderm and appears generally during the first year of growth in a species-specific manner. The first phellogen arises in most species of dicotyledons and conifers in the subepidermal layer, but in some as in *Nerium oleander* or *Pyrus* it comes from epidermal cells. It is also possible that the epidermis and the subepidermis participate in the formation of the phellogen. Characteristic of the phellogen is that it consists of only one cell type which is rectangular-flat in shape. A special type of phellogen can be found in the polyderm of roots and underground portions of certain plants, *e.g.,* Myrtaceae. Phelloids, phellem-like cells without suberin content may occur. The regaining of the embryonal potential in fully differentiated tissues is a process which occurs not only during abnormal growth processes as in galls and real unlimited autonomous growth processes in plants, but also under normal processes during the formation of phellogen. K. Esau states:

> The cells of the epidermis, the collenchyma, or the parenchyma that initiate periderm are living cells, and their change into phellogen is an expression of their ability to resume meristematic activity under appropriate conditions. These cells are usually indistinguishable from neighboring cells. (3)

Histoid Galls. Histoid galls, characterized by cell and tissue abnormalities, are the types of abnormal growth processes in non-animal organisms most significant for the comparative oncologist.

The cells of histoid galls are characterized by a remarkable increase in size when compared to normal parent tissues. The relation of nucleus and cytoplasm has changed as is the case for this relationship in the neoplastic cells of animals. It is important that the large nuclei of the cells of histoid galls correspond to the meristematic cells of primary origin from which they derive. The singular characteristics of the cells of the histoid galls are summarized in Table 2.7.

Neoplasms Deriving from or Involved with Meristems. *Neoplasms of Apical Meristems.* Certain galls at the shoot axis are profoundly influenced by the primary meristems. The simplicity of bud galls is at least partially explained by primary meristems. Acroceadia show a typical arrest of the growth of the tip.

Neoplasm of the Lateral Meristem or Cambium. Galls at the shoot axis and at the root axis are at least influenced by their relation with the cambial cylinder.

To this group of galls which are involved with the lateral meristem, belong the galls of Leguminosae produced at their roots by bacteria which stimulate the resting lateral meristem to change into fast growing parenchymal cells as well as collenchyma and other tissues.

The galls at the shoot axis exhibit a tremendous dependence on the primary meristem of the shoot and the lateral meristem. Details are omitted due to the large number of those types of abnormal growth (see Mani (11)).

Neoplasm of the Succeeding Meristems. Succeeding meristems play a very important role in the development of galls and galls with unlimited growth. The majority of galls involved with fully differentiated tissues develop in reality through a change from the fully differentiated tissues to a succeeding meristem and to the gall. We have to note, also, that some tumors of the short axis and those where cork cambium is involved may belong to this category at least partially. The tissues of concern, the secondary tissues in gall development are those from which the newly formed gall meristems derive. The gall

meristem as a special type, let us say, a pathological type of succeeding meristem leads to the development of different inhibition of fully differentiated gall tissues, as, for example, to the enormous production of parenchymal cells or an increase of growth of phloem or xylem.

Neoplasms of the Meristemoids. Meristems which are constantly involved in plant galls are those of stomata and trichomes. These structures play an important role in leaf galls, the majority of galls, and in epidermal galls as seen from the histologic aspect. They will be discussed in the section of this book dealing with the galls of the epidermis.

Meristems as Topographic and Functional Portions of Fully Differentiated Plant Tissue. The distinction of animal tissues on the basis of morphological characteristics and of plant tissues by temporal distinction is artificial. Fully differentiated animal tissues as they occur in the adult body are able to enter unlimited cell division in the case of malignant development. Plant cells of fully differentiated tissues are able to undergo limited or unlimited cell differentiation by developing a secondary meristematic or embryonal potential when forced to do so by a particular stimulus.

Characterization of Fully Differentiated Plant Tissues

In contrast to meristematic tissues fully differentiated tissues of plants have been termed permanent tissues. It is my belief that these tissues should be called fully differentiated plant tissues because these tissues are not really permanent in the sense of the word. In this book therefore, the functionally nonliving tissues of plants such as the acting or functioning sclerenchyma are considered permanent tissues. Only the precursors of these tissues are able to produce neoplasms, comparable to the situation in cell-invariable animal tissues.

Covering and Protective Tissues. *Epidermis.* Characteristics of Normal Epidermis and Rhizodermis. The epidermis derives from the outermost layer of the "Urmeristem," the protoderm, and is therefore the outermost layer of cells on the primary plant body. The epidermis is the primary surface tissues of the entire plant. In its typical arrangement it is a simple layer of cells, composed of longitudinal or elongated living cells which often show undulated or jagged outlines. With the exception of the roots it is always covered by a cuticle. The meristematic activity

Table 2.7
Selected Characteristics of the Cells of Histoid Galls

1. Increased size of cell
2. Increased water content
3. Increased number of vacuoles
4. Disintegration of plastids and mitochondria as well as fusion
5. Arrest of plastids and mitochondria formation
6. Inhibition of plastid division
7. Depletion of chromatin in nucleus
8. An increase of up to 250 times in the size of the nucleus (e.g., as in galls caused by *Synchitrium* sp.)
9. Increase in the number of nucleoli, in nematode-produced galls up to 500
10. Canal-like structures in nucleus toward position of gall producer
11. Abnormalities of chromosomes
12. General decrease of chlorophyll content

is resumed after certain needs in normal development and after injury. This latter fact is important in relation to gall development.

1. *Cells.* The cells of the epidermis exhibit a simple type of flat platelike cells on one hand and many different cell types on the other, when seen comparatively, according to different plant groups such as dicotyledons, monocotyledons, graminae, species and specific plant parts (see Linsbauer (9)).

The general cells of plant epidermis shall be discussed first, followed by a short review of certain peculiarities. The general squamous-like cell may show variations by building either a simple layer of cells or a multiple structure from 2 to 16 layers of cells which may originate from their epidermis or the underlying parenchyma which is known as hypodermis. But it must be stressed that the typical epidermis is a simple layer, composed of polygonal or elongated cells. The same principle is observed in the integument of all metazoans where the epidermis is simple; but beginning with chaetognatha it changes at least regionally to a stratified type of integument, which is typical for the stratified integument of vertebrates.

The relationship of different diameters of epidermal cells changes as, for example, in the case of the epidermis of seeds or in elongated plant portions where the epidermal cells also may be elongated in accordance with the elongation of the organ as in stems or certain leaves. The contour of epidermal cells may be wavy in appearance or zigzag. In graminae different cell types are present, namely the elongated, so-called long cells, two types of short cells, the silica and cork cells. Again the short cells may develop such appendage structures as hairs, bristles, and spines. Another cell type of monocotyledons are the bulliform cells. In a comparative sense the principle is similar to the eumetazoan epidermis or integument with the appearance of sweat glands, hairs, sebaceous glands, etc. in its highest diversification in the vertebrate integument; but it is also found in the invertebrates, for example, as nettle cells in coelenterates.

2. *Stomata.* The stomata are epidermal holes at the aired portions of the plants serving gaseous exchange, disposal of water vapor, etc. They are surrounded by two guard cells, which by changes in their volume open and close the aperture; in this way, they expose the spaces of the plant to the environment. These cells are bean-like in shape. In some cases they also occur as the supporting cells. The stomata are rare at the flowers and lacking at the roots.

3. *Trichomes.* The trichomes or hairs (a misnomer in the comparative sense) are unique multicellular appendages of the epidermis on aerial plant parts, and variations, known from roots are to be discussed in the next paragraph. Trichomes are formed exclusively from the epidermal cells, in contrast to emergences where subepidermal tissues may participate in the formation. Transition stages exist. We distinguish among protective, supporting and glandular hairs, sacs and papillae. They may be persisting or temporary structures and play an important role in many plant galls. The development starts with the initial elongation of an epidermal cell.

4. *Root hairs.* Root hairs are absorbing structures, originating from the rhizodermis to expand the surface of the root. They develop also at other plant parts; they are unicellular at the root in the soil and multicellular on adventitious roots in the air.

Galls (Neoplasms, as in the Case of Crown Gall) Involving the Epidermis. General characteristics of the gall epidermis: the epidermal tissues of galls arise either from the normal epidermis or from the subepidermal parenchyma. The first case is more common and the cells in the second case may resemble more or less the parenchymal cells they derived from. The cells are generally much larger than normal epidermal cells and in certain galls such as the fungal galls of *Synchitrium* spp. they show a remarkable heterogeneity. We can even find a stratified epidermis as in the galls produced by *Copium tenceii* on *Teucium capitulum* and of *Janetiella* (*Oligotrophus*) *lemeei* on *Ulmus*. This is a remarkable case because a more specialized condition is reached through a pathological process. (This is not a pathophylogenetic progression because the same happenings occur under normal conditions, as in the epidermis of xerophyta or fruits/seeds.)

The number of stomata is generally decreased or they are totally absent. The guard cells of the stomata are often very swollen and lose their functional capacity. Constant closure of the stomal opening, or a constant open condition, as well as the development of irregular stomata in patches are common.

The trichomes of galls are strongly and densely developed in a number of galls initiated by Acarina, Diptera, Hymenoptera, and some aphids. The trichomes may be changed into glandular structures if they are modified, or they may remain similar to those in the normal tissues. A large diversity in size, shape, and structures characterizes newly developed hairs of galls. Trichomes may not only arise from epidermal cells but also from parenchymal units as in the case of *Hartigiola* (= *Oligotrophus*) *annalipes* on *Fagus silvatica*.

The epidermal cells of "leaf margin roll galls" are mainly hypertrophic, without or with deformed stomata; characteristic are hairy outgrowths especially on the inner side.

In the case of the *Lenticula* galls, the tissue of the epidermis is characterized by thickened epidermal cells.

In nematode galls which affect leaves the epidermal cells are highly enlarged. Thickening of cell walls of epidermal cells occurs also in pouch galls.

One group of leaf galls is directly known as epidermal galls. These galls, which comprise quite a large number, originate from simple epidermal cells, which are attacked by gall-initiating organisms. In most cases the galls start from a number of epidermal cells, which produce hairy outgrowths or fleshy emergences. The cells of these latter matted galls are highly enlarged epidermal cells. In some cases narrow patches of some cells are highly enlarged epidermal cells. Many types of these abnormal galls are known, and for further decision of the involvement of epidermis by crown gall (9) see Chapters 49–52.

Periderm. The Characteristics of Normal Periderm. The periderm is a secondary, protective tissue, replacing the epidermis in the case of increased thickness growth. This tissue occurs on stems and roots of gymnosperms and dicotyledons undergoing secretory increase in thickness. The periderm develops also around wounds. The secondary meristem or phellogen producing the periderm has already been discussed; the phellem is the second component growing toward the outside of the periderm and the phelloderm growing to the inside is the third. The cells of the phellem exhibit a prismatic shape which may be elongated and the radial diameter is shorter when compared to the tangential diameter. The shape of the phelloderm cells corresponds to the phellogen cells; structure and content of the cell walls are similar to that of the cortical cells. The outermost cell layers of the periderm are dead, the inner ones alive. The tissues outside the vascular cambium are called outer bark or *rhytidome*.

Galls (Neoplasms) Deriving from Periderm. Galls with external cecidozoa show, for example, an involvement of the periderm as in the case of *Asterolecanium variolosum* Ratzb. on *Quercus robur* Linn, which has unilateral swelling on one side and an exaggerated production of periderm.

Absorptive Tissue. The main, generally distributed, absorptive tissue of plants is the noncuticularized rhizodermis, the epidermis of the young root. It is a special type of epidermis as are some other types of absorptive structures, such as absorptive hairs or trichomes or the hydropotes of the aquatic plant. In addition, the velum radicum of certain monocotyledons, originating from the protoderm and the ligula of selaginellales, lepidodendrales, and isoetales belong to this tissue group.

The rhizodermis is specialized for active water intake and absorption. The root hairs are especially adapted for this purpose and may be compared functionally with such structures as the intestinal villi; the whole rhizodermis may easily be compared to the absorptive surface of lower organisms such as cestodes and others. The cells of the rhizodermis are known as trichoblasts which produce the extensions of the root hairs and the atrichoblasts of which the first ones are smaller. Sometimes, a secondary absorptive system occurs. Characteristic of the epidermis of the root are closely arranged cells which have thin walls. The rhizodermis of the underground roots is uniseriate in contrast to the velamen of air roots which is an example of the multiseriate epidermis.

Neoplasms Deriving from or with Involvement of Absorptive Tissue. The root galls are connected with changes of the epidermis, where the epidermis serves as transmitter of the stimulus to deeper laying tissues. It is there, that the first multiplication of bacteria starts, for example, in the case of root galls of leguminosae. Fungal galls occur also in the cortex. The best known root galls produced by a nematode are those of *Heterodera*. Root galls occur also as a product of organisms of aerial habitat. Finally, galls occur on aerial roots. But the changes in the rhizodermis are not as pronounced as in the case of the epidermis *per se*. Nearly nothing is known of galls of the other absorptive structures aside from the rhizodermis.

Secretory Tissues. Secretory tissues comprise two groups of structures, those which excrete to the outside and which are known as the glandular cells or tissues and those which deposit into cellular spaces and are known as excretory cells or tissues. Both groups may be found either as singular cell patches or in tissue formations among other tissues of the plant. The main types of these cells or tissues are summarized in the following. The structures show an interchange from one type to the other and we distinguish:

A. External structures:
  1. Trichomes
  2. Glands
  3. Nectaris   } glandular structures
  4. Osmophores
  5. Hydathodes
B. Internal structures:
  1. Secretory cells
  2. Secretory spaces
C. Lactifers

Trichomes. These were mentioned in the section of the epidermis. Some facts may be added. Secretory trichomes as well as glands may be of epidermal origin or they may arise from epidermal derivatives and deeper layers. Large areas of the epidermis may be glandular as happens in leaves and flowers. Different types of hairs are distinguished by a unicellular or multicellular head, others are the peltate hairs and so on. Glandular hairs secrete between the wall and cuticle, expanding the latter tremendously. Others as the stinging hairs of *Urtica* exhibit special mechanism for the release of their excretory product. Regarding glands we must not forget the glands of carnivorous plants. Their glands secrete even trypsin, just as animal glands.

Nectaris may be divided into floral nectaris, occurring on flowers, and extrafloral nectaris, occurring on other parts of the plants, for example, stems or leaves. The excretion of nectar occurs in the less specialized forms via the stomata and in higher forms through cell wall and cuticle. Osmophors are special glands of flowers as they occur in Araceae or Burmaniaceae. The hydathodes perform the discharge of water from the interior portion of the leaf to the surface, a process generally known as gutation.

As far as the internal structures are concerned, the secretory cells derive from parenchyma cells and contain certain substances such as resins or tannins. Oil cells belong to this group and the secretory product occurs in a distinct area of the cell surrounded by a limiting membrane. The canals or cavities known as secretory spaces are formed by schizogeny or lysigeny or both and are surrounded by a cellular epithelium. The breakdown of such an epithelium provides the spaces and may be compared with holocrine secretion in animals. The lactifers are either articulated or nonarticulated. The cells of lactifers contain a living protoplast.

Neoplasms Deriving from or with Involvement of Secretory Tissues. The involvement of trichomes in galls has already been mentioned.

1. *Glands.* Glands play a role in different types of galls as in those of leaves, buds and flowers (see Mani (11)). Nectaris play a role in the galls which develop from flowers.

2. *Osmophors.* They also play a role in flower-galls of Asclepiadaceae, Aristolochiaceae, Araceae, Burmaniaceae, and Orchidaceae.

3. *Hydathodes.* They may be of importance in leaf galls, by storing excretory products from gall producers. They may offer insight into gall-initiating processes if used in new comparative experiments.

4. *Secretory cells.* For a list of the distribution and different types of sensory cells, see Esau (4). They can be involved in most different gall types.

5. *Secretory spaces.* They occur in nearly every part of the plant and may be very useful for new experiments with chemical carcinogens in learning more about their role in abnormal growth processes in plants.

6. *Lactifers.* The same is true also for lactifers, which occur in different plants such as Cichoriaea, Campanulaceae, Cariaceae, Papaveraceae, Euphorbiaceae, Convolvulaceae, Liliaceae, Musaceae, Moraceae, and Urticaceae. They may be useful for studying the microinjection of compounds such as nitrosamines. They play a role in many galls of leaves.

Parenchymata. *Characteristics of Normal Parenchymata (Phytoparenchymata).* Parenchymata are also known as the basic tissue of the plant body. The parenchyma is nearly always a living tissue, which may arise from the basic meristem if it is a portion of the primary plant body. To this group belong the parenchymata of the cortex, the pith, the mesophyll of leaves and parenchyma of the flower. Parenchyma connected with vascular tissues derive from procambium and vascular cambium; it may also emerge from phellogen (the phelloderm). The main types of parenchyma are assimilatory parenchyma or chlorenchyma, storage parenchyma, conducting parenchyma or aerenchyma. Parenchyma may contain aerial spaces. The collenchyma is also a type of parenchyma, but will be discussed later as a separate tissue.

In the Table 2.8 the parenchyma is compared to the connective tissues of animals.

The parenchyma is responsible for many vegetative functions of the plant. The term comes from the Greek and means the tissue poured beside the earlier formed ones. Parenchyma as tissue may compose entire plant parts or the parenchyma cells may be intermingled heterogenously with other distinct plant tissues. The cells are living, relatively undifferentiated, with thin walls and are of polyhedral shape. Pith and cortex of stem and roots, mesophyll of leaves, the flesh of succulent fruits, and the endosperm of seeds are more or less totally composed of parenchyma, which surrounds such structures as sclerids in leaf mesophyll. According to function, assimilatory parenchyma or chlorenchyma, storage parenchyma, conducting parenchyma, and aerenchyma may be distinguished.

Galls, Including Plant Neoplasms Deriving from Plant Parenchymata, or Those in Which Parenchymata Are Involved. Parenchymata are distinctly involved in the galls of leaves, buds, flowers, fruits, the shoot axis and the root; in other words, in galls of all major topographic types of the plant body. Since its is impossible

to mention here all the types involved, some examples have been selected. The most common group and the most complicated are the parenchyma galls of the leaf blade. Examples are: the pockengall caused by the midge *Cystiphora pilosellae* Kieff, on the leaf of *Hieracium* spp.; the fold gall of *Schizomyia meruae* Felt. on the leaf of *Maerua arenaria* Hook. & Bl.; the lenticular gall of the cynipid *Neuroterus* on *Quercus*, in which the disc itself is made up of simple parenchyma cells; the Mark-gall of an unknown gall midge on the underside of the leaf blade of *Machilus* sp.; the complex leaf gall of *Asphondylia trichocecidarum* Mani on the leaf of *Acacia leucophloea* Willd and the cylinder-piston gall of *Lobopteromyia* sp. on *Acacia suma* Ham.-Buch. in which the gall tissue consists of greatly hypertrophied and elongated parenchyma cells. Role galls can be cited as another typical example.

Supporting Tissues. *Collenchyma.* Collenchyma is a plant tissue characterized by living cells elongated in the direction of the structure concerned. This tissue has only one cell type. It is always of primary origin and the cell walls are only partially thickened. The cells of the collenchyma resemble, at least partially, the parenchyma cells but they are differentiated from them by the thickening of certain portions of the cell wall. By the development of lignified secondary walls collenchyma may change into sclerenchyma.

Galls (Plant Neoplasms), in Which Changes of Collenchyma Are Involved. Characteristic of the remarkable petiole gall of *Pemphigus spirothecae* on Populus "Spirallockengall" is the total absence of collenchyma which normally appears in the healthy petiole. The main portion of the gall originates from a strong proliferation of peripheral cortical parenchyma.

Sclerenchyma. Sclerenchyma is a nonliving tissue which takes over the duties of fully grown plant organs from collenchyma. In general, stone cells or sclereids and sclerenchyma fibers are distinguished. In particular, brachysclereids or stone cells, macrosclreids or rodlike cells, osteosclereids or bone-shaped sclereids, astrosclereids, literally starsclereids, filiform sclereids of elongated shape, and trichosclereids of branched shape can be distinguished. Due to the fact that sclerenchyma is a fully differentiated nonliving and therefore permanent tissue, it is not able to produce neoplasms but it may be involved either by its precursors (*e.g.*, the before-mentioned collenchyma) or by other involvement in gall formation.

Table 2.8
Parenchym Comparison with Animal Connective Tissue

Types of Connective Tissues in Animals	Comparable Plant Tissues
A. CONNECTIVE TISSUES PER SE	A. PHYTOPARENCHYMATA
I. *Connective tissues rich in cells*	I. *Parenchyma*
1. Mesenchyme	
2. Spinocellular connective tissue with variations	
3. Reticular connective tissue with variations and the deriving hematogenic tissues	3. Chlorenchyma
II. *Connective tissues with abundant fibers*	
1. Gelatinous connective tissue	
2. Loose interstitial connective tissue	
3. Pigmented connective tissue	
4. Fibrillar connective tissue	4. Sclerenchyma (fibers)
B. SUPPORTING TISSUES	
I. *Supporting tissues rich in cells*	
1. Adipose tissue	1. Collenchyma
2. Chordoid tissue	
3. Chondroid tissue	
II. *Supporting tissues rich in matrix*	
1. Cartilage	
2. Bone	2. Sclerenchyma (sclereids)

Galls (Neoplasms) Deriving from Precursors of Sclerenchyma and Sclerenchyma Involved in Gall Development. Galls which involve the sclerenchyma are root galls, shoot axis galls, leaf galls, and galls on flowers. Sclerotic cells occur in lenticular galls on *Quercus* as those produced by *Diplolepis longiventris*. The root gall of *Biorrhiza pallida* and *Andricus quercus-radicis* on *Quercus* also develop sclerenchyma. The same holds true for the gall of *Aylax latreillei* on the rectangular stem of *Glechoma hederacea*. Sclerenchyma composes the outer zone in the gall of *Mikiola fagi* on the leaf of *Fagus silvatica* Linn. One to three layers of sclerenchyma cells with very much thickened walls especially at the outer side of the gall occur on the lenticular galls produced by the cynipid *Neuroterus* on *Quercus*. In the flower galls of *Oxsphondylia floricola*, on the flowers of *Indigofera gerardiana* from the Himalaya, and in the gall on *Amajoua guinensis traxiliensis* from South America, the entire swollen spongy mass into which the whole flower has been transformed contains an axial larval cavity which is surrounded by a 1-mm thick sclerenchyma zone.

Vascular Tissues. *Xylem*. Xylem is the water-conducting tissue of the plant. It is a complex tissue composed of living and nonliving cells. We distinguish between the primary xylem of the primary plant body and the secondary xylem developing from vascular cambium. The primary xylem can again be divided into protoxylem and metaxylem depending on the time of development of vascular differentiation. Regarding the cells, we distinguish between fibers and parenchyma cells. Two types of fibers occur in the xylem: the fiber tracheids and the libriform fibers. The living cells are the parenchyma cells which are either axial parenchyma or reparenchyma, which can again be separated into procumbent ray cells and upright ray cells. Since the parenchyma has already been described it is not necessary to elaborate on it in more detail as far as the cells are concerned. As for the nonliving cells, only the living precursors are able to participate actively in gall development and those have already been described for the case of the lateral meristem or cambium.

Neoplasms Deriving from Xylem or Involvement of Xylem in Gall Development. Galls in which the xylem is involved belong most commonly to shoot and root galls and especially leaf galls. But xylem occurs also in other galls, as the gall of *Glechoma hederacea* produced on its stem by *Aylax latreillei*.

Phloem. Characteristics of Normal Phloem.

Phloem is the most important food-conducting tissue of the tracheophyta. It is a complex tissue exhibiting several types of cells and is also divided in primary and secondary phloem. The main components are the sieve elements, different types of parenchyma cells, fibers and sclereids, and in some plants lactiferous elements. The primary phloem originates from the procambium as the primary xylem. The sieve elements show two types of structure, the sieve cells and the sieve tube members. The sieve cell is a long and slender cell with a sieve area on both ends and attached next to the sieve cell. The sieve tube members are of similar form and the sieve area is higher specialized. Parenchyma cells, fibers and sclereids as well as lactiferous elements and other components have been described before.

Neoplasms Deriving from Phloem, or Phloem Involved in Gall Production. Phloem is either altered by way of suppression or excessive development involving primary tissues: a rich development of phloem occurs in the gall of *Mompha* on *Epilobium*; vascular elements built only of phloem appear in the gall of *Ustilago maydis* on *Zea mays* and a duplication of vascular bundles occurs in the gall of *Baizongia pistaciae* on *Pistacia*. There also exists a new formation or alteration of secondary phloem tissue in galls.

Reproductive Structures. In contrast to the animal, we consider here the whole structure of the flower, not just the germinative tissues of the plant such as the ovary. The flower is often thought of as the real organ of the angiosperm and can be seen as the sex organ of the plant.

Neoplasms or galls of reproductive structures are the galls of flower and fruit. The following main types can be distinguished: (a) galls in which the cecidogenetic reaction is localized, (b) galls in which the cecidogenetic reaction is not localized (c) galls on the inflorescence, and (d) galls on fruits.

SUMMARY

In this chapter on histogenesis it was shown that the different tissues exhibit a more or less broad comparability. A comparison of the histogenesis of the different types of tumor growth in animals and plants is possible and justified on this basis. Tumors or abnormal growth processes with limited growth capability occur in both kingdoms of the two- or six-kingdom approach such as the benign neoplasms in animals or the majority of galls in plants. In addition to growth processes with limited potential we have growth processes with unlimited growth potential such as the malignant neoplasms in man and animals or the plant neoplasms with unlimited growth which can be considered as being malignant. The best studied example is the widely distributed crown gall or the genetic plant tumors such as those found in tobacco plant hybrids, certain virus diseases and surely many more not properly investigated up to now. The tissues which are easily comparable in animals and plants provide the center and fundament of the comparison whereas the more or less noncomparable tissues between animals and plants may open new avenues of research by adding specific information to the topic of histogenesis. The comparative value of meristems, permanent plant tissues, tissues with endocrine hormone production in both kingdoms, and muscle and nervous tissues belong to this group.

Final Comparative Remarks on Histogenesis of Human, Animal, and Plant Neoplasms

In benign neoplasms of man and animals the histogenesis of abnormal growth reaches only the condition of limited abnormal growth. This is also the case for most plant galls. Some thoughts on the histology and histogenesis as well as the life span of stem, root, leaf, flower, fruit, and seed and concerning the tissues involved and their relation to the neoplasms developing therefrom may provide further understanding. In the case of plant galls, such as that of the flower and certain parts of the organs such as that of the petal permit generally only such a change because of the often very short life span of the structure. We have to think especially of infiltrative growth and the other limitation imposed by the plant body which make metastatic growth unable to occur, that is, in contrast to the animal body, that floating cells do not exist in the plant body. The survival of cells in the sap of the plant (body fluids) may only be possible for a very limited time, in the case of the wounding of the plant. But the cells will never be able to settle naturally as, for example, in the case of the wounding of a crown gall tumor.

But in animals as well as plants the same tissues which support benign neoplasms can also develop malignant ones. Finally, experiments have proven that quite often chemical carcinogens have the potential to produce a similar reaction in plants as they do in animals. Benzo[a]pyrene is as toxic in the plant as in the animal, but benzo[e]pyrene is only weakly carcinogenic in plants just as in animals (Kaiser, unpublished data). The crown gall initiating *Bacterium tumefaciens* with its wide variation in plants is said to be responsible also for the production of vertebrate and invertebrate tumors. This seems likely if we look at the newest discoveries on plastids and their role in crown gall formation as summarized by Lippincott *et al.* (10).

The cell with ability to undergo malignant transformation in an animal or plant tissue first has to react to the initiating or promoting stimuli; this is then followed by the more or less partial metabolic interaction of the stimulus in the cells resulting in cellular changes which provoke limited or unlimited growth. Histogenesis may vary tremendously in the reaction of different cell types and the aggressiveness of the resulting neoplasms, due to the cells affected, but the reaction to the seven causes of neoplasms, (chemical carcinogens, physical carcinogens, radioactive emissions, virus, bacteria, parasites, and genes) boils down to intercellular processes in which the cell reacts metabolically with chemical and physical factors. This is the case because even viruses are only chemical entities for example, parasites have only a chemical or physical effect.

How the problem of neoplastic growth can be illuminated from the different oncologic aspects is shown in the various sections of the book which have been contributed by different specialists. But first the distribution and comparability of normal tissues and the variation in the phenomenon of normal growth as it occurs in the different types of ontogenetic development, have to be discussed and this is done in the following three chapters. Only in this way will it be possible to reach a proper evaluation of the variations and particularities of the phenomenon of abnormal growth and especially of autonomous growth in the different organisms.

References

1. Boonyanit, S., and Kaiser, H. E. (1977): Malignant neoplasms of the vulva. *Anat. Rec.,* 187:538–539.
2. Boonyanit, S., and Kaiser, H. E. (1977): Geographic variation in the occurrence of cancer in Thailand compared with other countries. *Cancer Research,* AACR, Abstract 726.
3. Dawe, C. J., and Harshbarger, J. C. (1975): Neoplasms in feral fishes: their significance to cancer research. In: *The Pathology of Fishes,* pp. 876–894, edited by W. E. Ribelin and G. Migaki. The University of Wisconsin Press, Madison, Wisc.

4. Esau, K. (1966): *Anatomy of Seed Plants*. John Wiley & Sons, New York.

5. Esau, K. (1965): *Plant Anatomy*, Ed 2. John Wiley & Sons, New York.

6. Evans, R. W. (1966): *Histological Appearances of Tumours*. Williams & Wilkins, Baltimore.

7. Janovski, N. A., and Paramanandhan, T. L. (1975): *Ovarian Tumors: Tumors and Tumorlike Conditions of the Ovaries, Fallopian Tubes and ligaments of the Uterus*. W. B. Saunders, Philadelphia.

8. Kent, Jr., G. C. (1954): *Comparative Anatomy of the Vertebrates*. Mc-Graw-Hill, New York.

9. Linsbauer, K. (1930): Die Epidermis. In: *Handbuch der Pflanzenanatomie, Vol. 4*. Gebrüdrer Borntraeger, Berlin.

10. Lippincott, J. A., Lippincott, B. B., and Starr, M. P. (1980): The genus *Agrobacterium*. In: The Prokaryotes, edited by M. P. Starr, H. Stolp, H. G. Truper, A. Balows, and H. G. Schlegel. Springer Verlag, New York.

11. Mani, M. S. (1964): *Ecology of Plant Galls* (Monographiae Biologicae, Vol. XII). Dr. W. Junk, The Hague.

12. Masson, P. (1970): *Histologic Diagnosis of Human Tumors* (translation by D. Kobernick). Wayne State University Press, Detroit, Mich.

13. Starck, D. (1965): *Embryologie*, Ed. 2. George Thieme Verlag, Stuttgart.

14. *Strasburger's Textbook of Botany* (1980): Translated by P. R. Bell and D. E. Coombe. Longman Group Ltd., London.

15. Von Albertini, A. (1974): *Histologische Geschwulstdiagnostik* George Thieme Verlag, Stuttgart.

16. Von Mayersbach-Reale (1973): *Grundriss der Histologie des Menschen, Vol. 1*, edited by H. von Mayersbach: Allgemeine Histologie. Gustav Fischer, Stuttgart.

II

Distribution and Function of Normal Tissues

3

Distribution of True (Real) Tissues in Organisms: A Preliminary Condition of Neoplastic Growth

Hans E. Kaiser

INTRODUCTION (10, 124, 184, 234, 345)

The presence of true tissues, which occur in the majority of organisms, seen from the species-specific point of view, is a necessary precondition for an understanding of neoplastic growth. The major changes have been observed in the lower organisms, with the beginning of tissue development while the eumetazoans, representing the animals with true tissues and the vascular plants, have remained stable in their taxonomic position. The lower organisms are significant for the phylogenetic development of neoplastic growth because they show certain preliminary conditions and sidelines, e.g., fungi.

Considering the phyla of organisms from the point of view of tissue development and distribution the whole group of organisms can be divided into two categories: (a) organisms without true tissues which may be termed Nonhistonia and (b) organisms with true tissues which may be termed Histonia.

From the time of Aristotle (384–322 B.C.) and his pupil Theophrastus to Carolus Linnaeus (1707–1778) only two kingdoms were distinguished, animals and plants. The unicellular organisms were raised to kingdom status by J. Hogg (1860) and E. Haeckel (1866), a move which resulted in the three-kingdom approach; animals, plants, and protoctista or protista. In 1938, A. D. Copeland raised the number of kingdoms to four by dividing the unicellular organisms into two kingdoms. The first one, the mychota or monera, is characterized by prokaryotic cells and comprises the bacteria and blue-green algae, the second one, the protoctista, have eukaryotic cells and comprise the algae, with the exception of the blue-green algae, the protozoans, the slime molds and the fungi. The third kingdom is that of the higher plants and the fourth kingdom that of the multicellular animals. Thirty years later Whittaker suggested a five-kingdom approach by raising the fungi to a kingdom in their own right. Jahn and Jahn in 1949 and Kaiser in 1980 proposed a six-kingdom approach by raising the viruses to kingdom status. One- (Walter, 1930) or seven-kingdom approaches (Jeffrey, 1971) have also been recommended (300, 352).

The historical taxonomic extension to six kingdoms (Table 3.1) provides an opportunity for more logical and definitive categorization with regard to cell and tissue evaluation. We distinguish: (a) subcellular organisms, (b) organisms with prokaryotic cells, (c) unicellular or uninucleated organisms with eukaryotic cells (d) multicellular organisms without true tissues, (e) multicellular organisms with restricted differentiation of true tissues, and (f) multicellular organisms with true tissues. The eumetazoans, the phyla taxonomically superior to porifera, build the majority of animal species characterized by true animal tissues. Comparable is the case concerning the tracheophyta or vascular plants composing the stock of species with true plant tissues. Mesozoans, placozoans, and sponges in animals can be seen as the first steps in which restricted tissue development occur similar as in certain fungi, highest rhodophyta, phaeophyta, chlorophyta, charophyta and bry-

43

Table 3.1
The Six-Kingdom Approach According to Structural Makeup

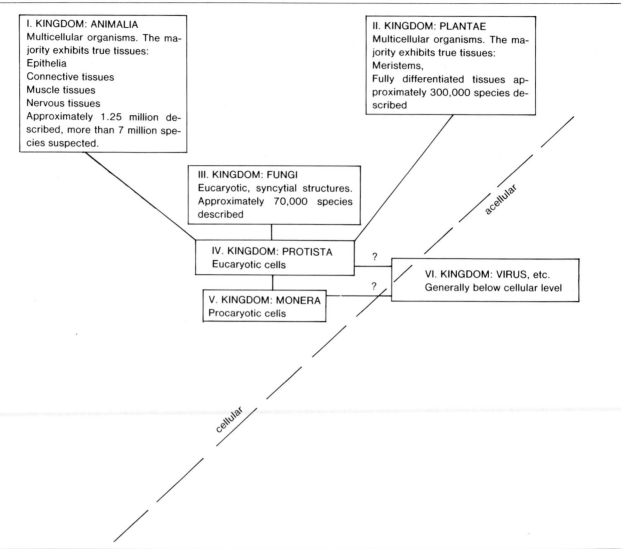

ophyta as far as plant tissues are concerned. In view of neoplastic differentiations eumetazoans and vascular plants stand in the lime light.

The Kingdoms of the Organisms with Cellular Characteristics

1. KINGDOM ANIMALIA: Animals

Cellular Characteristics. Multicellular, cells without walls and plastids, no photosynthesis; eukaryotic; digestive nutrition; sometimes absorptive nutrition; nerve and muscle tissues; mostly sexual reproduction.

Animal Phyla. Mesozoa, mesozoans; Porifera, sponges; Cnidaria, coelenterates; Ctenophora, comb jellies; Platyhelminthes, flatworms; Nemertea (Rhynchocoela), ribbon worms; Gnathostomulida, gnathostome worms; Entoprocta, pseudocoelomate polyzoans; Acanthocephala, spiny-headed worms; Rotifera (rotifers), wheel animalcules; Gastrotricha, gastrotrichs; Kinorhyncha, kinorhynch worms; Nematoda, roundworms; Nematomorpha, hairworms; Priapulida, priapulid worms; Mollusca, molluscs; Sipuncula (Sipunculida), peanut worms; Echiura, spoon worms; Annelida, segmented or annelid worms; Arthropoda, arthropods; Echinodermata, echinoderms; Chaetognatha, arrow worms; Pogonophora, beard worms; Hemichordata, acorn worms; Cephalochordata, lancelets; Vertebrata, vertebrates.

2. KINGDOM PLANTAE: Plants

Cellular Characteristics. Multicellular, cells walled, often vacuolated and photosynthetic pigments present; nutrition mainly photosynthesis, sometimes absorptive. Meristematic and fully differentiated tissues, some of which are nonliving while performing function; propagation mainly sexual with haploid and diploid stages.

Plant Phyla (Divisions). Rhodophyta, red algae; Phaeophyta, brown algae; Chlorophyta, green algae; Charophyta, stoneworts; Bryophyta, liverworts, hornworts, and mosses; Tracheophyta, vascular plants.

The development of tissue-like structures and of true tissues occurred in convergent lines and in phylogenetically different periods during the history of the earth.

The structural makeup shows that in plants a larger number of organisms remained at the level of cell accumulations, that is multicellular organisms without true tissues. Thus, there exist at least 33,000 algae, 10,000 fungi and lichens, and 26,000 mosses as lower plants, and 50 species of mesozoans, and perhaps 4,000 sponges regarding animals. Some of these multicellular organisms without true tissues reached dimensions of up to 300 feet in length as in the largest algae. But the majority of the animal and plant species, in the two-kingdom approach, is composed of organisms with true tissues. About 1.5 million animal species and about 370,000 plant species with true tissues have been described. The number of living animal species is estimated at 5–7 million the majority of which are insects, and that of plants, at half a million the largest group of which are dicotyledones with more than 200,000 species.

Multicellular organisms with limited differentiation of true tissues in the highest or most advanced forms belong to the phyla Rhodophyta (red algae), Phaeophyta (brown algae), Bryophyta (mosses), and Porifera (sponges). In the highest forms of Rhodophyta or Phaeophyta meristematic zones, reproductive zones, special regions for photosynthesis and storage, and in the highest Phaeophyta even conducting structures and tissues are found. In mosses, only roots are missing (therefore the rhizodermis). The majority of species of these groups shows no formation of true tissues. The first animal epithelia developed in the Porifera. A separation of the reproductive structures from the other somatic cells occurs in higher fungi; this may be considered as a lower type of tissue separation.

The plectenchymata best developed in highest fungi and rhodophyta by interweaving of cells and the pseudotissues can be seen as sidelines of development; whereas the apical cells and resulting tissues of bryophyta are intermediate stages between the highly developed thalli of highest algae and the cormus of vascular plants. The organs of the thallus of highest phaeophyta are known as phylloids, cauloids, or rhizoids.

3. KINGDOM FUNGI: Mushrooms

Cellular Characteristics. Mainly multinucleate syncytial (nuclei eukaryotic), without photosynthesis, absorptive nutrition; asexual and sexual reproduction.

Phyla (Divisions) of Fungi. Myxomycota, syncytial or plasmodial slime molds; Acrasiomycota, cellular or pseudoplasmodial slime molds; Labyrinthulomycota, cell-net slime molds; Oomycota, oosphere fungi; Chytridiomycota, true chytrids and related fungi; Zygomycota, conjugation fungi; Zygomycota, conjugation fungi; Ascomycota, sac fungi; Basidiomycota, club fungi.

4. KINGDOM PROTISTA: Eukaryotic Colonies, Unicells

Cellular Characteristics. Mainly unicellular or colonial unicellular organisms; cells eukaryotic, diverse nutritive modes, and varying reproductive cycles.

Phyla (Divisions). Euglenophyta, euglenoid organisms; Chrysophyta, golden algae; Pyrrophyta, dinoflagellates and cryptomonads; Hyphochytridiomycota, hyphochytrids; Plasmodiophoromycota, plasmodiophores; Sporozoa, sporozoans; Cnidosporidia, cnidosporidians; Zoomastigina, animal flagellates; Sarcodina, rhizopods; Ciliophora, ciliates and suctorians.

5. KINGDOM MONERA: Prokaryotic Unicells/Colonies

Cellular Characteristics. Cells are prokaryotic without nuclear membranes, plastids, mitochondria and advanced flagella. The organization is unicellular or colonial-unicellular. Nutrition mainly absorptive and reproduction generally asexual.

Phyla (Subdivisions). Cyanophyta, blue-green algae; Myxobacteriae, gliding bacteria; Eubacteriae, true bacteria; Ascomycota, mycelial bacteria; Spirochaetae, spirochetes; Rickettsiae.

6. KINGDOM VIRUS, CHLAMYDIAE: Bedsoniae

Structural Characteristics. Obligate intracellular parasites, below cellular level.

Phyla (Divisions). Viruses; Chlamydiae.

HISTOLOGIC REVIEW OF THE STRUCTURES DEALING WITH THE MAIN LIFE FUNCTIONS IN PARAZOA (PORIFERA) AND EUMETAZOA (EUMETAZOANS)[1] (41, 115, 145, 158a, 177, 335)

General Selected Aspects (Table 3.2)

Species-specific ionic and osmic regulation in Atlantic crustaceans (91) may serve as an example of a comparison of closely related species and their similarities and differences concerning a specific problem. Special structural types may be found only in the tissue of a few particular species, such as an unusual type of continuous junction in *Limulus* revealed by electron microscopy (EM) (183) which may be compared to annelid septate junctions (346) or the cell junctions of *Hydra* as viewed by freeze fracture replication (354). Cell junctions are important for comparative oncology but need to be investigated species-specifically. They may be the one key issue to the characteristic of most malignant neoplasms: metastasis. How do the age changes of cell junctions compare in different organisms? (See also Kelly and Skipper (161) about age changes of human fibroblasts.)

The effects of vitamin A deficiency on ultimobranchial cysts in the thyroid gland (175) serve as another example of the many factors, *e.g.*, nourishment, that may play a role in an accurate species-specific comparison of the

same tissue as the base for neoplastic development. With regard to carcinogens, see Lee *et al.* (188) concerning the effects of protein diet on the reaction of a carcinogen in the rainbow trout.

The relationship of specialized cells, capillaries, and intermedian cytofibrillary elements was discussed by Marza (197). See also Rizki *et al.* (262) on the modification of *Drosophila* cell surfaces by concavalin A.

The phyla in this chapter are treated in the same sequence throughout. Described are structures of wide distribution and/or great diversification as the integuments or structures of sensitivity, and each phylum is treated separately. In dealing with structures of limited distribution such as those of gaseous exchange or excretion, the section is written as general text but in the same sequence of phyla. Only in the case of compilations of negative facts (missing a type of structure such as excretory systems) has the author left (in a few cases) this sequence for purposes of summarization.

Integuments (274)

0. Phylum Porifera. Simple epithelia of flat cells (pinakocytes) appear in highest forms.

1. Phylum Cnidaria.[2] Simple epithelium is found, flat, squamous cell epithelium in exumbrella of medusae, sometimes flagellated in medusae; cubic epithelium in *Hydra*; columnar or columnar ciliated in *Anemonia*; specialized cells are desmocytes, epitheliomuscular cells, cnidoblasts and nettle cells (penetrants, volvents and glutinants). Also cuticles occur in some members (Coantharia) of the phylum or syncytial structures; a caenosarg covers the ectoderm in *Gorgonaria*. The ultrastructure of the nematocysts of *Chryasora quinquecirrha* was described by Burnett (49) and Sutton and Burnett (309).

2. Phylum Ctenophora. The epithelium is simple comparable to cnidarians. Specialized cells are sticky colloblasts, grasping cells and glandular cells.

3. Phylum Platyhelminthes. The epithelium is composed of submerged cells. In turbellarians the epithelium is simple and sometimes syncytial; the cell form is squamous, cuboidal or columnar. An ectodermal basement membrane may occur, mesenchymal goblet cells are comparable to those in mammals. Glandular cells (rarely multicellular glands) appear for the first

---

[1] Additionally the sponges are included, because they exhibit incipient tissue level.

[2] With exception of Porifera all other phyla, characterized by true tissues belong to the eumetazoans.

Table 3.2
Short Characteristics of Porifera and Eumetazoan Phyla

Phylum	Classes	Popular Name	Macroscopic Appearance and Distinguishing Characteristics	Characteristic Species
0. Porifera		Sponges	Sessil, mostly marine	*Sycon* sp.
1. Cnidaria		Jellyfish, sea anemones, corals, *Hydra*, hydroids	Sessil polyps or free-swimming medusae	*Hydra littoralis, Metridium senile*
2. Ctenophora		Comb jellys, sea walnuts	Football, bell- or rim-shaped	*Cestum veneris* (Venus girdle), *Beroe* sp.
3. Platyhelminthes		Flatworms		
	Turbellaria	Planarians	Vermiform undivided	*Microstomum* sp., *Tugesia* sp.
	Trematoda	Flukes	Vermiform undivided	*Polystoma nearcticum, Fasciola hepatica*
	Cestoda	Tapeworms	Vermiform divided	*Taenia saginata*
4. Nemertinea		Nemertini, rhynchocoela, ribbon or proboscis worms	Vermiform	*Tubulanus annulatus, Prostoma rubrum*
5. Gnathostomulida			Vermiform, minute size head, trunk and tail	*Gnathostomula paradoxa*
6. Entoprocta or Camptozoa			Vermiform, calyx, crown, tentacles stalk and substrate	*Loxosoma* sp., *Barentsia* sp., *Urnatella* sp.
7. Acanthocephala		Thorny- or spiny-headed worms	Vermiform animals composed of proboscis and trunk	*Gigantorhynchus* sp., *Gorgorhynchus* sp.
8. Rotifera	—	Wheel animalcules	Minute unsegmented pseudocoelomates, ciliated corona, head, flat trunk, and foot	*Philodina* sp., *Epiphanes senta*
9. Gastrotricha	—	—	Minute forms, wormlike body with bristles	*Chaetonotus* sp.
10. Kinorhyncha	—	—	Wormlike minute forms, with body of 13–14 zonites	*Campyloderes* sp.
11. Nematoda	—	Roundworms	Wormlike cylindrical body of uniform makeup in different species, strong cuticle	*Ascaris megalocephala*
12. Nematomorpha	—	Horsehair worms	Long and slender body, smooth cuticle	*Gordius* sp.
13. Priapulida		—	Inversible proboscis (presoma) and trunk	*Priapulus caudatus*
14. Mollusca		Molluscs	Main body mass, mantle and shell(s)	
	Polyplacophora		Large foot, 8-valve shell	*Cryptochyton stelleri*
	Aplacophora		Rudimentary foot, reduced shell	*Chetoderma* sp.
	Monoplacophora		Bilateral body, ventral foot, one pieced shell	*Neopilina* sp.
	Gastropoda	Snails, slugs	Head, body, mantle, foot, and shell	*Helix pomatia* (vineyard snail)
	Scaphopoda	Tusk shells	Elongated shell, open on both ends, encloses the body	*Dentalium* sp.
	Bivalvia, Pelecypoda	Mussels, oysters, scallops, clams	Uncoiled, bilateral body, shell with two symmetric, middorsally connected lateral halves and bilobed mantle; head missing	*Unio* sp., *Mytilus edulis, Crassostrea gigas*
	Cephalopoda	Squids, cuttlefish, octopuses	With external (*Nautilus*), internal shell or without, foot (tentacles), body and mantle	*Sepia officinalis, Octopus* sp.
15. Sipunculida	—	Peanut worms	Wormlike body, with retractile proboscis and tentacle crown and elongated body	*Sipunculus nudus*

Table 3.2—*continued*

Phylum	Classes	Popular Name	Macroscopic Appearance and Distinguishing Characteristics	Characteristic Species
16. Echiurida	—	—	Nonretractile proboscis and cylindrical or ovoid body	*Echiurus* sp.
17. Annelida		Segmented worms, annelids		
	Polychaeta		Head with tentacles, segmented (externally and internally) body, with parapodia and setae	*Nereis diversicolor*
	Oligochaeta	Earthworms and others	Reduced head, externally and internally segmented body, no parapodia	*Lumbricus terrestris*
	Myzostomida	—	Disc-shaped body, 5 pairs of parapodia and setae	*Myzostoma* sp.
	Hirudinea	Leeches	Flattened body, head with 4 segments and posterior sucker	*Hirudo medicinalis*
18. Onychophora	—	—	One pair of antennae, and one pair of oral papillae on anterior end (indistinct head); unsegmented elongated body, with paired appendages	*Peripatus torquatus*
19. Pentastomida (Linguatulida)	—	Tongue worms	Elongated unsegmented body, composed of short cephalothorax and long abdomen	*Porocephalus* sp.
20. Tardigrada	—	Water bears	Cylindrical, unsegmented body with rounded ends and four pairs of legs; animals belong to the smallest metazoans	*Echiniscus scrofa*
21. Arthropoda			Segmented body with appendages; main body portions composed of head, thorax, and abdomen which may or may not be fused; chitinous exoskeleton	
	Merostomata	King crabs, horseshoe crabs	Two pairs of eyes, compound and simple; big dorsal carapace, two types of leg appendages, telson	*Limulus polyphemus*
	Arachnida	Scorpions, spiders, mites and ticks	Cephalothorax and abdomen, 4 pairs of walking legs. Chelicerae, pedipalps	*Lycosa carolinensis, Scorpio* sp., *Pandinus imperator*
	Pycnogonida	Sea spiders	Head fused to first segment of reduced body; 4–6 pairs of long walking legs	*Pycnogonum* sp.
	Crustacea	Crustaceans (crayfish, etc.)	Head (2 pairs of antennae and maxillae, 1 pair of jaws); body usually has head, thorax, and abdomen; body ends with telson	*Homarus* sp., *Callinectes sapidus*
	Myriapoda	Myriapods (centipedes and millipeds)	Head and segmented body with one, chilopoda, or two, diplopoda pair of extremities on each segment	*Lithobius* sp., *Julus* sp.
	Insecta	Insects	Body divided into head, thorax, and abdomen. Three pairs of walking legs at thorax. Many variations from the general plan in	*Apis mellifera, Musca domestica*

Table 3.2—*continued*

Phylum	Classes	Popular Name	Macroscopic Appearance and Distinguishing Characteristics	Characteristic Species
22. Phoronida			details according to a tremendous number of species. Wings occur as outgrowths of the exoskeleton	*Phoronis* sp.
23. Ectoprocta:Bryozoa		Moss animals	Body composed of lophophore and slender trunk, surrounded by a secreted tube	*Paludicella articulata*
24. Brachiopoda		Lamp shells	Colonial coelomates characterized by lophophore and body	*Lingula unguis*
25. Echinodermata		Echinoderms (sea stars, sea urchins, brittle stars, sea cucumbers, sea lilies)	Lophophore, bivalved shell secreted by mantle and pedicle are distinguishable	
	Crinoidea	Sea lilies	Body usually contains 5 fields with ambulacra and 5 fields of interambulacra, is unsegmented and uncephalized, exhibit oral-aboral axis	*Metacrinus superbus*
	Holothuroidea	Sea cucumbers	Body bearing arms is cup-shaped; stalked and nonstalked species exist	*Cucumaria planci*
	Echinoidea	Sea urchins, sand dollars, heart urchins	Elongated body without arms, spines, or pedicellariae; anterior mouth and posterior anus	*Echinus esculentus*
	Asteroidea	Sea stars, starfish	Rigid skeleton, body hemispherical or like disc, no arms	*Asterias rubens*
	Ophiuroidea	Brittle stars	Body composed of disc and arms, tube feet with suckers	*Ophiura albida*
26. Chaetognatha		Arrow worms	Disc and sharply separated arms of slender shape	*Sagitta elegans*
27. Pogonophora: Brachiata		Beard worms	Body is divided into head, with mouth, teeth, chaetae and eyes; and trunk with lateral and caudal fins	*Siboglinum ekmani*
28. Hemichordata		Acorn worms	Long cylindrical body is composed of protosome with anterior cephalic lobe and tentacles, mesosome, and metasome	*Balanoglossus gigas*
29. Tunicata (Urochordata)		Sea squirts	Body is divided into protosoma, mesosoma, and metasoma. One or more pairs of gill slits connect pharynx and exterior	*Salpa* sp., *Ciona intestinalis*
30. Cephalochordata		Lancelets, amphioxus	Body is divided into thorax, abdomen, and postabdomen and characteristic tunic. Animals are solitary, social, or colonial	*Branchiostoma californiense*
31. Vertebrata		Vertebrates	Laterally compressed body, spindle-like, naked, depigmented and without head	
			Body is divided in head, trunk, and tail; generally paired appendages are present	

Table 3.2—*continued*

Phylum	Classes	Popular Name	Macroscopic Appearance and Distinguishing Characteristics	Characteristic Species
	Agnatha		Body is eel-like without paired appendages but exhibits median dorsal, median ventral, and caudal fin and is covered by slimy skin without scales	*Myxine glutinosa*
	Chondrichthyes	Cartilaginous fishes; sharks, rays, etc.	Body is streamlined as in sharks or flattened as in rays and skates	*Chimaera sp.*
	Osteichthyes	Bony fishes; trout, cichlids, anabatids, etc.	Skeleton is composed of bone and cartilage produces different forms of varying species. Body exhibits head and trunk with tail and paired and unpaired appendages, fins; operculum covers gill slits	*Esox lucius, Lebestes reticulatus, Beta splenders*
	Amphibia: Caudata	Salamanders, newts, etc.	Cold-blooded vertebrates with gilled aquatic larvae and air-breathing adults, with tail persisting throughout lifetime, mainly 2 pairs of extremities in adult	*Desmograthus fuscus, Ambystoma maculata*
	Anura	Frogs, toads	Cold-blooded vertebrates with no tail, with gilled aquatic larvae and air-breathing adults	*Rana pipiens*
	Reptiles	Alligators, crocodiles, lizards, snakes, turtles	Body of these air-breathing vertebrates is generally covered with scales or bony plates and is totally supported by ossified skeleton	*Alligator mississippiensis, Crocodilus acutus, Chelonia midas*
	Aves	Birds	Warm-blooded vertebrates characterized by lightly built skeleton and beak; body more or less covered with feathers and fore-limbs developed into wings	*Columba livia, Falco peregrinus, Grus canadensis*
	Mammalia	Mammals	Warm-blooded vertebrates characterized by mammary glands with which to nourish their young with its secretion, milk; body more or less covered with hair; four chambered heart	
	Mammalian orders: Monotremata	Monotremes: Duck-billed platypuses and spiny anteaters	Lay eggs; reptile-like skeletal features	*Tachyglossus aculeatus*
	Marsupialia	Marsupials: Opossums, kangaroos, etc.	Aplacentalia; nearly as diversified as placental orders	*Didelphis virginiana*
	Insectivora	Insectivores: Tenrecs, hedgehogs, shrews, etc.	This, and all following orders are placental mammals. Small animals, with long, narrow snout; primitive teeth	*Erinaceus europaeus; Microsorex hoyi*
	Dermoptera	Gliding or flying lemures	Unique lower incisor teeth; gliding membrane from head and neck to side of body	*Cynocephalus volans*

Table 3.2—*continued*

Phylum	Classes	Popular Name	Macroscopic Appearance and Distinguishing Characteristics	Characteristic Species
	Chiroptera	Bat: Insectivorous bats, fruit eating bats, etc.	According to species they are second largest order after rodents; fingers of hand adapted to form wings; only truly flying mammals	*Myotis myotis* (widest distribution)
	Primates	Primates: Tree shrews, monkeys, baboons, gibbons, orangutans, gorillas, chimpanzees and man, etc.	Great development of cerebral hemispheres is the most pronounced characteristic in higher forms	*Macaca mulatta; Papio hamadryas*
	Edentata	Edentates: Sloths, anteaters, armadillos	Slugginess characterizes sloths; type of elongated head and claws, anteaters; hornlike skin modifications, armadillos	*Myrmecophaga tridactyla*
	Lagomorpha	Lagomorphs: Pikas, rabbits, hares	Dental details are more diagnostic than external characteristics	*Lepus europaeus*
	Rodentia	Rodents: Mice, rats, hamsters, guinea pigs, gerbils, squirrels, chinchillas, lemmings, gophers, beavers, etc.	Rodents with 351 live genera form largest order of mammals; clearly characterized by four incisor teeth (two above and two below). Other characteristics are peculiarities of bones of forearm, generalized brain and inguinal or abdominal testes	*Mus musculus, Rattus rattus Mesocricetus auratus, Tamiasciurus hudsonicus, Chinchilla laniger, Lemmus trimucronatus, Geomys bursarius, Castor canadensis, Aplodontia rufa*
	Cetacea	Cetaceans: Whales, dolphins, porpoises	Wholly aquatic mammals, of which toothed whales and whalebone whales can be distinguished. Blue whale is largest animal. No hind legs; no sebaceous glands; no sweat glands. Adaptation for diving	*Physeter catodon, Balaenoptera musculus*
	Carnivora	Carnivores: Dogs, wolves, weasels, civets, cats, bears	Small to large mammals with well-developed canines that are primarily adapted to carnivorous diet	*Canis familiaris, Mustela nigripes, Viverricula indicor, Leo leo, Ursus arctos*
	Pinnipedia	Pinnipeds: Seals, sea lions, walruses	Streamlined body, all limbs modified to flippers. Outer ears reduced or absent; teats and external genitalia mostly invisible	*Otaria flavescens, Odobenus rosmarus, Phoca vitulina*
	Tubulidentata	Tubulidentates: Aardvarks or earth hogs (one species only)	Long head and snout with piglike muzzle; adapted for digging for termites and ants	*Orycteropus afer*
	Proboscidea	Proboscideans: African elephant, Asiatic elephant	Elongated, flexible and muscular trunk: huge head; large body	*Loxodonta africana, Elephas maximus*
	Hyracoidea	Hyraxes	External appearance similar to lagomorphs and rodents, but dentition entirely different and more closely related to proboscideans	*Dendrohyrax dorsalis*
	Sirenia	Sirenians: Dugongs, sea cows, manatees	Aquatic mammals adapted to shallow water; massive, spindle-shaped body form; no hind limbs; horizontal tail fin. Pachyostotic skeleton; extreme topography of body cavity	*Trichechus senegalensis, Dugong dugon*
	Perissodactyla	Horses, tapirs,	Odd-toed hoofed mammals,	*Equus caballus, Tapirus*

Table 3.2—*continued*

Phylum	Classes	Popular Name	Macroscopic Appearance and Distinguishing Characteristics	Characteristic Species
		rhinoceroses	adapted to running; medium to large size; nonruminating stomach	*indicus, Diceros bicornis*
	Artiodactyla	Pigs, hippopotamuses, camels, deer, giraffes, okapis, sheep, goats, cattle, antelopes and others	Even-toed hoofed mammals. Foot is uniting characteristic of members of this order. Many species have complex four-chambered stomachs which enable them to consume hard grasses, etc.	*Sus scrofa, Bos indicus, Odocoileus virginianus, Antilocapra americana*

time in phylogeny. A ciliated variation of epithelium is found in small members.

For scanning electron microscopic investigations of the epidermis of the turbellar *Dugesia tigrina*, see Smales and Blankespoor (295) and for interstitial structures, see Pedersen (237). For the tegument of trematoda, see Matricon-Gondran (199). A cuticle occurs in some cases. Typical is the polychord *Discolides longi* with a one-layered ciliated epidermis on a basement membrane and broad papillae at the border (237). Characteristic structures are the rhabdoids. In the early stages, three types of cytogenic cells can be distinguished from the adult tegumentary cells as in *Cercaria pectinada* (199). A true epidermis is missing in trematodes, but a covering cuticle is found instead, perhaps produced by mesenchymal cells. The body coverings in turbellarians is simply ciliated. In cestodes, the epidermal cells are invaginated into the mesenchyme. An epidermis-like membrane does not exist. The ontogenetic origin is open to question.

4. Phylum Nemertinea. The epidermis is simple columnar ciliated, intermingled with serous or mucous glandular cells, multicellular glands exist in the epidermis or below in the underlying hypodermis.

5. Phylum Gnathostomulida. Epithelium of simple flagellated cells is found.

6. Phylum Entoprocta. The epidermis is columnar cuboidal with a different degree of ciliation and many glandular cells. A cuticle covers the epidermis and the musculature of the body wall underlies it.

7. Phylum Acanthocephala. A cell-constant syncytial epidermis, occasionally composed of four layers as in *Echinorhynchus gadi* covered by a thin cuticle and with underlying connective tissues and muscle is present.

8. Phylum Rotifera. In the adult, the epidermis is syncytial, but it develops from initially individual cells. Two types of glandular cells exist partially ciliated with microvilli or with a cuticle. For the ultrastructure see 282a.

9. Phylum Gastrotricha. A syncytial epidermis of different height according to the different subgroups is found with epidermal glands and covered by a cuticle.

10. Phylum Kinorhyncha. The epidermis appears syncytial using light microscopy, but electron microscopy shows individual cells with narrow intercellular spaces.

11. Phylum Nematoda (24, 34). The epidermis is cellular or syncytial. The size of the nuclei depends on location and age. Gland cells often appear in groups; the cuticle is complex and generally composed of three layers. The integumental condition in such areas as the vulva varies in members of different genera.

12. Phylum Nematomorpha. The epidermis shows cuboidal or columnar cells; the cuticle has two layers.

13. Phylum Priapulida (213). A syncytial epidermis is made up of tall columnar cells covered by a cuticle composed of two layers.

14. Phylum Mollusca. The epidermis is generally simply ciliated with large variations. In Amphineura-Polyplacophora the epidermal cells are cuboidal to tall columnar, but also flat. They are cuboidal or columnar with glandular cells in Amphineura-Aplacophora and flat or high columnar, with interspersed mucus-producing cells in Conchifera-Monoplacophora.

For Gastropoda a ciliated epidermis with many glandular cells is characteristic. In Opisthobranchia the epithelial cells are flat or cuboidal columnar; cilia or a cuticle are present. Glands are intraepidermal, subepidermal or multicellular with mucous secreting and eosinophilic cells. The conditions in Prosobranchia are similar to the former group. Epidermal cells of pulmonates are of different height; cilia and a cuticle are present. All glands are superepidermal, mucous-producing or calciferous. Pigmented cells occur.

Scaphopoda contain simple ciliated cells with sensory endings and glandular structures.

In Lamellibranchiata ciliated or nonciliated integuments appear with sensory endings, including ocelli and glandular structures.

Columnar cells with glandular and sensory structures are characteristic for Cephalopoda. For the ultrastructure of Koelliker's organs, see Brocco et al. (40).

15. Phylum Sipunculida. The epidermis is generally cuboidal, but also columnar and ciliated. Uni-, bi-, or multicellular gland cells open through a single or common duct; many sensory organs are present (213).

16. Phylum Echiurida. The epidermis contains many gland cells and produces a tender cuticle; cilia occur occasionally.

17. Phylum Annelida. The epidermis has high columnar cells and invaginated glands underlined with connective tissue and covered by a cuticle. For the histochemistry of mucous cells of the epidermis of some lumbricillid enchytraeids (Oligochaeta), see Richards (259).

18. Phylum Onychophora. The simple epidermis exhibits cells comparable to those in arthropods, covered by a cuticle and underlain by a dermis of connective tissue.

19. Phylum Pentastomida. An epidermis of tall cells, with multicellular glands and covered by a cuticle is present.

20. Phylum Tardigrada. The simple epidermis exhibits flat rectangular to polygonal cells. The nucleus of the squamous cells bulges out in the main areas. Glands are missing and the cuticle generally shows three layers. The fine structure of the integument of the heterotardigrad *Echiniscoides sigismundi* (118) shows that the cuticle (comparable to the one in eutardigrada) consists of an outer multilayered epicuticle, a homogenous inner epicuticle, a trilaminated layer, an intracuticle, and a fibrous procuticle. The cuticles on the legs and near the claws resemble those of other heterotardigrada. The epidermis exhibits a simple cell layer without glands.

21. Phylum Arthropoda. The one-layered epidermis secretes the exoskeleton or cuticle. The shape of the epidermal cells ranges from columnar, cuboidal, to flat with indistinct boundaries. Epidermal glands of many types and sensory structures occur. The epidermis is underlain by a basement membrane. The epidermis

in merostomata is a simple columnar epithelium. In Arachnida, the epidermal cells assume variable shapes depending on species, function, and body region; silk and toxin glands are known. In crustacea the epidermal cells are twice as tall as they are wide, and therefore equal columnar, but with wide variations. The fine structure of cuticle and epidermis in the crayfish, *Oronectes limnosus* changes during the moulting cycle (178). Variations appear similar to those as in other groups in the myriapoda. Insecta have a very thin epidermis with flat to tall columnar as well as glandular and sensory cells. Few examples may be given concerning some very common or rare specializations. Macrotrichia, secreted by the trichogenic cells is one type of differentiation, the tumorigenic cells another, forming the ring which gives flexibility to the hair. Tegumentary pygidial glands, which secrete the posterior shield in the sessil plant parasitic insect, *Aoimidiella aurantii* (Homoptera, Diaspididae) are composed of seven cells (241), namely "a principal unpaired secretory cell which produces an abundant glycoproteinaceous secretion; a small associated cell with a secondary reservoir for this secretion; two accessory secretory cells which have very abundant tubular extensions coming from the plasma membrane, and a flocculant secretion gathered in a large subcuticular space; two cells forming an enlarged part of the excretory canal, functioning like a spinneret; and finally a single cell forming the tubular duct of this complex gland."

22. Phylum Phoronida. The epidermal cells are flat to columnar, sensory and glandular cells occur. The cuticle is thin, cilia are present, especially at the tentacles.

23. Phylum Ectoprocta. Simple ciliated cells are typical. In certain regions of some genera an extremely thick cuticle occurs. The epidermis secretes a zooecium.

24. Phylum Brachiopoda. The epidermis is cuboidal to columnar, sometimes ciliated, even striated upon nerve masses; cilia and setae are present; gland cells are intermingled. The epidermis is underlain by connective tissue.

25. Phylum Echinodermata. In Crinoidea, the epidermis is poorly developed; the cells are tall, sometimes ciliated. Glandular and sensory cells are present. In Holothuroidea, a nonciliated epidermis of tall cells, with underlaying connective tissue, is covered by a thin cuticle. Flagellated columnar epidermal cells, two types of glandular cells, and neurosensory cells appear in Asteroidea. In Echinoidea, cuboidal, columnar, ciliated, and glandular epidermal cells as well as a dermis are present. In Ophiuroidea, the cellular epidermis of young animals changes later into a syncytial structure; ciliated cells exist in certain regions.

26. Phylum Chaetognatha. The epidermal cells are flat to highly prismatic. The epidermis is stratified in certain species, at the rostral body region.

27. Phylum Pogonophora. The epidermis consists of columnar cells and a cuticle.

28. Phylum Hemichordata. The epidermis is cuboidal to tall-columnar-ciliated with gland cells.

29. Phylum Tunicata. The epidermis has flat to cuboidal cells covered by a thick extracellular layer. The dermis is inconspicuous as in some other invertebrates and composed of collagen fibrils and fibroblasts. For the attachment of the tunic see Katow and Watanabe (159).

30. Phylum Cephalochordata. Simple cuboidal to low prismatic cells make up the epidermis; the dermis is composed of connective tissue.

31. Phylum Vertebrata. In fishes (130, 131) the epidermis is stratified, exhibits two to more than 60 cell layers, cuboidal prismatic (and uppermost sometimes flattened cells). Glands and sensory structures have been observed. Epidermal, glandular, mucus- or slime-producing, serous granulated, clavate (club-shaped), chemoreceptor, excretory delanide (photoreceptor), free blood cells, sensory cells, and free nerve endings can be distinguished. For the ultrastructure of the integumental melanophores of the coelacanth, *Latimeria chalumnae*, see Lamer and Chavin (181); for the integumental melanophores of the Australian lungfish, *Neoceratodus forsteri*, see Imaki and Chavin (147), and for pigment movements in fish melanophores, see Schliwa and Bereiter-Hahn (277) (as well as Chapter 29). For the ultrastructure of the skin of the teleost *Hippoglossoides elassodon*, see Brown and Wellings (43).

The integument of amphibia starting from the outside shows a stratum corneum, a transitional layer of polygonal cells and a stratum germinativum of low columnar cells. The dermis is three-layered, and tubular, acinar, mucous and granular glands are abundant. The epidermis of embryos consists of a simple columnar epithelium.

Reptiles have a stratum corneum, a stratum granulosum, and a stratum germinativum. Paucity of glands is characteristic. Holocrine glands are the musk glands of crocodiles and the femoral glands of lizards.

Birds have a stratum germinativum and a stra-

tum corneum (192). Glands are the rump gland of which the outer zone ducts are comparable to the sebaceous glands in mammals. Feathers are cornified appendages, as are beaks, claws, etc.

The epithelium in mammals consists of stratified squamous cells as in reptiles and birds. Glands are: (a) coiled or sweat glands; merocrine or apocrine, missing in whales, sea cows, and some others such as dogs; two-cell types. The epithelium in the ducts is double-layered cuboidal; (b) odoriferous glands: apocrine, e.g., in axilla, related to sexual cycle; (c) sebaceous glands: holocrine, they originate from hair primordia and are associated with hairs except in the angle of the mouth, on lips, and labia minora; they are also lacking in the nude mouse (for gap junctions in the human, see Kitson *et al.* (168)); (d) perigenital glandular organs of rodents and bovids and antorbital glands of artiodactyla, with holocrine and apocrine portions; (e) mammary glands are tuboalveolar, open separately in monotremata, at the nipple in the other orders. The epithelium in ducts and alveoli is simple cuboidal.

Langerhans cells are additional epidermal components of the mammalian skin as the keratinous structures, such as hair, nails, horns, sheaths of horns in bovids and antilocaprids, horn(s) of rhinoceroses, and claws.

In addition, the integument often serves other functions undertaken by the animal body, for example, by the respiratory and excretory organs, the intestines, etc. The tracheae of the tracheata in the majority of animals are an epidermal outgrowth showing epidermal characteristics. The anterior and posterior portion of the digestive tube in many animals is ectodermal in origin, with typical characteristics of the ectoderm, sometimes even a cuticle.

Digestive System

Lining Membranes

0. Phylum Porifera. Choanocytes or collar cells form a digesting epithelium only in sponges. They are columnar ciliated cells with a collar surrounding the long cilium.

1. Phylum Cnidaria. The lining of the gastric cavity consists of an entodermal epithelium of tall columnar and sometimes ciliated myoepithelial cells containing mucous and absorptive and glandular cells, and sometimes nematocysts.

These structures vary also in polyp and medusa.

2. Phylum Ctenophora. The presence of ciliated, glandular, and sensory cells varies with the region. *Berriam*, for example, exhibits a range from low unciliated cells to high ciliated ones.

3. Phylum Platyhelminthes. In Turbellaria, a columnar epithelium, with lower absorptive and higher secretory cells, a basal membrane, mesenchyme, and underlining musculature occurs. Trematoda exhibit columnar and goblet cells in the intestinal epithelium. Functionally secretory and lower absorptive cell types have been observed. No digestive system is present in cestoda.

In the majority of higher animals a digestive tract exists with mouth and anal opening. The anterior and posterior portion are lined by ectodermal epithelium, the medial portion with endodermal ones. The food transport is undertaken by ciliary beating in most protostomians and deuterostomians, with the exception of nematodes and arthropods where cilia are generally lacking; another exception are the vertebrates. The movement of the intestinal musculature is pronounced in arthropods and vertebrates.

4. Phylum Nemertinea. Cells beginning at the intestine are similar to ectodermal epithelium; in general a ciliated epithelium, containing also large subepithelial or intraepithelial glandular cells, is present.

5. Phylum Gnathostomulida. The conditions are comparable to gastrotricha; new studies, especially concerning ultrastructure, are urgently needed.

6. Phylum Entoprocta. Nonciliated and ciliated cuboidal to columnar and granular cells (regional differences) are found. At the endintestine, tall to flat cells, and some muscular elements of the intestinal tract are revealed.

7. Phylum Acanthocephala. The digestive function is performed by the integument.

8. Phylum Rotifera. The ciliated or nonciliated mixed epithelium may be covered by a cuticle of cellular or syncytial character. The epithelium secretes trophi; cell invariability occurs also; the musculature underlies certain regions. The digestive system of the rotifer *Habrotrocha rosa* exhibits the alimentary tract, composed of oral cavity, pharynx, esophagus, mastax, stomach-hose, syncytium of intestine, and terminal intestine; as well as five digestive glands and another gland closely related to the intestinal syncytium (282c).

9. Phylum Gastrotricha. Cuboidal or columnar epithelium with cuticle; cross-striated muscle fibers and glandular cells; partially circular musculature in the midgut are observable.

10. Phylum Kinorhyncha. The lining membranes are similar to those of gastrotricha.

11. Phylum Nematoda. Invaginated cells appear in the frontal part of the intestinal tract, connected by tubes with the surface. Cell invariability, syncytial cuboidal to columnar epithelium, a cuticle in certain regions; glandular structures, microvilli and cilia occur occasionally. The beginning of extracellular digestion is phylogenetically remarkable. The ventral gland on the ventral surface appears in the case of intestinal parasites. Regarding the fine structure of the intestine of the nematodes, *Ancylostoma canium* and *Phocanema decipiens*, see Andreassen (8) and for *Heterakis gallinarum*, see Zmoray and Guttekova (362). Recent studies (232) on the intestinal epithelium of nematodes also include those of *Ascarida galli*. Cilia occur in the intestine of nematodes digesting solid food. The intestine of nematodes exhibits no musculature capable of peristalsis (361).

12. Phylum Nematomorpha. Degenerated cells in the form of an epithelial tube, cords, or syncytia are present.

13. Phylum Priapulida. The epithelium is columnar and partially lined with a cuticle.

14. Phylum Mollusca. Species number and different food sources explain the diversification of structures. Jaws occur in cephalopods; odontoblasts are important cells for radula development. The odontophore is composed of cartilaginous tissue and is the supporting structure of the radula with three cell types. The intestinal epithelium is ciliated and innervated; salivary glands are composed of protein-synthesizing secretory cells; and ion and fluid transporting cells. The hepatopancreas is the largest intestinal gland.

Amphineura. The monoplacophora have been excluded from this review.

Polyplacophora. Generally a radula is present in these chitons. The mouth leads into the alimentary canal divided into esophagus, stomach, and intestine. A portion of the alimentary canal is ciliated. For the ultrastructure of the subradular organ of *Lepidochitona cinereus*, see Boyle (36). The digestive tract is simple and a radula sometimes present in Aplacophora.

Gastropoda. The digestive system of gastropods consists mainly of a mouth, a buccal cavity, nearly always containing a radula, the long esophagus which may have a gizzard, the stomach, sometimes bearing a cuticle, and the intestine terminating with the anus. The hepatopancreas enters the stomach with two ducts. Cartilage occurs in the radula as skeleton. A review of the nudibranch *Acanthodoris pilosa* was made by Morse (215). The degradation of the radula in the pulmonate snails *Biomphalaria glabrata* and *Limnea stagnalis* is described by Peters (243) and the scanning and transmission electron microscopy of the rectal ridge of the pulmonate snail *Biophalaria glabrata* by Sullivan *et al.* (308).

Scaphopoda. The mouth exhibits radula and mandibles, and continues into the esophagus where the ducts of digestive glands and piloric cecum enter. The following intestine arising from the anterior portion of the stomach terminates with the anus. The *Lammelibranchiata* are tongueless mollusks which exhibit labial palps. The digestive tract follows the general molluscan plan. Fine structure and histochemistry of the digestive diverticula of the protobranchiate bivalve *Nucula sulcata* exhibit nonciliated main ducts with one cell type, secondary ciliated ducts with one cell type, and blind ending tubules with pyramid shaped basophilic cells and columnar digestive cells (231). The arms of *Cephalopoda* surround the mouth. Cup-shaped suckers at the arms contain mucus-secreting cells and a particular horny cornification is important for seizing the prey. The buccal cavity, enveloped by the buccal mass containing the beaks, exhibits a radula. One cell layer is involved in the secretion of the beaks in octopods and squids, and is composed of tall columnar cells known as beccublasts. Three subtypes of cells can be distinguished, those with cell-long fibrils, those with masses of abundant endoplasmic reticulum, and those with a mixture of fibrils and secretory organelles (73). The epithelium of the digestive tract is columnar in type with a cuticle in certain regions, while ciliated in others. The esophagus is chitinized, the following stomach exhibits a strong muscular wall, the mucosa is columnar ciliated. Ciliated areas also occur in the cecum. The intestine again exhibits a cuticle and leads via the rectum to the anus. The ink sac is a rectal diverticulum and expels its content through the anus. The ink sac belonging to the glandular structures is lined with a cuboidal epithelium, with underlaying circular and longitudinal muscle cells and connective tissue.

15. Phylum Sipunculida. The intestinal wall consists of columnar ciliated epithelium (enzymatic cells in the posterior region), connective tissue, muscle, and peritoneum.

16. Phylum Echiurida. The intestinal wall is composed of nonciliated or ciliated intestinal epithelium (pigmented in the rectum) and musculature.

17. Phylum Annelida. *Polychaeta.* The anterior intestine varies greatly according to the species. For details of the pharyngeal bulb (muscles and myoepithelial junctions) and the stomodeal cuticle of *Protodrilus* sp., consult Jouin (156, 157).

Midintestine. Ciliated epithelium appears in the pharynx (?) and the stomach exhibits columnar epithelium as well as musculature and peritoneum.

Hind-intestine. A columnar epithelium with various types of differentiations is found.

Oligochaeta. The earthworm serves as an example. A buccal cavity is present. Nonciliated columnar cells with cuticle, in diverticulum without cuticle, appear. The pharynx exhibits columnar ciliated and columnar nonciliated cells with or without cuticle. Glandular cells occur also. The esophagus exhibits dilatations, crop, calciferous glands, ciliated epithelium, thin musculature, and abundant vascularization.

Hirudinea. The intestine of Hirudinea consists of ciliated columnar epithelium and glandular cells as well as circular and longitudinal musculature. Many variations exist. The epithelium in pharynx and esophagus is simple columnar and exhibits a cuticle. Salivary unicellular glands occur. The pharynx exhibits radial, circular, and longitudinal muscle fibers. The midintestine is characterized by diverticula. Epithelium is low columnar, with microvilli, and the epithelium of the end intestine is high prismatic (columnar). The epithelium of the diverticula (alimentary tract) of *Hirudo medicinalis* exhibits low columnar cells, with large accumulations of lipid granules and mitochondria close to the surface. The apical surface of the cells shows microvilli. The nuclei are intensely folded and the Golgi complex is poorly developed (126). The epithelial cells of the intestine are highly columnar, exhibit microvilli, a complex basal labyrinth, two different populations of mitochondria and an elaborate Golgi complex (127).

18. Phylum Onychophora. Fore-, mid-, and endgut can be distinguished. Fore- and endgut are ectodermal and exhibit a cuticle. Paired tubular salivary glands enter into the foregut characterized by one buccal cavity. In a cross section of the pharynx a cuticle, epithelial columnar lining, radial muscles with intermingled gland cells and endothelium can be distinguished. The midgut is lined with a tall columnar epithelium and has no digestive glands.

19. Phylum Pentastomida. Mouth, pharynx, esophagus, midintestine, and rectum are discernable. The epithelium exhibits cuboidal to columnar absorptive and glandular cells. Only the midintestine lacks a cuticle.

20. Phylum Tardigrada. Cell invariable columnar epithelium and salivary glands are present. The midgut epithelium of the eutardigrade *Isohypsibius augusti* (216) is a convoluted monolayer of a single cell type (with striated border, some basal infoldings, cytosis vesicles, abundant mitochondria, and rough endoplasmic reticulum in the cells held together by apical zonulae continue) (117).

21. Phylum Arthropoda. The anterior intestine is ectodermal: low epithelial cells with basement membrane appear. The other portions of the intestine shall be discussed according to the different groups.

Merostomata. The intestine has an arthropod-like appearance (158a).

Arachnida. The midintestine has a low to columnar epithelium; the hindgut a cuticle, epithelial layer, basement membrane and musculature.

Crustacea (Malacostraca). Columnar cells (developed in ducts of hepatopancreas) and loose connective tissue are present. The midintestinal epithelium is one-layered cylindrical. Cardia, pylorus, and endintestine exhibit a cuticle which is missing in the midintestine the dorsal diverticulum and the ducts of the hepatopancreas. Four cell types are present in the hepatopancreas: embryonic, absorbing, fibrillar, and vacuolated cells.

The midgut of the copepod *Centropages typicus* exhibits three main zones, with four principal cell types (comparable to the cells in the midgut of malacostracans especially the hepatopancreas of decapod crustaceans): R cells with the function of absorption exhibit smooth endoplasmic reticulum and high microvilli; F cells, providing synthesis and secretion of predigestive enzymes, show a rough endoplasmic reticulum and short microvilli; and B cells for enzyme synthesis, intracellular digestion and extrusion, with a large vacuolar apparatus (12). Studies with the intracellular junctions in the posterior cecal epithelium of the crustacean *Orchestris*, indicated that it is necessary to distinguish between the P-type gap in vertebrates and the E-type gap in arthropods (114). The junctions between epithelial cells in different phyla are of great importance for an evaluation of distribution ability of neoplastic cells deriving from these epithelia when undergoing metastasis. For the fine structure and function of the alimentary epithelium in *Artemia salina* Nauplii, see Hootman and Conte (140).

Myriapoda. The pharynx and the end intestine are ectodermal. In the midintestine resorptive and secretory cells are found.

Insecta. Simple squamous cell epithelium occurs in the anterior portion of the gut; in the midgut a columnar epithelium with underlaying thin musculature (inner circular and outer longitudinal cross-striated components). Larvae, e.g., of *Drosophila*, exhibit in the midgut four cell types: prismatic interstitial cells, cuprophilic cells, flat cells, and cuboidal cells. In the posterior gut squamous cell epithelium with a cuticle occurs; rectal papillae and the subgroup of anal papillae may be characteristic in certain developmental stages and species. For the structure of the rectal papillae in the parasitic hymenopteron *Nasonia vitripennis*, see Davis and King (67). Morphometric differences were detected in the midgut epithelial cells between two strains of female *Aedes aegypti*. One strain was recently isolated from nature and the other of an old laboratory strain. These studies (132) indicated strong deterioration processes in the old laboratory strain. Care should be taken with too much trust in unnatural cell and animal breeding in strains for oncology which may result in artificial findings.

22. Phylum Phoronida. In the proventriculus, cuboidal to tall columnar cells, gland cells, and a basal nervous layer occur. The character of the circular and longitudinal musculature depends on the region. Feeding behavior in the phoronid *Phoronopsis viridis* was recently investigated (267).

23. Phylum Ectoprocta. Columnar cells appear in the pharynx.

24. Phylum Brachiopoda. Commonly, a ciliated (flagellated) tall columnar pseudostratified epithelium, with basement membrane, musculature and peritoneum is present. The midgut diverticula have two types of epithelial cells.

25. Phylum Echinodermata. Crinoidea have tall ciliated or nonciliated cells (rectum). Also goblet cells occur in the rectum. The intestinal mucosa is surrounded by connective tissue and musculature. A cross section of the intestinal wall in Holothuroidea shows from the inside to the outside columnar ciliated to low ciliated epithelium, connective tissue, circular and longitudinal musculature, connective tissue and peritoneum with cilia. In the epithelium of the stomach abundant intermingled goblet cells are found. In Echinoidea, a ciliated epithelium, with tall columnar cells, cuboidal and glandular cells (mucous), and secretory cells which are variable according to the regions, is present. Variations in the epithelium of the intestinal wall exist. The pharynx exhibits mucous glands and secretory cells; the esophagus, cuboidal cells and glandular crypts; the stomach, secretory cells, and the rectum, gland cells. Additional components of the intestinal wall are connective tissue, musculature, and the peritoneum. In Asteroidea, the intestinal epithelium exhibits tall cells (columnar flagellated, mucous gland cells, and zymogen cells) and a subepidermal (subepithelial) underlying nerve cell layer in the anterior portion. Epithelial cells are basally permeated by axons. The wall of the pyloric ceca of *Asterias rubens* has a high columnar epithelium, basally permeated by abundant axons, the basal lamina, a layer of smooth muscle cells, thin nerve fibers, and a coelomic epithelium. The very simple digestive system in Ophiuroidea is composed only of mouth and stomach but no anus, and an intestinal epithelium with flagella and brush border. The stomach wall is significant and exhibits a flagellated epithelium, with a brush border; a nervous layer exists. Additional components of the intestinal wall are a layer of connective tissue, musculature, and the coelomic epithelium of cuboidal cells with flagella.

26. Phylum Chaetognatha. In general ciliated and nonciliated cuboidal to columnar absorptive and glandular cells are present. The esophagus shows secretory granular and vacuolated cells, a basement membrane, and longitudinal and circular musculature.

27. Phylum Pogonophora. A digestive tract is lacking.

28. Phylum Hemichordata. The digestive epithelium in members of this phylum is low columnar ciliated to high columnar, including glandular cells.

29. Phylum Tunicata. They possess a mouth, pharynx, esophagus, stomach and anus; ciliated or nonciliated columnar cells (depending on the region), with scarce musculature (?). Argyrophilic and argentaffin cells occur in the gut of *Ciona intestinalis* (98), mucous, endocrine, and plicated cells in the gastric epithelium of *Botryllus schlosseri* (48), and two types of endocrine cells in the gut of *Styela clava* (312), an insulin immunoreactive cell type in the esophageal epithelium of the same species (30) of which the gastric epithelium shows three distinct cell types (311).

30. Phylum Cephalochordata. The digestive tract of cephalochordates consists of buccal cavity, pharynx, esophagus, midgut, intestine, and anus, with a single layer of ciliated (?) epithelium containing tall columnar secretory cells. Basically large vacuoles occur in the cells.

31. Phylum Vertebrata. *General Review.* The oral cavity is covered by stratified nonkeratinizing squamous epithelium in land-living tetrapods. Outer enamel epithelium—a simple squamous or cuboidal epithelium and ameloblasts (=gonoblasts)—occurs at the inner wall of the enamel organ as a tall columnar epithelium. Special conditions occur in marsupials. The musculature is smooth or cross-striated: in the esophagus of fishes it is cross-striated; in other species such as in mammals it is divided. The serosa exhibits a simple layer of mesothelial cells. Esophageal mucous cells are present in fishes, and/or ciliated cells in amphibians and reptiles. The epithelium is stratified columnar, but in birds and mammals it is stratified squamous, in some mammals it is keratinized. The stomach has tall epithelial cells and an exocrine cell occurring as the principle cell in the species up to and including the birds. The midgut is simple prismatic epithelium; the main cells are enterocytes, paneth cells, intermediate cells in insectivores and bats, bush cells in insectivores and rodents, and ciliated in petromyzon. The end intestine shows generally abundance of goblet cells.

Chondrichthyes. The oral cavity and pharynx have a squamous stratified epithelium with lamina propria and supporting connective tissue; mucus secreting cells; rarely multicellular glands are found. Fish teeth consist of outer enamel, inner dentine, and a pulp. The esophagus has a stratified cuboidal or columnar epithelium, often ciliated, many goblet cells, and basement membrane. Smooth muscle fibers build the muscularis mucosae. Musculature and a cuboidal mesothelium are present. The stomach is highly variable and not present in all forms. Columnar cells, ciliated cells, special goblet cells and wandering granular cells, comparable to eosinophils, connective tissue (lamina propria), and multicellular gastric glands occur. Fundic glands are tubular, prismatic, like goblet cells, cuboidal to columnar. Pyloric glands range from cuboidal to low columnar. The submucosa is of loose areolar tissue. The muscularis is smooth or cross striated in type. The remaining components are the serosa (connective tissue), and the cuboidal mesothelium is simple. In the intestine, the mucosa consists of columnar cells, lamina propria and connective tissue, sometimes a muscularis mucosae. A submucosa is generally present and areolar in type. Outer longitudinal and inner circular musculature (?) appears. The serosa is made up of connective tissue, the mesothelium of simple squamous or cuboidal cells. The cloaca exhibits a stratified or cuboidal epithelium with connective tissue adjusting to the condition of the skin; smooth muscle changes to cross-striated.

Osteichthyes. No large variation exists in the histology of the oral cavity in teleost species. There occurs no tongue in the sense of mammals. Filiform and fungiform papillae have been observed. The enamel of teleosts is mesodermal. The esophagus is characterized by a stratified cuboidal to columnar epithelium. Goblet cells are abundant, cilia may occur. Changes of the esophageal epithelium of the eel during adaptation to seawater are observable (357). Characteristic of the fish (teleost) stomach is its large variability. Rugae and gastric pits can be observed. The crypts of the stomach are composed of high columnar cells and goblet cells may be found. Two portions of the stomach—fundic and pyloric—may be distinguished, and some fishes even show no stomach. Fundic and pyloric stomach are lined by a variation of cell forms, including glands. Submucosa, muscularis, and serosa show no peculiarities. The histologic make-up of the intestine is also quite simple. Multicellular glands occur only very seldom and show no important variations between the species. Ceca as outpocketings of the intestinal wall, the spiral valve (a long fold, composed of mucosa and submucosa) and intestinal villi occur only in a few genera. The cloaca, the termination of the excretory, genital, and digestive system, is characterized by a lining of cuboidal cells, underlain by connective tissue and striated musculature.

In the oral cavity and pharynx of amphibia the mucosa is stratified with columnar or cuboidal cells, often ciliated or with a striated border, seldom cornified. The alveolar capillary network serves respiration; mucous glands exist. The tunica propria consists of nerve bundles and connective tissue, the filiform and fungiform papillae of lymphoid tissue. The teeth are formed from dentine and enamel. The mucosa of esophagus and stomach is built from one or two layers of cuboidal to columnar cells, the upper row being ciliated and containing goblet cells. Some species have multicellular glands, the smooth muscle of the mucosa is incomplete.

An alveolar submucosa, muscularis, and serosa appear. In the stomach mucosa, tunica propria, muscularis mucosae, areolar submucosa, muscularis, and serosa can be distinguished. The small intestine has columnar and goblet cells, lamina propria, muscularis mucosae, areolar submucosa, muscularis and serosa; the large intestine has epithelial goblet and columnar cells, poor tunica propria, poor muscularis mucosae, submucosa and muscularis; the cloaca has two to three layers of cuboidal cells.

The lining of oral cavity and pharynx in reptilia differs from species to species. Simple ciliated columnar epithelium exists in snakes or young turtles, stratified squamous in old turtles, cornified in the lizard; all have many goblet cells. The epithelium of the tongue consists of stratified squamous cells as in land turtles and some snakes; of pseudostratified columnar cells as in some lizards, of stratified columnar cells also in lizards, and of simple columnar cells as in sphenodon. In addition, goblet cells and multicellular alveolar glands are present. Teeth are usually of dentine and enamel. The mucosa of the esophagus is formed from one or two layers of cuboidal or columnar ciliated epithelium with included goblet cells. The stomach exhibits a columnar epithelium as in the amphibia. The intestinal wall is characterized by an epithelium of nonciliated tall columnar and goblet cells, lamina propria, muscularis mucosae. The epithelial cells of the cloaca range from columnar and goblet cells to stratified ones.

The digestive tract of *birds* shows two characteristic peculiarities: (a) the beak and (b) the crop with a different development in the individual species. Both are extremely important with respect to weight with limitation and, therefore, the ability to fly. The mucosa of the mouth and pharynx are comparable to the skin and are composed of stratified squamous epithelium. The esophagus also has a stratified squamous epithelium with different types of glands and various amounts of lymphoid tissue depending on the development of the crop. A crop is lacking in owl, woodpecker, penguin, gull, goose, duck, and petrel. In the crop, glands are reduced and lymph nodes increased. The stomach exhibits the proventriculus and the ventriculus. The stomach glands contain cuboidal cells. The ventriculus has columnar cells. The epithelial lining of the bird intestine is simple columnar with goblet cells. In the cloaca, the epithelium shows a change assuming the character of the outer skin.

The epithelium of the oral cavity in mammals is composed of stratified squamous cells, with intermingled mucous cells. Filiform, fungiform, circumvallate and foliate papillae occur on the tongue. The epithelium of the esophagus is stratified squamous. Tubular mucous glands with cuboidal or columnar cells are present. In the stomach of insect-eating marsupials, some edentates, most carnivores and man, glandular columnar cells occur. In artiodactyls, perissodactyls, edentates, herbivorous marsupials, cetaceans, some monotremes and lower primates, the stomach lining exhibits in its upper portion stratified squamous epithelium; a condition which also holds true in a few monotremes and marsupials as well as many rodents. Surface mucous cells, parietal cells, mucous neck cells, argentaffin cells, and chief cells occur in the gastric glands of mammals. The stomach of mammals can be simple, it is more highly developed in the cardiac region as for example, in the pigs, it extends to a saclike part in whales, becomes two-chambered in hamsters, and multichambered in ruminant artiodactyls. In the latter the rumen is covered by stratified squamous epithelium, the reticulum by a stratified squamous epithelium, the omasum by a cornified stratified squamous epithelium, and the abomasum by a columnar epithelium. The small intestine contains columnar cells with striated border and glands of Lieberkühn which contain Paneth cells at their base. Lymphoid tissue is present depending on the location of the intestinal portion. The muscularis is double-layered. The large intestine has tubular mucous glands and is lined by a columnar epithelium with goblet cells at the base, lymphoid tissue and the muscularis mucosae and a strong muscularis which is especially pronounced in carnivores.

Glands of the Digestive System

A short review of the most important glands of the digestive tract in the different eumetazoan phyla is provided in Table 3.3. Some selected points about some digestive glands may be added.

Four cell types, undifferentiated epithelial cells, digestive cells, secretory cells, and excretory cells occur in the hepatopancreas (liver) of the opisthobranch gastropod *Trinchesia granosa* (279). The epithelial organization in digestive gland tubules of two species of bivalve molluscs was autoradiographically investigated (253), as well as the histological structure of the posterior

salivary glands in the blue ringed octopus *Hapalochlaena maculosa* (105). The catecholaminergic salivary glands in the amphipod crustacean *Gammarus pulex* (87) and the segmented head glands of *Scutigerella* sp. (Symphyla, Myriapoda) were also investigated (129). The salivary glands of the cockroach *Nauphoeta cinerea* are dually innervated, from both the ventral nerve cord and the stomodeal nervous system (35). For the differentiated regulation of the synthesis of ribosomal RNA, 5S RNA and 4S RNA in the polytenic salivary gland cells of the blowfly *Calliphora erythrocephala* see Griffith (119), for alterations of the pancreas of the aging Syrian golden hamster see Takahasha and Pour (310), and for the occurrence of argyrophil and argentaffin cells in salivary glands (submandibular, sublingual, and parotid) of 9 mammalian species (mouse, spiny mouse, gerbil, rat, guinea pig, Chinese hamster, rabbit, cat and dog), see Carlsöö and Östberg (53). The ultrastructural and histochemic diagnosis was applied for the identification of the polypeptid-producing cell of the human pancreas (16). Argyrophil cells in rat parotid gland intercalated ducts gave a positive staining (?).

STRUCTURES OF GASEOUS EXCHANGE (209, 234)

O. Throat flagellar cells are present in Porifera.

1–13. Phylum. Respiration is performed by surface epithelia in the phyla Cnidaria, Ctenophora, Platyhelminthes, Nemertinea, Gnathostomulida, Entoprocta, Acanthocephala, Rotifera, Gastrotricha, Kinorhyncha, Nematoda, Nematomorpha, Priapulida, Pentastomida, and Tardigrada.

In **14. Phylum Mollusca**, the integument, the gills, and lungs participate in breathing. Feather-like gills with ciliated epithelium and shaft appear in placophora, also gills in monoplacophora and polyplacophora. In gastropoda, the respiration is performed by surface epithelium especially in aquatic forms, or lungs in pulmonata and prosobranchia (the epithelium of the lungs is composed of cuboidal to squamous cells; goblet-like cells and underlain by a network-like pattern of blood vessels), otherwise gills are commonly distributed. The surface epithelium performs the function in Scaphopoda. In Bivalvia, gills are filibranch (*Mytilus edulis*) or eulamellibranch (*Anodonta* sp.). The epithelium is simple cuboidal to columnar, partially ciliated

Table 3.3
Selected Examples of the Occurrence of Digestive Glands in Metazoans (16, 51)

Phylum	Subgroup	Type of Gland	Example of Species
Mesozoa	—	—	—
Porifera	—	—	—
Cnidaria	—	Intermingled gland cells	Hydra, *Metridium* sp.
Ctenophora	—	Intermingled gland cells	*Pleurobrachia* sp.
Platyhelminthes	Turbellaria	—	*Dugesia* sp.
	Trematoda	—	*Polystoma* sp.
	Cestoda	—	*Dibothriocephalus latum*
Nemertini	—	Intermingled gland cells	*Gorgonorhynchus* sp.
Kamptozoa	—	Regions of intermingled glands in stomach	*Lophopus crystallinus*
Rotifera	—	Salivary glands, gastric glands	Philodinae
Gastrotricha	—	Pharynx glands	*Chaetonotus* sp.
Kinorhyncha	—	Salivary glands and pancreatic glands	*Pycnophyes* sp.
Nematoda	—	Intermingled glands	*Ascaris megalocephala*
Nematomorpha	—	—	*Parachordode tolosa*
Priapulida	—	—	*Priapulus* sp.
Mollusca	Amphineura	Salivary glands, digestive glands	*Chaetopleura* sp.
	Gastropoda	Midintestinal gland	*Helix pomatia*
	Lamellibranchiata	Midintestinal gland (234)	*Pecten* sp.
	Scaphopoda	Midintestinal gland	*Dentalium* sp.
	Cephalopoda (98)	Two pairs of salivary glands, liver and pancreas	*Architeutis* sp.
Sipunculida	—	Rectal glands	*Sipunculus* sp.
Echiurida	—	—	*Echiurus* sp.
Annelida	Polychaeta	Esophageal glands	*Lumbricus terrestris*
	Clitellata		*Arenicola cristata*
	Oligochaeta	Pharyngeal salivary glands, calc. glands-intestine, glandular	
	Hirudinea	Salivary glands	*Hirudo medicinalis*
Onychophora	—	Salivary glands	*Peripatus capensis*
Pentastomida	—	—	*Pentastomum* sp.
Tardigrada	—	Salivary and intestinal glands	*Macrobiotus* sp.
Arthropoda (118)	Xiphosura	Midintestinal glands	*Limulus polyphemus*
	Scorpions	Midintestinal glands	*Pandinus imperator*
	Araneae	Midintestinal glands	*Teraphosa leblondi*
	Crustacea (81)	Hepatopancreas	*Astacus fluviatilis*
	Chilopoda	Salivary glands	*Lithobius* sp.
	Diplopoda	Salivary glands	*Julus terrestris*
	Insecta	Salivary glands (34, 112, 284)	*Apis mellifera*
Tentaculata			*Phoronopsis californica*
Branchiotremata			*Balanoglossus gigas*
Echinodermata	Crinoidea	Intermingled glands	*Heliometra glacialis*
	Asteroidea	Digestive glands	*Asterias rubens*
	Ophiuroidea	—	*Gorgonocephalus* sp.
	Echinoidea	Intermingled glands and stomach	*Holothuria tubulosa*
Pogonophora	—	—	*Siboglinum* sp.
Hemichordata			
Chaetognatha			*Sagitta gazellae*
Urochordata	Tunicata	"Liver"	*Amoroucium* sp.
Cephalochordata	Acrania	"Liver"	*Branchiostoma* sp.

Table 3.3—*continued*

Phylum	Subgroup	Type of Gland	Example of Species
Vertebrata	Pisces	Intermingled glands	*Esox lucius*
	Amphibia	Salivary glands, liver, and pancreas	*Rana ridibunda*
	Reptilia	Salivary glands, liver, pancreas, and intermingled glands	*Lacerta agilis*
	Mammalia	Salivary glands, liver, pancreas, and intermingled glands	*Mus musculus*
	Aves	Salivary glands, liver, pancreas, and intermingled glands	*Gallus domesticus*

and supported by connective tissue elements, including blood spaces. For the excretion of acidic phosphatase by the goblet cells of the gills of *Mytilus edulis*, see Pasteels (233), and for the fine structure and innervation of gill-lamellae in *Anodonta*, see Nakao (219). In Cephalopoda, appear bipectinate gills with a highly diversified blood supply. Breathing in the members of **15. Phylum Sipunculida** is performed through the body surface in cooperation with thin-walled blood vessels enclosed approximately beneath the skin. In **16. Phylum Echiurida**, respiration takes place through the surface epithelium. In the species of the **17. Phylum Annelida** the function of respiration is undertaken by the body surface, segmental appendages, gills, or tentacular crowns. In polychaeta, respiration is performed by the surface epithelium as main source combined with capillaries underlaying epithelia, tentacle crowns, and lobes of parapodia. Especially in the case of larger polychaeta, a rich capillary network of the circulatory system underlines the skin. In oligochaeta respiration depends on the body surface. Gills occur in some aquatic genera. Others exhibit a type of lung as in the case of the slow-worm, *Anguis fragilis*, with specialized respiratory epithelium (202). The skin assumes the respiratory function in Hirudinea and is widely underlined by capillary plexuses. No respiratory organs occur in Myzostomida, the respiratory function is performed by the body surface. The respiratory organs in the members of **18. Phylum Onychophora** are tracheids (with invaginated epidermal epithelium). They are tubelike invaginations of the epidermis with a cuticle but no stigmata. No specialized respiratory organs appear in **19. Phylum Pentastomida** and **20. Phylum Tardigrada**.

21. Phylum Arthropoda. The most widely distributed structures of respiration in these organisms are the most common organs of arthropods, the tracheids. But the conditions in this largest phylum are very diversified. Approximately 150 leaves of book gills occur in Merostomata. Book-lungs (stigmata, cavity) and/or tracheae are the respiratory organs of Arachnida. The same arrangement occurs also in isopodes characterized by a tender epithelium with thin cuticle. Breathing pockets show low columnar epithelial cells. Tracheid walls from the inside to the outside exhibit basement membrane, an epithelial layer of cuboidal/columnar cells and a tender chitinous intima. Ventral sacs occur in palpigradi and whip scorpions. In crustaceans, the most common respiratory structures with great variability (gills) are characterized by a differentiated epidermis. Epipodites of leaf legs serve the function in Anacostraca, double layered structures of the back, under tender skin in Ostracoda; epipodites working as gills in Leptostraca; epipodial gills in Euphausiacea; and gills, rarely lungs especially in terrestrial forms, in Decapoda. A thin cuticle, a one-layered epithelium, a third layer of connective tissue, and gland cells are present.

The gills of the brown shrimp, *Penaeus aztecus* are composed of a central axis with biserially arranged branches subdividing into bifurcating filaments. The lumina of these structures are divided by a septum into afferent and efferent channels. Additionally, the gill is permeated by numerous blood vessels. The epithelium which secretes the cuticle is separated from the hemolymph by a basal lamina. Subcuticular lacunae are formed by pillar processes of the epithelial cells. To the cells of the epithelium also belong granular cells with elaborate Golgi apparatus and several types of granules. The efferent channels are lined by nephrocytes resembling glomerular podocytes. The septum in the axis is traversed by a large nerve (96). The medial wall of the carapax serves gaseous exchange in Cumacea and epipodial structures in Amphipoda.

Insecta (297). Gills are found in aquatic insects, especially larvae; tracheid gills in Trichoptera with simple squamous epithelium as in tracheae. The tracheid epithelium in insects is a direct continuation of the epidermis. The epithelium secretes the cuticle. Tracheid end cells are present, and even project in some cases into the mitochondria of the host tissue.

No special respiratory organs are found in **22. Phylum Phoronida**, but lophophore tentacles seem to oxygenate the blood. The epidermis especially of the tentacles serves the respiratory function in members of **23. Phylum Ectoprocta**. No special respiratory organs exist in **24. Phylum Brachiopoda** where the function is performed by lophophore and mantle.

Body surface, especially papulae and tube feet of the water vascular system in species generally not supplied with a special respiratory system, undertakes respiration in **25. Phylum Echinodermata**. Gills occur only in regular echinoids with the exception of the order Cidaroidea. The histology of these appendages is similar to the body wall, composed of the columnar ciliated epidermis, the dermis, and the coelomic lining characterized by flagellae. Many coelomocytes are found in the first two layers. Papulae and tube feet in asteroidea are simple or branched. The wall of the tube feet is similar to the body wall without skeletal components. From the outside to the inside the epidermis, dermis, longitudinal musculature, circular musculature, and flagellated coelomic epithelium can be distinguished. Some authors consider the papulae of asteroids, the peristomal gills of regular echinoids, and the respiratory podia of irregular echinoids altogether as simple gills. In the red sea star *Asterias rubens*, the tube feet consist of a cuticle composed of two layers: an external layer of mixed acid mucoids, and an internal layer of sulfated acid mucopolysaccharides. The tissue *per se* is composed of five layers: the external epithelium, a nervous zone, a layer of connective tissue, a layer of musculature, and a hydrocele epithelium. The external epithelium contains different cells according to location: revestment cells, mucocytes, cells with lipoprotein granules, inserted cells, and granulous cells with acid mucoids (221). The respiratory trees occurring in only three orders of holothurians with regard to their epithelium are similar to the intestinal epithelium. They are found in the intestine at the border in the cloaca.

In the **26. Phylum Chaetognatha** and **27. Phy-**

lum Pogonophora, respiratory organs are lacking. In **28. Phylum Hemichordata**, a branchial apparatus or gill intestine, with columnar ciliated or cuboidal epithelium and glandular cells, are found.

29. Phylum Cephalochordata. In *Branchiostoma* sp. occur differences in the epithelium in the regions of the gill arches. Near the atrium are large gland cells; at the medial side, ciliated and nonciliated cells, at the lateral side it is multilayered, and the uppermost layer consists of tall columnar ciliated cells. Members of the **30. Phylum Tunicata** have a branchial apparatus.

31. Phylum Vertebrata. Agnatha (lamprey) have gills covered by cuboidal or columnar epithelium; chondrichthyes (sharks) exhibit gills of which the second lamellae show simple stratified epithelium of cells. In the osteichthyes (40, 132, 199, 282), the epithelium is in general: The swim bladder can be considered an accessory organ. The following examples are intended to give a few samples of variations of the respiratory structures in these lower vertebrates. For the morphology of the gill epithelium of the lung-fish *Lepidosiren paradoxa*, see Wright (355); for comparative studies of the ultrastructure of the water-blood pathway in the secondary lamellae of teleost and elasmobranch fishes, see Hughes and Wright (144). For arteriovenous anastomoses in gill filaments of *Tilapia mossambica*, see Vogel *et al.* (331), and for those in the rainbow trout, Vogel *et al.* (332); for the fine structure of the physostomatous swim bladder of the rainbow trout (*Salmo gairdneri*), see Brooks (42), and of the toadfish (*Psanus tau*) see Morris and Albright (214). The gas gland in *Myxine* corresponds to the bladder in fish. The histology of the wall of the gas gland exhibits columnar epithelium with basement membrane, papulae, and muscular mucosa above the submucosa (loose connective tissue). The gill epithelium of the lamellae is simple squamous or cuboidal with basement lamella and an underlying bicapillary network. Gill filaments are supported by cartilage or bone. The respiration in amphibia is performed by the body surface, air swallowing and the lungs. Gills also occur as in tadpoles. The air conducting portion in the lungs of reptiles has a pseudostratified ciliated epithelium. The lungs of Aves are more or less assisted by air sacs. The air conducting portion is characterized by a pseudostratified ciliated epithelium. The air conducting portion in the lungs of mammals exhibits a pseudostratified ciliated epithelium.

Structures Dealing with Excretion and Waste Removal

No special excretory cells occur in **0. Phylum Porifera**. Pulsating vacuoles are present. Contractile vacuoles in fresh water sponges (38) may serve the excretory function. In the first eucoelomate phylum (**Cnidaria**) no special excretory organs are present. The mouth can also be considered as an expelling structure. Sometimes phagocytic cells occur. In **2. Phylum Ctenophora**, special excretory organs are lacking. The excretory function may be served by the cell rosettes. Protonephridia (closed tubes) in **3. Phylum Platyhelminthes** exhibit the flame cell (flame bulb), one or more ciliated cells, and a simple, nonciliated, cuboidal or syncytial epithelium. The ultrastructure of the protonephridial system in the common fresh water planarian *Dugesia tigrina* exhibits flame cells, the cyrtocytes, comparable to those in other phyla (201) and the nonciliated cells of ductules and the ciliated cells of collecting ducts with pronounced polarity. The cells of the osmoregulatory ducts finally are characterized by abundant mitochondria (201). A protonephridial system occurs generally in **4. Phylum Nemertinea**, with terminal flame bulbs. Certain specialized cells are ciliated and cuboidal. Excretory structures are lacking in **5. Phylum Gnathostomulida**. The upper portion of the stomach acts as excretory organ. Protonephridia occur only in the Archiacanthocephala of **7. Phylum Acanthocephala** which exhibits otherwise no excretory organs. Protonephridia with flame bulbs are observable in **8. Phylum Rotifera**. The tissue is syncytial. A urinary bladder may be present. Two protonephridia compose the excretory system of *Habrotrocha rosa* (282b). Seven tubules lead from each of them to a terminal organ, formed by a single cell known as a cyrtocyte. Its basket contains structures which resemble ciliary rootlets. A syncytial layer of cytoplasm borders the lumen of the excretory system. In the upper region of the trunk, the channel is twisted several times, and this is the only place where cells are found. In **9. Phylum Gastrotricha**, protonephridia occur only in Chaetonodoidea living in fresh water. Protonephridia characterized by a large single, multinucleated solenocyte with one flagellum are the excretory structures of **10. Phylum Kinorhyncha**. One single or a few large cells, never cilia or flagella, are involved in excretory processes of **11. Phylum Nematoda**. In **12. Phylum Nematomorpha**, no particular excretory organ exists; the gut may serve as such. The urogenital system of the species of **13. Phylum Priapulida** occurs on both sides of the intestine. The protonephridia are formed by several terminal cells, each equipped with one cilium.

In **14. Phylum Mollusca** metanephridia exist, with podocytes and in general columnar epithelium. In the renopericardial duct, the ciliated columnar epithelium is underlain by musculature. The kidney sac has cuboidal to columnar epithelium; the cells are known as nephrocytes. The cells of the ureter are prismatic. For a review on excretion in molluscs, see Potts (250). Kidneys in placophora are composed of ciliated funnels and tubes. Large variations in genera are present. In polyplacophora, metanephridia with columnar epithelium are found. Ciliated nephrostomes, mainly only one kidney, a duct with expanded channel, the nephroporus, and a primary or secretory ureter releases the urine. The funnel is ciliated and cilia occur in the duct as well as secreting epithelial cells and pericardial glands. The epithelium of metanephridia is cuboidal or columnar, sometimes a ciliated urinary bladder occurs in certain members. The kidney is not united with the pericard in scaphopoda. In bivalvia the kidney starts with a ciliated funnel from pericard; a ureter is present. The epithelium is folded and underlined by connective tissue; the epithelial cells are the excretory ones. The kidney in cephalopoda starts with a ciliated funnel; the pericardial glands seem to be excretory organs also. The excretory epithelium is closely related to the veins and their extensions.

Characteristic excretory organs, only comparable to those in certain holothurians, are the ciliated urns in **15. Phylum Sipunculida**. In some species the wall contains chloragogen cells. Either one pair of metanephridia, or one metanephridium is present. The epithelium is underlined by the musculature. Columnar cells, the chloragogen cells, are phagocytic and developed from the cells of the coelomic cover. In **16. Phylum Echiurida**, two long anal tubes with ciliated epithelium and numbering from a few up to 200 metanephridia with ciliated funnel are present at the base.

Metanephridia are characteristic in **17. Phylum Annelida**, starting with the open funnel and continuing into an excretory tube; each metanephridium develops from a single cell known as nephroblast which divides into a cord of cells. A few species of polychaeta have protonephridia with solenocytes. The tube of the metanephridium in larger forms of polychaeta is surrounded by a capillary network. For the histology of the excretory system of the maldanid *polychaetes Clymenella* torquata and *Eucly-mene oerstedi*, see Pilgrim (246). The nephridia are generally metanephridia; the tube is often surrounded by blood capillaries. In the megas-colecidae mesonephridia occur. Chloragogen cells are present. The peritoneum is important for excretion. As possible sites of ultrafiltration in the oligochaete *Tubifex tubifex* (242) the endothelia occur consisting of myoendothelial cells, chloragocytes and podocytes. The inside of the endothelium is lined by a basement membrane which is the only continuous layer of blood vessels and capillaries. Ultrafiltration is the first process in excretion. Modified metanephridia of Hirudinea are composed of a ciliated funnel, a capsule with amoebocytes, and a nonciliated nephridial tube, which are the structures of concern. Besides the nephridia, bothryoid cells developing from the coelothelium work as excretory units. The nephridial activity in the horse-leech *Haemopis sanguisuga* exhibits a neural regulation based on a rich network of nerves, terminating on or between the cells of the tubules. In the urinary bladder, only the mural muscles are innervated. The nerve cells near the nephridia are multipolar (93).

The metanephridia of **18. Phylum Onychophora** are composed of a long narrow and ciliated funnel, a following tube and a contractile urinary bladder. The nephridia of the third segment differentiate to salivary glands, a condition comparable to arthropods. In contrast to the annelida, the ontogenesis of nephridia does not start from the nephroblasts.

Excretory organs have not been observed in **19. Phylum Pentastomida**. Perhaps the skin glands act instead. In **20. Phylum Tardigrada**, organs with excretory functions are the epidermis, portions of the rectum, the Malpighian vessels, salivary glands, and midintestinal cells. Different organs participate in the excretion of **21. Phylum Arthropoda**. They are composed of the remainder of a coelomic cavity of the particular segment, a sacculus, a small unciliated funnel, a nephridial tube, and sometimes a bladder.

Chelicerata. Excretion in merostomata is undertaken by one pair of coxal glands of very complicated structure and active red color. In arachnida coxal glands and Malpighian vessels are in most species the excretory organs. Deposition of pigments in the epidermis and other structures has to be seen as a type of passive excretion.

According to developmental stage and species, the excretion in crustaceans differs. The epithelium of the midintestinal gland and of the gills,

thin portions of the integument, and nephridia are structures dealing with excretion. The nephridia known as antennal or maxillary glands comparable to the coxal glands in chelicerata are composed of a sacculus, an excretory tube, and sometimes a bladder. A green or antennary gland is known in the adult decapoda, mysidiacea, amphipoda, and euphausiacea, whereas a maxillary gland is present in all nonmalacostraca as well as the hoplocarida, cumacea, tanaidacea, and isopoda. Both types of glands seldom develop or occur as a rudiment as in the lophogastrida of the mysidacea. Phagocytes and nephrocytes seem to be the most significant sources of excretion in crustaceans. For detailed histology see Gnatzy (109), Hyman (145), and Kuekenthal and Krumbach (177). Freshwater species develop hypotonic urine and differ from the marine crayfish, such as *Homarus* sp., that secretes isotonic urine.

Tracheata. In myriapoda, the chilopoda and diplopoda exhibit Malpighian tubules as excretory organs. As in insects, Malpighian vessels develop as a differentiation of the intestinal epithelium. The maxillary glands appear as paired nephridia and are composed of the sacculus, the excretory duct, and sometimes a bladder. Besides these organs of excretion, nephrocytes and the intestinal epithelium itself acts as such. The epithelium of the Malpighian vessels is simple, the epithelial cells of the duct are striated. The Malpighian tubules of *Drosophila* consist of a thickened proximal portion, a short transitory portion, the long main portion, and the ureter which enters into the intestine. The cells exhibit a typical polarity.

Many electron microscopic investigations of the cells of the Malpighian tubules have shown a similar cell structure among different groups of insects and in the nephrons of the vertebrate kidneys.

An example of a cell of the Malpighian tubule as a resorbing cell is found in *Drosophila*. Three regions are distinguishable: the apical region, the intermediary region, and the basal region. All three are connected by the channels of the endoplasmic reticulum uniting the polar cell borders. A brush border of microvilli with central channels leading to the endoplasmic reticulum is characteristic for the apical region. The intermediary region contains generally the nucleus and storage areas of lipids and other compounds. Infoldings of the basal cell membrane and a basal membrane are observable in the basal region. Mitochondria are abundant, especially in the upper and lower regions of the cell (348).

Metanephridia in **22. Phylum Phoronida** which shall develop from the larval protonephridia are exhibiting ciliated epithelium and solenocytes. Special excretory organs are not present in **23. Phylum Ectoprocta**, but excretion was observed through the skin, the wall of the stomach, intestine, and the different parts of the tentacles. Cells of coelomic walls and amoebocytes are also active. In **24. Phylum Brachiopoda**, metanephridia (ciliated cells in funnel as well as excretory cells in tube) and also coelothelium and amoebocytes in the coelomic fluid are active. Excretory organs are missing in **25. Phylum Echinodermata**, but thin portions of the integument, such as tube feet, the coelomoporus and the coelomocytes seem to be involved in excretory functions. No special excretory system occurs in **26. Phylum Chaetognatha**, but in certain species subepidermal glandular excretory cells are acting. In **27. Phylum Pogonophora**, an excretory system is missing. Excretory organs are lacking in **28. Phylum Hemichordata**, the walls of the coelomic cavity seem to act in enteropneusta. **30. Phylum Cephalochordata** possess 100 or more protonephridia with solenocytes. Some excretion occurs through the surface of the tunic in ascidiacea. There participate also nephrocytes which build excretory storage areas in the intestine and gonads in waste removal.

31. Phylum Vertebrata. In agnatha (cyclostomata) the larval pronephros, adult opisthonephric mesonephros and salt secretory glands exist. The epithelium of the nephrostome is ciliated. The mesonephros, the nephron of chondrichthyes, shows the glomerulus as an important part and Bowman's capsule as well as the tubular system. The lining of Bowman's capsule is simple squamous. The epithelium of the rectal glands of elasmobranchs is stratified cuboidal. Cyclostomes and young fish exhibit protonephridia in osteichthyes, adult animals meso- or metanephridia characterized by flat to tubular cells. Besides opisthonephric kidneys, gills act in the excretory process. The mesonephros of amphibia, characterized by Bowman's capsule and a glomerulus, is the main source of excretion, but the skin, lungs, and gills play an additional role depending on the stage of the animal. Metanephric kidneys and orbital salt glands are present in reptilia. Metanephric kidneys and orbital salt glands are the excretory organs in aves. The epithelium of the salt glands is columnar (234). In mammalian metanephric kidneys, the skin and lungs participate in excretion as well as sweat glands (293). Accessory organs of the excretory system are the urinary bladders in fishes, amphibians, reptiles, mammals and birds (ostrich), as well as ureters and urethras.

Structures Dealing with Reproduction

The description is given in Chapter 6.

Structures Dealing with the Production and Storage of Hormones

0. Phylum Porifera. Certain bi- and multipolar cells in porifera with the character of neurons around the osculum of such species as *Sycon ciliatum* are considered neurosecretory in character (189a).

1. Phylum Cnidaria. Hormone production is restricted to nettle cells and neurosecretion (351).

2. Phylum Ctenophora. Neurosecretion seems to occur.

3. Phylum Platyhelminthes. Neurosecretory cells are found in the brain and near the ovaries and testes of several species in platyhelminthes (184).

4. Phylum Nemertinea. Neurosecretory cells occur sometimes separated as cerebral organ in the brain in nemertinea. These worms may also exhibit more or less simultaneously the lowest condition of a neurohemal organ developed during phylogeny (286, 287).

5–13. Neurosecretory cells may occur in **Gnathostomulida, Entoprocta, Acanthocephala, Rotifera, Gastrotricha, Kinorhyncha, Nematoda, Nematomorpha,** and **Priapulida.** For example, *Ascaris lumbricoides* and *Phocanema decipiens* (nematodes) exhibit neurosecretory cells in their ganglia (65).

14. Phylum Mollusca. Extensive hormone production performed by different structures is known from molluscs (135a). Neurosecretory cells, neurosecretory glands, neurohemal organs, neuroendocrine glands, and independent endocrine glands are distinguishable in the various groups. In polyplacophora the "organes juxtacommissural" occurs which may be comparable to the "organes juxtaganglionnaires" in the prosobranchia and the opisthobranchia as well as to the dorsal bodies in the pulmonate gastropods. *Lymnaea stagnalis* is a relatively well investigated species of which recently a special type of neurosecretory cell has been identified by physiologic and ultrastructural characteristics (167) and neurosecretion in the periphery described (135a).

Neurosecretory cells are present in all ganglia of pelecypod molluscs. They may also appear in scaphopoda but new studies are needed.

The most important endocrine organs in cephalopods (octopus, squid) are the optic glands which control the genital organs. Cephalopod molluscs and arthropods are the only invertebrates which exhibit epithelial endocrine glands. The whole endocrine system of cephalopods and arthropods is comparable in its complexity to the endocrine system in vertebrates.

15. Phylum Sipunculida. Neurosecretory cells, neurohemal organs, and neurosecretory glands are present in Sipunculida.

16. Phylum Echiurida. They exhibit neurosecretory cells.

17. Phylum Annelida. The segmented worms are characterized by neurosecretory cells, perhaps the beginning of a neurohemal organ in the form of the cerebrovascular complex, and the infracerebral gland, considered to be a glandular portion of the system (135a).

18. Phylum Onychophora. Neurosecretion can be assumed as well as more complex structures than neurosecretory cells (neurosecretory glands). The members of this phylum have not been sufficiently investigated.

19. Phylum Pentastomida. Hormone-producing structures are unknown in Pentastomida.

20. Phylum Tardigrada. Neurosecretion in Tardigrada can be assumed, particular structures are not known.

21. Phylum Arthropoda. They exhibit a wide variety of hormone-producing and hormone-storing structures comparable only to vertebrates as a diversified group. Neurosecretory cells, neurosecretory glands, neurohemal organs, neuroendocrine glands, and independent endocrine glands are distinguishable from the main arthropod groups, the merostomata, the arachnida, the crustacea, the myriapoda, and the insecta; the crustacea and the insecta are the two best investigated groups.

In merostomata, neurosecretory cells are abundantly scattered throughout the central nervous system. Cerebral neurosecretory cells and neurohemal organs are present in arachnida (115, 345).

Moulting, reproduction, and heart beat are hormonally controlled main processes in crustacea. The involved organs are: epithelial endocrine glands, the Y-organs, located in the head and comparable to the thoracic glands of insects. Male crustacea exhibit in the region of the sperm ducts the androgenic glands as a second type of epithelial endocrine glands. The main neurohemal organs are the sinus glands, the postcommissural organs, and the pericardial organs. The question of whether neurosecretory cells in the central nervous system of which special groups

are known as X-organs exist is still unresolved. For a general review including hormonal action, see (135a).

The sinus gland in the eyestalk of crayfish consists of aggregated axon terminals ending near the blood space. Proximal cell bodies occur only in the region of the X-organ. Non-neurosecretory cells are intermingled in this region (9). In freshwater prawn *Palaemon paucidens*, two types of neurosecretory fibers occur (138; see also 136, 137, 217). They occur in the fiddler crab *Uca pugnax* (289) and in the shore crab *Carcinus maenas* (299). In myriapoda, protocerebral neurosecretory cells are present, and the cerebral glands represent neurohemal organs comparable to the sinus gland of crustacea and corpora cardiaca of insecta.

The endocrine system of insects exhibits four structural entities: neurosecretory cells in the brain; the corpora cardiaca, transformed ganglia which produce their own hormones but are also the most important neurohemal organs; the corpora allata; and thoracic glands, comparable and homologous to the ventral glands in certain species. Some insects such as cockroaches have ventral and thoracic glands together. The neurosecretory cells in the brain and the corpora cardiaca compose together the cerebral neurosecretory system; whereas the corpora allata and the thoracic (ventral) glands represent epithelial endocrine glands.

Neurosecretory Cells in the Brain. For liberation of hormones from neurosecretory neurons, the lack of a glial envelope is a precondition.

The detailed description of neurosecretory cells of some species may serve as examples to initiate further studies in comparative oncology. These species are *Locusta migratoria migratorioides* (Orthoptera) (107); *Pecilocerus pictus* (Orthoptera) (254); *Calliphora erythrocephala* (Diptera) (164); *Galleria mellonella* (Lepidoptera) (341); *Leptinotarsa decemlineata* (Coleoptera) (281).

The extrusion of neurosecretory material in the corpora cardiaca of *Leucophaea maderae* (Orthoptera) occurs in a considerable speed (276). Steroid transport through the cell surface of giant polyploid prothoracic gland cells in the last larval instar of *Galleria mellonella* seems to occur by macropinocytosis during the feeding period, and release of the steroids produced by the gland occurs by reverse micropinocytosis generally on the 5–7th day of the instar (31).

Corpora Cardiaca. The neuron-like cells differ from those of the brain by small, rough endoplasmic reticulum, cisternae, and ribosomes.

Corpora Allata. Neurosecretory axons from the brain, passing the corpora cardiaca, terminate in the corpora allata. The corpora allata contain various nonneuronal glandular cells (68).

Prothoracic Glands. Cells with long interdigitating processes which communicate with the hemolymph appear. Few organelles, rough and smooth endoplasmic reticulum cisternae, and few mitochondria of crista type are seen. Special hormone-producing cells in insects are oenocytes thought to be responsible for the production of steroid hormones.

22. Phylum Phoronida. Neurosecretory cells may be present; the knowledge on this phylum needs to be expanded.

23. Phylum Ectoprocta. Neurosecretory cells can also be assumed in Ectoprocta, but new studies are urgently needed.

24. Phylum Brachiopoda. Neurosecretory cells may be present in brachiopoda; special neuroendocrine organs have not been identified.

25. Phylum Echinodermata. Neurosecretory cells are present in echinoderms. Certain topics such as the production of a possible evisceration factor need further clarification.

26. Phylum Chaetognatha. Neurosecretory cells occur in Chaetognatha; the gonads may also act.

27. Phylum Pogonophora. The Pogonophora have neurosecretory cells.

28. Phylum Hemichordata. Neurosecretory cells and cells of the gonads are found in the Hemichordata.

29. Phylum Tunicata. Neurosecretory cells and other endocrine cells are present. Endocrine cells occur for example in the gut of *Styela clava* (312). The esophageal epithelium in the same species shows two types of endocrine cells (30).

30. Phylum Cephalochordata. Neurosecretory cells and the gonads are structures of significance in Cephalochordata.

31. Phylum Vertebrata. The Vertebrata exhibit the highest peak of endocrine development. As in cephalopods and arthropods, single endocrine cells, neurosecretory glands, neurohemal organs, and independent endocrine glands can be discerned. The morphological and functional comparability to the other aforementioned groups is not sufficiently established yet. The functional approach of such a comparison is the most promising one. For a general review see Patt and Patt (234). Discussion of some detailed recent studies is in order. At least four types of endocrine-like cells in the mucosa of the human colon and rectum are present (46); endocrine cells appear at the 16th day of gestation of mouse embryos and in the small intestine with the formation of villi (51); also the tracheal mucosa of man and other mammals contains endocrine cells (64); the digestive tract of the teleost *Barbus conchonius* exhibits also enteroendocrine cells (265).

Sensitivity (47)

The nervous system is composed of two major types of cells, the nerve cells or neurons themselves and the cells associated with the neurons also considered supporting cells. This second group of cells is known as the glia or the nonnervous cells typically associated with nerve cells. The glia or neuroglia occur in both vertebrates and invertebrates. In mammals the best known glial elements are the astrocytes, the oligodendroglia or the microglia. The special elements of the glia vary to a certain extent among the phyla. Some authors believe that astrocytes are not known from invertebrates. There exists no direct counterpart of the vertebrate autonomic nervous system in invertebrates; it is wrong to consider the stomodeal or stomatogastric system as such.

0. Phylum Porifera. The simple nervous system in porifera, e.g., in *Sycon* shows two types of neurons, spindle-shaped bipolar and multipolar cells.

1. Phylum Cnidaria. The nervous system in cnidaria is subepidermal. Bipolar (in region of the foot of polyps) or multipolar nerve cells compose a network. Bipolar neurons with short and bi- and multipolar neurons with long processes can be distinguished. Many neurons are neurosecretory in character. Spindle-shaped sensory cells look nearly like bipolar neurons. Comparable nerve nets occur as a primitive type in flatworms, echinoderms, and hemichordates, appearing as ring nerve and ganglia in medusae. Diffuse and synaptic nerve nets are found in the coelenchymal mesoglea and ectoderm of *Muricea* and *Lophogorgia* colonies. Plasmid sensory cells from ciliary cone complexes seem to activate or modify nematocyst discharge (272). Statocysts occur in hydromedusae (291) and the fine structure of the neuromuscular system of *Polyorchis penicillatus* (Hydromedusae, Cnidaria) is somewhat comparable to the aforementioned species and contains outer, inner (with some giant axons exhibiting infolded plasma membranes and annular gap junctions), and endodermal nerve rings (292).

2. Phylum Ctenophora. One nerve net can be found in ctenophora. Isopolar ganglion cells are mainly multipolar. Unipolar neurons occur beneath the complex. Two kinds of sensory nerve cells are present as well as sense cells, statocysts, ocelli with pigment, and sensory cells. The ciliated cells, compared with the comb plates of *Pleurobrachia bachei* and of those in the ciliated grooves, are separated by intercellular gap junctions which are lacking between the cells of the ectodermal tissue and the comb rows (273).

3. Phylum Platyhelminthes. Uni-, bi-, or multipolar neurons and medullary rays occur. Fibers are generally unmyelinated. Tactile receptors, chemoreceptors, rheoreceptors, photoreceptors, and statocysts have been observed.

Some turbellarians have a primitive nerve net. Others possess cerebral ganglion, longitudinal and transverse medullary rays and submuscular and subepithelial plexus. Unipolar neurons are present and bi- and multipolar neurons are more branched. The organization of the peripheral nervous system of flatworms as of the polyclad, *Notoplana acticola* seems to have developed from a diffuse network of fibers (171), with many properties of the CNS of higher animals. The synaptic junctions are important for such action (172). Sense organs from *Dugesia tigrina* are well known by scanning electron microscopy (295). Some glial cells occur in the cerebral ganglion. Type G cells are believed glial in character inside the capsule and along peripheral trunks; they are spindle-shaped with fine processes. Glial cells are also seen in cestodes.

4. Phylum Nemertinea. The neurons of nemertinea are unipolar and in many species giant neurons are observable. Statocysts, papillae, and photoreceptors occur; cerebral organs are for chemoreception, the system is basiepithelial. With the exception of lower genera, a capsule or ganglionic neurolemma of connective tissue appears in most nemertineans.

5. Phylum Gnathostomulida. The nervous tissue in gnathostomulida is concentrated at the anterior end and occurs also beneath the epithelium.

6. Phylum Entoprocta. Neurons in entoprocta are histologically very simple. Sense organs are unicellular bipolar receptors (128).

7. Phylum Acanthocephala (75). Cell invariability occurs in acanthocephala. Neurons are characterized by a constant nuclear number (eutely). *Hamaniella* has 80 nuclei in the cerebral ganglion and 30 in the genital ganglion. The neurons are mainly bi- or unipolar; sense receptors are tactile; sense organs consist of three simple spots. The male *Moniliformis moniliformis* exhibits paired genital ganglia composed of

an externally located soma and a poorly developed internal neuropile. The ganglia are connected by a dorsal commissure and each one is characterized by 19 cells (80).

8. Phylum Rotifera. Cell constancy is typical for rotifera. Eutely: *Epiphaenes senta* has approximately 280 nerve cell nuclei. Neurons thought to be uni- and bipolar. There are four types of ganglion cells; no neural glia; cilia motor and muscular motor innervation occurs; sensory cells are unicellular. Photoreceptors are present and five types of ciliary sense organs: membranelles, sensory hairs, sensory bristles, rods in patches, and ciliary grooves. The combinations are abundant. Other receptors are palpal organs, statocysts, and free nerve endings.

9. Phylum Gastrotricha. Neurons are not well known, especially with regard to electron microscopy. Tactile hairs, lateral sense grooves, and sometimes ocelli are present.

10. Phylum Kinorhyncha. Neurons in Kinorhyncha are awaiting new studies similar to those done to gastrotricha. Sense organs are simple ocelli and palpating structures, sensory bristles, innervated by epidermal sensory nerve cells.

11. Phylum Nematoda. The neurons of nematoda are mainly unipolar but multipolar and a few bipolar ones occur, too. Sense organs have bipolar cells. Cell constancy is developed in different portions of the nervous system. The ganglion cells exhibit special features. The anterior sense organs of *Gastromermis boophthorae* exhibit a particular pattern composed of a cuticular channel and a proximal amphidial gland (47). Cilia, rare in nematode nervous system, play an important role in these sensory structures. The nematode nervous system contains also glial structures.

12. Phylum Nematomorpha. Neurons are uni- or bipolar, giant bipolar in nematomorpha. Also multipolar neurons occur. The giant nerve cell of the cephalic ganglion could prove significant for research, especially its precursors (youth stages). Neuroglia are prominent, sensory organs are not well known. Many receptors degenerate together with the digestive tract in various degrees during the life cycle. Bristles, spines, and papillae have been described.

13. Phylum Priapulida. The neurons of the epidermal nervous system of Priapulida are not well enough known for the exact definition of types. Sense organs are not clearly defined. Sense receptors are very simple.

14. Phylum Mollusca. The nervous system and the sense organs of this second largest animal phylum exhibit a wide variety, from relatively simple structures to very high developed ones. The general plan presents six pairs of well-defined ganglia with certain exceptions as in the case of brain and sense organs of the cephalopods; the histology of the nervous system of this phylum is not well enough known. The differentiation of the neuropile in cephalopods reaches the level of the highest arthropods or of fishes.

Amphineurans are the only molluscs which exhibit no statocysts. Uni- and multicellular sensory structures as the osphradium, cyathiform bodies, olfactory, subradular, and branchial organs, and appendages of the mantle, including so called esthetes occur (36, 37, 47).

The gastropods follow the general plan of six major ganglionic groups. The best known and most highly developed brain is that of *Helix*. The large nerves are ensheathed in glial processes and the glia may produce longitudinal indentations in these layers. The sense organs range from unicellular to complex structures (47, pp. 1284 *ff*.). Due to the fact that the histology of this large class is relatively neglected, some remarks on the newer studies are in order. *Lymnaea* sp. and *Aplysia* sp. are, beside *Helix pomatia*, the more often investigated species (340); for the giant neurons, see Pogorelaya (249); concerning serial synapses in *Aplysia*, see Graubard (116), and for sensory cells in the chemoreceptor of the ommatophore of *Helix pomatia*, see Wondrak (353). Price (251) reported on the histology of the CNS in the pulmonate *Melampus bidentatus* and Robbes and Fisher (263) discussed the special features in neurons of the opisthobranch *Bulla gouldiana*. The snail brain is frequently used in pharmacological research (163). For a review on pharmacology, toxicology, and immunology in relation to the distribution of tissue structures, see the summarization by Kaiser (158a).

The nervous system in scaphopoda is typically molluscan, shows no torsion, and is of medially advanced development. Statocysts osphradia, the subradular organ, and captacula are the sense organs, eyes are lacking; the cells of the nervous system show no peculiarities.

Microscopic anatomy and histology of bivalvia and pelecypoda are barely known and seem to show no peculiarities. The visceroparietal ganglion of *Pecten* exhibits the most advanced neuropile. The receptors are generally unicellular structures. Some mechanisms of fast transport in the CNS of *Anodonta cignea* (141), the innervation of the byssus retraction muscle in *Mytilus edulis* and *galloprovincialis*, artificial degeneration in the myenteric plexus of *Mytilus* sp. (269), the ultrastructure of peripheral neurons and associated nonneuronal structures in the bivalve *Spisula solidissima*, and the ultrastructure of the ciliated receptors of the long tentacles in the giant scallop, *Placopecten magellanicus* (211), have been recently investigated.

In cephalopoda, the pattern and differentiation in the neuropile are very highly developed. Granule and giant cells are present. The majority of cells are unipolar but cephalopods also exhibit multipolar cells which are comparable by their heteropolarity to vertebrate neurons. The receptors (3) exhibit a high development, including stretch receptors and olfactory organ, rhinophores, statocysts, and the highly developed eye (7). The glial elements of the nervous system are very specialized and present different types. Opinions vary regarding whether astrocytes occur which are comparable to those in vertebrates. It is assumed that nothing like microglia is present. Some of the glia cells are large, others small, or elongated. The retina of the cephalopods consists of two main cell types, the visual sense cells and the supporting cells (47, pp. 1434 *ff*.).

15. Phylum Sipunculida. Multipolar giant cells, small multipolar globulet cells, and neural secretory cells occur in the brain of sipunculida. Receptors are either unicellular (bipolar), or simple multicellular and perhaps centralized sensory cells. The brain is covered by connective tissue (glia?).

16. Phylum Echiurida. Primary sense cells are bipolar sensory neurons.

17. Phylum Annelida. The histology of the ventral cord in annelida is unlike that of the spinal cord in the vertebrates; neurons are unipolar but also multipolar; globulet cells appear in the brain of polychaeta, first optical ganglia occur in annelids. Few motor neurons are present. *Aphroditides* displays the highest annelid brains, together with related forms. A review of the histology of the maldanid *polychaetes Clymenella torquata* and *Euclymene oerstedi* can serve as an example of selected species (246). The subesophageal ganglion of the lugworm *Arenicola marina* was investigated by Howie (142), as was the distribution of neurons and fiber pathways of leeches (92). The CNS of leeches contains Retzius cells (189). Annelid worms exhibit glial cells, as in the case of the earthworm (162). Neuroglia resemble ordinary connective tissue of perhaps one or more types: giant fiber system, epidermal sense cells, deep sense cells, isolated cells as photoreceptors; shadow and light detectors, and statocysts. Nuchal organs are dorsal pits, grooves, or folds. Slow and fast muscle control exists as well as a stomodeal system.

18. Phylum Onychophora. Neurons are simpler but comparable to those in arthropods. The synapses of the ventral nerve cord of *Peripatoides leuckarti* are asymmetric and differ from those of annelids and insects. They show a well developed synaptic cleft of 300 Å, pre- and subsynaptic election, dense apposition. Frequently an assay of presynaptic projections and subsynaptic cisternae characterize the endoplasmic reticulum (284). Sense organs are simple papillae, and the eye is composed of receptor neurons, sensory cells, corneal cells, and subcorneal cells.

19. Phylum Pentastomida. The histology of Pentastomida, including the neurons, is reminiscent of arthropods. Simple sensory organs are sensory papillae.

20. Phylum Tardigrada. The neurons in Tardigrada are unipolar at the ring of ganglia; no consistency of cell number occurs; sensory papillae exist. The histology of the nervous system is not well known. Ciliary structures occur in the sensory cells of *Macrobiotus hufelandi* and the cilia patterns are unusually modified (11 + 0; 12 + 0; 17 + 0) (339).

21. Phylum Arthropoda. The distribution of the elements of the nervous system (neurons and glia) of the arthropods, comprising more species than all other phyla together and the highest degree of activity, shows a great variability of structures which nevertheless can be attributed to a general plan. This general image exhibits a dorso-anteriorly located brain with circumesophageal connectives: a ventral cord with segmental ganglia, commissures, and nerves. There exists additionally a peripheral nervous system and a stomodeal or stomatogastric system for the anterior digestive tract. Motor neurons and interneurons and a wide variety of different neuron types occur. There are dozens of types of axons partially still unknown. Superficial glial cells ensheathe the neurons with their cytoplasm. The most common receptors of arthropods are cuticular hairs but there occur also many others, such as short hairs known as sensilla basiconica characteristic for insect antennae. Internal mechanoreceptors are the chordotonal organs, campaniform sensilla, hypopharyngeal sense organs. The campaniform sensilla are important for sensitivity with regard to the movements of joints, and hypopharyngeal sense organs are found in the pharynx of many arthropod species. Arachnids exhibit lyriform organs or slit sensilla; each slit has a bipolar neuron and is significant for cuticular strain. Arthropods have two types of photoreceptors, the simple eyes and the compound eyes. The simple eyes have a cuplike retina and a lens in chelicerata and are characterized by dorsal ocelli in insecta. The compound eyes exhibit ommatidia usually composed of 6–8 receptor cells. There are also many other types of photoreceptors including larval organs, such as nauplius eyes of crustaceans. A proper comparison of the ganglia, neurons, sense organs and glia is injured because "every study has been made from a different aspect, using different techniques" (47, p. 1166). Some details shall be given based on more recent studies.

Merostomata (4, 74, 84, 158). Neurons are encapsulated unipolar (two types of secretory unipolar cells) encapsulated bipolar cells, neuroglandular bipolar cells, and small nonencapsulated cells; sense cells are photoreceptors, glia occur; small and large axons exist. The peripheral nerve of *Limulus polyphemus* is ensheathed in the artery which is a very peculiar distribution (79). The *Limulus* visual system shows in the lateral eye eccentric cells, which have the ability to accumulate indole amines (4) and retinula cells (170). The ocelli of the median eye contain 155 retinula cells and 26 arhabdomeric cells (secondary sensory neurons) each (90).

Arachnida. Arhabdomeric cells occur in the eye of the scorpions (94). Certain compounds are known from the CNS of arachnids and these studies give a link from the morphologic aspects to the biochemical aspects (204), urgently needed for comparative oncology.

The distribution and characteristics of different neurons are investigated in several crustacean species as, for example, of monoaminergic neurons in non-malacostracan species (11); fast-axon synapses in the leg muscle of the crab, *Pachygrapsus crassipes* (13); neuromuscular synapses of pyloric muscle, arising via an axon of the stomatogastric ganglion in the blue crab, *Callinectes sapidus* (14); developmental abnormalities are known from neurons of *Procambarus simulans* (20), as well as crayfish interneurons (108). Synapse-like structures occur in peripheral nerves of *Cambarus* and *Procambarus* spp. during regeneration (224). Five classes of neurons are found in the lamina of the compound eye of the branchiopod crustacean, *Artemia salina* and *Daphnia magna*: photoreceptor axons, monopolar, centrifugal, tangential, and amacrine neurons (218). Each compound eye of *Munida irrasa* contains approximately 12,500 ommatidia of which each is composed of a typical cornea, corneagenous cells, crystalline cone cells, crystalline cone, crystalline cone tract, and eight retinula cells; distal pigment cells are present (50). Photoreceptor cells occupy approximately 42% of the lateral eye of the barnacle, *Balanus eburneus* (174). The shape of the rhabdom differs during light and dark adaptation of the shrimp, *Palaemonetes* (148). Differences also occur between the larval and adult eye of the western rock lobster, *Panulirus longipes* (205). It can be assumed from these few samples how great the variations in the different species alone of one arthropod group are. These facts have to be considered in experimental comparative oncological studies in arthropods, as well as those with crayfish mechanoreceptors (360).

Myriapoda. Petit and Sahli (244) studied paraesophageal bodies and related nerves in the diplopod, *Schizophyllum sabulosum.* Two axonal types are present. The sensory hairs of the millipede, *Polyxenus* sp., showed an unusual fine structure of these mechanoreceptors when compared to other animals (313).

Insecta. Sensory neurons of the CNS in *Drosophila* recognize defined pathways if, for example, an adult nerve has been experimentally misrouted and is able to develop a normal projection (104). The lateral ocellar nerve projections have been studied in the brain of the dragonfly (56). The frontal ganglion of *Periplaneta americana* contains approximately 60–80 neurons and five groups of fibers can be distinguished (320). The neurons in the metathoracic ganglion of the locust, *Schistocerca gregaria*, and the grasshopper, *Romalea microptera*, exhibit large cell bodies (143). Individual visual cells of the bee, *Apis mellifera* were identified by Sommer and Wehner (300). The large and medium size ocellar afferent neurons within the brain of the locust, *Schistocerca gregaria*, terminate in the brain and their cell bodies are located in the protocerebrum (111). The retina of the male scale insect, *Ericoccus* sp., a homopteran, exhibits no microvilli but shows membrane stacks with an analogous configuration to the stacked plates of vertebrate cones (78). Three different cell stages could be distinguished in the paramedian neurosecretory cells in the subesophageal ganglion of the cricket, *Teleogryllus commodus* (81). Ovariectomy increases the neurosecretory secretion into the cerebral neurohemal organ (135a). Neurons and fiber tracts in the frontal ganglion of *Periplaneta americana* are directly connected with different regions of the CNS and with more caudal regions of the stomodeal nervous system (121). The ultrastructure of stimu-

lated and nonstimulated mechanoreceptors in the taste hair of the blowfly, *Phaenicia serricata*, was compared (200), and the auditory responsiveness in the large fibers of the ventral nerve cord of the cricket, *Acheta domesticus*, and the cockroach, *Periplaneta americana*, investigated (135a).

The neoplasms of the nervous system can be divided into those deriving from precursors of neurons (because cell consistency of the neurons in mammals such as man and other groups) and those deriving from glial elements. Specific experimental studies using invertebrates as models remain scarce and histologically superficial but it should be kept in mind that, for example, the nervous cell of the coelenterate *Hydra* sp. shows high regeneration capacity and that recent studies of insects added important details. The invertebrates between these two extremes of specializations may contribute to a new understanding of basic problems in comparative oncology. The following details may help to stimulate new research. (See also Chapter 6 for other developmental questions.)

Different morphologic types of antennal hair sensilla can be distinguished in *Periplaneta americana* which change according to postembryonic development and in relation to sex (wall structure, number of sensory cells). In the adult male, approximately 54% of the antennal sensilla are long, single walled, and composed of four sensory cells. Half of this number are newly formed by imaginal ecdysis, the other half derives from shorter sensilla of the nymph. These short type SW B sensilla are present in all larval stages of both sexes and in adult females. The number of sensory fibers exhibits an increase from 14,000 in the first larval instar to about 270,000 in the adult male. Approximately 90% of this increase takes place in the last developmental stage (275).

In comparison to the aforementioned exhibit, in the filiform hairs on the cerci of *Gryllus bimaculatus* which are mechanoreceptors, there are six stages of development during the last larval stage. The cytoplasm of the sense cells points to an intensive protein synthesis of cell metabolism and intercytoplasmic material exchange via glial imagination (109). The ultrastructure of the compound eye of the haploid male and diploid female beetle, *Xyleborus ferrugineus*, shows sex differences, such as number of facets (19–33 facets in the male, 70–100 in the female) to the distribution of rhabdomeric microvilli (59, 60). See also Duelli (78) concerning an insect retina without microvilli.

The glial cells of the photoreceptor of the

retina of the drone, *Apis mellifera*, seem to participate in the regulation of K⁺ activity and stimulate cellular metabolism (318).

The neural sheath in the brain of the midge, *Chironomus riparius*, is composed of neural lamella and an underlying perineurium, exhibiting two cell types. The cortical layer beneath presents cell bodies of neurons and glial cells and ensheathes the centrally located neuropiles. Three types of glia cells, five types of neurons, and four types of axons have been observed (274).

22. Phylum Phoronida. In Phoronida, nerve cells are interepithelial and a true nerve net is present; connection of neurons is unknown; three types of nerve cells occur: (a) large, unipolar cytoplasmic rich cells which are most abundant; (b) bipolar cells with horizontal processes; and (c) a third type varies from the second but is otherwise similar. No sense organs but sensory epithelia occur; sense cells are bipolar with short bristle; giant fibers are present. In the nervous system of the body wall, four types of nerve cells exist: vertically bipolar sense cells, large unipolar ones with short axons, large horizontal bipolar cells, and motor neurons.

23. Phylum Ectoprocta. A nerve net is present in Ectoprocta comparable to *Hydra*; multipolar neurons occur (tentacle sheath and body wall); sense organs are simple unicellular receptors. The histology of the brain is typical for small lower order invertebrates. In the cerebral ganglia, the neurons are unspecialized bipolar. Few or no glia occur apart from the vesicle wall of flat cells.

24. Phylum Brachiopoda. It is questionable whether ganglion cells are unipolar, bipolar, or both. The ganglion cells in the periphery are generally multipolar and isopolar. Giant nerve cells occur in the subesophageal ganglion of *Lingula*. Statocyst is the only sensory organ. Certain similarities exist between the setae of brachiopods and polychaetes (122).

25. Phylum Echinodermata. The neurons in Echinodermata are small (3–12 μm); the disoriented internuncial plexus is extensive. The ectoneural nervous system exhibits sensory cells and basiepithelial, internuncially degenerating neurons. The sensory cells and the basiepithelia plexus form the ectoneural system: (a) the superficial plexus—multipolar neurons (12 μm in diameter), with very short processes (20–30 μm). Bipolar cells occur only rarely; (b) the fiber layer of plexus—product of bipolar neurons, 6–12 μm in length. Fibers especially well developed at the tube feet; (c) the radial cord and nerve ring—it is the CNS of echinoderms. Multipolar and bi-

polar ganglion cells are 6–20 μm in size. Only one type of glia tissue and no real sheath of cords are found. Thyponeural system includes motor nerve, and hyponeural centrally connected neural fibers. The peripheral motor system includes nerve processes of bipolar neurons in the echinoid spine. Hyponeural motor systems include unipolar neurons in clusters of 20. They are about 12 μm long and are the primary distribution neurons for the tube feet; others are unipolar or bipolar. The ribbon axons, known for asteroids and holothuroideae but not described for echinoids, ophiuroids, and crinoids, are flat, ribbon-like widenings of the axon at their final end (synapsis). Unicellular sensory cells are generally bipolar, sometimes multipolar. Unipolar cells have not been found in the sensory system. Common to all echinoderms are: neuron size and form, patterns of fiber association and the mode of excitation and circuiting. The aganglionic nervous system has medullary strains which are unsheathed. Their fibers are very fine (approximately 0.1 μm); the plexus is basiepithelial; the sensory cells are bipolar and spindle-shaped (cell body 2–5 μm).

Sensory cells are spindle-shaped and bipolar in asteroidea, 6–10 μm in length and 1.5 μm in diameter. For further details of ophiuroidea, echinoidea, holothuroidea, and crinoidea, see Bullock and Horridge (47).

26. Phylum Chaetognatha. The neurons in Chaetognatha are uniform and unspecialized. Sense organs consist of eyes exhibiting retinula cells and bristle receptors. Ciliary loop and retrocerebral organ are only scarcely known.

27. Phylum Pogonophora. Neurons are multipolar and unipolar with ample cytoplasm and large nucleus in Pogonophora. Bipolar sense cells exhibit elongated nuclei.

28. Phylum Hemichordata. Neurons are giant unipolar cells similar to Mauthner and Müller neurons in lower vertebrates. In addition, though less frequently, multipolar and bipolar cells are found. The preoral ciliary organ is the only sense organ. Sensory neurons, bipolar sense cells occur; the preoral ciliary organ of Brumbell and Cole is a receptor organ; sensory nerve cells are found.

29. Phylum Cephalochordata. A nerve net is present in cephalochordata.

30. Phylum Tunicata. The cord in the class larvaceae and the larvae of metamorphosis groups is homolog to the neural tube in invertebrates. The cerebral ganglion of ascidians and thaliaceans is a typical invertebrate ganglion, with cells mainly unipolar, generally characteristic in invertebrates. Bipolar and multipolar cells occur; glial nuclei are present. It is reported that the dorsal cord of appendicularians exhibits eutely. Regeneration of the dorsal strand may give rise to a new excretory canal, normal gland, and cerebral ganglion (39). Receptors are eyes, statocysts, specialized epidermal, and unicellular structures; simple and multicellular layers occur.

31. Phylum Vertebrata. Vertebrate histology is reviewed by Patt and Patt (234) and several excellent textbooks exist concerning the histology of man. Therefore only a few recent publications may be mentioned. Additionally, most scientists in the field of comparative oncology are well aware of the histology of vertebrate models.

Cell invariability of neurons of vertebrates brings some restriction to the development of neoplasms deriving from those cells. Some studies may be of interest, such as concerning the brain of *Lampetra planeri* (337); olfactory epithelium in the goldfish, *Carassius auratus* (146); taste buds in *Xiphophorus helleri* (258); photoreceptors of the cave salamander (29); taste buds of anurans (268); the subcommissural organ of *Rana esculenta* (135); the hypothalamus and infundibulum of the squirrel monkey (23); neuronal cell bodies of rat dorsal root ganglion (76); mechanoreceptors in the raccoon, *Procyon lotor* (134); ventricles of the female armadillo (149); endoneural mast cells of peripheral nerves in the armadillo (53); and the structure of brain neurons due to swelling in man and other mammals (180).

Structures Dealing with Motion

The structures of motion can be divided into active and passive ones. The most significant ones are the different types of musculature; but also specific structures such as the comb plates of ctenophorans occur.

Passive structures in form of exo- or endoskeletons are present only in the species of certain phyla. Exo- and endoskeletons may occur side by side. These passive structures are either tissues such as cartilage and bone or secretion products such as the endoskeletons of sponges, or exoskeletons of arthropods.

Active structures of motion are myoepithelial musculature, type A, and ciliated comb plates in **2. Phylum Ctenophora**; myoepithelial musculature, type A, in **6. Phylum Entoprocta**; smooth musculature (possibly oblique striated musculature) in **3. Phylum Platyhelminthes, 5. Phylum Gnathostomulida, 7. Phylum Acanthocephala, 9. Phylum Gastrotricha, 10. Phylum Kinorhyncha,**

22. Phylum Phoronida; smooth musculature in **4. Phylum Nemertinea, 12. Phylum Nematomorpha**, and **15. Phylum Sipunculida**; oblique striated musculature (smooth musculature?) in **11. Phylum Nematoda**; oblique striated musculature (?) in **16. Phylum Echiurida** and **19. Phylum Pentastomida**; smooth, partly striated musculature in **13. Phylum Priapulida**. Striated musculature with thick and thin myofilaments comparable to flight muscles in insects occurs in *Sagitta elegans* and *Sagitta setosa* (213, 345) of **26. Phylum Chaetognatha**. The muscles are myomesothelial in type in *Siboglinum fiordicum* (**27. Phylum Pogonophora**) and exhibit thick and thin filaments in both the body wall and the vessels. The passive support in these phyla is generally given by internal body pressure.

Active and passive structures of motion are found in the remaining phyla. In the Porifera active cells are the choanocytes and myocytes. The endoskeleton is composed of spicules, or organic fibers. In only a few forms is a skeleton missing. In the Cnidaria, as the first eumetazoan phylum, myoepithelial musculature type A is present. The fine structure of the neuromuscular system is known from *Polyorchis penicillatus* (292) and striated musculature has been reported from anthomedusa (280). As endoskeleton exists the mesoglea and the secreted epidermal exoskeleton as in anthozoans. In **8. Phylum Rotifera** the active structures are represented by smooth and striated musculature as well as the ciliated wheel organ (corona). The trophi of the jaws can be considered as endoskeletons. The **14. Phylum Mollusca** exhibits smooth or striated musculature (penis retractor muscle of *Helix pomatia* (336); heart musculature of cuttlefish, *Rossia macrosoma* (155)). Exoskeletons appear in form of shells. Endoskeletons as shells are rare but cartilage is found as radular support or in the form of the head cartilage in squid which is an equivalent to hyaline vertebrate cartilage. The musculature in **17. Phylum Annelida** is smooth or oblique striated and cartilaginous skeletons are known (176). **18. Phylum Onychophora** has striated musculature (?) and the cuticle can be seen as a type of exoskeleton. The musculature in *Macrobiotus hufelandi* and *Milnesium tardigradum* (**20. Phylum Tardigrada**) exhibits a particular type which may be best considered as a variation of oblique striated musculature (338). A cuticle is present.

The musculature in the **21. Phylum Arthropoda** is striated. The general type is cross-striated but cardiac musculature type A is found in such decapod crustaceans as *Homarus* sp. (298). The proximal accessory flexor of the myochordotonal organ in the meropodite of crayfish walking legs exhibits thick and thin muscle fibers (89). For crustacean muscle, see Castel and Papir (54) and Zacharova and Uhrik (358) and for crustacean stomach muscle, see Jahromi and Govind (150). A method for the preparation of enriched cultures of *Drosophila* myoblasts (28) may spur new research in comparative oncology; see Reinecke and Walther (257) concerning the turnover and biogenesis of synaptic vesicles at locust neuromuscular junctions.

Smooth, possibly oblique striated musculature and zooecia as passive structures exist in **23. Phylum Ectoprocta**. Also in the **24. Phylum Brachiopoda** the musculature is smooth, perhaps oblique striated and the mantle epithelium secretes the shells. **Echinodermata (25. Phylum)** have smooth musculature and tube feet of the water vascular system and as endoskeletons calcit plates. The muscles in *Asterias rubens* are fixed to the skeleton by tendinous loops which run around the skeletal beamlets. The tendons arise from a basement membrane enveloping the terminal processes of the muscle cell and are composed of tender parallel filaments (322).

The determination of the musculature of the **28. Phylum Hemichordata** seems questionable and the passive structure is the notochord (234, 343). **Phylum 29. Tunicata** exhibits striated and smooth musculature (55). The notochord appears at least in a certain period of development. **30. Phylum Cephalochordata** shows striated and smooth musculature as well as notochord and cartilage-like reinforcements as thin rays. In **Phylum 31. Vertebrata** different types of musculature such as striated musculature (115, 124), smooth musculature (52, 99), cardiac musculature, type B, and myocpithelial musculature, type C (basket cells), occur as active structures (see also 10, 27, 41, 173, 177, 354). Certain types of connective tissue *per se*, the notochord or its remnants, and adipose tissue, cartilage, and bone are the passive structures.

The characterization of invertebrate musculature and connective tissues is due to the historic development of light and electron microscopy as well as the number of investigated species, sometimes not clearly definable. This also holds true for some aspects of the system of body fluids to be described next.

Systems of Body Fluids

The **Phyla 0-3 and 5-12** (Porifera, Cnidaria, Ctenophora, Platyhelminthes, Gnathostomulida, Entoprocta, Acanthocephala, Rotifera, Gastro-

tricha, Kinorhyncha, Nematoda, and Nematomorpha) have no circulatory system. A closed circulatory system with vessels exhibiting an endothelium, blood corpuscles, and amebocytes occurs in **4. Phylum Nemertinea**; and an open circulatory system with round cells occurs in the **13. Phylum Priapulida**.

Generally an open circulatory system occurs in **14. Phylum Mollusca**; in pulmonates and cephalopods there is a mixed circulatory system. Blood cells vary in the species. Pericard shows simple cuboidal epithelium. The amebocyte is the only floating cell type in pulmonates. Pore cells in the freshwater snails, *Biomphalaria glabrata* and *Planorbarius corneus*, produce hemoglobin (296), whereas interstitial cells in the body wall of the gastropod, *Limax* sp., synthesize hemocyanin by merocrine secretion. The hemocyanin secretion in the merostome arthropod, *Limulus polyphemus*, in contrast is performed by holocrine secretion (256). Hemocyanin synthesis in the cephalopod *Octopus* seems to occur in cells of the branchial gland (72). The fine structure of cephalopod blood vessels reveals two main types in retina and arms of *Octopus* and the lip of *Sepia*. One type of vessel exhibits complete basement membrane, incomplete endothelial lining, and complete envelope of pericytes. In the second type, myofilaments are scarce and the endothelium more simple (21).

The fibroblast differentiation of amebocytes in molluscs such as the common snail *Lymnea stagnalis* exhibits several phases (271). In **15. Phylum Sipunculida** the circulatory system is open, the coelom acts respectively. The coelomic lining is composed of flat, granular ciliated chloragogue cells and fixed urns occur. In the body fluid red corpuscles, hyaline amebocytes, granulocytes, floating urns, and multinucleated cells are present.

The simple circulatory system in **16. Phylum Echiurida** is the closed type; the coelomic cavity exists also. Phagocytic amebocytes appear in the circulatory system and erythrocytes and leukocytes in the coelomic cavity. **17. Phylum Annelida** have a closed circulatory system. A portion of the main vessel may act as a heart (151). In some species, the vessels are without endothelium, but with endothelium similar to vertebrates in leeches, such as *Hirudo medicinalis* (125-127). The coelomocytes of the earthworm *Lumbricus terrestris* permit the distinction of four to five subtypes: basophils, acidophils, neutrophils, granulocytes, and chloragogen cells. It has not been decided whether these are distinct subtypes, if developmental stages may be included, or if all subtypes are developmental stages of one type of coelomocytes (34, 191, 302, 316).

In **18. Phylum Onychophora**, an open circulatory system is present and the amebocytes occur as free cells. The fluid-filled remnant of the body cavity in **19. Phylum Pentastomida** contains floating cells. No circulatory system exists in **20. Phylum Tardigrada**.

The circulatory system of **21. Phylum Arthropoda** is open with different cell types. The blood is also known as hemolymph. The body fluid of *Limulus* (merostomata) contains only one type of blood cell.

Arachnida. Different blood cells in spiders are produced in the circular musculature of the heart, but in scorpions in lymphocytic organs.

Crustacea. Phylogenetically the first appearance of the cardiac musculature, type A, takes place in crustacea (298). This type of cardiac musculature appears similar to vertebrate cardiac musculature if observed with the light microscope but the electron microscope reveals differences, for example concerning innervation. Hemocytes of the blue crab, *Callinectes sapidus*, exhibit three subtypes: hyaline cells, intermediate cells, and granulocytes, which seem to be different stages of the cytogenetic process. The functional complexity is expressed by the cytoplasmic occurrence of three to four types of inclusion bodies, other membrane-bound compartments, such as lysosome-like structures, autophagic vacuoles, and peroxisome-like bodies (32).

Insecta. The open circulatory system contains hemocytes. One basic type of hemocyte occurs in six developmental or functional stages: prohemocytes, blasmotocytes, granular cells, spherule cells, cystocytes, and oenocytoids. Intermediate stages are also present in the fly *Calliphora* sp. An additional type was observed: thrombocytoid (easy fragmentation as in mammalian platelets). Special conditions occur in larvae. The heart lacks endocardial epithelium. An external layer of connective tissue is present, but no special pacemaker tissue.

A well-developed closed circulatory system with nucleated blood corpuscles exists in **22. Phylum Phoronida**. No circulatory system but a comparable action of the coelomic fluid with ameboid cells is found in **23. Phylum Ectoprocta**. In **Phylum 24. Brachiopoda** an open circulatory system occurs—no blood cells or corpuscles, but sometimes coelomocytes have been observed. **25. Phylum Echinodermata** have open systems of body fluids with coelomocytes; the hemal system exists with different types of amebocytes. The wall of the dorsal hemal vessel of the sea cucumber, *Parastichopus tremulus*, is composed from the inside to the outside of an inner connective tissue layer, a medial circular muscle layer, and an outer flagellated epithelium (152).

26. Phylum Chaetognatha are provided with an open circulatory system, not well known. The movement of body fluids is performed by ciliated cells. The circulatory system is closed in **27. Phylum Pogonophora**; and an open circulatory system, with floating cells and vessel endothelium in **28. Phylum Hemichordata. 29. Phylum Tunicata** exhibits an open circulatory system. The heart is provided with pacemakers on both ends; no respiratory pigment occurs but there are several types of blood cells. **30. Phylum Cephalochordata** have a closed circulatory system comparable to other lower chordates; no respiratory pigment has been detected. **31. Phylum Vertebrata** are characterized by a closed circulatory system.

Interstitial Tissue Structures (61, 197, 263)

Interstitial tissue structures in sponges and eumetazoans comprise for oncology a very important tissue group, details of which deserve additional investigations. Interstitial tissues are the origin of such significant diseases as sarcomas and leukemias. One of the first questions is whether the origin is one of the mesenchymal stem cell, or perhaps stem cells, with a varying value in different phyla. This variability is given through the differing capability in the production of precursor tissues. The mesenchymatic stem cell of coelenterates is able to produce nerve cells, which are not cell invariable, as well as nematocytes. The equivalent cell of platyhelminth worm parenchyma is comparable to loose connective tissues in vertebrates, molluscs, annelid worms, and arthropod cartilage. The stem cell of vertebrates is able to produce bone as the highest type of connective tissue. Some parallel may exist to the phylogeny of glia as envisaged in lower invertebrates on one side and perhaps annelids but surely higher arthropods and higher molluscs on the other; some intermediaries between glia and connective tissue can be assumed.

There exist certain variations but the most important one among the different phyla is the fact that the number of subgroups of connective and related tissues increased phylogenetically. Main characteristics, such as the presence of collagenous fibers or reticular fibers, conditions of the matrix, and the cell types can be generalized. Additionally, a wide comparison to the plant parenchymata is possible.

Mesenchyme with ameboid cells, such as collencytes, scleroblasts, spongioblasts, archeocytes, and gland cells, is found in the phylum **O. Porifera**. Six species of marine sponges exhibited remarkable variations of the connective tissue elements, especially with regard to the fibers (63). A mesenchymal stem cell in *Hydra* (33, 66, 193) and a nearly acellular mesoglea can be mentioned in the hydrozoa of **1. Phylum Cnidaria**. The cells with fluid-filled vacuoles and fibers are distinguishable in several species. The axial skeleton of *Veritillum cynomorium* is composed of a fibrillar collagenous matrix with calcifications (187). In the polyps of *Cordylophora* anchoring cells exist, known as desmocytes (194). The synthesis of collagen in relation to the mesogleal organization was studied in the sea anemone, *Aiptasia diaphana* (290). A mesoglea with connective tissue comparable to cartilage has been observed in the **Phylum Ctenophora**.

The parenchyma in the **3. Phylum Platyhelminthes** is comparable to loose connective tissue with reticulated fibers in vertebrates. Free ameboid cells with fluid-filled vacuoles are present in turbellarians. The character of the connective tissue can be called syncytial. The connective tissue of the polyclad turbellarian, *Discocelides langi* exhibits large amounts of ground substance. The filaments are considered collagenous (237). **4. Phylum Nemertinea** are the second group of the acoelomate animals, the body of which is also filled with mesenchyme (parenchyme). But they are also the phylogenetic first group of animals with a closed circulatory system. The direction of this development can be compared to the trend in vascular plants; recalling the relationship of plant parenchymata, phloem, and xylem development. Free cell types, filaments of collagenic character and ground substance, can be distinguished in the parenchyma in *Amphiporus pulcher*, *Lineus bilineatus*, and *Lineus ruber* (238).

In **5. Phylum Gnathostomulida** the parenchyma is scanty, and mesenchyme occurs in **6. Phylum Entoprocta**. In **7. Phylum Acanthocephala** the ligament sac, ligaments, and subepidermal connective tissue are present, and in the **8. Phylum Rotifera** a syncytial type of mesenchyme is present. The conditions are similar in **9. Phylum Gastrotricha** and **10. Phylum Kinorhyncha**. In **11. Phylum Nematoda**, mesenchyme cells are present. The formation of collagen in *Panagrellus silusiae* during postembryonic development is discontinuous. The collagen produced during a peak period is later lost, but collagen material synthesized during nonpeak periods is retained (190). The cuticle of nematodes contains collagen (222). Mesenchyme occurs in **12. Phylum Nematomorpha**. In the case of **13. Phylum Priapulida** fluid-containing amebocytes should be mentioned with reservation. New studies are urgently needed for this phylum.

14. Phylum Mollusca. The molluscs show a wide variation of connective tissue types. Supportive structures are associated with the radula of *Limax maximus* (collostyle). These structures are macroscopically but not microscopically similar to vertebrate cartilage. The capsule is composed of connective tissue. The closest relationship may be to vertebrate mucoid connective tissue. The subesophageal ganglion of *Helix aspersa* has an epidermal connective tissue sheath (264). Fibroblasts seem to be precursors of amebocytes in *Lymnea stagnalis* (271). Pore cells in connective tissue of the kidney of *Achatina achatina* and *Arion hortensis* produced hemocyanin in the second species (293, 294). Aragonite crystals surrounded by organic matter occur in crystal sheath from bivalve hinge ligaments (195). For the byssal apparatus, see Bairati and Vitellaro-Zuccarello (18, 19) and Ottosen (230). The structure is here included because of the "fiber" production.

Ligament can be compared to the shell of the mollusc as well as vertebrate dental enamel. The cutis in cephalopods is of mesodermal origin, mesenchyme occurs, and cartilage surrounding the central nervous system, known as head cartilage in cephalopods, is characterized by branching cells.

In **15. Phylum Sipunculida** and **16. Phylum Echiurida**, subepidermal connective tissue is present. In **17. Phylum Annelida** subepidermal connective tissue occurs but not in all species. In leeches mesenchymatic connective tissue narrows the coelom (69). Tentacular cartilage is found in polychaetes, such as *Sabella penicillum* (176). *Nereis* cuticle collagen is resistant to proteolysis by bacterial collagenase (165, 166). In **18. Phylum Onychophora** there exists a dermis of connective tissue. New studies are necessary for **19. Phylum Pentastomida**. With regard to **20. Phylum Tardigrada**, the conditions in the heterotardigrad, *Echiniscoides sigismundi*, may serve as an example (118). The large **21. Phylum Arthropoda** has been thoroughly investigated and conditions have been found to be quite complicated (113). The thick layer of connective tissue surrounding the mesenteron of *Periplaneta americana* exhibits many collagen fibrils, elastic fibers, fibroblasts, and a small number of hemocytes (97). Especially large forms of arthropods such as *Limulus polyphemus* and others contain cartilage. Finally, the fat body in insects, either of larval stages (261) or of adult animals, is of interest. The direct comparability to mammalian fat tissue is improper (100, 356). As an example for the three lophophorate phyla, **22. Phylum Phoronida, 23. Phylum Ectoprocta**, and **24. Phylum Brachiopoda**, the connective tissue of the articulate brachiopod, *Terebratalia transversa*, has been selected. The tentacles contain an acellular connective tissue cylinder of collagen fibrils and amorphous ground substance (255). The **25. Phylum Echinodermata** exhibits mesenchymal cells producing skeletal elements. The inner structures of the echinoid, *Sphaerechinus granularis*, contain (with regard to the axial complex) a connective tissue matrix (15). New studies are needed for **26. Phylum Chaetognatha** and **27. Phylum Pogonophora**. In **28. Phylum Hemichordata**, the notochord and connective tissue of the body wall are present. The stomochord is enveloped by a basement lamina and connective tissue fibers; the question of whether stomochord and notochord are homologous is still open. The investigated species are the enteropneusts, *Harrimania kupfferi* and *Ptychodera flava* (343). A notochord appears at least at one stage of development in the members of **29. Phylum Tunicata**. Additionally, connective tissue is present (95). **30. Phylum Cephalochordata** exhibits notochord and cartilage-like supporting structures. **31. Phylum Vertebrata** shows the largest number of connective tissue specializations. A review of the phylogenetic peak of this development is provided in Chapters 2 and 43. Some details are of interest. In elastic ligaments, the longitudinally elastic fibers are surrounded separately by a layer of spirally oriented collagen fibrils with a thin layer of microfibrils between (285). Adipose tissue appears also functionally nearly incomparable to this one of arthropods in two versions, the white and brown adipose tissue, as in the rodent *Citellus lateralis* (120) and other hibernators. The variations of the cells of body fluids known as the hematogenic system, deriving in vertebrates from reticular connective tissue precursors, but from several sources in invertebrates, is comparable to this questionable comparability of fat tissues. In contrast, cartilage exhibits a relative uniform character in all phyla where present. Certain peculiarities are found in vertebrates themselves. Cartilage is the supporting tissue of the adult agnatha, and remains in decreasing frequency in adult skeletons of amphibians, reptiles, mammals, and birds. With the presence of elastic fibers, cartilage takes part in the formation of such body portions as the eustachian tube in reptiles, birds, and mammals and also in the external ear, the epiglottis, and tracheal rings in certain mammalian species. Calcified cartilage is an end tissue in some species of chondrichthyes (234), whereas it is pathologic in mammals. The characteristic and highest supporting tissue of vertebrates is bone, which composes the adult skeleton in man. In other vertebrates this tissue appears in other body locations also: the armored plates in fossil fishes and reptiles; the adlacrimal bone in the upper eyelid of alligators, sclerotic plates around the cornea in certain reptiles and birds, the epipubic bone in monotremes and marsupials, in the gizzard of one species of dove, the bone in the tongue of one bat species, the rostral bone in the snout of the pig, and in the penis as the penis bone of several insectivores, bats, rodents, carnivores, whales, and nonhuman primates. In rodents and other otters, bone occurs as the os clitoris. Bone is also found in ungulates as the skeleton of the heart (162a).

Structures with Functional Peculiarities and Specific Characteristics

To these group of cells or tissues belong structures with very limited distribution and no particular interest for comparative oncology. An exception could be seen in the nettle cells of the first phylum **Cnidaria** because they are the highest developed cells in the animal kingdom (49, 309). The colloblasts of **2. Phylum Ctenophora**, the light and electricity producing cells as they occur in arthropods and fishes, or the alarm substance cells in fishes such as *Phoxinus phoxinus*, are other examples.

DISTRIBUTION OF TRUE REAL TISSUES AMONG ORGANISMS: A PRELIMINARY CONDITION OF NEOPLASTIC GROWTH

The general tissue distribution in the phyla is given as follows. This is not to be considered a complete survey but the main general appearances are given. Note that Sections 48 and 49 dealing with the nervous systems show a slight variation between Chapters 3 and 43 due to a varying discussion of the topics.

1. Simple Squamous Epithelium. This type of epithelium occurs in the integument of: porifera, cnidaria, ctenophora, platyhelminthes, mollusca, tardigrada, arthropoda, chaetognatha, and tunicata; as digestive epithelium in ctenophora and arthropoda; as respiratory epithelium in mollusca, arthropoda, and vertebrata; as excretory epithelium in vertebrata and in the circulatory channels of nemertinea.

2. Stratified Squamous Epithelium. With the exception of the rostral integumentary region of chaetognatha is this type of epithelium restricted to vertebrata where it occurs as integument, as lining of the digestive and excretory tract and in the genital and sensory systems.

3. Simple Cuboidal Epithelium. Cuboidal epithelium has a wide distribution in invertebrates and vertebrates alike. It comprises the integument of cnidaria, ctenophora, platyhelminthes, entoprocta, nematomorpha, mollusca, sipunculida, arthropoda, brachiopoda, echinodermata, chaetognatha, hemichordata, tunicata, cephalochordata; digestive epithelia in entoprocta, gastrotricha, kinorhyncha, nematoda, mollusca, pentastomida, arthropoda, phoronida, echinodermata, chaetognatha, and vertebrata. Structures of gaseous exchange are lined by this type of epithelium in mollusca, echinodermata, hemichordata, and vertebrata; those of excretion in platyhelminthes, arthropoda and vertebrata; structures of propagation and sensitivity in vertebrata and those of circulation in mollusca.

4. Simple Columnar Epithelium. Columnar epithelium is especially widely distributed in the form of integuments and lining membranes of digestive structures. It is found in the integuments of cnidaria, ctenophora, platyhelminthes, nemertinea, entoprocta, nematomorpha, priapulida, mollusca, sipunculida, annelida, pentastomida, arthropoda, phoronida, brachiopoda, echinodermata, chaetognatha, and pogonophora. Digestive linings of this epithelium occur in cnidaria, platyhelminthes, nemertinea, entoprocta, gastrotricha, kinorhyncha, nematoda, priapulida, mollusca, sipunculida, annelida, pentastomida, tardigrada, arthropoda, phoronida, ectoprocta, brachiopoda, echinodermata, chaetognatha, hemichordata, tunicata, cephalochordata, and vertebrata. Structures of gaseous exchange exhibiting this type of epithelium occur only in hemichordata and vertebrata; those of propagation and sensitivity only in vertebrata.

5. Pseudostratified Columnar Epithelium. This is present in digestive structures of brachiopoda and vertebrata. It is also found in lining dealing with gaseous exchange, excretion and propagation of vertebrata.

6. Stratified Cuboidal Epithelium. It is only present in integuments, digestive, excretory structures and propagation and sensitivity linings of vertebrata.

7. Stratified Columnar Epithelium. This occurs only in the integuments, the digestive tract and structures of gaseous exchange and propagation of vertebrata.

8. Transitional Epithelium. It is only found in the structures of excretion and propagation of vertebrata.

9. Exocrine Appendage Glands of Skin (I), Sebaceous and Sweat Glands. These structures are found only in the vertebrate class mammalia.

10. Epithelia of Exocrine Glands (II), Mammary Gland. Again, the epithelia of this glandular type exist only in the vertebrate class of mammalia.

11. Epithelia of Exocrine Glands (III), Salivary Glands. Epithelia of salivary glands have been found in rotifera, gastrotricha, kinorhyncha, nematoda, mollusca, annelida, onychophora, tardigrada, arthropoda, and vertebrata.

12. Epithelia of Exocrine Glands (IV), Liver. Epithelia of this type and function are present in mollusca, arthropoda, echinodermata, tunicata, cephalochordata, and vertebrata.

13. Exocrine Glands (V), Exocrine Portion of Pancreas (Hepatopancreas). Exocrine pancreatic tissue is found in the three phyla of mollusca, arthropoda, and vertebrata.

14. Epithelia of Endocrine Glands (I), Islets of Langerhans. Islets of Langerhans are present only in vertebrata.

15. Epithelia of Endocrine Glands (II), Pineal Gland. These are found only in vertebrata. The same holds true for 16–20.

16. Epithelia of Endocrine Glands (III), Pituitary Gland.

17. Epithelia of Endocrine Glands (IV), Thyroid Gland.

18. Epithelia of Endocrine Glands (V), Parathyroid Gland and Ultimobranchial Gland, respectively.

19 and 20. Epithelia of Endocrine Glands (VI, VII), Adrenal Cortex, and Medulla (Inter-renal and Chromaffin Tissues).

21. Germinal Epithelium and Organ-related Structures (VIII), Testis. All phyla exhibit those, but there occur differences in hormonal influence.

22. Germinal Epithelium and Organ-related Structures (IX), Ovary. They are also found in all phyla, but exhibit differences in hormonal influence in the different phyla.

23. Endocrine Glands of Invertebrata. These are present in mollusca, annelida, arthropoda.

24. Neurohemal Organs of Invertebrata.

25. Desmal Epithelium of Serous Membranes (Coelomic Epithelium) and Pseudoepithelia of

Vessels. These are found in nemertinea, priapulida, mollusca, sipunculida, echiurida, annelida, onychophora, pentastomida, tardigrada, arthropoda, phoronida, ectoprocta, brachiopoda, echinodermata, chaetognatha, pogonophora, hemichordata, tunicata, cephalochordata, and vertebrata.

26. Desmal Epithelia (Synovial Origin). These occur only in vertebrata.

27. Connective Tissue (Rich in Cells—1. Mesenchyme). This is represented in porifera, cnidaria, ctenophora, entoprocta, nematoda, mollusca, onychophora, arthropoda, brachiopoda, echinodermata, chaetognatha, and vertebrata.

28. Connective Tissue (Rich in Cells—2. Spinocellular Connective Tissue). This occurs only in vertebrata.

29. Connective Tissue (Rich in Cells—3. Reticular Connective Tissue). This is exhibited with regard to support and motion in vertebrata only; with regard to body fluids in nemertinea, priapulida, mollusca, sipunculida, echiurida, annelida, onychophora, pentastomida, arthropoda, phoronida, echinodermata, pogonophora, hemichordata, tunicata, and vertebrata (cephalochordata?).

30. Connective Tissue (Rich in Fibers—1. Gelatinous Connective Tissue). This occurs only in vertebrata.

31. Connective Tissue (Rich in Fibers—2. Loose Connective Tissue). This is found in members of all animal (eumetazoan) phyla from porifera and cnidaria to vertebrata.

32. Connective Tissue (Rich in Fibers—3. Fibrous (Fibrillar) Connective Tissue). With regard to support and motion, the main function of connective tissues, it is found in echinodermata and vertebrata.

33. Melanocytes (Melanogenic System). It is the characteristic of the cells of this system to contain or produce the pigment melanin and its relatives, either intra- or extracellular. With regard to animals, these cells have been found in the integuments of mollusca, arthropoda (also extracellular), and vertebrata; from digestive structures of mollusca; and from sensitivity structures of vertebrata. But they are also seen in the plectenchymata of fungi and in fully differentiated tissues of vascular plants (601). The system occurs therefore in plants and animals alike (see also Chapter 28 by Lima-de-Faria and Table 38.1 in the chapter by Giordano et al.).

34. Adipose Tissues. They are present regarding support and motion mainly in arthropoda (also important for hormone production) and vertebrata in the form of white and brown adipose tissues.

35. Chordal Tissue. This is present in the chordate phyla, hemichordata, tunicata, cephalochordata, and vertebrata.

36. Chondroid Tissue. This is a supporting tissue, present only in vertebrates.

37. Cartilage. This occurs in mollusca, annelida, arthropoda, and vertebrata.

38. Bone. Bone occurs in integuments of vertebrata, in propagative structures of vertebrata (penis bone in ruminants and carnivores), as supporting endoskeleton, and in the heart of certain large mammals (skeleton of heart).

39. Osteoid Tissue. Osteoid tissue is a type of supporting tissue found in certain fish species (Carangidae), but has no implication for man. Malignant neoplasms are not known in this tissue but a condition called pachyostosis has been described.

40. Myoepithelial Musculature. This is exhibited by cnidaria, ctenophora, and entoprocta (type A),[1] ectoprocta (type B), and vertebrata (basket cells in mammals/salivary glands and mammae/or type C).

41. Smooth Musculature. This is found in porifera, platyhelminthes, nemertinea, gnathostomulida, entoprocta, acanthocephala, rotifera, gastrotricha, kinorhyncha, nematoda, nematomorpha, priapulida, mollusca, sipunculida, annelida, echinodermata, hemichordata, tunicata, cephalochordata, and vertebrata. The musculature of many invertebrates considered to be smooth in type may proof to be oblique striated if investigated according to its ultrastructure.

42. Oblique Striated Musculature. This is found in plathyhelminthes, gnathostomulida, acanthocephala, gastrotricha, kinorhyncha, nematoda, and annelida.

43. Transverse Striated or Skeletal Musculature. This is present in rotifera, mollusca, arthropoda, pogonophora, hemichordata, tunicata, cephalochordata, and vertebrata.

44. Cardiac Musculature. This occurs in two types: arthropoda and vertebrata.

45. Neurons of the Central Nervous System. Neurons, as found in mollusca, annelida, arthropoda, and vertebrata, are unipolar in annelida, brachiopoda, tunicata; they are bipolar in ectoprocta, brachiopoda, and echinodermata, and multipolar in sipunculida, annelida and echinodermata, and of the giant type of sipunculida, to give only these few examples.

46. Different Types of Neurons in the Peripheral Nervous System. Unipolar neurons occur in

---

[1] The subtypes A, B, and C have been established to designate the big gaps with regard to phylogenetic appearance.

ctenophora, platyhelminthes, nemertinea, acanthocephala, rotifera, nematoda, nematomorpha, tardigrada, arthropoda, phoronida, echinodermata, pogonophora, hemichordata, and vertebrata(?); bipolar neurons occur in porifera, cnidaria, platyhelminthes, acanthocephala, rotifera, nematoda, nematomorpha, arthropoda, phoronida, echinodermata, hemichordata, and vertebrata; multipolar neurons occur in porifera, cnidaria, ctenophora, platyhelminthes, nematoda, nematomorpha, ectoprocta, brachiopoda, echinodermata, pogonophora, hemichordata and vertebrata; giant neurons occur in nemertinea and sipunculida; nonmyelinated ones occur in platyhelminthes.

47. The Sensory Receptors According to Function in the Different Phyla. Free nerve endings are found in ctenophora, rotifera, and annelida; mechanoreceptors in ctenophora, platyhelminthes, gnathostomulida, rotifera, gastrotricha, kinorhyncha, and annelida; chemoreceptors in platyhelminthes, nemertinea; photoreceptors in ctenophora, platyhelminthes, gnathostomulida, rotifera, gastrotricha, kinorhyncha, annelida, and onychophora; thermoreceptors, hygroreceptors in platyhelminthes.

48. Autonomic Nervous System and Chromaffin Tissue. Embryonal elements of retina, nasal cavity and carotid body are found in the vertebrata.

49. Meninges. These are found in vertebrata, the comparison to structure of the squid or arthropod brain are questionable.

50. Choroid Tissue. Choroid is found in vertebrata.

51. Glia of the Central Nervous System. This is present in mollusca, annelida, onychophora, arthropoda, and vertebrata.

52. Peripheral Glia. This appears in mollusca, annelida, onychophora, arthropoda, and vertebrata.

53. Plectenchymata. These tissues compose integuments, digestive, respiratory, excretory, hormone productive structures and those of sensitivity, support, and motion, as well as parenchymata in rhodophyta and phaeophyta.

54. Pseudoparenchymata. These tissues play a role as structures of hormone production, sensitivity, support and motion, as well as parenchymata in rhodophyta and phaeophyta.

55. Phylloid, cauloid, or rhizoid true tissues of algae. These occur in rhodophyta, phaeophyta, chlorophyta, and charophyta.

56. The True Tissues of Bryophyta. These are characteristic of this taxonomic group.

57. Succeeding Meristems. "Folgemeristeme" are found in integuments, digestive structures,

structures of gaseous exchange, excretion, propagation, hormone production, sensitivity, support and motion as well as body fluids and parenchymata of tracheophyta.

58. Meristemoids. These occur in the integuments, structures of gaseous exchange, excretion, sensitivity, and support and motion of tracheophyta.

59. Apical Meristems. These play a role in the integumentary structures, hormone producing structures and parenchymata of tracheophyta.

60. The Cambium or Lateral Meristems. These are found in integumentary structures, structures of sensitivity, support and motion and parenchymata of tracheophyta.

61. Phellogen. This is found in the integument of the tracheophyta just as

62. Phytoepidermis.

63. Rhizodermis. This is the integument of the root in tracheophyta.

64. Phyto-Parenchymata. These occur as structures of gaseous exchange, excretion or plain parenchymata in tracheophyta.

65. Collenchyme. This is a tissue of support and motion in tracheophyta.

66. Sclerenchyme. This is a tissue of support and motion in tracheophyta.

67. Xylem. Xylem is a tissue of the system of body fluids in tracheophyta.

68. Phloem. As described for xylem.

69. Secretory Structures. These are of excretory type in tracheophyta.

70. Periderm. This is an integumentary tissue in tracheophyta.

THE PHYLOGENETIC AGE OF TISSUES

Two questions are of fundamental importance: Why are the true tissues in animals according to the old definition more widely distributed with respect to the number of species on the one hand and the relative number of animals and plants on the other and why are the true tissues of animals more highly differentiated? By considering the phylogenetic evolution we can give at least a partial answer.

The trilobites, distant relatives of the more recent *Limulus polyphemus* and other chelicerates, were the key fossils of the Cambrian period of about 540 million years ago. These animals belong to the arthropods, the pinnacle in the development of the protostomians. Thus, they are highly developed invertebrates whose development must have lasted several hundred million years.

We must assume that animals with true tissues appeared about from 500 to 1000 or more million years earlier than the Cambrian trilobites. There exist singular, animal fragments from the pre-Cambrian period but their position and value are not certain. The oldest plants with true tissues, belonging to the vascular plants, are the Rhyniophytina from the lower Devonian, perhaps even from the upper Silurian period. They appeared about 380 million years ago. This simple confrontation shows that true animal tissues on the basis of the known fossil content of the earth's crust appeared at least 160 million years earlier than the true plant tissues. We cannot expect that the picture will change drastically if we consider the origin of true tissues in the highest forms of brown and red algae. The mosses do not contribute anything to this question, because they appear so much later in the history of the earth than could be expected on the basis of their phylogenetic and taxonomic position. Another point to consider is: Why are animal tissues more highly specialized and more widely distributed than those of plants? In part, the answer can be found in the adaptation of living things to their surroundings. The oldest organisms, plants as well as animals, were restricted to life in water. The main nutritional process in plants is performed through photosynthesis, a process which restricted possible plant life to a limited region in surface water layers. As soon as they no longer transmitted light, the lower strata in waters became uninhabitable for plants. But nonplant organisms did develop in the benthos. The plants had no reason for developing more advanced histological systems before they adapted to life on land. The most important contribution to the life process, photosynthesis, was already developed in unicellular types or cell clusters.

References

The references on comparative histology and ultrastructure of the different organisms accumulated so tremendously in the last decade that some measures had to be taken to give a review which will help the scientist but which at the same time keeps the number of citations reasonable:

1. Much emphasis was put on invertebrates because they comprise the majority of living species and offer new avenues for cancer research. With their large species number they exhibit more variations in solving certain physiological problems by structure variation of their tissues and other modes than the other groups of living organisms. Mollluscs, for example, inhabit the regions from the mountain peaks to the deep sea and similar is the range of adaptation of arthropods. Additionally, with the functional and developmental capability, they occupy an intermediate position between vertebrates and plants (especially meristematic and larval tissues).

2. Those phyla, easy to obtain but rarely investigated because limitation in species number, have been preferred. They are the ones to offer new avenues of research.

3. Very few older references of treatise character have been included. These older references are basic with regard to light microscopic studies.

4. When available, most recent studies have been used.

5. If one author has published several papers in a series, only the last one available will be cited. The same holds true if several articles by the same author or author group appeared in different journals because the unmentioned publications may be retrieved with the available computer systems (see Appendix II).

1. Abolins-Krogis, A. (1975): A study of ^{14}C-proline and ^{14}C-hydroxyproline incorporation in different homogenate fractions of the hepatopancreas of the snail, Helix pomatia L. Cell Tissue Res., 156:217–221.
2. Abraham, M., Dinari-Lavie, V., and Lotan, R. (1977): Quantitation of fiber growth in transplanted central monoamine neurons. Cell Tissue Res., 179:285.
3. Adelman, W. J., Jr., Moses, J., and Rive, R. V. (1977): An anatomical basis for the resistance and capacitance in series with excitable membrane of the squid giant axon. J. Neurocytol., 6:621–646.
4. Adolph, A., and Ehinger, B. (1975): Indoleamines and the eccentric cells of the Limulus lateral eye. Cell Tissue Res., 163:1–14.
5. Amsellem, J., and Nicaise, G. (1976):Distribution of the glio-interstitial system in molluscs; II. Electron microscopy of tonic and phasic muscles in the digestive tract of Aplysia and other opisthobranchs. Cell Tissue Res., 165:171–84.
6. Amsellem, J., Nicaise, G., and Baux, G. (1973): Distribution du systeme glio-interstitiel chez les Mollusques; Les parties tonique et phasique du muscle adducteur posteriour chez Anodonta. Experientia, 29:1274–1276.
7. Anderson, R. E., Benolken, R. M., Kelleher, P. A., Maude, M. B., and Wiegand, R. D. (1978): Chemistry of photoreceptor membrane preparations from squid retinas. Biochim. Biophys. Acta, 510:316–326.
8. Andreassen, J. (1968): Fine structure of the intestine of the nematodes, Ancylostoma caninum and Phocanema decipiens. Z. Parasitenkd., 30: 318–336.
9. Andrew, R. D., Orchard, I., and Saleuddin, A. S. (1978): Structural reevaluation of the neurosecretory system in the crayfish eyestalk. Cell Tissue Res., 190:235–246.
10. Andrew, W. (1959): Textbook of Comparative Histology. Oxford University Press, New York.
11. Aramant, R., and Elofsson, R. (1976): Distribution of monoaminergic neurons in the nervous system of non-malacostracan crustaceans. Cell Tissue Res., 166:1–24.
12. Arnaud, J., Brunet, M., and Mazza, J. (1978): Studies on the midgut of Centropages typicus (Copepod, Calanoid); I. Structural and ultrastructural data. Cell Tissue Res., 187:333–353.
13. Atwood, H. L., and Jahromi, S. S. (1978): Fast-axon synapses of a crab leg muscle. J. Neurobiol., 9:1–15.
14. Atwood, H. L., Govind, C. K., and Kwan, I. (1978): Nonhomogeneous excitatory synapses of a crab stomach muscle. J. Neurobiol., 9:17–28.
15. Bachmann, S., and Goldschmid, A. (1978): Fine structure of the axial complex of Sphaerechinus granularis (Lam.) (Echinodermata: Echinoidea). Cell Tissue Res., 193:107.
16. Baetens, D., De Mey, J., and Gepts, W. (1977): Immunohistochemical and ultrastructural identification of the pancreatic polypeptide-producing cell (PP-cell) in the human pancreas. Cell Tissue Res., 185:239.
17. Baid, I. C., and Gorgees, N. S. (1977): On the neurosecretory system of Dendrobaena atheca Cernosvitov. J. Morphol., 153:163–85
18. Bairati, A., and Vitellaro-Zuccarello, L. (1974): The ultrastructure of the byssal apparatus of Mytilus galloprovincialis; II. Observations by microdissection and scanning electron microscopy. Mar. Biol., 28:145–158.
19. Bairati, A., and Vitellaro-Zuccarello, L. (1976): The ultrastructure of the byssal apparatus of Mytilus galloprovincialis. Cell Tissue Res., 166:219–234.
20. Ballinger, M. L., and Bittner, G. D. (1978): Developmental abnormalities of identifiable neurons in the crayfish Procambarus simulans. J. Neurobiol., 9:301–307.
21. Barber, V. C., and Graziadei, P. (1965): The fine structure of cephalopod blood vessels; I. Some smaller peripheral vessels. Z. Zellforsch., 66:765–781.
22. Barnes, S. N. (1971): Fine structure of the photoreceptor and cerebral ganglion of the tadpole larva of Amaroucium constellatum (Verrill) (Subphylum: Urochordata; class: Ascidiacea). Z. Zellforsch., 117:1–16.
23. Barry, J., and Croix, D. (1978): Immunofluorescence study of the hypothalamo-infundibular LRH tract and serum gonadotropin levels in the female squirrel monkey during the estrous cycle. Cell Tissue Res., 192:215.
24. Barus, V., Kotrla, B., and Tenora, F. (1978): Scanning electron microscopic study of the vulva of some trichurids (Nematoda). Folia Parasitol. (Praha), 25:31–34.
25. Baskin, D. G. (1974): Further observations on the fine structure and development of the infracerebral complex ("infracerebral gland") of Nereis limnicola (Annelida, Polychaeta). Cell Tissue Res., 154:519–531.
26. Batson, B. S. (1978): Ultrastructure of the anterior sense organs of adult Gastromermis boophthorae (Nematoda: Mermithidae). Tissue Cell, 10: 51–61.
27. Benchimol, M., De Souza, W., and Machado, R. D. (1977): An electron

microscopic investigation of the surface coat of the electrocyte of *Electrophorus electricus. Cell Tissue Res., 183:239.*

28. Bernstein, S. I., Fyrberg, E. A., and Donady, J. J. (1978): Isolation and partial characterization of *Drosophila* myoblasts from primary cultures of embryonic cells. *J. Cell Biol., 78:856–865.*

29. Besharse, J. C., and Hollyfield, J. G. (1977): Ultrastructural changes during degeneration of photoreceptors and pigment epithelium in the ozark cave salamander. *J. Ultrastruct. Res., 59:31.*

30. Bevis, P. J., and Thorndyke, M. C. (1978): Endocrine cells in the oesophagus of the ascidian *Styela clava,* a cytochemical and immunofluorescence study. *Cell Tissue Res., 187:153–158.*

31. Blazser, I., and Mala, J. (1978): Steroid transport through the surface of the prothoracic gland cells in *Galleria mellonella* L. *Cell Tissue Res., 187:507–513.*

32. Bodammer, J. E. (1978): Cytological observations on the blood and hemopoietic tissue in the crab, *Callinectes sapidus;* I. The fine structure of hemocytes from intermolt animals. *Cell Tissue Res., 187:79–96.*

33. Bode, H. R., and David, C. N. (1978): Regulation of a multipotent stem cell, the interstitial cell of *Hydra. Prog. Biophys. Mol. Biol., 33:189–206.*

34. Bonner, T. P., Menefee, M. G., and Etges, F. J. (1970): Ultrastructure of cuticle formation in a parasitic nematode, *Nematospiroides dubius. Z. Zellforsch., 104:193–204.*

35. Bowser-Riley, F. (1978): The salivary glands of the cockroach *Nauphoeta cinerea* (Olivier). A study of its innervation by light and scanning electron microscopy. *Cell Tissue Res., 187:525–534.*

36. Boyle, P. R. (1974): The aesthetes of chitons; II. Fine structure in *Lepidochitona cinereus* (L.). *Cell Tissue Res., 153:383–398.*

37. Boyle, P. R. (1975): Fine structure of the subradular organ of *Lepidochitona cinereus* (L.), (Mollusca, Polyplacophora). *Cell Tissue Res., 162: 411–417.*

38. Brauer, E. B., and McKanna, J. A. (1978): Contractile vacuoles in cells of a fresh water sponge, *Spongilla lacustris. Cell Tissue Res., 192:309.*

39. Brien, P. (1932): Contribution a l'etude de la regeneration naturelle chez les spongillidae *Spongilla lacustris* (L.); *Ephydatia fluviatilis* (L.). *Archs. Zool. Exp. gen., 74:461–506.*

40. Brocco, S. L., O'Clair, R. M., and Cloney, R. A. (1974): Cephalopod integument; the ultrastructure of Kölliker's organs and their relationship to setae. *Cell Tissue Res., 151:293–308.*

41. Bronn, H. G. (ed.): *Klassen und Ordnungen des Tierreichs.* Akademische Verlagsgesellschaft, Leipzig.

42. Brooks, R. E. (1970): Ultrastructure of the physostomatous swimbladder of rainbow trout (*Salmo gairdneri*). *Z. Zellforsch., 106:473–483.*

43. Brown, G. A., and Wellings, S. R. (1970): Electron microscopy of the skin of the teleost, *Hippoglossoides elassodon. Z. Zellforsch., 103:149–169.*

44. Budelman, B.-U. (1976): Equilibrium receptor systems in molluscs. In: *Structure and Function of Proprioceptors in the Invertebrates,* pp. 529–565, edited by P. J. Mill. Chapman & Hall, London.

45. Budelmann, B.-U., and Wolff, H. G. (1976): Mapping of neurons in the gravity receptor system of the Octopus statocyst by iontophoretic cobalt staining. *Cell Tissue Res., 171:403–406.*

46. Buffa, R., Capella, C., Fontana, P., Usellini, L., and Solcia, E. (1978): Types of endocrine cells in the human colon and rectum. *Cell Tissue Res., 192:227.*

47. Bullock, T. H., and Horridge, G. A. (1965): *Structure and Function in the Nervous Systems of Invertebrates, Vols. I and II.* W. H. Freeman, San Francisco.

48. Burighel, P., and Milanesi, C. (1975): Fine structure of the gastric epithelium of the ascidian *Botryllus schlosseri.* Mucous, endocrine and plicated cells. *Cell Tissue Res., 158:481–496.*

49. Burnett, J. W. (1971): An ultrastructural study of the nematocytes of the polyp of *Chrysaora quinquecirrha. Chesapeake Sci., 12:225–230.*

50. Bursey, C. R. (1975): The microanatomy of the compound eye of *Munida irrasa* (Decapoda: Galatheidae). *Cell Tissue Res., 160:505–514.*

51. Calvert, R. (1978): Sequential differentiation of intestinal endocrine cells in the fetal mouse. *Cell Tissue Res., 192:267.*

52. Campbell, G. R., and Chamley, J. H. (1975): Thick filaments in vertebrate smooth muscle. *Cell Tissue Res., 156:201–216.*

53. Carlsöö, B., and Östberg, Y. (1976): On the occurrence of argyrophil cells in salivary glands. *Cell Tissue Res., 167:341–350.*

54. Castel, M., and Papir, D. (1975): The ultrastructure of normal and glycerol treated muscle in the ghost crab, *Ocypode cursor. Cell Tissue Res., 159:369–378.*

55. Cavey, M. J., and Cloney, R. A. (1976): Ultrastructure and differentiation of ascidian muscle; I. Caudal musculature of the larva of *Diplosoma macdonaldi. Cell Tissue Res., 174:289–313.*

56. Chappell, R. L., Goodman, L. J., and Kirkham, J. B. (1978): Lateral ocellar nerve projections in the dragonfly brain. *Cell Tissue Res., 190:99–114.*

57. Chi, C., and Carlson, D. (1976): The large pigment cell of the compound eye of the house fly *Musca domestica. Cell Tissue Res., 170:77–88.*

58. Chi, C., and Carlson, S. D. (1976): High voltage electron microscopy of the optic neuropile of the housefly, *Musca domestica. Cell Tissue Res., 167:537–545.*

59. Chu, H., and Norris, D. M. (1976): Ultrastructure of the compound eye of the haploid male beetle, *Xyleborus ferrugineus. Cell Tissue Res., 168: 315–324.*

60. Chu, H., Norris, D. M., and Carlson, S. S. (1975): Ultrastructure of the compound eye of the diploid female beetle, *Xyleborus ferrugineus. Cell Tissue Res., 165:23–36.*

61. Cobb, J. L., and Pentreath, V. W. (1977): Anatomical studies of simple invertebrate synapses utilizing stage rotation electron microscopy and densitometry. *Tissue Cell, 9:125–135.*

62. Colmers, W. F. (1977): Neuronal and synaptic organization in the gravity receptor system of the statocyst of *Octopus vulgaris. Cell Tissue Res., 185:491.*

63. Cowden, R. R. (1970): Connective tissue in six marine sponges; A histological and histochemical study. *Z. Mikrosk. Anat. Forsch., 82:557–569.*

63a. Curtis, S. K., and Cowden, R. R. (1973): Effects of antimetabolites on reconstituting fragments of the calcareous sponge, *Sycon ciliatus. Acta embryol. Exp. (Palermo), 3:299–311.*

64. Cutz, E., Chan, W., Wong, V., and Conen, P. E. (1975): Ultrastructure and fluorescence histochemistry of endocrine (APUD-type) cells in tracheal mucosa of human and various animal species. *Cell Tissue Res., 158:425–437.*

65. Davey, C. B. (1966): Temperature dependent anomalies in growth of micro-organisms. *J. Bacteriol., 91:18–27.*

66. David, C. N., and MacWilliams, H. (1978): Regulation of the self-renewal probability in *Hydra* stem cell clones. *Proc. Natl. Acad. Sci. U.S.A., 75: 886–890.*

67. Davis, I., and King, P. E. (1975): The structure of the rectal papilla in a parasitoid hymenopteran *Nasonia vitripennis* (Walker) (Hymenoptera, Pteromalidae). *Cell Tissue Res., 161:413–419.*

68. Deleurance, S., and Charpin, P. (1978): Ultrastructural dynamics of the corpus allatum of *Choleva angustata* Fab. (Coleoptera, Catopidae). *Cell Tissue Res., 191:151–160.*

69. Desser, S. S., and Weller, I. (1977): Ultrastructural observations on the body wall of the leech, *Batracobdella picta. Tissue Cell, 9:35–42.*

70. Dilly, P. N. (1975): The dormant buds of *Rhabdopleura compacta* (Hemichordata). *Cell Tissue Res., 159:387–397.*

71. Dilly, P. N. (1977): Further observations of transport within paddle cilia. *Cell Tissue Res., 185:105–113.*

72. Dilly, P. N., and Messenger, J. B. (1972): The branchial gland: A site of haemocyanin synthesis in *Octopus. Z. Zellforsch., 132:193–201.*

73. Dilly, P. N., and Nixon, M. (1976): The cells that secrete the beaks in octopods and squids (Mollusca, Cephalopoda). *Cell Tissue Res., 167: 229–241.*

74. Doering, G. N., and Palincsar, E. E. (1978): Acid phosphatase during the life cycle of the nematode, *Panagrellus silusiae. Biol. Bull., 154:374.*

75. Doyle, W. L., and McNiell, G. F. (1964): The fine structure of the respiratory tree in *Cucumaria. Q. J. Microsc. Sci., 105* (Pt. 1):7–11.

76. Duce, I. R., and Keen, P. (1977): An ultrastructural classification of the neuronal cell bodies of the rat dorsal root ganglion using zinc iodide-osmium impregnation. *Cell Tissue Res., 185:263.*

77. Ducros, C. (1975): An electron microscopic radioautographic study of the uptake of tritiated serotonin by nerve fibres in the posterior salivary duct and gland of cephalopods. *Cell Tissue Res., 161:351–371.*

78. Duelli, P. (1978): An insect retina without microvilli in the male scale insect, *Eriococcus* sp. (Eriococcidae, Homoptera). *Cell Tissue Res., 187: 417–427.*

79. Dumont, J. N., Anderson, E., and Chomyn, E. (1965): The anatomy of the peripheral nerve and its ensheathing artery in the horseshoe crab, *Xiphosura* (*Limulus*) *polyphemus. J. Ultrastruct. Res., 13:38–64.*

80. Dunogan, T. T., and Miller, D. M. (1978): Anatomy of the genital ganglion of the male acanthocephalan, *Moniliformis moniliformis. J. Parasitol., 64:431–435.*

81. Durnberger, H., and Pohlhammer, K. (1978): The paramedial neurosecretory cells of the suboesophageal ganglion in the cricket, *Teleogryllus commodus* (Walk.); II. Electron microscopic studies in normal and ovariectomized females. *Cell Tissue Res., 187:495–506.*

82. Durnberger, H., Pohlhammer, K., and Weinbormair, G. (1978): The paramedial neurosecretory cells of the suboesophageal ganglion of the cricket, *Teleogryllus commodus* (Walk.). *Cell Tissue Res., 187:489–494.*

83. Dyer, R. F. (1978): Endoneurial mast cells in peripheral nerves of the armadillo dermis. *Cell Tissue Res., 192:97.*

84. Eastwood, A. B., Wood, D. S., and Reuben, J. P. (1978): Unusual thick and thin filament packing in a crustacean muscle. *J. Cell Biol., 77:48–58.*

85. Eaton, J. L., and Pappas, L. G. (1977): Synaptic organization of the cabbage looper moth ocellus. *Cell Tissue Res., 183:291.*

86. Eichelberg, H. (1977): Fine structure of the drum muscles of the piranha (Serrasalminae, Characidae). *Cell Tissue Res., 185:547.*

87. Elofsson, R., Myhrberg, H., Aramant, R., Lindvall, O., and Falck, B. (1978): Catecholaminergic salivary glands in *Gammarus pulex* (Crustacea, Amphipoda); An electron microscopic and microspectrofluorometric study. *J. Ultrastruct. Res., 64:14–22.*

88. Emery, D. G. (1974): Ciliated sensory neurons in the lip of the squid

Lolliguncula brevis Blainville. *Cell Tissue Res.*, 157:323–329.

89. Emery, D. G. (1975): Ciliated sensory cells and associated neurons in the lip of *Octopus joubini* Robson. *Cell Tissue Res.*, 157:331–340.

90. Fahrenbach, W. H., and Griffin, A. J. (1975): The morphology of the *Limulus* visual system. VI. Connectivity in the ocellus. *Cell Tissue Res.*, 159:39–47.

91. Felder, D. L. (1978): Osmotic and ionic regulation in several western Atlantic callianassidae (Crustacea, Decapoda, Thalassinidea). *Biol. Bull.*, 154:409.

92. Fernandez, J. (1978): Structure of the leech nerve cord: Distribution of neuron and organization of fiber pathways. *J. Comp Neurol.*, 180:165–191.

93. Fischer, E. (1969): Morphological background of the regulation of nephridial activity in the horse leech (*Haemopis sanguisuga* L.). *Acta Biol. Acad. Sci. Hung.*, 20:381–387.

94. Fleissner, G., and Siegler, W. (1978): Arhabdomeric cells in the retina of the median eyes of the scorpion. *Naturwissenschaften*, 65:210–211.

95. Flood, P. R. (1975): Scanning electron microscope observations on the muscle innervation of *Oikopleura dioica* Fol. (Appendicularia, Tunicata) with notes on the arrangement of connective tissue fibres. *Cell Tissue Res.*, 164:357–369.

96. Foster, C. A., and Howse, H. D. (1978): A morphological study on gills of the brown shrimp , *Peneus aztecus. Tissue Cell*, 10:77–92.

97. Francoís, J. (1978): The ultrastructure and histochemistry of the mesenteric connective tissue of the cockroach *Periplaneta americana* L. *Cell Tissue Res.*, 189:91–107.

98. Fritsch, H. A. (1976): The occurrence of argyrophilic and argentaffin cells in the gut of *Ciona intestinalis* L. *Cell Tissue Res.*, 175:131–135.

99. Gabella, G. (1974): Special muscle cells and their innervation in the mammalian small intestine. *Cell Tissue Res.*, 153:63–77.

100. Gardner, P. J., and Weidler, D. J. (1975): Ultrastructural study of the neural fat-body system in the cockroach *Periplaneta americana. Cell Tissue Res.*, 159:485–491.

101. Geisert, B., and Altner, H. (1974): Analysis of the sensory projection from the tarsal sensilla of the blow-fly (*Phormia terraenovae* Rob.-Desv., Diptera. *Cell Tissue Res.*, 150:249–259.

102. Georges, D. (1977): Functional analysis of the neural complex in *Ciona intestinalis* (Tunicia, Ascidiacea). The role of the ganglion cell. *Gen. Comp. Endocrinol.*, 32:454–473.

103. Gerould, J. (1896): The anatomy and histology of *Caudina arenata. Proc. Boston Soc. of Natl. Hist.*, Vol. 27.

104. Ghysen, A. (1978): Sensory neurones recognise defined pathways in *Drosophila* central nervous system. *Nature*, 274:869–872.

105. Gibbs, P. J., and Greenaway, P. (1978): Histological structure of the posterior salivary glands in the blue ringed octopus *Hapalochlaena maculosa* Hoyle. *Toxicon*, 16:59–70.

106. Gilloteaux, J. (1978): Innervation of the anterior byssus retraction muscle (ABRM) in *Mytilus edulis* L. and in *Mytilus galloprovincialis* LMK. V. Cytochemical localization of cholinesterase activities. *Histochemistry*, 55:209–224.

107. Girardie, A. (1974): Study on physiological significance of protocerebral lateral neurosecretory cells of *Locusta migratoria migratorioides* (insect Orthoptera). *Zool. Jahrb. Physiol.*, 78:310–326.

108. Glantz, R. M. (1978): Crayfish antennal neuropil; II. Periodic bursting elicited by sensory stimulation and extrinsic current in interneurons. *J. Neurophysiol.*, 41:1314–1327.

109. Gnatzy, W. (1978): Development of the filiform hairs on the cerci of *Gryllus bimaculatus* Deg. (Saltatoria, Gryllidae). *Cell Tissue Res.*, 187:1–24.

110. Gnatzy, W., and Weber, K. M. (1978): Tormogen cell and receptor-lymph space in insect olfactory sensilla. Fine structure and histochemical properties in *Calliphora. Cell Tissue Res.*, 189:549–554.

111. Goodman, L. J., Patterson, J. A., and Mobbs, P. G. (1975): The projection of ocellar neurons within the brain of the locust, *Schistocerca gregaria. Cell Tissue Res.*, 157:467–492.

112. Goossens, N., Dierickx, K., and Vandesande, F. (1978): Immunocytochemical study of the neurohypophysial hormone producing system of the lungfish, *Protopterus aethiopicus. Cell Tissue Res.*, 190:69.

113. Gouin, F. J. (1970): Morphologie, Histologie und Entwicklungsgeschichte der Insekten und der Myriapoden; VI. Cuticula; Basalmembran; Binde-, Hüll- und Stützgewebe. *Fortschr. Zool.*, 20:301–317.

114. Graf, F. (1978): Structural diversity of communicating intercellular junctions (gap junctions) in the posterior cecal epithelium of the crustacean Orchestis. *C. R. Acad. Sci. D (Paris)*, 187:41–44.

115. Grassé, P. (1949–1965): *Traité de Zoologie.* Masson & Cie, Paris.

116. Graubard, K. (1978): Serial synapses in *Aplysia. J. Neurobiol.*, 9:325–328.

117. Greven, H. (1976): Some ultrastructural observations on the midgut epithelium of *Isohypsibius augusti* (Murray, 1907) (Eutardigrada). *Cell Tissue Res.*, 166:339–351.

118. Greven, H., and Grohe, G. (1975): Die Feinstruktur des Integumentes und der Muskelansatzstellen von *Echiniscoides sigismundi* (Heterotardigrada). (The fine structure of the integument and the muscle attachments in *Echiniscoides sigismundi* (Heterotardigrada.) *Helgol. Wiss. Meeresunters.*, 27:450–460.

119. Griffith, J. K. (1978): The differential regulation of the synthesis of ribosomal RNA, 5 S RNA, and 4 S RNA in the polytenic salivary gland cells of the blowfly, *Calliphora erythrocephala. Dev. Biol.*, 65:353–371.

120. Grodums, E. I. (1977): Ultrastructural changes in the mitochondria of brown adipose cells during the hibernation cycle of *Citellus lateralis. Cell Tissue Res.*, 185:231.

121. Gundel, M., and Penzlin, H. (1978): The neuronal connections of the frontal ganglion of the cockroach *Periplaneta americana.* A histological and iontophoretical study. *Cell Tissue Res.*, 193:353.

122. Gustus, R. M., and Cloney, R. A. (1972): Ultrastructural similarities between setae of brachiopods and polychaetes. *Acta Zool.*, 53:229–233.

123. Halvarson, M., and Afzelius, B. A. (1969): Filament organization in the body muscles of the arrowworm. *Ultrastruct. Res.*, 26:289–295.

124. Ham, A. W. (1974): *Histology*, Ed. 7. J. B. Lippincott, Philadelphia.

125. Hammersen, F., and Staudte, H.-W. (1969): To the fine structure of invertebrate blood vessels; I. The lateral sinus of the leech, *Hirudo medicinalis* L. *Z. Zellforsch.*, 100:215–259.

126. Hammersen, F., and Pokahr, A. (1972): Epithelial ultrastructure of the alimentary tract of *Hirudo medicinalis* L.; I. Epithelium of the diverticula. *Z. Zellforsch.*, 125:378–403.

127. Hammersen, F., and Pokahr, A. (1972): Epithelial ultrastructure of the alimentary tract of *Hirudo medicinalis* L.; II. Epithelium of the intestine. *Z. Zellforsch.*, 125:532–552.

128. Harmers (1886): On the life history of pedicellina. *Q. J. Microsc. Sci.*, 27:239–263.

129. Haupt, J. (1976): Die segmentalen Kopfdrüsen von *Scutigerella* (Symphyla, Myriapoda). *Zool. Beitr.*, 22:19–37.

130. Hawkes, J. C. (1974): The structure of fish skin; I. General organization. *Cell Tissue Res.*, 149:147–158.

131. Hawkes, J. C. (1974): The structure of fish skin; II. The chromatophore unit. *Cell Tissue Res.*, 149:159–172.

132. Hecker, H., and Brun, R. (1975): Morphometric differences in midgut epithelial cells between strains of female *Aedes aegypti* (L.) (Insecta, Diptera). *Cell Tissue Res.*, 159:91–99.

133. Herbert, D. C. (1978): Identification of the LH and TSH-secreting cells in the pituitary gland of the rhesus monkey. *Cell Tissue Res.*, 190:151.

134. Herron, P. (1978): Somatotopic organization of mechanosensory projections to SII cerebral neocortex in the raccoon (Procyon lotor). *J. Comp. Neurol.*, 181:717.

135. Hess, J., Diederen, J. H. B., and Vullings, H. G. B. (1977): Influence of changes in composition of the cerebrospinal fluid on the secretory activity of the subcommissural organ in *Rana esculenta.* A quantitative histochemical and autoradiographic study by means of scanning cytophotometry. *Cell Tissue Res.*, 185:505.

135a. Highnam, K. C., and Hill, L. (1977): *The Comparative Endocrinology of the Invertebrates*, Ed. 2. University Park Press, Baltimore.

136. Hisano, S. (1976): The ultrastructure of the sinus gland of the freshwater prawn, *Palaemon paucidens. J. Fac. Sci. Hokkaido Univ. Ser. VI, Zool.*, 20:167–176.

137. Hisar, S. (1976): Neurosecretory cell types in the eyestalk of the freshwater prawn *Palaemon paucidens. Cell Tissue Res.*, 166:511–520.

138. Hisano, S. (1978): Synaptic junctions in the sinus gland of the freshwater prawn *Palaemon paucidens. Cell Tissue Res.*, 189:435–440.

139. Honegger, H.-W., and Schürmann, F. W. (1975): Cobalt sulphide staining of optic fibres in the brain of the cricket, *Gryllus campestris. Cell Tissue Res.*, 159:213–225.

140. Hootman, S. R., and Conte, F. P. (1974): Fine structure and function of the alimentary epithelium in *Artemia salina* Nauplii. *Cell Tissue Res.*, 155:423–436.

141. Howes, E. A., McLaughlin, B. J., and Heslop, J. P. (1974): The autoradiographical association to fast transported material with dense core vesicles in the central nervous system of *Anodonta cygnea* (L.). *Cell Tissue Res.*, 153:545–558.

142. Howie, D. I. (1977): On the fine structure and distribution of secretory cells in the supradesophageal ganglion of the lugworm (*Arenicola marina* L.). *Gen. Comp. Endocrinol.*, 31:350–363.

143. Hoyle, G. (1978): The dorsal, unpaired, median neurons of the locust metathoracic ganglion. *J. Neurobiol.*, 9:43–57.

144. Hughes, G. M., and Wright, D. E. (1970): A comparative study of the ultrastructure of the water-blood pathway in the secondary lamellae of teleost and elasmobranch fishes—benthic forms. *Z. Zellforsch.*, 104:478–493.

145. Hyman, L. H. (1940–1967): *The Invertebrates.* McGraw-Hill, New York.

146. Ichikawa, M., and Ueda, K. (1977): Fine structure of the olfactory epithelium in the goldfish, *Carassius auratus.* A study of retrograde degeneration. *Cell Tissue Res.*, 183:445.

147. Imaki, H., and Chavin, W. (1975): Ultrastructure of the integumental melanophores of the Australian lungfish, *Neoceratodus forsteri. Cell Tissue Res.*, 158:363–373.

148. Itaya, S. K. (1976): Rhabdom changes in the shrimp, *Palaemonetes. Cell Tissue Res.*, 166:265–273.

149. Jacobs, J. J., and Monroe, K. D. (1977): A scanning electron microscopic survey of the brain ventricular system of the female armadillo. *Cell Tissue Res.*, 183:531.

150. Jahromi, S. S., and Govind, C. K. (1976): Ultrastructural diversity in motor units of crustacean stomach muscles. *Cell Tissue Res.*, 166:159–166.

151. Jensen, H. (1974): Ultrastructural studies of the hearts in *Arenicola marina* L. (Annelida: Polychaeta). *Cell Tissue Res.*, 156:127–144.

152. Jensen, H. (1975): Ultrastructure of the dorsal hemal vessel in the sea-cucumber, *Parastichopus tremulus* (Echinodermata: Holothuroidea). *Cell Tissue Res.*, 160:355–369.

153. Jensen, H. (1976): Ultrastructure of the aortic diverticula of the adult dragonfly *Sympetrum danae* (Odonata: Anisoptera). *Cell Tissue Res.*, 168:177–191.

154. Jensen, H., and Myklebust, R. (1975): Ultrastructure of muscle cells in *Siboglinum fiordicum* (Pogonophora). *Cell Tissue Res.*, 163:185–197.

155. Jensen, H., and Tjonneland, A. (1977): Ultrastructure of the heart muscle cells of the cuttlefish *Rossia macrosoma* (Delle Chiaje) (Mollusca: Cephalopoda). *Cell Tissue Res.*, 185:147.

156. Jouin, C. (1978): Anatomical and ultrastructural study of the pharyngeal bulb in *Protodrilus* (Polychaeta, Archiannelida). I. Muscles and myo-epithelial junctions. *Tissue Cell*, 10:269–287.

157. Jouin, C. (1978): Anatomical and ultrastructural study of the pharyngeal bulb in *Protodrilus* (Polychaeta, Archiannelida); II. The stomodeal and its cuticles. *Tissue Cell*, 10:289–301.

158. Juberthie, C., and Juberthie-Jupeau, L. (1974): Ultrastructure of neuro-hemal organs (paraganglionic plates) of *Trogulus nepaeformis* (Scopoli) (Opiliones, Trogulidae) and release of neurosecretory material. *Cell Tissue Res.*, 150:67–78.

158a. Kaiser, H. E. (1980): Comparative functional histology. In: *Species Specific Potential of Invertebrates for Toxicological Research.* University Park Press, Baltimore.

159. Katow, H., and Watanabe, H. (1978): Fine structure and possible role of ampullae on tunic supply and attachment in a compound ascidian, *Botryllus primigenus* OKA. *J. Ultrastruct. Res.*, 64:23.

160. Kaul, S., and Vollrath, L. (1974): The goldfish pituitary; I. Cytology. *Cell Tissue Res.*, 154:211–230.

161. Kelley, R. O., and Skipper, B. E. (1977): Development of the aging cell surface: Variation in the distribution of intramembrane particles with progressive age of human diploid fibroblasts. *J. Ultrastruct. Res.*, 59:113.

162. Kensler, R. W., Brink, P., and Dewey, M. M. (1977): Glial cells in the earthworm ventral nerve cord make an A-type nexus. *Am. J. Anat.*, 149:605–611.

162a. Kent, G. C., Jr. (1954): *Comparative Anatomy of the Vertebrates.* McGraw-Hill, New York.

163. Kerkut, G. A. (1978): The snail brain in pharmacological screening and research. *Gen. Pharmacol.*, 9:79–80.

164. Khan, T. R., Singh, S. B., Singh, R., Singh, R. K., and Singh, T. K. (1978): Ontogenic fate of cerebral neurosecretory cells in *Calliphora erythrocephala* Meig.) (Cyclorhapha: Diptera). *Folia Morphol.* (Praha), 26:117–121.

165. Kimura, S., and Tanzer, M. L. (1977): *Nereis* cuticle collagen; isolation and characterization of two distinct subunits. *Biochemistry*, 16:2554–2560.

166. Kimura, S., and Tanzer, M. L. (1977): Nereis cuticle collagen. Isolation and properties of a large fragment resistant to proteolysis by bacterial collagenase. *J. Biol. Chem.*, 252:8018–8022.

167. Kiss, I., and Benedeczky, I. (1977): Physiological and ultrastructural investigations of an identified neurosecretory cell of *Lymnaea stagnalis*. *Acta Biol. Acad. Sci. Hung.*, 28:355–360.

168. Kitson, N., Van Lennep, E. W., and Young, J. A. (1978): Gap junctions in human sebaceous glands. *Cell Tissue Res.*, 190:115.

169. Koefoed, B. M. (1975): The cryptonephridial system in the mealworm *Tenebrio molitor*; Transport of radioactive potassium, thallium and sodium; a functional and structural study. *Cell Tissue Res.*, 165:63–78.

170. Kong, K. L., and Wasserman, G. S. (1978): Temporal summation in the receptor potential of the *Limulus* lateral eye; comparison between retinula and eccentric cells. *Sens. Processes*, 2:9–20.

171. Koopowitz, H., and Chien, P. (1974): Ultrastructure of the nerve plexus in flatworms. *Cell Tissue Res.*, 155:337–351.

172. Koopowitz, H., and Chien, P. (1975): Ultrastructure of nerve plexus in flatworms; II. Sites of synaptic interactions. *Cell Tissue Res.*, 157:207–216.

173. Korneliussen, H., and Nicolaysen, K. (1975): Distribution and dimension of the T-system in different muscle fiber types in the Atlantic hagfish (*Myxine glutinosa*, L.). *Cell Tissue Res.*, 157:1–16.

174. Krebs, W., and Schaten, B. (1976): The lateral photoreceptor of the barnacle, *Balanus eburneus*. *Cell Tissue Res.*, 168:193–207.

175. Krupp, P. P., and Frink, R. (1978): Effects of vitamin A deficiency on ultimobranchial cysts in the thyroid gland. An electron microscopic study. *Cell Tissue Res.*, 190:181.

176. Kryvi, H. (1977): The fine structure of the cartilage in the annelid *Sabella penicillum*. *Protoplasma*, 91:191–200.

177. Kuekenthal, W., and Krumbach, T. (eds.) (1926): *Handbuch der Zoologie.* Walter de Gruyter, Berlin.

178. Kümmel, G., Claasen, H., and Keller, R. (1970): The ultrastructure of

179. Kustin, K., Levine, D. S., McLeod, G. C., and Curby, W. A. (1976): The blood of *Ascidia nigra*; blood cell frequency distribution, morphology, and the distribution and valence of vanadium in living blood cells. *Biol. Bull.*, 150:426–441.

180. Kvitnitsky-Ryzhov, Yu. N. (1978): Brain neuron structure variation in man and in other mammals due to edema and swelling of brain substance. *Tsitologiya*, 20:27.

181. Lamer, H. I., and Chavin, W. (1975): Ultrastructure of the integumental melanophores of the coelacanth, *Latimeria chalumnae*. *Cell Tissue Res.*, 163:383–394.

182. Lane, N. J., and Abbott, N. J. (1975): The organization of the nervous system in the crayfish *Procambarus clarkii*, with emphasis on the blood-brain interface. *Cell Tissue Res.*, 156:173–187.

183. Lane, N. J., and Harrison, J. B. (1978): An unusual type of continuous junction in *Limulus*. *J. Ultrastruct. Res.*, 64:45–51.

184. Leake, L. D. (1975): *Comparative Histology.* Academic Press, New York.

185. Leatherland, J. F., and Percy, R. (1976): Structure of the nongranulated cells in the hypophyseal rostral Pars distalis of cyclostomes and actin-operygians. *Cell Tissue Res.*, 166:185–200.

186. Leatherland, J. F., and Ronald, K. (1978): Structure of the adenohypophysis in parturient female and neonate harp seals, *Pagophilus groenlandicus*. *Cell Tissue Res.*, 192:341.

187. Ledger, P. W., and Franc, S. (1978): Calcification of the collagenous axial skeleton of *Veretillum cynomorium* Pall. (Cnidaria: Pennatulacea). *Cell Tissue Res.*, 192:249–266.

188. Lee, D. J., Sinnhuber, R. O., Wales, J. H., and Putnam, G. B. (1978): Effect of dietary protein on the response of rainbow trout (*Salmo gairdneri*) to aflatoxin B. *J. Natl. Cancer Inst.*, 60:317.

189. Lent, C. M. (1977): The Retzius cells within the central nervous system of leeches. *Prog. Neurobiol.*, 8:81–117.

189a. Lentz, T. L. (1966): Histochemical localization of neurohumors in a sponge. *J. Exp. Zool.*, 162:171–175.

190. Leushner, J., and Pasternak, J. (1975): Programmed synthesis of collagen during postembryonic development of the nematode *Panagrellus silusiae*. *Dev. Biol.*, 47:68–80.

191. Linthicum, D. S., Stein, E. A., Marks, D. H., and Cooper, E. L. (1977): Electronmicroscopic observations of normal coelomocytes from the earthworm, *Lumbricus terrestris*. *Cell Tissue Res.*, 185:315–330.

192. Lucas, A. M., and Stettenheim, P. R. (1972): *Avian Anatomy Integument*, Parts I and II. U.S. Government Printing Office, Washington, D.C.

193. Marcum, B. A., and Campbell, R. D. (1978): Developmental roles of epithelial and interstitial cell lineages in *Hydra*; analysis of chimeras. *J. Cell Sci.*, 32:233–47.

194. Marcum, B. A., and Diehl, F. A. (1978): Anchoring cells (desmocytes) in the hydrozoan polyp *Cordylophora*. *Tissue Cell*, 10:113–124.

195. Marsh, M., Hamilton, G., and Sass, R. (1978): The crystal sheaths from bivalve hinge ligaments. *Calcif. Tissue Res.*, 25:45–51.

196. Martin, R., and Miledi, R. (1978): A structural study of the squid synapse after intraaxonal injection of calcium. *Proc. R. Soc. (Lond.) Biol.*, 201:317–333.

197. Marza, V. D. (1978): Relationships between specialized cells, capillaries and intermediary cytofibrillary elements; X. Biological evolution of the emonctory subsystem and stereotype in invertebrates. *Morphol. Embryol.* (Bucur), 24:13–17.

198. Mathieu, O., Claasen, H., and Weibel, E. R. (1978): Differential effect of glutaraldehyde and buffer osmolarity on cell dimensions. A study on lung tissue. *J. Ultrastruct. Res.*, 63:20.

199. Matricon-Gondran, M. (1971): Origin and differentiation of the tegument of digenetic trematodes: Ultrastructural study of *Cercaria pectinata*. *Z. Zellforsch.*, 120:488–524.

200. Matsumoto, D. E., and Farley, R. D. (1978): Comparison of the ultrastructure of stimulated and unstimulated mechanoreceptors in the taste hairs of the blowfly *Phaenicia serricata*. *Tissue Cell*, 10:63–76.

201. McKanna, J. A. (1968): Fine structure of the protonephridial system in planaria; II. Ductules, collecting ducts, and osmoregulatory cells. *Z. Zellforsch.*, 92:524–535.

202. Meban, C. (1978): The respiratory epithelium in the lungs of the slow-worm, *Anguis fragilis*. *Cell Tissue Res.*, 190:337–347.

203. Metuzals, J., and Tasaki, I. (1978): Subaxolemmal filamentous network in the giant nerve fiber of the squid (*Loligo pealei* L.) and its possible role in excitability. *J. Cell Biol.*, 78:597–621.

204. Meyer, W., and Idel, K. (1977): The distribution of acetylcholinesterase in the central nervous system of jumping spiders and wolf spiders (Arachnida, Araneida: Salticidae et Lycosidae). *J. Comp. Neurol.*, 173:717.

205. Meyer-Rochow, V. B. (1975): Larval and adult eye of the western rock lobster (*Panulirus longipes*). *Cell Tissue Res.*, 162:439–457.

206. Meyer-Rochow, V. B. (1978): The eyes of mesopelagic crustaceans; II. *Streetsia challengeri* (Amphipoda). *Cell Tissue Res.*, 186:337.

207. Mikami, S.-ichi, Kurosu, T., and Farner, D. S. (1975): Light- and electronmicroscopic studies on the secretory cytology of the adenohypo-

physis of the Japanese quail, *Coturnix coturnix japonica*. *Cell Tissue Res.*, 159:147–165.

208. Mikami, S.-ichi, Kawamura, K., Oksche, A., and Farner, D. S. (1976): The fine structure of the hypothalamic secretory neurons of the white-crowned sparrow, *Zonotrichia leucophrys gambelii* (Passeriformes: Fringillidae); II. Magnocellular and parvocellular nuclei of the rostral hypothalamus. *Cell Tissue Res.*, 165:415–434.

209. Mill, P. J. (1972): *Respiration in the Invertebrates*. Macmillan St. Martin's Press, London.

210. Mill, P. J. (ed.) (1976): *Structure and Function of Proprioceptors in the Invertebrates*. Chapman & Hall, London.

211. Moir, A. J. (1977): Ultrastructural studies on the ciliated receptors of the long tentacles of the giant scallop, *Placopecten magellanicus* (Gmelin). *Cell Tissue Res.*, 184:367–380.

212. Monpeyssin, M., and Beaulaton, J. (1978): Hemocytopoiesis in the oak silkworm *Antheraea pernyi* and some other lepidoptera; I. Ultrastructural study of normal processes. *J. Ultrastruct. Res.*, 64:35–45.

213. Moritz, K., and Storch, V. (1970): The fine structure of the integument of priapulids and sipunculids (*Priapulus caudatus*, *Phascolion strombi*). *Z. Zellforsch.*, 105:55–64.

214. Morris, S. M., and Albright, J. T. (1975): The ultrastructure of the swimbladder of the toadfish, *Opsanus tau* L. *Cell Tissue Res.*, 164:85–104.

215. Morse, M. P. (1968): Functional morphology of the digestive system of the nudibranch mollusc *Acanthodoris pilosa*. *Biol. Bull.*, 134:305–319.

216. Murray, J. (1907): Arctic tardigrada collected by Wm. S. Bruce. *Trans. R. Soc. Edinb.*, 45:669–681.

217. Nässel, D. R. (1975): The organization of the Lamina ganglionaris of the prawn, *Pandalus borealis* (Kröyer). *Cell Tissue Res.*, 163:445–464.

218. Nässel, D. R., Elofsson, R., and Odselius, R. (1978): Neuronal connectivity patterns in the compound eyes of *Artemia salina* and *Daphnia magna* (Crustacea: Branchiopoda). *Cell Tissue Res.*, 190:435–437.

219. Nakao, T. (1975): The fine structure and innervation of gill lamellae in *Anodonta*. *Cell Tissue Res.*, 157:239–254.

220. Nakauchi, M., and Kawamura, K. (1978): Additional experiments on the behavior of buds in the ascidian, *Aplidium multiplicatum*. *Biol. Bull.*, 154:453.

221. Newell, P. F., and Skelding, J. M. (1973): Studies on the permeability of the septate junction in the kidney of *Helix pomatia* L. *Malacologia*, 14:89–91.

222. Noble, S., Leushner, J., and Pasternak, J. (1978): In vitro translation of nematode cuticular collagens. *Biochim. Biophys. Acta*, 520:219–228.

223. Noirot-Timothe, E. C., Smith, D. S., Cayer, M. L., and Noirot, C. (1978): Septate junctions in insects; comparison between intercellular and intramembranous structures. *Tissue Cell*, 10:125–136.

224. Nordlander, R. A., and Singer, M. (1976): Synaptoid profiles in regenerating crustacean peripheral nerves. *Cell Tissue Res.*, 166:445–460.

225. Nordmann, J. J. (1977): Ultrastructural appearance of neurosecretory granules in the sinus gland of the crab after different fixation procedures. *Cell Tissue Res.*, 185:557.

226. Nuesch, H., and Stocker, R. F. (1975): Ultrastructural studies on neuromuscular contacts and the formation of junctions in the flight muscle of *Antheraea polyphemus* (Lep.); II. Changes after motor nerve section. *Cell Tissue Res.*, 164:331–355.

227. Ohly, K. P. (1975): The neurons of the first synaptic region of the optic neuropil of the firefly, *Phausis splendidula* L. (Coleoptera). *Cell Tissue Res.*, 158:89–109.

228. Oldfield, S. C. (1975): Surface fine structure of the globiferous pedicellariae of the regular echinoid, *Psammechinus miliaris* Gmelin. *Cell Tissue Res.*, 162:377–385.

229. Orida, N., and Josephson, R. K. (1978): Peripheral control of responsiveness to auditory stimuli in giant fibres of crickets and cockroaches. *J. Exp. Biol.*, 72:153–164.

230. Ottosen, P. D. (1978): Ultrastructure and segmentation of microdissected kidney tubules in the marine flounder, *Pleuronectes platessa*. *Cell Tissue Res.*, 190:27–45.

231. Owen, G. (1973): The fine structure and histochemistry of the digestive diverticula of the protobranchiate bivalve *Nucula sulcata*. *Proc. R. Soc. (Lond.) (B)*, 183:249–264.

232. Parshad, V. R., and Guraya, S. S. (1978): Morphological and histochemical observations on the intestinal epithelium of *Ascardia galli* (Nematoda: Ascaridida). *Z. Parasitenkd.*, 55:199–208.

233. Pasteels, J. J. (1969): Excretion de phosphatase acide par les cellules mucipares de la branchie de *Mytilus edulis* L. (Excretion of acidic phosphatase by the Goblet-cells of the gill of *Mytilus edulis* L.). *Z. Zellforsch.*, 102:594–600.

234. Patt, D. I., and Patt, G. R. (1969): *Comparative Vertebrate Histology*. Harper & Row, New York.

235. Pearce, R. B., Cronshaw, J., and Holmes, W. N. (1977): The fine structure of the interrenal cells of the duck (*Anas platyrhynchos*) with evidence for the possible exocytotic release of steroids. *Cell Tissue Res.*, 183:203.

236. Pedersen, K. J. (1961): Studies on the nature of planarian connective tissue. *Z. Zellforsch.*, 53:569–608.

237. Pedersen, K. J. (1966): Comparative organization of the connective tissue of

238. Pedersen, K. J. (1968): Some morphological and histochemical aspects of nemertean connective tissue. *Z. Zellforsch.*, 90:570–595.

239. Perpeet, Ch., and Jangoux, M. (1973): Contribution to the study of the tube feet and ampulla of *Asterias rubens* (Echinodermata, Asteroidea). *Forma Functio*, 6:191–209.

240. Perron, F. E. (1978): Seasonal burrowing behavior and ecology of *Aporrhais occidentalis* (Gastropoda: Strombacea). *Biol. Bull.*, 154:463.

241. Pesson, P., and Foldi, I. (1978): Fine structure of the tegumentary glands secreting the protective "shield" in a sessile insect (Homoptera, Diaspiddae). *Tissue Cell*, 10:389–399.

242. Peters, W. (1977): Possible sites of ultrafiltration in *Tubifex tubifex* Müller (Annelida, oligochaeta). *Cell Tissue Res.*, 179:367.

243. Peters, W. (1978): Degradation of the radula in the snails *Biomphalaria glabrata* Say and *Limnaea stagnalis* L. (Gastropoda, Pulmonata). *Cell Tissue Res.*, 193:283.

244. Petit, J., and Sahli, F. (1975): Cytochemical and electron-microscopic study of the paraoesophageal bodies and related nerves in *Schizophyllum sabulosum* (L.) Diplopoda Julidae. *Cell Tissue Res.*, 162:367–375.

245. Petrzilka, G. E., Graf-de-Beer, M., and Schroeder, H. E. (1978): Stereological model system for free cells and base-line data for human peripheral blood-derived small T-lymphocytes. *Cell Tissue Res.*, 192:121.

246. Pilgrim, M. (1978): The anatomy and histology of the nervous system and excretory system of the maldanid polychaetes *Clymenella torquata* and *Euclymene oerstedi*. *J. Morphol.*, 155:311–325.

247. Plate, L. (1898): Über primitive (*Pythia scarabeus*) und hochgradig differenzierte (*Vaginula gayi*) Lungenschnecken. *Verh. Dtsch. Zool. Ges.*, 7.

248. Plesch, B. (1977): An ultrastructural study of the innervation of the musculature of the pond snail *Lymnaea stagnalis* (L.) with reference to peripheral neurosecretion. *Cell Tissue Res.*, 183:353–369.

249. Pogorelaya, N. K., Elekes, K., and Kiss, I. (1977): Electron microscopic investigation of a giant neuron identified in the right parietal ganglion of *Lymnaea stagnalis* (L.). *Acta Biol. Acad. Sci. Hung.*, 28:451–460.

250. Potts, W. T. W. (1967): Excretion in the molluscs. *Biol. Rev.*, 42:1–41.

251. Price, C. H. (1977): Morphology and histology of the central nervous system and neurosecretory cells in *Melampus bidentatus* Say (Gastropoda: Pulmonata). *Trans. Am. Microsc. Soc.*, 96:295–312.

252. Prior, D. J., and Lipton, B. H. (1977): An ultrastructural study of peripheral neurons and associated non-neural structures in the bivalve mollusc, *Spisula solidissima*. *Tissue Cell*, 9:223–240.

253. Punin, M. Yu. (1978): An autoradiographical study of the epithelium organization in digestive gland tubules of two species of bivalve molluscs. *Tsitologiya*, 20:58.

254. Raziuddin, M., Kahn, T. R., and Singh, S. B. (1978): Studies on the neuroendocrine system of the grasshopper, *Poecilocerus pictus* Fabr. I. The protocerebral neurosecretory cells and their axonal pathways in the adult insect. *Folia Morphol. (Praha)*, 26:16–27.

255. Reed, C. G., and Cloney, R. A. (1977): Brachiopod tentacles; ultrastructure and functional significance of the connective tissue and myoepithelial cells in Terebratalia. *Cell Tissue Res.*, 185:17–42.

256. Reger, J. F. (1973): A fine structure study on hemocyanin formation in the slug, *Limax* sp. *J. Ultrastruct. Res.*, 43:377–387.

257. Reinecke, M., and Walther, C. (1978): Aspects of turnover and biogenesis of synaptic vesicles at locust neuromuscular junctions as revealed by zinc iodid-osmium tetroxide (ZIO) reacting with intravesicular SH-groups. *J. Cell Biol.*, 78:839–855.

258. Reutter, K., Breipohl, W., and Bijvank, G. J. (1974): Taste bud types in fishes; II. Scanning electron microscopical investigations on *Xiphophorus helleri* Heckel (Poeciliidae, Cyprinodontiformes, Teleostei). *Cell Tissue Res.*, 153:151–165.

259. Richards, K. S. (1978): The histochemistry of the mucous cells of the epidermis of some lumbricillid enchytraeids (Annelida, Oligochaeta). *Cell. Mol. Biol.*, 22:219–225.

260. Ridgway, S. H., and Patton, G. S. (1971): Dolphin thyroid; some anatomical and physiological findings. *Z. Vergl. Physiol.*, 71:129–141.

261. Rizki, T. M., and Rizki, R. M. (1978): Larval adipose tissue of homoeotic bithorax mutants of *Drosophila*. *Dev. Biol.*, 65:447–461.

262. Rizki, R. M., Rizki, T. M., and Andrews, Ch. A. (1977): Modification of *Drosophila* cell surfaces by concanavalin A. *Cell Tissue Res.*, 185:183.

263. Robbes, L. J., and Fisher, S. K. (1975): Acid phosphatase localization in neurons of *Bulla gouldiana* (Gastropoda: Opisthobranchia). *Cell Tissue Res.*, 157:217–225.

264. Rogers, D. C. (1969): Fine structure of the epineural connective tissue sheath of the subesophageal ganglion in *Helix aspersa*. *Z. Zellforsch.*, 102:99–112.

265. Rombout, J. H. W. M. (1977): Enteroendocrine cells in the digestive tract of *Barbus conchonius* (Teleostei, Cyprinidae). *Cell Tissue Res.*, 185:435.

266. Romijn, H. J., Mud, M. T., and Wolters, P. S. (1977): A pharmacological and autoradiographic study on the ultrastructural localization of indoleamine synthesis in the rabbit pineal gland. *Cell Tissue Res.*, 185:199.

Discocelides langi (Turbellaria, Polycladida). *Z. Zellforsch.*, 71:941–1017.

267. Ronan, T. E., Jr. (1978): Food-resources and the influence of spatial pattern on feeding in the phoronid *Phoronopsis viridis. Biol. Bull., 154:* 472.

268. Sagmeister, H., Gubo, G., Lametschwandtner, A., Simonsberger, P., and Adam, H. (1977): A new cell type in the taste buds of anurans. A scanning and transmission electron microscopic study. *Cell Tissue Res., 183:*553.

269. Salhananthan, A. H. (1977): Degeneration of possible serotonergic nerves in the myenteric plexus of *Mytilus* induced by 5,7-dihydroxy-tryptamine (5,7-DHT). *Cell Tissue Res., 179:*393.

270. Sassaman, C., and Rees, J. T. (1978): The life cycle of *Corymorpha* (= *Euphysora*) *bigelowi* (Mass, 1905) and its significance in the systematics of corymorphid hydromedusae. *Biol. Bull., 154:*485.

271. Satdykova, G. P., Starostin, V. I., and Khrushchov, N. G. (1978): Electron microscopic analysis of the fibroblast differentiation of amebocytes in the common snail, *Lymnaea stagnalis* L. (Mollusca, Gastropoda) in a lesion focus. *Ontogenez, 9:*91–94.

272. Satterlie, R. A., and Case, J. F. (1978): Neurobiology of the Gorgonian coelenterates, *Muricea californica* and *Lophogorgia chilensis. Cell Tissue Res., 187:*379–396.

273. Satterlie, R. A., and Case, J. F. (1978): Gap junctions suggest epithelial conduction within the comb plates of the ctenophore *Pleurobrachia bachei. Cell Tissue Res., 193:*87.

274. Scales, M. D., and Credland, P. F. (1978): The ultrastructure of the non-neurosecretory components in the brain of the midge, *Chironomus riparious* Mg. (Diptera: Nematocera). *Cell Tissue Res., 187:*355–366.

275. Schaller, D. (1978): Antennal sensory system of *Periplaneta americana* L.: Distribution and frequency of morphologic types of sensilla and their sex-specific changes during postembryonic development. *Cell Tissue Res., 191:*121–239.

276. Scharrer, B., and Wurzelmann, S. (1978): Neurosecretion; XVII. Experimentally induced release of neurosecretory material by exocytosis in the insect *Leucophaea maderae. Cell Tissue Res., 190:*173–180.

277. Schliwa, M., and Bereiter-Hahn, J. (1975): Pigment movements in fish melanophores; morphological and physiological studies. *Cell Tissue Res., 158:*61–73.

278. Schmekel, L. (1972): An electron-microscope study of "cellules speciales" in normally nourished and starved aeolids (Gastr. Nudibranchia). *Z. Zellforsch., 124:*419–432.

279. Schmekel, L., and Wechsler, W. (1968): Feinstruktur der Mitteldarmdrüse (Leber) von *Trinchesia granosa* (Gastropoda Opisthobranchia). *Z. Zellforsch., 84:*238–268.

280. Schmid, V. (1978): Striated muscle; influence of an acellular layer on the maintenance of muscle differentiation in anthomedusa. *Dev. Biol., 64:*48–59.

281. Schooneveld, H. (1974): Ultrastructure of the neurosecretory system of the Colorado potato beetle, *Leptinotarsa decemlineata* (Say). *Cell Tissue Res., 154:*275–288.

282. Schramlov, A. J. (1978): Microscopical anatomy of larva of *Cheladonia costulata* (Acarina: Trombiculidae); I. Glands. *Folia Parasitol. (Praha), 25:*61–65.

282a. Schramm, U. (1978): Studies on the ultrastructure of the integument of the rotifer *Habrotrocha rosa* Donner (Aschelminthes). *Cell Tissue Res. 189:*167–177.

282b. Schramm, U. (1978): On the excretory system of the rotifer *Habrotrocha rosa* Donner. *Cell Tissue Res. 189:*515–523.

282c. Schramm (1978): Studies on the ultrastructure of the rotifer *Habrotorocha rosa* Donner (Aschelminthes). The alimentary system. *Cell Tissue Res., 189:*525–535.

283. Schubert, Chr., and Welsch, U. (1976): Temperature dependent changes in the thyroid gland of *Mertensiella caucasica* (Urodela, Amphibia). *Cell Tissue Res., 165:*467–475.

284. Schürmann, F. W. (1978): A note on the structure of synapses in the ventral nerve cord of the onychophoran *Peripatoides leuckarti. Cell Tissue Res., 186:*527–534.

285. Serafini-Fracassini, A., Field, J. M., Smith, J. W., and Stephens, W. G. S. (1977): The ultrastructure and mechanics of elastic ligaments. *J. Ultrastruct. Res., 58:*244.

286. Servettaz, F., and Gontcharoff, M. (1976): Cytochemistry of apparent neurosecretory cells in the central nervous system of heteronemerteans, Lineidae). *Gen. Comp. Endocrinol., 30:*285–291.

287. Servettaz, F., and Gontcharoff, J. (1976): The possible endocrine function of the cerebral organs of the Heteronemertian, Lineus). *C. R. Acad. Sci. (D) (Paris), 282:*369–372.

288. Shaw, S. R. (1978): The extracellular space and blood-eye barrier in an insect retina; an ultrastructural study. *Cell Tissue Res., 188:*35–61.

289. Silverthorn, S. U. (1975): Neurosecretion in the sinus gland of the fiddler crab, *Uca pugnax.* Short communication. *Cell Tissue Res., 165:* 129–133.

290. Singer, I. I. (1974): An electron microscopic and autoradiographic study of mesogleal organization and collagen synthesis in the sea anemone *Aiptasia diaphana. Cell Tissue Res., 149:*537–554.

291. Singla, C. L. (1975): Statocysts of hydromedusae. *Cell Tissue Res., 158:* 391–407.

292. Singla, C. L. (1978): Fine structure of the neuromuscular system of *Polyorchis penicillatus* (Hydromedusae, Cnidaria). *Cell Tissue Res., 193:*163.

293. Skelding, J. M. (1973): The fine structure of the kidney of *Achatina achatina* (L.). *Z. Zellforsch., 147:*1–29.

294. Skelding, J. M., and Newell, P. F. (1975): On the functions of the pore cells in the connective tissue of terrestrial pulmonate molluscs. *Cell Tissue Res., 156:*381–390.

295. Smales, L. R., and Blankespoor, H. D. (1978): The epidermis and sensory organs of *Dugesia tigrina* (Turbellaria: Tricladida). A scanning electron microscope study. *Cell Tissue Res., 193:*35.

296. Sminia, T., Boer, H. H., and Niemantsverdriet, A. (1972): Haemoglobin producing cells in freshwater snails. *Z. Zellforsch., 135:*563–568.

297. Smith, D. S. (1968): *Insect Cells.* Oliver and Boyd, Ltd., Edinburgh.

298. Smith, D. S. (1972): The disposition of membrane systems in cardiac muscle of a lobster, *Homarus americanus. Tissue Cell, 4:*629–645.

299. Smith, G. (1974): The ultrastructure of the sinus gland of *Carcinus maenas* (Crustacea: Decapoda). *Cell Tissue Res., 155:*117–125.

300. Sommer, E. W., and Wehner, R. (1975): The retina-lamina projection in the visual system of the bee, *Apis mellifera. Cell Tissue Res., 163:*45–61.

301. Spearman, R. I. C. (1973): *The Integument—A Textbook of Skin Biology.* Cambridge University Press, Cambridge.

302. Stein, E., Avtalion, R. R., and Cooper, E. L. (1977): The coelomocytes of the earthworm *Lumbricus terrestris*; morphology and phagocytic properties. *J. Morphol., 153:*467–477.

303. Steinacker, A. (1978): The anatomy of the decapod crustacean auxiliary heart. *Biol. Bull., 154:*497.

304. Storch, V., and Welsch, U. (1974): Epitheliomuscular cells in *Lingula unguis* (Brachiopoda) and *Branchiostoma lanceolatum* (Acrania). *Cell Tissue Res., 154:*543–545.

305. Storch, V., and Herrmann, K. (1978): Podocytes in the blood vessel linings of *Phoronis muelleri* (Phoronida, Tentaculata). *Cell Tissue Res., 190:*555.

306. Stowe, S. (1977): The retina-lamina projection in the crab *Leptograpsus variegatus. Cell Tissue Res., 185:*515.

307. Stretton, A. O., Fishpool, R. M., Southgate, E., Donmoyer, J. E., Walrond, J. P., Moses, J. E., and Kass, I. S. (1978): Structure and physiological activity of the motoneurons of the nematode *Ascaris. Proc. Natl. Acad. Sci. U.S.A., 75:*3493.

308. Sullivan, J. T., Rodrick, G. E., and Cheng, T. C. (1974): A transmission and scanning electron microscopical study of the rectal ridge of *Biomphalaria glabrata* (Mollusca: Pulmonata). *Cell Tissue Res., 154:*29–38.

309. Sutton, J. S., and Burnett, J. W. (1969): A light and electron microscopic study of nematocytes of *Chrysaora quinquecirrha. J. Ultrastruct. Res., 28:*214–234.

310. Takahashi, M., and Pour, P. (1978): Spontaneous alterations in the pancreas of the aging of Syrian golden hamster. *J. Natl. Cancer Inst., 60:*355.

311. Thorndyke, M. C. (1978): Evidence for a mammalian thyroglobulin in endostyle of the ascidian *Styela clava.* Nature, 271:61–62.

321. Thorndyke, M. C., and Bevis, P. J. (1978): Endocrine cells in the gut of the ascidian *Styela clava. Cell Tissue Res., 187:*159–165.

313. Tichy, H. (1975): Unusual fine structure of sensory hair triad of the millipede, *Polyxenus. Cell Tissue Res., 156:*229–238.

314. Tjoa, L. T., and Welsch, U. (1974): Electron microscopical observations on Kölliker's and Hatschek's pit and on the wheel organ in the head region of Amphioxus (*Branchiostoma lanceolatum*). *Cell Tissue Res., 153:*175–187.

315. Tombes, A. S. (1977): Type 2 neurosecretory axons (secretory end-feet) at the base of the cerebral ganglion of *Perinereis cultrifera* Grube (Annelida: Polychaeta). *Gen. Comp. Endocrinol., 32:*407–410.

316. Toupin, J., Marks, D. H., Cooper, E. L., and Lamoureux, G. (1977): Earthworm coelomocytes in vitro. *In Vitro, 13:*218–222.

317. Tramu, G., and Dubois, M. P. (1977): Comparative cellular localization of corticotropin and melanotropin in Lerot adenohypophysis (*Eliomys quercinus*). An immunohistochemical study. *Cell Tissue Res., 183:*457.

318. Tsacopoulos, M., and Coles, J. A. (1978): The role of the glial cells in the maintenance of the ionic environment of the photoreceptors of the retina of the drone. *Klin. Monatsbl. Augenheilkd., 172:*449–451.

319. Tsuneki, K., Adachi, T., Ishii, S., and Oota, Y. (1976): Morphometric classification of neurosecretory granules in the neurohypophysis of the hagfish, *Eptatretus burgeri. Cell Tissue Res., 166:*145–157.

320. Ude, J., Eckert, M., and Penzlin, H. (1978): The frontal ganglion of *Periplaneta americana* L. (Insecta): An electron microscopic and immunohistochemical study. *Cell Tissue Res., 191:*171–182.

321. Uehara, A., Toh, Y., and Tateda, H. (1978): Fine structure of the eyes of orb-weavers, *Argiope amoena* L. Koch (Aranea: Argiopidae). 2. The anterolateral, posterolateral and posteromedial eyes. *Cell Tissue Res., 186:*435–452.

322. Uhlman, K. (1968): On the connection between skeletal muscles and skeleton of the echinoderm, *Asterias rubens* L. *Z. Zellforsch., 87:*210–217.

323. Unnithan, G. C., and Nair, K. K. (1977): Ultrastructure of juvenile hormone-induced degenerating flight muscles in a bark beetle, *Ips*

paracontusus. Cell Tissue Res., 185:481.

324. Vagnetti, D., and Farnesi, R. M. (1978): Morphological and ultrastructural study of the ventral nerve cord in *Branchiobdella pentodonta* Whitman (Annelida, Oligochaeta). *J. Comp. Neurol., 178:365–382.*

325. Valvassori, R., De Eguileor, M., and Lanzavecchia, G. (1978): Flight muscle differentiation in nymphs of a dragonfly Anax imperator. *Tissue Cell, 10:167–178.*

326. Vandermeulen, J. H., and Reid, R. G. (1969): Digestive tract enzymes in phoronida. *Comp. Biochem. Physiol., 28:443–448.*

327. Van Lennep, E. W., Kennerson, A. R., and Compton, J. S. (1977): The ultrastructure of the sheep parotid gland. *Cell Tissue Res., 179:377.*

328. Verma, V., and Pecot-Dechavassine, M. (1977): A comparative study of physiological and structural changes at the myoneural junction in two species of frog after transection of the motor nerve. *Cell Tissue Res., 185:451.*

329. Vernick, S. H., Thompson, S., Sonenshine, D. E., Collins, L. A., Saunders, M., and Homsher, P. J. (1978): Ultrastructure of the foveal glands of the ticks, *Dermacentor andersoni* Stiles and *D. variabilis* (Say). *J. Parasitol., 64:515–523.*

330. Vitellaro-Zuccarello, L. (1973): Ultrastructure of the byssal apparatus of *Mytilus galloprovincialis*; I. Associated fungal hyphae. *Mar. Biol., 22:225–230.*

331. Vogel, W., Vogel, V., and Schlote, W. (1974): Ultrastructural study of arteriovenous anastomoses in gill filaments of *Tilapia mossambica*. *Cell Tissue Res., 155:491–512.*

332. Vogel, W., Vogel, V., and Pfautsch, M. (1976): Arterio-venous anastomoses in rainbow trout gill filaments. *Cell Tissue Res., 167:373–385.*

333. Von Ewijk, W., Rozing, J., Brons, H. C., and Klepper, D. (1977): Cellular events during the primary immune response in the spleen. A fluorescence-, light- and electronmicroscopic study in germfree mice. *Cell Tissue Res., 183:471.*

334. Von Gaudecker, B., and Schmale, E.-M. (1974): Substrate-histochemical investigations and ultrahistochemical demonstrations of acid phosphatase in larval and prepupal salivary glands of *Drosophila melanogaster*. *Cell Tissue Res., 155:75–89.*

335. Von Möllendorf, W. (1929-1962): *Handbuch der Mikroskopischen Anatomie des Menschen*. Springer, Berlin.

336. Wabnitz, R. W. (1975): Functional states and fine structure of the contractile apparatus of the penis retractor muscle (PRM) of *Helix pomatia* L. *Cell Tissue Res., 156:253–265.*

337. Wächtler, K. (1974): The distribution of acetylcholinesterase in the cyclostome brain. I. *Lampetra planeri* (L.). *Cell Tissue Res., 152:259–270.*

338. Walz, B. (1973): Zur Feinstruktur der Muskelzellen des Pharynx-Bulbus von Tardigraden. (The fine structure of muscle cells of the pharyngeal bulb of tardigrada.) *Z. Zellforsch., 140:389–399.*

339. Walz, B. (1975): Modified ciliary structures in receptor cells of *Macrobiotus huflandi* (Tardigrada). Short communication. *Cytobiologie, 11: 181–185.*

340. Warton, S. S., and Borovjagin, V. L. (1977): Ultrastructural organization of giant neurones of the mollusc *Lymnaea stagnalis* under different environmental temperatures. *Acta Biol. Acad. Sci. Hung., 28:429–441.*

341. Warton, S., and Dutkowski, A. B. (1978): Ultrastructural analysis of the action of reserpine on the brain neuroendocrine system of the wax moth, *Galleria mellonella* L., Lepidoptera. *Cell Tissue Res., 192:143.*

342. Weihe, E., and Kalmbach, P. (1978): Ultrastructure of capillaries in the conduction system of the heart in various mammals. *Cell Tissue Res., 192:77.*

343. Welsch, U., and Storch, V. (1970): The fine structure of the stomochord of the enteropneusts *Harrimania kupfferi* and *Ptychodera flava*. *Z. Zellforsch., 107:234–239.*

344. Welsch, U., and Schubert, Ch. (1975): Observations on the fine structure, enzyme histochemistry and innervation of parathyroid gland and ultimobranchial body of *Chthonerpeton indistinctum* (Gymnophiona, Amphibia). *Cell Tissue Res., 164:105–119.*

345. Welsch, U., and Storch, V. (1976): *Comparative Animal Cytology and Histology*. Sidgwick & Jackson, London.

346. Welsch, U., and Buchheim, W. (1977): Freeze fracture studies on the annelid septate junction. *Cell Tissue Res., 185:527.*

347. Wessing, A. (1966): Die Exkretion der Insekten. *Naturwiss. Rundsch., 19:139–147.*

348. Wessing, A. (1967): Funktionsmorphologie von Exkretionsorganen bei Insekten. *Verh. Dtsch. Ges. Pathol.*, pp. 633–81.

349. Wessing, A., and Polenz, A. (1974): Structure, development and function of the protonephridia in trochophores of *Pomatoceros triqueter* (Annelida, Polychaeta, Sedentaria). *Cell Tissue Res., 156:21–33.*

350. West, D. L. (1978): Comparative ultrastructure of juvenile and adult nuchal organs of an annelid (Polychaeta: Opheliidae). *Tissue Cell, 10: 243–257.*

351. Westfall, J. A., and Kinnamon, J. C. (1978): A second sensory—motor—interneuron with neurosecretory granules in *Hydra*. *J. Neurocytol., 7: 365–379.*

352. Whittaker, R. H. (1977): Broad Classification: The Kingdoms and the Protozoans. In: *Parasitic Protozoa, Vol. 1*, edited by J. P. Kreier. Academic Press, New York.

353. Wondrak, G. (1975): The ultrastructure of the sensory cells in the chemoreceptor of the ommatophore of *Helix pomatia* L. *Cell Tissue Res., 159:121–140.*

354. Wood, R. L. (1977): The cell junctions of *Hydra* as viewed by freeze-fracture replication. *J. Ultrastruct. Res., 58:299.*

355. Wright, D. E. (1974): Morphology of the gill epithelium of the lungfish, *Lepidosiren paradoxa. Cell Tissue Res., 153:365–381.*

356. Wuest, J. (1978): Histological and cytological studies on the fat body of the cockroach *Nauphoeta cinerea* during the first reproductive cycle. *Cell Tissue Res., 188:481–490.*

357. Yamamoto, M., and Hirano, T. (1978): Morphological changes in the esophageal epithelium of the eel, *Anguilla japonica*, during adaptation to seawater. *Cell Tissue Res., 192:25.*

358. Zacharova, D., and Uhrik, B. (1978): Kinetics of functional and morphological changes during decoupling and recoupling induced by glycerol in isolated muscle fibres of the crayfish. *Cell Tissue Res., 192:167.*

359. Zachary, D., Brehelin, M., and Hoffmann, J. A. (1975): Role of the "thrombocytoids" in capsule formation in the dipteran *Calliphora erythrocephala. Cell Tissue Res., 162:343–348.*

360. Zaguskin, S. L., and Kaminski, I. (1978): Relationship between the spike responses of crayfish mechanoreceptor neurons and the initial functional state and degree of aggregation of their nissl substance. *Neirofiziologiia, 10:84–91.*

361. Zmoray, I., and Guttekova, A. (1969): Ecological conditions for occurrence of cilia in intestines of nematodes. *Biologia (Bratisl.), 24:97–112.*

362. Zmoray, I., and Guttekova, A. (1978): Ultrastructure of intestinal cells of *Heterakis gallinarum. Angew. Parasitol., 19:106–111.*

4

Comparability of Animal and Plant Tissues: The Nine Principal Life Functions with Associated Structures

Hans E. Kaiser

INTRODUCTION

A comparison of animal and plant tissues should begin with the species number of animals and plants. The significance of this endeavor is indicated by the large number of species involved. In both animals and plants (two-kingdom approach), the majority of species is characterized by organisms having true tissues. Animal species with true tissues by far outnumber vascular plant species. The majority of animal species are the insects, of which approximately 1 million species have been described and whose total number of phylogenetically recent species may be estimated as 7 million. Some 10–20 thousand species of nematode worms alone have been described; Hyman (7) has estimated, however, that there exist a half million species. To date, more than 370,000 living plant species are known in which the seed plants (spermatophytes), with approximately 800 species of gymnosperms and 226,000 species of angiosperms (172,000 dicotyledons and 54,000 monocotyledons), constitute the majority of plants. In regard to the vascular plants with true tissues, an additional number of 12,000 species of ferns, equisetums, club-mosses, mosses, etc. must be added. The highest red and brown algae also exhibit incipiencies of true tissues, just as do the mosses that lack true roots. The mosses made their phylogenetic appearance later than we might have expected based on their taxonomy. It can

be estimated that due to the annual increase in the recorded species number, especially of angiosperms and fungi, approximately half a million plant organisms are in existence if viewed from the two-kingdom approach. Therefore, animal species with true tissues dominate with respect to species numbers.

This domination must not be considered as representing a higher value attached to the animal organism, but rather a difference in the lifestyle of the plant related to a later development of plant tissues in their phylogeny. It may be concluded that: (a) The cells of the animal and nonanimal tissues are primarily eukaryotic. (b) Certain morphologic and functional differences between the tissues of animal and plant cells and their subcellular units may be seen, such as the plastids, as well as their related autotrophic metabolism, the cell wall of the plant cells, and the particularly large vacuoles of the plant cells. These variations are not found in all cell types. (c) In histology the concept of two organismic kingdoms remains valid, thus we deal in general only with the eumetazoans and vascular plants. (d) The characteristic life functions of animals and plants are mostly similar and thus permit the broadest comparison in a functional histology. (e) Animal tissues are older, as they already emerged in Cambrian time, whereas the plant tissues did not appear before the uppermost Silurian/lowermost Devonian. As far as the animals are concerned, the trilobites, as members of the arthropods, and, in the plants, the Rhyniophytina[1], as the most primitive tracheo-phytes, constitute the characteristic representatives. (f) In the differentiation of the tissues of animals and plants, two major considerations apply. First, six major tissue groups can be distinguished: the animal epithelia; the connective, muscular, and nervous tissues of animals; the plant meristems or building tissues with at least theoretically unimpaired embryonal potential; and the topographical differentiation, if we deny the meristems of the plants the status of a tissue group but consider them instead to be no more than cell accumulations, as a number of botanists believe (we would then distinguish only among the fully differentiated tissues of animals and plants). In either event, the cells of the fully differentiated tissues display a group-specific life-span. In such a comparison it is essential to bear in mind the unlimited embryonal potential of meristematic cells, the functional binding of characteristic plant tissues to nonliving cells, and the differing or totally absent regenerative potential of typical animal tissues with cell invariability or nonliving plant tissues. (g) In animals and plants there exists not only a characteristic principle in the constitution of tissues peculiar to each, but also there are other particularities of makeup which separate them, just as there are between the single subgroups in the animal kingdom and the single subgroups in the plant kingdom. (h) In their latest conceptions, biochemistry and biophysics emphasize comparability of true tissues of the organisms. It may be firmly postulated that together with subcellular biology a comparative functional histology constitutes a supporting pillar of a comparative pathology. (i) Taking the above into consideration, it can be argued that a comparative functional histology may form the basis of a comparative histogenesis. (j) With reference to the number of species and the degree of specialization, the true tissues of animals dominate in comparative histology in comparison with those of vascular plants.

INFLUENCE OF METHODOLOGIES ON CONCEPTS OF ANIMAL AND PLANT HISTOLOGY

The methodologies in animal and plant histology differ, a fact which has hampered the com-

parison of animal and plant tissues. The main difference exists in the fact that the animal tissues have been investigated and classified by the use of structural characteristics such as space. We divided them therefore into the well-known categories such as epithelial connective tissues, muscular, and nervous tissues. On the contrary, the investigators of plants divided the tissues and classified them according to time elements, to developmental steps. This resulted in the division of embryonal tissues with unlimited embryonal potential which appear first but remain also in the adult plant as precursors of the fully differentiated or permanent tissues. These are the meristems. The term permanent tissues is misleading if used for all fully differentiated tissues and should be reserved for functionally nonliving tissues such as the sclerenchyma. These two approaches of methodology in zoology and botany hampered the comparison of animal and plant tissues.

The Life Functions

The majority of organisms of animals and plants are composed of specialized tissues. These tissues perform similar functions in all organisms. They may be compared from different points of view.

The sole rationale for the presence of the tissues in organisms is to fulfill the life functions of these organisms at a high level of effectiveness. Assessment of this level of performance permits the broadest possible comparisons of tissue qualities. (Table 4.1) presents the principal

Table 4.1
The Principal Life Functions

1. Functions of integuments and body coverings
2. Functions of digestion and metabolism
3. Functions of gaseous exchange
4. Functions of excretion and waste removal
5. Functions of reproduction and propagation
6. Functions of hormone-producing structures
7. Functions of sensitivity
8. Functions of motion and support
9. Functions of body fluids
10. Functions of interstitial tissues
11. Functions of unique tissues[a]

[a] Digesting and metabolizing structures in carnivorous plants; nettle cells in cnidarians; electrical organs as a special type of musculature in fishes; spinnerets of spiders; illuminating organs in insects; and other structures.

---

[1] See H. P. Banks: The early history of land plants. In: *Evolution and Environment*, edited by E. T. Drake. Yale University Press, New Haven, Conn., 1968.

life functions of the organisms possessing true tissues.

The tissues serve the completion and specializations of functions which are also present at a lower level in organisms without true tissues. The broadest basis of comparison is achieved by a functional approach. There exists, of course, a different value and comparability of the various functional principles. The comparison of the tissue structures among animals and plants provides the basis for a comparative understanding of neoplastic growth (Table 4.2). The purpose of histologic differentiation and of neoplastic histogenesis can be best understood functionally. The improved functions and the increase of performance have to be seen as the purpose of phylogenetic development. However, the complication and specialization result also in a higher neoplastic readiness. This is the reason why the approach presented here is understood as a functional comparative histology or histopathology.

Comparability on the Basis of Tissues

Let us examine the performance of the life functions by the tissues of the histonia animalia and the histonia plantae (mainly, the eumetazoa and vascular plants).

The Functions of Integuments and Body Coverings

The basic element of body coverings is a simple cell layer which may become stratified in eumetazoans, as well as in vascular plants such as xerophyta. In both cases this lining cell layer is covered by a cuticula and may be underlain by hypodermis, continuing in or followed by interstitial tissues (connective tissue or plant parenchyma). In both cases various auxiliary arrangements occur that must be understood as a further development of the general principle. Such auxiliary arrangements comprise exoskeletons, glands, scales, feathers, hairs, horns, antlers, and hoofs in the eumetazoans and stomata, trichomes, excrescencies, and glands in the vascular plants. The functions, such as protection, absorptive selection, respiratory exchange, absorption, temperature control, and sensitivity, among others, are similar in both groups.

Table 4.2
Comparability of the Tissues of the Organisms

I. Comparable tissues in both kingdoms in the sense of the two-kingdom approach
  1. Epithelial or lining membranes and glandular structures
    a. In animals: lining epithelia, glandular epithelia, reproductive epithelia, desmal epithelia, endothelia
    b. In plants: epidermis, rhizodermis (in part periderm), reproductive epithelia, secretory structures (including glands and lactifers)
  2. Group of connective tissues in animals—phytoparenchymata in plants: connective tissues, phytoparenchymata, collenchyma, hematopoietic tissues, xylem, phloem, supporting tissues (in part periderm), sclerenchyma.
II. Partially comparable tissues in animals and plants
    Meristematic tissues in plants with at least theoretically unlimited embryonal potential, embryonal larval tissues of invertebrates with long-lasting embryonal potential, tissues of invertebrates with primary and secondary embryogenesis
III. Noncomparable tissues in the sense of the two-kingdom approach
  1. Muscle tissues[a] of animals with no counterpart in plants
  2. Nerve tissues of animals with no counterpart in plants

[a] The uniform function of muscle tissues should be stressed.

Digestion and Metabolism and the Tissues Serving These Functions

The primary tissue is again the absorbing membrane, as we find in coelenterates in the wider sense, constituting the entoderm of the gastrula. In the lower acoelomate parasites, such as the cestodes, the membrane forms the body surface, but in most eumetazoans it covers the intestinal tract. In vascular plants, the principal tissue involved is the absorbing rhizodermis of the root. Glands are widely distributed among eumetazoans, but only rarely in vascular plants; however, they do occur here also and once again exhibit the same principle of structural constitution, being composed of secretory and supporting cells. The chief functional purpose remains the intake of nutritional substances into the body. As in the animal, not all glands in the plant, however, are concerned with food intake and related metabolism.

Gaseous Exchange and the Structures Serving This Function

Gaseous exchange occurs in the organelle, in the cell, and in the tissue, always associated with a membrane separating two media. This concept is basic to an understanding of the comparability of metazoans and vascular plants. The structures in the various organisms may be different, but the principle remains the same. That the term "organ" is of little value in this connection can be especially clearly demonstrated, since the function of respiratory exchange is associated in eumetazoans with widely differing structures of various organ systems.

In the vascular plants, the primary element of respiratory exchange lies in the membrane of the epidermis, especially the lower side of the green blade of the leaf with its stomata. Stomata may be opened and closed actively. By the stomata the outer environment is connected with the internal air spaces of the plant. During the transformation of meristematic to resting cells, the median lamellae at the edges of the cells are dissolved. Intercellular spaces develop this way, building a connecting system of fine channels. These channels penetrate the tissues and are important for the respiration of the cells located inside the plant. This system is comparable to the tracheal system of the tracheata, especially that of the insects. Swamp and aquatic plants have the aerenchymata, which can be considered as a peak of this development. The plant vessels are nonliving tubes with the main purpose of water transport. If they are nonfunctional, they may contain air. They serve sometimes for the storage of water and in the case of the gymnosperms also for support. (Tables 4.3 and 4.4).

Excretion and the Structures Serving this Function

The metabolism of organisms generally produces chemical compounds and other products useless or toxic to the organism (Tables 4.5–4.7). These compounds must be eliminated from the active metabolism, a process involving two principles in all organisms. First, the active elimination, or excretion per se, and second, storage (deposition) or passive excretion. Generally, both principles occur together, with a higher percentage of active excretion in animals but a higher percentage of passive excretion in plants. Active excretion, comparable to the function of

Table 4.3
Structures Dealing with Gaseous Exchange in Eumetazoans[a]

Type of Structure	Distribution in Eumetazoan Group
a. Plain body surfaces	In low or parasitic types, such as cnidarians, cestodes, gnathostomulida, acanthocephalans and various larval types
b. Body appendages and other surface duplications	e.g., in entomostracans
c. Body surfaces especially supplied with blood vessels	e.g., in annelids
d. Tentacle crowns especially supplied by the circulatory system (transport mechanism)	Tentacle crowns of sedentary annelids, the lophophores of lophophorata, specially constructed tentacles of chaetognatha or pogonophora
e. Further development of the principle of surface enlargement (external)	Gills of molluscs, crustaceans, fishes
f. Invertebrate lungs	Pulmonate snails
g. Tracheal system	Tracheata
h. Tracheal gills	Certain larvae of arthropods
i. Book lungs	Chelicerates
j. Ambulacral feet	Echinoderms
k. Papulae	Echinoderms
l. Respiratory trees	In intestine of holothuriae
m. Lungs of vertebrates	Amphibians, reptiles, birds, and mammals

[a] In animals, the dominant structures of respiratory exchange as well as those of excretion are associated with separating membranes.

gaseous exchange, is dependent upon separating membranes. Animal organisms that lack a respiratory system often lack an excretory system also.

Reproduction and Propagation and the Structures Serving This Function

The principle of sexual multiplication by the unification of two parent cells prevails alongside asexual multiplication by division, budding, or fission in animal and plant organisms. In the case of sexual reproduction, the two parent cells form the zygote from which the embryo results and, consequently, the total organism of the particular species. Thus, in both kingdoms, in the sense of the two-kingdom approach, it is possible to distinguish between those tissues producing the sexual cells and those that simply play a supportive role, as is the case with nutritive cells and certain other cells (see chapter 6 for details). The floating endosperm of the coconut palm (*Cocos nucifera*) can be compared to the amniotic fluid of amniota (reptiles, birds, and mammals).

Endocrine Systems

Structures that produce hormones are found in both plants and animals. In the plant are cells or cell groups, such as those cells which produce growth hormones near the tips of shoots and roots. Hormone production in plants does not attain the status of hormone-producing tissues or organs. Even in the lower vertebrates the relevant organ formation is less well developed as is known from chromaffin tissues or equivalent tissues of the mammalian adrenal cortex and adrenal medulla. The same applies to other endocrine structures. Single cells producing hormones are also found in highly developed animals, as in the intestinal tract of mammals. The general action of hormones in plants and animals is, in principle, comparable, but the producing structures above the cellular level are

not. Hormones occur in plants, invertebrates, and vertebrates. Their action differs somewhat but shows a continued trend in these groups. Actually, plant hormones are very largely involved in the growth and development of the organism whereas in animals such as the mammal, the hormones we know most about are regulators of the functions of the adult organism. This difference is a reflection of the role that meristematic tissues with at least theoretically embryonal potential play in the plant in contrast to the ceasing of the embryonal potential in vertebrates. Neurosecretory cells are the only hormonal coordinators in low invertebrates. In invertebrates hormones are widely involved in growth and reproduction as the hormones dealing with growth and regeneration in turbellarians or in annelids, and with reproduction in molluscs but also osmotic control. In crustaceans hormones dealing with moulting and controlling heart beat and color change can be found. In insects the moulting hormones, the juvenile hormones but also those dealing with peristalsis, hyperglycemia, and lipid transport are present. In vertebrates, as in man, the majority of hormones deals with the performance of the functions in the adult in addition to reproduction and growth.

As has already been mentioned, there are no hormone-producing organs as such in the plant, and hence we are unable to make direct com-

Table 4.4
Evaluation of the Comparability of Structures of Gaseous Exchange

Type of structure	Fungi (Protista, Monera)			Animalia	Plantae
Intercellular membranes	+	+	+	+	+
Cell membranes	+	+	+	+	+
Surface integumental areas, serving gaseous exchange	+(?)			In small organisms without resp. system, such as tardigrada	e.g., algae
Special appendage				Such as tentacle crown in polychaeta, extremities in crustacea	Aerial roots
Gills				As in mollusca, merostomata, crustacea, insect larvae, pisces, amphibian larvae	
Book lungs				Arachnida	
Tracheids				Onychophora, arthropoda (brachnida, tracheata)	
Tracheid-gills				Aquatic insect larvae	
Pulmonate lungs				Pulmonata (snails)	
Lungs				Amphibia, reptilia, avis, mammalia	
Respiratory trees				Holothuria	
Lophophore				Lophophorata phyla	
Leaves					Vascular plants

Table 4.5
Comparability of the Structures Dealing with Waste Removal (Selected Examples)

Organelles	Excretion at Subcellular Level Alone, such as in the Case of Protista and Lower Algae

Special Cells
  (a) As only source of excretion
    (1) unspecialized
    (2) specialized
  (b) Excretory function of certain cells occurs as an additional type of excretion
	
	Mesozoa
	Cnidaria, procaryotic cells; Acnidaria "Zellrosetten"
	Sipunculida; free urns (ciliated cells); holothurians; coelomocytes; different types of crustaceans; nephrocytes; chaetognatha; additional action of otherwise specialized cells

Lack of Excretory System Functions performed by other structures in phyla or subgroups of those	Porifera Linguatulida Lower forms of crustacea Branchiodermata Echinodermata Pogonophora Chaetognatha

Nephridia
  Protonephridia
  Mesonephridia
  Metanephridia
Modified Nephridia
	
	Platyhelminthes; Chordate Phyla
	Chordates
	Sipunculida; echiurida; annelida; onychophora; tentaculida; chordata
	Depending on subgroup of arthropoda: antennal glands; coxal glands; maxillary glands in crustacea

Malphighian Tubules	Insects and other arthropod groups
Inactivation from Active Metabolism and Storage in Animals and Plants	Intra- and extracellular storage of compounds in different animal groups during aging, with storage of compounds as in exoskeletons (and cuticles); storage most intensively in nonliving plant tissue (wood)
Loss of Body Portions	Such as leaves and bark in vascular plants. Less common in animals as the loss of antlers in deer
Excretion by Excretory Organs of Vascular Plants	Trichomes and glands; nectaries; osmophoers; hydathodes and laticifers (classification of excretion and secretion depends partially on the opinion of the researcher and needs new investigations, especially concerning the different compounds of the plant and their usefulness for the plant body)
Accessory Structures of Excretion	In this category belong especially only transmitting structures such as the renal pelvis, the ureters, urinary bladder, and urethra as we find them in different invertebrates and vertebrate species, varying from case to case concerning the plant; internal spaces could be considered here

parisons with incretory glands, such as the branchial gland of cephalopods, the molting glands of harvest-men, the Y-organ of the crustaceans, the prothoracal gland of insects, or the hypophysis of vertebrates. As noted previously, the plant tissues made their appearance during the history of the earth later than that of animals. It is repeatedly apparent that convergent lines of development among animals and plants or among different animals or various plants begins with relatively simple arrangements of the structures involved in acting to serve the chief life functions. Later, these solutions diverge more and more.

Sensing of the Environment

Perception of and reaction to endogenous or exogenous stimuli is a basic phenomenon of living matter. This fundamental characteristic of life is found in both plants and animals, with the difference being that in plants the reaction, *i.e.*, the response to irritants, is accomplished at the cellular level, often by a growth response. In the animal, however, beginning with a cellular arrangement, there gradually appear specialized tissues and organ systems. These include the tissues of the nervous system and tissues of the sensory apparatus, resulting in the construction of complex organs at the highest level of accomplishment. In both kingdoms, in the sense of the two-kingdom approach, the same principle applies but at a totally different hierarchical level. Thus, the nervous tissue with its supporting structures is a tissue type restricted entirely to the *Histonia animalia*.

Table 4.6
Structures Dealing with Active Excretion in Eumetazoan

Type of Structure	Distribution in Eumetazoan Groups
1. Excretion by structures other than excretory system, e.g., integument	Phyla without excretory systems, such as rotifera, tardigrada
2. Malpighian tubules	Insecta, therefore majority of species
3. Nephridia	Majority of eumetazoan phyla
a. Protonephridia	Platyhelminthes, nemertinea, certain aschelminth phyla, polychaeta among annelida, priapulida, cephalochordata, and cyclostomata of vertebrata
b. Mesonephridia	Fishes and amphibia of vertebrata
c. Metanephridia	Mollusca, sipunculida, echiurida, annelida, onychophora, tentaculata and certain chordata, as the mammalia
d. Coxal glands of arthropods as modified nephridia	Arthropoda
Antennal gland Coxal glands per se Maxillary glands	Crustacea
4. Rectal glands	Elasmobranchii among vertebrata
5. Salt glands	Birds

Table 4.7
Removal of Waste Products from Active Metabolism by Plants

1. Deposition of metabolic end-products without excretion in nonliving tissues of plants
2. Deposition with later removal (change of foliage in moderate climates, continued change of foliage in tropical regions, decelerated change of foliage in gymnosperms)
3. Removal of water vapor and gases via leaves
4. Excretion or secretion by excretory structures, for example, by uni- or multicellular glands

Moving and Supporting Structures

In the case of plants, the function of motion is performed either on the cellular level or achieved by different rates of growth. In addition, in some nonliving plant tissues, certain mechanisms of motion, such as the ejection of seeds by the splitting of dried seed capsules, among other actions, are accomplished by application of mechanical laws. By way of contrast, animals have developed intercellular fibrils occurring originally in unicellular organisms into a tissue group characteristic for the eumetazoan phyla. These are the muscle tissues (Tables 4.8 and 4.9).

Sooner or later, a higher development of living matter requires a supporting function which, in certain organisms, may be combined with the function of motion. Supporting structures are already found in highly organized unicellular organisms, as well as in organelles serving motion. In the animal and the plant, the structures of support follow the same principle, but are morphologically noncomparable, as we know already from the supporting tissues or structures of animals. As mentioned earlier with regard to protozoans, the lowest group of supporting structures is found in organelles. In both animals and plants, turgor pressure of living tissues serves as support, for example in wormlike organisms (earthworms), or in the herbaceous members of vascular plants. Loss of liquid in the tissues leads to flaccidity in the animal and wilting of the plant. Similar conditions are also known in aging organisms, taking the form of a relaxation of tissues. In the plant, both living and nonliving tissues serve a supporting function. In an earlier section of this volume (Chapter 3), the living collenchyma and the nonliving sclerenchyma have been mentioned. In the animal, the nonliving cell secretions of the endo-

Table 4.8
Evaluation of Processes and Structures Involved in Motion (a Selection)

Type of Movement	Type of Structure	Distribution
1. Movement of structures at the organelle level	Movement of cell sap Intercellular fibers and fibrils	All cells Many unicells
	Pseudopodia	Protozoans, myxomycetes, cells of body fluids, as leukocytes in mammals
	Cilia	Nearly in all animal phyla, with general exception of nematoda and arthropoda—in plants known from flagellae of algae
	Flagellae	Protozoa, male sex cells of most animal phyla (eumetazoans) unicellular algae, movable developmental stages (zoospores and gametes etc.) of higher algae, fungi, mosses, fern and some gymnosperms (spermatocoides)
2. Movement by uneven growth in cell populations (tissues): tropisms such as phototropism, geotropism, haptotropism, chemotropism. Certain nastic movements, depending on growth, e.g., in the case of the tentacles of carnivorous plants such as *Drosera* sp.; autonomous movements; also certain cohesive mechanisms	Involvement of different plant tissues	Especially well known from vascular plants.
3. Movement of body fluids	Common in plants and animals but forced by totally different sources: plant and animal cells; xylem, phloem and muscular tissues:	
	Intercellular movement of body fluids	Common in all organisms

	Circulatory systems in eumetazoans: Open circulatory system, e.g., arthropoda
	  Mixed circulatory system as in pulmonata and cephalopoda
	  Closed circulatory system as in nemertini, annelida, vertebrata	

	System of body fluids in vascular plants: water-conducting xylem and food-conducting phloem	
4. Movement by muscle		Common only in animals

	Myoepithelial musculature:
	  type A
	  type B
	  type C
		e.g., cnidaria
		e.g., ectoprocta
		e.g., mammalia

Table 4.8—*Continued*

Type of Movement	Type of Structure	Distribution
	Smooth musculature	*e.g.,* mollusca
	Oblique striated musculature	*e.g.,* nematoda
	Transverse striated (skeletal) musculature	*e.g.,* arthropoda, vertebrata
	Cardiac musculature	
	type A	*e.g.,* Decapod crustacea, vertebrata
	type B	
5. Movement by pure physical means of living and nonliving tissues		Common only in plants
Nastic movements depending on turgor changes	Seismonastic movements of stamen of *Berberis vulgaris*; or petiole of *Mimosa pudica*; nastic movements are also those of stomata	
Hygroscopic movements	Opening and closure of spore cases and capsules	
Some cohesion mechanisms:	Elaterophores of mosses; special cells of fern sporangia	

and exoskeletons exist, especially in such invertebrates as the corals, echinoderms, or insects. There is also with the living tissues that perform a supporting function, such as the cartilages of invertebrates and vertebrates, the chorda tissue of chordate phyla, and, as the highest type, the supporting bone of vertebrates. It is apparent from these considerations that in both animals and plants, the same principle of a supporting function is accomplished by totally different tissues or tissue products (as summarized in Table 4.8).

The Function of Body Fluids

The apparatus of body fluids and their supporting structures in animals and plants permit only a more or less limited comparison. The intake of fluid is achieved in both kingdoms via limiting membranes. This function is performed by the rhizodermis of the roots in vascular plants, a surface structure such as the absorbing membranes, for example, in cestodes, and acanthocephalans. These absorbing structures are comparable to the intestinal epithelium of higher animals.

In the lower forms of plants, as well as in those of animals, water is absorbed via the body surface. Absorptive structures are hence found in both kingdoms, but fluid transport is performed by totally different mechanisms. In the plant there is a clear distinction between separate xylem and phloem systems; there is no true circulatory system. In general, an upward movement of water in the xylem and a movement in both directions in the phloem facilitate the transport of nutritional compounds. Fluid movement from cell to cell is accomplished via the plasmodesmata.

In the animal kingdom, on the other hand, several systems operate. Especially in small animal forms, there are no special circulatory organs. An open circulatory system may exist, as in the arthropods; a mixed circulatory system, as in the cephalopods and pulmonates, or a closed circulatory system, as in the nemertines, annelids, and vertebrates. The variations in the systems of body fluids, including the lymphatic system, cannot be discussed here in detail, but it can be stated that the basic principles of this function in animals and plants are comparable but diverge more sharply during higher development. A typical difference between animals and plants lies also in the fact that floating cells do not generally occur in the body fluids but even should they be found there as, for example, through injury, they survive for only a very short time. The floating cells of the body fluids of

Table 4.9
Evaluation of Comparability of the Organisms Supporting Structures (A Selection)

Type of Supporting Structures	Taxonomic Distribution	Remarks
Groups of epidermal (cuticular) structures/exoskeletons	Coelenterata (esp. corals)	Way of secretion of skeletal material is species specific
	Mollusca	In gastropoda, for example, the periostrocum and several chalk layers can be distinguished.
	Arthropoda	Pro- and epicuticle can be distinguished; in insects the layers are endocuticle, exocuticle, and epicuticle (four layers)
	Brachiopoda	Periostrocum and inner chalk layer ($CaCo_3$) are discernable
	Vertebrata	Certain structures, such as the shells of turtles and the exoskeletons of fossil fishes, as well as the armor of the scaly anteater should be mentioned
Groups of internal structures/endoskeletons	Porifera	Little skeletal needles develop in scleroblasts, larger ones are formed by several cells
	Coelenterata	Mesoglea can be considered an endoskeleton
	Rotifera	The jaws can be seen as a type of focal skeleton
	Mollusca	An internal shell is present in cephalopodes, others in *Nautilus*. Cartilage occurs in the other parts of the skeleton such as the head of animals.
	Arthropoda	An internal skeleton of cartilage is found in the gill arches of *Limulus* sp. (horseshoe crab). Cartilage-like connective tissue occurs as endoskeleton in arachnida.
	Echinodermata	Mesenchymal cells producing the skeletal elements permit growth of those throughout its life. The sclerit starts as granular in a single mesenchymal cell; growth bulges the cell walls out, mainly attaining a pre-axonal form. Then the neighboring mesenchymal cells fuse with building cell to form a syncytium, and the sclerit continues to grow
	Hemichordata, tunicata, cephalochordata	Internal skeleton composed of chordal tissue at least, as in tunicates, during certain periods of individual life.
	Vertebrata	Bone is the most important supporting tissue; in some fishes osteoid substance of Koellicker occurs instead. The different types of cartilage, chordal tissue, chondroid tissue, and adipose tissue are other supporting elements. In chordal and adipose tissue, the internal cell pressure is important, comparable to the following two groups of functional skeletons.
Body fluids in widest sense acting as skeleton	Herbaceous plants (wilting), including collenchyma	The wilting is produced by loss of tissue pressure according to the decrease of water content. This is also the case in

Table 4.9—*Continued*

Type of Supporting Structures	Taxonomic Distribution	Remarks
		the living cells of collenchyme. The role of plant parenchyma is also especially important.
Supporting structures of vascular plants	Living collenchyma with ability to stretch Nonliving sclerenchyma	The main supporting tissue in herbaceous plants is the collenchyme. Sclerenchyma is the supporting firmer tissue in stems, limbs, and roots of trees and shrubs, in capsules of seeds, or in stones of fruits (plum stone). The main groups of sclerenchymatous cells are sclereids and fibers.

Table 4.10
Evaluation of the Structure and Functions of Body Fluids

Type of Body Fluid	Organism			
Cell Sap	General distribution, large vacuoles in plants			
Tissue sap	Generally not present in nonliving plant tissues			
Circulatory System in Animals	Three subgroups			
No Circulatory System	*Open Circulatory System*	*Mixed Circulatory System*	*Closed Circulatory System*	
Porifera	Priapulida	Mollusca	Nemertinea	
Cnidaria	Mollusca	Pulmonata	Echiurida	
Ctenophora	Sipunculida	Cephalopoda	Annelida	
Platyhelminthes	Onychophora		Pogonophora	
Rotifera	Linguatulida		Hemichordata	
Gastrotricha	Arthropoda		Urochordata	
Kinorhyncha	Phoronida		Cephalochordata	
Gnathostomulida	Ectoprocta		Vertebrata	
Nematoda	Brachiopoda			
Nemamorpha	Branchiotremata			
Acanthocephala	Echinodermata			
Entoprocta	Chaetognatha			
Tardigrada				
Food- and water-conducting systems of vascular plants	Tracheophyta			
Liquid endosperm comparable to allantoic fluid	Coconut			

animals, on the other hand, can be considered as a type of connective tissue. They derive from reticular connective tissue, and hence we may consider the blood of vertebrates and the other body fluids of invertebrates as a liquid tissue. As is generally known, the fibers characteristic of animal connective tissues appear during the coagulation of blood. A comparative similarity exists insofar as the plant parenchymata, the ground tissues of the plants contain the respiratory pigments as occurs in the cells or corpuscles (e.g., erythrocytes) of connective tissue. The connective tissues themselves can be considered as the ground tissue of the animal body, a condition best demonstrated in the acoelomate animals. In the case of the plant, however, it is not defensible to consider the content of the paths of fluid conduction as tissue because no floating cells occur. The paths, in fact, contain only nutritional substances or a salt solution. Table 4.10 provides a summary of these findings.

Integration

The majority of eumetazoans are bilateral-symmetrical. In the bilateral-symmetrical animals, three main groups can be distinguished: the acoelomates, the pseudocoelomates, and the coelomates. The acoelomates have no body cavity. In their case, the spaces between the single organs are occupied by connective tissue. The platyhelminthes offer a typical example. The pseudocoelomates lack a proper body cavity but have certain spaces between the organs. The nematodes and rotifers belong to this group. Finally, the coelomates exhibit a body cavity which walls are lined by an epithelium. The coelomates may be divided into schizocoelomates, such as the molluscs or arthropods, and the enterocoelomates, such as the echinoderms and vertebrates. It is apparent that the connective tissues or parenchyma of the acoelomates

Table 4.11
Comparability of Integrating (Connective and Interstitial) Tissues as such and the Correlating Functions of the Other Animal and Plant Tissues

Animals	Integrating tissues	Plants
	1. The mesenchymatic stem cells in their different taxonomic capacity	
	2. Connective tissues and interstitial tissues per se	
Loose and other connective tissues in animals		Plant parenchymata
	3. Hematopoietic tissues	
Reticular connective tissues in animals		Limited comparability to phloem, xylem, and chloroplasts in plants
	4. Supporting tissues	
Dense connective tissue, adipose, chondroid, chordal tissues, cartilage and bone in animals		Collenchyma and sclerenchyma in plants

Selected Correlative Functions of Other Tissue Systems		
Animals	Epithelia	Plants
Covering membranes, structures with endocrine function		Plant epidermis and rhizodermis
	Nervous tissues	
Conduction Neurosecretion Glial functions		Not present above cellular level
	Muscular tissues	
Myoepithelial, smooth, oblique striated, cross striated, cardiac		Not present above cellular level in plants
Larval tissues	Meristems	Types of meristems

ᵃ The different types of fully differentiated plant tissues are subgroups according to function.

can be readily compared with the ground tissues (phytoparenchymata) of herbaceous plants. As the different groups of animals specialize more and more away from each other during phylogeny, the higher members of the animal and plant kingdoms diversify more and more. The arrangement of the different types of parenchymata in plants, as it occurs beneath the epidermis in the blade of the leaf, reminds us principally of the arrangement of animal connective tissues also in higher organisms. The closest comparison, of course, is possible among acoelomates and highly developed algae and herbaceous plants (Table 4.11).

Functions of Unique Structures

There are a number of exceptional functions performed by special structures. They are characteristic for narrowly circumscribed groups of organisms in both kingdoms. Thus, they are group specific; they stand isolated, as it were. They comprise such structures as the glands of carnivorous plants, the spinnerets of spiders, the feathers of birds, and the hairs and mammary glands of mammals. The glands of carnivorous plants are in turn composed of secretory and supporting cells, just as in all other glands of the organisms. The digestive juices of these organisms are specific and may even contain trypsin, as in animals. At the cellular level, nettle cells of the coelenterates can be in principle compared to nettle cells in plants, e.g., of the species *Urtica*.

References

1. Andrew, W. (1959): *Textbook of Comparative Histology*. Oxford University Press, New York.
2. Bronn, H. G. (1862): *Klassen und Ordnungen des Tierreichs*. Akademische Verlagsgesellschaft, Leipzig.
3. Bullock, T. H., and Horridge, G. H. (1965): *Structure and Function in the Nervous Systems of Invertebrates*. Freeman, San Francisco.
4. Esau, K. (1977): *Plant Anatomy*, Ed. 3. John Wiley & Sons, New York.
5. Grassé, P. (1949–1965): *Traité de Zoologie*. Masson & Cie, Paris.
6. Ham, A. W. (1974): *Histology*. J. B. Lippincott, Philadelphia.
7. Hyman L. H. (1940–1966): *The Invertebrates*. McGraw-Hill, New York.
8. Kaiser, H. E. (1979): *Species Specific Potential of Invertebrates for Toxicological Research*. University Park Press, Baltimore.
9. Kükenthal, W. (1923–1941): *Handbuch der Zoologie*. Walter de Gruyter, Berlin.
10. Leake, L. (1976): *Comparative Histology*. Academic Press, New York.
11. Strasburger, E. (1980): *Textbook of Botany*, Translated by P. R. Bell and D. E. Coonbe. Langman Group Ltd. London.

III

General Review of Normal Growth

5

Circadian Time Structure of *Euglena*: A Model System Amenable to Quantification

Leland N. Edmunds, Jr., and Franz Halberg

INTRODUCTION

Temporal organization along an approximately 24-hour (circadian) scale is not restricted to multicellular organisms. Overt persisting circadian rhythms have been documented in a number of unicellular forms, including the green algae *Acetabularia, Chlamydomonas,* and *Chlorella,* the marine bioluminescent dinoflagellate *Gonyaulax,* the algal flagellate *Euglena,* the ciliates *Paramecium* and *Tetrahymena,* and the bacterium *Escherichia coli.* The variables exhibiting rhythms include cell division, mating type reversal, luminescence, pattern formation and enzymatic activity (reviewed by Bruce and Pittendrigh (7); Edmunds (20); Ehret and Wille (28); Halberg and Connor (34); Hastings (37); Vanden Driessche (55)). In each of these different microorganisms, furthermore, several different circadian rhythms have been observed concurrently (in some cases even in individual cells as well as in synchronous populations), with the attendant implication that many or all of the overt rhythms in a unicell may represent "hands" of a single underlying master pacemaker mechanism (see particularly McMurry and Hastings (43)). These organisms, therefore, constitute attractive systems for the experimental investigation of the fine structure of circadian rhythms and the mechanism(s) whereby they are generated.

In particular, *Euglena gracilis* Klebs (strain Z) has been intensively studied in a number of laboratories over the past 20 years (reviewed by Edmunds (20, 21)), and along with *Gonyaulax* and *Tetrahymena,* form a trio that provided evidence for the so-called "G-E-T effect" described by Ehret and Wille (28). This organism can be grown on a variety of different completely defined media (58) either autotrophically in the presence of CO_2 or organotrophically in the light or dark on carbon sources ranging from acetate, ethanol, lactic and glycolic acid to glutamic and malic acids over a wide pH range (alkaline to acidic pH <3.0). This versatility in growth mode, in conjunction with the fact that cell division can be easily synchronized by appropriate 24-hour lighting schedules (14, 16) and temperature cycles (53), has made *Euglena* a key experimental organism for a variety of physiological and biochemical investigations (9). Another important consideration is that populations of *Euglena* can be maintained in the stationary phase of growth (the so-called infradian growth mode (28)) for days, weeks, and even longer time spans with little or no net increase in cell concentration; circadian outputs can thus be monitored while divorced from the driving force of the cell cycle (which itself can be modulated or gated by a circadian oscillator (20)). Finally, a number of photosynthetic mutants (or even completely bleached strains devoid of their chloroplast genome) have been isolated. These strains also exhibit light-entrainable circadian rhythms, but now with the problem of the dual use of imposed light spans and signals—as an energy source for growth on the one hand, and

Table 5.1
Circadian Rhythms in *Euglena gracilis* Klebs

A. PHYSIOLOGICAL

Rhythm[a,b]	Strain[c]	Phase Marker	ϕ^d	Reference[e]
Cell division	Z	Onset	CT 12–13 [180–195°]	Edmunds (15, 16, 20, 21) Edmunds and Funch (24, 25)
	P₄ZUL	Onset	CT 10–12 [150–180°]	Edmunds (19, 21), Edmunds et al. (22, 26, 27), Jarrett and Edmunds (38)
	P₇ZNgL	Onset	CT 10–12 [150–180°]	Mitchell (44)
	W₆ZHL	Onset	CT 10–12 [150–180°]	Edmunds (21), Edmunds et al. (26)
	WₙZUL	Onset	CT 10–12 [150–180°]	Mitchell (44)
	Y₉ZNalL	Onset	CT 10–11 [150–165°]	Edmunds et al. (26)
Cell volume	Z	Maximum	CT 18–21 [270–315°]	K. Brinkmann and U. Kipry (unpublished)
Flagellated cells (%)	Z, 1224-5/9 (Göttingen)	Maximum	CT 03 [45°]	Brinkmann (2)
Motility, random (dark) *Dunkelbeweglichkeit*	Z, 1224-5/9 (Göttingen)	Minimum	CT 18–21 [270–315°]	Brinkmann (2, 3), Schnabel (49)
	WₙZHL, 1224-5/25 (Göttingen)	Minimum	CT 12 [180°]	Kirschstein (40)
Photokinesis (photoactivation of random (motility)	Z	Maximum	CT 18–21 [270–315°]	Brinkmann (5)
Photosynthetic capacity ¹⁴CO₂ uptake	Z, ZR	Maximum	CT 06–08 [90–120°]	Walther and Edmunds (57) (*cf.* Codd and Merrett (10); Laval-Martin et al. (41)
O₂ evolution		Maximum	CT 04–06 [60–90°]	Walther and Edmunds (57) (*cf.* Cook (13); Lonergan and Sargent (42))
Phototaxis (capacity)	Z	Maximum	CT 04–08 [60–120°]	Bruce and Pittendrigh (6, 8), Brinkmann (2), Feldman (29), Pohl (46)
Settling	Z	Maximum	CT 21–09[f] [315–135°]	Terry and Edmunds (54)
			CT 15 [225°]	Kiefner et al. (39)
Shape	Z, 1224-5/9 (Göttingen)	Maximum elongation	CT 03–09 [45–135°]	Brinkmann (5)

B. BIOCHEMICAL

Amino acid incorporation [DL-phenylalanine-3-¹⁴C]	Z	Maximum	CT 10–12 [150–180°]	Feldman (30)
Gross metabolic variables[g]				
Carotenoids	Z	Onset	ST 0 [0°]	Cook (12), Edmunds (17)
Chlorophyll *a*	Z	Onset	ST 0 [0°]	Cook (12), Edmunds (17)
Dry weight	Z	Onset	ST 0 [0°]	Cook (11), Edmunds (17)
Total protein	Z	Onset	ST 0 [0°]	Cook (12), Edmunds (17)
Total cellular RNA	Z	Onset	ST 0 [0°]	Cook (12), Edmunds (17)
Total cellular DNA	Z	Onset	ST 08–09 [120–135°]	Edmunds (15, 17) (*cf.* Cook (12))
Enzymatic activity[h]				
Acid phosphatase	Z	Peak	ST 06–08 [90–120°]	Sulzman and Edmunds (51), Edmunds (20)
Alanine dehydrogenase	Z	Peak	CT 06–08 [90–120°]	Sulzman and Edmunds (51)

Table 5.1—*continued*

B. BIOCHEMICAL

Rhythm[a,b]	Strain[c]	Phase Marker	ϕ^d	Reference[e]
Glucose-6-P-dehydrogenase	Z	Peak	ST 06 [90°]	Sulzman and Edmunds (51), Edmunds (20)
Glutamic dehydrogenase	Z	Peak	ST 06–08 [90–120°]	Sulzman and Edmunds (51), Edmunds (20)
Glyceraldehyde-3-P-dehydrogenase [NADP-and NADPH-dependent]	Z	Peak	ST 05–08 [75–120°]	Walther and Edmunds (57)
Lactic dehydrogenase	Z	Peak	ST 06 [90°]	Sulzman and Edmunds (51), Edmunds (20)
L-Serine deaminase	Z	Peak	ST 06 [90°]	Sulzman and Edmunds (51), Edmunds (20)
L-Threonine deaminase	Z	Peak	ST 08 [120°]	Sulzman and Edmunds (51), Edmunds (20)
Susceptibility				
Ethanol (pulses)	Z [1224-5/9, Göttingen]	Maximum	CT 03–06 [45–90°]	Brinkmann (4)
Trichloroacetic acid	Z [1224-5/9, Göttingen]	Maximum	CT 03–06 [45–90°]	Brinkmann (5)

[a] All rhythms listed have been shown to persist macroscopically with a circadian period in DD (or LL) and constant temperature following prior synchronization or initiation unless otherwise indicated.

[b] All cultures were essentially nondividing (stationary or long infradian), except for those in which the cell division rhythm itself was monitored. Consult reference for precise culture conditions.

[c] The wild-type strain is designated as Z strain. Unless otherwise noted, it was originally obtained from the American Type Culture Collection (No. 12716) and maintained at the State University of New York at Stony Brook since 1965 or at Princeton University. Also available from the Algal Collection at Indiana University (No. 753) and the Algensammlung Pringsheim at Göttingen (No. 1224-5/9). All other strains are photosynthetic mutants or completely bleached strains incapable of photosynthesis.

[d] Phase given in circadian time (CT, hours or degrees after subjective dawn, where the onset of light would have occurred had the synchronizing light cycle been continued). Synchronizing light cycles were either LD: 12,12 or LD: 10,14 (except in the case of the settling rhythm where the cultures were synchronized by a 12:12 temperature cycle [18°/25°, LL] before release into LL, and CT 0 = onset of lower temperature). In those instances where a free-run was not monitored, phase is given in synchronizer time (ST 0 = onset of light).

[e] Only key references are given; no attempt is made to survey all relevant or derivative publications.

[f] Rhythm synchronized by a 12:12 temperature cycle (18°/25°) in either dividing or nondividing cultures maintained in LL before release into constant conditions (25°, LL). CT 0 = onset of lower temperature.

[g] These variables have been monitored only in light-synchronized (LD: 14,10), synchronously dividing cultures. The phase marker, onset, here refers to the stage in the rhythm when values start to increase.

[h] Although all of the enzymes indicated undergo oscillations in activity in nondividing cultures in LD: 10,14, only alanine dehydrogenase has been investigated in sufficient detail to demonstrate conclusively, if macroscopically, that its activity persists for long time spans in DD and constant temperature.

as a cue for the timing mechanism on the other—effectively eliminated (26, 27, 38, 40, 44).

These important and useful characteristics prompt us to (a) tabulate a number of the circadian rhythms reported for *Euglena* throughout the literature, (b) quantitate the data where possible, and (c) determine by rhythmometry the relations among a number of these rhythms as has been done for multicellular organisms, including human beings (32).

TABULATION OF CIRCADIAN RHYTHMS IN *EUGLENA*

Many circadian rhythms that have been documented in *Euglena* are tabulated in Table 5.1. As is evident, a number of variables have been studied by repeated sampling (usually every 1 or 2 hours). For the sake of convenience, they have been grouped arbitrarily (and somewhat artificially) into physiological and biochemical rhythms. In the majority of studies, the Z strain of *Euglena gracilis* Klebs was utilized, though in several cases (such as the investigations of cell division and mobility rhythms) various photosynthetic mutants or bleached strains—obligate organotrophs—were used.

In each instance, the variable has been measured in synchronously dividing cultures held under conventional, full-photoperiod, 24-hour cycles of light and darkness (e.g., LD: 8,16, LD: 10,14, LD: 12, 12 and LD: 14,10) or of temperature (e.g., 18°/25°C: 12, 12), and in certain cases, as for the rhythm of cell division, under more exotic illumination regimens (e.g., LD: 1,3, LD: 12,36, and so-called two-point symmetric skeleton photoperiods, as <u>L</u>D: <u>3</u>,6, <u>3</u>:12).[1] Although some of the key gross metabolic factors (e.g., total protein, RNA, and DNA) are given for the sake of reference, no attempt has been made to include *all* such reported rhythms since there are innumerable reports of biochemical variables that change across the cell cycle of *Euglena*. Rather, emphasis is given to those 24-hour rhythms which not only occur in synchronously dividing cultures, but which also (a) appear in nondividing (stationary, or long infradian) populations as well; and (b) persist for extended time spans under conditions held constant with respect to illumination (or darkness), temperature, and other culture variables such as pH and aeration.

Under these circumstances, then, we have tabulated circadian rhythms (*sensu stricto*) that free-run with a period which usually only approximates 24 hours following removal of the synchronizer (also referred to as an entraining agent, or *Zeitgeber*). The exceptions given include the persisting rhythm of cell division itself which, of course, must be monitored in a dividing culture, and certain biochemical variables (e.g., DNA, RNA, enzymatic activities (see footnotes g and h of Table 5.1)) whose long-term assays are quite laborious. It is important to note, however, that in these cases it is quite likely that the oscillations would have been found to persist had the variables in question actually been measured, if for no other reason than that they *have* all been shown to exhibit 24-hour fluctuations across the cell cycle in <u>L</u>D: <u>10</u>,14, <u>L</u>D: <u>12</u>, 12, and <u>L</u>D: <u>14</u>,10, and that cell division itself manifests a persisting circadian rhythmicity in LL or DD. Further, all enzyme activities listed oscillate in nondividing cultures subjected to appropriate LD cycles. Finally, the common enzyme alanine dehydrogenase has been selected for detailed study (51, 52) and was shown to undergo rhythmic changes in activity of relatively large amplitude for at least 14 days in DD (but not in LL) in nondividing cultures of *Euglena* grown organotrophically and initially synchronized by an imposed <u>L</u>D: <u>10</u>,14 cycle.

Lastly, it is evident even from the qualitatively determined time relations of the rhythms (correlated in Table 5.1 to the onset of the light, *i.e.*, synchronizer time zero (ST 0, also referred to as ZT 0) under synchronizing regimes, or circadian

time zero (CT 0, *i.e.*, "subjective dawn" (45)) under constant illumination or darkness during a free-run) that they scan the entire time span of 24 hours (=360°). It is important to note that in this tabulation the phase marker on a rhythm (feature chosen to indicate phase relations, sometimes referred to as phase reference point) is arbitrarily and often visually selected by the experimenter (usually, *but not always*, the peak or maximum value of the oscillation, or its onset). The timing of such markers is not necessarily equal to the quantitatively defined and determined acrophase (ϕ) described in the following sections. Indeed, the phase marker for the cell division and the phototaxis rhythms is taken usually as the onset and the maximum value, respectively. In contrast, acrophase values computed with the cosinor method are directly compared because they indicate the timing of high values in the rhythm as approximated by a cosinor model. The acrophases thus determined for each of the tabulated rhythms of *Euglena* will be displayed in an acrophase chart permitting the convenient visualization of the time relationships among the several rhythms and their phase angle to an imposed light cycle during synchronization.

QUANTIFICATION OF TIME RELATIONS BY RHYTHMOMETRY

As we have seen in Table 5.1, a number of variables in *Euglena* has been studied by repeated sampling of cell populations under synchronizing conditions with conventional 24-hour light and temperature cycles; data are available also for many of these variables under conditions of continuous light (or darkness) and constant temperature. It is thus possible to attempt to quantify the time relations among these diverse circadian rhythms in order to determine which processes are roughly coincident or "in phase" and which are out of phase during synchronization. Such quantitative examination of the circadian time structure of *Euglena* is particularly important for determining whether any of these phase angles are altered with statistical significance under conditions of presumed constancy with regard to environmental inputs (*i.e.*, "free-running" conditions). Indeed, internal desynchronization of a number of free-running physiological circadian rhythms—with attendant implication of a spectrum of different frequencies—has been demonstrated under certain

---

[1] The term "LL" will be used to denote continuous illumination, "DD" continuous darkness, and "<u>L</u>D: <u>10</u>,14" a repetitive, 24-hour light cycle (period $T = 24$ hours) consisting of 10 hours of light followed by 14 hours of darkness; "D/L" refers to a single transition from darkness to light (1).

experimental conditions in man and several other mammals, but not in a unicell. The demonstration of circadian dyschronism (or dysphasia) at the cellular level of organization would be most provocative.

One widely used method of quantitative and objective assessment of time relationships inherent in time series data is the so-called *cosinor analysis* developed by Halberg and his colleagues (35, 36), whose aim is to estimate statistically the "microscopic" parameters of a biological rhythm by the least squares fit of a cosine curve. This statistical method enables one to compute values for the circadian *mesor* (M, rhythm adjusted average midway between the highest and lowest values of the fitted curve); *amplitude* (A, half the peak-to-trough difference of the fitted curve, *i.e.*, the difference between the maximum and the mesor); and *acrophase* (ϕ, the lag of the *peak* in the fitted curve from an arbitrarily chosen zero time—which may be local midnight or some other time-point—expressed in hours or degrees, with $360° \equiv$ period of fitted curve; *e.g*, 24 hours. In the cases to be discussed here, this zero time will be designated as the onset of the light in an imposed LD cycle (usually LD: 10,14) on the basis of both computational and biological considerations). The values for M, A, and ϕ are usually expressed together with their 95% confidence limits (CL) or standard errors (SE), together with the probability (p) that the rhythm is statistically significant (so regarded if an F-test of zero-amplitude for the fitted curve yields a p-value < 0.05) and the *percent rhythm*, PR (percentage of variability accounted for by the fitted curve).

Although Pöppel (47) has argued that cosinor analysis can lead to biased parameter estimations if the circadian function as represented by the raw data in actuality is *not* a sinusoidal oscillation, we note that this criticism is true of virtually all approaches and that in most instances the cosine approximation has proved a useful and successful first step in the statistical analysis of biological rhythms. It is certainly more desirable than simply relying on an intuitive, cursory visual analysis of the "macroscopic" raw data.

COSINOR ANALYSIS OF CIRCADIAN RHYTHMS IN *EUGLENA*

Accordingly, a number of the circadian rhythms tabulated for *Euglena* in Table 5.1 were analyzed by the cosinor method (34). Similar or related rhythms have been grouped in the following six sets of figures for convenience and to facilitate the comparison of their acrophases[2] and other parameters. In each set, first the individual time plots are shown (with references to the published data), and then the cosinor display for most or all of the grouped rhythms is presented together with the computed values for ϕ, M, A, p and PR. These cosinors constitute statistical summaries, displayed on polar coordinates, of a rhythm's amplitude and acrophase relations as represented by the length and the angle, respectively, of a directed line. Further, these plots indicate the bivariate statistical confidence region (typically circular or elliptical) at the tip of the vector computed (a) to detect a rhythm (by non-overlap of the pole) and (b) to estimate conservative (95%) confidence intervals for ϕ and A.

Some Major Categories of Rhythms

One of the most intensively studied persisting circadian rhythms in *Euglena* is that of *cell division*. Figure 5.1A shows a typical population growth curve in a culture of *Euglena* synchronized by a LD: 10,14 light cycle under photoautotrophic conditions at 25°C. As is evident from the raw data the mean period ($\bar{\tau}$) of the observed cell division rhythm is 24.0 hours, thus matching that (T) of the imposed synchronizer, with divisions being confined to the dark intervals. Similar data are presented in Figure 5.3A.

In these experiments the length of the light interval was chosen empirically so that an approximate doubling of cell number (factorial increase, or stepsize, $\bar{\bar{ss}}$, of 2.0) of cell number occurred every 24 hours (16). If 24-hour LD cycles having L <10 hours are employed, the stepsize will be <2.0. Thus, with LD: 8,16, the average stepsize is 1.68, indicating that only about ⅔ of the cells divide during any one burst (25). Such cultures, therefore, are developmentally asynchronous since a one-to-one correspondence does not exist among all the constituent cell cycles. In this case, it can be calculated from the

---

[2] Note that ϕ represents the so-called "external acrophase" and in this review relates the peaks of the fitted curve to the onset of light in the synchronizing LD cycle (33) and to "subjective dawn" in DD or LL when the lights would have come on had the synchronizer been continued. This notation corresponds to ψ (phase angle difference between the entraining *Zeitgeber* and the biological oscillation) in the "circadian vocabulary" introduced by Aschoff *et al.* (1).

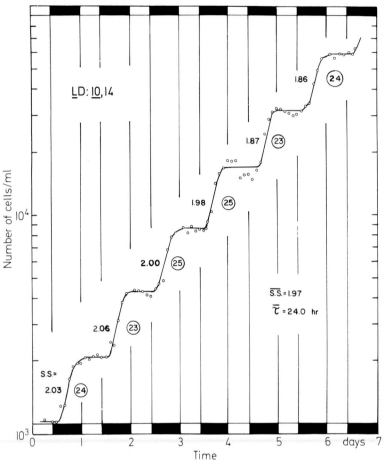

Figure 5.1A. Synchronization of cell division in a population of *Euglena gracilis* Klebs (Z strain) grown photoautotrophically at 25°C in LD: 10, 14. *Ordinate*: cell concentration (cells per milliliter); *abscissa*: elapsed time (days). Step-sizes (ratio of number of cells per milliliter following a division burst to that just before the onset of divisions) are indicated for the successive division bursts. The period of the rhythm is also given in hours (encircled just to the right of each burst). The average period ($\bar{\tau}$) of the rhythm in the culture is essentially identical to that of the synchronizing cycle, and a doubling of cell number usually occurs every 24 hours (25).

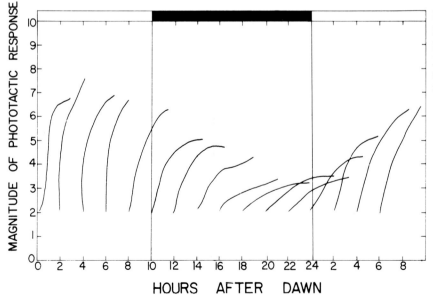

Figure 5.1B. Rhythm of phototactic response of *Euglena* during synchronous photoautotrophic growth in LD: 10, 14. The rhythm persists with a circadian period in *DD* (L. N. Edmunds, unpublished data).

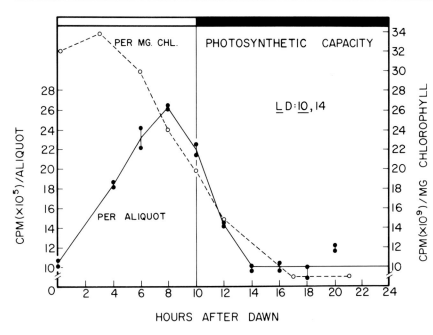

LD:10,14

Figure 5.1C. Photosynthetic capacity during an LD: 10, 14 cycle. Aliquots (10 ml) of the master culture were exposed to 1 μc of $NaH^{14}CO_3$ for 10 min in saturating light. Photosynthetic capacity per aliquot, *solid line*; per mg chlorophyll, *dashed line*. Double points indicate duplicate determinations (57).

Figure 5.1D. Single cosinor displays of circadian rhythms of (*A*) cell division (data from Fig. 5.3A); (*B*) phototactic response (see Fig. 5.1B), and (*C*) photosynthetic capacity (see Fig. 5.1C). The length and direction of the lines (vectors) directed outward from the center of the figure respectively represent a given rhythm's amplitude (*A*) and its acrophase (ϕ) in relation to the synchronizing light cycle as read in degrees (middle circular scale; 0° = onset of *L*). The circular or elliptical regions at the tip of the vectors indicate the joint 95% confidence regions for ϕ and *A*. Mesors and amplitudes expressed as (*A*) $\log_{10}$ (cells/ml) (mantissa only); (*B*) relative magnitude on scale of 1 to 10; and (*C*) CPM ($\times 10^5$)/aliquot. See text for further explanation of cosinor analysis.

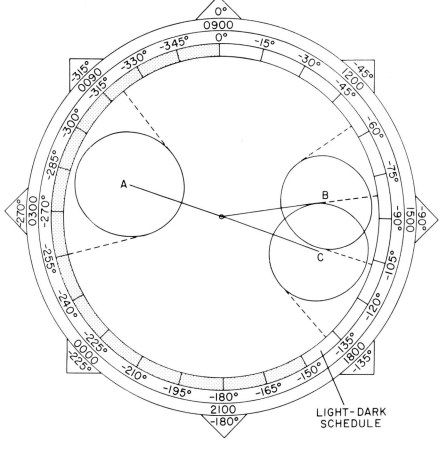

ID	VAR	N	P	PR	M ± SE	A (95% CL)	$\emptyset$° (95% CL)
A	DIV	13	0.002	71.9	0.5 ± 0.02	0.15 (0.07, 0.24)	-287 (-255, -321)
B	TAX	16	<0.001	76.6	4.9 ± 0.22	1.96 (1.13, 2.80)	- 82 (- 56, -107)
C	CO2	12	<0.001	81.2	15.1 ± 0.85	7.50 (4.00, 11.00)	-109 (- 82, -138)

data that the doubling time (g) of the culture is approximately 36 hours; therefore, the length of the *average* individual cell cycle is also by inference about 36 hours.[3] On the other hand, the cells that *do divide* during any given burst do so every 24 hours during a relatively narrow, 6- to 10-hour bandwidth, or "gate," occurring each dark period. Consequently, there is a synchrony with regard to simultaneity of event.

These data suggest, therefore, that the endogenous, light-sensitive, self-sustaining circadian oscillation (pacemaker) hypothesized to underlie the overt circadian population rhythm[3] (by way of analogy, a "hand" of a clock) has been synchronized to a 24-hour period by the imposed 24-hour LD cycle and that this pacemaker then allows cells that are prepared to divide to do so when the "gate" is open (permissive conditions); and, conversely, those cells that do not quite make this gate are prevented from doing so until the next gate opens some 24 hours later. In other words, the cellular pacemaker blocks (or differentially promotes) the progress of cell cycles in a predictable manner by an as yet unknown mechanism (20, 21). We shall return to this rhythm shortly and examine its persistence in DD and LL.

Another major class of circadian rhythms in *Euglena* comprises those involving different types of *cell mobility*. One of these, phototaxis (oriented reponse to a light source), is illustrated in Figure 5.1*B* and can occur in both dividing (L. N. Edmunds, unpublished) and in nondividing cells in the so-called "stationary" phase of growth (2, 6, 8, 29, 46) under both entraining (LD) and free-running (DD) conditions. As is shown, the maximum response to an assaying test light occurs approximately midway into the photofraction (light span) of an LD: 10,14 cycle. In addition to the rhythm of phototactic response, *Euglena* displays persisting circadian rhythms of random (dark) motility in both the wild-type (2, 49) and a bleached mutant (40) and of cell settling (39, 54). This latter rhythm may also

entail oscillations in cell adhesiveness or charge (54).

Yet a third category of persisting circadian rhythms in this unicell include those in *photosynthetic capacity* as assayed by measuring the incorporation of radiolabeled $^{14}CO_2$ into aliquots (exposed to a saturating light source) taken from either synchronously dividing cultures of *Euglena* (Fig. 5.1*C*) or from nondividing cultures (Fig. 5.6*B*); or by monitoring O_2 evolution (Fig. 5.3*B*) (57). In all cases peak capacity occurs midway or later in the L span. These rhythms, too, will be discussed subsequently in greater detail (*cf.* Codd and Merrett (10) and Cook (13)).

Examples of circadian rhythms from each of these classes—cell division, phototactic response, and photosynthetic capacity—have been analyzed by the cosinor method, and, together with the estimation of the various rhythm parameters, are summarized in a single cosinor display (Fig. 5.1*D*). Despite variations due to differing experimental conditions and methodology employed by different workers, it is clear that the *maximum* of the cell division rhythm in the wild type (Z strain) occurs toward the latter part of the scotofraction (dark span) in LD: 10,14 (with the onset occurring at the beginning of darkness), whereas the phototactic and photosynthetic rhythms have their acrophases during the photofraction, nearly in antiphase with the cell division rhythm. All three oscillations are statistically significant ($p < 0.002$) and have relatively large amplitudes.

The Rhythm of Cell Division

Let us now return to the cell division rhythm and examine it in more detail. The evidence obtained under 24-hour full-photoperiod cycles in which $\overline{ss} < 2.00$ is consistent with a pacemaker gating hypothesis, yet by itself does not demand such a mechanism. One could argue that light directly inhibits cell division in an LD cycle (or that darkness promotes it via some cell division factor). Shifts between two sets of environmental conditions occur every 24 hours. Experiments involving the manipulation of various light regimes, however, make this seemingly straightforward hypothesis of direct inhibitory effects of light on mitoses an unlikely—or at the least inadequate—explanation. (Indeed, the notion of light inhibition as a *cause* of division synchrony would appear to be negated by the observations

---

[3] It is important to distinguish an LD cycle from the division cycle as observed in the *population* of cells (some or all of which may divide at about the same time), and from the *individual* cell cycle, whose period can only be inferred from the stepsize of the division bursts and from their period (τ). Thus, in LD: 8,16 the *synchronizer* $T = 24$ hours, $\overline{\tau}_{pop} = 24$ hours, but $\overline{\tau}_{cell} = 36$ hours (although it is assumed that the period of the cellular gating oscillation is 24 hours, matching T (20, 21)). It is possible, of course, that the g's of individual cells are not distributed continuously but rather are distributed discontinuously and multimodally, perhaps clustered at nodal points, around the average value of g seen in the population (21).

that $\overline{ss}$ increases with increasing L spans and that $\overline{g}_{pop}$ is lowest (fastest) in LL.)

These other lines of evidence include: (a) synchronization by LD cycles having $T \neq 24$ hours (e.g., LD: 10,10) may also occur within certain limits (25); (b) appropriate temperature cycles (e.g., 18°/25°C: 12,12 or 28°/35°C: 12,12) will synchronize the rhythm in cultures maintained in LL (53); (c) "skeleton" photoperiods comprising the framework of a normal, full-photoperiod cycle (e.g., LD: 4,4,4:12 or LD: 3,6,3:12) will also synchronize the rhythm to a precise 24-hour period (25); (d) high-frequency (e.g., LD: 1,2) LD cycles and even "random" illumination regimes induce circadian division periodicities (24, 25); and (e) rhythmic cell division will persist for a number of days with $\tau \simeq 24$ hour in the autotrophically grown wild-type batch-cultured under dim LL (18).

This last series of experiments is perhaps the most definitive for autotrophically grown cultures but was restricted by the low light intensities (800 lux) that had to be utilized.[4] Nevertheless, although the division bursts were relatively small (on the average only 17% of the population underwent fission in a given step), those cells that did divide did so during their "subjective night" at the times when they would have experienced darkness had the LD regime been continued. The average width of any given "gate" was approximately 12 hours (the duration of the fission burst in the population), while the time of occurrence of the midpoint of a gate relative to the onset of the light period (*i.e.*, the D/L transition) in the previously imposed, synchronizing LD cycle could be calculated from the expression

$$t_d = k + n\tau$$

where t_d is the midpoint of the observed fission burst, k is a constant (empirically determined to be approximately 12 hours), n is an integer denoting the nth free-running circadian cycle in LL, and τ is the calculated free-running period of the cell division rhythm as exhibited by the *population*. In contrast, the overall generation or doubling time (g) of the culture under these light-limiting conditions (LL$_{dim}$) was about 5½ days. Consequently, if possible cell death is ig-

nored, it can be deduced that the *individual cell cycle*[3] has an average duration of 134 hours.

The results summarized thus far have dealt only with photoautotrophically cultured wild type *Euglena*, and their interpretation is thus necessarily complicated by the dual role of imposed light regimes and signals: as an energy source for photosynthesis, cell growth and division on the one hand, and as a timing cue for the putative circadian pacemaker on the other. This problem has been effectively eliminated by utilizing light-entrainable, nonphotosynthetic mutants of *Euglena* (19, 20, 22, 26, 27, 38).

One such strain is the obligate organotroph, ultraviolet light-induced P_4ZUL photosynthetic mutant of *Euglena* isolated and characterized by Russell and Lyman (48) and later by Schwelitz *et al.* (50). This mutant has reduced amounts of chlorophyll and appears to have a block in the electron transport chain between photosystem I and II and to lack plastoquinone, the postulated primary electron acceptor of PS II. The synchronizing effects of an LD: 10,14 cycle on long term *continuous cultures* (techniques described by Terry and Edmunds (53) of P_4ZUL followed by DD and LL free-runs are shown in Figure 5.2*B* (22, 27). (These data should be compared to a synchronized, continuous culture of the wild type [Z strain] in LD: 10,14 as illustrated in Figure 5.2*A*.) Clearly, the light cycle is synchronizing the cell division rhythm, which then persists with $\overline{\tau} \neq 24.0$ hours for extended time spans in constant conditions with no signs of decaying or damping out. The difference in the wave form of curves A and B (Fig. 5.2*B*) is probably due to a superimposed circadian rhythm of cell settling in the latter (54).

More recently these studies of the cell division rhythm have been extended to the nalidixic acid-induced Y_9ZNalL photosynthetic mutant (26) and to the completely (heat-)bleached W_6ZHL mutant that is totally devoid of chloroplasts (20, 26). A set of results for the latter strain batch-cultured in LD and LL is presented in Figure 5.2*C*; here, the culture generation time (g) is about 48.1 hours while $\overline{\tau}_{LD} = 24.0$ hours and $\overline{\tau}_{LL} = 21.0$ hours. These data are consistent with those of Mitchell (44) for the white, UV-bleached W_nZUL mutant and the pale green, nitrosoguanidine-mutagenized P_7ZNgL mutant (isolated by Russell and Lyman (48)). In the studies for all 5 different photosynthetic mutants of *Euglena*, cell division is confined primarily to the dark spans of LD cycles (or to subjective night in DD or LL). This timing agrees with findings of other workers on the algae *Chlamydomonas, Chlo-*

---

[4] Because of the requirement of light for photosynthesis, one cannot use DD; nor can one impose LL of those moderate intensities normally comprising the L portions of the synchronizing LD cycle (L$_{bright}$ = 3500 lux or 7000 lux) because the population reverts to asynchronous, exponential growth.

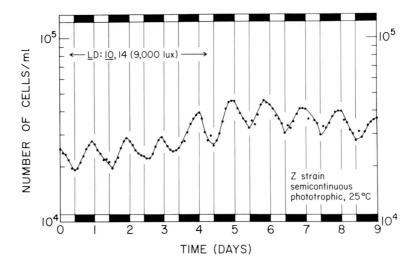

Figure 5.2A. Circadian rhythm of cell division in *Euglena* (Z strain) grown photoautotrophically at 25°C in LD: 10, 14 in semicontinuous culture (compare with Fig. 5.1A). Note that the rate of dilution with fresh medium approximately balances the overall growth rate of the culture (L. N. Edmunds, unpublished data).

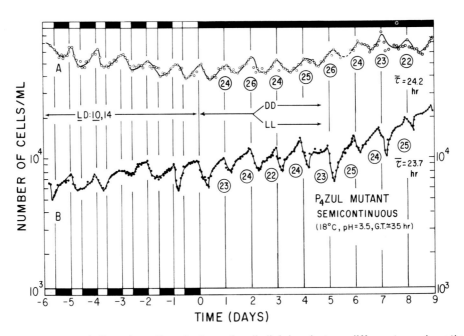

Figure 5.2B. Long term, persisting circadian rhythm of cell division in two different semicontinuous cultures of the P$_4$ZUL photosynthetic mutant of *Euglena* grown on low pH glutamate-malate medium at 18°C. The cultures were first synchronized by LD: 10, 14 (6 monitored days shown) and then placed either in *DD* (*top, curve A*) or in *LL* (*bottom, curve B*); the first nine cycles under constant conditions are indicated. The overall generation time (G.T.) of both cultures was calculated from the known dilution rate to be about 35 hours. Successive period lengths are encircled just below each "free-running" cycle and the average period (τ̄) is given to the right for each curve (27).

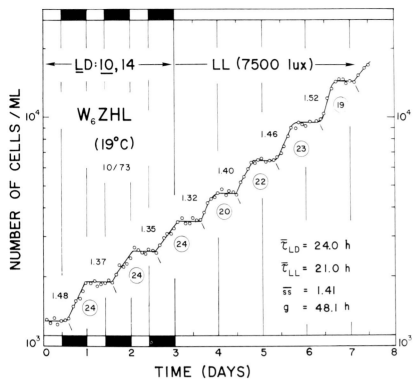

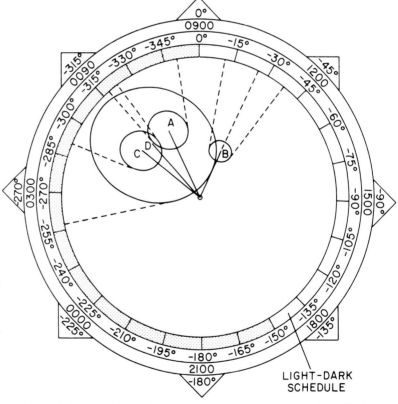

Figure 5.2C. Synchronization of the cell division rhythm and its persistence for at least 5 days under constant illumination in the aplastidic, heat-bleached W_6ZHL mutant of *Euglena gracilis* batch-cultured photoorganotrophically at 19°C under a LD: 10, 14 cycle and subsequently released into *LL* (3500 lux). Labels and notation as for Figure 5.2B. Note that although the period of the population rhythm is about 24 hours, the period of the individual cell cycle is approximately 48 hours (21).

Figure 5.2D. Single cosinor displays for synchronized rhythms of cell division in *Euglena*: (*A*) Z strain (Fig. 5.2A); (*B*) P_4ZUL mutant (Fig. 5.2B, *upper curve A*); (*C*) P_4ZUL mutant (Fig. 5.2B, *lower curve B*); and (*D*) W_6ZHL mutant (Fig. 5.2C). Mesors and amplitudes expressed as $\log_{10}$ (cells/ml) (mantissa only).

ID	VAR	N	P	PR	M ± SE	A (95% CL)	$\emptyset°$ (95% CL)
A	Z	14	<0.001	90.8	0.4 ± 0.00	0.07 (0.05,0.08)	-334 (-318,-351)
B	P4/A	14	<0.001	94.7	0.6 ± 0.00	0.05 (0.04,0.06)	- 24 (- 10,- 39)
C	P4/B	14	<0.001	89.8	0.6 ± 0.00	0.07 (0.05,0.08)	-306 (-291,-323)
D	W6	14	0.031	46.8	0.2 ± 0.01	0.06 (0.01,0.12)	-316 (-256,- 25)

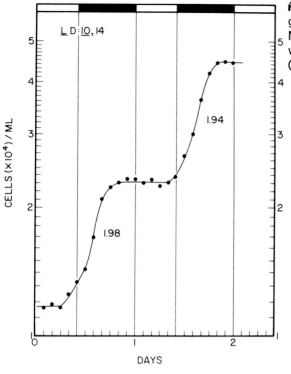

Figure 5.3A. Synchronous cell division of *Euglena gracilis* (Z) grown photoautotrophically at 25°C in LD: 10, 14 cycles. Numbers by division curves indicate step-sizes (factors by which cell concentration increases). Compare with Figure 5.1A (57).

Figure 5.3B. Circadian rhythm of photosynthetic capacity (oxygen evolution) during synchronous growth of *Euglena* (Z) cultured photoautotrophically at 25°C in LD: 10, 14. Compare with CO_2-fixation rhythm depicted in Figure 5.1C (57).

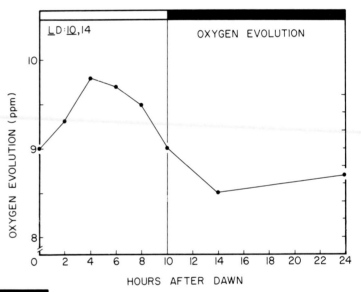

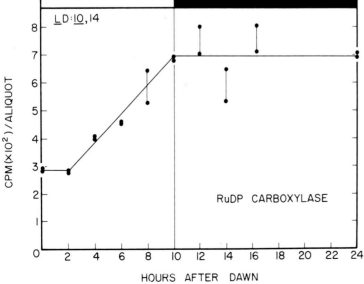

Figure 5.3C. Activity of RuDP carboxylase during synchronous growth of *Euglena* in LD: 10, 14. Two-liter aliquots were removed from the master culture every 2 hours, and the pellets were frozen for later analysis. After sonication the crude supernatant was tested directly for enzyme activity; duplicate determinations are shown (57).

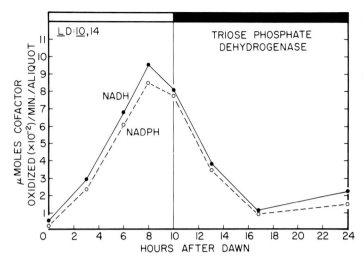

Figure 5.3D. Activity of glyceraldehyde-3-P-dehydrogenase (triose phosphate dehydrogenase) over the cell cycle in synchronized *Euglena* cultures. Both the NADPH and the NADH enzymes were assayed (57).

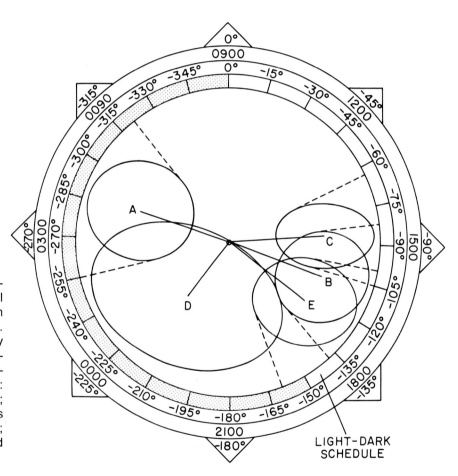

Figure 5.3E. Single cosinor displays of circadian rhythms of (*A*) cell division (Fig. 5.3A), (*B*) CO_2 fixation (Fig. 5.1C), (*C*) O_2 evolution (Fig. 5.3B), (*D*) RuDP carboxylase activity (Fig. 5.3C), and (*E*) glyceraldehyde-3-P-dehydrogenase (Fig. 5.3D). Mesors and amplitudes expressed as: (*A*) $\log_{10}$ (cells/ml) (mantissa only); (*B*) CPM ($\times 10^5$)/aliquot; (*C*) parts per million; (*D*) CPM ($\times 10^2$)/aliquot; and (*E*) μM NaDP(H) oxidized ($\times 10^{-2}$)/min/aliquot.

ID	VAR	N	P	PR	M ± SE	A (95% CL)	$\emptyset°$ (95% CL)
A	DIV	13	0.002	71.9	0.5 ± 0.02	0.15 (0.07,0.24)	-287 (-255,-321)
B	CO2	12	<0.001	81.2	15.1 ± 0.85	7.50 (4.0 ,11.0)	-109 (- 82,-138)
C	O2	8	0.003	90.0	8.8 ± 0.08	0.84 (0.41,1.26)	- 85 (- 63,-105)
D	RuDP	10	0.056	56.1	5.7 ± 0.47	1.68 ( )	-217 ( )
E	GPD	8	0.004	89.3	3.6 ± 0.49	4.5 (2.12,6.9)	-127 (- 99,-160)

Table 5.2
Linear Rhythmometry of Cell Division[a]

Series	N	τ	PR	M ± SE	A ± SE	ϕ ± SE
Z (LD)	108	26.0	8.0	0.494 ± 0.009	0.036 ± 0.012	
		24.4	21.4	0.493 ± 0.008	0.059 ± 0.011	
		24.2	21.9	0.493 ± 0.008	0.060 ± 0.011	
		24.0	22.0	0.494 ± 0.008	0.060 ± 0.011	−337.1° ± 11°
		23.8	21.5	0.494 ± 0.008	0.060 ± 0.011	
		23.6	20.4	0.494 ± 0.008	0.058 ± 0.011	
		22.0	2.7	0.494 ± 0.009	0.021 ± 0.013	
P₄ZUL (LD)	141	26.0	3.9	0.617 ± 0.005	0.017 ± 0.007	
		24.2	26.7	0.617 ± 0.004	0.044 ± 0.006	
		24.0	29.0	0.617 ± 0.004	0.045 ± 0.006	−319° ± 8°
		23.8	29.1	0.617 ± 0.004	0.047 ± 0.006	
		23.6	32.3	0.617 ± 0.004	0.048 ± 0.006	
		23.4	33.0	0.617 ± 0.004	0.049 ± 0.006	−351° ± 7°
		23.2	33.0	0.617 ± 0.004	0.049 ± 0.006	
		23.0	32.4	0.617 ± 0.004	0.048 ± 0.006	
		22.0	18.0	0.617 ± 0.005	0.037 ± 0.07	
P₄ ZUl (LL)	174	26.0	4.4	0.727 ± 0.006	0.023 ± 0.008	
		24.2	20.6	0.728 ± 0.005	0.051 ± 0.008	
		24.0	21.9	0.729 ± 0.005	0.053 ± 0.008	−292° ± 8°
		23.8	22.5	0.729 ± 0.005	0.054 ± 0.007	
		23.6	22.5	0.728 ± 0.005	0.054 ± 0.007	−315 ± 8°
		23.4	21.9	0.728 ± 0.005	0.053 ± 0.008	
		23.2	20.7	0.728 ± 0.005	0.051 ;± 0.008	
		22.0	5.8	0.726 ± 0.006	0.023 ± 0.008	

[a] Least squares fit of trial periods at 1-hour intervals in the spectral region from 20 to 28 hours describes consolidate periods of the cell division rhythm in the Z strain and the P₄ZUL photosynthetic mutant of *Euglena* (see Fig. 5.2 for the time plots of the original data). Only a portion of the computer printout is tabulated in each case.

rella, Gonyaulax, and *Gymnodinium* and the ciliates *Paramecium* and *Tetrahymena* (see review by Edmunds (20, 21)).

To summarize the foregoing data conveniently, a cosinor display for these long term persisting cell division rhythms in the Z strain and the P₄ZUL and W₆ZHL photosynthetic mutants is shown in Figure 5.2*D* together with the key rhythm parameters. The *p* values for the rhythms of cell division monitored in continuous culture are all *p* <0.001. It should be noted that these long trains of data enable one to perform a more thorough frequency analysis by the least squares method. One can carry out a chronobiologic "*serial section*" by fitting a fixed-period cosine curve to consecutive data intervals displaced by increments throughout the time series so as to ascertain continuously (by moving point estimates) the mesor, amplitude, and acrophase of a rhythm (31, 34, 36).

Thus, if one applies least squares frequency analysis to the cell division rhythm of Z strain in continuous culture (Fig. 5.2*A*) for the periods between 20.0 and 28.0 hours (at intervals of 0.2

hour), the best fit (highest PR) yields a period of 24.0 hours, a 22% rhythm, an amplitude of 0.060 (±0.011 SE) (log₁₀ cells/ml, mantissa only), a mesor of 0.494 (±0.008 SE), and an acrophase of −337 (±11° SE). A portion of the computer printout is shown in Table 5.2. This analysis objectively confirms and quantifies the subjective impression given by the raw data that the rhythm is synchronized to τ = 24 hours under LD: 10,14. The acrophase (peak cell division almost at end of the scotofraction) approximates that seen for the batch culture shown in Figure 5.1*A*, but occurs about 3 hours later than the culture shown in Figure 5.3*A* (acrophase = −287°; see corresponding cosinor display in Figure 5.1*D*).

Table 5.2 also gives some of the results obtained by frequency analysis of the long train of data for the cell division rhythm in the P₄ZUL mutant in LD: 10,14 (Fig. 5.2*B*, curve B) and also during the LL free-run. If the LD cycle is assumed to synchronize the culture to τ = 24 hours, the values of the rhythm parameters are as follows: 29% rhythm, mesor of 0.617 (±0.004 SE), amplitude of 0.045 (±0.006), and acrophase of −319° (± 8° SE). (It is interesting to note that a slightly higher amplitude is found at $\tau = 23.4$, probably due to the fact that only 6 days of data were utilized.) In LL, the curve having the highest amplitude (0.054 ± 0.007) corresponds to a τ of 23.6 hours over the 9 days examined, with a 22.5% rhythm, a mesor of 0.728 (±0.005), and an acrophase of −315° (±8°). The "microscopic" analysis agrees rather closely with the visually determined, "macroscopic" τ_{FR} of 23.7 hours (Fig. 5.2*B*, curve B). The acrophase of this curve somewhat leads that found by single cosinor analysis (Fig. 5.2*D*) for the P$_4$ZUL mutant in another experiment (Fig. 5.2*B*, curve A, $\phi = -24°$) under slightly different conditions with sampling at 2-hour intervals instead of every hour (curve B).

The Rhythm of Photosynthetic Capacity

The oscillation in photosynthetic competence in *Euglena* (Z strain) has also been examined intensively in photoautotrophic cultures synchronized by LD: 10,14. Photosynthetic capacity, as measured by the ability of an aliquot of cells to incorporate $NaH^{14}CO_3$ in saturating white light (7500 lux) for 10 min, was found to vary in a cyclic manner (Fig. 5.1*C*) during the cell cycle (Fig. 5.3*A*), reaching a peak 2 hours before the onset of darkness (55). Alternatively, if oxygen evolution (Fig. 5.3*B*) were measured across the LD cycle as an assay of photosynthetic capacity (55), a peak was found to occur at about 4 hours after the onset of light. Similar studies have been conducted by Codd and Merrett (10) and Cook (13), although there was some variation in the results obtained. More recently, Lonergan and Sargent (42) have found persisting circadian rhythms of both CO_2-uptake and O_2-evolution in continuous dim illumination in nondividing cultures (the rhythms peak in the mid-subjective day), and Laval-Martin, Shuch, and Edmunds (41) have discovered a persisting circadian rhythm of CO_2-uptake in nondividing cultures maintained in high frequency LD:⅓, ⅓ (T = 40 min) LD cycles in both Z and ZR strains.

Several of the photosynthetic light reactions were investigated during the cell cycle to determine what role they played in the control of the observed rhythmic changes in capacity. Light-saturation curves showed no major change in the light-limited region. No fluctuations were found in Hill reaction activity or photoreduction

of methyl red during the cell cycle. These results suggest that the reactions comprising photosystems I and II themselves do not generate the capacity rhythm (57)(but see Lonergan and Sargent (42)).

Some of the photosynthetic dark reactions were also followed during the cell cycle in an attempt to determine their possible role in the control of the rhythm of photosynthetic capacity (55). The step activity of ribulose-1,5-diphosphate carboxylase showed no correlation with the rhythm (Fig. 5.3*C*). On the other hand, the activity of glyceraldehyde-3-phosphate dehydrogenase was found to parallel the change in photosynthetic rate under certain conditions of growth (Fig. 5.3*D*). The rhythm in photosynthetic capacity could be effectively divorced from the cell cycle itself by placing cultures in high frequency light cycles (LD: 2,4) or in stationary growth phase conditions. Indeed, under nondividing conditions the close correlation of the rhythmic changes in glyceraldehyde-3-P dehydrogenase (as contrasted, for example, with the pattern observed for ribulose-1,5-diphosphate carboxylase) with the circadian rhythm of photosynthetic capacity is particularly striking; this enzyme may play a role in the mediation and control of the overt rhythmicity (see Fig. 5.6*B*), although other mechanisms are also probably involved (41, 42).

The results of a single cosinor analysis (Fig. 5.3*E*) objectively, succinctly, and quantitatively portray the time relations among these related rhythms and the entraining LD: 10,14 cycle while indicating also some of the corresponding uncertainties. The acrophases progress as follows: O_2 evolution (−85°), CO_2 incorporation (−109°), glyceraldehyde-3-P-dehydrogenase (−127°), ribulose-1,5-diphosphate carboxylase (−217°), and finally, cell division (−287°). Note in the cosinor plot for RuDP carboxylase a *p*-value of 0.056; the corresponding error ellipse slightly overlaps the pole. The time plot (Fig. 5.3*C*) shows the nonsinusoidal steplike form of changes in the activity of this enzyme: macroscopically, it has been called a "step enzyme" rather than a "peak enzyme."

Circadian Rhythms in Gross Metabolic Parameters

The general patterns of biosynthesis of gross biochemical constituents have been mapped across the cell cycle in cultures of *Euglena* syn-

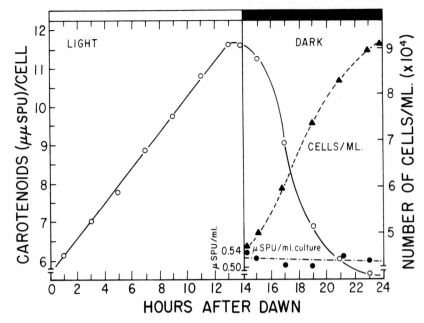

Figure 5.4A. Carotenoid content of *Euglena gracilis* (Z) during synchronous growth in L̲D: 1̲4, 10. (17).

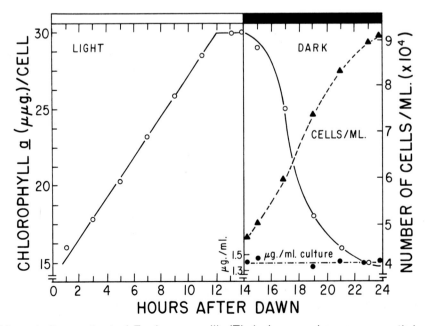

Figure 5.4B. Chlorophyll *a* content of *Euglena gracilis* (Z) during synchronous growth in L̲D: 1̲4, 10. (17).

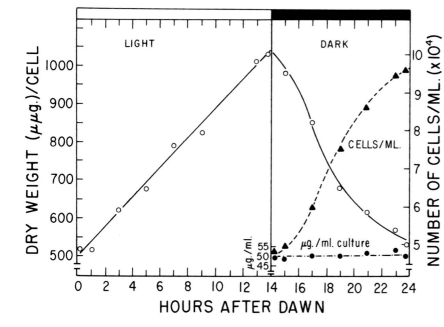

Figure 5.4C. Dry weight of *Euglena gracilis* (Z) during synchronous growth in LD: 14, 10. Cell number was constant throughout the light period and doubled during the dark period (*dashed line*); the number of cells/ml is given on the right ordinate. The dry weight per average cell (*left ordinate*) is plotted on the abscissa as a function of time (hours after the onset of light). Dry weight/ml culture during the dark period is indicated also in the *lower right corner* of the graph (17).

Figure 5.4D. Single cosinor display of circadian rhythms in metabolic parameters in *Euglena* grown photoautotrophically in synchronous culture in LD: 14, 10. (*A*) Cell concentration, (*B*) total carotenoids (Fig. 5.4A), (*C*) total chlorophyll *a* (Fig. 5.4B), (*D*) dry weight (Fig. 5.4C). Mesors and amplitudes for each variable expressed in units identical to those given in their respective figures; cell concentration given as percent of the mean value (cells [×10⁴]/ml).

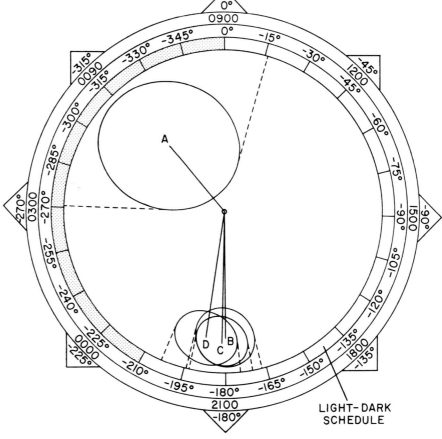

ID	VAR	N	P	PR	M ± SE	A (95% CL)	Ø° (95% CL)
A	DIV	14	0.015	53.3	5.9 ± 0.38	1.93 (0.39, 3.5)	-319 (-270,- 16)
B	CAR	13	<0.001	93.8	8.4 ± 0.17	2.86 (2.19, 3.5)	-180 (-166,-194)
C	CHL	13	<0.001	95.7	22.2 ± 0.37	7.5 (6.1 , 9.0)	-181 (-170,-193)
D	DWT	14	<0.001	94.3	763. ±13.0	226. (179. , 273.)	-189 (-175,-203)

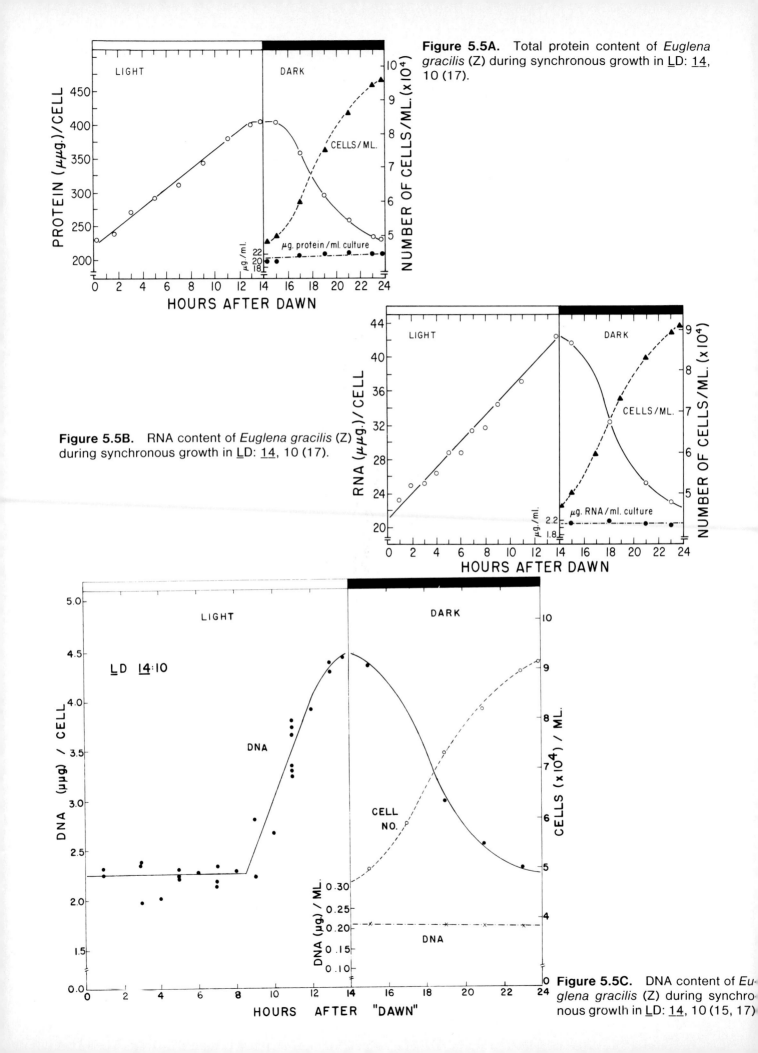

Figure 5.5A. Total protein content of *Euglena gracilis* (Z) during synchronous growth in LD: 14, 10 (17).

Figure 5.5B. RNA content of *Euglena gracilis* (Z) during synchronous growth in LD: 14, 10 (17).

Figure 5.5C. DNA content of *Euglena gracilis* (Z) during synchronous growth in LD: 14, 10 (15, 17).

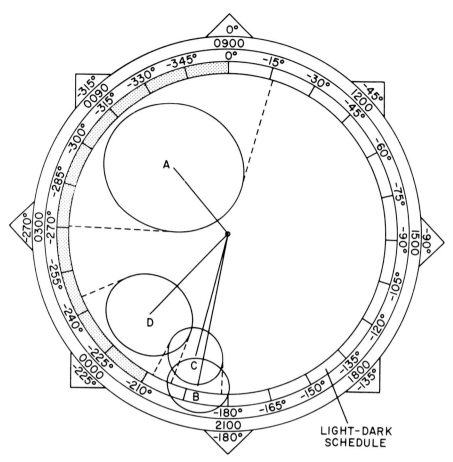

Figure 5.5D. Single cosinor displays of circadian rhythms in metabolic variables in *Euglena* grown photoauto-trophically in synchronous culture in L̲D: 1̲4, 10 (*A*) cell concentration; (*B*) total cellular protein (Fig. 5.5A); (*C*) total cellular RNA (Fig. 5.5B), and (*D*) total cellular DNA (Fig. 5.5C). Mesors and amplitudes expressed in picograms/cell for cell rhythms except cell concentration (percent of the mean value of cell concentration, measured as cells [×10⁴]/ml).

ID	VAR	N	P	PR	M ± SE	A (95% CL)	Ø° (95% CL)
A	DIV	14	0.015	53.3	5.9 ± 0.38	1.93 (0.39, 3.5)	-319 (-270,-376)
B	PRO	15	<0.001	95.6	315. ± 4.1	86. (86. ,86.)	-191 (-179,-198)
C	RNA	15	<0.001	93.1	31.4 ± 0.49	8.5 (6.7 ,10.4)	-195 (-182,-208)
D	DNA	17	<0.001	81.0	2.9 ± 0.10	1.04 (0.67, 1.41)	-223 (-201,-245)

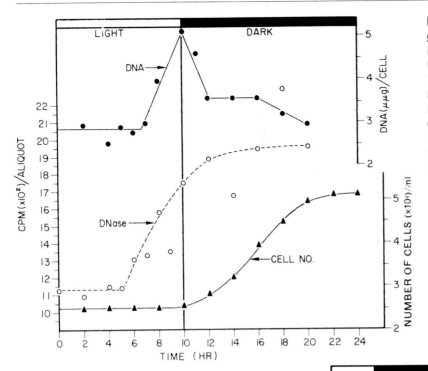

Figure 5.6A. Periodic activity of *Euglena* DNase (single-stranded DNA substrate) and discontinuous synthesis of DNA. DNA synthesis (●) begins about 6–7 hours after the beginning of the light span. DNase activity per aliquot (○) approximately parallels DNA synthesis. Cell concentration (▲) was determined at 2-hour intervals and indicates that the culture had been synchronized by the imposed LD: 10, 14 cycle (56).

Figure 5.6B. Circadian variations in photosynthetic capacity (NaH $^{14}CO_3$ incorporation) and in the activity of glyceraldehyde-3-phosphate dehydrogenase (TPD) activity in nondividing, stationary cultures of *Euglena* in LD: 10, 14 at 25°C on minimal salt medium (57).

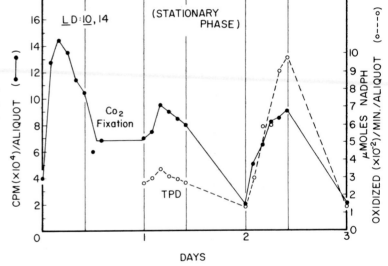

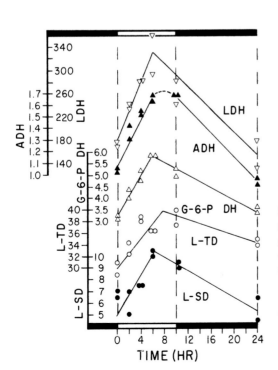

Figure 5.6C. Circadian variations in the activities of several enzymes in nondividing, stationary cultures of *Euglena* in LD: 10, 14 at 19°C on low pH glutamate-malate medium. Enzyme activities are given on the ordinates. ●, L-serine deaminase (L-SD) activity (μmoles pyruvate produced/min); ○, L-threonine deaminase (L-TD) activity (μmoles α-ketobutyrate produced/min); △, glucose-6-phosphate dehydrogenase (G-6-P DH) activity (μmoles $\times$ 10^2 NADH oxidized/min); ▲, alanine dehydrogenase (ADH activity μmoles $\times$ 10^2 NADH oxidized/min); ▽, lactic dehydrogenase (LDH) activity (μmoles $\times$ 10^2 NADH oxidized/min) (F. M. Sulzman and L. N. Edmunds, unpublished) (20).

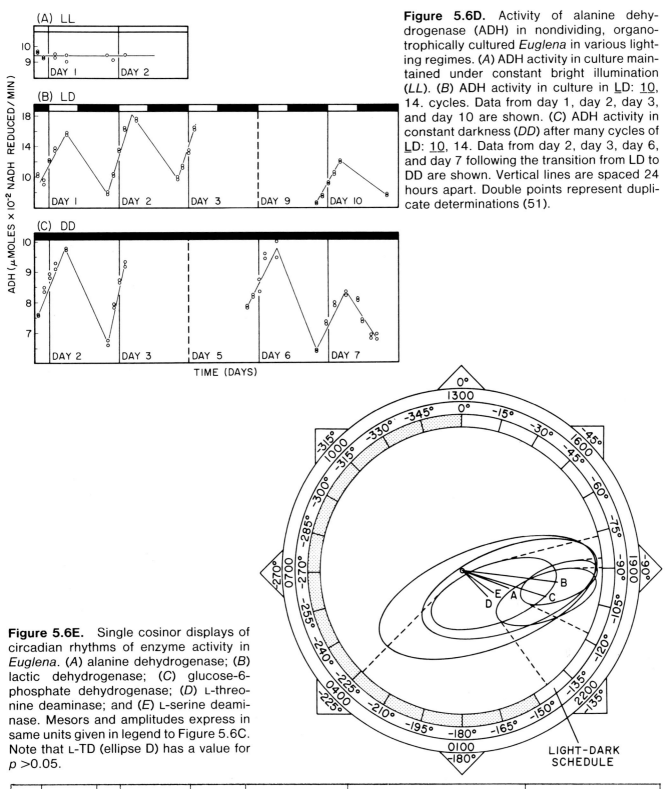

Figure 5.6D. Activity of alanine dehydrogenase (ADH) in nondividing, organotrophically cultured *Euglena* in various lighting regimes. (*A*) ADH activity in culture maintained under constant bright illumination (*LL*). (*B*) ADH activity in culture in LD: 10, 14. cycles. Data from day 1, day 2, day 3, and day 10 are shown. (*C*) ADH activity in constant darkness (*DD*) after many cycles of LD: 10, 14. Data from day 2, day 3, day 6, and day 7 following the transition from LD to DD are shown. Vertical lines are spaced 24 hours apart. Double points represent duplicate determinations (51).

Figure 5.6E. Single cosinor displays of circadian rhythms of enzyme activity in *Euglena*. (*A*) alanine dehydrogenase; (*B*) lactic dehydrogenase; (*C*) glucose-6-phosphate dehydrogenase; (*D*) L-threonine deaminase; and (*E*) L-serine deaminase. Mesors and amplitudes express in same units given in legend to Figure 5.6C. Note that L-TD (ellipse D) has a value for $p > 0.05$.

ID	VAR	N	P	PR	M ± SE	A (95% CL)	Ø° (95% CL)
A	ADH	6	0.061	84.5	1.1 ± 0.19	0.68 ( )	-112 ( )
B	LDH	6	0.002	98.6	185. ± 8.5	132. (85. ,183.)	- 98 (- 86,-117)
C	G6PDH	6	0.003	97.8	4.0 ± 0.16	1.71 (0.94, 2.60)	-109 (- 90,-144)
D	LTD	6	0.122	75.4	35. ± 1.91	4.1 ( )	-137 ( )
E	LSD	6	0.034	89.6	7.2 ± 0.67	2.60 (0.33, 8.9)	-127 (- 77,-224)

chronized by LD: 14,10 under photoautotrophic conditions of growth (17). Dry weight, total protein, chlorophyll *a*, carotenoids, soluble protein, RNA, DNA, and total phosphorus were determined at intervals of two hours during synchronous growth of *Euglena* at a cell concentration of 5–10 × 10⁴ cells/ml maintained by periodic dilution. Detailed analyses of the soluble proteins (DEAE-cellulose fractionation) and of the intracellular distribution of phosphorus were made also.

In general, a linear doubling of each of the major components occurred during the photofraction, as illustrated in Figures 5.4*B*–*D* and 5.5*B*–*D*. There was no net synthesis during the dark. Since cell number doubled during the scotofraction (Figs. 5.4*A* and 5.5*A*), a halving of the amounts of the variables in each cell occurred. It is apparent that not all patterns of biosynthesis proceed in the same manner. Different absolute rates of synthesis were found for the different compounds, with a doubling of a given substance sometimes being completed *before* the end of the photofraction (e.g., carotenoids, chlorophyll *a*; Fig 5.4 *A* and *B*). In most work subsequent to these earlier experiments we have reduced the photofraction from LD: 14,10 to LD: 10,14. The most notable exception to the linear increase observed for most variables was the discontinuous synthesis of DNA (Fig. 5,5*C*) during the photofraction in LD: 14,10. DNA replicated only during the last 6 hours of the photofraction, commencing approximately at 8 hours after the onset of light. Although DNA replication is a necessary condition for cellular division, it is not necessarily a sufficient one in *Euglena* (15). Most of the foregoing results agree well with those of Cook (11, 12).

The single cosinor displays shown in Figures 5.4*D* and 5.5*D* indicate that these circadian rhythms are highly significant (with values for $p < 0.001$). All the variables (except for DNA) have their acrophases clustered at about −180° to −195°, toward the end of the synthetic (light) span and just preceding the onset of cell division in the population. These results suggest that the G_1 phase of the cycle lasts about 8 hours, that the S phase is approximately 6–7 hours, and that the G_2 phase is relatively short. *Individual* cells, of course, show considerable variation in the timing of these processes.

Presumably similar biosynthetic temporal patterns would obtain under free-running conditions inasmuch as the overt rhythm of cell division persists under constant dim LL (18). Their assay, however, would be complicated by the fact that in the population only a small number of cells divide during any given 24-hour time span with the result that the culture is developmentally asynchronous. Better results might be achieved with the photosynthetic mutants where stepsizes of 2.0 can be routinely attained (26, 38).

Periodic Changes in Enzyme Activity during the Cell Cycle

In addition to temporally mapping the patterns of various gross cellular constituents, the activities of a number of enzymes have been monitored during synchronous growth of wild-type *Euglena* photoautotrophically batch-cultured in LD: 10,14; certain of these enzymes might contribute to some of the concomitant overt physiological rhythms routinely observed (20). Furthermore, a circadian oscillation in enzyme activity can quite validly itself be considered as an index of an underlying biological pacemaker. Some of these periodic enzymes are listed in Table 5.1.

Although the activity of many of these enzymes increases more or less linearly throughout L and then levels off (on a per aliquot basis) with the onset of D and ensuing cell division in the synchronized population, this is not always the case. Thus, deoxyribonuclease activity (Fig. 5.6*A*) remains at nearly the same level for about 5–6 hours after the onset of L and then sharply increases until the onset of D some 5 hours later, at which time it levels off (56). This discontinuous increase parallels that of total DNA (15, 17) (see Fig. 5.5*C*) though occurring slightly before the latter; the two events are possibly associated. Likewise, both NADH- and NADPH-dependent glyceraldehyde-3-phosphate dehydrogenase (= triose phosphate dehydrogenase) exhibit periodic increases during the cell cycle (57) (see Fig. 5.3*D*). In this case, the activity of the enzyme peaks between 6 and 8 hours after the onset of L in LD: 10,14 and then commences to decrease well before the onset of D and cell division back to its base level (on an aliquot basis). The close correlation of the rhythmic changes in GPD with the circadian rhythm of photosynthetic capacity, as we have already noted, is particularly striking (especially in stationary culture) (see Fig. 5.6*B*). This enzyme may play a role in the mediation and regulation of the overt rhythmicity. It seems likely that most, if not all, of the enzymes listed in Table 5.1 will continue to oscillate under LL (or DD) and constant temperature if one can draw a parallel from the persistence under these conditions of the circadian rhythm in cell division.

Circadian Oscillations in Enzyme Activity in Stationary Cultures

Periodic changes in enzyme activity during the cell cycle of *Euglena* have already been discussed (see Table 5.1). The system has been simplified by divorcing autogenous enzyme oscillations from those directly generated by the driving force of the cell cycle itself (whereby replication of successive genes would lead to an ordered, temporally differentiated expression of enzyme activities). This was accomplished by using light-synchronized, photoorganotrophically batch-cultured wild-type *Euglena* that had reached stationary growth stage where essentially no net change in cell number occurs (20, 21). These cultures had been previously grown and were then subsequently maintained in LD: 10,14 at 19°C.

Relatively large amplitude oscillations were found in the activities of alanine, lactic and glucose-6-P dehydrogenases, and L-serine, and L-threonine deaminases (with maxima usually occurring during light) entrained to a 24-hour period by the imposed LD cycle (Fig. 5.6C). Similar findings have been made (57) for glyceraldehyde-3-P dehydrogenase in stationary cultures of *Euglena* photoautotrophically grown and maintained in LD: 10,14 at 25°C (Fig. 5.6B). These rhythmic changes in enzyme activity, therefore, were effectively divorced from the cell cycle and periodic replication of the genome. Even more interesting, however, was our finding (27, 51, 52) that the activity of alanine dehydrogenase (ADH) continues to oscillate in these nondividing (infradian) cultures for at least 14 days in DD (but not in LL), and thus constitutes an overt circadian rhythm in itself (Fig. 5.6D).

The time relations and other rhythm parameters for the enzymatic oscillations shown in Figure 5.6C are presented in the single cosinor display of Figure 5.6E. The variations in threonine deaminase (L-TD) barely approach the 10% level of statistical significance ($p = 0.122$; note ellipse extends beyond pole). If one macroscopically reexamines the time plot for this enzyme (Fig. 5.6C), one observes that of all 5 curves obtained, L-TD had the smallest amplitude (the range extends from about 30 to only 38 units of

enzymatic activity) and the last point did not return back to the original level, while the other enzymes exhibited close to a doubling in activity. Clearly, additional data are needed on this variable. Additional data, also desirable for alanine dehydrogenase ($p = 0.061$), are furnished in Figure 5.6D (51) and by a complete 24-hour curve with sampling at 2- to 3-hour intervals (52).

AN ACROPHASE CHART FOR THE CIRCADIAN SYSTEM OF *EUGLENA*

A convenient way to illustrate the time relationships of the various circadian rhythms (listed in Table 5.1) in *Euglena* to the LD cycle imposed during synchronization (usually LD: 10,14) is by means of an *(external) acrophase* (ϕ) *chart* (Fig. 5.7). Such a chart also allows one to visualize the synchronized time relations among the various rhythms.

In this presentation, actual acrophases[5] (computed by cosinor analysis or subjectively estimated from published chronograms) are utilized rather than the variable phase reference points given in Table 5.1. In addition, similar types of rhythms are grouped. Thus, cell division rhythms in the wild type and the several mutants all show ϕ's in the latter part of the dark span (or during late subjective light in LL or DD), while most synthetic activities (gross metabolic variables and enzymatic activity) show high values towards the end of the light span (or in the late subjective day in the case of alanine dehydrogenase, which was also monitored under free-running conditions of constant illumination and temperature).

Clearly, then, the *Euglena* system provides an excellent case for *temporal differentiation*: a large number of diverse behavioral, physiological, and biochemical activities are partitioned in time—24-hour time—thus providing dimensions for both environmental adaptation and, what is at least equally important, functional integration in time. One would like next to examine several rhythms concurrently in LL or DD to see whether desynchronization can occur in a uni-

---

[5] Further standardization has been attempted by reference to a LD: 10,14 cycle throughout, although in several cases measurements were made in an LD: 12,12 or LD: 14,10 regimen. In these instances ϕ could differ possibly by an hour or so (especially if the rhythm were not keyed to the onset of light but rather to the light-to-dark transition) from the values that would be obtained in LD: 10,14.

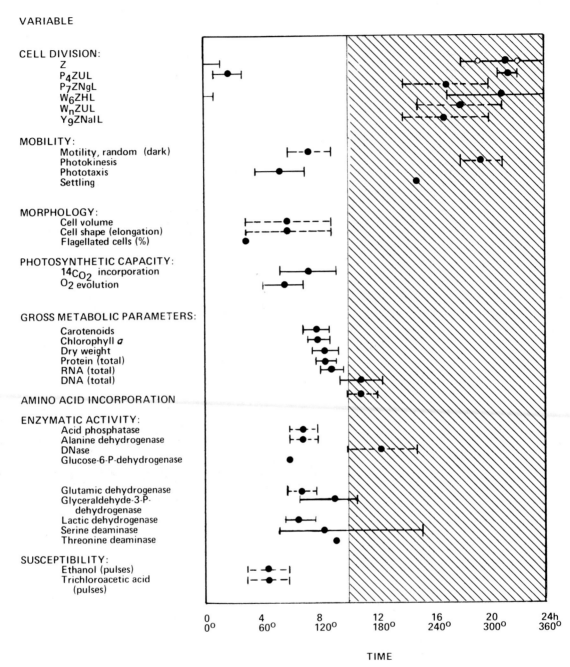

Figure 5.7. Circadian system of *Euglena*. Acrophase (φ) chart for *Euglena* showing the time relations among the circadian rhythms listed in Table 5.1. The *bars* extending to the right and left of the acrophase points give the 95% confidence interval where calculated by cosinor analysis. In all cases acrophases are used (in contrast to the variable and arbitrarily chosen phase markers for timing itemized in Table 5.1). Single points or points with *dashed lines and brackets* indicate subjective estimates of the acrophase from published data without benefit of statistical analysis. (The data for gross metabolic variables, although originally obtained in LD: 14, 10, have been adjusted to correspond to a synchronizing LD: 10, 14 cycle used for most of the other rhythms.) By convention, the sign of the degree indications on the abscissa is negative.

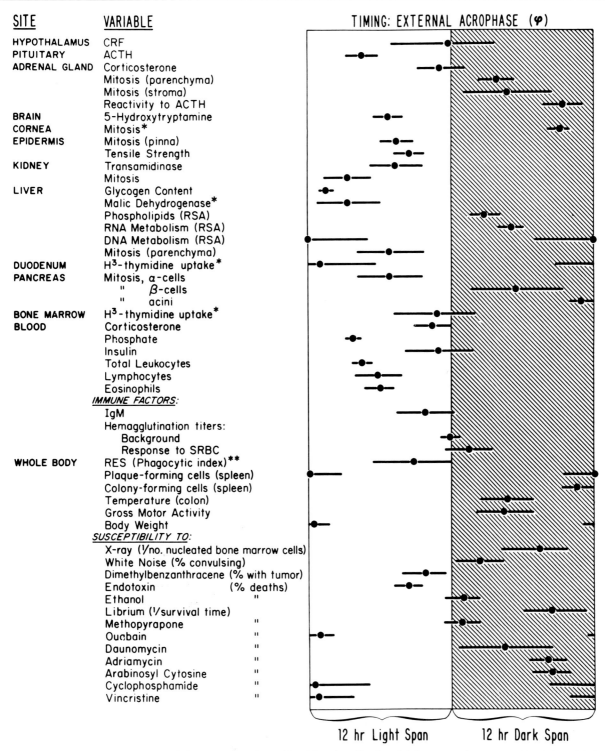

Figure 5.8. Circadian system of the mouse, described by the fit of a 24-hour cosine curve to data obtained in most instances by serially independent sampling as to individuals. Point estimate of the acrophase, defined as lag from zero time of the peak in cosine function best approximating the data, shown as a *dot*, while *horizontal bars* denote 95% confidence arc of acrophase. Circadian rhythms characterize many variables in this rodent and their timing is quite similar for some of these variables, whereas there are marked differences in acrophase for other variables. Nonoverlapping confidence intervals indicate the statistical significance of the differences in acrophase. Such can be found for the same variable, mitosis, in different tissues, as in the adrenal gland on the one hand or the ear pinna, cornea, or liver parenchyma on the other hand. The near ubiquity of circadian organization in this mammal (and others) can be aligned with the importance of these rhythms: they determine susceptibility-resistance cycles to many agents, ranging from physical ones (x-ray or white noise) to bacteriologic ones (endotoxin) and to drugs. (Original data from Chronobiology Laboratories of Minnesota, Minneapolis, * Department of Anatomy, Little Rock, Arkansas, and ** University Medical School of Szeged, Hungary.)

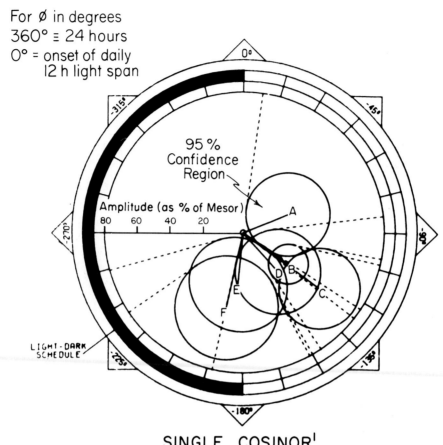

For ∅ in degrees
360° ≡ 24 hours
0° = onset of daily
　　12 h light span

SINGLE COSINOR[1]

KEY TO ELLIPSES	Drug Tested	# Studies	Total # Mice	p[2]	% Rhythm[3]	Amplitude[4] (95% C.L.)	Acrophase;∅ (95% C.L.)
A	DAUNOMYCIN	4	690	.021	31	29 (4,54)	- 67° (- 8,-127)
B	ADRIAMYCIN	6	1072	<.001	60	33 (21,45)	-124° (-103,-146)
C	ARA-C	2	480	<.001	76	56 (32,80)	-126° (-100,-151)
D	MELPHALAN	4	456	.015	33	31 (18,57)	-138° (- 83,-193)
E	CYCLOPHOSPHAMIDE	6	826	.027	18	32 (3,60)	-185° (-123,-255)
F	VINCRISTINE	2	239	.007	67	46 (15,76)	-193° (-150,-235)

Figure 5.9. Circadian rhythms in resistance of mice to anticancer drugs (evaluated from data on percentage survival vs. treatment-timing). Acrophase differences and differing amplitudes (potential gains) and corresponding variabilities of murine circadian susceptibility rhythms to carcinostatic drugs (from fit of 24-hour cosine to data from 6 time points, 4 hours apart, on mice kept in LD: 12, 12. 1) Results from least-square fitting of 24-hour cosine curve, 2) from test of zero-amplitude hypothesis, 3) percent rhythm = percent of total variability attributable to fitted cosine, and 4) expressed as percent of mesor.

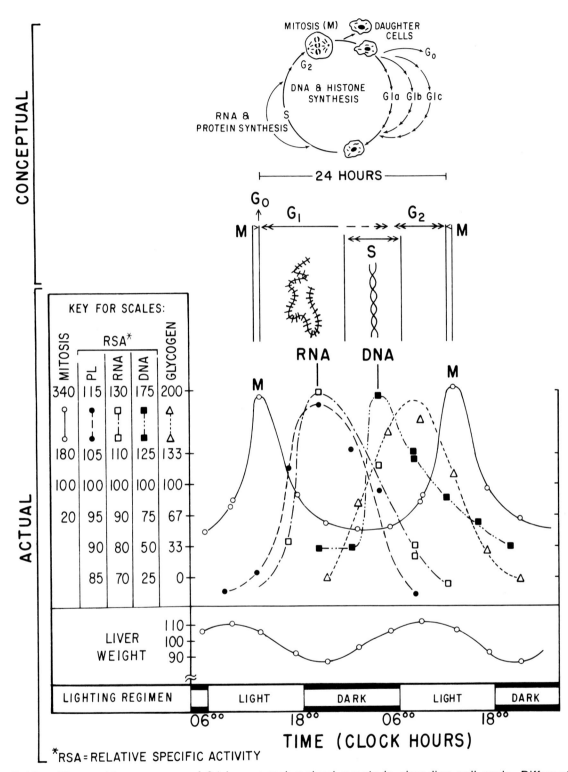

Figure 5.10. Observable sequence of 24-hour synchronized events in circadian cell cycle. Different cellular processes in growing mouse liver: labeling of phospholipid (PL), RNA and DNA, glycogen content and mitosis (as well as liver weight) in relation to a LD: 12, 12 regime.

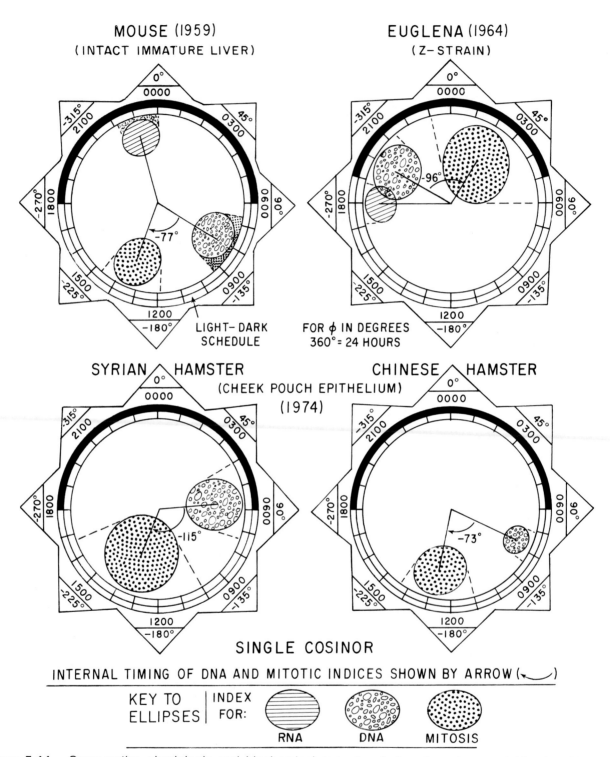

Figure 5.11. Comparative physiologic and biochemical aspects of circadian chronocytokinetics. Note time relations between indices for RNA, DNA, and mitosis in unicell and mouse liver and more limited information on hamsters. A web of cellular rhythms underlying responses to hormones and drugs, in many species, can be described *in vivo* with time specification for a given event; pertinent information in various models of disease, notably of cancer, awaits exploitation for chronotherapy.

cellular system; a demonstration of circadian dysphasia would have important implications as to the multiple pacemaker problem and the nature of the time-keeping mechanism or mechanisms.

IMPLICATIONS AT HIGHER LEVELS OF ORGANIZATION

It is instructive to compare the acrophase chart for *Euglena* (Fig. 5.7) with that developed for a more highly organized system such as a mammal. A rhythmometric analysis of the relations among a number of murine rhythms is shown in Figure 5.8 (32). That such studies have great practical significance is well illustrated by the documentation of circadian rhythms in the resistance of mice to anticancer drugs, some of which are shown in the single cosinor plot given in Figure 5.9. Rhythmicities in therapeutic efficiency in the case of tumor-bearing animals may be due not only to variations in general physiological and systemic sensitivity to the drug of choice, but also to circadian oscillations in the rate of cell division in the neoplasm itself (just as has been observed for populations of *Euglena*). Chronochemotherapy, therefore, must take into account both host resistance to a drug as well as tumor susceptibility, both of which may oscillate (32). It may well be that a comparison between the circadian time structure—particularly chronotolerance—of lower microorganisms and higher animals will be useful in this regard (Figs. 5.10 and 5.11).

Acknowledgments. Dr. Klaus Brinkmann kindly provided some of the data on rhythms that he and his colleagues have studied; Robert Sothern aided in the computer analyses.

This work was supported by a National Science Foundation Research Grant (PCM 75-13125) to L.N.E. and by U.S. Public Health Service (5-K6-GM-13981), National Cancer Institute (CA-14445) and U.S. Environmental Protection Agency (R804512) grants to F.H.

References

1. Aschoff, J., Klotter, K., and Wever R. (1965): Circadian vocabulary. In: *Circadian Clocks*, pp. x–xix, edited by J. Aschoff. North-Holland, Amsterdam.
2. Brinkmann, K. (1966): Temperatureinflüsse auf die circadiane Rhythmik von *Euglena gracilis* bei Mixotrophie und Autotrophie. *Planta (Berl.),* 70:344–389.
3. Brinkmann, K. (1971): Metabolic control of temperature compensation in the circadian rhythm of *Euglena gracilis.* In: *Biochronometry,* pp. 567–593, edited by M. Menaher. National Academy of Science, Washington, D.C.
4. Brinkmann, K. (1976): The influence of alcohols on the circadian rhythm and the metabolism of *Euglena gracilis. J. Interdisc. Cycle Res.,* 7:149–170.
5. Brinkmann, K. (1976): Circadian rhythm in the kinetics of acid denaturation of cell membranes of *Euglena gracilis. Planta (Berl.),* 129:221–227.
6. Bruce, V. G., and Pittendrigh, C. S. (1956): Temperature independence in a unicellular "clock." *Proc. Natl. Acad. Sci. U.S.A.,* 42:676–681.
7. Bruce, V. G., and Pittendrigh, C. S. (1957): Endogenous rhythms in insects and microorganisms. *Am. Nat.,* 91:179–196.
8. Bruce, V. G., and Pittendrigh, C. S. (1958): Resetting the *Euglena* clock with a single light stimulus. *Am. Nat.,* 92:294–306.
9. Buetow, D. E. (Ed.): *The Biology of Euglena: Vol. I. General Biology and Ultrastructure; Vol. II. Biochemistry.* Academic Press, New York, 1968.
10. Codd, G. A., and Merrett, M. J. (1971): Photosynthetic products of division synchronized cultures of *Euglena. Plant Physiol.,* 47:635–639.
11. Cook, J. R. (1961): *Euglena gracilis* in synchronous division; I. Dry mass and volume characteristics. *Plant Cell Physiol.,* 2:199–202.
12. Cook, J. R. (1961): *Euglena gracilis* in synchronous division; II. Biosynthetic rates over the light cycle. *Biol. Bull.,* 121:277–289.
13. Cook, J. R. (1966): Photosynthetic activity during the division cycle in synchronized *Euglena gracilis. Plant Physiol.,* 41:821–825.
14. Cook, J. R., and James, T. W. (1960): Light-induced division synchrony in *Euglena gracilis* var. *bacillaris. Exp. Cell Res.,* 21:583–589.
15. Edmunds, L. N., Jr. (1964): Replication of DNA and cell division in synchronously dividing cultures of *Euglena gracilis. Science,* 145:266–268.
16. Edmunds, L. N., Jr. (1965): Studies on synchronously dividing cultures of *Euglena gracilis* Klebs (strain Z); I. Attainment and characterization of rhythmic cell division. *J. Cell. Comp. Physiol.,* 66:147–158.
17. Edmunds, L. N., Jr. (1965): Studies on synchronously dividing cultures of *Euglena gracilis* Klebs (strain Z); II. Patterns of biosynthesis during the cell cycle. *J. Cell. Comp. Physiol.,* 66:159–182.
18. Edmunds, L. N., Jr. (1966): Studies on synchronously dividing cultures of *Euglena gracilis* Klebs (strain Z); III. Circadian components of cell division. *J. Cell. Physiol.,* 67:35–44.
19. Edmunds, L. N., Jr. (1971): Persisting circadian rhythm of cell division in *Euglena:* some theoretical considerations and the problem of intercellular communication. In: *Biochronometry,* pp. 594–611, edited by M. Menaker. National Academy of Science, Washington, D.C.
20. Edmunds, L. N., Jr. (1975): Temporal differentiation in *Euglena:* Circadian phenomena in non-dividing populations and in synchronously dividing cells. In: *Les Cycles Cellulaires et Leur Blocage chez Plusieurs Protistes,* pp. 53–67. Colloques Int. C. .N. R. S., No. 240. Centre National de la Recherché Scientifique, Paris.
21. Edmunds, L. N., Jr. (1978): Clocked cell cycle clocks. In: *Aging and Biological Rhythms,* pp. 125–184, edited by H. V. Samis, Jr. and S. Capobianco, Plenum Publ. Corp., New York.
22. Edmunds, L. N., Jr., Chuang, L., Jarrett, R. M., and Terry O. W. (1971): Long-term persistence of free-running circadian rhythms of cell division in *Euglena* and the implication of autosynchrony. *J. Interdisc. Cycle Res.,* 2:121–132.
23. Edmunds, L. N., Jr., and Cirillo, V. P. (1974): On the interplay among cell cycle, biological clock and membrane transport control systems. *Int. J. Chronobiol.,* 2:233–246.
24. Edmunds, L. N., Jr., and Funch, R. R. (1969): Circadian rhythm of cell division in *Euglena;* effects of a random illumination regimen. *Science,* 165:500–503.
25. Edmunds, L. N., Jr., and Funch R. (1969): Effects of "skeleton" photoperiods and high frequency light-dark cycles on the rhythm of cell division in synchronized cultures of *Euglena. Planta (Berl.),* 87:134–163.
26. Edmunds, L. N., Jr., Jay, M. E., Kohlmann, A., Liu, S. C., Merriam, V. H., and Sternberg, H. (1976): The coupling effects of some thiol and other sulfur-containing compounds on the circadian rhythm of cell division in photosynthetic mutants of *Euglena. Arch. Microbiol.,* 108:1–8.
27. Edmunds, L. N., Jr., Sulzman, F. M., and Walther W. G. (1974): Circadian oscillations in enzyme activity in *Euglena* and their relation to the circadian rhythm of cell division. In: *Chronobiology,* pp. 61–66, edited by L. E. Scheving, F. Halberg, and J. E. Pauly. Igaku Shoin, Tokyo.
28. Ehret, C. F., and Wille, J. J. (1970): The photobiology of circadian rhythms in protozoa and other eukaryotic microorganisms. In: *Photobiology of Microorganisms,* pp. 369–416, edited by P. Halldal. Wiley-Interscience, New York.
29. Feldman, J. F. (1967): Lenghtening the period of a biological clock in *Euglena* by cycloheximide, an inhibitor of protein synthesis. *Proc. Natl. Acad. Sci. U.S.A.,* 57:1080–1087.
30. Feldman, J. F. (1968): Circadian rhythmicity in amino acid incorporation in *Euglena gracilis. Science,* 160:1454–1456.
31. Halberg, F. (1969): Chronobiology. *Ann. Rev. Physiol.,* 31:675–725.
32. Halberg, F. (1974): Protection by timing treatment according to bodily rhythms—an analogy to protection by scrubbing before surgery. *Chronobiologia,* 1(Suppl. 1):27–72.
33. Halberg, F., Carandente, F., Cornelissen, G., and Katinas, G. S. (1977): Glossary of chronobiology. *Chronobiologia,* 1, Supplement 4, 189 pp.
34. Halberg, F., and Connor, R. L. (1961): Circadian organization and micro-

biology; variance spectra and a periodogram on behavior of *Escherichia coli* growing in fluid culture. *Proc. Minn. Acad. Sci.*, 29:227–239.

35. Halberg, F., Johnson, E. A., Nelson, W., Runge, W., and Sothern, R. (1972): Autorhythmometry. Procedures for physiologic self-measurements and their analysis. *Physiol. Teacher*, 1:1–11.

36. Halberg, F., Tong, Y. L., and Johnson, E. A. (1967): Circadian system phase, an aspect of temporal morphology. Procedures and illustrative examples. In: *The Cellular Aspects of Biorhythms. Symposium on Rhythmic Research*, pp. 20–48, edited by H. Von Mayerbach. Springer-Verlag, Berlin.

37. Hastings, J. W. (1970): The biology of rhythms from man to microorganism. *N. Engl. J. Med.*, 282:435–441.

38. Jarrett, R. M., and Edmunds, L. N., Jr. (1970): Persisting circadian rhythm of cell division in a photosynthetic mutant of *Euglena. Science*, 167:1730–1733.

39. Kiefner, G., Schliessmann, F., and Engelmann, W. (1974): Methods for recording circadian rhythms in *Euglena. Int. J. Chronobiol.*, 2:189–195.

40. Kirschstein, M. (1969): Das rhythmische Verhalten einer farblosen Mutante von *Euglena gracilis. Planta (Berl.)*, 85:126–134.

41. Laval-Martin, D., Shuch, D., and Edmunds, L. N., Jr. (1979): Cell cycle-related and endogenous, circadian photosynthetic rhythms in *Euglena gracilis. Plant Physiol.*, 63:495–502.

42. Lonergan, T. A., and Sargent, M. L. (1978): Regulation of the photosynthesis rhythm in *Euglena gracilis*; I. Carbonic anhydrase and glyceraldehyde 3-phosphate dehydrogenase do not regulate the photosynthesis rhythm. *Plant Physiol.*, 61:150–153.

43. McMurry, L., and Hastings, J. W. (1972): No desynchronization among four different circadian rhythms in the unicellular alga, *Gonyaulax polyedra. Science*, 175:1137–1139.

44. Mitchell, J. L. A. (1971): Photoinduced division synchrony in permanently bleached *Euglena gracilis. Planta (Berl.)*, 100:244–257.

45. Pittendrigh, C. S. (1965): On the mechanism of the entrainment of a circadian rhythm by light cycles. In: *Circadian Clocks*, pp. 277–297, edited by J. Aschoff. Elsevier North Holland, Amsterdam.

46. Pohl, R. (1948): Tagesrhythmus im phototaktischen Verhalten der *Euglena gracilis. Z. Natursforsch.*, 3b:367–374.

47. Pöppel, E. (1975): Parameter estimation or hypothesis testing in the statistical analysis of biological rhythms? *Bull. Psychon. Soc.*, 6:511–512.

48. Russell, G. K., and Lyman, H. (1968): Isolation of mutants of *Euglena gracilis* with impaired photosynthesis. *Plant Physiol.*, 43:1284–1290.

49. Schnabel, G. (1968): Der Einfluss von Licht auf die circadiane Rhythmik von *Euglena gracilis* bei Autotrophie und Mixotrophie. *Planta (Berl.)*, 81:49–63.

50. Schwelitz, F. D., Dilley, R. A., and Crane, F. L. (1972): Biochemical and biophysical characteristics of a photosynthetic mutant of *Euglena gracilis* blocked in photosystem II. *Plant Physiol.*, 50:161–165.

51. Sulzman, F. M., and Edmunds, L. N., Jr. (1972): Persisting circadian oscillations in enzyme activity in non-dividing cultures of *Euglena. Biochem. Biophys. Res. Commun.*, 47:1338–1344.

52. Sulzman, F. M., and Edmunds, L. N., Jr. (1973): Characterization of circadian oscillations in alanine dehydrogenase activity in non-dividing populations of *Euglena gracilis* (Z). *Biochim. Biophys. Acta*, 320:594–609.

53. Terry, O., and Edmunds, L. N., Jr. (1969): Semi-continuous culture and monitoring system for temperature-synchronized *Euglena. Biotechnol. Bioeng.*, 11:745–756.

54. Terry, O. W., and Edmunds L. N., Jr. (1970): Rhythmic settling induced by temperature cycles in continuously-stirred autotrophic cultures of *Euglena gracilis* (Z strain). *Planta (Berl.)*, 93:128–142.

55. Vanden Driessche, T. (1970): Les rythmes circadiens chez les unicellulaires. *J. Interdisc. Cycle Res.*, 1:21–42.

56. Walther, W. G., and Edmunds, L. N., Jr. (1970): Periodic increase in deoxyribonuclease activity during the cell cycle in synchronized *Euglena. J. Cell Biol.*, 46:613–617.

57. Walther, W. G., and Edmunds, L. N., Jr.: Studies on the control of the rhythm of photosynthetic capacity in synchronized cultures of *Euglena gracilis* (Z). *Plant Physiol.*, 51:250–258.

58. Wolken, J. J. (1967): *Euglena. An Experimental Organism for Biochemical and Biophysical Studies*, Ed. 2. Appleton-Century-Crofts/Meredith, New York.

Addendum. A detailed review by L. N. Edmunds, Jr. of "Circadian and Infradian Rhythms" in *Euglena* will appear in *The Biology of Euglena*, Vol. III (Chapter 3), edited by D. E. Buetow, Academic Press, New York. For additional details of method, the reader is referred to papers by W. Nelson, Y. L. Tong, J. K. Lee, and F. Halberg (Methods for cosinor rhythmometry. *Chronobiologia*, 6:305–323, 1979) and by G. Cornelissen, F. Halberg, J. Stebbings, E. Halberg, F. Carandente and B. Hsi (Data acquisition and analysis by computers and pocket calculators. *Ricerca in Clinica e in Laboratorio*, 10:1980, in press). The latter paper provides means for the computation of the single cosinor and of the population mean cosinor on a pocket calculator.

Recent single cosinor analysis in collaboration with H.

-G. Schweiger of original data (M. W. Karakashian and H. -W. Schweiger, *Proceedings of the National Academy of Science, U.S.A.* 73:3216–3219, 1976) revealed a rhythm below the 5% level of macroscopically observed cycloheximide-induced delays in peak values of oxygen production in the unicellular green alga *Acetabularia mediterranea* maintained in continuous illumination. The response was temperature-dependent, exhibiting a statistically significant difference in acrophase between algae kept at 20°C and 25°C, respectively. Schweiger interprets these results as being consistent with the role of protein synthesis in generating circadian rhythms with translation occurring on 80 S (cytosol) but not 70 S (organellar) ribosomes.

6

Fundamental Aspects of Normal Organismal Growth in Animals

Hans E. Kaiser

The importance of ontogenetic life processes (in porifera and eumetazoa) for comparative oncology lies in the fact that, with rare exceptions,[1] neoplasms may develop from any stage of the life cycle of a multicellular organism with true tissues.—H. E. K.

INTRODUCTION

One of the main characteristics of life is growth; organisms are characterized by a certain species-specific life span. A large variety of general and group-, genus-, and species-specific growth processes occur during the life span of the organisms, resulting in important variations of organismic size.

For species-specific size of selected members of eumetazoan phyla, see Chapter 13. These conditions are recognized by convergent lines of individual chains of which each one has its own ontogeny. A great number of ontogenies build the chains of generations known as phylogeny. Ontogeny and phylogeny together are called hologeny.

Individuals of one species develop either from one cell as in asexual reproduction or in parthenogenesis, or through sexual reproduction from at least two parent cells. In the latter case, the zygote splits into a large number of cells and separates simultaneously into different tissues, resulting in a growth of the new organism, mainly by increase of cell number. The timely preservation of the embryonal growth potential varies according to the capability, species, cell types, and tissues. This is true of eumetazoans

and vascular plants. Under abnormal conditions and in unicellular organisms, a second type of growth takes place: the increase in the size of single cells. This simple process of organismic multiplication and growth exhibits a large variety of growth and ontogenetic patterns, with many specializations, complications, and detours which will be discussed in this chapter. Abnormal growth may develop at each phase of this process.

According to ontogenetic growth, two types of cells may be distinguished: germ cells and somatic cells. The tissues involved in the ontogenetic growth processes are practically the same as are found in the adult organisms. The many exceptions to this rule will be discussed briefly. The problems involved concerning somatic cells can be summarized as follows:

1. There exist cells, which, although less differentiated than other cells, possess multiple potential in their early ontogenetic stages. They can be found in mammals, or during certain periods of larval development in crustaceans and insects, or during a whole life span, as in the meristems of vascular plants.

2. There remain nests of undifferentiated cells with embryonal potential more or less comparable to meristematic tissues in plants, such as intercalated discs in holometabolic insects.

3. During certain developmental stages, e.g., during asexual reproduction, highly differentiated cells of particular tissues change back into a simpler form; they resume differentiation after the reproductive process.

4. Tissues may undergo histolytic or decomposition processes during normal ontogeny as in catastrophic development.

These are the most important points which

---

[1] See Chapter 13 (cell invariability and regeneration).

warrant attention. Degenerative processes during metamorphosis are known in the catastrophic developments in nemertini, holometabolic insects, echinoderms, and others (see Table 6.5).

A study of the behavior of tissues of *non-adult growing structures* during ontogeny should be highly rewarding and should produce new insights into normal as compared to pathological autolysis.

COMPARATIVE ASPECTS OF NORMAL GROWTH

General Aspects

Normal growth and development take place in an ordered manner, in a species-specific pattern, regulated through inheritance to the parent organism or organisms. This is the guarantee for the continuous existence of the species involved. Phylogenetic changes of the characteristics of the species can be neglected here, because we are not dealing with long geological time intervals. This typical pattern of normal growth in its multitude of variations must be first understood, before we are able to attempt to understand the problem of abnormal growth. Normal growth is therefore the preliminary condition of abnormal growth. If the normal growth potential has stopped, as in the human nervous system of which the neurons are cell constant (cell-invariable), neoplastic development cannot occur. The same holds true for the totally cell-invariable organisms as well as nonliving plant tissues. Normal growth is controlled by hormones in both animals and plants, and by the nervous correlation and/or neurosecretion in animals. Abnormal (especially malignant) growth on the other hand is autonomous and uncontrolled. Whereas in normal growth the cells show the necessary differentiations with continued tissue growth and specialization, the neoplastic cells and tissues are characterized by a decrease in specialization. Here, the only increase occurs in the growth potential which grows inversely with the decrease in specialization. It is well known that the less specialized malignant cells, such as those found in spindle or round cell sarcomas, are the most malignant, fastest growing, and the ones with the highest metastasizing potential. But metastatic growth depends also on the im-

mune reaction of the whole body to those cells as a second fundamental factor.

Neoplasms are able to develop in each stage of an organism's life. We know, for example, of intrauterine neoplasms in mammals. It is the purpose of this section to show with a few selected examples how the normal ontogenetic growth in animals provides a variety of backgrounds for the platform and development of abnormal growth.

Life Cycles

Each species exhibits a characteristic life cycle just as it has a species-specific age limit and size. Neoplastic growth may develop in each section of the life cycle of a given species. For a meaningful evaluation of the neoplasms in the different phyla, it is important to understand the main problems of the species-specific factors of normal growth processes.[2] The life of an organism can start from the fertilized diploid zygote, from egg cells as in parthenogenesis (haploid), or from larger amounts of different tissue accumulations, as in asexual reproduction. The life cycle may be directly continuing or it may proceed via one or more larval and even pupal stages or the development of placentae. This should be called "indirect continuation." But it can also be catastrophic as in holometabolic insects, where a total rebuilding of organs during ontogeny occurs. As far as the tissues are concerned, the indirect, second way, may be continuous or catastrophic. In the latter case tissues or whole organs may be discarded and replaced by others. It is known, for example, that the larvae of certain insects may be adapted to aquatic life, whereas the adults are adapted to terrestrial life. Discarding old, primary organs may be necessary when the change from one stage to another occurs. This necessitates that whole new organs must be rebuilt, in most cases, from unspecialized tissues with embryonal potential. Important differences in the normal growth processes in the various animal phyla occur. This chapter provides a short informative review of sexual reproduction, asexual reproduction, organ differentiation after sexual and asexual reproduction (selected examples), and detours in development such as placentae and larval metamorphosis with continued and catastrophic development.

---

[2] The lack of an understanding of these factors of normal growth may be a reason why we know so little about and where to look for abnormal growth, particularly in the invertebrates.

In the following, we shall discuss in detail those processes which are especially important for an understanding of comparative oncology.

To this complicated picture in animals is added the problem of the embryonal potential of meristematic tissues in vascular plants. They can be considered as the culmination of the lifelong embryonal potential in the form of cells or tissues in the world of organisms.

In both kingdoms, animals and plants, organisms occur which exhibit alternation of generations.

In invertebrates undifferentiated tissues with continued embryonal potential over a long life span, occur in certain species. These larval tissues, which are not present in vertebrates, have the closest resemblance to meristems (Table 6.1).

Reproduction in the animal kingdom is either sexual or asexual. In a phylogenetic comparison, asexual reproduction is more widely distributed, as it is the case with regeneration, in the lower

Table 6.1
Review of Growth Processes Seen from the Six-Kingdom Approach

I.	Animalia:	Eucaryotic multicellular, digestive nutrition, nerve and muscle tissues, sexual reproduction dominating but also asexual, direct and indirect development, either continued or catastrophic (hystolysis). Mainly ceasing of growth potential, long remaining embryonal potential in larval tissues, special conditions in placentae
II.	Plantae:	Multicellular cell walls, photosynthesis, main source of nutrition; meristematic tissues with at least theoretically unlimited embryonal potential during the life of the plant and fully differentiated tissues. Regaining of embryonal growth potential of fully differentiated tissues possible (succeeding meristems or "Folgemeristeme" of German literature). Some fully differentiated tissues ("permanent tissues") lose all living protoplasm before they become fully functional. Propagation mainly sexual with haploid and diploid stages (change of generations)
III.	Fungi:	Mainly multinucleate syncytia, no photosynthesis, absorptive nutrition dominating in contrast to two former groups. Asexual and sexual reproduction. Pseudotissues, known as plectenchymata, and characterized by fusion of before separated cells in the course of their development appear especially in the highest members of the group (Basidiomycetes)
IV.	Protista:	Unicellular or colonial unicellular eucaryotic, varying ways of nutrition and reproductive cycles
V.	Monera:	Unicellular or colonial, but procaryotic forms. Absorptive nutrition. Mainly asexual reproduction
VI.	Virus:	Below cellular level. Multiplication only in cells

phyla. This is evident especially if we look at the chordates, in which asexual reproduction is found only in the tunicates. The majority of phyla show the dioecious form of sexual reproduction with the exception of ctenophora and chaetognatha in which forms only hermaphroditic reproduction occurs. Several phyla show asexual as well as sexual reproduction. There are no phyla in the animal kingdom without sexual reproduction. A few phyla, such as of the superphylum aschelminthes, of annelida, and echinodermata, are also protandric. Annelida and arthropoda show also the parthenogenetic variation of sexual reproduction (Table 6.2).

Reproduction from mesozoans to chordates shows a tremendous variation, starting with a few reproductive cells, medially located in mesozoans to highly specialized organs accompanied by supporting structures and secondary sex characteristics in the higher forms. The sex cells may be nearly equal in lower forms, but generally the female sex cells are larger and nonmotile, whereas the male ones are small and generally characterized by a motile apparatus in form of a flagellum. But differences occur here also and will be described later. Besides the sex cells, highly specialized organ systems for their production and protection often have developed. It is interesting to note that one of the most complicated reproductive systems, in terms of arrangement, is found in the phylum of flatworms. The adult stages of certain insects, for example, exhibit in the male, a total degenerative type of organism which is not able to take in and digest food. The purpose of those forms as in certain diptera lays solely in the fulfillment of the sexual function. It must be mentioned that the larval stages of these forms prolong duration of life.[3] In certain wormlike genera, the males are also highly degenerated, very small, and may even live in the vagina of the female. Many insects are characterized by different larval forms or the condition of parthenogenesis in which case generations without males are responsible for reproduction. This type of reproduction may last for a certain amount of time, according to species, and afterward be replaced by sexual reproduction. These changes occur periodically. Conditions, which are found in the human being only in pathology, such as hermaphroditism, are found in certain forms, such as molluscs, as normal conditions of animal organization.

---

[3] The larval stage is the growth stage and the emerging adult the nongrowing sex stage with short duration of life span.

Table 6.2
Review of Types of Reproduction in Porifera and Eumetazoa

Taxonomy			Sexual Reproduction				Asexual Reproduction		Special Conditions of Reproduction
Phylum	Class	Order	Dioecious	Hermaphroditic	Protrandry	Partheno-genesis	Fission	Budding	
Porifera			+	+ (majority)				+	
Cnidaria			+ (majority)	?				+	
Ctenophora			−	+	−	−	+	−	
Platyhelminthes	Turbellaria			+ (usually)		−		+	
	Trematoda		+	+ (usually)			+	−	
	Cestoda			+ (majority)					
Nemertina			+ (usually)	+					
Gnathostomulida			+	+					
Entoprocta			+		+			+	
Acanthocephala			+						
Rotifera	Bdelloidea		+	−		+ (only)			
	Monogononta		−			+ (usual)			
Gastrotricha			+	+	+ (few)	+	−	−	
Kinorhyncha			+						
Nematoda			+ (usually)				−	−	
Nematomorpha			+					−	
Priapulida ?			+	+		+	−	−	
Mollusca	Monoplacophora								
	Amphineura		+					−	
	Gastropoda		+	+				−	
	Bivalvia		+ (usually)	+				−	
	Scaphopoda		+						
	Cephalopoda		+					−	
Sipunculida			+					−	
Echiurida			+					−	
Anelida	Polychaeta		+ (usually)	+	+		+	+	
	Clitellata	Oligochaeta	−	+			+	−	
		Hirudinea		+				−	
Onychophora			+					−	
Pentastomida			+					−	
Tardigrada			+			+		−	
Arthropoda	Merostomata		+					−	
	Pycnogonida		+					−	
	Arachnida	Scorpionida	+ (majority)			(+)		−	
		Araneae	+ (majority)			−		−	
		Acarina	+ (majority)			(±)		−	
	Crustacea		+	+		+		−	
	Ostracoda					(+)		−	
	Copepoda							−	
	Cirripedia		−	+		+1 or 2 species		−	
	Malacostraca	Decapoda	+ (majority)		+		−	−	

Special Conditions of Reproduction:

1. Reduction bodies are masses of amebocites surrounded by epidermal cells, which persist from original sponge
2. Gemmules are cystlike bodies of fresh water sponges able to withstand winter conditions and to germinate a new sponge, when conditions are favorable
3. Frustules are nonciliated, planulalike buds that develop into a polyp in some hydrozoans
4. Epitoky is a seasonal modification in the posterior part of a marine polychaete, which becomes swollen with gonads and eggs or sperms
5. Polyembryonid is the production of two or more embryos from one egg. This condition is known in insects
6. Paedogenesis, also known in insects, is the node of reproduction of young or larval animals

	Col.		Col.	Col.	Notes
Phoronida	−	−	−	−	+
Ectoprocta	−	−	−	−	+
Brachiopoda	−	−	−	−	+
Echinodermata	−	−	−	−	+
Chilopoda				+	+
Diplopoda				+	+
Pauropoda				+	+
Symphyla	+			+ almost all	+
Insecta	+			(+)	−
Asteroidea	+			−	+ (majority)
Ophiuroidea	+			+ (majority)	(+)
Ophiuroidea		+		+ (majority)	
Echinoidea				+	+ (individual exception)
Holothuroidea				+ (majority)	(+)
Crinoidea				+	+ (abnormality)
Chaetognatha				−	(+)
Hemichordata				+	+
Enteropneusta				+	+
Pterobranchia				+	+
Pogonophora				−	−
Cephalochordata			(+)	−	−
Tunicata	+			+	+
Ascidiacea				+	
Thaliacea	+			+ (abnormality)	
Vertebrata	−			−	+ (abnormality)

Some of the hermaphroditic forms may be able to use both sex organs at the same time, as is well known in the copulation of earthworms.

Reproductive organs in the animal kingdom show an interesting diversification reflected in a histologic description based on function. As in the plant kingdom, asexual propagation occurs, especially in lower forms such as cnidaria, ctenophora, wormlike animals, and especially colony-building forms. The majority of animals are characterized by the development of sexual reproduction and the separation of the sexes. But we also find conditions which are normal in the groups concerned; if they occur in human beings, these conditions are abnormal. One of the most striking examples is the hermaphroditism as we observe it in the pulmonates such as the vineyard snail *Helix pomatia* or annelids such as the earthworm *Lumbricus terrestris*. Hermaphroditism may occur in one way when the male and female sex organs are fully developed at the same time, or when, for example, the male organs are fully developed in the young animal and change later on to female conditions. If we remember that both sex glands develop from undifferentiated so-called germ layers, these facts are easy understood. Those particular changes offer interesting histologic problems. Another condition is the so-called parthenogenesis in which for a certain amount of time only female organisms develop which are replaced by a bisexual generation after several generations.

Sexual Reproduction

Structures of sexual reproduction in certain species of animals can be divided into the gonads with the sex cells including nourishing cells of the ova and spermatids. To the accessory structures belong the duct system such as oviduct, uterus, vagina, and the copulatory organs as external sex organs in the female dioecious apparatus, and ductus ejaculatorious, vas deferens, prostata, male urethra as the duct system, and the copulatory organ or penis if present. A tremendous variation of structures exist. If we recall that the sex cells of both sexes in man develop from the same germinal epithelium, we understand that the different variations of sexual structures found in the human and mammalian body as pathological conditions, occur normally in different phyla or their subgroups. The most important types of sexual structures are:

1. In the dioecious condition, the single

organism of the particular species is either a male one with testes or a female one with ovaries as gonads.

2. In the hermaphroditic condition, both gonads of which are found in one organism of the particular species act with both gonads of another individuum of this species during copulation. Sexual maturity of male and female organs may be reached at different times.

3. There exists in certain genera only one type of gonad which in the young organism produces sperm and in the older one ova. This special condition is known as protandry.

4. If in an otherwise dioecious species, a number of generations consisting only of female organisms occur and produce eggs which need not be fertilized, these forms are called parthenogenetic. In those animals the eggs are able to develop into new organisms without fertilization. In these forms, generally generations dioecious in character are followed by parthenogenetic generations.

Variations of sexual reproduction in the animal kingdom can be compared in propagation in the plant kingdom, especially with regard to Groups 1 and 2: dioecious animals and plants; hermaphroditic animals and monoecious plants.

Sexual reproductive structures of the different phyla will be discussed in the following sequence:

1. A review of female and male gonads with their sex cells.

2. Description of histological features, including most recent accounts of ultrastructure.

3. Comparative histology of accessory structures (Table 6.3).

The most commonly distributed mode of sexual reproduction is the dioecious type, in which the individuals of the species concerned possess either male or female characteristics and, in higher forms, organs. In most individuals there occur, beside the reproductive organs, so-called secondary sex characteristics, including differences in body size, color etc.

Structures of Dioecious Reproduction

Mesozoa. The tube of the somatic cells or syncytium contains the male or female sex cells.

Porifera. Sponges exhibit no gonads. The male sex cells of sponges develop from amoebocytes, archeocytes, or choanocytes. Choanocytes or amoebocytes act as supporting cells carrying them to the amoeboid ova, which develop from amoebocytes. Trophocytes, as well as amoebocytes, act as nurse cells for the ova.

Cnidaria. Gonads in cnidaria occur generally in the medusae and the sex cells develop from the interstitial cells. The gonads are really accumulations of sex cells; their topographic location depends on the genus concerned. Accessory structures do not occur. The development of the sex cells exhibits no peculiarities if compared with the development of other phyla. The spermatozoa are flagellated, the ova either rich in yolk or small.

A. L. Burnett et al. (16) concluded in 1966 that there exists no specific germinal cell line in *Hydra* because isolated gastrodermal gland cells after isolation are capable of differentiation into interstitial cells and those are able to form normal gametes.

Growth and fusion of oocytes is known in *Hydra* (2).

Platyhelminthes. The family schistosomatidae of trematods, for example, exhibits functionally dioecious forms.

In the class cestodes the genus *Dioecocestus* is dioecious.

Entoprocta. *Urnatella* is an example of a dioecious genus with hermaphroditic and protandrous forms. The conditions of the three types of reproduction are not well known. Gonads are supplied with short gonoducts. The ova and sperms show no peculiarities, the spermatozoa are flagellated. The epithelium of the gonoducts is glandular in type. New investigations are needed.

Nemertini. Most nemertini are dioecious. Exceptions are the hermaphroditic *Prostoma* or some species of the genus *Lineus* which are able to reproduce asexually by transverse fission.

The simple reproductive system lacks in general accessory organs and is composed of saclike gonads located close to the intestine or over the mesenchyme. The epithelium of the gonads, deriving from mesenchyme, may be enforced by musculature. The gonads open by short ducts to the exterior of the animal.

Rotifera. Rotifers are dioecious but reproduce parthenogenetically also, as in the case of the order Bdelloidea, where only females have been observed. This will be described further under the subheading of parthenogenesis.

The female organs exhibit a syncytial ovary and vitellarium, covered by a membrane which continues as an oviduct. In some genera the organs may be paired structures. In the male, testis, generally unpaired, a sperm duct, often ciliated with cirrus, and a prostate may be distinguished. Two types of sperm, the flagellated with oval head and undulating membrane and the atypical rod-shaped, may be discerned.

Gastrotricha. A single or paired ovary is characteristic for the female and the number of ova seems to be, in certain cases, predetermined. A uterus and oviduct are present. The whole female organ system of this group is poorly understood. This holds true also for the male system comprised of single or paired testes, sperm duct, and sometimes a penis as an accessory structure.

Nematoda. Nematodes are dioecious, with the exception of a few parasites which are always hermaphroditic for a few generations. In the female, two ovaries with oviduct and uterus are present. The covering of the ovary, comparable to that of the testis, continues to the female duct system consisting of oviduct and uterus. The epithelium is at first columnar and becomes cuboidal or flat in the uterus and underlain by circular and longitudinal musculature. In the male the singular or double testes and bursae, genital papillae, and spiculae as accessory structures, may be distinguished. Sperm duct, seminal vesicle, and ejaculatory duct are present. Musculature is exhibited in the ejaculatory duct in addition to the epithelium in its wall. The covering epithelium of the gonad is composed of flat cells. Therefore, in both sexes, the musculature joins the epithelium in the composition of the sexual ducts. In the uterus, this portion, acting as seminal receptacle, has in certain genera a phagocytic epithelium. The vagina, following the uterus, has an additional cuticle; glands occur in some species. The spermatozoa of nematodes exhibit no flagella.

The epithelial cells of the uterus of *Ascaris lumbricoides*, arranged in a single sheet, permits detailed study of cell function. These cells may be important for experimental studies dealing with polyploidy (22). The nucleoli in 4-celled embryos of *A. lumbricoides* are concerned with the production of ribosomal RNA (29).

Kinorhyncha. The exclusive dioecious animals show the following characteristics. The developing gonad is first syncytial. The paired ovaries exhibit the initiating apical cell, the germ cells, the vitelline cells, and the cells of the epithelial wall. Besides this, an oviduct occurs along with a seminal receptacle leading to the gonophores.

The testis shows an epithelium of flat cells and different stages of the development of spermatozoa. Spermatic duct, gonophorus, and accessory structures as bristles also occur.

Nematomorpha. Our knowledge regarding the genital organs of these animals is very scarce. Little is known about the histology. In the female, paired ovaries, uteri, oviducts, and seminal receptacle have been observed. The continuation

of the ovaries has a glandular epithelium. Paired testes, a seminal vesicle, and accessory spines in the cloaca have been seen. The spermatozoa are composed of a head and tail and appear relatively simple. In Gordioidea the sperm is rod-shaped (20).

Acanthocephala. The reproductive system of these endoparasites is closely related to the ligament sacs which are remnants of the digestive system, being an unnucleated structure. The ovaries have been described in one species only and our knowledge is very limited. So many peculiarities exist, a study dealing with different species of the group could provide rewarding results.

The male organs are the testes, with divided and later united sperm duct, seminal vesicle, cement glands, bursa, and penis. The sperms have no head. Flagellogenesis with special emphasis positioning and disorganization of the spermatic axonema has been investigated (39).

The female organs are one or two ovaries, uterine bell, uterine duct (characterized by large cells), uterus with well-developed musculature, and vagina.

Priapulida. The dioecious structures consist of the gonads and ducts. The ducts are really components of the urogenital system. There occur no other accessory structures. The sexual portion of the urogenital organ exhibits in the lobular arranged gonad the spermatozoa or ova and is covered by a peritoneal epithelium. New histologic and embryologic studies are urgently needed.

Mollusca. The majority of molluscs exhibits the dioecious type of sexual reproduction.

Polyplacophora. Polyplacophora are dioecious with exception of the hermaphroditic *Trachydermon raymondi.* The gonads and gonoducts may be distinguished. The sex glands are surrounded by musculature and connective tissue. The epithelium of the ovary is folded. The epithelium of the gonoduct is ciliated changing to glandular in the more final portion. In the area where the epithelial change occurs, appears the slime sac. The testis and ovary are similar in appearance with regard to makeup of epithelium. The epithelium of the sperm duct is also cuboidal ciliated.

In the chiton, *Sympharochiton septentriones,* one primary and two secondary egg membranes occur around the oocyte. The follicle cells deposit a spiny chorion around each oozyte. The inner acid mucopolysaccharide layer, secreted by the Golgi apparatus of the oocyte, represents the primary egg membrane. The intermediate protein layer and the outer lipid layer represent

Table 6.3
Review of Primary and Secondary (Accessory) Reproductive Organs, with Tissue Characteristics in Eumetazoans

Phylum	Subunit (Class)	♀ Reproductive Organ(s), with Tissue Characteristics	Accessory ♀ Organ(s) with Tissue Characteristics	♂ Reproductive Organ(s) with Tissue Characteristics	Accessory ♂ Organs with Tissue Characteristics	Type of Reproduction[a]	Remarks
Cnidaria		Mostly germ cell development in interstitial positions	—	Mostly germ cell develop in interstitial positions	—	bi	
Ctenophora		Ovary, low to high ciliated epithelium (glandular epithelum), oocytes—nerve cells	Oviduct, gonopore(s), seminal receptacles, brood chambers	Testes, low to high ciliated epithelium, testicular membrane	Sperm ducts	her	
Platyhelminthes	Turbellaria	Ovary (2 types)	Oviducts, yolk ducts	Testis(es)	Sperm duct, ejaculatory ducts, prostate apparatus, penis	her	
	Trematoda	Ovary	Yolk glands (?)	Testis(es)	Sperm ducts, copulatory complex: muscular cirrus sac, seminal vesicle, prostatic glands, prostatic vesicles	her, bi	
	Cestoda	Ovary	Uterus-uterine sac, uterine partition, vagina, yolk gland, Mehlis gland, seminal receptacle	Testis		her	
Nemertinea		Ovaries	—	Testis			
Gnathostomulida		Ovaries	Vagina-bursa system	Testis	Accessory glands, penis	her	
Entoprocta		Ovaries (2)	Ducts	Testis (2)	Ducts	di, her, par	
Acanthocephala		Ovary (ies) egg balls	Ligament sac, uterine bell	Testis (2)	Sperm ducts, seminal vesicle, cement glands, penis	di	
Rotifera		Ovary proper (germanium), vitellarium, syncythial yolk	Oviduct(s)	Testis	Sperm duct (ciliated)	di, par	
Gastrotricha		Ovary(ies)	Oviduct	Testis (2)	Sperm duct, bursa	her (prot), par	
Kinorhyncha		Ovary (syncytial) ova and nutritive cells	Oviduct	Testis	Sperm duct	di	
Nematoda		Ovary(ies) (3 zones)	Uterus-vagina, seminal receptacle, vulva	Testis (3 zones)	Sperm duct, seminal vesicle, ejaculatory duct,		

[a] di, dioecious; her, hermaphroditic; prot, protandry; par, parthenogenesis; sep,

Table 6.3—*Continued*

Phylum	Subunit (Class)	♀ Reproductive Organ(s), with Tissue Characteristics	Accessory ♀ Organ(s) with Tissue Characteristics	♂ Reproductive Organ(s) with Tissue Characteristics	Accessory ♂ Organs with Tissue Characteristics	Type of Reproduction[a]	Remarks
					prostatic gland, spicular pouches, bursa		
Nematomorpha		Ovary	(Uterus) 2 oviducts, seminal receptacle	Testis	Seminal vesicle, sperm duct, cloaca		
Priapulida		Ovaries	Urogenital duct	Testis	Urogenital duct	di, her, par	
Mollusca	Monoplacophora						
	Aplacophora	Ovotestis		Ovotestis		her	
	Polyplacophora	Ovary		Testis		bi	
	Gastroproda (Prosobranchs)	Ovary	Gonopericardial canal, gonoduct, albumin gland, seminal receptacle, hermaphroditic duct, hermaphroditic pore, ciliated channel, pallial duct, penis, accessory glands	Testis	Gonoduct, penis	her	
	Opisthobranchia (Pulmonates)	One gonad					
	Pelycopoda	Ovary	Gonoduct	Testis	Gonoduct	di, her	
	Scaphopoda	Ovary	Gonoduct	Testis	Gonoduct	bi	
	Cephalopoda	Ovary	Oviduct, glands, nidamental glands	Testis	Sperm duct, seminal vesicles, prostate, Needham's sac	bi	
Sipunculida		Ovary (peritoneal outgrowth)		Testis (peritoneal outgrowth)		bi, her	
Echiurida		Ovary	Celomic cavity duct and storage system	Testis	Celomic cavity duct and storage system	sep (bi)	
Annelida	Polychaeta	Gonad or mass of sex cells also nerve cells	Ciliated gonoducts	Gonad or mass of sex cells	Gonoducts, ciliated	di, her, par, prot	Epigony, schizogony in several groups
	Clitelliata Oligochaeta	Ovary(ies)	Celomic pouch, gonoducts, seminal receptacle	Testis(es)	Celomic pouch, gonoducts	her	
	Hirudinea	Ovaries (1 pair)	Ovisac, oviduct, vagina, gonopore	Many with penis and testis	Vas deferans (seminal vesicle, muscular	her	

Phylum	Subunit (Class)	♀ Reproductive Organ(s), with Tissue Characteristics	Accessory ♀ Organ(s) with Tissue Characteristics	♂ Reproductive Organ(s) with Tissue Characteristics	Accessory ♂ Organs with Tissue Characteristics	Type of Reproduction[a]	Remarks

Table 6.3—*Continued*

Phylum	Subunit (Class)	♀ Reproductive Organ(s), with Tissue Characteristics	Accessory ♀ Organ(s) with Tissue Characteristics	♂ Reproductive Organ(s) with Tissue Characteristics	Accessory ♂ Organs with Tissue Characteristics	Type of Reproduction[a]	Remarks
					ejaculatory duct, anetrun gland, penis		
Onychophora		Paired ovaries	Genital tract, seminal receptacle, uterus with chambers	Paired testes, ejaculatory tube (lower tract of nephiridium)		sep (bi)	Ovivivíparaous or viviporous with placenta development
Linguatuliva		Ovary	Oviduct, seminal receptacle, accessory gland, uterus/vagina	Testis	Seminal vesicle, ejaculatory duct cirrus sac	sep (bi)	
Tardigrada		Simple ovary	Single oviduct seminal receptacle (heterotardigrades)	Simple testis	Pair of sperm ducts		
Arthropoda	Chelicerates, Merostomata	Simple gonad (ovary)	Paired gonoducts, paired gonopores		Simple testis, paired gonoducts, paired gonopores	bi	
	Arachnida	Paired ovaries	Copulatory ducts, seminal receptacles, oviduct (vagina, gonopores)	Paired testes	Sperm ducts, gonopores		
	Crustacea	Paired ovaries	Gonoducts	Paired testes	Clasping organ (most appendages) (penis)		di, her, part, alteration of generation in low forms
	Chilopoda	Single tubular ovary	Single oviduct	1–24 testes	1 pair of sperm ducts, urogenital opening, penis	bi	
	Diploda	Single tubular ovary	Oviduct, uterus, 2 vulvas, seminal receptacle	Paired testes	Sperm duct, penis(es), gonopods	bi	
	Chilopoda	Single tubular ovary	Single oviduct	1–24 testes	1 pair of sperm ducts, urogenital opening, penis	bi	
Diploda	Single tubular ovary	Oviduct, uterus, 2 vulvas, seminal receptacle	Paired testes	Sperm duct, penis(es), gonopods	bi		
	Insecta	Paired ovaries (ova)	Pair of oviducts, one vagina, one vulva, special glands, spermatheca	Paired testes	Paired vasa deferentia, seminal vesicle, one ejaculatory tube	bi	Parthenogenesis, polyemdrynom, and paedogensis are exceptions

144

Table 6.3—*Continued*

Phylum	Subunit (Class)	♀ Reproductive Organ(s), with Tissue Characteristics	Accessory ♀ Organ(s) with Tissue Characteristics	♂ Reproductive Organ(s) with Tissue Characteristics	Accessory ♂ Organs with Tissue Characteristics	Type of Reproduction[a]	Remarks
Phoronida		Ovary (sex cells)	—	Testis (sex cells)	—	her (bi)	
Ectoprocta		Ovary (peritonem and sex cells developing from it)	—	Testis (peritonem and sex cells developing from it)	—	her	Largest variation of types of reproduction. Dioecism—polyembryony, proandry, brood bodies alteration of generations?
Brachiopoda		4 ovaries	Metanephridia functions as gonoducts, brood pouches occur in some	4 ovaries	Metanephridia functions as gonoducts	di	
Echinodermata	Asteroidea	Ovaries in genital sac		Testis in genital sac		di	Occasional hermaphroditism
	Ophiuroidea	Saclike ovaries	—	Saclike testis	—	di(her)	
	Echinoidea	3–5 ovaries, peritoneal germinal epithelial	Gonoducts, brood pouches in some	3–5 testes, peritoneal germinal epithelial	Gonoducts	(di) her	
	Holothuroidea	Ovaries (?) peritoneal and germinal epithelial	Duct of ciliated and connective tissue	Testis? peritoneal epithelial	Duct, ciliated and connective tissue	bi/her, prot	
	Crinoidea	Ovaries, brood pouches in some (?)		Testis		bi	
Chaetognatha		Pair of ovaries	2 oviducts, 2 seminal receptacles, vagina, gonophore	Pair of testes	2 sperm ducts, 2 seminal vesicles	her	Celomic completion of spermatonia
Pogonophora		Pair of ovaries	Oviducts	Pair of testes	Pair of sperm ducts	sep (bi) (di)	
Hemichordata	Enteropneusta	Ovaries	—	Testis	—	sep (bi)	
	Pterobranchia	Ovary		Testis			
Cephalochordata		25–33 pair of ovaries		25–33 pair testes		sep (bi)	
Tunicata (Urochordata)	Ascidiacea	Single ovary (pairs in some)		Single testis (paired in some)	Sperm duct	her, prot	
Vertebrata		Ovaries: medulla, cortex, and covering epithelium		Testes: compound tubular glands, covered by celomic epithelial and fibrous capsule septa; seminiferous tubules spermatogonic cells; Sertoli cells; interstitial tissue			
	Cyclostomata	No oviducts			No vas deferens		

Table 6.3—*Continued*

Phylum	Subunit (Class)	♀ Reproductive Organ(s), with Tissue Characteristics	Accessory ♀ Organ(s) with Tissue Characteristics	♂ Reproductive Organ(s) with Tissue Characteristics	Accessory ♂ Organs with Tissue Characteristics	Type of Reproduction[a]	Remarks
	Chondrychthyes		Elasmobranchs have shell gland		Claspers, siphon in sharks		
	Osteichthyes		Salmonid fishes lack oviducts		Salmonidae lack vas deferens, some telosts have a gonopodium		
	Amphibia		Primitive oviducts				Lack intromittant organs
	Reptilia		Uterus (stratified cuboidal epithelium) clitoris,		Vasa afferentia (cuboidal and/or low columnar cells)		Snakes and lizards (except Sphenodon) have hemipenes. Crocodilians, chelonians and ostrichs and some anseriformes have phallus. Carnivores lack seminal vesicle. Prostatic and bulbourethral glands in marsupials and placental mammals with exception of edentata and cetacea
	Aves		Clitoris		Epididymis (columnar or pseudostratified epithelium)		
	Mammalia		Uterus: mucosa, muscularis, serosa; vagina, external genital organs	Testes of proboscidea, cetacea and sirenia remain in body cavity	Vasa deferentia (columnar pseudostratified epithelium)		

secondary egg membranes, secreted by the follicle cells (56).

Monoplacophora are also dioecious, the makeup of the sex organs is comparable to that of polyplacophora.

Gastropoda. The animals concerned are the prosobranchia. The majority of the animals are dioecious. Single gonads and ducts with accessory glandular structures occur. In the female, the duct system is composed of the gonoduct terminating in a uterus and the accessory glandular structure. The lining of the uterus with the attached seminal receptacles exhibits columnar cells above a muscular coat. In general, the lining in the female epithelial tract is composed of columnar cells. The male gonoduct, known as the sperm duct, is also supplied with glandular structures and a penis. In the prostate, columnar cells occur as lining intermingled with glandular cells. The epithelium of the sperm duct is columnar ciliated and, in the penis which the sperm duct penetrates, it is surrounded by musculature, connective tissue, and blood vessels. The cells of the epithelial cover are cuboidal in shape. In this group of gastropods two types of sperm, the normal with flagella and the abnormal degenerated one, are produced. The first kind is able to fertilize eggs; the function of the second type is not known. The architectural pattern of the wall of the egg capsule of the snail *Urosalpinx cinerea* consists of four laminae, three anisotropic and one isotropic (63).

Scaphopoda. The dioecious animals exhibit either one ovary or one testis; there are no accessory structures.

Pelecypoda. The majority are dioecious. The

gonads occur as paired organs, and gonoducts may be present.

Ultrastructural changes during the differentiation of the sperm in the clam *Spisula solidissima* showed that, during early development of the spermatids, proacrosomal vesicles start from the Golgi complexes, form one acrosomal vesicle which moves to the anterior region of the nucleus, elongates, and makes a cone-shaped figure with an invagination at the nuclear side. The axial rod occurs as fiber structure in the older spermatid. The nucleus of the early spermatids shows aggregations and filaments of chromatin in the periphery. The mitochondria show a reduction in number from many to four during spermiogenesis (37, 38).

Cytoplasmic constituents of the ovarian *Mytilus* egg showed cytoplasmic constituents as described by Worley (71) and pallial substances as described by Urbani-Mistruzzi and Scollo-Lavizarri (66) and Reverberi 1967 (49). Similar findings were made in the oocyte of *Bankia australis* (46).

Cephalopoda. The animals are dioecious. In the female reproductive system of cephalopods, a single ovary (the germ cells proper and nourishing cells may be distinguished) and a single or paired oviduct (depending on the genus concerned) occur. Accessory glandular structures have been found. The male system exhibits the testis, the duct system (sperm duct, seminal vesicle, prostate, and Needham's sac for sperm storage), and other accessory organs.

Sipunculida. The gonads of sipunculids lack accessory structures. Comparable to priapulids the immature sex cells ripen in the coelomic fluid and are then shed by the excretory system into the ocean. The mechanism of the transport from the gonads to the release from the body as well as most of the details of the sexual morphology and physiology of the sipunculida are unknown.

Echiurida. The gonads of both sexes are unpaired cellular clusters. Sexual dimorphism is remarkable; the males are small and degenerated. Of particular interest is the fact that the foregut of the degenerated intestinal tract acts as a sperm duct. The immature oocytes of *Urechis caupo* develop as single cells floating in the coelomic fluid. They are free of associated nurse or follicle cells (41).

Annelida. The majority of polychaeta are dioecious, but some protandric hermaphrodites occur, as well as parthenogenetic forms. The two other major groups of annelids, the oligochaeta, on one hand are hermaphroditic, and the hirudinea are protandric on the other. Remark-

able is the fact that, in polychaeta, the posterior portion of the body may separate from the anterior one during spawning. Phagocytosis of structures, such as gut and musculature, in coelomocytes changes the tissues, and the transformed body portion dies after the sexual purpose is fulfilled. This occurs, of course, under hormonal influence and leads to new insight into sexual and endocrine function in invertebrates. Endocrine function in invertebrates has not been proven in those forms until now. The gonads are cell clusters. In some cases nutritional cells of the ova occur. No sex ducts have been observed; they may be modified nephridia.

Lipid and yolk inclusions occur only in the cytoplasm of oocytes of *Nereis pelagical.* (Annelida, Polychaeta) with a diameter less the 100 μm. Maturity starts with the appearance of acid mucopolysaccharides, the dilatations of the distal saccules of the Golgi apparatus, and the release of Golgi vacuoles. The mucopolysaccharides form, during further ripening, a cortical layer. The dictysomes move toward the center of the cytoplasm and start to degenerate. All mature oocytes contain intranuclear annulate lamellae. A fast growth of oocytes occurs if brain hormone is absent, and the mucopolysaccharides form a cortical layer, but less abundant under normal conditions. The endoplasmic reticulum is increased, cytoplasmic and intranuclear lamellae show a pronounced augmentation. Vesicular and membranous formations characterize the structure of the yolk bodies (19).

Testes in the microannelid *Enchytraeus fragmentosus* once thought to reproduce only asexually, have been reported by Vena and Palumbo (67).

Distinguishable stages occur in early oogenesis of *Platynereis dumerilii* (21) and acrosome formation is seen in the spermatozoa of *Sabella penicillum* (35).

Onychophora. The onychophora are always dioecious. The paired ovaries continue in a genital tract of modified nephridia, seminal receptacle (not present in all species), and uterus (wall: nonciliated epithelium, longitudinal musculature, circular musculature, connective tissue) leading to the gonophore. The paired testes (the epithelium shows high ciliated cells and we find musculature and connective tissue) continue in a tube system composed of a modified nephridium. The paired sex ducts of both sexes unite and lead to the gonophore. The young animals are born alive. Details concerning the placenta are given at the end of the chapter.

Linguatulida. The histologic knowledge of the reproductive system of this phylum is scarce.

We know that the female organs are composed of ovarium, oviduct, the copulatory vesicle, and the uterovaginal tube. The testes exhibit special gland cells and the musculature is remarkably abundant in the germinal epithelium.

Tardigrada. The ovary and the oviduct which opens into the cloaca compose the simple female sexual system of the animal. The male system consists of a singular testis and two sperm ducts. Our knowledge concerning the history of the system is very poor.

Arthropoda. The overwhelming majority of arthropods are dioecious.

Amandibulata. Chelicerata; Merostomata. In the female of the horseshoe crab, *Limulus polyphemus* L., an ovary and a pair of oviducts occur; in the male, the testis and the vasa deferentia but no accessory structures. The sex glands have a network-like structure.

Chelicerata; Arachnida. The araneae or spiders may serve as an example. The female organs consist of paired ovaries and oviducts, unpaired uterus and vagina. The male organs exhibit the paired testes and vasa deferentia and a singular seminal vesicle. A particularity of the spiders is the fact that the male copulatory organs (pulpi) are separated from the reproductive system proper. The tubular testes of 6 among 25 species of spiders exhibit giant polyploid cells (61). Spermatoblasts and oocytes of *Eudendrium racemosum* differentiate from ectodermal I-cells (24).

Mandibulata. Crustacea, Crayfish. The majority of crayfish are dioecious and the main organs in the female are paired ovaries with oviduct and in the male, paired testes with sperm ducts. The male uses appendages for transformation during copulation and some crayfish exhibit a penis. Accessory structures in the female are the seminal receptacles. Because of the variation in the class and the diversified pattern in the dioecious structures of crustaceans, four histologic examples have been chosen.

During spermiogenesis of spermatids of the ostracod *Cypridopsis* sp., the nucleus undergoes elongation and segregation into two compartments. Two mitochondria become aligned along the largest portion of the length of mature spermatozoons. Nuclear membrane, endoplasmic reticulum, and Golgi apparatus give rise to unique bilaterally located membranous organelles (47).

Mature spermatozoa of the ostracod *Cypridopsis* sp. are 1 mm long, filiform and spirally patterned cells. The spiral pattern is composed of an arrangement of the mitochondria, intracellular membranous organelles, and the outer plasma membrane. The cristae of the mitochondria, tubular in shape, always contain one 40–60 Å thick filament (47). The secretory product of the epithelial cells in the vas deferens of crayfish is rich in protein carbohydrate. Inosine-5'-diphosphatase was found in the vesicles of muscle cells which surround the vas deferens (30). Scanning electron microscopy of the egg shell in some anostraca has been reported (23).

Myriapoda (Chilopoda, Diplopoda, Pauropoda and Symphila). The animals are characterized by separate sexes and, in contrast to the crayfish and insects, the sex glands are unpaired structures. The gonoducts are paired as well as the seminal receptacles.

Insecta. The majority of insects are dioecious and exhibit a relatively general plan of the sex structures. The main organs are the female or male paired gonads, the paired gonoducts, which unite in both sexes to a median singular duct, as well as accessory structures. The male sex gland exhibits, from the beginning or anterior portion to the posterior one, the spermatozoa in continuing developmental stages. The testes in insects are composed of coiled tubelike structures. The general plan of the spermatozoon is similar to that of vertebrates. The vasa deferentia may exhibit a seminal vesicle for storage of spermatozoa.

The ovaries exhibit a similar sequence of the ripening sex cells in the tubular structure of the organ as was described for the testes. Nourishing cells occur in some forms, in others, they do not. An important difference concerning the development of the ova is that ripening and rupture of the follicle is noted. No hormone action in the insect occurs after the rupture, as in the case of the corpus luteum in the mammal.

The spermatheca or receptaculum seminis in insects can be considered as an extension of the body surface and exhibits a lining and cuticle. A more or less columnar cell epithelium as well as glandular or secretory cells can be distinguished (60).

Distinguishable stages of oogenesis also occur in insects, as in the proturan *Acerentomon gallicum* (12).

The Lophorate Phyla

Ectoprocta. The ectoprocta, also known as bryozoans, show the largest variation of reproductive methods in a particular animal group, including peculiar types of regeneration. Most of the animals are hermaphroditic. Dioecious forms have distinct ovaries and testes. The gonads are clusters of developing sex cells, surrounded by a peritoneal cover. No accessory structures are found.

Phoronida. Only a few species are dioecious, the majority are hermaphroditic. The gonads develop from peritoneal cells which are usually flat. (These flat peritoneal cells enlarge, become columnar during this development or pyramidal with nutritional inclusions to nourish the sex cells. The sex cells among them develop from peritoneal cells which do not undergo such changes.) Sex cells are cell clusters and are generally released by the nephridia to the outside or develop fertilized at the tentacles.

Brachiopoda. Brachiopods (except *Argyrotheca* sp.) are dioecious and generally exhibit four gonads. In some, the gametes are discharged through the metanephridia, in others breeding occurs in particular brood pouches. The gametes are developed from the peritoneum. No accessory structures exist. The fine structure of brachiopod spermatozoa reveals that they belong to the primitive type. *Jerebutulime-caput serpentis* resembles epemretossous of lower denterortonniaus and *Crana ahomala* comes closer to lower protortormiaus (1).

Echinodermata. Recent echinoderms are, in general dioecious. Certain exceptions occur, such as the starfish *Asterina gibbosa* which is hermaphroditic. In addition, it is not uncommon that, in particular genera, hermaphroditic or protandrous animals are found. These are considered as anomalies.

Crinoidea. The gonads are an accumulation of sex cells located in arms or pinnulae escaping by rupture of the pinnulae. The cement glands play a role in fixation. The development of the sex cells starts in the genital canal at the genital cords. The canal, as a portion of the coelom, is lined by endothelium.

Holothuroidea. The sex organs in the holothurians are comparable to those in crinoids. The wall of the tubes is composed of the flat to columnar epithelium of the coelom, circular and longitudinal musculature, and connective tissue. The innermost layer of epithelium gives rise to the sex cells, the usual condition found in echinoderms.

Echinoidea. In the gonads of this group, we find again a similar arrangement of the layers: coelomic epithelium, musculature, connective tissue, and epithelium from which the sex cells develop.

It was shown by ruthenium red staining procedures that gametes of the sea urchin *Paracen-trotus lividus* exhibit an extraneous coat on the surface of the plasmalemma containing acid mucopolysaccharide or mucoprotein (5). Spermatozoa of the sea urchin *P. lividus* contain, in their mitochondria, glycogen, glucose-6-phosphatase, and adenosine triphosphatase (5).

The ribosomes of sea urchin eggs show amino acid incorporation after fertilization.

Asteroidea. The gonads in asteroids show the usual picture of echinoderms, with walls surrounded by a coelomic cover underlain by connective tissue, musculature, and again connective tissue followed by the germinal epithelium as the innermost structure. Between the musculature and the second connective tissue layer the genital sinus occurs, enabling us to distinguish between a genital wall composed of all layers and the genital wall proper composed of two latter layers only.

Ophiuroidea. The wall of the sex organs again exhibits the coelomic epithelium, connective tissue with interspersed musculature, and layer of germ cells. Ciliated gonoducts have also been observed. The comparative ultrastructural study of spermatozoa of *Ophiocoma echinata* and *Ophiocoma wendti* showed that these cells of oplinoid species resemble those of other nonechinoid echinoderms (28).

Pogonophora. The female genital system of these dioecious animals is composed of paired ovaries and attached oviducts. A pair of testes occurs in the male with sperm ducts. The histology of this rarely investigated phylum is nearly unknown. The epithelium of the sperm ducts is ciliated. The sperms become enclosed in spermatophores.

The Chordate Phyla

Hemichordata. The gonads are simple saclike structures which open by a gonophore, is relatively direct. There are no accessory structures.

Cephalochordata. Ovaries as well as testes are paired structures but their appearance is simple when compared to the higher chordates. The paired gonads consist of 25–33 entities on each side. No accessory structures occur.

Vertebrata. In vertebrates, dioecious reproduction is generally found. The reproductive system usually consists of paired gonads, tubes, accessory glands, and other accessory structures.

The ontogenetic development of the gonads begins with the indifferent gonads (genital ridges, with germinal epithelium containing presumptive germ cells). The gonadal medulla is composed of the primary sex cords, the rete cords, and interstitial cells. The tunica albuginea appears.

The course of the basic gonadal development explains why the various types of neoplasms derive from the different cells in a comparable fashion in male and female gonads.

In vertebrates, seasonal breeders and those which are able to breed continuously, if sexually mature, are distinguished. Different intermittent phases occur. No regeneration of the testes is found in migratory salmon which die following fertilization.

Male reproductive tracts are missing in cyclostomes and salmonidae; sperm are excreted into the body cavity and leave through genital pores. The male genital ducts show a large variation in teleosts. The vasa efferentia are present in fishes and amniotes. The epididymis is as large or larger than the testes in reptiles, relatively small in birds, and of considerable size in mammals. In primates, certain carnivores, and most rodents, sperm ducts appear as enlargements of the vas deferens. The ampulla is then followed by the ejaculatory duct. Placentalia among mammals, with the exception of carnivores, have a seminal vesicle. In the chondrostei claspers and siphon, in some teleosts the gonopodium, in reptiles and birds hemipenis, crocodilians and others a phallus, and in mammals the penis is the intermittent organ.

The main accessory glands in mammals are the prostate and the bulbourethral (Cooper's) glands. Only marsupials and placental mammals exhibit a prostate; it is missing in edentates and cetaceans.

Hermaphroditic Structures of Sexual Reproduction

Porifera. Most sponges exhibit hermaphroditism. The cell types involved in the sexual process have been described previously. No gonads occur in sponges, only scattered sex cells occur in the mesenchyme.

Ctenophora. In ctenophora only hermaphroditic reproduction is found. The sex cells develop from the gastrodermal cells. The mouth acts as a gonophore or the germ cells are released through the epidermis. The gonads lay side-by-side in the meridian canal as longitudinal structures. Sperm ducts may occur.

Platyhelminthes. The hermaphroditic mode of sexual reproduction is the most common type of reproduction in general and of sexual reproduction in particular of this phylum. In contrast to structures of other low organism groups which often are simple, the genital organs of flatworms are highly complicated structures.

The sex cells may be freely produced by mesenchymal cells, a condition observed in lower phyla, or gonads may exist. A tremendous number of variations occurs. As already stated, the majority of these animals are hermaphroditic as such or may be protandric, a condition which has to be considered as a protection against self-fertilization.

The female system consists in general of:
1. The reproductive gland in form of one or two ovaries
2. The duct system composed of:
   a. Oviduct
   b. Uterus
   c. Accessory ducts
   d. Genital antrum for sperm storage
3. Accessory glands:
   a. Yolk or vitelline glands. A special condition in platyhelminthes is that the yolk necessary for the nourishment of the egg is not stored in the egg itself, but in special cells. Composition of these glands and variations of different development depend on the genera involved
   b. Mehlis gland.

The male system is in general composed of:
1. Abundant testes as reproductive gland
2. The duct system
   a. Sperm ducts
   b. Ejaculatory duct
3. Accessory glands and copulatory organ
   a. Prostate
   b. Penis.

There occur many structural, functional as well as topographical variations.

Turbellaria. The ovaries are either single or double structures with one or two ducts. The lining, a one-layered epithelium, shows variations according to area or functional condition. Ciliated or glandular cells are found. Main portions of the latter may be located in the underlying tissues of the epithelium. The gland cells are often topographically united, forming the so-called cement sac. The tubular portions of the female sexual system are also characterized by circular and longitudinal musculature. The yolk or vitelline glands are of particular interest because they are unique in the animal kingdom and are known only in this phylum of platyhelminthes.

The testes occur as single, paired, or abundant structures. The sperm cells exhibit no particularities but show certain variations. The seminal vesicle and the penis exhibit tremendous variations and have been described in the literature about parasites. The prostate is composed of glandular cells. Instead of a penis, cirrus may be present.

Trematoda. The sexual structures of trematoda follow in general the common plan given above. There are variations of the subgroups which have been extensively described in zoological journals because of the economic importance of those worms.

Cestoda. The sexual structures of the cestodes also follow the common plan of the phylum. The highly complicated sexual structures are of great importance for taxonomy. With exception of the genus *Dioecocestus*, which is dioecious, all members of the class are hermaphroditic. The development of the sex organs starts from the mesenchyme followed by a differentiation into the lining epithelium which may be replaced by a cuticle and the supporting musculature.

Nemertini. Hoplonemertini exhibit hermaphroditic genera. This is considered an exception because most of the nemertini are dioecious, as already mentioned.

Gastrotricha. The majority of the animals, whose genital system is not well understood, are hermaphroditic. This is the main concept. We find variations such as the degeneration of the male system leading to parthenogenesis, protandry or even male, female or hermaphroditic forms in mixed occurrence, depending on genus, species, or individuum.

Mollusca. In molluscs, where the majority of animals are dioecious, the aplacophora, opisthobranchia, and pulmonata are hermaphroditic. This also holds true for some other gastropods and genera such as the pelecypods *Ostrea*, *Pecten*, *Unio*, and *Venus*.

Opisthobranchia (54). This group is composed of hermaphroditic animals (exceptions are *Microhedyle* and *Strubellia paradoxa*). The histology of the reproductive system of opisthobranchs is not well known. The ovotestis is a follicular organ. There is great variation in the topography of female and male components which may be intermingled, one component central and the other peripheral or separated, depending on the genera concerned. All thinkable combinations occur. The glands may produce both sex cells simultaneously or in the protandric way. The hermaphroditic duct leads to the ampulla (which is an enlargement with glandular epithelium, characterized by ciliated or at least partially nonciliated columnar epithelium, connective tissue and musculature) acting as a

seminal vesicle. It continues in the gonoduct and generally a sperm duct (ciliated and with musculature) with prostate (columnar cells making up the lining) as well as a penis, through which the sperm duct may run. The glands of the female components are known as albumen gland and mucous gland. Their similar histology may be discussed. The epithelial lining is characterized by columnar cells with granular inclusions. Ciliated cells are intermingled. In certain genera different regions according to the mucus type may be discerned (15).

Pulmonata. Pulmonates are generally simultaneous hermaphrodites. We are able to distinguish among the hermaphroditic portion proper, the female components, and the male components. The hermaphroditic portion proper is composed of the ovotestis and the hermaphroditic duct characterized by cuboidal or columnar ciliated epithelium and a muscle coat. The female components are the fertilization pouch exhibiting an epithelium of columnar cells which may be mixed with ciliated cells; the albumen gland is generally tubular and characterized by columnar epithelium; then follows the oviduct with its enlargement, the uterus (with glands such as the mucous gland), characterized again by tall ciliated cells and in certain species surrounded by strong circular muscles. Several regions may be discerned histologically. The lining of the vagina is ciliated and surrounded by musculature. The bursa copulatrix may enter here and additional glandular structures have been described.

The male structures are the sperm duct seen as a continuation of the hermaphroditic duct and are characterized by cuboidal to columnar ciliated cells, or similar unciliated cells with ciliated intermingled cells which are surrounded by circular and often longitudinal musculature and covered by connective tissue. Granulated epithelial cells and ciliated cells characterize the prostate. Goblet cells are found in the glandular epithelium of the muscular penis.

Mature spermatozoa of the gray field slug *Agriolimax reticulatus* (Pulmonata, Stylomatophora), as a typical pulmonate sperm type, show a simple acrosome and spiral nucleus, a head, and a tail ensheathed by mitochondria (11).

Annelida. Myzostomida and oligochaeta are hermaphroditic, the polychaeta described before and generally dioecious, and the hirudinea or leeches to be described later are protandric.

Myzostomida. They are hermaphroditic animals. The ova are free-lying in the celomic cavity and are fertilized by the sperm which are transported by a sperm syncytium, composed of a combination of sperm and podocytes, building a sperm syncytium, changing in a sperm rhizome from which the sperms are freed for fertilization.

Oligochaeta. The female organs are the ovaries, paired oviducts, and seminal receptacles. The male organs consist of the paired testes, sperm duct; a prostate and penis may also be present. The sex organs of oligochaeta are restricted to certain body segments, varying according to the species.

Arthropoda. The arthropoda exhibit hermaphroditic genera only as rare exceptions. An example of this exception occurs in the order of acari (arachnid). In crustaceans, hermaphroditic forms occur in cirripeds and some isopods.

Tentaculata, the Lophophorate Phyla. *Ectoprocta.* The majority of the animals are hermaphroditic. The organs have been described under "Dioecious Structures of Reproduction." Not much has to be added, insofar as the gonads are merely cell clusters or accumulations with a peritoneal cover.

Phoronida. The majority of the phoronids are hermaphroditic, in which case the ovary is generally dorsally located, the testis ventrally located; in some, gonadal position is reversed. The histology has been discussed under the "Dioecious Structures of Reproduction."

Echinodermata. Hermaphroditic forms occur among some cucumarids in the dendrochirotes, aspidochirotes, synaptides of the holothuroidea; whereas in asteroidea some hermaphroditic individuals of normally dioecious genera occur. In echinoidea hermaphroditic forms have been found as rare anomalies. In ophiuroidea, hermaphroditic forms occur among the ophiurae. Some species of these echinoderms may also be occasionally dioecious. We observe in these deuterostomians the crystallizations of conditions which will be phylogenetically later pathologic as in vertebrate hermaphroditism, especially humans.

Chaetognatha. These animals are hermaphroditic, with paired ovaries anteriorly and paired testes posteriorly. The ovaries, filled with ova of different developmental stages, continue in an oviduct characterized by cuboidal to columnar epithelium (surrounding the seminal receptacle), then into the vagina. The testes are supplied with the ciliated sperm ducts and funnel as well as seminal vesicle (the wall is composed of epidermis and a one-layered internal epithelium). New studies on the function of the organs are necessary.

Vertebrata. True hermaphroditism is known in teleosts (serranidae). For the structures involved, see the description of dioecious structures in teleosts (p. 150).

Protandric Structures of Sexual Reproduction

Aschelminthes. Protandric structures in aschelminthes are found in **gastrotricha,** belonging to the macrodasyoidea. New histological studies on the whole reproductive system are urgently needed from a functional point of view.

Mollusca (Prosobranchia). The transformation from the male to the female organs in the genus *Crepidula* is well known.

Annelida. A few species such as *Brania* sp. or Ophrytrocha sp. are protandric. The biggest group of protandric hermaphrodites in annelid worms is the order of Hirudinea or leeches.

Echinodermata. This type of reproduction occurs occasionally in starfish. *Asterina gibbosa* and *Frana ghardaqana* are protandric. In the first, the young animals behave as males and the older as females. Ova may be found in the gonads of young individuals, and sperm may be present in the gonad of older animals, however.

Vertebrata. Cyclostomes and several species of teleosts as the Menidae, Sparidae, and Serranidae exhibit protandry. It is generally an exceptional condition. The structures show no peculiarities if compared to normal dioecious forms.

Parthenogenetic Structures of Sexual Reproduction

Aschelminthes. Rotifera. Parthenogenetic reproduction in aschelminthes is known in rotifers and gastrotricha as well. In the rotifer order, bdelloidea have only parthenogenetic females. Males have never been observed. This is one of the rare examples of permanent parthenogenesis. The organs and their histology have been described on page 140.

Gastrotricha. In the class gastrotricha, the chaetonotoidea, with the exception of *Xenotrichula*, are parthenogenetic. But in contrast to the Bdelloidea, in which the parthenogenetic forms developed from dioecious ones, they have developed these parthenogenetic forms from hermaphroditic ones.

Annelida. Some polychaeta exhibit parthenogenesis.

Tardigrada. Parthenogenesis occurs in many genera.

Arthropoda. *Crustaceans.* Parthenogenesis occurs in only a few groups of arthropods, such as crustaceans and insects. In crustaceans some branchiopods of the order notostraca are parthenogenetic, whereas parthenogenesis occurs quite commonly in the order cladocera. Generations of females change with those of both sexes. In ostracoda, parthenogenetic genera occur also, but are not very common.

Insects. Parthenogenesis in insects appears in aphids (aphidae) belonging to the order Homoptera.

Some Remarks on Spermiogenesis, Oogenesis, Egg Types, Cleavage, and Germinal Layers

These general topics are well known among biologists, but there occur certain peculiarities or exceptions to the rule which may be of interest in comparative oncology. Spermatozoa are generally flagellated structures and follow a common plan of development. Nevertheless, aflagellate spermatozoa are known in crustaceans and acarina, and spermiocytogenesis differs from that seen with flagellate spermatozoa. The spermiocytogenesis of the North American river crayfish *Procambarus clarkii* is a typical example. The spermatozoa of this species are flattened and exhibit armlike appendages in one plane. The mitochondria are not involved in the makeup of this akinetic cell. The centriole degenerates, the acrosome is well developed, the nucleus is flat and invaginates the armlike processes (59). The nourishment of spermatozoa during development occurs by syncytia, anucleated protoplasma masses, or special nourishing cells (15, 59). The development of the egg cells is comparable.

Oogenesis exhibits similar variations in nourishing the egg cells and the developmental stages in members of different phyla. Mesodermal connective tissues of the ovary appear only in cephalopoda and vertebrata (54, 59). Different egg types exist with regard to the amount of yolk as well as a different pattern of cleavage. Cleavage may totally or partially affect the germ. The most widely distributed type of cleavage in protostomian is spiral, and in deuterostomians it is radial. In porifera, cnidaria, and ctenophora, two germ layers are present; in all other metazoans there are three.

Asexual Reproduction

Porifera (Sponges). Three types of asexual reproduction (in addition to the sexual one) are known in sponges: (a) budding, (b) gemmulae, and (c) asexual larvae. In all three cases the archeocytes are the cells responsible for the process. In the case of budding, clumps of archeocytes are released; in the case of gemmulae, clumps of the same multipotent cell type are surrounded by a coat including archeocytes. Some genera of sponges develop from the gemmulae (see under larvae; pages 155, 160, 173) as asexual larvae. Archeocytes, very common in the body of the sponge, are characterized by a large nucleus and nucleolus.

Mesozoa. Under certain conditions, fragmentation occurs in the orthonectida.

Cnidaria. Fission and budding are the types of asexual reproduction in cnidarians. Fission may be longitudinal or transverse. In the case of budding, both epithelia, ectoderm and entoderm, including mesogloea and interstitial cells, are involved. A special form of budding is the separation of small, nonciliated structures which may develop into a new organism.

Platyhelminthes. The question of regeneration comes into the picture if we are looking at asexual reproduction of plathyhelminthes, where transverse fission or fragmentation occur, in addition to some still debatable types of asexual reproduction. Those are polyembryony as well as larval budding in some forms.

Entoprocta. The type of asexual reproduction of entoprocta is budding and several types of tissues are involved. Our knowledge regarding the different types of tissues and their involvement in the asexual process of reproduction is rather scarce and new investigations should be undertaken.

Nemertini. Transverse fission or fragmentation is a mode of asexual reproduction in these forms, which are otherwise generally dioecious. Interestingly the regenerative ability in this phylum is not limited to the tissues concerned, but to the body region. Differences in the regenerative capacity between the anterior and posterior portion of the animal's body exist.

Annelida. In polychaeta asexual reproduction has been observed in the form of transverse fission (fragmentation) or budding. This type of fragmentation may be the only type of reproduction, as in *Zeppelina monostyla*. Asexual reproduction occurs especially under culture growth conditions.

Tentaculata, the Lophophorate Phyla. In tentaculata, asexual reproduction is found only in ectoprocta and phoronida; it is uncommon in brachiopoda.

The two types of asexual reproduction in ectoprocta are budding and the production of statoblasts. In the case of budding, indifferent basal epidermal cells produce the bud and the basement membrane, and muscle cells disappear in the particular area of budding.

Each statoblast can be considered as a cell cluster surrounded by a shell-like layer. The cell types of the cell cluster of the statoblasts are peritoneal cells and basal cells of the epidermis similar to those occurring in the buds.

Asexual reproduction in phoronida (*P. ovalis*) occurs in the form of transverse fission in the area of the body where musculature is missing. Fission never occurs in the muscular portion of the body.

Branchiotremata. Asexual reproduction occurs only in the enteropneust *Balanoglossus capensis* in the form of automatous fragmentation of the tail end. These small pieces regenerate into total animals.

Chordata. Asexual reproduction in this superphylum can be considered as a carryover from ancestors in an earlier period of history of the earth. Asexual reproduction occurs only in low chordates, namely urochordata or tunicata, in the classes of ascidiacea and thaliacea. The type of asexual reproduction is budding, found in all developmental stages. It is initiated (as in certain other groups mentioned before) by the epidermis, as in ascidiacea. Asexual reproduction in thaliacea appears also in the form of budding.

Selected Aspects of Normal Organismic Growth, Especially Important for Comparative Oncology: Roundabouts (Detours) in Ontogenetic Development

Detours in ontogenetic development have been neglected in oncology, with the exception of investigations of human placental neoplasms. They also have been neglected in comparative oncology, with the exception of studies dealing with larvae of a few species such as *Drosophila* sp. The roundabouts in ontogenetic development can be seen as an organismic attempt to increase the adaptation to specialized and differing environments during the ontogenetic life span. This is the case in holometabolic insects whose larvae may be aquatic organisms and the imago a terrestrial organism. At the same time prolonged larval stages represent the ontogenetic growth period, whereas the imago is the sexual period without growth. Therefore, these ontogenetic developments are an important and, until now, neglected, reservoir for experimental comparative oncology. Other typical larval structures are those which free the embryo from the egg, or locomotory devices not seen in the adult. The same is true in the case of different types of respiratory organs in larvae and imagines, etc. Some of the structures can be explained only as phylogenetic remnants, for example, the tooth bud in the embryonal head of whalebone whales. At least theoretically, neoplasms may develop from all of these structures. We know from human placental or embryonic tumors that a spread of the tumor to the mother organism or vice versa is possible. The same possibility exists, at least theoretically, for the other structures of ontogenetic detours and the later resulting imagines.

Metamorphosis may be distinguished into embryonal and larval.

Embryonal Metamorphosis

Egg (Vitelline) Membranes. Vitelline membranes must be distinguished from embryonal sheaths. Vittelline membranes occur in the egg cell during its development, often not before ripening and seldom before fertilization. They are noncellular structures, secreted either from the egg cell or the different tissues contacting the egg cell during its development (ovary, oviduct, accessory glands) (31, 59).

Embryonal Sheaths. The embryonal sheaths are composed of material which belongs to the embryo. They may be cellular or acellular; one type can be transformed into the other as is known of cestodes in which the inner embryonal sheath changes from its cellular structure to a cuticular one. Embryonal sheaths are found in cestodes where they exhibit two cell layers, in oligochaeta where they result from a large portion of the germ, in nemertines, in pentastomida, and in echinoderms. The highest form of embryonal sheath occurs in arthropoda and amniotes (59).

Placenta. Placentae are embryo-maternal exchange organs. This transitional organ gave the name to a big group of mammals, the placental mammals or placentalia (all mammals except monotremes and marsupials). But placentae are also found in metatheria as in the opossum and in other groups besides the mammals, vertebrates and invertebrates alike. Invertebrate placentae are present in onychophora, arthropoda, ectoprocta, and urochordata, and in the vertebrate sharks and reptiles. The different placental types are reviewed in Table 6.4. Comparison of embryonal and larval metamorphosis shows that in the case of embryonal metamorphosis destruction is more dominant, whereas in larval metamorphosis synthesis and reconstruction prevail. These facts are one reason why larval metamorphosis and its processes are so important for comparative oncology.

Larval Metamorphosis

Larval metamorphosis can proceed under greatly varying circumstances. It may be continuing or catastrophic, the latter characterized by far reaching histolytic processes. A review of larval stages of porifera and eumetazoa is given in Table 6.5 and general organ characterization of selected larvae in Table 6.6.

Selected Cases of Organ Development. The following short section is intended to give a few examples of basic differences in cells and tissues of varying stages of ontogenetic detours. These variations may be exploited to solve certain questions of comparative oncology which cannot be answered by only using adult forms.

Comparative organ development exhibits a tremendous variety in the different phyla (7, 59, 62). It is well known that the ontogenesis in the most important groups of protostomians, the arthropods, is totally different from the most important group of deuterostomians, the chordates. With regard to the circulatory system of coelomates, a primary and a secondary one may be discerned. Certain similarities appear with regard to body fluid cells insofar as they all are derivatives of the mesoderm.

The actinotrocha (a modified trochophora) of the phoronidea develops protonephridia which are later replaced by the metanephridia of the adult. The phylogeny of embryonal and larval development produced similarities and dissimilarities. In the case of holometabolic insects, metamorphosis becomes more differentiated parallel to the increase of the varying environment in which the larvae and imagines live. This is necessary because the differences in organization of larvae and imagines provide a greater

efficiency. Synthetic and destructive processes increase in severity; remodeling without destruction becomes rare, and totally unchanged organs are extremely rare. New cells and cell groups appear in the place of histolytically discarded cells of larval organs. These cells, known as imaginal cells, are unaffected by the surrounding histolytic processes and fill the places of the old discarded tissues. These occasions seem to be the most essential contribution for comparative oncology holometabolic insects are able to offer. Pupal conditions and the so-called processes of internal metamorphosis, not only of holometabolic insects, but also of cirriped crustaceans or marine ectoprocta, enlarge this scope. Embryonal and larval metamorphoses exhibit the same path. The variation occurs in cases of the roundabouts of metamorphosis. New findings, including facts of cell cloning and experiments with different types of reproduction, are of interest for a comparison of the path of development in structures serving the same function, but in different organisms of porifera and eumetazoans.

Integument. During ontogeny of holometabolic insects the larval epidermis is histolyzed in the path of inner metamorphosis (pupa) (59). Regarding the integument of aquatic larvae, new studies are urgently needed. They will not only give basic information with regard to the influence of carcinogens, but also a practical evaluation of pollution of the aquatic environment.

Digestion. The fine structure of the midgut epithelium in the mite (Acarina, Argasidae) *Ornithodores papillipes* nymphs in the blood assimilation period exhibits three cell types: reserve, digestive, and secretory cells (6). The response of lysosomes and other cell organelles of the digestive cells of the mussel, *Mytilus edulis* (42) and related studies are of comparative interest.

Respiration. With regard to respiration, the changes from one type to another between different larval stages, and larval stages to adult organisms, as changes from tracheid gills to tracheids in certain holometabolic insects (with respiration of the larvae using hemoglobin) to gaseous exchange by diffusion, need new studies.

Excretion. Noticeable questions of the development of excretory structures have been touched upon. Investigations concerning the renal sac in ascidia are important (51).

Reproduction. Comparative studies of the development of spermatozoa and ova in their re-

Table 6.4: Placentae[a]

Type of Placenta	Systematic Unit of Appearance	Characteristic Species	Remarks
A. INVERTEBRATE PLACENTAE			
1. Placentae of Onychophora	Onychophora	*Peripatus edwarsii, P. torquatus, Peripatopsis capensis, Peripatopsis balfouri, P. sedgwicki*	These placentae start from neck region. They are either simple or voluminous neck-bladders or embryonal covers surrounding the whole body. Reduction of yolk in different species of *Peripatopsis* goes parallel with improvement of breeding care. Umbilical cord remains on back
2. Placentae of Arthropoda	Arthropoda Class: Arachnida Scorpiones, scorpions	*Hormurus australasiae*	Placenta somewhat similar to those of Onychophora and Eutheria
	Pseudoscorpiones, pseudoscorpions	*Pselaphochernes* sp.; *Chelifer* sp.	Main portions of this nutritional mechanism are nourishing fluid of female, embryonic sheath, and pumping organ of embryo. Pumping organ will later be discarded, process reminding us of metamorphosis
	Class: Insecta Hymenoptera (Family: Chalcididae, chalcid wasps)	*Platygaster* sp.	In this mechanism, composed of host tissue and tissue of embryonic parasite (embryonal paranuclear mass, trophamnion, and cover from host), epitheloid layer, above the embryonic sheath can be distinguished.
3. Placentae of Bryozoa (Ectoprocta)	Bryozoa, Ectoprocta	Freshwater species	Girdle-like thickening surrounds embryo
4. Placentae of Tunicata	Tunicata, Urochordata Class: Thaliacea	*Salpa primata, Thalia democratica*	Placentation starts from ovarial tissue, which develops to functional uterus. Placenta bud develops surrounding embryo and its ectoderm. Blood circulates in placenta. Placenta degenerates after birth and material serves for nourishment
B. VERTEBRATE PLACENTAE			
1. Placentae of Chondrichthyes	Class: Chondrichtyes	*Mustelus laevis*	Vitelline sac infiltrates folds of uterus, making possible metabolic exchange
2. Placentae of Reptilia	Class: Reptilia		Periostracum is preserved in some species. White egg is reduced but allantois produces with its vessels via allantochorion an organ of exchange
a. Epithelio-chorial placenta of reptilia		*Seps* sp.	
b. Endothelio-endothelial placenta of reptilia		*Lygosoma* sp.	

3. Placentae of Mammalia
  a. Placentae of Metatheria
   (1) Placenta omphaloides
	Class: Mammalia	*Didelphis* sp.	Production of amnion occurs by folding. Sinus terminalis is at equator. Extraembryonal celom remains small. Chorion produces folds invaginating identations of uterine mucosa. Allantois plays no role in nutrition of embryo

[a] Prepared with the assistance of S. E. Nawab, M.D., Department of Obstetrics and Gynecology, Holy Cross Hospital, Silver Spring, Maryland.

Table 6.4—*Continued*

Type of Placenta	Systematic Unit of Appearance	Characteristic Species	Remarks
(2) Placenta allantoides		*Perameles* sp.	Placenta exhibits during implantation some remarkable similarities to placenta of the Eutheria. Allantois and chorion coalesce to allantochorion. In contrast to Eutheria occurs fixation at uterine wall with this melting region, not with embryonal pole. This placental type is endothelio-endothelial placenta, never occurring in Eutheria. In this species maternal and fetal epithelium unite to functional unity
b. Placentae of Eutheria			Placenta, as fetomaternal exchange organ, serves functions of excretion, resorption and respiration. Placentae of Eutheria exhibit tremendous variation. They can be classified according elimination of fetus, histological layers, external shape, and finally based on whether maternal blood vessels are opened during expulsion of fetus

1. Classification of Eutherian placentae based of conduct of uterine mucosa during elimination of fetus

Placenta of Deciduata	Deciduata		Portions of uterine, maternal mucosa are torn away at partition
Placenta of Adeciduata	Adeciduata		Maternal tissues are undisturbed at parturition
Placenta of contradeciduate type		*Talpa europea*	After parturition placenta is absorbed by uterus

2. Classification of Eutherian placentae according to histological layers by which maternal and fetal tissues border each other

Placenta epitheliochorialis	Perissodactyla	*Equus caballus*	Histological layers between maternal and fetal blood: (1) maternal vessel wall, (2) maternal connective tissue, (3) maternal uterine epithelium, (4) chorionic epithelium, (5) chorionic connective tissue, (6) fetal vessel endothelium
	Artiodactyla	*Sus scrofa* *Hippopotamus amphibius* *Bos taurus*	
	Cetacea Pholidota Primates: Lemuroidea with exception of Tarsus		
	Insectivora (secondary)	*Scalopus* sp.	Chorionic and maternal epithelium are intact, no tissue disintegration takes place
Placenta syndesmochorialis	Artiodactyla	Many species	Fetal epithelium invaginates maternal tissue more and more, and leads in this and following types of placentae to reduction to maternal tissues. These placentae are known as invasive types. Placenta syndesmochorialis shows following tissue layers between maternal and fetal blood: (1) maternal vessel wall, (2) maternal connective tissue, (3) chorionic epithelium, (4) chorionic connective tissue, (5) fetal vessel endothelium

Table 6.4—_Continued_

Type of Placenta	Systematic Unit of Appearance	Characteristic Species	Remarks
Placenta endotheliochorialis	Edentata Carnivora Some Chiroptera	_Bradypus_ sp. _Sorex_ sp.	Placenta endotheliochorialis shows following tissue layers between maternal and fetal blood: (1) maternal vessel wall, (2) chorionic epithelium, (3) chorionic connective tissue, (4) fetal vessel endothelium
Placenta haemochorialis	Insectivora Insectivora Chiroptera (?)	_Tupaia_ sp. Majority of species	Placenta haemochorialis shows following tissue layers between maternal and fetal blood: (1) chorionic epithelium, (2) chorionic connective tissue, (3) fetal vessel endothelium. Border layers between maternal and fetal blood are only of fetal origin
	Primates Lagomorpha Rodentia Edentata Proboscidea Hyracoidea Sirenia	_Tarsius_ sp., _Homo sapiens_ _Dasypus_ sp. (?) _Elephas indicus_ _Procavia capensis_ _Trichechus_ sp.	

3. Classification of Eutherian placentae according to whether maternal blood vessels are opened during parturition

Semiplacentae			Opening of maternal vessels does not take place
Placentae verae			Maternal blood spaces are opened during parturition (compare with Classification 1)

4. Classification of Eutherian placentae based on the external form

A. Placentae covering a large areal, stretched placentae: Placenta diffusa	Primates Pholidota Certacea Perissodactyla Artiodactyla	 _Sus scrofa, Hippopotamus amphibius, Camelus_ sp., _Tragulus_ sp.	Whole surface of blastocyst is addressed as placenta facet
B. Placentae covering a diffused but localized area, diffusely localized placentae: Placenta multiplex or cotyledonaria	Artiodactyla	_Bos taurus_	Placental fields cover wide areal
C. Placentae covering a localized area, localized placentae:			
Placenta zonaria	Carnivora	_Canis familiaris, Vulpes vulpes, Gulo gulo, Felis cattus, Panthera tigris_	Placenta surrounds fetus in girdle-like fashion
Placenta zonaria incompleta	Carnivora	_Procyon lotor_	Placenta surrounds fetus in girdle-like but incomplete fashion
Placenta bidiscoidalis	Primates	_Gorilla gorilla_	Two placental fields are present
Placenta discoidalis	Primates Carnivores	_Homo sapiens_ _Ursus_ sp.	One placental field remains

5. Classification of normal human placentae

Placenta dispersa	Primates	_Homo sapiens_	Umbilical arteries divide in dichotomous manner and diminish rapidly in caliber
Placenta magistralis	Primates	_Homo sapiens_	Umbilical arteries release small side branches, but show nearly no decrease in size before almost reaching placental margin

Table 6.4—*Continued*

Type of Placenta	Systematic Unit of Appearance	Characteristic Species	Remarks
6. Classification of abnormal human placentae			
Placenta ovalis Placenta membranacea (diffusa) Placenta pseudozonaria Placenta bidiscoidalis Placenta lobulata Placenta multilobulata Placenta succentoriatae	Primates	*Homo sapiens*	Human placentae may show abnormal location and abnormal form. They should be considered as pathologic conditions but not as phylogenetic setback. Terms are self-explanatory
			Additional placenta occurs in 1% of cases and is clinically especially important; they remain after parturition in uterus, causing bleeding and inflammations
Placenta praevia			Placenta is attached to lower cervical portion of uterus
Placenta praevia centralis			Placenta covers completely internal os of uterus
Placenta praevia lateralis			Placenta covers partially internal os of the uterus
Placenta praevia marginalis			Part of placenta lies in lower region of uterus but internal os is not covered

lation to nourishing cells and organelle development give new insights (35).

Hormone Production. The ultrastructure of the larval corpus allatum of *Hyphantria cunea* (Insecta, Lepidoptera) revealed

Sensitivity. The structures of sensitivity are intensively investigated. But the variation of cell capacity is wide, ranging from highly regenerative neurons in the coelenterates *Hydra* sp. to cell-invariable neurons in man.

Postembryonic development of the visual system of the locust, *Schistocerca gregaria* (the formation of the retina lamina projection (4)); the fine structure of the photoreceptor of the ascidian tadpole during development (9); the development of the auditory tympana in the cricket, *Telleogryllus commodus* were the first changes in connection with the tympana start (8); the relationship of tympanum and underlying trachae (due to the withdrawal of epidermal cells) (8); the ontogeny of photoreceptor pattern in the compound eyes of mucoid flies (65); and the fine structure of juvenile and adult nuchal organs of annelids (69) are questions which may open new avenues for research in comparative oncology. Knowledge could be gained through such studies.

Body Fluids. With regard to such neoplasm and/or systematic diseases as leukemias, etc., the importance of studies dealing with the differentiation of hemocytes in the embryo of *Oncopeltus fasciatus* (Insecta, Heteroptera) (19a) and youth stages of other species cannot be overestimated.

Motion. The normal changes occurring in the fine structure of muscle insertions on the larval shell and operculum of the nudibranch, *Phestilla sibogae* (mollusca, gastropoda) (13), before and during metamorphosis; the metamorphosis of larval adhesive organs in ascidians, *Distaplia occidentalis* (17); the development of muscle cells of larvae of the ascidian, *Botryllus schlosseri* (52); or of *Cyclosalpa affinis* (64) may stimulate new research concerning experimental benign and malignant rhabdomyomas in different developmental stages of the derivatives of the mesenchymal stem cell.

Interstitial Structures. It was stated elsewhere in this book that the mesenchymal stem cell has a different potential in the organism of various taxonomic levels. Only in the vertebrates, especially the mammal, it can be considered multipotential in the true sense of the word. The neoplastic potential should also vary, at least theoretically. New studies are urgently needed.

Primary and Secondary Larvae. Great differences may exist between one or more larval stages and the adult; but also between larval stages before the development proceeds to the adult in an organism during catastrophic development. Generally larvae become less complicated by the environmental change of the organism to freshwater whereby they may return to the direct development. In some groups there occur intermediate stages with structures not found in the adult organism. These developmental stages are also to be considered as larvae. The secondary larva is closer to the adult than

Table 6.5
General Structural Characterization of Selected Larvae

Type of Larvae	Subtype of Larvae	Taxonomic Units Where Known	Larval Characteristics	Remarks
Blastula	Coeloblastula	Porifera, *Oscarella lobularis, Clathrina blanca*	Usually hollow mass of cells. Cells are ciliated	Specific larval characteristics are often missing
	Amphiblastula	Porifera, *Leucosolenia variabilis, Sycon raphanus*	Cellstructure and ciliation vary in different regions	
	Coeloblastula	Cnidaria (metagenetic Hydrozoa); e.g. *Tiara pileata, Clytia flavidula, Laodice cruciata*	As above	
	Blastula/Gastrula	Echinoderms		Preceding Dipleurula
Planula	—	Cnidaria	Planula is gastrula, which exhibits as larval characteristics glandular and some sensory cells at animal pole	As secondary larvae appears in certain hydrozoa, actinula, and arachnactis
Parenchymula	—	Porifera	Parenchymula is characterized by internal ectoderm and external ciliated entoderm	Largest portion of prospective, ciliated entoderm may undergo hystolysis as in freshwater sponge, *Spongilla* sp.
Trochophora		Protostomia	Characteristic of the trochophora is ciliated girdle (ring), prototroch, running circulary around larval body and separating anterior region, episphere, from posterior region or hyposphere. Prototroch serves locomotion and sometimes nutrition. Cells which produce prototroch are trochoblasts. Prototroch may be pre- or postorally located. Occasionally occurring are additional ciliated girdles in hyposphere, known as telotroch and paratroch. Additional characteristics are apical (neural) plate often with tuft of cilia; larvale protonephridia; nerve rings beneath ciliated bands; simple intestinal tract with mouth and anus; primary body cavity, between body wall and intestine which will be replaced later by larval mesenchymal structures such as musculature	Trochophora theory (originally described by Hatschek in 1878) looked for tracing back of all bilateria to an original form, trochozoon, which passed postembryonal to trochophora

Table 6.5—*Continued*

Type of Larvae	Subtype of Larvae	Taxonomic Units Where Known	Larval Characteristics	Remarks
	Müller's or Götte's larvae	Platyhelminthes (Polycladida, Turbellaria)	Apical plate with tuft of cilia, ciliated lobes, brain, eyespot, mouth opening leading to intestinal tract and yolk should be mentioned	
	Pilidium	Nemertini (Heteronemertini)	Apical plate and complicated ciliary circle are present. Missing are protonephridia, intestine, and anus. Ciliated lobe and embryonal anlage	Metamorphosis of this larva is complicated and exceptional to other trochophorae
	Veliger	Mollusca	Veliger exhibits apical plate with ciliary tuft, prototroch, mesenchyme, intestinal tract with mouth and radular pouch, foot anlage, and shell gland	Atypical larva of unionid bivalves is Glochidium, which follows veliger-like development in egg
	Trochophora S. Str.	Entoprocta, Sipunculida, Annelida	Modified trochophora of entoprocta is similar to cyphonautes of ectoprocta. Preoral organ is connected to apical plate by paired nerves. Another dissimilarity to cyphonautes is presence of protonephridium	Autolytic processes during metamorphosis concern apical plate, ciliary circle, and generally preoral organ. Other transformation occurs by displacement
		Sipunculida	Trochophora of this phylum shows apical plate with tuft of cilia, prototroch, intestinal tract with mouth and anus, larval nephridium and circular and retractor muscles	
		Echiurida	Trochophora of Echiurida exhibits apical plate with tuft or cilia. Mouth leads into intestinal tract. Episphere and hyposphere are separated by prototroch	
		Annelida, Polychaeta	Trochophora of *Polygordius* sp. presents apical plate, tuft of cilia, episphere and hyposphere separated by prototroch, metatroch, telotroch, intestinal tract with mouth and anus, larval nephridium, mesenchymatic musculature and	Variations of trochophora of annelida are found in trochophora known as Mitraria or trochophora of myzostomida

Table 6.5—_Continued_

Type of Larvae	Subtype of Larvae	Taxonomic Units Where Known	Larval Characteristics	Remarks
			mesoteloblast. As in case of _Plathymereis dumerilii_ during metamorphosis, larval stages of trochophora (protrochophora in other species), metatrochophora, nectochaeta and metamorphic stage of worm may be distinguished	
	Actinotrocha	Phoronidea	Trochophora of phoronidea and actinotrocha displays apical plate, larval lobes, ciliated tentacles, three mesodermal portions (mesenchyme in prosoma, hydrocele and somatocele as paired coelomic sacs), suctorial disc, intestinal tract with mouth and anus, and pair of larval protonephridia	
	Cyphonautes	Ectoprocta	Trochophora of ectprocta (marine Bryozoa). Cyphonautes exhibits apical plate, tuft of cilia, ciliary circle, larval shell, suctorial disc, preoral vestibule, mouth, stomach, preanal vestibule, pear-shaped organ, and proctadeum. Hyposphere is small, hystolysis extensive	
Nauplius	—	Arthropoda, Crustacea: Anostraca, Ascothoracida, Cirripedia, Copepoda, Decapoda (Penaeidae), Euphausiaceae, Ostracoda, Phyllopoda	Nauplius exhibits three nauplius segments, carrying all extremities (antenna, mandible), nauplius-eye, often chewing lobe at 2nd antennae, schizopodial leg structure, mandible, and excessive upper labrum	The segments of the nauplius resemble those of the metatrochophora. The continued metamorphosis of the different groups is characterized by additional species specific larval stages or types
	Metanauplius	Copepoda	Two nauplius stages are followed by 4 metanauplii: (1) maxilla, (2) maxilla, (1) thoracal leg and maxilliped, (2) thoracal leg and maxilliped	
		Cirripedia	_Balanus improvinus_ starts development	

Table 6.5—_Continued_

Type of Larvae	Subtype of Larvae	Taxonomic Units Where Known	Larval Characteristics	Remarks
			with nauplius (three stages) followed by three metanauplii	
Cypris	Cypris (larva)	Cirripedia	Two-lobed shell is characteristic. Nauplius eye, one pair of complex eyes, reduced mouth parts, massive first antenna, thorax has six segments, abdomen has no extremities and is composed of four segments, and large carapax. This larva settles soon with first antennae, changing to the cypris—pupa	
	Cypris (pupa)	Cirrepedia	Anterior end and first antennae become stalk or floor plate. Body makes rotation of 180°. Copepodoit extremities are prolonged to richly articulated cirri	Especially interesting for oncology is radical degradation processes of complex eyes and abdomen
		O. Rhizocephala: _Sacculina_ sp.	Metamorphosis is more severe in these endoparasites. Nauplius and cypris have no intestine; cypris no complex eyes. Cypris endoparasite exhibits ectoderm surrounding mass of undifferentiated cells. Together are known as "Kentrogen." Discarded become: the Cypris-exuvie, extremities, remaining musculature, pigment, nauplius-eye and rests of yolk. In antenna, fixed to host, develops hollow stalk. "Kentrogon" enters host body via this hollow stalk as sacculina interna. Embryonal cell material gives rise to two typical parts: (1) in all directions grow the rootlike ramifications with characteristic histologic makeup, surrounding host organs. (2) Voluminous center, known as tumor, remains, with forma-	

Table 6.5—*Continued*

Type of Larvae	Subtype of Larvae	Taxonomic Units Where Known	Larval Characteristics	Remarks
			tion of nucleus. This structure reminds us of non-parasitic cirriped; with mantle, mantle cavity, surrounding body with testes and ovaries, as well as ganglion. This structure, the sacculina interna, leaves host at place of original infection, at border of thorax and abdomen. It shows more clearly organization of nonparasitic cirriped. Especially important is fact that during metamorphosis there remains mass of embryonal cells from which, after all specialized tissues have been discarded, new organism originates, which exhibits characteristics comparable to nonparasitic cirriped	
Calyptis-, Furcilia-, Cyrtopia-stages		Crustacea: Euphausiacee	They develop in this taxonomic unit after 2 nauplii and 1 metanauplius	
Protozoea		Crustacea: Decapoda: Penaeidae	Two pairs of antennae, three pairs of thoracopods (3rd as anlage), abdominal segments, additional appendages. Development continues into mysis stage	3 Metazoea stages proceed from metanauplius. Metazoea is intermediate larva
Zoea	(Metazoea)	Crustacea decapoda (zoea is a common larval type)	Anterior thoracopods, carapax and long segmented abdomen with buds of extremities are present. Outside of zoea of *Thia polita* exhibits rostrum back thorn, complex eyes, 1–3 maxillipeds, pereiopods	
Mysis		Crustacea, Natantia, Penaeidea	Mysis can originate from protozea as in *Penaeopsis stebbingi* with fully developed thoracal extremities and anlage of abdominal extremities; but it can also originate from zoea	
	Phyllosoma	*e.g.*, Scyllaridae	Special type (subtype) of Mysis	

Table 6.5—*Continued*

Type of Larvae	Subtype of Larvae	Taxonomic Units Where Known	Larval Characteristics	Remarks
Megalopa		Brachyura	Zoea is able to reach megalopa stage via metazoea	
Manca stage	Peracarida (Isopoda, Tanaidacea, Cumacea)	Peracarida (Isopoda, Tanaidacea, Cucea)	Embryo, in direct development which originates directly from the egg, may differ from adult by lack of last pair of thoracal legs	
		Arthropoda—Insecta Ametabola (Apterygota) Protura, Collembola, Diplura, Thysanura	—	True metamorphosis is absent
		Metabola (Pterygota)	Usually wings; larva develops with full complement of adult segments; genitalia and cerci are only abdominal appendages. This group includes most insects	Incomplete or complete metamorphosis
	Nymphs	Hemi- and Paurometabola	Gradual or incomplete metamorphosis; nymphs with compound eyes; externally developing wings	
		Orthoptera, Dermaptera, Isoptera, Embioptera, Odonata, Ephemeroptera, Mallophaga, Anoplura, Psocoptera, Thysanoptera, Zoraptera, Hemiptera, Homoptera	A. Aquatic larvae: *Prometabola* (Ephemeridae). Exhibit tracheal gills. Two imaginal stages are present in contrast to other insects *Archimetabola* (Odonata, Plecoptera, e.g.). Tracheal gills are present, subimago is missing B. "Larvae" and imago in similar environment: *Paurometabola* (Heteroptera, several Homoptera). Stepwise transformation of adult-like larvae. *Homometabola* (e.g., Phylloxeridae). Nymph exhibits wing	

Table 6.5—_Continued_

Type of Larvae	Subtype of Larvae	Taxonomic Units Where Known	Larval Characteristics	Remarks
			anlage at exterior	
			Remetabola (Thysanoptera). Two wingless larval stages are followed by pronympha and one or two (half-resting) nymphae	
			Parametabola (of Coccidiae). Two to three wingless larvae are succeeded by motile or nonmotile pronymphae or nymphae. (Males of Coccidiae exhibit no food intake and are without functional intestine)	
			Allometabola: In case of Aleurodines, fourth wingless larval stage transforms directly to imago with wings	
	Holometabola (Endopterygota): Mecoptera, Trichoptera, Neuroptera, Lepidoptera, Diptera, Siphonaptera, Coeloptera, Strepsiptera, Hymenoptera	C.	Larvae without compound eyes, internally developing wings; complete metamorphosis including pupa: _Eoholometabola._ Tracheal gills are present, larva looks similar to imago, pupa is motile (_Sialis_ sp., (Megaloptera)) _Euholometabola._ Larvae	Metamorphosis is concentrated at two moultings at end of larval life: pupal and imaginal. Anlage of wings and genitalia appear externally first. This process is known as external metamorphosis. During pupal resting stage inner metamorphosis occurs; some larval organs as epidermis or intestine perish, others remain (Malpighian tubules) and are transformed as nervous system or differentiated (Siewing)

Table 6.5—*Continued*

Type of Larvae	Subtype of Larvae	Taxonomic Units Where Known	Larval Characteristics	Remarks
			and imago show remarkable differences (majority of holometabolic insect species), e.g., in mouth parts and abdominal extremities of larvae. Succeeding larvae differ essentially only by size (e.g., Lepidoptera)	
			Polymetabola. Larval stages differ strongly if they exhibit different life styles, e.g., free-living and parasitic larvae in succession (e.g., certain Coeloptera and Hymenoptera)	Histolytical processes play more or less important role. Histolysis and involvement of tissues with embryonal potential during these transformations make metamorphosis of holometabolic insects important as additional leads in chain of events to understand comparative pathology of growth. Pupa is resting system in which structures are reconstructed in time they must not function
			Hypermetabola. In certain Coeloptera appear one to two free-living larvae, followed by two grub-of-cockchafer-like larvae, followed by pseudo-pupa (larva coarctata), then again free larva and finally pupa	
			Cryptometabola. Whole larval development occurs in eggshell; larva pupates immediately after hatching	
Oligopod	Campodeiform	Neuroptera, Trichoptera, Strepsiptera, some Coeloptera	Prognathous head, long legs, dorsoventrally flattened and	

Table 6.5—*Continued*

Type of Larvae	Subtype of Larvae	Taxonomic Units Where Known	Larval Characteristics	Remarks
	Scarabaeiform	Some Coeloptera	well sclerotized Inactive, poorly sclerotized thorax and abdomen; short legged and fat	
Polypod	—	Lepidoptera, Mecoptera, certain Hymenoptera	Thoracic legs, abdominal prolegs and poor sclerotization are the characteristics	
Apodous			No legs, very poor sclerotization. Subtypes can be distinguished according to head sclerotization	
	Eucephalous	e.g., Nematocera, Buprestidae	Head capsule is well sclerotized	
	Hemicephalous	e.g., Brachycera	Reduced head capsule can be retracted into thorax	
	Acephalous	e.g., Cyclorrhapha	Head capsule is missing	
Protopod		Parasitic Hymenoptera	First instar larva of abnormal type	
Dipleurula		Echinodermata	As in all larvae of echinoderms, characteristic ciliated bands on body elevations are typical. Ciliated field like trapezoid surrounds mouth which is located in vestibulum	
	—	Echinodermata	Apical ciliary tuft may be present, underlain by nervous tissue. Larva is comparable to Tornaria of hemichordata	In general, echinoderm larvae are bilateral in shape and exhibit intestinal tract with mouth and anus
Auricularia	—	Holothuroidea	Ciliated bands are on four corners and extended. Ciliated field is before mouth and one before anus	
Bipinnaria	—	Asteroidea	Preoral aereal. Ciliar arrangement is similar to this one of the Auricularia. Fixation plate shows changes. Three processes develop cup-shaped suckers. This stage, not known for all	
Brachiolaria	—	Some Asteroidea	Asteroidea, is termed Brachiolaria	
Pluteus		Echinoidea, Ophiuroidea	Distance from mouth to anus is, in comparison to Bipinnaria and Auricularia types, shortened. Ciliated field surrounding mouth develops slender, fragile processes, supported by	

Table 6.5—*Continued*

Type of Larvae	Subtype of Larvae	Taxonomic Units Where Known	Larval Characteristics	Remarks
	Ophiopluteus		special skeletal bars Anterolateral, postero-lateral, postoral and transverse lateral arms are typical	
	Echinopluteus		Anterolateral, postero-lateral, preoral arms are typical	
Doliolaria	—	Crinoidea	It is most typically keglike larva of echinoderms. Tuft of cilia is located at apical pole, under-lain by nervous api-cal plate. Four cil-iated bands encircle the body	
Tornaria	—	Hemichordata, Enter-opneusta		Preliminary stages are compara-ble with dipleurula
Tadpole larva	—	Urochordata, Ascidi-acea	Eye and statocyst are present in cerebrale vesicle and papillae of attachment be-neath mouth open-ing. Generally tail portion is present, containing dorsally located neural tube and musculature	During metamorphosis, central nervous system and tail with all its organs is eliminated. Mouth and anus of larva are closed. Number of organs are rotated (180° in case of intes-tinal tract)
	Subtypes are "anuran larvae" with lack of tail	Ascidiacea		
	Anuran tadpole	Anura	Shape of mouth, horny teeth, long in-testinal tract, shape of aortic arch, gills, gill clefts, peribran-chial cavity, tail and tail fins are charac-teristic features of larva	As in other forms, where larvae and adult differ in mastering environment, differences of larva and adult are more pro-nounced in anuran than uro-deles. Anuran tadpoles are herbivorous in contrast to an-urans which are carnivorous. In urodeles tadpole and adult are carnivorous. This relation-ship is reflected in intensity of metamorphosis; pronounced in anurans, less pronounced in urodeles. Metamorphosis in anurans is short (days), and extended in urodeles (weeks)
	Tadpole of Urodela	Urodela	Larval characteristics are pronounced branchial apparatus, external gills, gill clefts, pronounced visceral skeleton, shape of head, con-dition of skin	
Ammocoete	—	Vertebrata, Cyclosto-mata		

Table 6.6
Taxonomic Appearance of Larvae

Phylum	Subgroup	Larva	Subtype of Larva	Most Common Type of Larva	Other Larvae
Porifera		Blastula	Coeloblastula Amphiblastula	Blastula	
		Parenchymula		Parenchymula	
Cnidaria		Planula		Planula	Actinula, Scyphiostoma, Strobila; Edwardsia and Halcampoides (developmental stages)
Ctenophora		Planula		Planula	Cydippid larva
Plathyhelminthes	Turbellaria (Plolycladida)	Götte's larva Müller's larva			
	Trematodes	Miracidium		Miracidium	Cercaria, Cysticercus, Redia, Sporocyst
	Cestodes	Onchosphaera			
Nemertinea		Pilidium		Pilidium	Desor's larva (only *Lineus viridis*)
Entoprocta		Trochophora		Trochophora	
Acanthocephala		Acantha		Acantha	Acanthella, Cystacanth
Kinorhyncha		Haploderes Centrophyes Habroderes Hyalophyes			
Priapulida		Three larval types similar to adult, not well known			
Mollusca	Polyplacophora Aplacophora Monoplacophora	Trochophora			
	Gastropoda	Trochophora and veliger			
	Lamellibranchiata	Trochophora and veliger		Veliger	Glochidium
	Cephalopoda	Larvae not well known			
Sipunculida		Trochophora		Trochophora	Lecitotrophic and planctrophic pelaguspheru larvae
Echiurida		Trochophora			
Annelida	Polychaeta	Trochophora		Trochophora	Metatrochophora, Nectochaeta
Pentastomida		Arthropod-like larva			
Arthropoda	Arachnida Scorpiones Acarina				
	Crustacea	Nauplius Zoea	Metanauplius Protozoea	Nauplius (Entomostraca) Zoea (Malacostraca)	Cypris of barnacles, Megalops of crabs, Mysis of lobsters, Phyllosoma of spiny lobsters, Calyptis-, Furcilia-, Cyrtopia stages in Euphausiaceae), Mancastage
	Insecta	Metabola, Paurometabola			
	Metabola: Paurometabola	Nymphae	Stages		
	Hemimetabola	Neiads	Stages		
	Holometabola	Oligopod larva	Campodeiform larva Scarabeiform larva		Protopod larva

a It is questionable if these types should be considered true larvae.

Table 6.6—_Continued_

Phylum	Subgroup	Larva	Subtype of Larva	Most Common Type of Larva	Other Larvae
		Polypod larva			
		Apodous larva	Eucephalus larva		
			Hemicephalous larva		
			Acephalous larva		
Phoronida		Actinotrocha			
Ectoprocta		Cyphonautes			
Brachiopoda		Larva			
Echinodermata		Dipleurula		Dipleurula	
	Holothuroidea	Auricularia			
	Asteroidea	Bipinaria			
	Echinoidea	Pluteus	Echinopluteus		
	Ophiuroidea	Pluteus	Ophiopluteus		
	Crinoidea	Doliolaria			
Hemichordata	Enteropneusta (Ptychodeidae, Spengelidae)	Tornaria			
Urochordata	Ascidiaceae	Tadpole larva	Anuran larva		Anuran larva
Vertebrata	Pisces, Cyclostomata	Ammocoete			
	Amphibia	Anuran tadpole			
		Tadpole of urodela			

the primary larva. For example, the primary larva of the marine lamellibranchiata is the veliger but in the case of the unionidae the glochidium appears as secondary larva. Similar cases are seen in freshwater ectoprocta and the echinoderms. The larvae of insects can be considered as secondary larvae (59).

Continued and Catastrophic Development: Selected Examples. Larval metamorphosis is characterized by two extreme types of development which are connected by intermediate phases. The first type of metamorphosis is known as continued metamorphosis in which destruction processes are minute. Changes of blastula larvae, metamorphosis of the trochophora to a polychaete annelid, in the case of myriapods, or in the case of the development of a nauplius to a crustacean are examples (59).

In the other extreme, known as catastrophic metamorphosis, extensive portions of the larva are discarded. Porifera, nemertini, marine ectoprocta, tunicates, or echinodermata are examples. The completion of this extreme is reached as in the pupa of cypris in cirripeds or of holometabolic insects.

Big taxonomic groups are not always characterized by the same type of metamorphosis. Instead, both types may occur in one species of a particular taxonomic group of animals (e.g., porifera—blastula). The individual development continues either in an invariable path in the case of continued metamorphosis, or during catastrophic metamorphosis, where the processes of development are concentrated at the end of the larval ontogeny. It is this adulteration of process, side by side in the taxonomic groups, that makes larval metamorphosis so valuable for comparative oncology.

Comparison in the Growth Potential of Larval and Meristematic Tissues. Multipotent cells occur in early stages of the development of vertebrates including man. The embryonal multiple growth potential ceases in general during early embryonic life. Some capacity for the ability to regenerate remains in most tissues, but no new organism can be built through these types of cells, which show a continued renewal in the mammalian body. Leukocytes, cells of the integument with appendages, and cells of holocrine glands are typical examples. The mesenchymatic stem cell has a rather wide range of embryonal potential in the early life stages. But pathologic study shows that even a metaplastic cell of one type of connective tissue can change only to another type of connective tissue, not to epithelial tissues; the same holds true for epithelial tissues which can alter only to other epithelial tissues.

In the large diversification of larval catastrophic development occur cells with different types of embryonal freedom which exhibit a variable capacity during various phases of development. The greatest potential is shown by cells of the so-called imaginal discs or buds, as they occur in holometabolic insects. It can be stated that this array of embryonal growth po-

Table 6.7
Selected Compounds Involved in Growth Stimulation

A. VERTEBRATES

Compound	Formula	Remarks
1. Somatotropin (growth hormone)		
2. Tri-iodothyronine	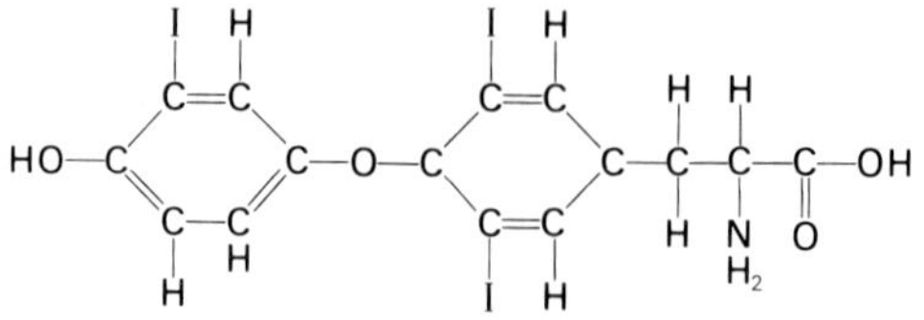	
3. Thyroxine	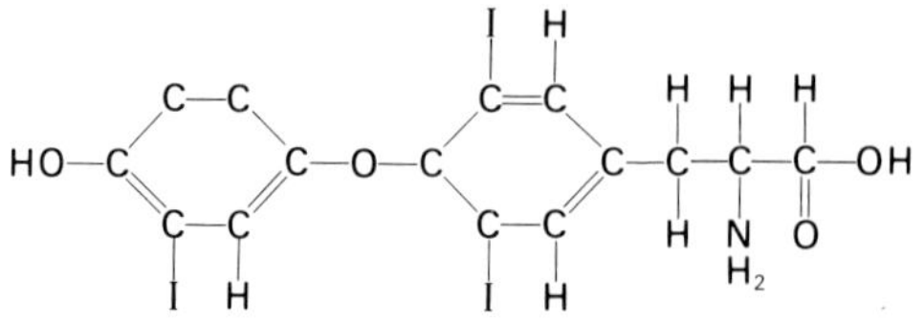	
4. Vitamin A	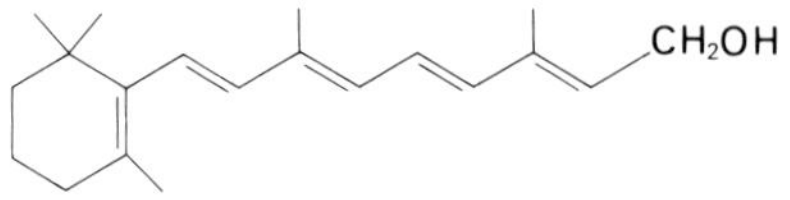 Vitamin A_1	

B. INVERTEBRATES

Compound	Formula	Remarks
1. Thoracotropic hormone (of insects)	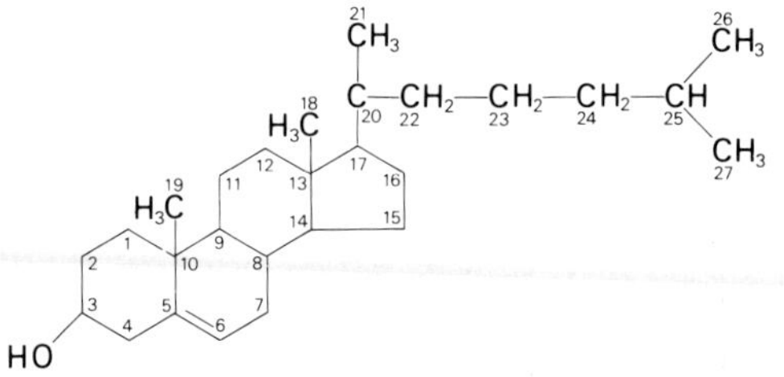	Growth hormones occur in coelenterates, nematodes, annelids.
2. α-Ecdysone	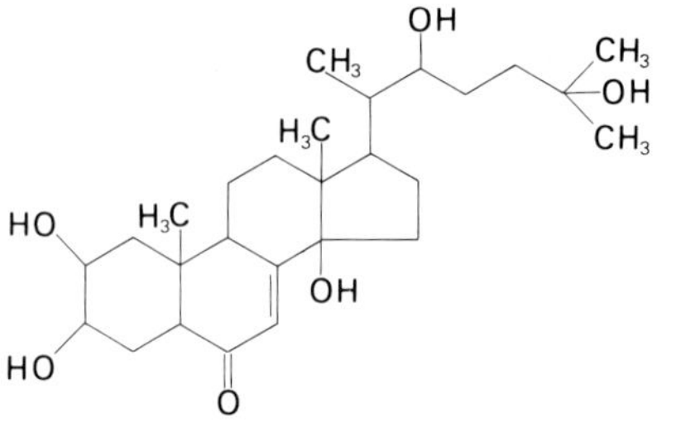	
3. 20-Hydroxyecdysone 4. 20,20-Dihydroxyecdysone 5. Crustecdysone 6. 2-Deoxycrustecdysone of *Jasus lalendi* 7. Callinecdysone A of *Callinectes sapidus* 8. Callinecdysone B of *Callinectes sapidus*	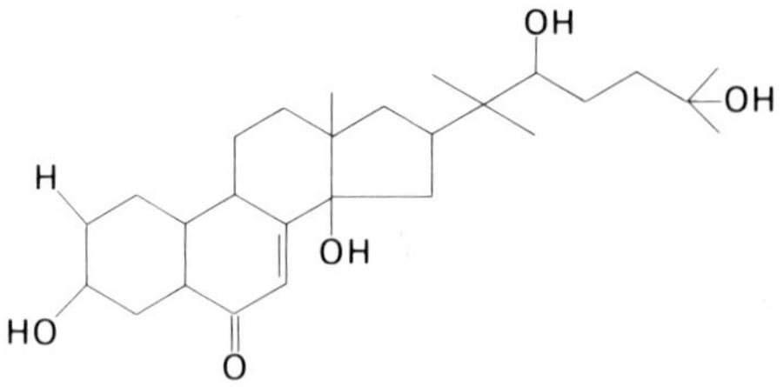	

9. Plant ecdysones:
  Ponasterone A
  Makisterone A
  Makisterone B
  Makisterone C
  Makisterone D
  Cystosterone
  Capitasterone
  Amasterone AA
  Amasterone B
  Polypodin BB
	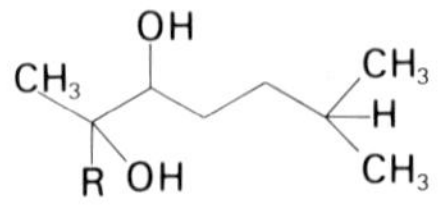	

Table 6.7—*Continued*

Compound	Formula	Remarks

10. Insect juvenile hormones:
  C_{18} juvenile hormone of *Hyalophora cecropia*
  C_{17} juvenile hormone of *H. cecropia*
  C_{16} juvenile hormone of *Schistocerca vaga* and
    S. gregaria		

11. Echinoderm hormones:
  Species-specific shedding hormone of *Asterias*
    anurensis
  1-Methyladenine or maturation-inducing
    substance of *A. anurensis*		

C. VASCULAR PLANTS

1. Auxin (β-indolacetic acid)		
2. Zeatin from *Zea mais*		

tential is already larger and of longer duration (considering the imaginal discs) in certain invertebrates than it is in vertebrates. This condition of growth potential of imaginal cell nests (imaginal tissues) can be compared most closely to the primary meristems in plants, especially the apical meristems. Other larval tissues should be comparable to the other types of meristems to a certain degree (57, 70).

SELECTED COMPOUNDS INVOLVED IN GROWTH STIMULATION

A group-specific review is given in Table 6.7; direct and indirect growth promotors can be distinguished.

SUMMARY

A review of the types of reproduction as the basic growth processes in porifera and eumetazoa and the structures involved has been provided. The validity of the different reproductive processes and structures is shown by the fact that they contain cells and tissues with a wide variation of growth potential. The appearance and expansion of the detours in development (e.g., placentae, larvae) gives researchers an arsenal of until now little used research possibilities. During the development of larval to adult structures, tissues occur in the same organism which are stable, (very rarely) undergoing remodeling with normal histolysis, and are derived mainly from imaginal cell groups. These cells are unique in that they are not involved in the deteriorating processes but instead exhibit only the ability to form new structures where the space becomes free of discarded larval tissues. Imaginal discs show the closest comparability to meristematic tissues. The experimental comparative pathologist will not find such an abundance of tissues with varying growth potential anywhere else in such a short time interval of growth, and in such a large number of different species than in ontogenetic developmental stages.

References

1. Afzelius, B. A., and Ferraguti, M. (1978): Fine structure of brachiopod spermatozoa. *J. Ultrastruct. Res.*, 63:308–315.
2. Aizenshtadt, T. B. (1978): Oogenesis in *Hydra*; III. The growth and fusion of the oocytes). *Ontogenez*, 9:115–123.
3. Altman, P. L., and Dittmer, D. S. (Eds.): *Biology Data Book*, Vols. 1–3, Ed. 2. Federation of American Societies for Experimental Biology, Bethesda, Md.
4. Anderson, H. (1978): Postembryonic development of the visual system of the locust, *Schistocerca gregaria*; II. An experimental investigation of the formation of the retina-lamina projection. *J. Embryol. Exp. Morphol.*, 46:1–7.
5. Anderson, W. A. (1968): Cytochemistry of sea urchin gametes. I. Intramitochondrial localization of glycogen, glucose-6-phosphatase and adenosine triphosphatase activity in spermatozoa of *Paracentrotus lividus*. *J. Ultrastruct. Res.*, 24:398.
6. Balashov, Iu. S., and Raikhel', A. S. (1978): Ultrastructure of the midgut in *Ornithodoros papillipes* (Acarina, Argasidae) nymphs in the blood

assimilation period. *Parazitologiia*, 12:21–26.

7. Balinsky, B. I. (1965): An Introduction to Embryology. W. B. Saunders Company, Philadelphia and London.

8. Ball, E. E., and Cowan, A. N. (1978): Ultrastructural study of the development of the auditory tympana in the cricket *Teleogryllus commodus* (Walker). *J. Embryol. Exp. Morphol.*, 46:75–87.

9. Barnes, S. N. (1974): Fine structure of the photoreceptor of the ascidian tadpole during development. *Cell Tissue Res.*, 155:27–45.

10. Bassemir, U. (1977): Ultrastructural differentiations in the developing follicle cortex of *Locusta migratoria*, with special reference to vitelline membrane formation. *Cell Tissue Res.*, 185:247.

11. Bayne, C. J. (1970): Organization of the spermatozoon of *Agriolimax reticulatus*, the grey field slug (Pulmonata, Stylommatophora). *Z. Zellforsch.*, 103:75–89.

12. Bilinski, S. (1977): Oogenesis in *Acerentomon gallicum* Jonescu (Protura) previtellogenic and vitellogenic stages. *Cell Tissue Res.*, 179:401.

13. Bonar, D. B. (1978): Fine structure of muscle insertions on the larval shell and operculum of the nudibranch *Phestilla sibogae* (Mollusca: Gastropoda) before and during metamorphosis. *Tissue Cell*, 10:143–152.

14. Bonar, D. B. (1978): Ultrastructure of a cephalic sensory organ in larvae of the gastropod *Phestilla sibogae* (Aeolidacea, Nudibrachia). *Tissue Cell* 10:153–165.

15. Buckland-Nicks, J. A., and Chia, F. S. (1977): On the nurse cell and the spermatozeugma in *Littorina sitkana*. *Cell Tissue Res.*, 179:347.

16. Burnett, A. L., et al. (1966):

17. Cloney, R. A. (1977): Larval adhesive organs and metamorphosis in ascidians; I. Fine structure of the everting papillae of *Distaplia occidentalis*. *Cell Tiss. Res.*, 183:423.

18. Colombo, L., and Burighel, P. (1974): Fine structure of the testicular gland of the black goby, *Gobius jozo* L. *Cell Tissue Res.*, 154:39–49.

19. Dhainaut, A. (1970): Etude cytochimique et ultrastructurale de l'évolution ovocytaire de *Nereis pelagica* L. (Annélide Polychète). *Z. Zellforsch.*, 104:375–404.

19a. Dorn, A. and Romer, F. (1976): Structure and function of prothoracic glands and oenocytes in embryos and last larval instars of *Oncopeltus fasciatus* Dallas (Insecta, Heteroptera). *Cell Tissue Res.*, 171:331–50.

20. Donin, C. L., and Cotelli, F. (1977): The rod-shaped sperm of Gordioidea (Aschelminthes, Nematomorpha). *J. Ultrastruct. Res.*, 61:193–200.

21. Fischer, A. (1974): Stages and stage distribution in early oogenesis in the annelid, *Platynereis dumerilii*. *Cell Tissue Res.*, 156:35–45.

22. Floyd, A. D., and Swartz, F. J. (1969): The uterine epithelium of *Ascaris lumbricoides* as a model system for the study of polyploidy. *Exp. Cell Res.*, 56:275–280.

23. Gilchrist, B. M. (1978): Scanning electron microscope studies of the egg shell in some anostraca (Crustacea: Branchiopoda). *Cell Tissue Res.*, 193:337.

24. Hanisch, J. (1966): Spermienentwicklung Cavolini. *Naturwissenschaften*, 53:587.

25. Harding, H. R., Carrick, F. N., and Shorey, C. D. (1975): Ultrastructural changes in spermatozoa of the brush-tailed possum, *Trichosurus vulpecula* (Marsupialia), during epididymal transit. *Cell Tissue Res.*, 164:121–132.

26. Harrigan, J. F., and Alkon, D. L. (1978): Larval rearing, metamorphosis, growth and reproduction of the eolid nudibranch, *Hermissenda crassicornis* (Eschscholtz, 1831) (Gastropoda: Opisthobranchia). *Biol. Bull.* 154:43.

27. Holland, N. D. (1978): The fine structure of *Comanthus japonica* (Echinodermata: Crinoidea) from zygote through early gastrula. *Tissue Cell*, 10:93–112.

28. Hylander, B. L., and Summers, R. G. (1975): An ultrastructural investigation of the spermatozoa of two ophiuroids, *Ophiocoma echinata* and *Ophiocoma wendti*; Acrosomal morphology and reaction. *Cell Tissue Res.*, 158:151–168.

29. Kaulenas, M. S., Foor, W. E., and Fairbairn, D. (1969): Ribosomal RNA synthesis during cleavage of *Ascaris lumbricoides* eggs. *Science*, 163:1201–1203.

30. Kessel, R. G., Panje, W. R., and Decker, M. L. (1969): Ultrastructural localization of inosine-5'-diphosphatase and glucose-6-phosphatase activities in the crayfish vas deferens. *J. Ultrastruct. Res.*, 27:319–329.

31. Kidd, P. (1978): The jelly and vitelline coats of the sea urchin egg; new ultrastructural features. *J. Ultrastruct. Res.*, 64:204.

32. Korschelt, E., and Heider, K. (1892): *Lehrbuch der vergleichenden Entwicklungs-geschichte der wirbellosen Tiere; spezieller Theil*. Gustav Fischer Verlag, Jena.

33. Korschelt, E., and Heider, K. (1902): *Lehrbuch der vergleichenden Entwicklungsgeschichte der wirbellosen Tiere; allgemeiner Theil*. Gustav Fischer Verlag, Jena.

34. Korschelt, E., and Heider, K. (1936): *Lehrbuch der vergleichenden Entwicklungsge-schichte der Tiere*. Gustav Fischer Verlag, Jena.

35. Kryvi, H., and Graebner, I. (1975): Acrosome formation and the centriolar complex in the spermatozoa of *Sabella penicillum* (Polychaeta). *Cell Tissue Res.*, 161:47–53.

36. Longo, F. J., and Anderson, E. (1970): Structural and cytochemical features of the sperm of the cephalopod *Octopus bimaculatus*. *J. Ultra-*

struct. Res. 32:94–106.

37. Longo, F. J., and Anderson, E. (1970): An ultrastructural analysis of fertilization in the surf clam, *Spisula solidissima*. *Ultrastruct. Res.*, 33:495–514.

37a. Longo, F. J., and Anderson, E. (1970): An ultrastructural analysis of fertilization in the surf clam, *Spisula solidissima*. *Ultrastruct. Res.*, 33:515–527.

39. Marchand, B., and Mattei, (1978): Spermatogenesis in acanthocephala. Flagellogenesis in an acanthocephala: positioning and disorganization of the spermatic axoneme. *J. Ultrastruct. Res.*, 63:41–50.

40. Melnikova, E. J., and Panov, A. A. (1975): Ultrastructure of the larval corpus allatum of *Hyphantria cunea* Drury (Insecta, Lepidoptera). *Cell Tissue Res.*, 162:395–410.

41. Miller, J. H. (1973): Studies of oogenesis in *Urechis caupo*; I. Method for separating different size classes of oocytes. *Dev. Biol.*, 32:219–223.

42. Moore, M. N.; Lowe, D. M.; Fieth, P. E. (1978): Responses of lysosomes in the digestive cells of the common mussel, *Mytilus edulis*, to sex steroids and cortisol. *Cell Tissue Res.*, 188:31.

43. Mukai, H., and Watanabe, H. (1976): Studies on the formation of germ cells in a compound ascidian *Botryllus primigenus* Oka. *J. Morphol.*, 148:377–382.

44. Mukai, H. (1977): Comparative studies on the structure of reproductive organs of four botryllid ascidians. *J. Morphol.*, 152:363–380.

45. Okamura, F., and Nishiyama, H. (1978): Penetration of spermatozoon into the ovum and transformation of the sperm nucleus into the male pronucleus in the domestic fowl, *Gallus gallus*. *Cell Tissue Res.*, 190:89.

46. Popham, J. D. (1975): The fine structure of the oocyte of *Bankia australis* (Teredinidae, Bivalvia) before and after fertilization. *Cell Tissue Res.*, 157:521–534.

47. Reger, J. F., and Florendo, N. T. (1969): Studies on motile, nontubule-containing, filiform spermatozoa of the ostracod *Cypridopsis*. *J. Ultrastruct. Res.*, 28:235–258.

48. Reinboth, R. (1968): Protogyny in parrotfishes (Scaridae). *Z. Naturforsch.* (B) 23:852–855.

49. Reverberi, G. (1967): Some observations on the ultrastructure of the ovarian *Mytilus* egg. *Acta Embryol. Morphol. Exp.*, 10:1–14.

50. Rosati, F., Monroy, A., and De Prisco, P. (1977): Fine structural study of fertilization in the ascidian, *Ciona intestinalis*. *J. Ultrastruct. Res.*, 58:261.

51. Saffo, M. B. (1978): Studies on the renal sac of the ascidian *Molgula manhattensis*; I. Development of the renal sac. *J. Morphol.*, 155:287–309.

52. Schiaffino, S., Burighel, P., and Nunzi, M. G. (1974): Involution of the caudal musculature during metamorphosis in the ascidian, *Botryllus schlosseri*. *Cell Tissue Res.*, 153:293–305.

53. Schiaffino, S., Nunzi, M. G., and Burighel, P. (1976): T system in ascidian muscle; organization of the sarcotubular system in the caudal muscle cells of *Botryllus schlusseri* tadpole larvae. *Tissue Cell* 8:101–110.

54. Schmekel, L. (1971): Histology and ultrastructure of the reproductive organs of nudibranchs (Gastropoda, Euthyneura). *Z. Morphol. Tiere*, 69:115–183.

55. Schmekel, L., and Fioroni, P. (1974): The ultrastructure of the yolk nucleus during early cleavage of *Nassarius reticulatus* L. (Gastropoda, Prosobranchia). *Cell Tissue Res.*, 153:79–88.

56. Selwood, L. (1970): The role of the follicle cells during ontogenesis in the chiton *Sypharochiton septentriones* (Ashby) (Polyplacophora, Mollusca). *Zeitschr. Zellforsch. Mikrosk. Anat.*, 104:178–192.

57. Seybold, W. D., and Sullivan, D. T. (1978): Protein synthetic patterns during differentiation of imaginal discs in vitro. *Dev. Biol.*, 65:69–80.

58. Shearn, A., Davis, K. T., and Hersperger, E. (1978): Transdetermination of *Drosophila* imaginal discs cultured in vitro. *Dev. Biol.*, 65:536–540.

59. Siewing, R. (1969): *Lehrbuch der vergleichenden Entwicklungsgeschichte der Tiere*. Paul Parey Verlag, Hamburg.

62. Starck, D. (197x): *Embryologie*, Ed. 3. Georg Thieme Verlag, Stuttgart.

63. Tamarin, A., and Carriku, R. (1967):

64. Toselli, P. A., and Harrison, A. R. (1977): The fine structure of developing locomotor muscles of the pelagic tunicate, *Cyclosalpa affinis* (Thaliacea: Salpidae). *Tissue Cell*, 9:137–156.

65. Trujillo-Cenoz, O., and Melamed, J. (1978): Development of photoreceptor patterns in the compound eyes of muscoid flies. *J. Ultrastruct. Res.*, 64:46.

66. Urbani-Mistruzzi and Scollo-Lavizarri (1954):

67. Vena, J. A., and Palumbo, M. (1967):

68. West, D. L. (1978): Ultrastructural and cytochemical aspects of spermiogenesis in *Hydra hymanae*, with reference to factors involved in sperm head shaping. *Dev. Biol.*, 65:139–154.

69. West, D. L. (1978): Comparative ultrastructure of juvenile and adult nuchal organs of an annelid (Polychaeta: Opheliidae). *Tissue Cell*, 10:243–257.

70. White, K., and Kankel, D. R. (1978): Patterns of cell division and cell movement in the formation of the imaginal nervous system in *Drosophila melanogaster*. *Dev. Biol.*, 65:296–321.

71. Worley, L. G. (1944): Studies of the vitally stained Golgi apparatus; II. Yolk formation and pigment concentration in the mussel *Mytilus californianus* Conrad. *Morphol.*, 75:77–98.

7

Circadian Time Structure of Vascular Flowering Plants

Willard L. Koukkari and Thomas K. Soulen

INTRODUCTION

In studies of the organization of vascular plants, the most emphasis has been placed on descriptive and developmental aspects of cyto-histological and morphological features. Yet, it is in the realm of temporal organization where morphological features take on added meaning in terms of the integrated functioning of the entire organism. A classic example of such integration can be found in photoperiodism, in which an external environment with a cyclic time structure interacts with the temporal organization (rhythms) of the plant to regulate the type of morphological structures produced, e.g., floral or vegetative buds. The capacity to respond via temporal organization enables plants —which do not possess the mobility of many animals—to measure, compensate, and prepare for maximum utilization of and protection from the environment. In some cases, the mechanism involved is sufficiently refined to detect very short changes in time span, e.g., minutes.

The temporal organization of plants is such a broad subject that the material covered here will be restricted primarily to the circadian time structure of vascular flowering plants (Angiosperms) and those rhythms which may relate to it. The limited selection of topics and examples in this chapter have been chosen to illustrate the overall importance of the circadian time structure of the vascular plant. Other perspectives on this general subject may be gained from a number of recent reviews (44, 47, 53, 64, 81).

INTERVAL AND PERIODIC TIME COMPONENTS

For the most part, vascular plants live in environmental conditions that are periodic. Days, lunar months, seasons, etc. recur at regular and predictable intervals. For a given plant, some portions of a particular cycle may, on the one hand, be absolutely necessary or, on the other, be extremely detrimental. Survival of vascular plants under these so-called "normal" conditions requires temporal organization, the components of which are very complex and variable. Even the categorizing of timing mechanisms for vascular flowering plants can often be more descriptive and prejudicial than actual. Nevertheless, it has been possible to propose a generalized scheme that includes two distinct categories, one being of the single interval type and the other having periodic characteristics (77). Perhaps the first type can be visualized as being more linear and the second as rhythmic. Both types may be very evident during plant growth and differentiation.

Single Intervals

There are morphological processes where only a single time span or interval needs to be measured. The timing mechanism which regulates these phenomena has been likened in the literature to an hourglass. Biologically, this type of temporal organization has been described for seeds of many species. For example, the seeds of freshly harvested apples (*Malus*) do not generally germinate until they have been exposed to several weeks of cold (ca. 5°C) temperature. The same is true for some aquatic plants, such as wild rice (*Zizania*). In the case of wild rice, the interval of cold can be overcome by removing portions of the seed coat before planting (17). The adaptive value to plants of the requirement for a span of cold temperature is very evident in the temperate climates where, for example, plants starting to grow from seeds that germinate in the fall could be destroyed by cold temperatures before they are mature enough to produce new seeds. The physiology of single-interval time measurements by plants can be quite intricate, for example, in such factors as permeability of the seed coat, inhibitors, and hormones.

Repeating Intervals

Many physiological processes once considered to be strictly linear in their time structure actually display rhythmicity. While linear time measurements focus on single spans, rhythms involve changes that occur systematically with specifiable patterns, probabilities, and frequencies (54). For example, the sensitivity of a plant to a factor such as light is not necessarily constant; rather, as has been predicted (8) and demonstrated in the photoperiodic response to flowering (20, 42, 51), circadian rhythmicity is present. In fact, rhythms are so prevalent that one could predict their potential involvement at most levels, ranging in complexity from the molecule to the complete organism or even beyond, to populations, communities, and ecosystems. Results obtained from studies with many different species suggest that a vascular plant conceivably displays a multiplicity of rhythms, including all three major types (ultradian, circadian, and infradian), which may occur simultaneously at various levels of the structural hierarchy (Fig. 7.1). With the potential existence of so many individual rhythms in a single plant, the question of how they coordinate through their interrelationships, networks, and a "master center" appears in order. This question has been addressed, at least in part, in a recent review (44). Some rhythms are definitely interrelated, purely because of their position in a metabolic sequence or developmental process. Likewise, different ones are entrained and synchronized by the same environmental cues. Yet, because the plant can retain many of its processes even at the isolated organ level, master organ type of synchronization is less likely than in mammals. However, this does not preclude temporal control at the cellular level.

The terms rhythm and oscillation are often used interchangeably in this chapter. Because an oscillation denotes just one cycle, and oscillations in a sequence may not necessarily have the same period length, it is sometimes a more applicable, if not "safer," term to select, particularly when discussing certain experimental results that are of a biochemical nature. This should not imply that processes referred to as oscillations are not also rhythms. Whenever possible, an attempt has been made to have rhythms denote oscillations with properties that do not directly reflect environmental fluctuations (44).

The circadian rhythms are those which have periods (τ) of approximately 24 hours (hr) that under constant conditions (CC) range from 20 to 28 hr. They are also relatively temperature independent (cf. Refs. 76 and 78). The ultradian rhythms have τ's less than 20 hr, often on the order of minutes, while the infradian rhythms are those usually longer than 28 hr.[1] Included with the infradian rhythms are the circannual (or approximately yearly) rhythms. Examples of these three types of rhythms in vascular plants are presented in Table 7.1. A more complete and comprehensive model for illustrating temporal-spatial organization in all organisms has been recently prepared (6).

SEEDLINGS AND TISSUES

A perennial plant that has developed and grown from a seed that germinated decades earlier may possess tissues and organs that range in age from days to years. Even though many stages of development are evident and the processes of growth and differentiation occur continuously, frequent cell division is in large measure restricted to special regions called meristems. Depending upon where the meristems are located, they are referred to as lateral, intercalary, apical, etc. Following cell division, growth

---

[1] These terms were coined with respect to frequency, *i.e.*, ultradian rhythms have frequencies higher than 1 cycle in 20 hr, and infradian rhythms have frequencies lower than 1 cycle in 28 hr (ultra = beyond, infra = below).

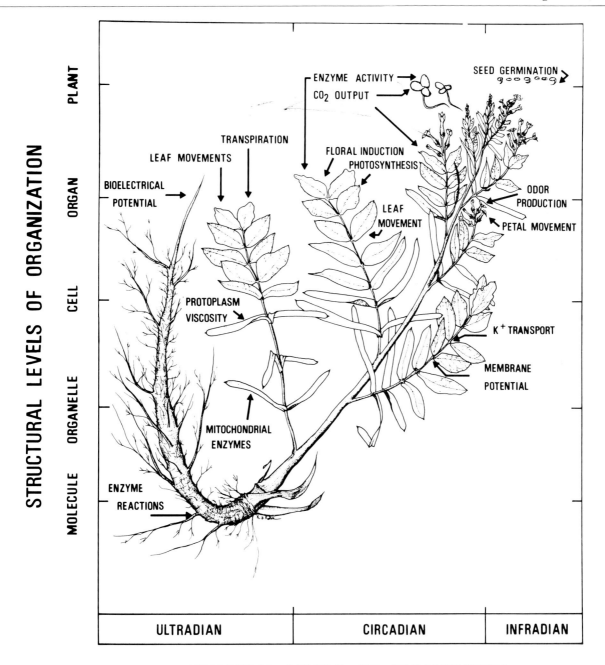

STRUCTURAL LEVELS OF ORGANIZATION

PLANT ORGAN CELL ORGANELLE MOLECULE

ENZYME ACTIVITY
CO₂ OUTPUT

SEED GERMINATION

TRANSPIRATION

LEAF MOVEMENTS

FLORAL INDUCTION
PHOTOSYNTHESIS

BIOELECTRICAL
POTENTIAL

ODOR
PRODUCTION

LEAF
MOVEMENT

PETAL MOVEMENT

PROTOPLASM
VISCOSITY

K⁺ TRANSPORT

MEMBRANE
POTENTIAL

MITOCHONDRIAL
ENZYMES

ENZYME
REACTIONS

| ULTRADIAN | CIRCADIAN | INFRADIAN |

TEMPORAL LEVELS OF ORGANIZATION

Figure 7.1 Diagrammatic illustration of the interrelationship between temporal and structural levels in the organization of vascular flowering plants. Period lengths (τ) for each of the three rhythms are: ultradian = less than a min to 20 hr; circadian = 20 to 28 hr; and infradian = over 28 hr to years. Actual examples within specific plants are presented in Table 7.1.

and differentiation occur and, depending upon the structure in question, cell division, growth, differentiation, and maturation may prevail until senescence. It is quite obvious, then, that a single living plant could, in one form or another, possess nearly all stages of development, including, at least at the organ level, senescence.

Cell Division

While circadian rhythmicity in mitotic frequency has been fairly well documented in animals and some nonvascular plants (Protista), it remains a questionable issue that needs to be

Table 7.1
Selected Examples of Vascular Plants and Their Processes That Have Been Shown to Display Rhythmicity or Oscillatory Behavior[a]

Process	Oscillation	Plant	References
Soluble enzyme reaction	Ultradian	*Armoracea rusticana* P. Gaertner[b]	Yamazaki *et al.* (89)
Bioelectric potentials	"	*Vicia faba* L.	Scott (69)
Enzyme activity (mitochondrial)	"	*Chenopodium rubrum* L.	Deitzer *et al.* (22)
		Glycine max L. Merr.	Duke *et al.* (23)
Viscosity of protoplasm	"	*Helodea densa*[c]	Stålfelt (74)
Transpiration	"	*Avena sativa* L.	Johnsson (46)
Leaf movements	"	*Gossypium hirsutum* L.	Miller (57)
Leaf movements	Circadian	*Phaseolus coccineus* L.	Bünning (10)
Enzyme activity	"	*Lemna perpusilla* Torr.[d]	Gordon & Koukkari (33)
Enzyme activity	"	*Glycine max* L. Merr.	Duke *et al.* (23)
Potassium transport	"	*Samanea saman* (Jacq.) Merrill[e]	Satter *et al.* (67)
Membrane potentials	"	*Samanea saman* (Jacq.) Merrill[e]	Racusen and Galston (65)
CO_2 output	"	*Lemna perpusilla* Torr.[d]	Hillman (43)
CO_2 output	"	*Bryophyllum fedtschenkoi* Hamet & Perrier	Wilkins (87)
Flower induction	"	*Chenopodium rubrum* L.	Cumming (20, 21)
Photosynthesis	"	*Arachis hypogaea* L.	Pallas *et al.*(61)
Flower induction	Circadian	*Sinapis alba* L.	Kinet *et al.* (51)
Odor production	"	*Cestrum nocturnum*	Overland (60)
Petal movements	"	*Kalanchoe blossfeldiana*	Bünsow (15) Engelmann *et al.* (27)
Seed germination	Infradian	*Gratiola officinalis* L.	Bünning and Müssle (14)

[a] Collectively, these examples provide the basis for the diagramatic illustration presented in Figure 7.1 of the interrelationship among temporal and structural levels in the organization of vascular flowering plants.
[b] In the article, only the common name "wild horseradish" was mentioned. Wild horseradish for peroxidase isolation in another biochemical paper was listed as *Cochlearia armoracia* L. (50).
[c] *Elodea densa* Casp.
[d] Species name has been recently changed.
[e] Genus changed to *Tricholobium* (cf. ref. 65).

resolved for vascular plants (44). Results from mitotic index studies with *Chenopodium rubrum* L. seedlings certainly have some circadian implications, since periods of ca. 20 hr have been monitored under CC (52).

Seedlings

Plants in the seedling stage, or portions thereof, can and do display circadian rhymicity at a very early age of development. However, there are strong indications that a daily entrainment cycle consisting of alternate light and darkness or variations in temperature is often a prerequisite before circadian rhythmicity can be effectively detected under CC. Sometimes, only a single change may be necessary, as in *Avena* coleoptiles, for which a growth rhythm was observed after, but not before, the young seedlings were transferred from continuous red light to constant darkness (DD) (4). The *Chenopodium rubrum* L. plant is very unique because it is able to flower in the laboratory setting while still a young seedling. It also has at this stage of development, as will be described later, a circadian rhythm of flower induction (20, 21).

Ultradian oscillations abound in young seedlings. As the young plant becomes taller or longer, it does so not in a straight vertical fashion, but rather in "rotating" motions called nutations. Organs of the young plant such as stems (3, 28), roots (73), hypocotyls (48), and coleoptiles (2) all appear to have these oscillations. On the other end of the spectrum of rhythms, a circannual infradian rhythm in seed germination may also exist (14).

Tissue Culture

A circadian rhythm of growth has been reported for tissue cultures of *Daucus carota* L. (25). At the metabolic level, pieces of mesophyll tissue isolated from *Bryophyllum fedtschenkoi* Hamet and Perrier display a rhythm in CO_2

output (87) as do cultures from *Bryophyllum* leaf callus (88). In all three studies the rhythms persisted for many cycles in DD.

PHOTOPERIODISM AND FLOWERS

Photoperiodism, the response of organisms to relative lengths of light (L) and darkness (D), is a basic biological phenomenon. Although flowering has received much of the emphasis in plants, tuber formation, winter hardening, bud dormancy, etc. are also photoperiodic. In regard to flowering, plants have been subdivided into three basic types according to L and D conditions necessary for floral induction: short-day plants, long-day plants, and the daylength-indifferent plants. Combinations and sequences of these three types, along with temperature requirements plus other quantitative and qualitative environmental features, form the basis for more elaborate systems of requirements for floral induction in many plants (ref. 82).

For those who may be less familiar with the physiological processes associated with these response types, it is worth noting that interrupting the long D span with L (e.g., 15 min) will, in short-day plants, inhibit floral induction. The quality of L necessary to accomplish this inhibition is red (660 nm), and with most plants the inhibition can be overcome by immediately exposing the leaves to far-red (730 nm). Playing a major role in such responses to L quality is the red, far-red absorbing, and photoreversible pigment, phytochrome. When first discovered, the transformational behavior of phytochrome was very suggestive of an interval time measurement system.

Early classical studies provided good systematic evidence for the existence of photoperiodism (29). An interval timing mechanism in photoperiodism (likened to an hourglass) was strongly emphasized at that time with little regard to rhythmicity. However, it is now fairly well established that circadian rhythmicity may play a major role in the photoperiodic time measurements of many plants (44). Some interesting comments concerning the historical events leading to the recognition of rhythmicity in photoperiodism have been presented in several articles (21, 36, 84).

An aquatic short-day flowering strain of *Lemna* (duckweed) can be readily cultured in flasks under minimal L by providing sucrose in the medium (42). Therefore, it has been possible to substitute a regular LD regime (daily schedule of 11 hr L followed by 13 hr of D) with a skeleton photoperiod (e.g., ¼ L:10½ D:¼ L:13 D) which in effect provides illumination only during the first and last 15 min of the normal L span. Such manipulations of L and D spans by skeleton photoperiods have made it possible to show that photoperiodic timing involves circadian rhythmicity (41, 45). Other results supportive of the presence of circadian components in photoperiodism have been demonstrated with the short-day flowering ecotype of *Chenopodium rubrum* L. (20, 21). In these experiments, seeds maintained on moist filter paper were subjected under constant light (LL) to a 12:12 temperature cycle and a light intensity cycle for 2 days, followed by 1 day CC of LL and temperature before being transferred to DD. At various intervals, groups of seed were removed and placed in CC of LL. The results of these superb experiments indicated a clear circadian rhythmic display of flowering (20). Circadian rhythmicity in the induction of flowering has been demonstrated with the long-day plant *Sinapis alba* L. (51) and also with some other species (19, 79).

In some plants, once the flowers have been formed, they themselves can display circadian rhythms both in the movements of the petals (15, 27) and in the production of odor (60). Recorded in the older literature are lists of plants which indicate the time of day when flowers of certain species open and close and thus supposedly provide a garden clock (cf. ref. 5) for observations of Linnaeus (7, 31).

Rhythms in the opening of flowers, nectar secretion, odor production, and insect interaction (10) have all the prerequisites for temporal studies at the community level.

HORMONES

Transport

The apical meristem and leaf primordia of the oat (*Avena*) embryo are enclosed by a sheath-like structure, called the coleoptile, resembling a thick finger of a glove. Because of its anatomical and physiological features, the coleoptile has been a classical structure for hormone studies, especially hormones of the auxin type (32, 86). Under certain experimental conditions it has been shown that auxin transport in coleoptiles may display ultradian oscillations (37, 58, 72). In movements of *Carica papaya* L. leaves, the daily changes have been attributed to the unequal distribution of auxin (90). However, the *C. papaya* studies were not designed to monitor circadian rhythmicity and are thus more suggestive of changes in auxin levels in relation to light-darkness (LD) cycles than CC.

Ethylene

Ethylene, a unique hormone in that it is a gas (C_2H_4), plays a major role in physiological processes, e.g., fruit ripening and stem thickening. In the leaves of tomato (*Lycopersicon esculentum* Mill.), the levels of ethylene not only display a 24-hr oscillation under LD, but also a circadian rhythm is suggested by its continuation under LL and DD (24).

Other Rhythm Involvements

Without distinguishing among the various manifestations of growth, the effects of hormones, and the mere presence of hormones *per se*, it can be stated in general terms that rhythmic components are, or can be related to, the following: electrical potential changes, tropisms, nutations, transport, and development and growth (53).

RESPONSE TO CHEMICALS

The response of a plant to a chemical may oscillate in relation to the time of day. Some chemicals may affect the characteristics of a rhythm. These are two separate issues and must be dealt with individually.

Time of Day

An interesting response of a plant to an inorganic chemical is that of *Lemna*, in which transferring plants from a nutrient medium to distilled water for a short span during a sensitive phase and then back to the medium will inhibit flowering (35). This effect has been shown to be partially reversed by supplementing the distilled water with $Ca(NO_3)_2$.

Sucrose is a primary carbohydrate in angiosperms and is transported in the vascular tissues. Recently, measurements with microelectrodes

implanted into *Samanea* leaf pulvini have indicated that membrane potentials were rhythmically sensitive to applications of sucrose (65). The nature of this sensitivity may be related to the circadian leaf movements of the plant.

The effects of auxins and herbicides may also display a 24-hr oscillation (53). Some of these effects may be related to environmental factors and others to experimental procedures and other rhythms (1), while still others cannot be attributed to such factors but do oscillate, at least under LD conditions (16, 34, 55) and single LL and DD cycles (16).

Effects on Rhythms

There are a limited number of chemicals which may affect the τ or phase of circadian rhythms in vascular plants (10). Included in this list, among others, are ethanol, theobromide, theophylline, and D_2O_2 (11, 49, 56), valinomycin (13); and lithium ions (26). When first reported, there is a great tendency to interpret the effects of certain chemicals to be more specific than they may later turn out to be. Alcohol could be just such an example, and its action may be much more diverse than on cellular membranes.

The effects of chemical agents on or during the phase or τ of rhythms, particularly ethanol (11), valinomycin (13), and potassium (66) have been selected as supporting evidence for the inclusion of membranes in hypothetical models that could comprise the circadian timing mechanism (cf. ref. 59).

ENZYMES

Peroxidase

At the level of enzymatic reactions, several types of periodic behavior have been observed. A variety of enzymes display very short-term oscillations in activity, with periods on the order of minutes or even less. It was a preparation from a vascular plant which provided the first clear report of such an ultradian oscillatory reaction for a soluble enzyme (see Table 7.1). This reaction involved an open system which included O_2, horseradish peroxidase (which in the presence of O_2 can act as an oxidase), and an electron donor: NADH or NADPH, dihydroxyfumarate, or indole-3-acetate (89, 91). Subsequent work on this and other oscillatory enzyme reactions has been discussed in considerable detail in several recent reviews (30, 38, 39). While some have questioned the significance of such short-term oscillations in relation to circadian time structure, it has been suggested that two or more suitably related enzyme reactions with short-term periodic variation in their activities, subject to appropriate allosteric and other controls, could provide a simple biochemical oscillator which might form the basis for circadian oscillatory behavior (62, 63, 70, 71). Whether or not such ultradian oscillations should prove ultimately to be related to circadian rhythms, they are of interest in their own right, and they do provide a periodic time structure.

In addition to the short-term ultradian oscillatory behavior just described, there have been observed in preparations from vascular plants a number of enzymes which display longer-term ultradian or circadian rhythmicity. Some of these enzymes occupy key positions in the metabolism of a plant, and their behavior and regulation thus might exert profound influence on its physiological activity and development. Two examples will serve to illustrate.

Phenylalanine Ammonia-Lyase

In the reaction catalyzed by phenylalanine ammonia-lyase (PAL), an amino acid is converted to *trans*-cinnamate, which then can serve as a precursor for synthesis of a wide variety of substances important in vascular plants, among them the chief pigments found in some flowers (anthocyanins) and a constituent of a very important structural component of the cell walls of woody species (lignin). It has been known for some time that PAL activity tends to be high during L spans and decreases in the D spans. Although it was suggested that these changes in activity were in response to L and D, Figure 7.2 illustrates the persistence of striking circadian rhythmicity in the activity of this enzyme in extracts prepared from plants maintained in LL (33). It is of interest to note that PAL activity remained relatively constant and low under DD.

Enzymes of Nitrogen Assimilation

The second example relates to the crucial process of assimilation of nitrogen (N) by plants. Vascular plants depend on the N supply of their

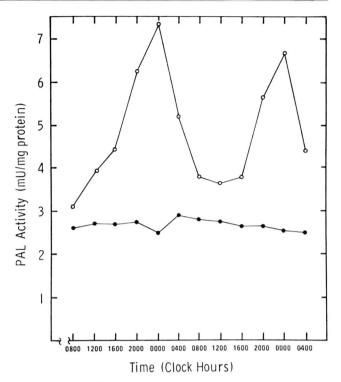

Figure 7.2 Phenylalanine ammonia-lyase activity in extracts from *Lemna perpusilla* 6746 maintained under LL (○) and DD (●). Plants entrained on a LD$_{16:8}$ regime before CC. (Reproduced with permission from W. R. Gordon and W. L. Koukkari: *Plant Physiology*, in press (33).)

immediate environment. Those species which cannot fix atmospheric N$_2$ via a symbiotic relationship with some microorganism (such as the one which exists in root nodules of legumes) must utilize other available forms of N, most commonly nitrate and ammonium. When the predominant form of N available is nitrate, the combined activities of the enzymes nitrate reductase (NR) and nitrite reductase (NiR) reduce the nitrate to ammonium. The next stage (or the first, if NH$_4^+$ happens to be the principal N source being utilized) is incorporation of NH$_4^+$ into the amino group of the amino acid glutamate. This assimilation of N can be accomplished directly via the enzyme glutamate dehydrogenase (GDH), or by the combined activities of two enzymes: glutamine synthetase (GS), which first incorporates the NH$_4^+$ into the amide group of glutamine, and glutamate synthetase (GOGAT), which then transfers the amide N of glutamine to α-ketoglutarate, with the resultant formation of two molecules of glutamate.

The activities of many of the enzymes involved in the assimilation of inorganic N by plants have been reported to show oscillations, frequently circadian. Results from the most comprehensive study to date have shown in soybean

(*Glycine max* Merr.) leaves a very interesting combination of rhythms and possible interactions among them (23). The peaks of activity of two of the enzymes, NR and GDH, are separated by 3–6 hr, with the NR peak occurring several hr into the L span and that of GDH occurring near the end of the D span. Perhaps even more interesting was the fact that these two enzymes, as well as the measured total soluble protein of the leaves, displayed both circadian and ultradian rhythms, with the period of the ultradian rhythms generally being about one-half that of the circadian rhythms. Thus the two types of rhythms appeared to reinforce each other.

The possible complexities of the status of enzymes of N assimilation in vascular plants are further underscored by the reported presence in pepper (*Capsicum*) leaves of three peaks of NR activity during the L span (75). Two of the three display circadian rhythmicity, but with differing times of maximum activity. Treatment of the plants with a spray of kinetin (which acts like a cytokinin type of hormone) brought about phase shifts of both rhythmic peaks of NR activity: one was advanced, the other delayed.

In addition to these and other studies of N assimilation, it is worth noting a report of fluctuations within the soluble N pool of leaves of field pea (*Pisum arvense* L.) of a number of amino acids. Such daily oscillations (LD regime) may be related to the overall process of N assimilation and possibly also to aging in plants, in which protein N may be mobilized in a senescing portion of a plant for utilization in growth and development in a meristematic or differentiating part of the plant (18).

Physiological Interactions

The activities of both PAL and NR have been shown to be subject at least in some plant tissues to modulation by different qualities of light via the protein pigment phytochrome. A recent review has discussed the current status of phytochrome control of these and other enzymes (68). When one considers the role believed to be played by phytochrome in control of photoperiodic phenomena (discussed in a pervious section), and of some leaf movements (66), it becomes increasingly clear that one must be alert to the possibility that the mechanism of any circadian time structure may involve the interaction of a number of components.

Yet another dimension is added to the possible complexity of such a structure by the suggestion—based on results of extensive studies with the seedlings of *Chenopodium rubrum* L.—that oscillations in the activity of a number of enzymes relating to energy metabolism may result in circadian rhythmicity in two very important aspects of the energy status of a plant: the redox state ($NADPH/NADP^+$) and the adenylate "energy charge" ($[ATP] + 0.5 [ADP]/[ATP] + [ADP] + [AMP]$). The amplitude of both of these reflections of energy status can be modulated by light via phytochrome, and it was suggested that all these components may interact to control temporal organization of development (83).

PATHOLOGY

Following the transfer of plants from a 24-hr LD regime to CC, many plant rhythms, though persisting for many cycles, begin to dampen, as evidenced by a reduction in amplitude. These oscillations in LL can be restored by a sufficiently long, e.g., 8–10 hr, D span (cf. ref. 9). Maintaining plants continuously under CC may eventually result in desynchronization of the rhythm, followed by pathological disturbances. The inflorescence (cluster of flowers) of *Cichorium intybus* L. may become deformed (9, 80) while the foliage of tomato (*Lycopersicon esculentum* L.) turns chlorotic (40). In the latter instance, in order for the plant to remain "healthy," either L or temperature may be kept constant, provided that the other is cycled. It has been superbly demonstrated with many plants that for normal or optimal development, a 24-hr environmental cycle, either L or temperature, is prerequisite (85). There is some experimental evidence that suggests that even the leaf movement rhythms, in relation to the day (L) and night (D) cycle, may have a protective role coinciding with the occurrence of "harmful" L (moon) that could interrupt or inhibit floral induction (12).

SUMMARY

Vascular plants, like other organisms, have a complex temporal organization that includes both interval (linear) and rhythmic timing. Rhythms have been observed at various levels of structural organization, ranging from the molecular to the whole organism, and have a potential involvement in most areas of physiological development. Collectively, they are an integral feature of the vascular plant and provide for its measurement of time in relation to the physical cycles of the natural environment.

Acknowledgments. The helpful comments of Dr. E. C. Abbe, Dr. D. C. Pratt, Dr. G. B. Ownbey and Ms. M. A. Johnson, and the artistic and photographic contributions of Ms. K. A. Kohn and Ms. A. A. Engels are sincerely appreciated.

References

1. Andersen, R. N., and Koukkari, W. L. (1978): Response of velvet leaf to bentazon as affected by leaf orientation. *Weed Sci.,* 26:393–395.
2. Arnal, C. (1953): Recherches sur la nutation des coléoptiles. I. Nutation et croissance. Ann. Univ. Sarav. *Scientia,* 2:92–105.
3. Baillaud, L. (1953): Physiologie Végétale. *C. R. Acad. Sci.* (Paris), 236: 1986–1988.
4. Ball, N. G. and Dyke, I. J. (1954): An endogenous 24-hour rhythm in the growth rate of the *Avena* coleoptile. *J. Exp. Botany,* 5: 421–433.
5. Blunt, W. (1971): *The Compleat Naturalist: A Life of Linnaeus.* W. Collins, London.
6. Bohlen, J. G. (1978): Manuscript in preparation, University of Minnesota, Minneapolis.
7. Brewer, E. C. (1898): *Dictionary of Phrase and Fable.* Henry Altemus, Philadelphia.
8. Bünning, E. (1936): Die endogene Tagesrhytmik als Grundlage der photoperiodischen Reaktion. *Ber. Dtsch. Botan. Ges.* 54:590–607.
9. Bünning, E. (1962): Mechanism in circadian rhythms: functional and pathological changes resulting from beats and from rhythm abnormalities. *Ann. N. Y. Acad. Sci.,* 98:901–915.
10. Bünning, E. (1973): *The Physiological Clock.* The English Universities Press Ltd., Springer-Verlag, London.
11. Bünning, E., and Baltes, J. (1962): Wirkung von Äthylalkohol auf die physiologische Uhr. *Naturwiss.,* 49:19.
12. Bünning, E., and Moser, I. (1969): Interference of moonlight with the photoperiodic measurement of time by plants, and their adaptive reaction. *Proc. Natl. Acad. Sci. U. S.,* 62:1018–1022.
13. Bünning, E., and Moser, I. (1972): Influence of valinomycin on circadian leaf movements of *Phaseolus. Proc. Natl. Acad. Sci.,* 69:2732–2733.
14. Bünning, E., and Müssle, L. (1951): Der Verlauf der endogenen Jahresrhythmik in Samen unter dem Einfluss verschiedenartiger Aussenfaktoren. *Z. Naturforsch. [B],* 6:108–112.
15. Bünsow, R. (1953): Endogene Tagesrhythmik und Photoperiodismus bei *Kalanchoe blossfeldiana. Planta,* 42:220–252.
16. Campiranon, S. and Koukkari, W. L. (1976): Circadian periodic response of *Phaseolus vulgaris* L. to 2,4-dichlorophenoxyacetic acid. *Chronobiologia,* 3:137–148.
17. Campiranon, S., and Koukkari, W. L. (1977): Germination of wild rice, *Zizania aquatica* seeds and the activity of alcohol dehydrogenase in young seedlings. *Physiol. Plant.,* 41:293–297.
18. Carr, D. J., and Pate, J. S. (1967): Ageing in the whole plant. *Symp. Soc. Exp. Biol.,* 21:559–599.
19. Chorney, W., Rakosnik, E., Jr., Diepert, M. H., and Dedolph, R. R. (1970): Rhythmic-flowering response in cocklebur. *Bioscience,* 20:31–32.
20. Cumming, B. G. (1967): Circadian rhythmic flowering responses in *Chenopodium rubrum;* effects of glucose and sucrose. *Can. J. Botany,* 45:2173–2193.
21. Cumming, B. G. (1969): Circadian rhythms of flower induction and their significance in photoperiodic response. *Can. J. Botany,* 47:309–324.
22. Deitzer, G. F., Kempf, O., Fischer, S., and Wagner, E. (1974): Endogenous rhythmicity and energy transduction. IV. Rhythmic control of enzymes involved in the tricarboxylic-acid cycle and the oxidative pentose-phosphate pathway in *Chenopodium rubrum* L. *Planta,* 117:29–41.
23. Duke, S. H., Friedrich, J. W., Schrader, L. E., and Koukkari, W. L. (1978): Cyclic activities of enzymes of nitrate reduction and ammonia assimilation in *Glycine max* and *Zea mays. Physiol. Plant.,* 42:269–276.
24. El-Beltagy, A. S., Kapuya, J. A., Madkour, M. A., and Hall, M.A. (1976): A possible endogenous rhythm in internal ethylene levels in the leaves of *Lycopersicon esculentum* Mill. *Plant Sci. Lett.,* 6:175–180.
25. Enderle, W. (1951): Tagesperiodische Wachstums- und Turgor-Schwankungen an Gewebekulturen. *Planta,* 39:570–588.
26. Engelmann, W. (1972): Lithium slows down the *Kalanchoe* clock. *Z. Naturforsch. [B],* 27:477.
27. Engelmann, W., Eger, I., Johnsson, A., and Karlsson, H. G. (1974): Effect of temperature pulses on the petal rhythm of *Kalanchoe:* an experimental and theroetical study. *Int. J. Chronobiol.,* 2:347–358.
28. Galston, A. W., Tuttle, A. A., and Penny, P. J. (1964): A kinetic study of

growth movements and photomorphogenesis in etiolated pea seedlings. *Am. J. Botany,* 51:853–858.
29. Garner, W. W., and Allard, H. A. (1920): Effect of the relative length of day and night and other factors of the environment on growth and reproduction in plants. *J. Agric. Res.,* 18:553–606.
30. Goldbeter, A., and Caplan, S. R. (1976): Oscillatory enzymes. *Annu. Rev. Biophys. Bioeng.,* 5:449–476.
31. Goldsmith, G. W., and Hafenrichter, A. L. (1932): *Anthokinetics: The Physiology and Ecology of Floral Movements.* Carnegie Institute of Washington.
32. Goldsmith, M. H. M. (1977): The polar transport of auxin. *Annu. Rev. Plant Physiol.,* 28:439–478.
33. Gordon, W. R., and Koukkari, W. L. (1978): Circadian rhythmicity in the activities of phenylalanine ammonia-lyase from *Lemna perpusilla* and *Spirodela polyrhiza. Plant Physiol.,* 62:612–615.
34. Gosselink, J. G., and Standifer, L. C. (1967): Diurnal rhythm of sensitivity of cotton seedlings to herbicides. *Science,* 158:120–121.
35. Halaban, R., and Hillman, W. S. (1971): Factors affecting the water-sensitive phase of flowering in the short day plant *Lemna perpusilla. Plant Physiol.,* 48:760–764.
36. Hamner, K. C. (1960): Photoperiodism and circadian rhythms. *Cold Spring Harbor Symp. Quant. Biol.,* 25:269–277.
37. Hertel, R., and Flory, R. (1968): Auxin movement in corn coleoptiles. *Planta,* 82:123–144.
38. Hess, B. (1977): Oscillating reactions. *Trends Biochem. Sci.,* 2:193–195.
39. Hess, B., and Boiteux, A. (1971): Oscillatory phenomena in biochemistry. *Annu. Rev. Biochem.,* 40:237–258.
40. Hillman, W. S. (1956): Injury of tomato plants by continuous light and unfavorable photoperiodic cycles. *Am. J. Botany,* 43:89–96.
41. Hillman, W. S. (1964): Endogenous circadian rhythms and the response of *Lemna perpusilla* to skeleton photoperiods. *Am. Naturalist,* 98:323–328.
42. Hillman, W. S. (1968): *Lemna perpusilla* Torr., Strain 6746. In *The Induction of Flowering,* edited by L. T. Evans. Macmillan, New York.
43. Hillman, W. S. (1970): Carbon dioxide output as an index of circadian timing in *Lemna* photoperiodism. *Plant Physiol.,* 45:273–279.
44. Hillman W. S. (1976a): Biological rhythms and physiological timing. *Annu. Rev. Plant Physiol.,* 27:159–179.
45. Hillman, W. S. (1976b): Calibrating duckweeds: light, clocks, metabolism, flowering. *Science,* 193:453–458.
46. Johnsson, A. (1973): Oscillatory transpiration and water uptake of *Avena* plants. I. Preliminary observations. *Physiol. Plant.,* 28:40–50.
47. Jones, M. B., and Mansfield, T. A. (1975): Circadian rhythms in plants. *Sci. Prog. [Oxford],* 62:103–125.
48. Karve, A. D., and Salanki, A. S. (1964): A feedback oscillation of a relatively high frequency in hypocotyls of *Carthamus tinctorius* L. *Z. Pflanzenphysiol.,* 52:98–102.
49. Keller, S. (1960): Über die Wirkung chemischer Faktoren auf die tagesperiodischen Blattbewegungen von *Phaseolus multiflorus. Z. Botanik,* 48:32–57.
50. Kenten, R. H., and Mann, P. J. G. (1954): A simple method for the preparation of horseradish peroxidase. *Biochem. J.,* 57:347–348.
51. Kinet, J. M., Bernier, G., Bodson, M., and Jacquard, A. (1973): Circadian rhythms and the induction of flowering in *Sinapis alba. Plant Physiol.,* 51:597–600.
52. King, R. W. (1975): Multiple circadian rhythms regulate photoperiodic flowering responses in *Chenopodium rubrum. Can. J. Botany,* 53:2631–2638.
53. Koukkari, W. L. (1979): Rhythms and their relations to hormones. In *Encyclopedia of Plant Physiology,* New Series. Vol. 3, edited by N. P. Kefford, R. P. Pharis and D. M. Reid. Springer-Verlag, Berlin.
54. Koukkari, W. L., Duke, S. H., Halberg, F., and Lee, J. K. (1974): Circadian rhythmic leaflet movements; student exercise in chronobiology. *Chronobiologia,* 1:281–302.
55. Koukkari, W. L., Johnson, M. A. (1979): Oscillations of leaves *Abutilon theophrasti* (velvet leaf) and their sensitivity to bentazone in relation to low and high humidity. *Physiol. Plant.,* 47:158–162.
56. Mayer, W., Gruner, R., and Strubel, H. (1975): Periodenverlängerung und Phasenverschiebungen der circadianen Rhythmik von *Phaseolus coccineus* L. durch Theophyllin. *Planta,* 125:141–148.
57. Miller, C. S. (1975): Short interval leaf movements of cotton. *Plant Physiol.,* 55:562–566.
58. Newman, I. A. (1963): Electric potentials and auxin translocation in *Avena. Aust. J. Biol. Sci.,* 16:629–646.
59. Njus, D., Sulzman, F. M., and Hastings, J. W. (1974): Membrane model for the circadian clock. *Nature,* 248:116–120.
60. Overland, L. (1960): Endogenous rhythm in opening and odor of flowers of *Cestrum nocturnum. Am. J. Botany,* 47:378–382.
61. Pallas, J. E., Jr., Samish, Y. B., and Willmer, C. M. (1974): Endogenous rhythmic activity of photosynthesis, transpiration, dark respiration, and carbon dioxide compensation point of peanut leaves. *Plant Physiol.,* 53: 907–911.
62. Pavlidis, T. (1973): *Biological Oscillators: Their Mathematical Analysis.* Academic Press, New York.

63. Pavlidis, T., and Kauzmann, W. (1969): Toward a quantitative biochemical model for circadian oscillators. *Arch. Biochem. Biophys.*, 132:338–348.

64. Queiroz, O. (1974): Circadian rhythms and metabolic patterns. *Annu. Rev. Plant Physiol.*, 25:115–134.

65. Racusen, R. H., and Galston, A. W. (1977): Electrical evidence for rhythmic changes in the cotransport of sucrose and hydrogen ions in *Samanea* pulvini. *Planta*, 135:57–62.

66. Satter, R. L., and Galston, A. W. (1971): Phytochrome-controlled nyctinasty in *Albizzia julibrissin*. III. Interactions between endogenous rhythm and phytochrome in control of potassium flux and leaflet movement. *Plant Physiol.*, 48:740–746.

67. Satter, R. L., Geballe, G. T., Applewhite, P. B., and Galston, A. W. (1974): Potassium flux and leaf movement in *Samanea saman*. I. Rhythmic Movement. *J. Gen. Physiol.*, 64:413–430.

68. Schopfer, P. (1977): Phytochrome control of enzymes. *Annu. Rev. Plant Physiol.*, 28:223–252.

69. Scott, B. I. H. (1957): Electric oscillations generated by plant roots and a possible feedback mechanism responsible for them. *Aus. J. Biol. Sci.*, 10:164–157.

70. Sel'kov, E. E. (1975): Stabilization of energy charge, generation of oscillations and multiple steady states in energy metabolism as a result of purely stoichiometric regulation. *Eur. J. Biochem.*, 59:151–157.

71. Sel'kov, E. E., and Sozinov, L. A. (1970): Stable circadian rhythms as a property of cell populations. In *Life Sciences and Space Research VIII*, pp. 157–167, edited by W. Vishiac and F. G. Favorite, Elsevier North Holland, Amsterdam.

72. Shen-Miller, J. (1973): Rhythmicity in the basipetal transport of indoleacetic acid through coleoptiles. *Plant Physiol.*, 51:615–619.

73. Spurny, M. (1968): Spiral oscillations of the growing radicle in *Pisum sativum* L. *Naturwissenschaften*, 55:46.

74. Stålfelt, M. G. (1946): The influence of light upon the viscosity of protoplasm. *Arkiv. Botanik*, 33:1–17.

75. Steer, B. T. (1976): Rhythmic nitrate reductase activity in leaves of *Capsicum annuum* L. and the influence of kinetin. *Plant Physiol.*, 57:928–932.

76. Sweeney, B. M. (1969): *Rhythmic Phenomena in Plants*. Academic Press, New York.

77. Sweeney, B. M. (1974): The temporal regulation of morphogenesis in plants, hourglass and oscillator. *Brookhaven Symp. Biol.*, 25:95–110.

78. Sweeney, B. M., and Hastings, J. W. (1960): Effects of temperature upon diurnal rhythms. *Cold Spring Harbor Symp. Quant. Biol.*, 25:87–104.

79. Takimoto, A., and Hamner, K. C. (1964): Effect of temperature and preconditioning on photoperiodic response of *Pharbitis nil*. *Plant Physiol.*, 39:1024–1030.

80. Todt, D. (1962): Untersuchungen über Öffnung und Anthocyangehaltsveränderungen der Blüten von *Cichorium intybus* im Litch-Dunkel-Wechsel und unter konstanten Bedingungen. *Z. Botanik.*, 50:1–21.

81. Vanden Driessche, T. (1975): Circadian rhythms and molecular biology. *Biosystems*, 6:188–201.

82. Vince-Prue, D. (1975): *Photoperiodism in Plants*. McGraw-Hill, New York.

83. Wagner, E. (in collaboration with G. F. Deitzer, S. Fischer, S. Frosh, O. Kempf, and L. Stroebele) (1975): Endogenous oscillations in pathways of energy transduction as related to circadian rhythmicity and photoperiodic control. *Biosystems*, 7:68–76.

84. Ward, R. R. (1971): *The Living Clocks*. New English Library, London.

85. Went, F. W. (1960): Photo- and thermoperiodic effects in plant growth. *Cold Spring Harbor Symp. Quant. Biol.*, 25:221–230.

86. Went, F. W., and Thimann, K. V. (1937): *Phytohormones*. The Macmillan Co., New York.

87. Wilkins, M. B. (1959): An endogenous rhythm in the rate of CO_2 output of *Bryophyllum*. I. Some preliminary experiments. *J. Exp. Botany*, 10:373–390.

88. Wilkins, M. B., and Holowinsky, A. W. (1965): The occurrence of an endogenous circadian rhythm in a plant tissue culture. *Plant Physiol.*, 40:907–909.

89. Yamazaki, I., Yokota, K., and Nakajima, R. (1965): Oscillatory oxidations of reduced pyridine nucleotide by peroxidase. *Biochem. Biophys. Res. Commun.*, 21:582–586.

90. Yin, H. C. (1941): Studies on the nyctinastic movement of the leaves of *Carica papaya*. *Am. J. Botany*, 28:250–261.

91. Yokota, K., and Yamazaki, I. (1965): Reaction of peroxidase with reduced nicotinamide-adenine dinucleotide and reduced nicotinamide-adenine dinucleotide phosphate. *Biochim. Biophys. Acta*, 105:301–302.

8

Organismic Time and Metabolic Control of Development

E. Wagner

Growth and differentiation of most living systems is tightly coupled to seasonal changes in environmental factors like light and temperature. The multiplicity of organismic responses to light and temperature signals from the environment is generally treated in plant and animal physiology under the headings of photo- and thermoperiodism. Both groups of phenomena reveal a rhythmic change in sensitivity which is endogenous in character and reflects an endogenous rhythm in metabolic activity. This sensitivity change has a period length of about 24 hr and is hence called circadian. By definition, circadian rhythms have the following features:

> They persist for some time in the absence of diurnal fluctuations in temperature and illumination; their phase can be altered by a brief disturbance of the constant regimen; and their period is relatively independent of the constant external temperature, at least within the physiological range (11).

The circadian rhythm is only a special case of the continuously increasing number of rhythms observed in living matter (18, 19). It seems therefore appropriate to assume that rhythmicity is an essential feature of physiology, development, and behavior to all living systems (3, 4). Circadian rhythmicity expresses itself at all levels of organization from unicellular systems to man.

There are good reasons to believe that circadian rhythmicity is based on common mechanisms and principles of biochemistry and biophysics. Thus, circadian rhythmicity results from the molecular properties of enzymes and multienzyme complexes with these allosteric control sites and the regulatory functions of biological membranes integrated into a feedback network of compartmental energy metabolism.

The network of eukaryotic energy transduction is conceived on an evolutionary adaptation to a cyclic energy supply from the environment (17). In the course of evolution, circadian metabolic activity became the innate timer of eukaryotes controlling growth, differentiation, and behavior. This view of circadian rhythmicity as a function of the metabolic control net of the whole cell is supported by the fact that circadian rhythms cannot be observed in isolated cell organelles, despite the fact that organelles as well as isolated metabolic sequences can display high-frequency (seconds to minutes) oscillations in their activities under *in vivo* and *in vitro* conditions (for review, see refs. 18 and 19). In contrast to these high-frequency oscillations, the circadian rhythm is temperature compensated and hardly susceptible to chemical manipulation. This stability of period length is a functional prerequisite for this oscillator to act as a precise physiological clock. The constancy or homeostasis of the circadian periodicity within an organism compensates for static and dynamic disturbances from the environment. From this point of view, homeostasis and rhythmicity can be considered as being just two aspects of one biological principle. Homeostasis protects living systems against *random* disturbances while circadian rhythmicity provides an optimal phase relationship between oscillatory metabolic sequences and cycle of the environment through entrainment to these environmental cycles.

Evidence is accumulating in favor of the concept that temporal organization of development might be coordinated through rhythmicity in energy transduction, through rate control of biological processes (6) at the level of membranes (13, 20). The energy source would assume the significance of an information factor, and the genome response would assume one of modulating the energy flux between the cell and environment (5, 10). The regulatory network of energy metabolism will strongly depend on membrane-bound transport or shuttle systems as the control sites for the coupling of compartmented metabolic sequences through transport systems.

The coupling functions of membranes might depend on manipulation of membrane-bound activities through (a) control of synthesis of membrane components; (b) assembly of membrane subunits; (c) metabolic feedback; (d) energy level and (e) turnover of membrane components.

The genetic determination of membrane components of cell organelles could be the basis for the genetically fixed period lengths of circadian rhythms. This might also be the key to ultimately understanding the timing of metabolic controls leading to normal and malignant growth (1, 2, 7–9, 12, 16).

Eventually, an understanding of biorhythmic controls and regulation could prove to be the basis for diagnostic and therapeutic success in medicine (14, 15).

References

1. Ayuso-Parrilla, M. S., and Parrilla, R. (1975): Control of hepatic protein synthesis. Differential effects of ATP on the initiation and elongation steps. *Eur. J. Biochem., 50*:309–316.
2. Bartalos, M. (1971): Time factor in cytogenetics and neoplasia. *Acta Genet. Med. Gemellol., 20*:350–358.
3. Bünning, E. (1973): *The Physiological Clock—Circadian Rhythms and Biological Chronometry.* Ed. 3 (rev. ed.). Springer, Heidelberg.
4. Bünning, E. (1977): *Die physiologische Uhr: Circadian Rhythmik und Biochronometrie.* 3. gründlich überarbeitete Auflage. Springer, Berlin-Heidelberg.
5. Daniel, J. W. (1966): Light-induced synchronous sporulation of a myxomcete—the relation of initial metabolic changes to the establishment of a new cell state. In *Cell Synchrony: Studies in Biosynthetic Regulation,* edited by I. L. Cameron and M. G. Padilla, pp. 117–151. Academic Press, New York and London.
6. Davies, D. D. (1973): Rate control of biological processes. *Symp. Soc. Exp. Biol., 27.*
7. Ehret, C. F. (1974): The sence of time; evidence for its molecular basis in the eukaryotic gene-action system. *Adv. Biol. Med. Phys., 15*:47–77.
8. Gedda, L. and Brenci, G. (1971): Chronology of the gene. *Acta Genet. Med. Gemellol., 20*:323–349.
9. Gilbert, D. A. (1973): The malignant transformation as a metabolic steady state transition: the possible significance of the phasing of enzyme synthesis and related aspects. *Biosystems, 5*:128–139.
10. Glass, L., and Kauffman, S. A. (1972): Co-operative components, spatial localization and oscillatory cellular dynamics. *J. Theor. Biol., 34*:219–237.
11. Hastings, J. W., and Schweiger, H.-G. (1976): *The Molecular Basis of Circadian Rhythms: Report of the Dahlem Workshop on the Molecular Basis of Circadian Rhythms, Berlin 1975.* Abakon Verlagsgesellschaft, Berlin.
12. Mahrle, G., and Orfanos, C. E. (1975): Ultrastructural localization and differentiation of membrane-bound ATP utilizing enzymes including adenyl cyclase in normal and psoriatic epidermis. *Br. J. Dermatol., 93*:
13. Nicolis, G., and Lefever, R. (1975): Membranes, dissipative structures, and evolution. *Adv. Chem. Physics, 29.*
14. Sinz, R., Amenda, G., and Fitzke, S. (1975): Kopplungscharkteristik minuten-rhythmischer Modulationsschwingungen physiologischer Funktionen unter Einwirkung von Diazepan (Faustan). *Acta Biol. Med. Ger., 34*:275–288.
15. Sinz, R., Goldhahn, S., Hendel, A., and Oehler-Beckert, P. (1975): Quantitative Bewertung von neurovegetativen Systemveränderungen anhand des minuten-rhythmischen Koppungsgrades und der Regulgute während akuter und chronischer Diazepan-therapie bei neurotischen Patienten. *Acta Biol. Med. Ger., 34*:289–301.
16. Smith, H. E., and Kenyon, D. H. (1973): A unifying concept of carcinogenesis and its therapeutic implications. *Oncology, 27*:99–105.
17. Wagner, E. (1976): Endogenous rhythmicity in energy metabolism: basis for timer photoreceptor interactions in photoperiodic control. In *The Molecular Basis of Circadian Rhythms: Report of the Dahlem Workshop on the Molecular Basis of Circadian Rhythms, Berlin 1975,* pp. 215–238, edited by J. W. Hastings and H.-G. Schweiger. Abakon Verlagsgesellschaft, Berlin.
18. Wagner, E. (1976): The nature of photoperiodic time measurement: Energy transduction and phytochrome action in seedlings of *Chenopodium rubrum.* In *Light and Plant Development,* (Proceedings of the 22nd Nottingham Easter School in Agricultural Sciences, pp. 419–443, edited by H. Smith. Butterworth, London.
19. Wagner, E. (1977): Molecular basis of physiological rhythms. In *Integration of Activity in the Higher Plant,* pp. 33–72, edited by D. H. Jennings. University Press, Cambridge.
20. Wolpert, L., and Lewis, J. H. (1975): Towards a theory of development. *Fed. Proc., 34*:14–20.

9

Fundamental Aspects of Normal Organismal Growth in Plants

J. A. Romberger

Introduction

The general subject of this book, the comparative pathology of abnormal growth, establishes a perspective. That perspective imposes limitations on what should be considered in a brief discussion of normal growth and development in plants. This is not the place for a detailed review of the literature on the physiological and biochemical aspects of plant growth. This is, though, a suitable place to consider the photosynthetic higher plant as a complex organism that, in its ontogeny from embryo to mature individual, copes with the necessity of control of growth and development in ways rather different from those characteristic of animals.

Certainly the control of growth and morphogenesis in both animals and plants is one of the major questions of biology. This major question includes within it many subsidiary and more specific questions. My objective here is to sort out and clarify some of the more significant questions that arise from our incomplete knowledge of the forces and processes underlying plant ontogeny. Formulation of clear and incisive questions may well be a greater contribution to the solution of major biological questions than are detailed answers to questions whose meanings and implications are poorly understood.

There are, of course, many biochemical, biophysical, and physiological similarities between plants and animals. Yet, the constituent processes and conditions of cellular and organismal growth and development in typical higher plants and higher animals differ fundamentally in three important ways.

Three Fundamental Differences between Growth in Plants and Animals

The Temporal Extent of Embryonal Growth

The first fundamental difference between growth in higher plants and higher animals is one of time and spatial localization. In higher animals, most cells are formed and differentiate into tissues and organs during a well-defined phase of embryonic growth, or during a limited juvenile period thereafter. Higher plants, though, generally continue to grow and to produce new tissues and organs, at least episodically, throughout their life cycles. This persistent embryogeny is mostly localized in the root and shoot tips and in a thin "vascular cambium" that ensheathes most stems and roots just inside the bark or cortex. These regions of continuing embryogeny are referred to as *meristems*. Collectively, the meristems usually constitute only a minute fraction of the total plant volume, but they are capable of producing new cells and tissues even while large volumes of older tissues are already senescent or dead. In most higher plants, there is no clear demarcation between embryonic development, juvenile stages, reproductive stages, and senescence. They can coexist in different parts of the same organism.

An inevitable consequence of the persistent nature of plant development is that it is more immediately susceptible to, and dependent upon, signals and stimuli from the external environment than is animal development. We find in plants beautiful examples of interactions between external environmental signals, such as the direction of gravity or the intensity and spectral quality of light, and the distribution or activity level of hormones that influence growth.

If we accept the mammal as the higher animal of central interest and the perennial woody plant, the tree, as the model higher plant, we can see that the long-continued embryonal growth of the perennial plant leads to progressive decentralization. In the mammal, the most significant morphogenesis is accomplished during a short, closely-regulated gestation. In contrast, the morphogenesis of the tree is very susceptible to the vagaries of the environment, in addition to being diffuse in time and space. Any sizeable tree has thousands of root apical meristems and thousands of shoot apical meristems. Each of these meristems has some autonomy, though it is dependent upon the rest of the tree for many of the essentials of survival. However, this kind of dependence of the individual upon the whole also applies to human and other societies. With regard to the physical aspects of size and form, the individual tree is much more a product of the environment to which it has responded, than is the mammal that happens to pass by. In a sense, a tree is a colony or a society, as much as it is an individual organism. Another aspect of persistent growth and organogenesis in plants is that the boundary between the individual organism and a colony of organisms can be lost, as, for example, in trees that send up shoot sprouts from roots (*Ailanthus, Robinia*) or put down roots from branches (*Ficus, Rhizophora*).

The differences between higher plants and animals in the temporal extent of embryonal and organogenic growth have a further consequence. This is manifested in basically different ways of responding to environmental stimuli. The day-to-day or moment-to-moment behavior of animals is mostly mediated through nerve-muscle systems. In contrast, the behavior (used in the same sense) of higher plants is mediated primarily through growth processes. In higher plants, the inciting stimuli are often integrated over appreciable time periods, and the resulting responses are typically irreversible or only partly reversible. In comparison to animal behavioral responses that are nerve-controlled and muscle-powered, plant response systems, being mostly growth-dependent, are slow and conservative. The basic question is: How, in view of their general decentralization, are plant growth processes controlled and integrated at the organism level?

Cell Walls and Extraneous Coats

The second fundamental difference between plant and animal growth is related to the nature of the extraneous coats that may envelop the protoplast of each cell. Some animal cells are surrounded by extraneous coats consisting of polymers of amino acids and uronic acids such as hyaluronic acid, chondroitin sulfate, and other mucopolysaccharides. Such coats or matrices, when they occur, become an important part of the microenvironment of the cells that produce them (11). In higher animal tissues, extraneous coats are not of general occurrence, include no cellulose or lignin, and seldom take the form of rigidly structured, form-limiting cell walls. In contrast, practically all plant cells are surrounded by walls consisting of pectins, cellulose, other polysaccharides, and lignins.

The wall of a plant cell is a product of the protoplast within it. The first formed layer, the primary wall, is in direct contact with the plasma membrane of the protoplast until a secondary layer of wall material is deposited inside the primary wall. Typically, the primary wall is thin and easily extended by the forces of cell volume growth. Deposition of secondary wall layers, because of their greater thickness and lesser extensibility, tends to limit or totally inhibit the cells' further growth in volume. Growth in dry weight due to accumulation of secondary wall materials may continue long after cell volume growth has stopped. As the cell goes through the changes in metabolism characteristic of its ontogeny, additional layers of wall material of varying chemical and physical properties may be deposited. Hence, plant cell walls generally have a laminated microstructure. This is further discussed in a following section.

Though the various wall layers are metabolic products of the cells they surround, once formed their constituents are seldom directly involved in further metabolic reactions (21), hence, they persist. Cell walls often continue to perform functions vital to the plant long after the cells that produced them are dead. For example, wood consists mostly of the walls of dead cells.

The origin of the primary walls that separate the daughter cells formed by cell division in plants is of interest. The formation of these walls constitutes a notable difference between the final stages of mitosis of plant and animal cells and also results in a process of cytokinesis that is basically different from the furrowing of animal cells. In plants, the establishment of a partition between sister cells has its visible beginnings during the metaphase or telophase of mitosis. Typically, a discoid *phragmosome* is organized in the central area of the equatorial plane; then a *cell plate* consisting of a back-to-back arrangement of the primary walls of both new cells solidifies within the phragmosome. The cell plate gradually extends across the equatorial plane and joins the existing walls, thus accomplishing cytokinesis.

With respect to the role of cell walls in plant growth control, there are two basic questions: What regulates the extensibility of the primary wall? What controls the onset and rate of deposition of secondary wall layers which, in turn, curtail the cell expansion phase of growth?

Generations, Seeds, and Other Complications

The third way in which the organismal growth and development of higher plants differs basically from that of higher animals is in the temporal, physiological, and genetic relations between "parent" and "offspring." There are several levels or classes of such differences.

First, vegetative propagation of plants is an everyday reality in nature as well as in the garden and laboratory. The persistent embryonal growth potential of a plant's meristems imparts a capability of asexual reproduction by natural fragmentation or by regeneration from artificial "cuttings." Such reproduction is unknown in higher animals.

A less obvious aspect concerns the totipotency that seems to be inherent in the somatic cells of the plant body. Such totipotency is seemingly repressed by signals or limiting conditions imposed upon each cell by its neighbors. A latent totipotency can sometimes be revealed experimentally by separating cells from their neighbors and culturing them in an artificial environment designed to imitate that in which a natural embryo develops. Such demonstrations were first achieved under the leadership of F. C. Steward with the production of thousands of embryoids from explants of very small pieces of carrot root tissue. These somatic embryoids were capable of growing into normal, fertile carrot plants (25, 64).

Wholly aside from considerations of persistent embryonal growth and somatic totipotency, "parent"-to-"offspring" relations in higher plants are complicated by the fact that reproduction by seeds is not as straightforward as it seems. This is so because the life cycles of higher plants include as a basic feature an alternation between asexual (diploid) and sexual (haploid) generations. Though well known in the academic sense, the alternation of generations in higher plants is often disregarded in physiological and developmental studies. To some this may seem justified because in most higher plants the sexual generation is only a microscopic vestige.

During the evolution of plants, the sexual, gamete-producing generation (the gametophyte) has been progressively reduced from the independently-living, leafy gametophytes of mosses and liverworts to the microscopic and parasitic gametophytes of flowering plants. Meanwhile, the asexual, spore-producing generation (the sporophyte), which in some algae exists only as a single-celled zygote, has become the dominant form that we recognize as the individual organism, the plant.

The higher plants that we see, classify, and utilize are sporophytes. As such they are diploid and asexual. When mature, these asexual plants may "flower." That is, they produce highly modified leaves which by further differentiation develop ovules (megasporangia) or pollen sacs (microsporangia). Within these organs, microenvironmental conditions and hormonal balances are such that some cells (archesporial cells) take developmental pathways different from those of their neighbors. These cells become enlarged, then undergo meiosis and produce haploid cells known as "spores." Such spores may be either of two types, megapsores or microspores, and the type seems to be mostly determined by the morphology of the sporangium and its position on the plant (28). Characteristically, megaspores differentiate within ovules and microspores within anthers. These haploid spores "germinate" to produce small or microscopic, and parasitic, plants of the gametophyte generation. These are sexual in the sense that when they mature they differentiate cells that function as male and female gametes. Microspores (pollen grains) yield microgametophytes, which produce male gametes (sperm cells). Megaspores yield megagametophytes (embryo sacs), which produce female gametes (egg cells).

Thus the flowering plant, technically asexual, has as "parasites" within its flowers (or strobili in gymnosperms) minute sexual plants of an alternate generation that produce sperm cells and egg cells. As a consequence of pollination, sperm cells are brought to the vicinity of egg cells. Fertilization, or syngamy, can then occur. When it does, the diploid condition is restored, and a new asexual sporophyte generation begins as a zygote. The zygote, without formation of a hollow blastula and gastrulation, develops directly into an embryo having distinguishable shoot and root apical meristems. This happens inside of ripening ovules within flowers. The tissues within which the ovule, the megaspore, the megagametophyte, and the egg cell differentiated become modified into the various tissues of the seed and fruit. Thus young embryonic organisms are packaged for dispersal.

The dispersal package, the seed, is a remarkable evolutionary development. Within it in a state of arrested development, and well protected from adverse environmental conditions, is an embryo, along with a reserve of metabolites. Seeds may be quiescent for decades, then when conditions become favorable, growth processes are reactivated, the seed germinates, and the embryo becomes a free-living plant. Morphogenically, the seed is much more complex than is superficially evident. Three "generations" are involved. Externally, the seed consists of diploid sporophyte tissue from the generation that bore it. Within these layers are remnants of the gametophyte generation that produced the egg cell. Embedded in these remnants, in turn, is the embryo, a diploid individual of the next sporophyte generation.

The suspension of development of the embryo in the maturing seed, the survival of the embryo over long dormant periods, and the reactivation of meristematic activity during seed germination pose interesting questions of control of growth and development. Other intriguing questions concern the basis and meaning of organism and cellular juvenility and aging in plants when vegetative preproduction is common, but rejuvenescence by sexual reproduction still seems necessary (54).

The Meaning of Continuing Embryonal Growth

The Concept of Meristems: Theories of Organization

On the time scale of the history of biology, the meristem concept is a relatively recent one, dating from the last half of the 19th century. In the early 19th century, the existence of cells was vaguely known, but the cell was not recognized as the basic structural unit of plants, and the origin of cells was not understood. By 1840, achromatic microscopes and precision microtomes were available, and the anatomical study of plants had become an active research area. The work of such men as Schleiden, Schwann, Von Mohl, Nägeli, and Hofmeister soon established that all plant organs and tissues are composed of cells, that cells arise by division of preexisting cells, and that plant growth results from cell division and cell enlargement in relatively localized regions.

By 1875, the term "meristem" was being applied to the region of dividing and enlarging cells at the tips of roots and shoots. It was recognized that the activities of these meristems produce the cells constituting the primary plant body, that is, the leaves and the tissues of the roots and shoots before secondary thickening growth begins. It was recognized, too, that, except for their very youngest extensions, roots and shoots of higher plants can grow in diameter (secondary growth) because a sheath-like layer of meristematic cells, the cambium, surrounds them just inside the bark. The outlines of our present ideas on the cambial meristem were, in fact, already evident in the work of Nägeli (43) in 1864.

The historical development of ideas on the organization and function of apical meristems is of continuing interest because each of the major theories advanced was partially correct and has some present usefulness. The *apical cell theory* (1850s) proposed that a single, large apical cell in each meristem, by divisions parallel to its several faces, gave rise to other cells of the meristem. Further divisions and development of these then constructed the plant. This theory seems valid for mosses and some other lower plants, and perhaps for embryos of some higher plants, but for higher plants generally it is inadequate. The *histogen theory*, advanced in 1868, proposed that root and shoot apical meristems consist of a central core of irregularly arranged cells covered by one or more mantle-like layers of regularly arranged cells. It proposed that each layer and the core were derived from a separately identifiable cell or small group of such cells, the *histogens* or tissue formers. The theory also proposed that cells derived from a specific histogen were predestined to become cells of the tissues characteristically derived from that histogen. This predestination aspect of the theory drew criticism that led to its eclipse. A modified histogen theory, however, has recently been invoked in interpretations of persistent cytochimeras of various plant shoots as manifested by variegated leaves (15, 65).

The more modern *tunica-corpus theory* (56) may be thought of as a simplified histogen theory in which only an outer layer, the *tunica*, and an inner core, the *corpus*, are recognized. Most angiosperm shoot apices can be described in tunica-corpus terms, though they are not generally applicable to gynosperms. Physiologically, the persistence of a tunica one or more cell layers in depth implies a control of the plane of cell division so that no divisions parallel to the apical surface occur in those layers. Whereas the tunica-corpus theory was not applied to roots, the related *Körper-Kappe theory* was specifically so applied (59). It offers a method of analyzing cell patterns and growth in root tips so that the location of the initial cells can be determined.

After 1930, increasing interest in the dynamic aspects of plant development led to a concept of *cytohistological zonation* within apical meristems. Zonation refers to the existence of regions distinguishable by differences in cell size, degree of vacuolation, relative nuclear volume, frequency of division, cell wall thickness, orientation of planes of cell division, and responses to histological staining. This concept came to fruition in Foster's (20) interpretation of the shoot apical meristem of *Ginkgo*. Applicability of these ideas has since been demonstrated for many other species. Details of zonation vary with the species, the individual plant, and the ontogenetic stage of the individual meristem. This is in agreement with the view that cytohistological zonation is a consequence of the different physiological conditions prevailing in local regions of a meristem at any one time.

More recent ideas on the organization of root apical meristems have taken a different course. One view that still has currency is that of von Guttenberg (24), whose ideas reveal an influence of the histogen theory. Von Guttenberg visualized two basic types of root apices, *open* and *closed*. The closed type has discrete histogens. This condition is common in roots of embryos and is retained in older roots of many species. In many others, though, the small groups of meristematic cells that could be called histogens lose their identity during postembryonic growth because there is open exchange of cells across previously closed boundaries of histogenic zones. Many root apices are open at all stages and never seem to have histogen-like groups of initial cells. In such apices, von Guttenberg

called the presumed initial cells *central cells*. Though these cells divide, subsequent divisions of their progeny generate most of the cells of the root. Thus, the central cells constitute a generative center, but not necessarily a center of great meristematic activity. The number of central cells can be small, sometimes even a single cell.

In another view, the number of totipotent and undifferentiated meristematic initial cells in a root apex is quite large, and the entire collection has been called the *promeristem* (8). According to Clowes, the promeristem need not be a compact mass with histogen initial cells or progenitor cells in its center. It is more likely to be a population of meristematically active cells on the periphery of a centrally located *quiescent center*. The latter is a spheroidal group of meristematically quiescent cells carried forward with the root tip by the growth and division of the active cells behind and around it. Cells of quiescent centers, though potentially meristematic, may be inactive because of their microenvironment. If surrounding active cells are cut away, the previously quiescent cells can become actively meristematic. Slender root meristems may never develop quiescent centers. Large root meristems can have quiescent centers having a thousand or more relatively inactive, but still potentially meristematic, cells. This is in agreement with the principle that large numbers of active meristematic cells cannot coexist en masse. Active meristems are always likely to be small masses, peripheral layers around larger masses, or thin plates.

Subordinate to the concept of meristems is that of meristemoids, these being small localized groups of meristematic cells scattered through differentiated tissue. The development of stomata in plant epidermis can be explained as an example of meristemoid activity that ends in the formation of a specific structure. In other instances meristemoids can persist for long periods, and under some conditions they can give rise to adventitious buds or roots within otherwise mature tissue.

Functional Types of Meristems

By definition, a meristem is a formative tissue made up of small cells capable of dividing indefinitely and thereby producing similar meristematic cells or cells that soon differentiate into the constituent cells of tissues and organs. Meristematic cells generally are also considered to be totipotent and "undifferentiated." This does not mean that all the meristematic cells of a plant are alike. There are differences in size, shape, and polarity, depending upon the position of the cell within the plant. Another way in which meristematic cells may be different is related to aging. There is some support for the idea that, along with the organism that their progeny have constructed, meristematic cells themselves may age. The real meaning of this in terms of cellular differentiation is not clear (54). With these qualifications, meristematic cells are undifferentiated and at least moderately active metabolically while being prone to divide. Being heterotrophic, metabolically active, and usually separated from functional vascular tissues by their differentiating progeny, meristematic cells are not adapted to accumulating in large masses. Cells that are successively displaced from the meristematic focus by cell divisions and growth become susceptible to differentiation. We can only speculate about the primary causes of this.

We can think of all meristematic cells as being subject to two rather opposite primal tendencies. One is to divide. That is the way of rejuvenescence and of potential immortality by maintenance of the meristematic function. The other is to differentiate. That is the way of structural and physiological specialization, of aging, and of death. Only a small minority of cells can maintain positions near the focus of meristematic activity. Those that do can be thought of as "inheriting" the initial function and as being repeatedly rejuvenated. Those many that do not maintain such positions contribute to the outward flux of differentiating progeny cells that is a feature of every active meristem.

Meristems can be functionally classified according to the characteristics of that flux of differentiating cells, the final state of those cells, and also according to where they are within the organism. Thus at the tip of every shoot with further growth potential is a *shoot apical meristem*. Its differentiating progeny cells typically become new leaves, and also contribute to the stem segments between leaves. At the tip of every root with further growth potential is a spheroidal or cup-like *root apical meristem* that contributes cells both to the expendable tissues of the root cap and to the permanent tissues of the primary[1] root. Ensheathing every segment of root and stem that is capable of secondary[1]

growth in thickness is a lateral meristem, the *vascular cambium*. Most perennial caulescent plants also have a more superficially located lateral meristem, the phellogen or cork cambium. This meristem is secondary in origin. It is of significance mostly in relation to periderm or bark characteristics and will not be further considered here.

All shoot apical meristems, though variable in size and shape, are similar in function. They generate new cells. Their terminal and superficial location determines that this flux of new cells is unidirectional, away from the base of the meristem. These cells contribute to the construction of the shoot in two quite different ways: in the initiation of foliar primordia, and in the establishment of cauline regions which become the internodes of the stem.

Foliar primordia begin as localized upwellings of growth around the lower flanks of the apical meristem. These begin as active sites within which a few cells divide more frequently and with greater control over the orientation of planes of division than is evident in neighboring cells. Such sites can become microscopically visible mounds within a few hours. These primordia soon become semiautonomous, develop ephemeral meristems at their tips and margins, and without further receipt of cells from the parent apical meristem, they begin developing into leaves. Each successive foliar primordium is initiated at a different point of the compass and a little higher than its predecessor. This means that along with each new primordium, the apical dome proper also leaves behind the cells in a thin disc-like volume that is, in effect, a primordial internode. The cells in this volume represent the second, and often the major, way in which the shoot apical meristem contributes to the construction of the shoot. The growing shoot tip, and especially the dormant bud with its embryonic shoot, contains as its central element a stack of such primordial internodes. Collectively, and there may be dozens or hundreds, these constitute a subapical meristem which is usually much more voluminous than the apical meristem itself. Further divisions of the cells in this subapical region give rise to most of the cells of the primary stem. These divisions, and the subsequent enlargement of the cells produced, account for most of the shoot extension growth that one sees and measures. The ultimate origin

---

[1] Primary tissues are those tissues derived directly from the embryo or from a root or shoot apical meristem. Primary growth refers to the multiplication and enlargement of the component cells of these tissues. Secondary tissues are those produced by the secondary meristems, that is, from the vascular cambium and the phellogen.

Multiplication and enlargement of the component cells of these tissues is called secondary growth. The meanings of "primary" and "secondary" with respect to cell walls are not directly related to the meanings of the same terms as they are applied to tissues.

of all, however, was from the few initial cells in the apical meristem.

Root apical meristems also have as their basic function the contribution of cells to the construction of the axes that bear them. Unlike their shoot counterparts, the meristematic initial cells of root apical meristems are located deep within the tissue mass of the tip. In most species the entire tip is covered by a superficial cap which is pushed through the soil by the growth behind it. Cap cells lost to abrasion are replaced by new cells from the meristematic zone. The outward flux of new cells from the root apical meristem, then, is multidirectional. There is a significant forward flux into the cap. These cap cells contribute nothing to the permanent structure of the root. There are also major lateral and backward fluxes of cells from the root apical meristem. These cells and their progeny become the tissues of the stele and cortex of the primary root. As in the shoot, there are many divisions among the enlarging and differentiating cells left behind by the advancing meristem. The root apical meristem does not contribute directly to the initiation of lateral branch roots. The latter arise some distance behind the advancing tip. The lateral root meristems are products of local activity near the stele-cortex boundary. The new root tips grow outward through the cortical tissue but form no physiological connection with it.

The third major functional type of meristem in higher plants is the vascular cambium. It is not involved in primary growth of the plant body because it is itself of secondary origin. The vascular cambium arises mostly from residual primary meristem cells left behind in the young plant axis by the advancing apical meristem. These cells are commonly elongate, arranged in provascular strands, and serve as the precursor cells from which primary vascular tissues (xylem and phloem) differentiate just behind growing root and shoot tips. In some plants, all the provascular cells differentiate into xylem and phloem elements, and no vascular cambium is formed. Such plants are likely to remain small, herbaceous, and annual. If strands of provascular meristematic cells remain after primary growth has ceased, they are collectively referred to as procambium. The procambial strands gradually develop into bands of vascular cambium lying between the primary xylem and phloem. In most higher plants, these bands soon extend themselves across intervening gaps and form a nearly continuous cambial sheath around the stem and roots. This pattern is basic to the development of large, woody, perennial plants.

The vascular cambium may also extend into the larger veins of leaves as a thin band.

There is, strictly speaking, only one vascular cambium in a tree, but it may be many square meters in area and involve billions of cells. Aside from a few exceptions such as palms, the woody plant is mostly constructed of cells generated by its vascular cambium, though the latter only thickens the root and stem segments already formed by the activities of the primary apical and subapical meristems. The vascular cambium is at most only a few cells deep, and arguments can be made that only one layer of cells includes most of the truly undifferentiated meristematic initials. There is unquestionably a narrow central zone within which cells divide to produce progeny that by subsequent divisions are displaced both inward and outward from the central zone. The derivative cells in the inward flux may divide a few more times and then differentiate into various components of the xylem as permanent tissues of the stem. The cells in the outward flux, usually fewer, may also undergo limited division and then differentiate into the components of phloem and related tissue. Phloem elements function briefly in translocation and then die and are crushed by growth pressure from within. Eventually, the dead remnants become part of the bark tissues and are gradually flaked off. Hence, in long-lived perennial plants, only the inward derivatives of the cambium become part of the permanent plant body (18, 47).

The vascular cambium is of significance only in plants that undergo extensive secondary growth. Monocotyledonous plants (grasses, lilies, etc.) do not have vascular cambia that form sheaths around their stems. Some of them, however, undergo primary growth of long duration. This commonly results from the activity of intercalary meristems. The latter term is used to designate a region of primary tissue growth in a shoot when that region is separated from the apical meristem by regions of greater cell differentiation and lesser division rates. The best examples of this are in grasses. Grass leaves, as are leaves of other plants, are initiated as primordia on the flanks of shoot apical meristems. The primordial internodes separating them are mostly very short. Elongation of these internodes may be initially slow and then rapid, or slow and of long duration. In either instance, cell division and elongation often become localized in the basal region of each internode. Some leaves, especially those of grasses, behave in this way and may grow from the base (as does a hair) for long periods. Intercalary meristems, however, always contain some differentiated differentiate, and the meristematic function is lost.

Cell Division and Growth in Meristematic Regions

In animal embryos at the cleavage stage, there can be many repeated cell divisions without appreciable cell growth. In sporophytes of higher plants this phase of ontogeny, if present at all, is limited to a very few divisions in the proembryo. Generally, plant cell divisions are cells. Eventually, their meristematic cells too closely related to growth. When there is no growth, there is also usually no division, but it does not follow that regions of rapid volume growth are regions of rapid cell division. Most cell divisions occur in meristematic regions, where growth is regulated in such a way that there is little change in mean cell volume despite cell divisions. Most cell volume growth occurs at the outer margins of the meristematic regions where divisions are infrequent and most cells become highly vacuolated.

The usual pattern is for a meristematic cell to divide by mitosis followed by cytokinesis. The "daughter" cells then grow back to the volume of the "mother" cell at division and soon undergo division themselves. It seems that division potentiates the metabolic situation that subsequently allows volume growth to occur, and that attainment of a critical nuclear and cytoplasmic volume is one of the conditions potentiating another division. In this limited view, cell division and growth are cyclical; hence, growth vigor can be assessed in terms of mean cell generation time.

Cell generation times have been estimated for root or shoot apical meristems of a modest number of higher plant species. For shoot meristems, times ranging from less than 30 to more than 1000 hr have been reported (35). The values of 50 to 80 hr found in *Picea abies* seedlings (55) are probably not atypical for woody plants. Many published times are averages for an entire apical meristem. At the cell level, generation times vary with position within the meristem (35). Cell generation times in root meristems seem to be shorter than those in shoot meristems (9).

Whereas the general outline of cell division in plants is similar to that in animals, there are significant differences. First, centrioles have no role in cell divisions in higher plants. These fiber-producing organelles seem to form the asters during animal cell mitosis, and by their position they may determine orientation of the spindle. Though centrioles are present in plant cells having flagellae, they are not detectable in higher plant somatic cells, even during mitosis (17). Organized spindles do, nevertheless, appear in dividing plant cells though they are barrel-shaped and not pointed at the poles as in animal cells.

The second notable departure of plant cell mitosis from that of animal cells is the appearance of a phragmoplast in the equatorial plane of the spindle during telophase. The phragmoplast is significant because the thin, discoid, and fibrous cell plate is organized in its plane. The cell plate initially consists of a thin layer of pectins, on both sides of which the primary walls of the new faces of the daughter cells are deposited. The margins of the cell plate gradually grow across the equatorial plane and join with the existing walls as the phragmoplast disappears.

Thus, the new cross wall of a daughter cell is made *de novo*, but the other walls are inherited from the mother, which in turn inherited most walls from its progenitors. Actually, there is evidence that primary wall lamellae are deposited not only on the cell plate, but also all around each protoplast. This can lead to a multilamellar primary wall structure of various thickness on various faces of the cell depending upon the planes of previous divisions (36, 42). In many meristems, the number of cell generations through which a cell wall has existed may be estimated by studying the lamellar ultrastructure (10), but it is often obvious upon even casual examination of sections with the light microscope that the various walls of meristematic cells have different origins and thicknesses. The thinnest walls will be the newest cross walls, and in that respect the two daughters cells of a division always have opposite polarities. In a sense, some differentiation of daughter cells is inevitable because the mitotic process cannot yield two really equal cells (5, 17).

The control of orientation of cell divisions is very significant in plant morphogenesis. This is because plant cell walls are generally anisotropic; hence, orientation of the partitioning wall between daughter cells has a great influence on the direction of the major growth axes of those cells. Orientation of the partitioning wall is generally determined by that of the cell plate, the phragmoplast, and the spindle. Spindle orientation, in turn, may be predicted (controlled?) by bands of microtubules existing in the cytoplasm even before prophase (48). Mechanical stresses may also influence orientation of planes of division (73). The basic question is: How are polarities, orientations of divisions, and growth in groups of cells integrated at the organism level so that characteristic and functional bodies are formed? Our knowledge is still not nearly adequate to allow one to attempt an answer.

Cells of apical meristems tend to be block-shaped and typically only 20–30 μm on a side. In any large woody plant, however, the apical meristem cells are far outnumbered by the meristematic cells of the vascular cambium that ensheathes its roots and shoots. Meristematic initial cells of the cambium are of two distinct types. One type, the ray initial, is roughly similar in size and shape to cells in the apical meristems; the other type, the fusiform initial, is extremely elongate and slender, and has pointed tips. These axially elongate initial cells are typically several hundred micrometers long, but have a tangential width usually less than 50 μm and a thickness of only 10–20 μm. Apical meristem cells usually have prominent nuclei and often are so densely cytoplasmic that they seem to be nonvacuolated. In contrast, cambial meristematic cells, especially the fusiform initials, have less prominent nuclei and are likely to be highly vacuolated.

Whatever the state of vacuolization in meristematic cells, vacuolar volume generally increases tremendously in the progeny cells in the regions where divisions are infrequent and cell expansion and differentiation dominate. Very roughly, the typical cell in the plant body has a volume of 20–200 times that of the meristematic cell that was its progenitor. Most of that volume growth is directly due to increase in vacuolar volume by water uptake.

The apical meristems proper and the cambial zone are the *ultimate* origins of all cells of the permanent plant body. Yet, the greatest number of cells may arise in the outer reaches of those meristems where the cells are already several generations removed from truly undifferentiated cells. Hence, the apical and subapical regions of shoot and root apical meristems are regions of cell generation, and behind them lie regions in which cell expansion, and especially elongation, predominate. In both roots and shoots, it is the elongation of previously formed cells that provides the major thrust of extension growth—pushing shoot tips upward or forward, and root tips downward or forward through the soil. In the cambial zone, relations are different, but still

similar. The cambial initial cells are the progenitors. The zones of xylem and phloem mother cells are characterized by further multiplication of cell types that are already partly differentiated. Further differentiation continues along with radial expansion. It is this final radial expansion, prior to the major phase of secondary wall deposition, that accounts for most of the radial growth of a stem.

One can reason that although most plant growth is the result of cell enlargement, such enlargement is normally stopped by secondary wall deposition. Thus organismal growth will soon stop unless new cells are being generated. The generation of new cells requires the doubling of nuclear materials in each cell generation. Hence, the extent of growth ultimately depends upon molecular events involving DNA synthesis and its control. These events are not yet well understood nor well correlated with the visible events of mitosis. This subject, the molecular events of the cell cycle, is of basic interest, but cannot be treated here. The review by Yeoman and Aitchison (72) is recommended.

Cell Walls, Growth, and Development

Primary and Secondary Cell Walls

The enlargement of cells to the volume of the mature and differentiated stage can be considered as a two-phase process. The first phase includes volume increases that are mostly related to the synthesis of additional cytoplasm and cell organelles in the daughter cell, while that cell is regaining the volume of its meristematic mother cell at the time of division. The second phase, including most of the volume increase that we recognize macroscopically as growth, is almost entirely due to the inflation of cell vacuoles by water—often to such an extent that the vacuoles occupy as much as 90% of the cell volume. This phase of water inflation coincides with a major increase in wall area.

It is emphasized, however, that all the cell wall synthesis that occurs during both these volume growth phases is of the primary type. It is only when cell expansion has practically stopped that new wall material, rather than appearing in microfibrils intermixed with the old, is deposited in discrete lamellae inside the old. We then speak of secondary wall synthesis. The latter limits rather than contributes to growth in cell volume, but it contributes very greatly to growth in terms of cell dry weight. What controls the shift from primary wall extension growth to secondary wall thickness growth? That basic question needs study.

With the usual minor exceptions, primary walls do not become thinner as the cells grow. What is the mechanism by which a cell wall maintains its thickness as it is extended by growth? In asking this question, it must be understood that a cell wall does not extend its area unless there is a hydrostatic pressure (turgor pressure) within the cell and that pressure is adequate to stress the wall beyond a critical threshold value. When that value is surpassed, the microfibrillary mesh of the primary wall opens up enough to allow intercalation of additional matrix and microfibrils of wall polymers. The exact mechanisms involved, and their controls, are still being investigated and debated (50). However, it seems likely that there is slow extension under near constant stress (creep).

The results of many experimental studies suggest that the rate of cell volume growth is generally proportional to the differences between the actual turgor pressure within the cell and some threshold turgor pressure that must be exceeded before cell volume growth can begin. Apparently, there are bonds in the primary wall that must be strained and broken before "creeping" growth is possible. There are indications too that the energies of these bonds, as well as the turgor pressure, are susceptible to metabolic control (50).

In digest, we can characterize extension growth of primary cell walls as a biochemically modulated creep driven by wall stresses induced by turgor pressures resulting from water uptake by vacuoles. Obviously, most of the questions we could ask cannot yet be answered. It would be a mistake, however, in any consideration of plant growth to regard the primary cell wall as a mere excretory product. Functionally, it is intimately involved with the living cytoplasm that produces it, almost to the extent of being an enveloping organelle.

The secondary wall that a plant cell protoplast usually deposits inside its primary wall is of interest for reasons different from those applicable to the primary wall. Either the secondary wall is deposited after primary expansion growth of the cell has stopped, or it is the deposition of secondary layers that makes the wall so strong that turgor pressures can no longer stress it to the point of yielding. In either case volume growth of the cell stops—in fact, in many cells, the accumulations of secondary wall materials can become so great that they substan-tially reduce the remaining volume available for cytoplasm and vacuoles. Consequently, growth in the sense of dry weight accumulation may show a great increase during secondary wall deposition. Normally, the material deposited in secondary cell walls is not involved in further metabolism. It remains in place through the life of the cell, and often far beyond that.

Though cause-and-effect relations are uncertain, secondary wall thickening involves a shift in the kinds of substances being deposited. The pectin (polyuronide) matrix of primary walls is replaced by hemicelluloses (xylan and galactomannan) in the secondary wall. At the same time, the proportion of matrix polysaccharides is reduced, and that of cellulose is increased. In some fibers, such as those in the cotton boll, secondary walls are largely cellulose, but usually there are some other polysaccharides and also an incrustation of lignin, suberin, and complex waxy materials. These materials, or their precursors, are synthesized in the cell cytoplasm. They, possibly still as precursors, then pass through the plasmalemma to be condensed or polymerized and deposited outside. Though the final deposition occurs outside the plasmalemma, it seems likely that the form and orientation of microfibrils in the lamellae being deposited are determined by organelles in the peripheral regions of the cytoplasm.

The secondary walls of higher plant cells are typically layered. The S (secondary) terminology of Bailey (4) is widely followed in referring to the layers. The first layer to be deposited, S_1, lies just inside the primary wall and often consists of four submicroscopic lamellae of polysaccharide microfibrils. The microfibrils in these lamellae run around the cell at a large angle to the cell axis with microfibrilar orientation in alternate lamellae inclined in opposite directions. The S_2 layer is usually much thicker, has many lamellae, and may constitute the bulk of total wall materials in mature cells. The microfibrils in the various lamellae of S_2 form small angles with the cell's major axis. These angles usually vary only slightly from lamella to lamella. The S_2 layer is thus typically anisotropic under polarized light. Though S_2 may also be a major site of lignin deposition, this occurs mostly after the polysaccharide lamellae are in place and hence at sites remote from the plasmalemma (31, 50). The next layer to be deposited, S_3, usually contributes little to the wall's mass and may sometimes hardly be detectable. When well developed, the S_3 layer consists of a few thin lamellae of microfibrils deposited at large and alternating angles with the major axis of the cell. Finally, inside S_3 there may be a "warty layer" that includes no cellulose. This may mostly be the remains of dead cytoplasm (68).

Secondary walls, because of their bulk and mechanical strength, typically inhibit growth in cell volume and substitute growth in dry weight. In highly differentiated cells, such as fibers and some tracheids, these walls may become so thick that the remaining cell lumen is much reduced in volume. Metabolically, these thickened walls are neutral, though they physically separate the plasmalemma from the primary wall, except in local unthickened areas referred to as pits.

The Functional Significance of Cell Walls

The plant cell wall is rich in carboxyl, hydroxyl, and other charged groups. It is, therefore, a micromosaic of sites reactive toward a broad range of solutes. In theory, the presence of the cell wall may in some situations have little effect upon the concentration of a specified solute at the plasmalemma, which is the cell's major permeability barrier. However, because of its many reactive sites and its netlike microstructure, the wall will usually have some effect on the concentrations of solutes at the plasmalemma. This wall effect may be large. Substances of high molecular weight may diffuse into and through the wall so slowly that for them the wall, rather than the plasmalemma, is the major permeability barrier of the cell.

Little is yet known concerning the changing contributions of the various wall constituents to ion binding as cells differentiate and mature. Among the polysaccharides, pectins and xylans might be expected to contribute most and cellulose least. Coordinate binding may sometimes be more important than ion binding, and cellulose would participate in the former. Cell walls also contain some protein, and that protein provides many positively charged binding sites. Some proteins may also be active in coordinate binding. In addition, most cell walls contain some lignin, though the amount and its relation to other components varies widely. The presence of lignin changes the effective dielectric constant.

If one gives consideration to the above relations, it seems inevitable that plant cell walls will affect the accessibility of metabolites and growth regulators to the cell membrane (plasmalemma). Thus, the cell wall probably has a regulating role in cell differentiation. Whereas its ultrastructure and composition vary with the state of differentiation of the cell, the wall attributes at any stage can also influence further differentiation.

The multicellular bodies of terrestrial plants must be able physically to support themselves in the atmosphere against gravity and the wind. The water-rich protoplasts of the metabolically active cells must be allowed to exchange gases with the atmosphere. They must, at the same time, not have too intimate contact with the atmosphere, lest evaporation losses of water be too great.

Cell walls allow plant cells to meet these rather divergent demands in somewhat different ways at different stages of cell differentiation and maturation. A rough analogy applicable to a thin-walled meristematic cell might be a toy balloon inflated inside of a tightly-fitting but somewhat stretchable cloth bag. Here, the rubber membrane of the balloon and the cloth bag would represent the plasmalemma and the primary wall, respectively. For a differentiated and more mature cell, a better analogy would be a balloon inflated inside a restraining tank having walls of crisscrossed multiple plies of fibers embedded in and encrusted with cementing substances (the tank representing a secondary wall). If the balloon in the first analogy were ruptured, its shriveled membrane would be left inside a collapsed and shapeless mesh bag. No structural rigidity would remain. Rupturing the balloon in the second analogy would have little effect on the shape and strength of the remaining empty tank. We can think that one of the general functions of cell walls is to provide structural rigidity either dynamically when held in tension by pressures within, or passively by mere stiffness and resistance to compression. The latter type of rigidity may persist long after the cell is dead and its protoplasm has been autolyzed. This is commonly the case in wood. Aside from their function of giving support and mechanical protection, cell walls also serve to keep the plasmalemma surrounded by a water-saturated microenvironment. The plasmalemma itself is almost never exposed to the drying effects of the atmosphere.

Meristematic cells usually have only thin primary walls. These consist of substances that are active in sorption and retention of water. However, as these cells or their progeny differentiate and mature, thick secondary walls are deposited inside the thin primary walls. Though these secondary walls consist largely of cellulose and other highly hydrated polysaccharides, they also include lignin-like substances that are less highly hydrated. Thus, the deposition of a secondary wall separates the plasmalemma from the primary wall and necessarily results in extensive changes in its external microenvironment.

Cell Walls in Relation to Communication and Translocation

The higher plant is a structural society of cells, the individuals of which live under several types of restraints. They are generally in some way dependent upon their neighbors: for water, mineral elements, metabolites, or access to atmospheric gases. In addition, they may be restrained by their age and developmental status, by their physical positions, and by their lineage with respect to ancestral cells. The degree of interdependence is always high, but the level of functional and morphogenic coordination is also high. The integrated development and function of organisms as complex as oak trees or corn plants requires effective communication between cells. Plants, of course, have no nervous systems and no truly circulatory vascular systems. How, then, is effective intercellular communication and well-coordinated behavior achieved?

The problems of communication and exchange of materials among the millions of cells of a plant must be viewed from the perspective of the basic organization of the plant body. The latter consists of two phases. Both are continuous. As mutually anastomosing systems, they pervade each other. At the cellular level these phases are readily distinguishable. One phase, the *symplasm* (3), is mostly liquid in the sense that cell contents are liquid. It includes the protoplasts with all their organelles and vacuoles, and with their various interconnections through micropores in the walls. As is discussed below, it is by such interconnections that all protoplasts (with a few exceptions) are joined into one continuous symplasm, or *symplast*, that is everywhere bounded by a plasmalemma membrane. The other continuous phase, the *apoplast*, consists of the cell walls surrounding the protoplasts. This phase, largely solid, is nevertheless water-rich and abounds in microcapillary spaces through which water and solutes can move (40). There is no membrane barrier between the apoplast and the ambient environment. However, the apoplast is everywhere interposed between

the environment and the plasmalemma, the limiting membrane of the symplast. Hence, most aspects of the transport and communication essential to plant growth and development necessarily involve both apoplastic and symplastic space within the plant body.

A significant fraction of the apoplast volume is water-filled space that is in barrier-free diffusive continuity with any external fluids. This space, the so-called "free space," is a major translocation pathway for water solutions (32). Experimental measurements yield results usually referred to as "apparent free space." This is because the values obtained vary greatly with the methods used, especially with the size and charge characteristics of the molecular or ionic substances in the test solutions. These variations are sometimes taken into account by dividing the total free space into two fractions: the water free space which is not under the electrical influence of wall charges and the Donnan free space which is under such influence and in which mobile cations exceed mobile anions. The relative values of these fractions change as wall compostion changes during growth and differentiation and as the transported entities change. Necessarily, then, the efficiency of translocation in the free space of the apoplast is variable.

The structural basis of the symplasm is cytoplasmic continuity through plasmodesmata. These almost ultramicroscopic channels between adjacent cells, passing through primary and secondary walls, have long been known (66) and a voluminous literature about them exists (23). Plasmodesmata are very numerous in most plant tissues. It seems likely that even a small meristematic cell will have from 1,000 to 100,000 such connections with its various neighbor cells. The numbers recorded vary greatly depending upon whether observations are made by optical or electron microscopy. There is still some question of how the two types of images are related to each other and of the ultrastructure of plasmodesmata in intact living cells. Plasmodesmata generally have a diameter of less than 0.1 μm; thus, in spite of their large numbers, the total cross-sectional area of all the plasmodesmata of a cell would be an exceedingly small fraction of the total wall area. In spite of the small dimensions of plasmodesmata, symplasmic continuity and transport through these minute channels has been experimentally demonstrated (62, 63).

In some tissues it seems that plasmodesmata are formed only during the final stages of cell division, perhaps as remnants of spindle fibers trapped in the new cell plate. Were that the case, we would expect plasmodesmata to be "diluted out" during wall expansion. Whether this happens is not certain. The spindle fiber hypothesis, however, also seems inadequate with regard to numbers. Other, yet unrevealed, mechanisms of formation must be invoked to account for the great numbers of plasmodesmata found in most cell walls.

Although typically each living cell of a higher plant body is in communication with its neighboring cells through thousands of plasmodesmata, no plasmodesmata have been found between maternal sporophyte reproductive structures and the gametophytic tissue within (16); nor have any been found between the egg, zygote, or developing embryo and the ambient gametophyte or endosperm tissue (44). Apparently, plasmodesmata do not cross boundaries between generations (52). Each generation, parent sporophyte, gametophyte, and embryonic sporophyte, is a symplast unto itself. Does this mean that isolation is necessary for embryo formation and other instances of divergent development in environments that are otherwise similar to ambient? It seems possible that isolation, either surgical or simulated by plasmolytic breaking of plasmodesmata, might cause some cells of an integrated part of an organism to revert to earlier ontogenetic stages and redevelop, for example, as zygotes (41, 73).

Our central concern here is intercellular transport and communication in relation to growth. As growing cells are sinks for a full range of metabolites and other substances usually carried to them in water from the soil, we know that both symplast and apoplast are involved. Unfortunately, we know little about the locations of the functional boundaries between the two systems with regard to transport of water or specific solutes. This is an area of study that may contribute significantly to understanding of the control of growth and differentiation. Ultimately, the actual expansion phase of the growth of any cell is powered by water uptake. A cell grows because it has a lower water potential than (some of) its neighbors and is able to take up water at their expense. Such water uptake can cause a chain reaction of water potential lowering, leading from cell to cell, to the roots, and to the water in the soil. Water moves along such gradients from regions of high to regions of low water potential. The water that is essential to growth may cross several symplast-apoplast boundaries in its migration to a growing cell,

and it is not likely that the final plasmalemma passage is the growth-controlling step.

Control of Growth and Morphogenesis

Hormones and Related Regulators

The higher animal is able to live as it does because its body includes a variety of specialized organs, the various activities of which are successfully coordinated and integrated by control systems. A central nervous system usually provides a means of rapid transmission of bioelectric signals to all organs, and the circulating blood and lymph permits hormonal substances produced by localized and specialized tissues to be distributed throughout the organism. We should notice, though, that in the animal body those substances that we know as hormones are better understood in relation to control of the physiological functioning of the adult organism than they are in relation to morphogenesis during embryogeny or to the growth of the juvenile stage.

In higher plants the situation is different in that hormonal substances are known primarily with reference to their effects upon processes of growth and morphogenesis—which continue throughout the life of the organism. The relation between plant hormones and plant growth and development is, in fact, so encompassing that the term "plant hormone" is essentially synonomous with "plant growth regulator." Furthermore, in the absence of both endocrine glands and a true circulatory system, the origins of the regulators themselves and the means by which they are translocated to the tissues in which they have their effects are not at all obvious. Also open to question is the extent to which the much-studied "hormones" of plants are only mute slaves of more basic systems that control the synthesis, translocation, and sensitivity of receptor tissues to such regulator substances.

For overview purposes here it must suffice to focus briefly on each of six classes of plant growth hormones or other regulating substances. These classes are: auxins, cytokinins, gibberellins, abscisins, ethylene, and phytochrome. The class designations should be considered only a convenience pending more thorough understanding (for more details see, for example, Leopold and Kriedemann (33) and Bonner and Varner (6)).

Auxins

Charles Darwin already knew the phototropic curvature response of the grass coleoptile to be induced by an "influence" originating in the apex and migrating downward. Further studies revealed that tropisms of plants generally are based on preferential elongation of cells on only one side of a shoot or root, thus causing curvature. These facts led to the search for the actual diffusible hormonal substance or *auxin* responsible for such localized growth. The existence of such a substance was demonstrated by Went (70), but because of its exceedingly low concentration, isolation and chemical identification were difficult. Somewhat ironically, the long-sought plant growth hormone, auxin, was first isolated from mammalian urine and was identified by Kögl et al. (30) as the rather simple compound, indole-3-acetic acid (IAA). Knowledge of the molecular structure of a substance giving the growth responses of natural auxin did not, however, lead to rapid clarification of the mode of action of auxin in regulating growth. That question is still very open.

The present stature of auxin, for which IAA is used almost as a synonym, as the preeminent plant growth regulator is based on a great mass of lore, data, and literature. It is, nevertheless, not firmly established that IAA is the major auxin in all higher plants. Because of the mere trace amounts present, usually along with oxidizing enzymes, rigorous chemical identification and quantification has only rarely been accomplished (22). The case for IAA as an important naturally occurring auxin rests on a great accumulation of indirect evidence, such as extraction and bioassay. It occurs in bound forms in many plants. Most plants tested have responded in some manner to exogenous synthetic IAA. In addition, work with ^{14}C has shown that plant tissues can synthesize IAA from tryptophan and related compounds (67). Even so, it seems likely that some plants contain nonindolic auxins (57).

Presumably, auxin is produced by meristematic cells, especially in the shoot apex. It is transported basipetally by an active polar transport system. Unequal transport of auxin in light and dark or in response to gravity is thought to explain phototropism and geotropism. Responses to auxin are also invoked to explain secondary root formation, enhanced elongation

of shoot internodes, apical dominance, and a variety of other growth phenomena. There is hardly any plant growth response or developmental phase discussed in the physiological literature that has remained free from auxin involvement.

Exogenous IAA can cause an increase in the elongation rate of sensitive tissues in as little as 10 min, even in the presence of cycloheximide; hence, its primary action need not involve protein synthesis (49). Beyond this, all is confusion. Though at least one of the natural auxins may be a simple compound, we cannot explain its promotion of cell elongation, much less understand the many other effects it induces in plants.

Somewhat related to auxins are the various indole derivatives and phenolic substances that are widely distributed in plants. Exogenously supplied phenolics commonly inhibit plant growth, but under some conditions, some of the phenolic acids and various indole derivatives stimulate growth. The natural role of such substances in regulating growth is unknown, but in *Prunus* a positive correlation has been reported between growth vigor and content of chlorogenic and coumaric acids (19).

Cytokinins

Evidence for the existence of cytokinesis-inducing substances, now referred to by the generic term *cytokinins,* first came from tissue culture studies. A very active fraction was isolated from commercial DNA preparations and was found to be 6-furfurylamino-purine. This compound, known as "kinetin," has been extensively used in experimental work. Many plant tissues respond to it by increased cell division and otherwise, though it has never been found to occur naturally. Hundreds of other biologically active synthetic cytokinins also are known. The most effective are N^6-substituted adenine derivatives (60, 67).

The first naturally occurring cytokinin to be isolated and identified was extracted from immature corn *(Zea)* kernels and was named zeatin (34). This compound, as well as other naturally occurring cytokinins found since, is a purine derivative. Zeatin and related natural cytokinins will promote the division of a variety of plant cells in culture, but their natural function may be more complex.

In general, cytokinins seem to promote cell division, enhance DNA synthesis, stimulate bud development, promote germination of some seeds, and counteract the senescence of isolated plant parts such as leaves. In many callus culture systems, the growth rate is determined by the ratio of cytokinins, auxins, and gibberellins.

We have little information on where and how naturally occurring cytokinins are synthesized within the plant, how they are translocated, or what their primary mode of action is in the cells where they exert their effects. The situation has been confused by the discovery of cytokinins in the transfer RNAs of many organisms. It is possible though that this role is unrelated to that of cytokinins as plant hormones (67).

It should be noted that cytokinins are not related to the polypeptide hormones known as bradykinins that are found in many animal fluids.

Gibberellins

Rice plants having "bakanae" disease are easily distinguishable from normal plants because they grow tall and spindly. The disease is caused by a fungus now called *Fusarium moniliforme*, but earlier called *Gibberella fujikuroi*. In 1926, E. Kurosawa succeeded in inducing tall growth in healthy rice plants by treating them with only the culture medium filtrate of the fungus. After much effort T. Yabuta and Y. Sumiki isolated several biologically active crystalline compounds from such culture media in 1938. They named these substances *gibberellins*, after the then current generic name of the fungus. This research was originally published only in Japanese and remained quite unknown in the West until the 1950s. Since then, a tremendous amount of research has revealed that gibberellin-type hormonal substances occur naturally in higher plants as well as in fungi. Almost 50 molecular species of gibberellins are now known. All are diterpenoid acids based on skeletons, including either 19 or 20 carbon atoms, and they are divided into two groups on that basis. The best known gibberellin is the C_{19} gibberellic acid, commonly known as GA_3. Gibberellic acid has long been commercially available; consequently its effects upon a great variety of plants have been studied under laboratory, greenhouse, and field conditions.

One of the most spectacular effects of the application of hormonal amounts of GA_3 and its close relatives is the induction of normal growth in otherwise dwarf varieties of plants. A related response is the conversion of rosette plants to tall forms by gibberellin treatment. Apparently,

these effects are due to gibberellin-induced promotion of cell division and elongation in the subapical meristem region of the shoot.

Present indications are that a single higher plant species may contain several or many types of gibberellins, some free and some in "bound" forms. This complement may vary with the organ examined and with the developmental stage. It also seems likely that root gibberellins may be different from shoot gibberellins or that root gibberellins may be converted into other types in the shoot. Additionally, there is the possibility that of the various gibberellins, some may be especially effective in promoting specific types of meristematic activity rather than others. All this, however, is still speculative. Unfortunately, the trend has been for research to generate more detail to be explained rather than contributing to general principles by which existing information about gibberellins and plant growth can be organized and understood (29, 67).

Abscisins

The discovery of the growth-regulating substance now known by the trivial name *abscisin* was the result of two separate lines of work. Osborne (46) provided the first good evidence of the existence in plants of diffusible substances that seemed to promote abscission of leaves and fruits. One such substance was eventually isolated from cotton fruits and was chemically characterized (45) under the designation of "abscisin II." About the same time, another group of workers who were studying dormancy in woody plants isolated a growth inhibitor and dormancy-inducing substance from maple leaves (12). They initially called this material "dormin," but it soon became obvious that dormin and abscisin II were chemically identical (13). This compound is now known as abscisic acid (ABA). It is a complex derivative of pentadienoic acid and has been chemically synthesized.

Abscisic acid is probably involved in control of seed germination, and may be identical with the inhibitors that can be leached out with water and which, when added back, will again inhibit germination. This same regulator is probably also involved with abscission of leaves and fruit and with senescence and dehiscence of some mature fruit (14). The most striking aspect of abscisic acid physiology, however, is its great and rapid increase in plants under water stress. This increase may be as much as 40-fold in 4 hr in wilted leaves (71), and only moderate stress is necessary to induce a marked increase in ABA. The increased ABA level somehow results in rapid closure of the stomates. Longer term effects may be general growth inhibition and leaf abscission. ABA can also in some situations reverse the effects of other growth regulators so that the balance of the various agents present is more significant than the absolute levels.

Ethylene

It can be argued that *ethylene* is not a hormone because it moves through tissue by diffusion rather than by a physiologically directed transport. In addition, it seems likely that in natural systems it has its greatest effects in the cells that produce it. Its questionable status as a hormone, however, does not detract from ethylene's ability to serve as an integrating regulator, once its synthesis is triggered. The possibility of such regulation by exogenous ethylene has long been recognized, but appreciation of the widespread involvement of endogenous ethylene in regulation of plant growth and development is recent.

Although details are not known, it is likely that ethylene is synthesized indirectly from methionine in a variety of plant tissues. Protein degradation in senescent tissues may lead to available methionine and hence may favor the increased ethylene synthesis that usually accompanies senescence (67). A similar explanation could be invoked to account for great increases in ethylene production by wounded tissues. Satisfactory explanations of why auxin treatment also enhances ethylene production and why the latter is almost an indicator of free auxin in some tissues are more difficult to construct (1).

The effects of ethylene on a great variety of growth and development processes have been described. These include promotion of abscission, retardation of elongation growth, induction of flowering, induction and acceleration of ripening, and counteraction of apical dominance. It seems that many responses to exogenous ethylene treatment, along with those to ABA, favor senescence. Hence, they tend to counter, in a general way, responses to auxins, gibberellins, and cytokinins. Half-maximal responses to ethylene are typically obtained at 0.1 ppm and saturation responses at 10 ppm (1). The ethylene receptor and the primary response to ethylene are not yet known. Nevertheless, the variety of rapid and measurable responses, the ease of plant treatment, and the lack of severe

toxic effects seems to offer a rich field for further study.

Phytochrome

During the early decades of this century, various plant species were studied with respect to the effects of differences in length of the daily photoperiod upon growth and flowering. The work of Garner and Allard (for summary, see Allard and Garner (2)) was especially important in establishing the principles of plant photoperiodism. These scientists, and others following them, learned that many plants can detect and respond to even small changes in the photoperiod, and that different species often respond in different ways. They also learned that the growth and flowering responses of many plants can be greatly altered by extending the natural photoperiod with artificial illumination of low intensity—and that different regions of the spectrum are not equally effective. It seemed quite clear that these light effects were not based on chlorophyll and photosynthesis, but upon some types of photomorphogenic receptor pigment. The results of these studies, along with evidence of the promotion of seed germination by red light and its inhibition by far-red light, led plant physiologists to begin searching for a photomorphogenic receptor pigment. By 1960, the existence of such a pigment was well confirmed (7, 26). It was named phytochrome.

Phytochrome is a blue-green protein present in very small amounts in many, perhaps all, higher plants. It exists in two interconvertible forms. The red-absorbing form, P_r, absorbs radiant energy maximally at 660 nm and by that absorption is converted to a far-red-absorbing form, P_{fr}, which is the physiologically active form of phytochrome. This active P_{fr}, however, is unstable and is susceptible to three types of depletion. Absorption of far-red radiation with a maximum at 730 nm converts it back to the stable, but inactive P_r; P_{fr} also spontaneously reverts back to P_r in the dark with a half-life of some minutes to several hours in various systems, and under most conditions it will also undergo slow, irreversible degradation into fragments of no further photochemical competence.

The reversion of P_{fr} to P_r in the dark was formerly looked upon to explain the timekeeping aspect of photoperiodism. This view, seemingly incompatible with some experimental data, is now regarded as inadequate. Instead, endogenous rhythms or "biological clocks" are invoked to explain the timekeeping. Whereas the reactions of phytochrome may indeed serve to entrain endogenous rhythms to cyclical light conditions, we can only speculate as to the nature of such interactions.

Because phytochrome can exist in two interconvertible forms of known spectral and biochemical properties, it can be detected in some living tissues by differential spectrophotometry. It has also been detected and localized by immunochemical techniques. As might be expected on the basis of its involvement in control of growth and development, the highest phytochrome levels are found in or near meristematic regions. It is, however, widely distributed in more mature plant parts also (61).

Phytochrome, strictly speaking, is not a hormone, and also not an enzyme in the usual sense, but it is probably the central component of a complex photomorphogenic control system. The range of observed responses to red versus far-red light treatments or to photoperiodic conditions is so vast that the question of *one* primary mode of action of phytochrome seems naive. There are two major hypotheses concerning the general mode of action. One is that the differing amounts of P_r and P_{fr} can lead to differential gene responses (38) or to enzyme induction or repression (39). The other is that P_{fr} alters the permeability of certain cell membranes, thus leading to differential physiological responses (27, 37). Superficially, it seems that most rapid responses (seconds) could be due to membrane effects, whereas growth and development responses (days or weeks) might also involve gene activation (51, 58). Real understanding, of course, is still distant.

Dormancy and Environmental Factors

The annual rhythm of growth and development of most higher plants is often thought of as a period of growth alternating with a period of dormancy. This seems obvious when we consider the winter-to-spring changes in field and forest. The actual physiological situation is much more complex. Whereas "dormancy" in the broad sense means a temporary suspension of visible growth, an accurate and complete technical definition of the concept is hard to achieve. As is especially true of trees, a state of dormancy need not apply to all meristems at the same time. Several types or levels of dormancy may prevail, even within the organs of a single twig at the same time. For example, the shoot apical meristems of a tree may be relatively inactive during the period of most rapid shoot elongation in spring. At the same time, the subapical meristem is highly active in producing new internodal cells, and cell growth by elongation is also pronounced. Likewise, cambial growth may continue into autumn, after shoots seem dormant to superficial inspection. In late summer, when the newly formed buds seem externally dormant and are not elongating, the initiation of new leaf primordia may be continuing rapidly within the buds.

Because of the coexistence of several types of dormancy and restricted growth, specific terms are needed for the various classes of physiological growth inhibition. The unqualified term *dormancy* may be used in all instances in which a tissue disposed to grow in some manner does not do so. *Quiescence* is a type of dormancy imposed by the external environment through unfavorable conditions such as cold or drought. *Correlated inhibition* is a type of physiological dormancy maintained by agents or conditions localized within the plant, but outside the affected organ. *Rest* is similar to correlated inhibition, except that it is maintained by agents or conditions localized within the organs affected themselves. This nomenclature should be regarded as a temporary expedient, for it is not really adequate to cope with the reality of differential growth limitations of various meristems in the same bud at the same time (53).

The complexity of integrated control of growth and dormancy in a large woody plant can only be suggested here by giving a few examples. The branching pattern, hence the shape and the light-intercepting ability of a plant, is greatly influenced by apical dominance—the way in which leading buds impose correlative inhibition upon the growth of positionally inferior buds. This is usually thought to be achieved by auxin-type hormones synthesized in large amounts by leading buds and transported basipetally in amounts that are supraoptimal for the buds below. The onset of various types of dormancy in the summer and fall in "preparation" for winter long before cold weather arrives is indirectly induced by phytochrome-mediated systems that perceive longer nights. The reduction of growth, perhaps to the level of quiescence, in response to summer drought is probably the result of increased ABA synthesis due to water stress. The bolting and flowering of rosette plants in late summer may be controlled by increased gibberellin synthesis which stimulates subapical meristem activity and internodal elongation. The point is that the interaction of the known hormonal control systems, especially from the perspective of our incomplete knowledge of what hormones and regulators even exist, is so complex (69) that no general explanation of dormancy and growth can yet be realistically attempted.

Summary

The organismal growth and development of the higher plant differs fundamentally from that of its animal counterpart in three ways: (a) Its embryonal growth is essentially unlimited, though not necessarily continuous. (b) Its cells are typically ensheathed by walls that are external to the living protoplasts. (c) The organismal body that we recognize as the plant is diploid and seemingly sexual, but actually is asexual and capable of vegetative reproduction. This asexual generation bears hidden within its floral organs an alternate generation of haploid, near microscopic, plants.

The continued embryonal growth of plants means that their meristems continue to generate new cells, which differentiate into new tissues and organs, after other parts of the same plants are mature, senescent, or dead. There are three major types of meristems. A shoot apical meristem is found at the tip of every shoot capable of further growth. It is usually a dome-like mound of a few thousand cells surrounded by primordial leaves or scales. Its meristematic initial cells are superficial or nearly so. A root apical meristem is similarly located at the tip of every root, but it is usually covered by a root cap, and its initial cells are, therefore, deep-seated. The third type of meristem, the vascular cambium, is sheath-like, thin, and extensive. Sandwiched between the bark and the wood, or cortex and stele, it is the source of cells contributing to thickness growth in roots and stems.

Meristems generate new cells and also sustain themselves. The new cells grow to mother cell size and then divide again. This cycle cannot continue indefinitely for all cells. Those that are displaced by even a few cell diameters from the meristematic center tend to differentiate and lose their meristematic function.

Appreciation of the structure and function of cell walls is basic to the comprehension of plant growth processes. Though cell walls are metabolically inactive, they are seldom inert physiologically. Each protoplast is surrounded by a limiting membrane, the plasmalemma, and the cell wall is constructed external to it. The primary wall is thin and extensible. It can grow enormously in area and still retain its near original thickness. During that extension growth phase, a cell may increase 200-fold in volume, primarily by water inflation of vacuoles. However, volume growth ends as the deposition of secondary wall lamellae inside the primary wall reduces extensibility. Thus, weight growth replaces volume growth, and secondary walls eventually make up most of the mass of plants as we know and utilize them.

While cell walls function as major structural elements, their microfibrous nature also allows them to serve as a continuous translocation pathway for water and solutes throughout the plant—thus, the walls constitute an apoplast. The cells walls and plasmalemma membranes do not generally, however, completely separate protoplasts from their neighbors. The walls are perforated by thousands of plasmodesmata. These minute intercellular channels unite most living cells of the organism into a single symplast. At certain stages of development, the plasmodesmatal connections may be broken or plugged, allowing local and isolated differential development. The dynamics of the symplast-apoplast boundary in relation to growth and morphogenesis needs more study.

At least six classes of hormones and regulators are involved in the control of plant growth. These are: auxins, cytokinins, gibberellins, abscisins, ethylene, and phytochrome. These substances may, in part, be only the messengers of other systems that are the more basic controls. Their interactions are many, complex, and confusing. There is a great gap between understanding some of the effects of growth regulators in isolated experimental systems and understanding the integrated growth and development of a whole plant in its natural environment.

Long-lived higher plants are much more likely to grow episodically than continuously. Periods of dormancy often alternate with periods of active growth. Several levels or types of dormancy or activity may exist at the same time in the various meristems of a plant. Phytochrome and ABA are probably involved in the induction of dormancy in response to changing environmental conditions. These same regulators, as well as all the others mentioned above, are also involved in regulation of growth and development in and near active meristems.

The subject of growth in plants is integral with that of morphogenesis and development.

The major blocks to better understanding lie in the areas of control of the plane of orientation of cell division, of the rate of cell division, of primary wall extension, and of deposition of secondary wall materials.

References

1. Abeles, F. B. (1973): Ethylene in plant biology. Academic Press, New York.
2. Allard, H. A., and Garner, W. W. (1940): Further observations on the response of various species of plants to length of day. U. S. Dept. of Agric. Tech. Bull. 727.
3. Arisz, W. H. (1956): Significance of the symplasm theory for transport across the root. Protoplasma, 46:5–62.
4. Bailey, I. W. (1957): Need for broadened outlook in cell wall terminologies. Phytomorphology, 7:136–138.
5. Brown, R. (1976): Significance of division in the higher plant. In Cell Division in Higher Plants, pp. 3–46, edited by M. M. Yeoman. Academic Press, London.
6. Bonner, J., and Varner, J. E. (eds.) (1976): Plant biochemistry, Ed. 3. Academic Press, New York.
7. Butler, W. L., Norris, K. H., Siegelman, H. W., and Hendricks, S. B. (1959): Detection, assay, and preliminary purification of the pigment controlling photoresponsive development of plants. Proc Natl. Acad. Sci. U. S., 45:1703–1708.
8. Clowes, F. A. L. (1961): Apical meristems. Botany Monograph 2. Blackwell, Oxford.
9. Clowes, F. A. L. (1976): The root apex. Cell Division in Higher Plants, pp. 253–284, M. M. Yeoman. Academic Press, London.
10. Clowes, F. A. L., and Juniper, B. E. (1968): Plant Cells. Blackwell, Oxford.
11. Cook, G. M. W., and Stoddart, R. W. (1973): Surface carbohydrates of the eukaryotic cell. Academic Press, London.
12. Cornforth, J. W., Milborrow, B. V., Ryback, G., and Wareing, P. F. (1965a): Chemistry and physiology of "dormins" in sycamore. Nature, 205:1269–1270.
13. Cornforth, J. W., Milborrow, B. V., and Ryback, G. (1965b): Synthesis of (±)-abscisin II. Nature, 206:715.
14. Davis, L. A., and Addicott, F. T. (1972): Abscisic acid; correlations with abscission and with development in the cotton fruit. Plant Physiol., 49: 644–648.
15. Dermen, H. (1969): Directional cell division in shoot apices. Cytologia, 34:541–558.
16. Diboll, A. G., and Larson, D. A. (1966): An electron microscopic study of the mature megagametophyte of Zea mays. Am. J. Bot., 53:391–402.
17. Dyer, A. F. (1976): The visible events of mitotic cell division. Cell Division in Higher Plants, pp. 49–110, edited by M. M. Yeoman. Academic Press, London.
18. Esau, K. (1977): Anatomy of seed plants, Ed. 2. Wiley, New York.
19. Feucht, W., and Nachit, M. (1976): Phenole und Indolderivate als Selektionsmerkmale für die Wüchsigkeit von Prunus-Gehölzen. Z. Pflanzenphysiol., 78:387–395.
20. Foster, A. S. (1938): Structure and growth of the shoot apex in Ginkgo biloba. Bull. Torrey Bot. Club, 65:531–556.
21. Frey-Wyssling, A. (1959): Die pflanzliche Zellwand. Springer-Verlag, Berlin.
22. Greenwood, M. S., Shaw, S., Hillman, J. R., Ritchie, A., and Wilkins, M. B. (1972): Indentification of auxin from Zea coleoptile tips by mass spectrometry. Planta, 108:179–183.
23. Gunning, B. E. S., and Robards, A. W. (eds.) (1976): Intercellular communication in plants; studies on plasmodesmata. Springer-Verlag, Berlin.
24. Guttenberg, H. von (1960): Grundzüge der Histogenese höherer Pflanzen. I. Die Angiospermen. In Handbuch der Pflanzenanatomie, Ed. 2, 3 Teil., Bd. VIII. Borntraeger, Berlin-Nikolassee.
25. Halperin, W., and Wetherell, D. F. (1965): Ontogeny of adventive embryos of wild carrot. Science, 147:756–758.
26. Hendricks, S. B., and Borthwick, H. A. (1959): Photocontrol of plant development by the simultaneous excitation of two interconvertible pigments. Proc. Natl. Acad. Sci. U. S., 45:344–349.
27. Hendricks, S. B., and Borthwick, H. A. (1967): The function of phytochrome in regulation of plant growth. Proc. Natl. Acad. Sci. U. S., 58: 2125–2130.
28. Heslop-Harrison, J. (1972): Sexuality of angiosperms. In Plant Physiology, a Treatise, Vol. 6, pp. 133–289. Academic Press, New York.
29. Jones, R. L. (1973): Gibberellins; their physiological role. Annu. Rev. Plant Physiol., 24:571–598.
30. Kögl, F., Haagen-Smit, A. J., and Erxleben, H. (1934): Über ein neues Auxin ("Heteroauxin") aus Harn. 11. Mitteilung über pflanzliche Wachstumsstoffe. Z. Physiol. Chem., 228:90–103.
31. Kremers, R. E. (1963): The chemistry of developing wood. In The Chemistry of Wood, pp. 369–404, edited by B. L. Browning. Interscience, New York.
32. Laüchli, A. (1976): Apoplasmic transport in tissues. In Encyclopedia of Plant Physiology, New Series, 2B, pp. 1–34, edited by U. Lüttge and M. G. Pittman.
33. Leopold, A. C., and Kriedemann, P. E. (1975): Plant growth and development. Ed. 2. McGraw-Hill, New York.
34. Letham, D. S., and Miller, C. O. (1965): Identity of kinetin-like factors from Zea mays. Plant Cell Physiol., 6:355–359.
35. Lyndon, R. F. (1973): The cell cycle in the shoot apex. In The Cell Cycle in Development and Differentiation, British Society for the Development of Biology Symposium, Cambridge Univ. Press.
36. Mahmood, A. (1968): Cell grouping and primary wall generations in the cambial zone, xylem, and phloem in Pinus. Aust. J. Bot., 16:177–195.
37. Marmé, D. (1977): Phytochrome; membranes as possible sites of primary action. Annu. Rev. Plant Physiol., 28:173–198.
38. Mohr, H. (1966): Differential gene activation as a mode of action of phytochrome 730. Photochem. Photobiol., 5:469–483.
39. Mohr, H. (1972): Lectures on photomorphogenesis. Springer-Verlag, New York.
40. Münch, E. (1930): Die Stoffbewegungen in der Pflanze. G. Fischer, Jena.
41. Murashige, T. (1974): Plant propagation through tissue cultures. Annu. Rev. Plant Physiol., 25:135–166.
42. Murmanis, L. (1970): Locating the initial in the vascular cambium of Pinus strobus L. by electron microscopy. Wood Sci. Tech., 4:1–14.
43. Nägeli, C. (K.). (1864): Dickenwachsthum des Stengels und Anordnung der Gefässstränge bei den Sapindaceen (Monograph.) München.
44. Norstog, K. (1972): Early development of the barley embryo; fine structure. Am. J. Bot., 59:123–132.
45. Ohkuma, K., Lyon, J. L., Addicott, F. T., and Smith, O. E. (1963): Abscisin II, an abscission-accelerating substance from young cotton fruit. Science, 142:1592–1593.
46. Osborne, D. J. (1955): Acceleration of abscission by a factor produced in senescent leaves. Nature, 176:1161–1163.
47. Philipson, W. R., Ward, J. M., and Butterfield, B. G. (1971): The vascular cambium; its development and activity. Chapman & Hall, London.
48. Pickett-Heaps, J. D. (1974): Plant microtubules. In Dynamic Aspects of Plant Ultrastructure, pp. 219–255, edited by A. W. Robards. McGraw-Hill, London.
49. Pope, D., and Black, M. (1972): The effect of indole-3-acetic acid on coleoptile extension growth in the absence of protein synthesis. Planta, 102:26–36.
50. Preston, R. D. (1974): The physical biology of plant cell walls. Chapman & Hall, London.
51. Quail, P. H. (1976): Phytochrome. In Plant Biochemistry, Ed. 3, pp. 683–711, edited by J. Bonner and J. E. Varner. Academic Press, New York.
52. Rodkiewicz, B. (1970): Callose in cell walls during megasporogenesis in angiosperms. Planta, 93:39–47.
53. Romberger, J. A. (1963): Meristems, growth, and development in woody plants. U. S. Dept. of Agric. Tech. Bull. 1293.
54. Romberger, J. A. (1976): An appraisal of prospects for research on juvenility in woody perennials. Acta Horticulturae, 56:301–317.
55. Romberger, J. A., and Gregory, R. A. (1977): The shoot apical ontogeny of the Picea abies seedling. III. Some age-related aspects of morphogenesis. Am. J. Bot., 64:624–632.
56. Schmidt, A. (1924): Histologische Studien an phanerogamen Vegetationspunkten. Bot. Arch., 8:345–404.
57. Schneider, E. A., and Wightman, F. (1974): Metabolism of auxin in higher plants. Annu. Rev. Plant Physiol., 25:487–513.
58. Schopfer, P. (1977): Phytochrome control of enzymes. Annu. Rev. Plant Physiol., 28:223–252.
59. Schüepp, O. (1926): Meristeme. In Handbuch der Pflanzenanatomie, Ed. 1. 1 Abt., 2 Teil, Bd. IV., Borntraeger, Berlin.
60. Skoog, F., and Schmitz, R. Y. (1972): Cytokinins. In Plant Physiology, A Treatise, Vol. 6, pp. 181–213. Academic Press, New York.
61. Smith, H. (1975): Phytochrome and photomorphogenesis; an introduction to the photocontrol of plant development. McGraw-Hill, London.
62. Spanswick, R. M. (1972): Electrical coupling between cells of higher plants; a direct demonstration of intercellular communication. Planta, 102:215–227.
63. Spanswick, R. M. (1976): Symplasmic transport in tissues. In Encyclopedia of Plant Physiology, New Series, 2B, pp. 35–53.
64. Steward, F. C., Mapes, M. O., Kent, A. E., and Holsten, R. D. (1964): Growth and development of cultured plant cells. Science, 143:20–27.
65. Stewart, N. N., Semeniuk, P., and Dermen, H. (1974): Competition and accommodation between apical layers and their derivatives in the ontogeny of chimeral shoots of Pelargonium x hortorum. Am. J. Bot., 61: 54–67.
66. Tangl, E. (1879); Ueber offene Communicationen zwischen den Zellen des Endosperms einiger Samen. Jahrb. wiss. Bot., 12:170–190.
67. Varner, J. E., and Ho, D. T.-H. (1976): Hormones. In Plant Biochemistry, Ed. 3, pp. 713–770, edited by J. Bonner and J. E. Varner. Academic Press, New York.

68. Wardrop, A. B. (1964): The structure and formation of the cell wall in xylem. In *The Formation of Wood in Forest Trees*, pp. 87–134, edited by M. H. Zimmermann. Academic Press, New York.

69. Wareing, P. F., and Saunders, P. F. (1971): Hormones and dormancy. *Annu. Rev. Plant Physiol.*, 22:261–288.

70. Went, F. W. (1928): Wuchsstoff und Wachstum. *Rec. Trav. Bot. Néerland.*, 25:1–116.

71. Wright, S. T. C., and Hiron, R. W. P. (1969): (+)-Abscisic acid, the growth inhibitor induced in detached wheat leaves by a period of wilting. *Nature*, 224:719–720.

72. Yeoman, M. M., and Aitchison, P. A. (1976): Molecular events of the cell cycle; a preparation for division. In *Cell Division in Higher Plants*, pp. 111–113, edited by M. M. Yeoman. Academic Press, London.

73. Yeoman, M. M., and Brown, R. (1971): Effects of mechanical stress on the plane of cell division in developing callus cultures. *Ann. Bot.*, 35: 1101–1112.

10

Selected Aspects of Human Development

Hans E. Kaiser

It is the author's desire to draw conclusions and make connections from the findings in the earlier chapters dealing with the developmental peculiarities of invertebrates, vertebrates, and mainly vascular plants in order to bring into line the comparative aspects of the ontogeny of these various organisms, characterized by true tissues, with development in man. This is particularly necessary because human neoplasms are the best established basis for a diagnostic platform of neoplasms in all organisms including plants. In Chapter 43 the bridge has been established to tumors in plants since these are the second single group of major importance for this question. The main growth processes take place during ontogeny, which varies so much in the different organisms.

To understand the basic problem of neoplasms fully, it is unavoidable to study several organisms and combine the gained knowledge from all of them. This becomes clear if it is realized that no knowledge about different chemical pathways in various organisms could have been investigated, or even detected, as described in Chapters 17, 18, and 19. It is similar with chronobiologic rhythms or the susceptibility to neoplastic transformation. It is often asked if cancer is hereditary, or if cancer is contagenous. The susceptibility of neoplastic transformation has a genetic background, as shown in those organisms such as the fish, *Xiphophorus*, in which it can be studied with meaningful contrast to the human situation (Chapter 29).

It is known from the most familiar plant tumor, the crown gall disease, that this tumor is caused by bacteria as described in Chapters 49 to 52. The relationship of genetics and viruses to different species has been pointed out, particularly in Chapters 23 and 27. The incorporation

of bacterial nucleic acids into the crown gall cell has been described in Chapter 52. These few examples explain the necessity of comparing selected aspects of human development with the ontogeny of other organisms.

1. The development of man is, in general, continuous. It leads from the zygote to the adult organism. The placenta as an accessory organ and its removal after giving birth cannot be considered as a typical indirect process of development. This is also proven by the fact that with certain chemical carcinogens the mother may transmit them via the placenta to the young, as is well known from urethane. Remaining and resting cell nests with masked embryonal and/or malignant potential are able to stay during adulthood.

2. A catastrophic development in man's ontogeny does not appear. No normal autolysis takes place.

3. Normal autolysis is missing in structures of man, as it occurs during detours of ontogeny in such forms as holometabolic insects in which whole gill systems may be replaced by tracheid systems and chemical hemoglobins by direct diffusion respiration via the tracheids.

4. The cessation of embryonal potential generally takes place in early life. In man, embryonal connective tissue is perhaps the tissue with the highest, most pronounced embryonal potential, whereas the embryonal potential in other tissues sooner or later ceases. The renewal during hematopoiesis, for example, cannot be compared because it is very limited in scope. There exists a direct difference in regard to the meristematic tissues in plants. Comparatively, three types of cessation of embryonal potential can be distinguished: (a) as early cessation in the vertebrate as in man; (b) the continued existence

of tissues with embryonal potential during a large part of ontogeny, as in the case of specific larval tissues in crustaceans and holometabolic insects; and (c) the retention of tissues with embryonal potential during the whole life-span, as in the event of the meristems in vascular plants.

5. Regeneration exhibits a very low degree in the body of man, with the exception of the liver, in contrast with such animals as annelids, echinoderms, and others in which regeneration of many parts occurs.

6. Cell invariability in comparison to such forms as many parasites, tardigrada, rotifera, etc., is very restricted in man, present only in the neurons of the nervous system and perhaps in the cardiac musculature. It is in contrast also to the permanent, nonliving, tissues in plants.

7. The same tissues or tissue types do not always have a similar potential of developing succeeding tissues in different taxonomic groups. The potential of mesenchyme, e.g., varies in coelenterates, acoelomates, articulates, and vertebrates.

8. Man's circulatory system is closed in type. It contains floating cells and corpuscles. A residue of the still open circulatory system can be observed in the circulatory sinuses of the spleen. Typical for mammals (crocodiles and birds) is the development of lymph nodes, very important in relation to metastatic spreading. The distribution and development of varying types of systems of body fluids in other organisms is able to broaden our knowledge and understanding of metastatic distribution of cells, especially if conditions of circulatory systems not present in man are investigated.

9. The highest correlation of the brain is characterized by its high diversification and its special condition of cell invariability. It brings interesting parallels with plants. These cell invariable tissues in the mammal or the nonliving tissues, such as sclerenchymas in vascular plants stand phylogenetically, ontogenetically, topographically, and functionally on a totally different level, but all are characterized by the fact that the precursors of these cells can, at least theoretically, transform into neoplastic cells.

These points, in a comparative sense of embryology, are given here to illustrate human development and to show man's particular ontogenetic stand among the organisms.

11

Toward a Molecular Chrono-oncology: Circadian Rhythms in RNA Polymerase Activities of Rat Liver[1]

Thomas Spelsberg and Franz Halberg

INTRODUCTION

A sequence of rhythmic metabolic and molecular events has been documented for the growing or regenerating liver of rodents (23, 25, 26). The sequence may be considered to start with a circadian bioperiodicity of phosphorus metabolism (29, 42) reflected in isotopic labeling of phospholipids (25, 51) and RNA (3, 4, 23). This in turn is followed on the energetic path by a peak in glycogen content and on the proliferative path by bioperiodic DNA synthesis (3, 10, 11, 18, 23; see also Chapter 15) and finally mitosis (18, 23, 40, 48). Complementing this background information of the 1950s and 1960s are more recent results, including work originally aimed at other problems (31). Glasser and Spelsberg in 1972 (15) described a circadian rhythm in the activities of two RNA polymerases: one (RNA polymerase I) synthesizes nucleolar (ribosomal) RNA, the other (RNA polymerase II) synthesizes nucleoplasmic (DNA-like) RNA, i.e., an RNA with a high content of adenine and uridine. Data previously presented macroscopically as time plots of enzyme activity are analyzed by the cosinor technique herein, with the aim of relating the information from our laboratories to data from other laboratories, covering in a broader context chronobiologic information on a mammalian cell cycle (23) and its complementary proliferative and energetic bioperiodic subsystems.

MATERIALS AND METHODS

Male Charles River rats, 8 weeks of age, were housed (6 per cage) in a room maintained at 22°C and 40% relative humidity, with light and darkness alternating at 12-hr intervals. Food and water were freely available at all times. After 3 weeks of standardization under these conditions, subgroups of four rats were killed at 1-hr intervals throughout a 24-hr span. Livers were removed, nuclei were isolated, and RNA polymerase activities were analyzed according to Glasser and Spelsberg (15), as verified by Glasser et al. (14). Data were placed on punch cards and analyzed by the single cosinor technique (27).

RESULTS AND DISCUSSION

Circadian Rhythms in RNA Polymerase Activities

Figure 11.1 shows, along with plots of data on the two RNA polymerases, the results of cosinor

[1] Supported by grants from U.S. Public Health Service 5-K6-GM-13981-16, National Cancer Institute (1RO1-CA-14445-05), National Institute of Aging (AG-00158), National Institute of Occupational Safety and Health (OH-00631), Environmental Protection Agency (R804512-01-0), and the Mayo Foundation.

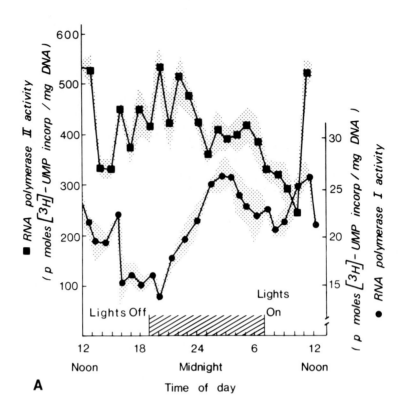

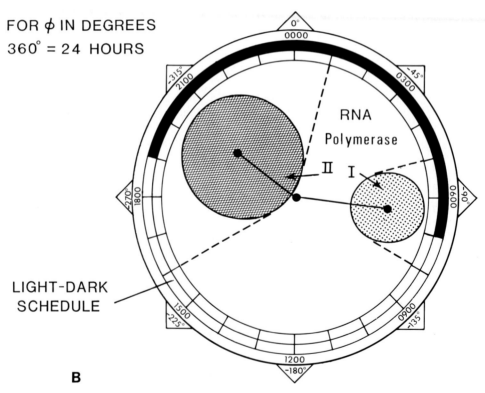

Figure 11.1. Sequence of events in hormone action on cell function and replication. *A* shows original data, *B* shows a cosinor summary, and *C* provides the context of the events as background to the finding of this summary of but one aspect of a broad molecular chronobiology.

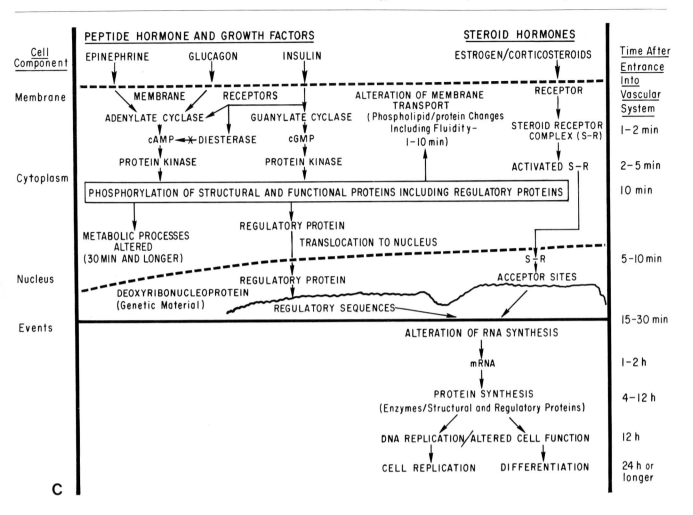

analyses, revealing 95% confidence regions that do not overlap the center of the plot, the so-called pole. This finding attests to the statistical significance of the circadian rhythms in these enzymes involved in RNA synthesis.

The timing of the rhythms in the two polymerases is different. This can be seen from the directed lines (vectors) pointing in different directions. Different point estimates of the acrophase (a measure of timing of peak enzyme activity) are associated with different interval estimates of the acrophases, each interval being delineated by an arc between radii drawn tangent to the 95% confidence regions shown around the tip of each vector. These arcs do not overlap one another, indicating that the difference in acrophases is statistically significant.

Etiology of the Rhythms in Polymerase Activities

In the absence of information on the rate-limiting factor(s) of transcription, circadian changes in the relative specific activity of RNA, presumably indicating a rhythm in RNA metabolism, may reflect circadian rhythms in (a) precursor labeling; and/or in (b) RNA polymerase activities; and/or in (c) rate of RNA degradation; and/or in (d) DNA template capacity of the chromatin (for RNA synthesis).

A circadian rhythm in isotopic labeling of RNA in mouse liver chromatin, possibly reflecting a rhythm in chromatin template activity, has been reported (49), and its behavior will have to be examined in the context of rhythms in RNA polymerase activities in rat liver (15)—perhaps by metarhythmometry. The latter is the study of rhythms before, during, and after manipulation of synchronizers, in an attempt to separate underlying mechanisms by their rates of travel, i.e., their adjustment times (21, 22, 24, 28).

The timing of high values in rat liver nucleoplasmic RNA polymerase II activity (presumably synthesizing messenger RNAs coding for proteins) also resembles that observed for the relative specific activity of RNA in mouse liver (3, 4) as well as the activities of several enzymes in the rat liver (5, 7, 9, 46, 47). Related to these studies are those of Letnansky (36), who demonstrated that the phosphorylation of the rat liver histone and nonhistone chromatin proteins follows a circadian rhythm. These chromosomal proteins are postulated to be involved in regulation of gene expression in the eucaryote chromatin and thus in chromatin template activities as well as in the transport of RNA from the cell nucleus to the cytoplasm. The different histone classes also exhibited enhanced phosphorylation at specific times along the 24-hr scale. All of the nuclear proteins undergo a complicated phosphorylation-dephosphorylation process during regulation of replication, transcription, and RNA transport. This process may represent the basis of circadian rhythms in RNA labeling (chromatin template capacity?) and RNA polymerase activities.

The exact factor(s) underlying these rhythms in RNA polymerase and/or chromatin template activities are unknown. Motor activity, food ingestion, or endogenous rhythmic biological webs acting through hormonal mediators may synchronize, modulate, or influence these rhythms. An intrinsic factor is supported by the persistence in continuous light of the labeling rhythms in hepatic phospholipids, RNA, and DNA (19). Interestingly, the acrophase of RNA polymerase II activity differs from that of RNA polymerase I with statistical significance, since the 95% confidence arcs do not overlap (Fig. 11.1). Any one factor could hardly account directly for the different timing of the two polymerase rhythms described here. The biological advantage of such rhythms is likely to be integrative within the organ, as it undergoes a division of labor in both space and time. Most certainly, similar rhythms exist in other organs of the rat and other animals.

Steroids and Other Hormones as Intrinsic Factors

Twenty years ago, certain studies involving labeling of RNA, DNA, and phospholipids demonstrated circadian rhythms in these processes (3, 4, 20, 23, 29). Today, the role of steroid and peptide hormones in biological rhythms is widely accepted (for review, see Hedlund et al. (30)). Indeed, steroid hormones are known to induce mitotic activity and cytodifferentiation during organogenesis and secondary organ development (8, 13, 34, 39, 43, 45). When steroids enter target cells, they interact with steroid receptor proteins in the cytoplasm. Two major responses occur. First, there is a rapid effect on membrane transport including histamine release (50) which does not appear to require transcriptional alterations. This is followed by alterations in RNA and protein synthesis (16, 34, 44, 45). Thus, rhythms in the amount of hormones or at some level in their mechanism of action could explain many other biological rhythms, especially membrane and transcriptional alterations. Rhythms in the amounts of estrogen receptors have been identified in a variety of mammalian organs (26, 32).

Relationship of Rhythms in Hepatic Transcription to Rhythms in DNA Replication and the Cell Cycle

Circadian rhythms in liver have been described for DNA synthesis (2, 23), RNA labeling (3, 4), the mitotic index (33), changes in the endoplasmic reticulum (6), and the activities of a number of enzymes (5, 7, 9, 41, 46, 47). Much earlier, mitotic rhythms in many tissues had been thoroughly documented to exhibit periods around 24 hr. Based on preliminary evidence, the role of adrenal corticosteroids as potential systemic regulators of mitosis was considered (3, 4, 17, 23, 29).

By the end of the 1950s, a combination of classical histology, radioactive tracer methods, and wet chemistry had led to the documentation of a circadian cell cycle in mouse liver. This entity summarized contributions from a small dividing subpopulation and a much larger nondividing one in the same organ. Nonetheless, one obtained a first temporal map of processes leading to energy storage and release, such as glycogen deposition and a sequence of phenomena related to phospholipid, RNA, DNA, and mitosis.

Early chronobiologic evaluations by Halberg et al. (29) and Barnum et al. (3, 4) suggested a sequence of phospholipid and RNA synthesis preceding DNA replication and mitosis. Today, this sequence, at least from RNA on, is known to exist. Figure 11.1C outlines the sequence. Briefly, DNA replication is, of course, required for mitosis. RNA synthesis, however, is required both as a primer RNA and as messenger RNA coding for protein factors required to initiate DNA synthesis (1, 35, 37). In addition, RNA synthesis is required to synthesize proteins involved not only as structural components but also as enzymes which synthesize other components for cell structure (e.g., phospholipids for membranes, etc.). Thus, studies of biological rhythms complement those of biochemical pathways in elucidating the events required for DNA synthesis and cell division. It is of great interest to focus upon such a sequence since it is known that circadian cycles can, in the organism as a whole, influence the function of an organ (such as liver) and can predict the outcome of the administration of agents such as proliferation-advancing hormones or oncostatic drugs (*cf.* Chapter 15) (22, 25, 38) among others (12).

SUMMARY

The activities of the RNA polymerases in Charles River rat liver have been documented to exhibit circadian rhythmicity by the fit of a 24-hr cosine curve and rejection of the zero-amplitude assumption. The timing of rhythms in two polymerases (I, for ribosomal RNA synthesis in the nucleolus, and II, for DNA-like RNA synthesis in the nucleoplasm) differs. In particular there is a statistically significant difference in the timing of the two rhythms, quite apart from differences in amplitude. The 95% confidence interval for the polymerase I acrophase extends clockwise from $-74°$ to $-119°$, whereas that for polymerase II extends from $-237°$ to $-15°$ (or $375°$), with $360° = 24$ hr, midnight as acrophase reference and darkness from 19^{00} ($-285°$) to 07^{00} ($-105°$). RNA polymerase I and II activities in rat liver tend to be higher during the animal's habitual activity span (the daily dark span) than during the habitual rest span. The relationship of these events with other processes in the hepatic cell is discussed.

References

1. Adams, R. L. P., Burdon, R. ., Campbell, A. M., and Smellie, R. M. S. (1976): *The Biochemistry of Nucleic Acids.* Academic Pres, New York.
2. Barbiroli, B., and Potter, V. R. (1971): DNA-synthesis and interaction-between controlled feeding schedules and partial hepatectomy in rats. *Science*, 172:738.
3. Barnum, C. P., Jardetzky, C. D., and Halberg, F. (1957): Nucleic acid synthesis in regenerating liver. *Tex. Rep. Biol. Med.*, 15:134–147.
4. Barnum, C. P., Jardetzky, C. D., and Halberg, F. (1958): Time relations among metabolic and morphologic 24-hour changes in mouse liver. *Am. J. Physiol.*, 195:301–310.
5. Black, I. B., and Axelrod, J. (1970): *Biochemical Action of Hormones*, p. 135, edited by G. Litwack. Academic Press, New York.
6. Chedid, A., Nair, V. (1972): Diurnal rhythm in endoplasmic reticulum of rat-liver electron microscopic study. *Science*, 175:(4018):176.
7. Civen, M., Ulrich, R., Trimmer, B. M. and Brown, C. B. (1967): Circadian rhythms of liver enzymes and their relationship to enzyme induction. *Science*, 157:1563–1564.
8. Clegg, P. C., and Clegg, A. G. (1969): *Hormones, Cells and Organisms.* Stanford University Press, Stanford.
9. Colas, A., Gregonis, D., and Mior, N. (1969): Daily rhythms in hydroxylation of 3-Beta-hydroxyandrost-5-en-17-one by rat liver microsomes. *Endocrinology* 84:165.
10. Echave-Llanos, J. M. (1967): Liver tissue growth factors and circadian rhythms in liver regeneration. In *Control of Cellular Growth in Adult Organisms*, edited by H. Teir and T. Tytomaa. Academic Press, London.
11. Echave-Llanos, J. M., and Nash, R. E. (1970): Mitotic circadian rhythm in a fast-growing and a slow-growing hepatoma: mitotic rhythm in hepatomas. *J. Natl. Cancer Inst.*, 44:581–585.
12. Ehret, C. F., Potter, V. R., and Dobra, K. W. (1975): Chronotypic action of theophyllin and of pentobarbital as circadian zeitgebers in the rat. *Science*, 188:1212–1215.
13. Frieden, E., and Just, J. J. (1970): Hormonal responses in amphibian metamorphosis. In *Biochemical Actions of Hormones*, Vol. 1, pp. 2–57, edited by G. Litwack, Academic Pres, New York.
14. Glasser, S. R., and Spelsberg, R. C. (1972): Early effects of estradiol-17 beta on chromatin and activity of deoxyribonucleic and dependent acid-dependent ribonucleic-acid polymerases (I and II) of rat uterus. *Biochem. J.* 130(4):947–957.
15. Glasser, S. R., and Spelsberg, R. C. (1972): Mammalian RNA polymerases I and II; independent diurnal variations in activity. *Biochem. Biophys. Res. Commun.*, 47:951–958.
16. Gurpide, E. (1977): Biochemical Actions of Progesterone and Progestins. *Ann. N. Y. Acad. Sci.*, 286:1–445.
17. Halberg, F. (1953): Some physiological and clinical aspects of 24-hour periodicity. *Lancet*, 73:20–32.
18. Halberg, F. (1957): Young NH-mice for the study of mitoses in intact liver. *Experientia* (Basel), 13:502–503.
19. Halberg, F., and Barnum, C. P. (1961): Continuous light or darkness and circadian periodic mitosis and metabolism in C and D_8 mice. *Am. J. Physiol.* 201:227–230.
20. Halberg, F., Barnum, C. P., Silber, R. H., and Bittner, J. J. (1958): 24-hour rhythms at several levels of integration in mice on different lighting regimens. *Proc. Soc. Exp. Biol. Med.*, 97:897–900.
21. Halberg, F., Cornelissen G., Carandente, F., and Katinas, G. S. (1977a): Glossary of chronobiology. *Chronobiologia*, 4 (Suppl. 1).
22. Halberg, F., Gupta, B. D., Haus, E., Halberg, E., Deka, A. C., Nelson, W., Sothern, R. B., Cornelissen, G., Lee, J. K., Lakatua, D. J., Scheving, L. E., and Burns, E. R. (1977b): Steps toward a cancer chronopolytherapy. In *Proceedings of the 14th International Congress on Therapeutics*, Montpellier, Paris, France, pp. 151–196.
23. Halberg, F., Halberg, E., Barnum, C. P., and Bittner, J. J. (1959): Physiologic 24-hour periodicity in human beings and mice, the lighting regimen and daily routine. In *Photoperiodism and Related Phenomena in Plants and Animals*, Publ. No. 55, pp. 803–878. Edited by R. B. Withrow. Washington, D. C., the American Association for Science.
24. Halberg, F., Halberg, E., and Carandente, F. (1976): Chronobiology and metabolism in the broader context of timely intervention and timed treatment. In *Diabetes Research Today*, Symposia Medica Hoechst 12, pp. 45–95. Edited by E. Lindenlaub. F. K. Schauttauer Verlag, New York.
25. Halberg, F., Haus, E., Cardoso, S. S., Scheving, L. E., Kuhl, J. F. W., Shiotsuka, R., Rosene, G., Pauly, J. E., Runge, W., Spalding, J. F., Lee, J. K., and Good, R. A. (1973): Toward a chronotherapy of neoplasia; tolerance of treatment depends upon host rhythms. *Experientia*, 29:909–934.
26. Halberg, F., Haus, E., and Scheving, L. E. (1978): Sampling of biologic rhythms, chronocytokinetics and experimental oncology. In *Biomathematics and Cell Kinetics*, pp. 175–190, edited by A. J. Valleron and P. D. M. MacDonald. Elsevier-North Holland Press, Amsterdam.
27. Halberg, F., Johnson, E. A., Nelson, W., Runge, W., and Sothern, R. (1972): Autorhythmometry—procedures for physiologic self-measurements and their analysis. *Physiol. Teacher*, 1:1–11.
28. Halberg, F., Reinberg, A., and Reinberg, A. (1977c): Chronobiological serial sections gauge circadian rhythm adjustments following transmeridian flights and life in novel environment. *Waking and Sleeping*, 1:259–279.
29. Halberg, F., Vermund, H., Halberg, E., and Barnum, C. P. (1956): Adrenal hormones and phospholipid metabolism in liver cytoplasm of adrenalectomized mice. *Endocrinology*, 59:364–368.
30. Hedlund, L. W., Franz, J. M., Kenny, A. D. (1973): Biological rhythms and endocrine function. *Adv. Exp. Med. Biol.*, 54:1–194.
31. Hopkins, H. A., Bonney, R. J., Walker, P. R., Yager, J. D., Jr., and Potter, V. R. (1973): Food and light as separate intrainment signals for rat liver enzymes. In *Advances in Enzyme Regulation*, Vol. II, pp. 169–191, edited by G. Weber. Pergamon Pres, New York.
32. Hughes, A., Jacobson, H. I., Wagner, R. K., and Jungblut, P. W. (1976): Ovarian-independent fluctuations of estradiol receptor levels in mammalian tissues. *Mol. Cell. Endocrinol.*, 5:379–388.
33. Jaffee, J. J. (1954): Diurnal mitotic periodicity in regenerating rat liver. *Anat. Rec.*, 120:935–954.
34. Jensen, E. V., and De Sombre, E. R. (1972): Mechanism of action of female sex hormones. *Annu. Rev. Biochem.*, 41:203–230.
35. Kornberg, A. (1974): *DNA Synthesis.* W. H. Freeman, San Francisco.
36. Letnansky, K. (1977): Chronobiology of gene activation. *Chronobiologia*, 3:129.
37. Lewin, B. (1974): In *Gene Expression-2, Eucaryotic Chromosomes.* John Wiley & Sons, New York.
38. Litman, R., Halberg, F., Ellis, S., and Bittner, J. J. (1958): Pituitary growth hormone and mitoses in immature mouse liver. *Endocrinology*, 62:361–364.

39. Lobue, J., and Gordon, A. S. (1973): *Humoral Control of Growth and Differentiation,* Academic Press, New York.

40. Mitchison, J. M. (1971): *The Biology of the Cell Cycle,* Cambridge, University Press, Cambridge, England.

41. Nechaev, A., Halberg, F., Mittelman, A., and Tritsch, G. L. (1977): Circannual variation in human erythrocyte adenosine aminohydrolase. *Chronobiologia,* 4:191–198.

42. Nelson, W. (1964): Aspects of circadian periodic changes in phosphorus metabolism in mice. *Am. J. Physiol., 20:* 191–198.

43. O'Malley, B. W., McGuire, W. L., Kohler, P. O., and Korenman, S. G. (1969): Studies on the mechanism of steroid hormone regulation of synthesis of specific proteins. *Recent Prog. Horm. Res.,* 25:105–160.

44. O'Malley, B. W., and Means, A. R. (1974): Female steroid hormones and target cell nuclei. *Science,* 183:610–620.

45. Pasqualini, J. (1976): *Receptors and Mechanisms of Action of Steroid Hormones.* Marcell Dekker, Inc., New York.

46. Radzialowski, F. M., and Bousquet, J. (1968): Daily rhythmic variation in hepatic drug metabolism in rat and mouse. *J. Pharmacol. Exp. Ther.,* 163:229.

47. Rapport, M. I., Feigin, R. D., Burton, J., and Beisel, W. R. (1966): Circadian rhythm for tryptophan pyrolase activity and its circulation substrate. *Science, 153:*1642.

48. Russo, J., and Echave-Llanos, J. M. (1964): 24-hour rhythm in the mitotic activity and in the water and dry matter count of regenerating liver. *Z. Zellforsch.,* 61:824–828.

49. Steinhart, W. L. (1971): Diurnal rhythmicity in template activity of mouse liver chromatin. *Biochim. Biophys. Acta,* 228:301.

50. Szego, C. M. (1976): Steroid-protein binding; from circulating blood to target cell nucleus. *Gynecol. Invest.,* 7:251–279.

51. Vermund, D. H., Halberg, F., Barnum, C. P., Nash, C. W., and Bittner, J. J. (1956): Physiologic 24-hour periodicity and hepatic phospholipid metabolism in relation to the mouse adrenal cortex. *Am. J. Physiol.,* 186:414–418.

52. Walker, P. R., Bonney, R. J., and Potter, V. R. (1974): Diurnal rhythm of hepatic carbohydrate metabolism during development of the rat. *Biochem. J.,* 140:523–529.

Addendum. A rhythm in total and messenger RNA content of human monocytes (about 95% lymphocytes) has been recently documented in blood from cancer patients and clinically healthy subjects (Hrushesky, W., Sanchez, S., Levi, F., Halberg, F., and Kennedy, B. J. "The RNA content of circulating mononuclear cells (MC) demonstrates marked circadian rhythmicity (CR)," *Clinical Research,* 28:349A (1980) and Hrushesky, W., Sanchez, S., Levi, F., Brown, H., Halberg, F., Haus, E., Sothern, R. and Kennedy, B. J. "Total RNA content of cancer patients' mononuclear cells demonstrate marked circadian rhythmicity," *Blood* (in press). These studies represent a follow-up of work by Heitbrock, H. W., Mertelsmann, R., Garbrecht, M. "Circadian rhythm of RNA polymerase B activity in human peripheral blood lymphocytes," *Int. J. Chronobiol.,* 3:255–261 (1976) by Mertelsmann, R., Heitbrock, H. W., Garbrecht, M.: "Circadian variations of -amanitine sensitive RNA-synthesis in normal human lymphocytes." In: *Modern Trends in Human Leukemia II,* edited by R. Neth, R. C. Gallo, K. Manweiler, W. C. Moloney, Lehmanns Verlag, Munich, pp. 106–111 (1977) by Mertelsmann, R., Heitbrock, H. W., Stein, E., Rehpenning, W., Kaupaun, W., Garbrecht, M. "Circadian variation of cyclophosphamide activation and lymphocyte RNA polymerase activity. A rational approach to reduce immunosuppression caused by cytostatic therapy." Proc. of the XII International Conference, of the International Society for Chromobiology, Washington, The Publishing House "Il Ponte," Milano, pp. 419–426, 1977. For further details of rhythms and their cellular mechanisms, consult Chapter 5 in this volume, L. N. Edmunds and F. Halberg: "Circadian Time Structure Underlying *Euglena:* A Model System Amenable to Quantification." An addendum to that chapter refers to a microscopic rhythmometric analysis of data by Karakashian, M. W., Schweiger, H. G., *Proc. Natl. Acad. Sci. U.S.A.,* 73: 3216–3219, 1976, on *Acetabularia mediterranea* studied macroscopically for consumption. These unicells were kept in continuous light of 2800 lux intensity at a stage just prior to cap formation for spans of weeks. Cycloheximide was applied for an 8-hr span. The delay of rhythms was judged by inspection of the original record on the second and third day. The studies carried out with two temperatures 25° and 20°C were analyzed by single-cosinor.

The sensitivity rhythm is clearly described at both temperatures at the 5% level for 25°C data and below the 1% level for the data at 20°C.

The percentage of the total variability accounted for by the single cosine fit to obviously non-sinusoidal data represents 92% and 70, respectively. There also was a lack of overlap in 95% confidence intervals—the most conservative demonstration of a very large difference in phase. The temperature-dependent difference was of 158°.

This work was done to raise the question whether protein synthesis plays a role in circadian rhythmicity. The description of the role of an adrenal corticoid pacemaker in phospholipid (29, 52) and RNA labeling (23) and DNA formation (23) would be compatible with this possibility in mammals. The demonstration of this phenomenon in a single cell is, of course, both elegant and was used to postulate that translation on 80 s-ribosomes may be a critical determination of the intracellular pacemaker, *i.e.,* of the pacemaker found in the cytosol and not (for translation on 70 s-ribosomes) in organelles. This line of thought will have to be aligned with the circadian rhythmicity reported by Rogers, L. H., and Greenbank, G. R., "The intermittent growth of bacterial cultures," *J. Bacteriol.* 19: 181–190 (1929) for *E. coli,* since a mechanism comparable to the one inhibited by cycloheximide is not known in prokaryotes. In this case, a different mechanism could account for the persistent bioperiodicity.

IV

Pathologic (Neoplastic) Growth

12

Cell Injury as a Basic Initial Phenomenon

Benjamin F. Trump, Irene K. Berezesky, Mary W. Smith, and
Raymond T. Jones

I. INTRODUCTION

The study of the cellular reaction to injury is fundamental to the study of disease in all plants and animals. The introduction of the cell theory of disease by Rudolf Virchow and the current renaissance of concepts and techniques in cell biology has meant that at the level of the cell and its organelles we can obtain the most fundamental understanding of disease processes including neoplasia. There is a fundamental similarity in the cellular reactions to injurious stimuli whether the cell is that of an amoeba, a radish, or a man. This conceptual simplification has lately led to the development of a much greater understanding of human disease. Cellular reactions to injury include acute reactions, which are sometimes lethal, as well as repair and regenerative reactions. Chronic altered steady states such as neoplasia are also included. While it is difficult to distinguish between an altered physiological stimulus and what we call an injury, for the purpose of the present discussion we will consider as an injury any effect, agent, or stimulus which perturbs the homeostasis of the cell, however transiently. Such injuries occur constantly during the lifetime of a uni- or multicellular organism and accordingly cells are constantly adapting to or succumbing to a variety of injurious stimuli. When these injuries are extreme, one sees marked changes in cell structure and function and the onset of what we call disease. When these reactions are mild and chronic, the changes in the cell may seem imperceptible; yet, over a period of years, or a lifetime, the cell and its descendants show many alterations sometimes resulting in what we call aging or neoplasia.

It can now be reasonably argued that alterations of cell division are the most important alterations in terms of human disease. Atherosclerosis (heart disease and stroke) and cancer are the most common causes of death in the United States. An atherosclerotic plaque is best described as a proliferation of medial smooth muscle cells in response to injury, a response that is in many ways akin to a benign smooth muscle tumor. It is important also to recognize that cellular reactions to injury are not specific for a given stimulus. There are many more stimuli or injurious agents than there are cellular reactions to injury. Therefore, it is much more important for the biologist or the physician to understand the altered pathophysiology of the cell and to grasp the significance of interrelationships between such altered patterns in order to prevent, diagnose, or treat the disease than it is to recognize a specific stimulus.

It is the purpose of this chapter to review the general principles of cellular reaction to injury and its repair. In Chapter 20 we will concentrate on subcellular changes in neoplasia. Space obviously precludes a comprehensive consideration of this large and expanding field. We will therefore attempt to give the reader a general feeling for the important principles and, hopefully, stimulate more research in this important area. Of all the areas in experimental pathology it is perhaps this area that most needs a comparative approach. This is because of the numerous advances in cell biology which reveal an essential unity in the cells of all living forms. Accordingly, it is a good tactic to employ, for research, the form in which the cellular differentiation features are most suitable for the study of a particular process. In the field of acute reactions to anoxic and ischemic injury, for example, much progress has been made with a relatively simple *in vitro* system consisting of the isolated kidney tubules of various marine flatfish.

In general there are two types of cells, dividing and nondividing. Dividing cells are in the mitotic cycle; nondividing cells are normally assumed to be in prolonged G_1 phase, although some of these cells such as adult neurons, are so-called "sterile" cells and apparently do not have the capability of reentering the mitotic cycle.

Dividing, nontransformed cells are constantly being injured by the stresses of life; ultimately they do undergo cycle arrest and become nondividing cells, mature or differentiate, age, die, and undergo necrosis. It is believed that dividing nontransformed cells normally have a limited number of divisions which are related to the life span of the animal. If the cell remains in the G_1 stage, the effects of the injury may continue as the cell attains altered homeostasis or may disappear in the case of reversible injury.

Now consider the effects of injury on nondividing cells. If an injury applied to dividing cells does not result in death, the mitotic cycle may be arrested and these cells become subject to the controls of nondividing cells. If cycle arrest does not occur, several possibilities again exist. These include malignant transformation where cells continue indefinitely as dividing cells; mitotic death, where the cells undergo death at a subsequent mitotic division; or continued division without transformation with the cells remaining subject to the controls applying to dividing cells. The entire interaction is depicted as a closed system where the only way cells can leave the cycle is by dying.

An example of an injury to a dividing cell that does not result in cycle arrest or immediate death but does result in mitotic death at a subsequent division is radiation injury.

ACUTE CELL DEATH AND NECROSIS

General

Acute cell death is a common event in many different disease processes including the effects of chemical carcinogens. In cell death which is a result of an approach to physicochemical equilibrium through degradative, predominantly hydrolytic reactions, a process called necrosis can occur. Although there are obviously various cellular functions represented by different cell organelles, which if sufficiently interrupted will result in acute cell death and necrosis, only two main functions will be discussed. These are interference with: (a) the integrity and function of the cell or plasma membrane, and (b) the system for bioenergetics including mitochondria and glycolytic phosphorylation. With either type of injurious interaction the cell progresses through a sequence of stages which typify the progression of lethal change followed by death and necrosis. The rate of change through this sequence and some of the details vary with the cell and the type of injury. However, in many respects it is possible to regard this as a common pathway of reactivity with certain exceptions as will be outlined below. With either interruption of cell membrane integrity or interference with bioenergetics, the initial changes are reversible; if the injurious stimulus is removed prior to the point of no return or point of cell death, the cell recovers. This sequence of changes is described as progressing from Stage 1, the normal cell, to Stage 7, the necrotic cell (47, 51, 54).

Interference with Bioenergetic Pathways

Interference with the bioenergetic pathways can result from interference with the supply of oxygen, interference with the supply of substrate, interference with both oxygen and substrate, or through the effects of metabolic inhibitors which interfere with specific enzymatic reactions. This would then include a variety of conditions: complete and partial ischemia, complete and partial hypoxia, substrate deprivation, and a variety of inhibitors including cyanide, antimycin, carbon monoxide, and dinitrophenol.

Complete Ischemia

We discuss here not only the morphology of the reactions but also their meaning in terms of altered function. The following phases are recognized: (a) initiation phase, (b) reversible phase, and (c) irreversible phase. Important differences in the patterns exist when the ischemia is partial rather than complete.

Initiation Phase

The initial events involve cessation of oxidative metabolism and substrate depletion. As the oxygen concentration rapidly falls to zero, mitochondrial function stops. Energy-requiring processes, such as ion transport and filament contraction, proceed for a time, and adenosine triphosphate (ATP) is rapidly depleted. Calcium increases in the cytosol since it can no longer be sequestered in mitochondria or microsomes, nor can it be excluded from extracellular space by the plasma membrane (Fig. 12.1).

The decreased ATP along with increased adenosine di- and monophosphate (ADP and AMP), and inorganic phosphate activates phosphofructokinase (PFK). The increased cytosol calcium stimulates phosphorylase to foster an increase in the breakdown of glycogen and increased flux through the glycolytic sequence. The activation of PFK results in increased amounts of fructose-1,6-diphosphate which activates pyruvate kinase with an accumulation of pyruvate. As reducing equivalents in the cytoplasm are rapidly increased, pyruvate is converted to lactate with a fall of cellular pH (10, 20, 23, 40). Ion shifts occur in response to changing proton gradients with a cessation of ion pumps. Increased calcium probably activates phospholipase A_2 of the plasma and mitochondrial outer membranes releasing fatty acids to accumulate along with those which would otherwise be oxidized.

Reversible Phase

During this phase the cell can recover from the injury if the damage is not severe. The duration of this phase varies with temperature, cell type, and collateral flow. This phase is characterized by a sequence of changes we have numbered Stage 1, 1a, 2, 3, 4, 4a, and 4b for purposes of discussion. Characteristics of these stages have been defined previously and will only be briefly summarized here (49, 53).

Stage 1. This represents normal conditions of the cell (Fig. 12.2).

Stage 1a. Nuclear chromatin is altered; glycogen concentration decreases; and mitochondrial granules disappear.

Stage 2. There is dilation of the endoplasmic reticulum; a distortion of the plasma membrane with small blebs developing, and in some instances a swelling of cytosol (Fig. 12.3).

Stage 3. In addition to the alterations in Stages 1 to 2 there is a prominent condensation of the inner mitochondrial compartments with the mitochondrial matrix appearing dense and the intracrystal space enlarged (Fig. 12.4).

Stage 4. In this stage, some mitochondria show an additional swelling of the inner compartment while others show condensation of this compartment. In cells such as the kidney proximal tubule cells, some mitochondria show both types of alterations.

Stage 4a. All mitochondria are swollen with expansion of inner compartments and often outer membranes are interrupted in this stage (Fig. 12.5).

Stage 4b. Tiny dense aggregates appear in an otherwise pale mitochondrial matrix (Fig. 12.6).

The rate of appearance of each stage is variable. Stage 3 may be transient in some cell types and Stage 4 is not always seen in every cell or at every temperature.

Significance of Organelle Alterations. *Nucleus.* Chromatin clumping appears to be associated with decreased cellular pH. This decrease is largely due to an accumulation of lactate (46). This clumping is probably associated with decreased RNA synthesis, since the condensed chromatin fibrils are inactive. This change is of

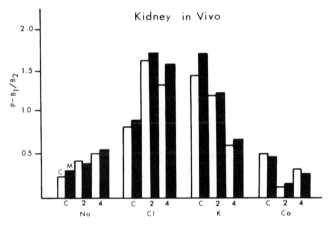

Figure 12.1. Bar graph illustrating P-B_1/B_2 ratios for Na, Cl, K, and Ca from x-ray measurements taken over cytosol (*C*) and mitochondria (*M*) from control and after 2 and 4 hr *in vivo* ischemic rat kidney proximal convoluted tubular cells. Note the progressive increases in Na and Cl both in the cytosol and mitochondria with a reciprocal decrease in K in ischemic measurements. Ca undergoes an early decrease followed by a gradual increase at the later time interval. (Reproduced with permission from B. F. Trump *et al.: Scanning Electron Microscopy,* 2:1027–1039, 1978.)

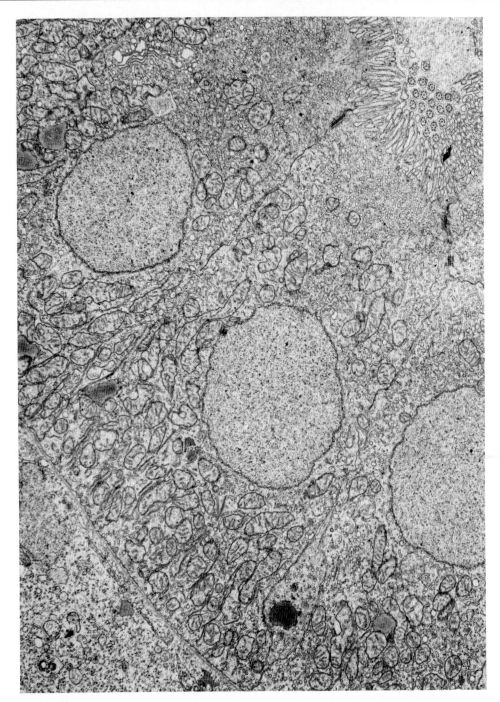

Figure 12.2. Electron micrograph of the isolated fish kidney tubule system which has been used to study cell injury. This is an example of Stage 1 or a normal cell.

no immediate lethal consequence to the cell and it is readily reversible.

Cell Membrane. These alterations include the formation of blebs and invaginations, distortion of the villous contours and changes in the histochemically demonstrable activity of plasma membrane enzymes (12, 14, 16). The scanning electron microscope (SEM) has been useful in visualizing these changes (Figs. 12.7 and 12.8).

Blebs may reflect changes in the contraction stage of cytoplasmic contractile filaments, as similar blebs are produced by cytochalasin and the calcium ionophore A23187 (Fig. 12.9). Apical vacuoles (invaginations) can be especially prominent in hepatic parenchymal cells in the form of hypoxic vacuoles and are typically surrounded by bundles of filaments. At this time, Na^+-K^+-ATPase has ceased pumping sodium and potassium ions due to the lack of ATP. However, there is no indication that this enzyme itself is rapidly inactivated, and it probably can recover following restoration of ATP synthesis.

Endoplasmic Reticulum (ER). Dilatation of both rough and smooth ER occurs in the reversible phase of cell injury. This dilatation often includes the Golgi cisternae and vesicles which may also form concentric lamellar profiles. This

dilatation is correlated with inward movement of water and ions into the cisternae following redistribution, possibly of potassium, and moreover is possibly related to potassium released from mitochondria with its subsequent movement into other compartments. Membrane-bound polysomes are sometimes maintained and often lose their orientation while maintaining membrane attachments. There are also indica-

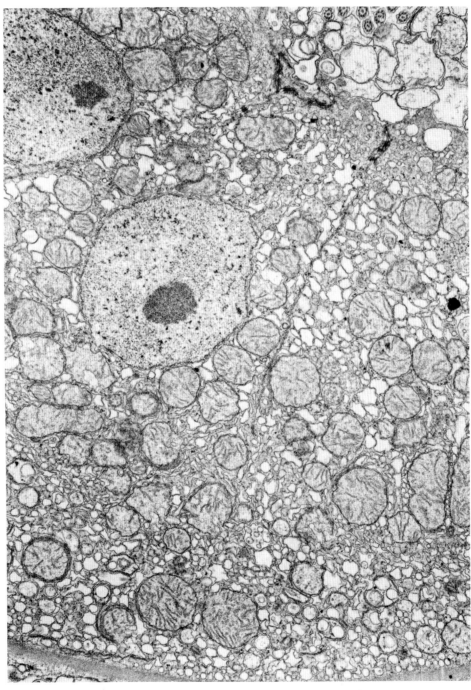

Figure 12.3. An example of Stage 2 of the cell injury stage. The mitochondria are swollen and the endoplasmic recticulum is dilated in these fish kidney cells which have been exposed to mercuric chloride.

tions of early defects in messenger RNA-polysome association (43). Defects of protein synthesis can readily be demonstrated by this time.

Mitochondria. Perhaps the earliest change is the loss or dispersal of normal mitochondrial matrix granules. Based upon techniques using frozen sections and x-ray microanalysis (Fig. 12.10) these granules are thought to represent sites of calcium localization. They appear to differ from calcium phosphate, which accumulates during deliberate loading, and may represent normal binding sites where calcium is normally sequestered in the mitochondrial matrix. The mitochondrial concentration of calcium may be some 1000 times that of the cytosol and is significant as a metabolic control mechanism (4). We have hypothesized that, concomitantly with loss of the granules, there is leak of calcium

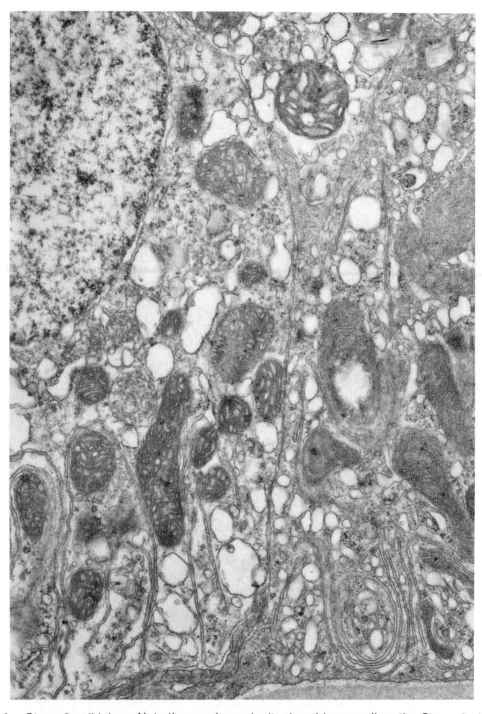

Figure 12.4. Stage 3 cell injury. Note the condensed mitochondria as well as the Stage 2 alterations.

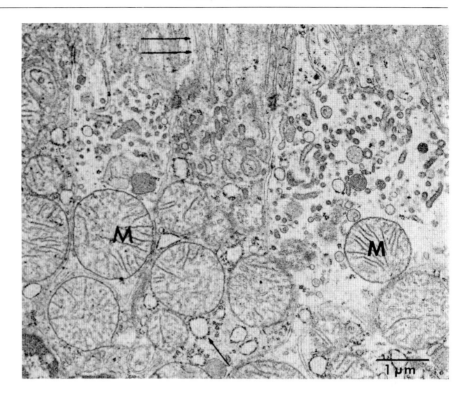

Figure 12.5. A portion of a proximal convoluted tubule cell after 30 min of *in vivo* ischemia. The mitochondria (*M*) are rounded and show swelling of the inner compartments. The RER is dilated (*arrow*), the microvilli swollen (*double arrow*), and the cytosol is less dense. Stage 4a. (Reproduced with permission from B. Glaumann *et al.*: *Virchows Àrchiv. B. Cell Pathology, 19*:281–302, 1975.)

across the outer membrane, activating mitochondrial phospholipases which then begin to attack the inner membrane lipid with release of fatty acids and subsequent deterioration of inner membrane function (33). The condensation that occurs during this reversible phase cannot yet be thoroughly explained, but it does correlate with the rapid loss of mitochondrial potassium.

Next, the condensed mitochondria begin to swell. Morphometric studies have demonstrated there is an increase in mitochondrial volume as a function of ischemic time. This change correlates with changes in the permeability of the inner membrane to chloride and perhaps other ions, resulting in an increased movement of these ions. Both the coupling and the respiratory control of mitochondria are becoming looser and there is an increased proton gradient with an oxygen pulse (34). The electron transport system of the inner membrane is maintained and may possibly be accelerated due to increased uncouplers such as fatty acids. Mitochondria contain much less potassium and gradually lose calcium along with a gradual increase in sodium while magnesium levels only slightly diminish (6).

In conditions of reflow, these mitochondria are able to accumulate enormous amounts of calcium (35). Small dense aggregates begin to appear in the matrix. These aggregates seem to be reversible unlike the larger apparently irreversible densities of the next phase. Recent studies show these densities are proteinaceous and we speculate that they may represent a reversible denaturation of matrix protein.

Lysosomes. During the reversible phase only slight swelling, increased fragility, and clearing of lysosomes occur. As the cellular pH drops, the hydrogen ion gradient between the interior of the lysosomes and the cytosol is dissipated. This can result in an efflux of materials such as the dye acridine orange that partition into the lysosomes because of their pK. Visible colloidal markers such as ferritin or Thorotrast added to lysosomes prior to reversible cell injury do not leak from the lysosomes (19).

Irreversible Phase (Stage 5)

The most characteristic morphological indicator of irreversible cell injury is the appearance of large flocculent densities in mitochondria. These flocculent densities are large, irregular, and electron dense (Fig. 12.11). They have no apparent internal fine structure nor do they appear to have a particular spacial relationship to the cristae. They are not extractable in acid solutions nor with lipid solvents, but they do disappear following pronase treatment, suggesting that they represent altered matrix proteins (5). Flocculent densities may also contain some bound divalent cations.

Functionally, mitochondria show loss of P/O ratio and loss of ability to maintain a proton gradient (34, 37). There is also great loss of cardiolipin as well as loss of other phospholipids (42). There is also evidence of irreversible damage to ATPase (36). This enzyme, the F_1 particle, which is visualized as spheres on short stalks on the matrix side of the inner membrane, disappears and cannot be isolated. We suspect that the critical event involves irreparable damage to the inner membrane, probably involving changes in phospholipids associated with preservation of the respiratory chain, which continues electron transport for a while though unable to generate energy. The formation of pentalaminar structures from cristae might result from attack by phospholipase.

Damage to other membrane systems of the

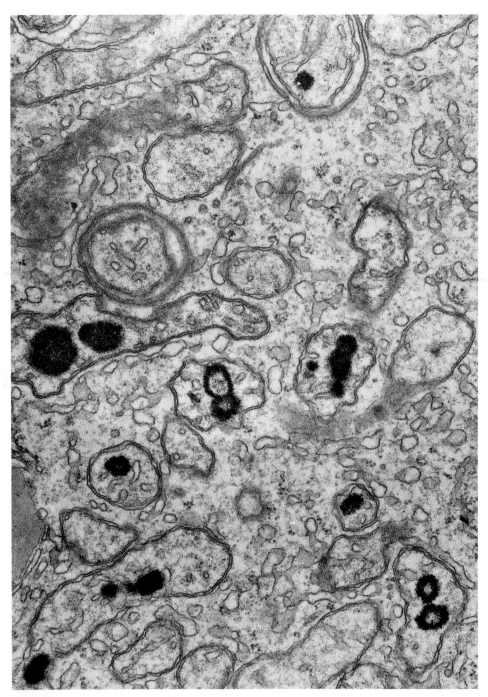

Figure 12.6. Stage 4b cell injury with examples of mitochondrial calcifications in a fish kidney tubule. (Courtesy of Dr. S. Sahaphong.)

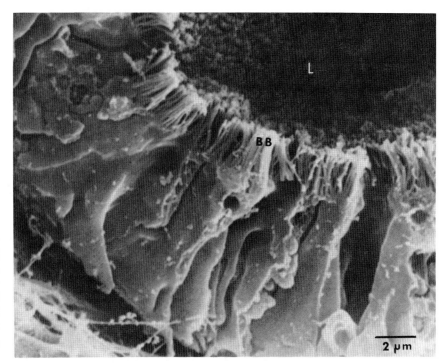

Figure 12.7. Scanning electron micrograph of a portion of a control rat kidney proximal convoluted tubule. The brush border (*BB*) with long slender microvilli is seen projecting into a patent lumen (*L*). (Reproduced with permission from B. F. Trump *et al.*: *Beitr. Path. Bd.*, *158:363–388*, *1976.*)

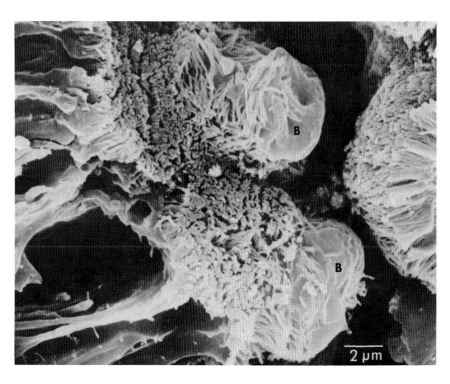

Figure 12.8. Scanning electron micrograph of a portion of rat kidney proximal convoluted tubule following 15 min of *in vivo* ischemia. Note the distortion of the microvillous border forming large apical blebs (*B*) which protrude into the lumen. Some lateral plasma membrane infoldings of the tubular cells appear greatly swollen. (Reproduced with permission from B. F. Trump *et al.*: *Beitr. Path. Bd.*, *158: 363–388, 1976.*)

cell is also severe. Fragmentation of the ER and Golgi apparatus continues along with distortion of the plasma membrane. Breaks in the plasmalemma can be observed in electron micrographs. This may represent increased membrane fragility and permeability which is also reflected by entry of vital dyes and sucrose and leakage of proteins such as lactate dehydrogenase into the extracellular space.

Phase of Necrosis (Stages 6 and 7)

The time this phase begins depends on the cell type and it extends until complete equilibration occurs.

During Stage 6, the rate of hydrolysis of the cell rapidly accelerates, as measured by increase in free amino acids, acid-soluble phosphorus, and decreased DNA and RNA. This is seen morphologically by the beginning of karyolysis and changes in the staining pattern of the cytoplasm, including an increased affinity for anionic dyes such as eosin (48). The disappearance of organized structure and persistence of lysosomal hydrolases, as compared with many other enzymes, strongly indicate that lysosomal leakage is followed by digestion. Cellular membranes display massive rearrangements including vesi-

culation, wrapping, elaboration of tubular structures in the inner mitochondrial compartments, disappearance of ribosomes from the membrane surface, alterations in nucleolus, clearing of microbody matrices, and frequent interruptions of the plasma membrane.

In Stage 7, large dense inclusions composed of homogeneous material with lamellar regions within lacunae form in the cytoplasm (Fig.

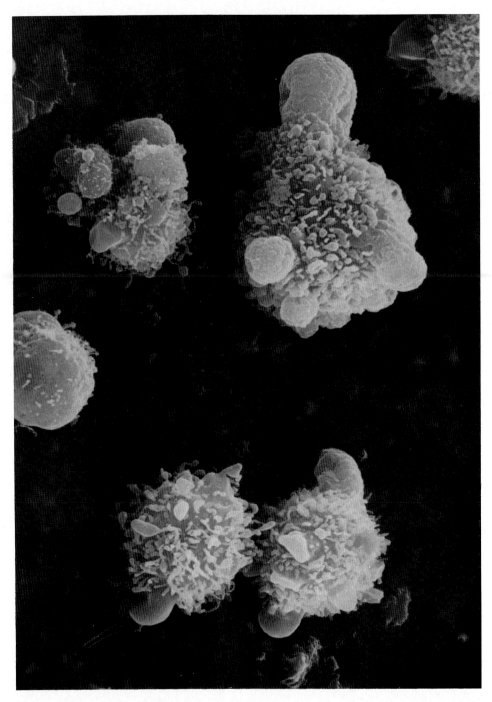

Figure 12.9. Ehrlich ascites tumor cells treated for 1 hr with 10^{-3} M calcium ionophore A23187 in PBS at 37°C. Large protuberances are seen and there is a loss of microvilli. (Courtesy of P. Phelps.)

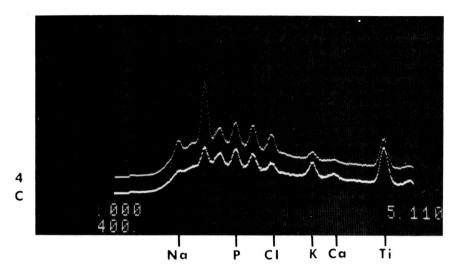

Figure 12.10. Typical x-ray spectra obtained over the cytosol from 4 hr *in vivo* ischemic (*4*) and control (*C*) rat kidney proximal convoluted tubular cell. Note the increases in Na and Cl and the decrease in K in the 4-hr spectrum. Titanium (Ti) is from the support grid. (Reproduced with permission from I. K. Berezesky et al.: *Proceedings of the 35th Annual Meeting of the Electron Microscopy Association*, pp. 524–525, 1977.)

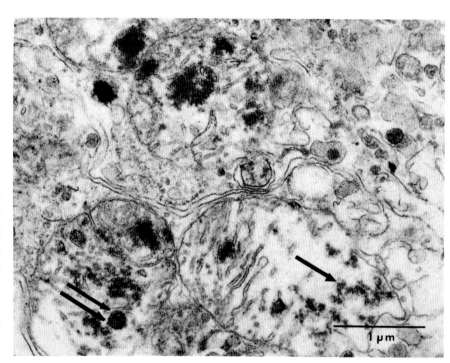

Figure 12.11. A portion of a rat kidney proximal convoluted tubule cell after 120 min of *in vivo* ischemia followed by 24 hr of reflow. The mitochondria are extremely swollen and contain large flocculent densities (*single arrow*) as well as intra-mitochondrial calcifications (*double arrows*). (Reproduced with permission from B. Glaumann *et al.*: *Virchows Archiv. B. Cell Pathology, 19:* 281–302, 1975.)

12.12). These periodic regions resemble stacks of membranes, but the fine structure within them has not actually been discerned. These bodies may correspond to the myelin described by Virchow. Although the precise chemical nature of these bodies has not been defined, they probably contain mixtures of lipid, including cholesterol, phospholipid, and fatty acids, and possibly some metal soaps. At this stage most enzymes, including lysosomal hydrolases, are inactive. Under the light microscope the cells resemble those in the center of an old infarct with eosinophilia, karyolysis, and indistinct cell outlines. Cells in an infarct become more or less stabilized in this condition, probably through the "fixation" effect of denaturation, unless other factors are present such as those occurring in caseous or gummatous necrosis. This can probably be explained in part on the basis that hydrolases and other enzymes are eventually inactivated and, unless other sources of enzymes such as those produced by microorganisms are present, the cells are stabilized for a relatively long period. Equilibration takes place in Stage 7 when extracellular pH approaches physiological levels. Intracellular calcium increases are possibly related to changes in pH and in reactive protein binding sites. The calcium concentration of mitochon-

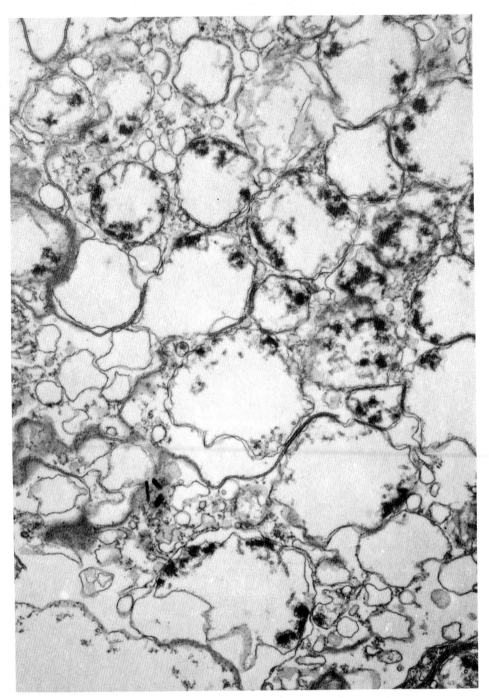

Figure 12.12. An electron microscopic example of necrosis. Note the disruption of the cell. Flocculent densities can still be observed in mitochondria. (Courtesy of Dr. S. Sahaphong.)

dria is probably small due only to energy-independent binding to molecules such as to glycoproteins which may still remain.

Complete Ischemia Followed by Reflow

The phase after blood flow is restored can be a very important one in infarcts *in vivo* and one in which increased cell damage can occur. The cell without ATP or an active energy generating system generally swells as it is exposed suddenly to extracellular fluid with which ion exchanges can occur rapidly. Magnesium and potassium are further lost and sodium, chloride, and calcium increase in the cytosol. Shrinking and/or swelling can occur, causing membrane damage, and in addition, mitochondria start sequestering calcium, causing further damage to that organelle (13, 14, 58). Most likely different cells respond differently to reflow and recovery (53).

One common pattern is shrinkage of the cells with increased density of the cytosol and dilatation of the ER. This may be due to a rapid loss of potassium in excess of sodium gained during this reflow phase, resulting in decreased value of cell water and lowered cation content (52). It is striking that in many cells mitochondrial restitution from the swollen or condensed phase to the orthodox phase can occur rapidly. In some cells, notably in those of the pars recta of the renal proximal tubule, recovery is accompanied by apparent turnover of organelles, especially the cell membrane, where striking invaginations of the apex including microvilli occur with breakdown of the sequestered microvilli so engulfed. This leads to an increase in the numbers of residual bodies, apparently as a part of the remodeling process that is proceeding. This seems to be followed by a period of increased prominence of rough ER and polysomes. This proliferation is probably involved in membrane and organ repair during the recovery phase.

Anoxia

The effects of virtually complete anoxia have been studied on a series of *in vitro* systems including isolated flounder tubules, Ehrlich ascites tumor cells (EATC), and transporting toad bladders. These studies with anoxia allow one to begin to dissociate between the effects of lack of oxygen and those due to lack of substrate. In most anoxic systems that have been studied, there is a remarkable protective effect imparted by addition of glucose to the medium presumably through stimulation of glycolysis which increases when mitochondrial ATP synthesis stops. The addition of glucose may permit survival for several additional hours or permit reversibility of complete anoxia with no added glucose in EATC for up to 3 hr. The effects of anoxia, although they resemble the sequence seen after complete ischemia, are different in the sense that the progression through the stages of cell injury mentioned above is less rapid and more prolonged in certain of the stages. For example, in anoxic flounder kidney tubules, EATC, or toad bladders, a prolonged Stage 3 with condensed mitochondria and dilated ER is typically seen. This is presumed to be due to the effects of ion shifts. Potassium leaks out of the mitochondria and from the cytosol to the extra-

cellular space, resulting in cell shrinkage. Calcification of mitochondria even during the phase of necrosis does not occur presumably because mitochondrial calcium accumulation is energy dependent. When glucose is added the progression through the stages is much less rapid, possibly the result of ATP production by the glycolytic sequence and subsequent protection of intracellular membrane systems. In anoxic cells, there is often a partial initial shrinkage of cells which correlates with the observed reduction of total cation content, principally because potassium escapes from the cells at a rate that is more rapid than the rate of sodium entry. This is reflected also in partial ischemia in cerebrovascular accident and myocardial infarcts where cell shrinkage may also be seen *in vivo*, probably because partial blood flow permits similar ion exchanges (11).

Metabolic Inhibitors

A variety of metabolic inhibitors of energy metabolism have been tested in a fashion similar to the above. These include such electron transport inhibitors as potassium cyanide, antimycin A, sodium azide, and uncouplers or inhibitors of oxidative phosphorylation including 2,4-dinitrophenol, and oligomycin. All of these agents have similar effects on the same *in vitro* systems mentioned above including EATC, flounder kidney tubules, and toad bladders. These effects include the rapid condensation of mitochondria, clumping of nuclear chromatin, and dilatation of the ER which presumably result from inhibition of ATP synthesis, and ion redistributions. In the late stages, mitochondrial swelling and flocculent densities occur which again are not accompanied by calcification. At the same time, during the early stages through Stage 4, the changes can be reversed in many instances by washing away the agent; glucose is frequently found to be protective.

Hypothesis of Progression

Table 12.1 illustrates our current working hypothesis of the interaction of various cellular events and changes following ischemia. As can be seen from the table, the principal changes involve cessation of ATP production, initiation of ion shifts, and a series of changes, which lead to irreversible membrane damage so that, when

Table 12.1
Working Hypothesis of Cellular Events following Ischemia

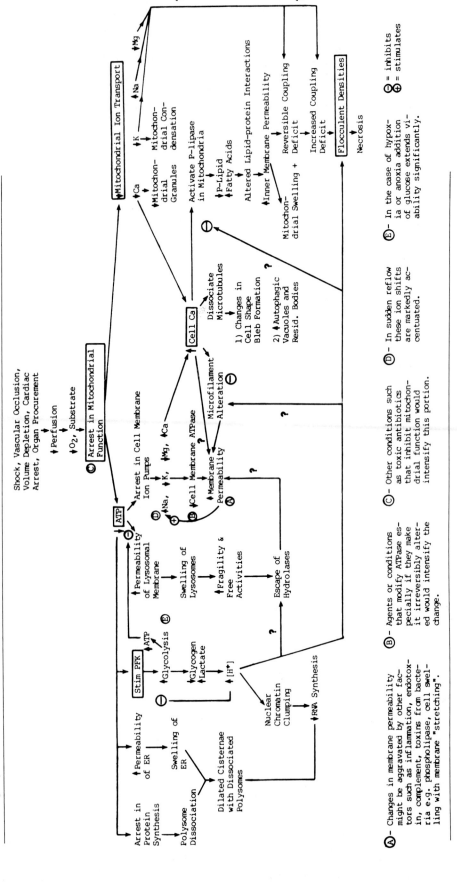

the injurious agents are removed, repair becomes impossible. There is some reason to believe that ion redistributions themselves may trigger the membrane damaging effects. In particular, we have been focusing on the possible role of a calcium redistribution in phospholipase activation with subsequent changes in membrane lipids and lipid-protein interactions. Since the restoration of bioenergetics in the cell is dependent on integrated membrane function, it could well be true that such alterations in membrane lipid components are responsible for the irreversibility. Earlier changes in membrane lipids apparently can be repaired but, after a certain point, the system appears to be irreparably damaged. A consideration of the sequence of events postulated in Table 12.1 leads one to propose a series of interventions which might be able to modify the course of cellular events. Such protective interventions could potentially be of great value in the treatment of heart disease, stroke, shock, spinal cord injury, head injury, and acute renal failure.

Direct Injury to the Cell Membrane

This is an important category of acute lethal cell injury because it includes not only the effects of a variety of toxic chemicals which either act directly or have metabolites which modify membrane permeability but also because it includes the whole category of immune damage to the cell through complement activation (26, 32). Guinea pig lymphotoxin seems to activate plasma membrane phospholipase A upon binding the cell surface receptors (24). When the cell membrane integrity is sufficiently violated, ion fluxes are rapid and extensive. The extreme case is mechanical violation through severing the cell membrane with a blade or puncturing with a microneedle or fibers of asbestos. Lesser degrees are seen with inorganic or organic mercurials or with antibody and complement. The resultant change in membrane permeability causes a rapid redistribution of ions—sodium and calcium rapidly leaking into the cell and potassium and magnesium rapidly leaking out. This typically results in rapid cell swelling and lysis and of course this is the most common cause of hemolysis of erythrocytes. Swelling and lysis are due to the Gibbs-Donnan effect and the swelling involves not only the cell itself but also the intracellular organelles including the ER and the mitochondria whose membranes are themselves damaged through the altered internal environ-

ment. Initially mitochondria condense through rapid loss of ions, presumably of potassium, but later mitochondrial swelling as well as calcification occur. After the primary injurious attack on the cell membrane, calcification of the swollen mitochondria is the rule, as the damaged mitochondria, in the face of increasing calcium concentrations, have a virtually unlimited supply of calcium. Very early marked conformational changes in the cell surface occur with irregular blebs, and protrusions possibly mediated by influx of calcium and microtubule-microfilament interactions. Later, the entire cell surface assumes a smooth contour presumably due to unfolding or irregular contours including those of microvilli (49).

Other Types of Cell Injury

There are obviously many other etiological agents which are important in cell injury besides the two principal types of acute lethal injury mentioned above. Each of these is discussed by major etiologic class and, in general, significantly less is known about the pathophysiology and histogenesis than in the above.

Chemical Injury

This is a very large class of etiologic agents including both carcinogenic and noncarcinogenic compounds. Many chemicals at the appropriate dose do cause acute lethal injury to cells resulting in necrosis. This includes many carcinogens whose metabolites are extremely cytotoxic. In the process of neoplastic transformation, usually in sites of regeneration and in a number of organs such as the liver, kidney, and pancreas, acute cell injury and cell death may lend "promoter-like" effects to the effects produced by the carcinogenic metabolites themselves. Most chemical agents have a number of metabolic effects on the cell including defects in energy metabolism, membrane transport, and macromolecular synthesis. It has generally been difficult to decide which of these is significant in terms of acute lethal injury. For reasons given above, however, we favor the hypothesis that chemicals producing acute cell killing do so by processes that interfere either with cell membrane transport and permeability or with the synthesis of ATP by mitochondria. Defects in macromolecular synthesis including protein synthesis do not seem to result in acute cell death though they can result in prolonged lack of cell division, that is, a prolonged G_1 phase with subsequent aging and accumulation of secondary lysosomes. One such agent is the commonly studied toxin, carbon tetrachloride, which produces acute hepatotoxicity within hours following a single dose administered in rats and humans. The necrosis is preceded by a number of changes including defective protein synthesis, mitochondrial swelling, mitochondrial uptake of calcium, and peroxidation of cell membranes. Available evidence, we feel, favors the view that cell membrane peroxidation is a probable limiting factor in cell survival.

Physical Agents

Although physical agents, principally radiation damage, have been widely studied in terms of long term cell effects and mutagenesis, much less is known about their acute lethal effects on the cell. Considerable work has, however, been done with ultraviolet irradiation which produces acute cell membrane damage including interference with permeability and with the sodium-potassium ATPase (7). In our laboratory, we have done a series of experiments with ultraviolet irradiation of isolated flounder kidney tubules in which the results are essentially similar to the acute cell membrane damage, produced by the compound p-chloromercuribenzene sulfonic acid (Figs. 12.1–12.5), or antibody and complement (41). Acute cell swelling is soon followed by dilatation of intracellular compartments including mitochondria and mitochondrial calcification.

Little still is known about acute cell injury and ionizing irradiation as it affects the cell cycle. Currently attention is being directed toward interventions including drugs and hyperbaric oxygen that minimize the effect of radiation therapy to patients with cancer.

Microbiologic Injury

Probably the most studied examples of acute lethal cell injury follows virus infection. Among the acute cytopathic effects of viruses are a series of proliferative and other organelle changes accompanied by marked cell surface changes preceding cell death and necrosis. Probably the best studied examples in this category are herpes simplex virus and poliomyelitis virus.

Both are accompanied by a variety of intracellular functional alterations including changes in macromolecular synthesis and conformational changes in the cell membrane which are sometimes dramatic. With poliomyelitis virus infection there is, in addition, marked proliferation of smooth membrane systems accompanied by membrane fusions which may relate to phospholipase action as it is also capable of forming pentalaminar configurations.

Another type of microbiologic agent that leads to acute lethal cell injury is the endotoxins released from clostridial organisms most commonly in human cases of gas gangrene. Patients suffering with such infections have serious acute lethal cell injury involving several organ systems including the heart, liver, kidney, and pancreas. In our experience this results in dramatic lethal changes in cells with swelling of mitochondria and appearance of mitochondrial flocculent densities at some point prior to somatic death of the patient. The mechanisms that are involved are not known; however, it is reasonable to suppose that a release of phospholipases into the circulation may cause this as a modification of the direct cell membrane injury mentioned above.

Genetic Injury

Genetic injury probably does not commonly result in acute cell death and necrosis because such modifications would result in fetal death in utero. There are, however, many examples of genetic modifications, especially identifiable enzyme deficits, which lead to chronic cell injury and adaptation as mentioned below.

CHRONIC CELL INJURY

General Considerations

The purpose of this section is to review sublethal injuries to cells which, although they are followed by marked alterations in cell structure and function, do not result in acute cell death and necrosis. They do, however, commonly result in marked adaptations of the cell and some of these changes may well be related to neoplastic transformation; indeed, some may represent endpoints in the process of carcinogen testing. In this section we will discuss first the reactions of individual organelles and then in the second section attempt to synthesize some of these changes as they occur in important overall cell and tissue reactions.

Organelle Changes

Cell Membrane

General. Changes in the cell membrane are among the most dramatic of those observed following chronic cell injury. These are especially striking, of course, because they can be readily visualized by light and electron microscopy and, furthermore, because such membrane changes could be in many instances important determinants of the overall cell functional change and, moreover, could be among the steps leading to neoplastic progression of injury. In the past, cell membrane alterations were often considered as separate entities. However, recently it has been increasingly clear that the cell membrane is not an independent entity but a structure which is engaged in important and intimate interactions with other macromolecular components in the cell, especially components of the cytosol including the microtrabecular network, contractile and noncontractile filaments, and microtubules. Therefore, many of the important cell membrane changes are related to alterations and are described below under "Cytosol and Cytoskeleton."

Among the more striking morphological changes characteristic of sublethal injury in the cell membrane are the changes in cell shape. These can result in alteration of microvillous borders converting them to smooth surface, ciliogenesis, and large bleb protrusions and related phenomena, variously known as podocytosis or zeiosis. These remarkable cell surface alterations are completely reversible initially and appear to be determined by as yet undisclosed interactions of contractile filaments, microtubules, and membrane proteins. The formation of long filopodia is especially characteristic of damaged cells in tissue culture monolayers. When retraction and movement occurs, foot processes adhere, leaving these long slender projections. Changes in surface macromolecules including glycoproteins and glycolipids may be important characteristics of malignant cell transformation, changing a number of cell surface properties including surface antigens. Such changes are

mentioned in Chapter 20 on the ultrastructure of neoplastic cells.

Junctional complexes can be dissociated by extracellular calcium depletion resulting in dramatic changes in cell shape and internal organization. Cell junctions appear to be important in the maintenance of cell shape, possibly serving as attachment sites for tonofilaments. Disruption of cell junctions affects electrical and ionic communications between cells. In malignant hepatomas, the electrical connection may be modified. Improper development of junctional complexes in neoplastic cells may also have significance in the explanation of tumor cell invasion and metastasis.

Intercellular Attachments. Mammalian cells may connect to adjacent cells by several different types of junctions. These include gap junctions (nexuses), desmosomes (macula adherens), intermediate junctions (zonula adherens) and tight junctions (zonula occludens). These are useful in electron microscopy in identifying and classifying cells as well as evaluating pathogenic change (57). For example, desmosomes are indicators of epithelial differentiation. The formation of intercellular desmosomes is sometimes quite evident in sites of increased keratinization, for example, in dysplasias and epidermoid carcinomas of the skin and bronchus. The complex of tight and intermediate junctions along a lumen or acinus is often characteristic of adenocarcinoma, as they form terminal bars that can be seen by light microscopy as a dark zone at the cell apex. Carcinoma, in general, is associated with decreased cell communication and may be reflected by a decreased number of gap junctions which appear to be the sites of intercellular communication.

Changes in Surface Antigens and Other Markers. Changes of the glycocalyx are just beginning to be deciphered but may result in many new types of morphological and biochemical tests for altered cell function. A number of observations have implicated the glycoproteins or glycolipids of the cell surface in the regulation of biological phenomenon, such as the processes of morphogenesis and malignant transformation (21, 22). Tumor-specific differences can be demonstrated through the use of lectins, since many transformed cells can be aggregated by lectins at concentrations much lower than those required for the agglutination of normal cells. Such changes in surface polysaccharides may also be involved in contact inhibition. Differences can be observed in different cell types and potentially between normal and abnormal subtypes.

In addition, migration of sites occurs following binding of concanavalin A and other lectins to normal membranes (3).

Abnormal Cilia. Abnormal cilia of several forms are frequently encountered in the respiratory epithelium and presumably represent a response to noxious environmental agents. In one extreme alteration, large protrusions containing up to 30 or 40 axonemes instead of the usual 1 axoneme results in a very unusual formation. Other abnormal forms include budding of basal bodies to form intracellular cilia or deviations from the 9 + 2 pattern normally seen. It is not clear whether or not these represent mutagenicity involving basal body DNA. Ciliogenesis may also be observed as part of normal repair as in the bronchial epithelium where damage to the epithelium results in loss of the ciliated cells, division of mucous cells, and formation of cilia in the newly formed mucous cells (30, 31, 53, 55).

Cytosol and Cytoskeleton

Changes in the component of the cytosol are doubtlessly very important in chronic cell injury as well as in neoplasia; however, their significance and range of variation is still being determined. Until recently the cytosol of the cell was considered to be largely a bag filled with proteins and other macromolecules in fluid compartments with communications between the membranous components. It is now becoming increasingly apparent that in addition to the membrane systems there is another system known as the cytoskeleton which is made up of networks of various fibrous proteins. Although some such filaments have been recognized since the introduction of electron microscopy, the recent introductions of specific antibody staining has led to the realization that these filaments are of three major types: microtubules, microfilaments, and intermediate filaments. (See recent reviews by Arstila *et al.* (1), Spooner (44), and Stephens and Edds (45).

The microtubules which are approximately 250 Å in diameter radiate outward from the cell center near the nucleus along straight or curved paths and terminate near the cell surface. These tubules help to maintain cell shape and guide the movement of organelles including pinosomes, phagosomes, mitochondria, and lysosomes. The microtubules change during mitosis at the beginning of cell division, being first or-

ganized into the mitotic spindle, and then reorganizing into the interphase pattern after the completion of mitosis. Since they are labile structures, they completely disappear after the use of certain fixatives or after fixation in the cold. Based upon their association with cellular movements, any abnormalities in their growth or function could seriously hamper cell function. Colchicine and vinblastine affect microtubules and their application to cells results in mitotic arrest at metaphase. Paracrystalline inclusions have also been found to appear following treatment with vinblastine. These inclusions measure several microns in diameter and may be composed of closely packed tubules measuring approximately 250 Å in diameter, each composed of globular 150 Å subunits. In the case of neurons, the vinblastine-induced inclusions may be associated somehow with a block of rapid axoplasmic transport, which supplies materials to the synapses.

The microfilaments which are approximately 60 Å in diameter are connected to the inner surface of the cell membrane. They are composed primarily of the contractile protein, actin, and certain other proteins including several types of myosin. They are organized into a meshwork or into bundles both of which are important for cell motility. These fibers are readily demonstrated with immunofluorescence and together with other poorly characterized components, form the so-called stress fibers which attach to the membranes and markedly change during alterations in cell shape as well as neoplastic transformation.

The so-called intermediate filaments are larger, about 100Å in diameter, and also form a rather wavy interwoven network through the cell exhibiting important interactions with the desmosomes. These are distinct from the other systems, may not be contractile, have to do with stabilizing cell shape, and interact with cell junctions especially the maculae adherens of desmosomes.

Recently, using high voltage electron microscopy and stereo pictures of rather thick sections, Porter and his colleagues have developed a new concept of a microtrabecular system which consists of a lacey network of fibers filling the entire cytoplasm (59). This network is composed of individual fibers which are thinner than microfilaments somewhere between 30 and 60 Å in diameter. Because of a topologic resemblance to the trabecular structure of spongy bone, Porter named it the microtrabecular system. It is currently believed to provide a kind of intracellular scaffolding to which the various organelles as well as the three major fiber systems are anchored. This microtrabecular network may also form as a type of cellular musculature constantly redistributing and reorienting the organelles as the cell goes about its other functions. The movement of cell components through this microtrabecular lattice seems to be achieved by extension and contraction of individual microtrabecular filaments with the energy being stored in the extended state. The nature of the proteins involved in the microtrabecular network is under study by Porter and others.

All of these systems although presently poorly characterized are undoubtedly of major importance in cellular reactions to injury. As the cytoskeletal elements closely interact with the cell membrane, changes in the cytoskeleton are closely paralleled by changes in membrane conformation. It has long been known that rapid modifications of cell shape occur following injury and elucidation of these will form an exciting chapter in the near future.

Cell sap exhibits marked changes in electron density following cell injury. An increase in density exhibited by the so-called dark cells has been observed in many nonspecific types of injury and suggests selective dehydration of individual cells. There may also be a decrease in the density of the cell sap, which can occur in conditions causing acute dilatation of ER cisternae. Changes in cell sap streaming and gelation, although common and possibly important in cell injury, are poorly understood. Some of these changes may relate to changes in divalent cation concentration. Another form of coagulation of cell sap occurs following denaturation of the cytoplasm in thermal burns or laser irradiation.

Endoplasmic Reticulum

Many quantitative and qualitative changes occur in the ER in altered steady states of the cell. These involve changes in volume, changes in ion content, changes in surface area, and changes in disposition of ribosomes. Closely allied with these are sometimes marked conformational changes in the arrangement and/or disposition of the reticulum within the cytoplasm. The factors responsible for these changes are currently being investigated and include changes in energy metabolism with altered ion and water gradients and consequent changes in volume, induced en-

zyme synthesis along with membrane synthesis causing increased membrane surface area, and changes in the chemical composition of the membranes sometimes related to ribosome detachment.

One of the most common changes in the ER following injury is dilatation of the ER cisternae apparently with a watery, presumably ion containing, solution. This occurs soon after acute cell injury and even apparently can be a chronic state. The exact ions included are not known though the change correlates with the altered sodium-potassium transport at the cell surface. Along with the increased electrolyte content of the reticulum, sparse flocculence can often be seen within the lumens. Other types of alterations in luminal content occur with retention of normally secreted material presumably synthesized on membrane polysomes which occur on the lumen wall. This is the case in the Russell body in which plasma cells develop hyaline cytoplasm due to the accumulation of glycoprotein. Somewhat similar changes occur in ethionine poisoning in hepatocytes where lipoprotein globules seem to persist within the ER cisternae possibly due to the effect of depleted ATP leading to alteration in transfer from ER cisternae to Golgi elements. Virus budding into ER cisternae has been identified and many other lamellar and other inclusions within the cisternae have been observed but not identified. Occasionally in iron overload, ferritin particles can be seen within the ER lumens possibly due to insertion across the membrane, although the mechanism of this remains unclear.

Alterations in the quantitative amount of ER are common in chronic adaptations, especially in the case of compounds which induce the mixed function oxidase along with ER membrane synthesis (Fig. 12, 13). These include compounds which are widely distributed in nature as well as man-made chemicals including drugs and carcinogens. Following induction there is often a significant proliferation of ER resulting in masses of tortuous cisterna within the cytoplasm visible often in inclusions known as ground glass cytoplasm by light microscopy. Quantitative measurements make it clear that this represents a hypertrophy which can be correlated with greatly increased specific activities of involved enzymes, including cytochrome P-450, as well as membrane protein and phospholipid. Following cessation of induction, turnover of the membrane occurs through autophagocytosis as mentioned below. When this change is severe, several large whorls of membrane appear

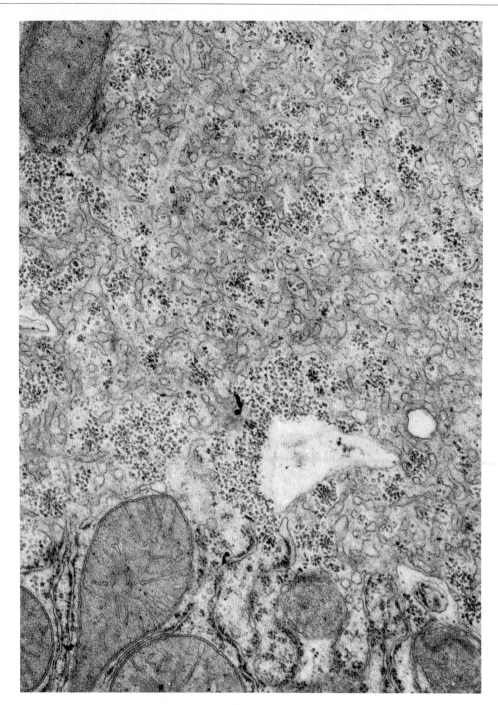

Figure 12.13. An example of proliferation of smooth endoplasmic reticulum in a hepatocyte from a rat which was fed safrole for 14 days. (Courtesy of Dr. M. Lipsky.)

in the cytoplasm forming dense cytoplasmic inclusions. These latter states of the ER may be enzyme deficient and are so-called hypotrophic hypoactive ER. Loss of characteristic marker enzymes occurs in the ER following other types of stimulation, especially by carcinogens. Well known in this regard is the enzyme glucose-6-phosphatase which often diminishes in activity during this hypertrophy. Similar proliferations of ER occur in hepatitis virus infection in the human and a somewhat similar ground glass appearance can often be found which is characteristic of hepatitis surface antigen.

Alterations of the chemical composition along with conformation of the ER membrane occurs with lipid peroxidation. After carbon tetrachloride poisoning or peroxidation of the ER microsomes *in vitro*, clumping and formation of dense material as well as alteration of conformation of the ER cisternae results. Treatment of ER fragments with phospholipases results in ultrastructural alterations of the membrane cell. Triglycerides are released and there is a reversible change in the activity of glucose-6-phosphatase which can be repaired with added phospholipid. In regenerating cells and cells treated with carcinogens, marked modifications in the conformation of the ER occur whereby normal organized cisternae are replaced by meandering cisternae which become fewer in number. Budding of organelles, including the ER, may occur. As described below under autophagocytosis, modification of the cytoskeleton of the cell including tubules and filaments may result in sequestration of organelles by ER, the first step in autophagocytosis. Alterations in the ribosome-membrane relationships are often observed either as prelethal changes following acute lethal injury or as parts of chronic sublethal interactions. Conditions that interfere with the ribosome-membrane interactions also result in the inhibition of protein synthesis, and polysome dissociation occurs. Ultimately, this results in a rather random dispersion of free ribosome units within the cell sap. In several experimental systems this has been shown to be reversible.

It should also be borne in mind that inhibition of protein synthesis itself does not necessarily result in membrane detachment of ribosomes. For example, the antibiotic cycloheximide that inhibits protein synthesis apparently does not promote such dissociation and in fact tends to stabilize the polysomes.

Golgi Apparatus

Morphologically, the Golgi apparatus of an injured cell shows dilatation, fragmentation, and wrapping. Hypertrophy of Golgi apparatus in denervated muscles has been described. During the process of squamous metaplasia in the bronchial epithelium, the cells undergoing regeneration and metaplasia are small mucous granule cells. These cells, which are capable of division and keratinization, exhibit marked hyperplasia and hypertrophy of the Golgi components. The Golgi apparatus can extend entirely across the apical half of the cytoplasm (30).

Secretory Granules

Secretory granules usually arise from the maturing face of the Golgi cisternae. These granules, which may contain a variety of products such as polypeptides, hormones, mucus, melanin, and other mucopolysaccharides, are usually typical for the particular cell differentiation. It has been found recently that the histogenesis of epidermoid metaplasia in the bronchus consists of a proliferation and keratinization in mucous cells.

Lysosomes

Lysosomes are digestive organelles which either serve as a means for organelle turnover (autophagy) or digestion of extracellular-derived material (heterophagy). See recent reviews concerning the role of lysosomes in injury and disease (9, 18).

Autophagic vacuoles form by exotrophy into a cisternae of ER or some other part of the cytocavitary network enclosing a portion of the cytoplasm, such as a mitochondrion in a double-walled sac. Digestive enzymes are added by fusion of endosecretory vesicles or digestive vacuoles with the outer membrane of the autophagic vacuole. The inner membrane thickens, resembling the membrane of other digestive vacuoles. It has been estimated that autophagy could account for the rate of mitochondrial turnover (half-life 10 days) in the liver (29). Glycogen turnover in liver also occurs within autophagic vacuoles. Autophagy may provide nutrition under injurious conditions such as starvation, specific dietary deficiencies, or inhibition of protein synthesis. Thus the cell is able to utilize its own substance to maintain homeostasis under these adverse conditions.

Multivesicular body (MVB) formation appears to represent a special case of autophagocytosis where budding of cytoplasm as small exotropic buds into phagosomes results in internal vesicles containing materials usually found within the cell sap. These vesicles, in contrast to the principal part of the MVB, contain autophagocytized material. The rest of the MVB may contain heterophagocytized material, and when the vesicles later breakdown, a mixed type of residual body is found. Multivesicular bodies occur as normal constituents of cells; however, they are found to increase in number following several types of sublethal injury.

Heterophagy refers to the esotropic uptake of particles such as macromolecules or macromolecular complexes from the external plasma membrane surface. This uptake is referred to as endocytosis or pinocytosis. The heterophagosomes formed carry ingested material toward the cell center where they acquire acid hydrolases by fusing with Golgi-derived vesicles or with preexisting vacuoles to form new digestive vacuoles. The material within the heterophagosome can then be hydrolyzed to soluble intermediates which can be reutilized or released to the cell. Some debris, mostly lipid, can remain and this frequently is auto-oxidized forming lipofuscin, or aging pigment. These indigestible materials are contained within structures with a single membrane and are now called residual bodies. Depending on the cell type they may either accumulate in the cells or fuse with the plasma membranes and discharge their debris.

Heterophagy is important in producing cellular changes in many disease processes. Normally phagocytosis results in a relatively rapid turnover of ingested material. However, in chronic injury extensive uptake of foreign material may deplete the reservoirs of acid hydrolases resulting in slow or incomplete digestion. The cell's ability to produce and transport acid hydrolases may be impaired leading to accumulation of materials inside these lysosomal systems. Lysosomal storage diseases may result from deficient digestion or synthesis of abnormal materials which cannot be digested by the cell's normal enzymes. Both heterophagy and autophagy are energy requiring processes and injury which interferes with bioenergetics also regulates their activity.

Peroxisomes

Peroxisomes or microbodies represent a distinct group of vacuoles that form as diverticula of the cytocavitary network in a variety of different cell types. Microbodies are limited by a single thin (65–70 Å) membrane. They also have a finely granular inner matrix and in some species an electron dense amorphous or paracrystalline core. Frequently peroxisomes contain a marginal plate, which is separated from the limiting membrane by a narrow space.

Microbodies contain a number of peroxidative enzymes such as catalase, urate oxidase, D-amino acid oxidase, and malatase synthetase. Their enzymes are thought to participate in cellular respiration, gluconeogenesis, and purine and lipid metabolism (39). Recently it has been shown that peroxisomes may play a major role in β-oxidation of fatty acids in cells (27).

Because the significance of peroxisomes in normal cells has not been completely elucidated,

their significance in injured cells is also unclear. Two diseases, however, have been classified as peroxisome related. These are acatalasemia and the cerebro-hepato-renal syndrome of Zellweger. In acatalasemia, there are very low concentrations of catalase in the liver as well as in other organs. In the cerebro-hepato-renal syndrome, the total concentration of liver catalase is similar to that found in normal liver, but peroxisomes are not able to be detected by histochemical techniques. Since, as mentioned above, peroxisomes appear to be ubiquitous, such diseases as hypercholesterolemia and hyperlipidemia could also be the result of peroxisomal defects.

Peroxisomal presence has also been used as an indicator of differentiation of tumor cells. Since much of the work involving peroxisomes in normal cells as well as in tumors has been done in experimental animals, we will need many more studies with human material in order to understand the role of the peroxisome in health and disease.

Mitochondria

The changes that mitochondria undergo after acute lethal cell injury are mentioned above. In this section we will consider changes associated with chronic sublethal injury.

Abnormally functioning cells often develop mitochondrial inclusions which may represent insoluble precipitations of ions, abnormal protein depositions, rearrangements of membranes or other phospholipids forming lamellar inclusions, or focal changes in the conformation of matrix proteins. Ion accumulation represents a common way in which the energized state is discharged through energized reactions supported by either ATP or substrate and oxygen. Often the phosphate is taken up simultaneously with calcium and results in the formation of insoluble phosphates within the mitochondrion. If both calcium and ADP are simultaneously introduced to a mitochondrion, calcium will be preferentially accumulated and ATP will not be phosphorylated until all calcium has been removed from the medium. Thus, if mitochondria are continually exposed to high concentrations of calcium, they will not phosphorylate ADP and will ultimately be destroyed. An example is the irreversible injury that occurs in mitochondria in which the permeability of the cell membrane has been altered, resulting in calcium leakage into the cell and reversal of the cytoplasmic ionic sodium to potassium ratio.

Deposits of iron salts in the inner compartment of mitochondria occur in a variety of sideroblastic anemias, which presumably have in common a block in the heme synthesis such as the inhibition of the enzyme ferrochelatase (50). These blockages result in transport of iron into the mitochondria but failure to incorporate it into heme, with accumulation of iron phosphate-type complexes. This can occur in lead poisoning and in pyridoxine deficiency, but it is commonly idiopathic. Many of these patients ultimately develop leukemia. The accumulation of these iron complexes results in the formation of the so-called ringed sideroblasts. This term refers to the ring of Prussian blue-positive cytoplasmic granules surrounding the nucleus.

Certain mitochondrial changes in disease are best understood in terms of alterations in mitochondrial growth and replication. Enlarged mitochondria (megamitochondria) are to be distinguished from mitochondrial enlargement due to swelling, in which the increased size is largely due to the uptake of water. Megamitochondria can be observed in liver cells in alcoholism as round eosinophilic inclusions often larger than the cell nucleus (25, 38). Treatment with copper chelating agents, essential fatty acid deficiency, vitamin E-selenium deficiency, cirrhosis, and nonhemolytic jaundice are some other conditions associated with enlarged liver mitochondria. Mitochondrial enlargement is also present in kidney tubules in tubular necrosis, and in tissue culture cells under abnormal growth conditions. Fusion of mitochondria or failure of mitochondrial fission may be involved in the pathogenesis of the enlargement. Mitochondria may show extreme pleomorphism with scalloping of mitochondrial margins, protrusions of one mitochondrion into another, and formation of crystal-like patterns within the mitochondria. Pleomorphism has been seen in neoplastic cells. Variation of the number of mitochondria can also be observed. Simple starvation of the rat results in a marked decrease in mitochondrial number within a few days; however, refeeding reverses this change.

Nucleus

Several types of inclusions located in the nucleoplasm have been described in chronically injured cells. The most common is crystalline arrays of virus particles. Intranuclear inclusions may also occur in the nuclei of renal tubules in bismuth or lead poisoning. Many other kinds of accumulation of vesicles, glycogen, concentric lamellar bodies, fibrillar structures, vacuoles, and tubular or filamentous inclusions have been described in nuclei. There are also pseudoinclusions which represent deep cytoplasmic indentations into the nucleus that, because of the plane of section, appear to reside within the nucleoplasm. As the nuclei become irregular, pseudoinclusions increase in number and they are often observed to occur in cells undergoing rapid turnover. However, breakdown of the envelope may occur after a period of time, resulting in true inclusions.

The nuclear membrane may have deep infoldings resulting in a marked redundancy of the nuclear envelope or cerebriform nucleus in mycosis fungoides and the Sezary syndrome. Herpes simplex infections cause extensive reduplication of the membrane where great protrusions of the envelope contain extremely attenuated portions of nucleoplasm and result in formation of multilayered structures.

Nucleolus

Many carcinogenic and antimetabolic agents induce changes in the structure and function of the nucleolus. Among these are actinomycin D, aflotoxin, and ultraviolet irradiation, all of which interfere with DNA-dependent RNA synthesis. These agents cause segregation or stratification of the nucleolar components into regions composed of particles, RNA-protein fibrils, and chromatin fibrils. There is also an altered RNA-protein component or dense plaque. They also apparently arrest the production of RNA subunits within the nucleolus (as well as in the nucleus).

In another category are agents exhibiting differential effects during the cell cycle, the so-called spindle poisons which include colchicine, griseofulvin, vincristine, and vinblastine. All these agents presumably interfere with the formation of the mitotic spindle, possibly by binding with specific microtubule proteins, thus blocking the process of mitosis in metaphase. Evidence indicates that microtubule subunit synthesis parallels mitosis but that subunits are stable and may persist in cells for several days.

Integrated Cell Reactions

In this portion of the chapter we will discuss reactions of the cell as a whole to chronic, sublethal injury. These reactions represent altered states, sometimes steady states, in which the cell maintains survival though sustaining continual injury or abnormal stimulation.

Atrophy

The term atrophy refers to decreased size of cell dry mass resulting from various factors. Etiologies include decreased work load, decreased nutrition, hypoxia, or decreased hormonal stimulation. The decrease in cell mass implies decrease in cell components. Typically, an increase in the number of autophagic vacuoles is found in cells undergoing atrophy as well as increasing numbers of residual bodies containing lipofuscin. Atrophic muscle may show breakdown and decrease in number of myofilaments, fragmentation of the endoplasmic reticulum, and swelling and degeneration of mitochondria.

Hypertrophy

One response to abnormal cell stimulation is hypertrophy, which refers to increased cell size. Ultrastructurally, it is often reflected by an increase in the size and number of organelles. Hypertrophy in muscle cells represents an adaptation to an increased workload. In the heart muscle cells, there is an increase in the amounts of sarcoplasmic reticulum, ribosomes, and numbers of myofilaments. The increase in organelles in turn increase the work capacity of the muscle. Mitochondria, in some instances, show a deficiency of cristal membranes which may relate to increased susceptibility of hypertrophied heart muscle to cardiac failure.

In the liver, many lipid-soluble compounds such as phenobarbital induce mixed function oxidases with the synthesis of endoplasmic reticulum membranes. The liver cell then undergoes hypertrophy which can be thought of as a protective adaptation as it substantially augments drug detoxifying ability.

Fatty Changes

The accumulation of lipid within the cell cytoplasm is a common sublethal reaction to injury. Although the appearance of the cells may be greatly changed, cells can exist with large amounts of triglyceride for long periods. Fatty changes occur in the liver cells, as a common accompaniment of many human diseases, especially chronic alcoholism. Lipids reach the liver mostly as alimentary chylomicrons or fatty acids from adipose tissue and are either utilized within the liver or secreted as lipoproteins. Small triglyceride droplets within the endoplasmic reticulum and the Golgi complex reflect the formation of lipoprotein particles. If the delivery of lipid to the liver is increased and the metabolic capacity of the liver is exceeded, as in conditions of fat mobilization, these triglycerides will accumulate.

Virus-Cell Interactions

Although many viruses are rapidly lethal to cells, other viruses have achieved variable degrees of adaptation, as in totally inapparent endosymbiotic infections, latent infections, slow virus infection, and malignant transformation of cells with disappearance of virus. Structural abnormalities in the infected cells may accompany these functional changes, depending on the type of virus and the type of infection. Large nuclear inclusions, often containing crystalline aggregates of virions, are typically seen with DNA viruses and cytoplasmic inclusions are seen with RNA viruses. Viral specified effects on cell membranes include changes in plasma membrane composition in the case of influenza virus, extensive fusion and redundancy of the nuclear envelope in herpes virus, proliferation of ER associated in vaccinia virus replication, and large filamentous cytoplasmic inclusions in measles virus (8, 17).

Aging

Specific cellular features of aging have not been identified; however, in many cells including neurons and heart muscle cells, the accumulation of lipofuscin segment exhibits a roughly linear increase with age (15). Changes in membrane lipid composition are thought to occur which reduce the fluidity and change functional characteristics (28). Other changes that may occur in aging are similar to those seen in atrophic cells. The neurons of some types of presenile dementia are typical. Although many theories of aging have been advanced, definite data have been difficult to obtain (56).

Regeneration and Repair

Undifferentiated cells occur in many pathologic reactions, such as regenerating epithelia or mesenchyme, many types of hyperplasia, embryonic tissue and hematomas, elements of the hematopoietic system, and neoplasia.

Undifferentiated cells are usually rounded or have only a few irregular processes, their shape depending on the environment and on adjacent structures. They often do not show typical membrane specializations of differentiated cells, such as microvilli or cilia. They are also characterized by a high ratio of nuclear to cytoplasmic volume. However, the cytoplasm is usually basophilic and pyroninophilic, owing to the high concentration of RNA expressed as numerous polysomes, which are predominantly free within the cell sap; relatively few profiles of rough endoplasmic reticulum are present. Mitochondria often are inconspicuous, probably reflecting well-developed systems for both aerobic and anaerobic glycolysis. Digestive vacuoles or lysosomes are usually not prominent, although early in regeneration in organs such as liver and kidney large autophagic vacuoles may indeed occur. Not all types of endoplasmic storage and secretory vacuoles are prominent. Nuclei are large, often because they are polyploid, and various abnormalities of mitotic division may occur. Nucleoli are numerous, large, and full of particles, presumably representing ribosome precursors and perhaps other forms of RNA.

These features probably reflect the fact that the transcription and translation systems are primarily directed toward the task of division. If differentiation occurs after division is completed, the appearance of the specialized organelles characteristic of the particular cell type can be readily followed, while in the case of malignant neoplasms, differentiation usually does not occur.

Metaplasia

The concept of metaplasia implies the replacement of one type of cellular differentiation by another. The usual explanation was that the new cell type differentiated from undifferentiated stem cells. Currently, it has become evident that in the bronchial epithelium and possibly in other cells as well there is direct conversion from one differentiated cell type to another (31). Mucous cells of the bronchus directly convert to stratified squamous epithelium. In the bronchus, epidermoid metaplasia is related to goblet cell hyperplasia which represents an early reaction to injury, later converted to squamous cells. Epidermoid metaplasia can follow either carcinogenic or noncarcinogenic stimuli.

References

1. Arstila, A. U., Hirsimäki, Y., Hirsimäki, P., and Sorvari, T. E. (1980): Cellular microtubules and microfilaments. Physiological and pathological aspects. In *Pathobiology of Human Disease*, edited by B. F. Trump, R. T. Jones, and A. Laufer. Fischer Verlag, New York (in press).
2. Berezesky, I. K., Chang, S. H., Pendergrass, R. E., Bulger, R. E., Mergner, W. J., and Trump, B. F. (1977): Applications of x-ray microanalysis to human and experimental pathology, pp. 524–525, edited by G. W. Bailey. 35th Annual Proceedings of the Electron Microscopy Society of America.
3. Brattain, M. B., Pittman, J. M., and Pretlow, T. G. (1976): The use of glutaraldehyde-conjugated horseradish peroxidase-bovine serum albumin in the visualization of concanavalin A binding to tissue sections of human colinic tumor. *Lab. Invest.*, 35:537–541.
4. Bygrave, and Fyfe, L. (1978): Mitochondria and the control of intracellular calcium. *Biol. Rev.*, 53:43–70.
5. Collan, Y., McDowell, E. M., and Trump, B. F. (1979): Studies on the pathogenesis of ischemic cell injury; VI. Mitochondrial flocculent densities of ischemia. *Lab. Invest.* (in preparation).
6. Collan, Y., Smith, M. W., and Trump, B. F. (1980): Ischemia-induced changes in potassium, sodium, magnesium, calcium and phosphate content in kidney mitochondria (in preparation).
7. Cook, J. S. (1975): Photopathology of the erythrocyte membrane. In *Pathobiology of Cell Membranes, Vol. I*, pp. 199–213, edited by B. F. Trump and A. U. Arstila. Academic Press, New York.
8. Dalton, A. J., and Haguenau, F. (1973): *Ultrastructure of Animal Viruses and Bacteriophages.* Academic Press, New York.
9. Ericsson, J. L. E., and Brunk, U. T. (1975): Alterations in lysosomal membranes as related to disease processes. In *Pathobiology of Cell Membranes, Vol. I*, pp. 217–254, edited by B. F. Trump and A. U. Arstila. Academic Press, New York.
10. Gaja, G., Ferrero, M. E., Piccoletti, R., and Bernelli-Zazzera, A. (1973): Phosphorylation and redox states in ischemic liver. *Exp. Mol. Pathol.*, 19:248–265.
11. Garcia, J. H., and Lossinsky, A. S. (1980): Cellular pathology of ischemic stroke. In *Pathobiology of Human Disease*, edited by B. F. Trump, R. T. Jones, and A. Laufer. Fischer Verlag, New York (in press).
12. Glaumann, B., Glaumann, H., Berezesky, I. K., and Trump, B. F. (1975): Studies on the pathogenesis of ischemic cell injury; II. Morphological changes of the pars convoluta (P_1 and P_2) of the proximal tubule of the rat kidney made ischemic in vivo. *Virchows Arch. B. Cell Pathol.*, 19: 281–302.
13. Glaumann, B., Glaumann, H., Berezesky, I. K., and Trump, B. F. (1977): Studies on cellular recovery from injury; II. Ultrastructural studies on the recovery of the pars convoluta of the proximal tubule of the rat kidney from temporary ischemia. *Virchows Arch. B. Cell Pathol.*, 24:1–18.
14. Glaumann, B., and Trump, B. F. (1975): Studies on the pathogenesis of ischemic cell injury; III. Morphological changes of the proximal pars recta tubules (P_3) of the rat kidney made ischemic in vivo. *Virchows Arch. B. Cell Pathol.*, 19:303–323.
15. Glees, P. (1975): Maturation and aging of vertebrate neurons. In *Metabolic Compartmentation and Neurotransmission*, p. 433, edited by S. Beri and D. D. Clarke. Plenum Press, New York.
16. Goldblatt, P. J., Trump, B. F., and Stowell, R. E. (1965): Studies on necrosis of mouse liver in vitro. Alterations in some histochemically demonstrable hepatocellular enzymes. *Am. J. Pathol.*, 47:183–208.
17. Grimley, P. M., and Demsey, A. (1980): Functions and alterations of cell membranes during active virus injection. In *Pathobiology of Cell Membranes, Vol. II*, pp. 93–168, edited by B. F. Trump and A. U. Arstila. Academic Press, New York.
18. Hawkins, H. K. (1980): Reactions of lysosomes to cell injury. In *Pathobiology of Cell Membranes, Vol. II*, pp. 251–285, edited by B. F. Trump and A. U. Arstila. Academic Press, New York.
19. Hawkins, H. K., Ericsson, J. L. E., Biberfield, P., and Trump, B. F. (1972): Lysosome and phagosome stability in lethal cell injury. *Am. J. Pathol.*, 68:255–287.
20. Hems, D. A., and Brosnan, J. T. (1970): Effects of ischemia on content of metabolites in rat liver and kidney in vivo. *Biochem. J.*, 120:105–111.
21. Hendrix, R. W., and Zwaan, J. (1975): The matrix of the optic vesicle-presumptive lens interface during induction of the lens in the chick embryo. *J. Embryol. Exp. Morphol.*, 33:1023–1049.

22. Hicks, R. M., and Wakefield, J. J. (1976): Membrane changes during urothelial hyperplasia and neoplasia. *Cancer Res.*, 36:2502–2507.

23. Kahng, M. W., Berezesky, I. K., and Trump, B. F. (1978): Metabolic and ultrastructural response of rat kidney cortex to in vitro ischemia. *Exp. Mol. Pathol.*, 29:183–198.

24. Kobayashi, Y., Sawada, J.-I., and Osawa, T. (1979): Activation of membrane phospholipase A by guinea pig lymphotoxin (GLT). *J. Immunol.*, 122:791–794.

25. Koch, O. R., Roatta de Conti, L. L., Bolanos, L. P., and Stoppani, A. D. (1978): Ultrastructure and biochemical aspects of liver mitochondria during recovery from ethanol induced alterations. Experimental evidence for mitochondrial division. *Am. J. Pathol.*, 90:325–344.

26. Laufer, A. (1980): Immune damage to the myocardium. In *Pathobiology of Human Disease*, edited by B. F. Trump, R. T. Jones, and A. Laufer. Fischer Verlag, New York (in press).

27. Lazarow, P. B. (1978): Rat liver peroxisomes catalyze the β oxidation of fatty acids. *J. Biol. Chem.*, 253:1522–1528.

28. Lenaz, G., Curatola, G., and Masotti, L. (1975): Perturbation of membrane fluidity. *J. Bioenerg.*, 7:223–299.

29. Locke, M., and Collins, J. V. (1980): Organelle turnover. In *Pathobiology of Cell Membranes, Vol. II*, pp. 223–248, edited by B. F. Trump and A. U. Arstila. Academic Press, New York.

30. McDowell, E. M., Barrett, L. A., and Trump, B. F. (1976): Observations on small granule cells in adult human bronchial epithelium and in carcinoid and oat cell tumors. *Lab. Invest.*, 34:202–206.

31. McDowell, E. M., Becci, P. J., Barrett, L. A., and Trump, B. F. (1978): Morphogenesis and classification of lung cancer. In *Pathogenesis and Therapy of Lung Cancer, Vol. 10*, pp. 445–519, edited by C. C. Harris. Marcel Dekker, New York.

32. Mayer, M. M. (1977): Mechanism of cytolysis by lymphocytes; a comparison with complement (Presidential Address to American Association of Immunologists). *J. Immunol.*, 119:1195–1203.

33. Mergner, W. J., and McDonnell, M. (1978): Phospholipase activity in normal aged and ischemic mitochondria. *Lab. Invest.*, 38:357.

34. Mergner, W. J., Smith, M. W., and Trump, B. F. (1977): Studies on the pathogenesis of ischemic cell injury; XI. P/O ratio and acceptor control. *Virchows Arch. B. Cell Pathol.*, 26:17–26.

35. Mergner, W. J., Smith, M. W., Sahaphong, S., and Trump, B. F. (1977): Studies on the pathogenesis of ischemic cell injury; VI. Accumulation of calcium by isolated mitochondria of ischemic rat kidney cortex. *Virchows Arch. B. Cell Pathol.*, 26:1–16.

36. Mergner, W. J., Chang, S.-H., Marzella, L., Kahng, M. W., and Trump, B. F. (1979): Studies on the pathogenesis of ischemic cell injury; VIII. ATPase of rat kidney mitochondria. *Lab. Invest.*, 40:686–694.

37. Mergner, W. J., Marzella, L., Mergner, C., Kahng, M. W., Smith, M. W., and Trump, B. F. (1977): Studies on the pathogenesis of ischemic cell injury; VII. Proton gradient and respiration of renal tissue cubes, renal mitochondrial and submitochondrial particles following ischemic cell injury. *Beitr. Pathol.*, 161:230–243.

38. Porta, E. A., Koch, O. R., and Hartoft, W. S. (1970): Recent advances in molecular pathology; a review of the effects of alcohol on the liver. *Exp. Mol. Pathol.*, 12:104–132.

39. Riede, U. N. (1980): Structure and function of peroxisomes and their role in disease processes. In *Pathobiology of Cell Membranes, Vol. II*, pp. 173–220, edited by B. F. Trump and A. U. Arstila. Academic Press, New York (in press).

40. Rovetto, M. J., Lamberton, W. F., and Neely, J. R. (1975): Mechanism of glycolytic inhibition in ischemic rat heart. *Circ. Res.*, 37:742–751.

41. Sahaphong, S., and Trump, B. F. (1971): Studies of cellular injury in isolated kidney tubules of the flounder; V. Effects of inhibiting sulfhydryl groups of plasma membrane with organic mercurials PCMB and PCM BS. *Am. J. Pathol.*, 63:277–288.

42. Smith, M. W., Collan, Y., Kahng, M. W., and Trump, B. F. (1980): Changes in mitochondrial lipids of rat kidney during ischemia. *Biochim. Biophys. Acta*, 618:192–201.

43. Smuckler, E. R., and Trump, B. F. (1968): Alterations in the structure and function of the rough-surfaced endoplasmic reticulum during necrosis in vitro. *Am. J. Pathol.*, 53:315–329.

44. Spooner, B. S. (1975): Microfilaments, microtubules, and extracellular material in morphogenesis. *Bioscience*, 25:440–451.

45. Stephens, R. E., and Edds, K. T. (1976): Microtubules: structure, chemistry and function. *Physiol. Rev.*, 56:709–777.

46. Trump, B. F., and Ginn, F. L. (1969): The pathogenesis of subcellular reaction to lethal injury. In *Methods and Achievements in Experimental Pathology, Vol. 4*, pp. 1–29, edited by E. Bajusz and G. Jasmin. S. Karger, Basel.

47. Trump, B. F., and Mergner, W. J. (1974): Cell injury. In *The Inflammatory Process, Vol. 1*, Ed. 2, pp. 115–257, edited by B. W. Zweifach, L. Grant, and R. T. McClusky. Academic Press, New York.

48. Trump, B. F., Goldblatt, P. J., and Stowell, R. E. (1965): Studies of necrosis in vitro of mouse hepatic parenchymal cells. Ultrastructural alterations of cytosomes, cytosegresomes, multivesicular bodies, and microbodies and their relation to the lysosome concept. *Lab. Invest.*, 14:1946–1968.

49. Trump, B. F., Jesudasen, M. L., and Jones, R. T. (1978): Ultrastructural features of diseased cells. In *Diagnostic Electron Microscopy, Vol. 1*, pp. 1–88, edited by B. F. Trump and R. T. Jones. John Wiley & Sons, New York.

50. Trump, B. F., Barrett, L. A., Valigorsky, J. M., and Jiji, R. M. (1975): Ultrastructural studies of sideroblastic anemia. In *Iron Metabolism and Its Disorders, Vol. 3*, pp. 251–263, edited by H. Kief. Elsevier-North Holland, New York.

51. Trump, B. F., Mergner, W. J., Kahng, M. W., and Saladino, A. J. (1976): Studies on the subcellular pathophysiology of ischemia. *Circulation*, 53(Suppl. 1): 17–26.

52. Trump, B. F., Berezesky, I. K., Chang, S. H., Pendergrass, R. E., and Mergner, W. J. (1979): The role of ion shifts in cell injury. In *Scanning Electron Microscopy III*, pp. 1–14, edited by O. Johari. SEM, Inc., A.M.F. O'Hare, Ill.

53. Trump, B. F., Berezesky, I. K., Collan, Y., Kahng, M. W., and Mergner, W. J. (1976): Recent studies on the pathophysiology of ischemic cell injury. *Beitr. Pathol.*, 158:363–388.

54. Trump, B. F., and Arstila, A. U. (1975): Cell membranes and disease processes. In *Pathobiology of Cell Membranes, Vol. I*, pp. 1–52, edited by B. F. Trump and A. U. Arstila. Academic Press, New York.

55. Trump, B. F., McDowell, E. M., Glavin, F., Barrett, L. A., Becci, P. J., Schürch, W., Kaiser, H. E., and Harris, C. C. (1978): The respiratory epithelium; III. Histogenesis of epidermoid metaplasia and carcinoma in situ in the human. *J. Natl. Cancer Inst.*, 61:563–576.

56. Walton, J. (1980): Mechanisms of biological aging. In *Pathobiology of Human Disease*, edited by B. F. Trump, R. T. Jones, and A. Laufer. Fischer Verlag, New York (in press).

57. Weinstein, R. S., Alroy, J., and Pauli, B. U. (1980): Pathobiology of cell junctions. In *Pathobiology of Human Disease*, edited by B. F. Trump, R. T. Jones, and A. Laufer. Fischer Verlag, New York (in press).

58. Whalen, D. A., Hamilton, D. G., Ganote, C. E., and Jennings, R. B. (1974): Effects of a transient period of ischemia on myocardial cells; I. Effects on cell volume regulation. *Am. J. Pathol.*, 74:381–397.

59. Wolosewick, J. J., and Porter, K. R. (1976): Stereo high-voltage electron microscopy of whole cells of the human diploid line WI-38. *Am. J. Anat.*, 147:303–323.

13

Ontogenetic and Complementary Aspects of Neoplastic Growth

Hans E. Kaiser

INTRODUCTION

Each organism undergoes different phases in its life cycle until it matures and dies. Growth abnormalities can occur in each of these phases. Neoplastic growth can take place in each developmental stage of an organism with true tissue development. It is the aim of this chapter to review the types of neoplasms and related disorders in the different organisms which develop from the transitional growth stages in direct or indirect development. In looking at these processes of neoplasms deriving from tissues with embryonal potential, several direct groups of neoplasms and several influencing factors important for their development may be distinguished. The group of tumors of this type includes: (a) embryonal tumors in man and in domesticated as well as laboratory animals (scarcely known in other species), (b) tumors of childhood, (c) teratomas, (d) tumors of the placentae (mammalian and nonmammalian), (e) tumors of larvae, and (f) tumors of, or with the involvement of, meristems.

The development of these neoplasms and related growth conditions, is in some organisms, restricted in their embryonal potential by the following factors: (a) cell replacement—life span of cells and tissues, (b) life span of organisms, (c) the species specific capacity of healing or repair from a wound to DNA repair, (d) capacity of regeneration, and (e) capacity of cell-invariability.

The last matter of concern and of theoretical and practical implication is the variability of the same neoplasms, deriving from the same type of tissue in the diversification of its malignancy in different species and the question of theoretical and practical malignancy, including premalignant conditions.

NEOPLASMS WITH EMBRYONAL POTENTIAL

If considered in a comparative sense, embryonal tumors have to be seen as tumors/neoplasms deriving from tissues with, at the time of tumor origin, persisting embryonal potential. The tumors may be typed as abnormal growths with limited growth potential (especially if the types of abnormal growth of plants are included). In this summarization the types of abnormal growth are arranged according to the duration of the theoretical embryonal potential of the tissues of origin (Table 13.1).

The term "embryonal tumors" in the medical sciences is used for tumors which develop between the zygote and before birth of the child or animal. The tumors of the youth stages are generally reviewed in medicine as tumors of childhood. Indirectly related to this kind of tumor are neoplasms of the placenta. With man, it is important to evaluate the embryonal cell theory of cancer by Joseph Cohnheim (the foremost student of Virchow). Cohnheim's theory states that remnants of embryonal cell nests in the adult organism may be able to develop into neoplasms. This theory about the cells, with at least theoretically persisting embryonal potential under abnormal conditions in the mammalian body, leads to those cell and tissue groups with normally, at least theoretically, unlimited em-

Table 13.1
Duration of the Embryonal Potential of Animal and Plant Tissues[a]

Selected Tissues or Tissue Groups	Life Expectancy										
	0	10	20	30	40	50	60	70	80	90	100%
Apical meristems	⊢————————————————————————————————————→
Residual meristems such as lateral meristems	⊢————————————————————————————————————→
Larval tissues such as imaginal discs of holometabolic insects	⊢——————————————————————————→ +/− (near 90)
Larval tissues of cirriped cypris: *Sacculina*	⊢———————————————→
Larval tissues of other invertebrates	⊢————————– – – – –?– – –→
Mammalian tissues in general	⊢→
Succeeding meristems originating from fully diffferentiated tissues such as phellogen	? ⊢———→ (from ~20 to ~40)
Red bone marrow deriving from yellow bone marrow	? ⊢– –?– –→ (from ~20 to ~30)

[a] ? = variability of embryonal reaction according to requirement; - - - - - = limited embryonal potential.

bryonal potential in higher plants, the so-called meristematic cells and tissues. Furthermore, comparable tissues exist in certain phases of invertebrate development, such as the embryonal buds and discs, for example in holometabolous insects. We know that, in cases of cellular injury, injury can be considered as the prerequisite of neoplastic growth (Virchow's theory) and leads either to repair by regeneration or neoplastic growth controlled more or less by hormones: ecdysones, the moulting hormones, and juvenile hormones and others, such as auxins in plants and in vertebrates. Carcinogens act with the primarily normal cell by interfering with metabolism through chemical pathways as described by Weisburger (Chapter 17). Interference in the metabolism of insects is caused by the hormonomimetic insecticides which mimic the effect of certain growth hormones and represent an inappropriate action of certain hormones at an inappropriate time for the organism. The result is a lethal interference which may lead a fifth instar insect to a seventh instar, followed by death instead of the development of the fifth instar into an adult insect or imago. Thousands of compounds have been detected and isolated and it is interesting to note that these compounds act either on whole families, certain genera of a family, or in a species-specific manner. But all interfere in the species-specific process of growth. The malignant melanoma is a tumor which is characterized by the dark pigment melanin (see Chapters 29 and 38). It was shown by Giordano et al. (Chapter 38) that this compound exists in vertebrates, invertebrates, and plants. The moulting hormones of insects and crustaceans are also found in plants but up to now have not been discovered in vertebrates.[1]

Neoplasms in larval stages, for example *Lepidoptera* and *Drosophila*, have been listed in Chapter 48.

Embryonal Tumors in Man

Not only the organisms, but also the organs, the tissues, and the cells exhibit development which is characterized by incompleted or youthful forms of the aforementioned structures. Accordingly it is possible to distinguish between neoplasms, such as those of whole organs or body portions as they occur in the teratomas, neoplasms of embryonal structures before birth such as embryonal tumors, tumors of the later gestation period, the fetal tumors, and finally tumors of childhood. Tumors from youth stages of cells, and also systemic diseases such as certain leukemias which develop from cellular youth stages, are not included here but are described in Chapter 43. The most important embryonal tumors in man are listed in Table 13.2.

Tumors of Childhood

Neoplasms of childhood are those which occur most frequently in young persons before reaching adolescence. Certain intestinal polyps of the human have even been called "children's

---

[1] A. Butenandt, personal communication.

Table 13.2
Tumors in Man

A. Embryonal Tumors (4, 70, 135, 349)

Type of Tumor	Site	Characteristics	Comparability Based on Embryonal Potential
Reinoblastoma	Eye	Embryonic tumors derive from embryonic precursors of different tissues	Comparable to man's embryonic tumors is abnormal growth processes of certain larval tissues in invertebrates and meristematic proliferations
Nephroblastoma	Kidney		
Embryonic tumors	Liver		
Embryonic sarcomas	Urogenital tract		

B. Mixed Tumors (29, 113, 349)

Type of Tumor	Site	Characteristics
Mixed tumor of skin	Skin	General: derive from pluripotential cells of one germ layer enabling them to differentiate in more than one tissue; result in mixed characteristics; no organ differentiation metastasize in most cases with sarcomatous component only
Mixed tumor of salivary glands	Salivary glands	
Hepatoblastoma	Liver	
Nephroblastoma	Kidney	
Mixed tumors of thyroid[a]		
Mixed tumors of uterus[b]	Uterine epithelium, uterine wall	
Mesenchymoma	Variable	
Mixed gliomas	Nervous system	
Mixed sarcoma and glioma	Nervous system	
Mixed meningeal tumors and sarcomas		

[a] Metastasizing mostly with sarcomatous tissue only.
[b] Some contain rhabdomyoblastic elements.

polyps" ("*Kinderpolypen*" in the German literature). One of the best known malignant neoplasm of this group is Wilms' tumor (embryoma or embryonal adenosarcoma) in which the average age of the patients is 3 years. Most of the neoplasms in childhood are of the mixed type because they derive generally from cells with multiple potentials, but from one germ layer in contrast to teratomas from several germ layers (Table 13.3).

Teratomas

The teratomas in man occur especially in the pineal body, the mediastinum, cystic or solid in the ovaries, and also in the testis. In the testis a lesion called teratocarcinoma may be also found. The characteristics are summarized in Table 13.4.

Tumors of Placenta

The tissues of the placenta can be indirectly considered as embryonal because they persist only so long as the embryo is in the womb. In the mammal placenta, neoplasms have been seen in several species but not in all and they are rarely described in species other than man (Table 13.5). To the author's knowledge, tumors in placentae of reptiles, thaliacea, and other invertebrates have not been observed.

Tumors of Larvae

Knowledge of tumors of larvae is still very scarce if the number of species with larval development and the number of tumors described from larvae are considered. According to the embryonal potential, several categories can be compared. It must be assumed that the purpose of larval development is a better and more efficient use of the environment. It will be useful to classify new findings according the following system, depending on the increase or decrease of structural and functional differences between larval and adult organisms. From the point of view of comparative pathology, two questions are essential: (a) where are the main growth processes taking place in the larval or in the

Table 13.3
Tumors of Childhood (Selected Aspects) (98, 173, 287, 349)

Diagnosis: Tumors of childhood are a heterogenous group of neoplasms characterized by frequency in early stages of life. Sarcomas prevail among malignancies of childhood. Phylogenetic parallel may exist (rule of Haeckel) because sarcomas are considered more frequent in lower vertebrates (fishes) than cancers in higher ones (especially mammals).

Reasoning: Prevalent sarcomas in youth stages may be attributed more to endogenous factors (or those exogenous ones transmitted by the mother), whereas carcinomas in adults and senile persons are attributed to a large extent to exogenous factors (epithelia exposed to environment).

Subgroups: Embryonic tumors, mixed tumors, teratomas, tumors with high percentage in children/young persons.

Selected Types of Malignant Tumors, According to Organ Systems and Organs

Organ system and/or organ	Frequent or most frequent type
I. Circulatory system: Leukemias	Acute lymphatic leukemia
II. Lymphatic system	Lymphosarcoma (Hodgkin's disease)
III. Neoplasms of central nervous system	Medulloblastoma
IV. Sympathic nervous system	Neuroblastoma
V. Retina	Retinoblastoma
VI. Kidney	Nephroblastoma
VII. Liver	Hepatoblastoma
VIII. Bone	Osteosarcoma
IX. Ovary	Dysgerminoma
X. Testis	Embryonal carcinoma
XI. Soft tissues	Rhabdomyosarcoma
XII. Melanogenic system	Melanoma

Histologic Characteristics of Neoplasms of Childhood (A Selection)

1. Neoplasms of cells with embryonal potential (characteristics)	2. Neoplasms of cells with the character of adult (fully differentiated) tissues		3. Others
Germinoma	Astrocytoma	Carcinoma of:	Ewing's tumor
Hepatoblastoma	Ependymoma	Bile ducts and	Histiocytoses
Malignant teratoma	Meningioma	liver cells	Lymphomas
Medulloblastoma	Neurofibroma	Bowel	Melanotic progonoma
Medulloepithelioma	Neurilemmoma	Endocrine glands	
Mesenchymoma	Oligodendroglioma	Salivary glands	
Nephroblastoma	Fibrosarcoma	Skin	
Neuroblastoma	Leiomyosarcoma	Renal pelvis	
Retinoblastoma	Haemangiosarcoma		
Rhabdomyosarcoma	Liposarcoma		
Yolk sac tumors	Osteosarcoma		

Selected Age Distribution of Predominant Occurrence				Review of Percentage of Malignancies According to Tissue Types[a]	
Age 0–4		*Age 5–9*		Leukemias	35%
Neuroblastoma	84%			Eye and CNS	25%
Nephroblastoma	81%	*Age 10–14*		Lymphomas	11%
Leukemia	49%	Neoplasms of bone	68%	Neuroblastoma	7%
Neoplasms of eye and CNS	44%	Lymphoma	42%	Soft tissue sarcomas	6%
Soft tissue sarcomas	40			Nephroblastoma	6%
				Miscellaneous	6%
				Bone neoplasms	4%

[a] The glandular polyp of children is an example of a benign tumor with 100% of appearance in childhood.

adult organism and which stages of this process can be recognized? and (2) which larval structures are dismissed by normal histolysis?

It is worthwhile to look at the crustaceans and insects. Probably the original development of insects was a continual one as may be observed in the lowest members of the class. This continued development led to a concentration of the larval transformation in those stages before the last moulting (homo-, para-, re-, allometabola); the pupa appears as the last youth stage (holometabola). This development results in a contin-

Table 13.4
Teratomas in Man (a Selection) (136, 264, 375) and Animals

A. Man

Place of Origin	Type	Remarks	References
Arteries	Primary teratoma of truncus pulmonalis (case of Joel, 1890) (172)	Extremely rare	(311)
Breast	Benign cystic teratoma (?)		(269)
Cardiac tumors			(174)
CNS	Dermoid cyst		(267)
Colon	Ovarian teratoma (?)		(120, 121)
Cranium	Malignant teratoma		(332)
Eye	Teratoid intraocular medullar epithelioma		(391)
Fallopian tube	Benign cystic teratoma		(157)
Hypothalamus	Hypothalamic tumors		(243)
Intracranial			(101)
Kidney	Dermoid cysts		
	Embryonal adenosarcoma		
	Embryonal teratomas		
	Intrarenal teratoma		(20)
Liver	Teratoid tumors		(81)
	True teratoma		(395, 379)
Lung	Dermoid cysts		
	Malignant teratomas		
Mediastinum	Extragonadal germ cell tumors		(297)
	Giant teratoma		(40, 270)
	Malignant teratoma		(56)
	Primary teratocarcinoma		(365)
Mesentery	Dermoid cyst	(61)	
Mouth, floor of nasopharynx	Dermoid cyst		(392)
	Malignant teratoma		(124)
	Teratoid tumors		(62)
	Teratoma		(12)
Nose	Teratoma of inner nose	Very rare	
Orbit	Teratoma		(158)
Ovary	Cystic teratoma		(126, 239)
	Cystic teratoma with melanocytes		(331)
	Foliculoma		(194)
	Germ cell tumors		(202)
	Malignant teratoma with extraovarian variation		(69, 89, 383)
	Metastatic teratoma with neuroblastoma		(356)
	Squamous cell cancer		(176, 201)
Pericard	Teratoma		(100)
Pharynx	Epignathes		
	Haired polyps		
	Mixed tumors	Rare	
	True teratomas	Extremely rare	

Table 13.4 continued

Place of Origin	Type	Remarks	References
Pineal	Teratoid tumor		(17, 238)
Retroperitoneal space	Extrarenal Wilms' tumor		(4)
	Organismoid teratoma		(124, 251)
	Teratoma		(74)
	Twin teratomas		(319)
Salivary gland	Teratoma		(31)
Spinal canal	Teratoma		(93)
	Teratomatous cyst		(308)
Stomach	Teratoma	Very rare	
	Teratoma		(290)
	Teratoma		(242)
	Teratoma		(254)
Testis	Metastasis of testicular teratoma		(141)
	Teratoma		(16)
	Teratoma		(264)
	Teratoma		(375)
	Teratoma deriving from malignant tumor		(146)
Thymus	Teratoma		(28)
Thyroid	Primary malignant teratoma		(187)
	Teratoma		(294)
	Teratoma		(348)
Tongue	Teratoma		(52)
Urachus	Squamous cell carcinoma		(214)
Urinary bladder	Dermoid cysts		
	Malignant teratomas		
Uterus	Cervix		
	Dermoid cysts	Extremely rare	(375)
	Fundus		
	Solid benign teratomas	Extremely rare	
	Malignant embryonal teratomas		
Vulva	Endodermal sinus tumor		(364)
Yolk sac			(47)

B. Comparable Animal and Experimental Data

Place of Origin	Special of Animal Teratomas	References
Ovary	Carp	(164)
Yolk sac derived teratoma *in vitro*	Gerbil	(304)
Ovarian teratoma	Guinea pig	(110)
Yolk sac derived teratoma	Hamster	(337, 338, 346)
Cell culture	Mouse	(54)
Extra gonadal teratoid carcinoma	Mouse	(18)
Teratocarcinoma cell stem *in vitro*	Mouse	(396)
Teratocarcinoma cells	Mouse	(87, 168–170, 275, 280, 335)
Intracranial teratoma	Rabbit, domestic	(34)
Human teratoma cell line		(144, 145)

ued increase in life span of the larvae and the adult organism. The larva, as the long living organism, performs the eating stage. The imago, the adult insect, develops wings but in general does not grow any more after this goal is reached. The value of the tissues which are able to give rise to tumors varies if we have only cell nests with high embryonal potential, as is the case during metamorphosis of endoparasitic crustaceans (rhizocephalan), e.g. *Sacculina*. A mass of embryonal cells remains from which a new organism develops after all specialized tissues have been discarded. The parasitic form is known as *Sacculina interna*, whereas the nonparasitic form is known as *Sacculina externa*. With this example, we approach the second question, that of histolysis of larval structures.

To the author's knowledge, no investigations exist which deal particularly with the effect of normal histolysis on tumor or metastatic development in invertebrates such as in ascidiacea, echinoidea, and others.

Tumors of larvae are most extensively known from studies of the fruit fly, *Drosophila melanogaster*. A review of neoplasms of larvae is given in Table 13.6.

Tumors of or with the Involvement of Meristems

The meristematic potential plays an important and basic role in the development of plant neoplasms and related growth disorders, known as

Table 13.5
Tumors of the Placenta in Man (108, 181)[a]

Origin	Type of Tumor	Frequency	Characteristic Features
Nonepithelial tissues	Fibromas	Very rare	
	Chorangiomas	Very rare	Make-up of capillary hemangioma
	Myxomas(?)		May belong to chorangiomas
	Myxofibromas(?)		May belong to chorangiomas
	Diffuse hemangiomatosis	Extremely rare	No real difference from chorangioma
	Dermoids	Extremely rare	
	Teratomas	Extremely rare	
	Sarcomas		Existence not satisfactorily proven
Melanogenic system	Secondary tumors		Maternal melanoma with metastasis in placenta and even fetus
Epithelial tissues	Hydatid mole	Quite common	Different stages with participation of the embryonal connective tissue and the epithelial layers can be distinguished
	Malignant chorionepithelioma	0.05–3.7% according to number of delivery	According to von Albertini, chorionepithelioma is the only malignant epithelial neoplasm which proliferates without stroma formation

[a] Placental neoplasms in other species, included domesticated ones, are most rarely observed. Placental neoplasms, other than from placental mammals, have not been observed.

Table 13.6
Tumors of Larvae (a Selection) (278)

Phylum	Type of Tumor	References
	Spontaneous	
Arthropoda	Int. imaginal disc neoplasm with compact mode of growth	(114a)
Class: Insecta		
Order: Diptera		
Drosophila sp.	Int. imaginal disc neoplasm with invasive mode of growth	
	Malignant blood cell neoplasm	
	Malignant neuroblastoma of the adult	
	Optic Neuroblast and ganglion-mother cells	
	Experimental	
Musca domestica sp.	9,10-dimethyl-1-2-dibenzanthracene, 1,2,5,6-dibenzanthracene, benzo(a)pyrene, methylcholanthrene, fluorenamine derivatives	(55a)
		(333a)

galls. The theory of cell stimulation of Rudolf Virchow can easily be applied. In tumor growth, the primary embryonal potential is the meristem. Secondary growth occurs where fully differentiated plant tissues regain their growth potential as is normally the case in succeeding meristems ("*Folgemeristeme*" in the German literature). The growth developments are either autonomous or limited. A review of some examples is given in Table 13.7.

FACTORS IMPAIRING THE GROWTH OF NEOPLASMS WITH EMBRYONAL POTENTIAL

Cell Replacement—Life Span of Cells and Tissues

Life would be impossible without repair, be it replacement of worn-out structures or repair following injury. The time element is essential when we compare cells, body structures, tissues, or whole organisms.

Cell replacement as well as life span of cells and tissues in the different organisms is widely dependent upon the species-specific management of growth. Also involved are roundabouts of ontogenetic development, life span of the organisms concerned, embryonal potential of tissues, regenerative capacity, cell invariability, change of generation, and ontogenetic autolysis (histolysis).

It was shown in Chapter 12 that the vascular plants, in particular, have tissues which are comparable to cell-invariable tissues in animals: from the meristems with at least theoretically unlimited embryonal potential, which are comparable to those larval tissues in the inverte-

brates such as the imaginal discs in insect larvae or the embryonal cell nests in the cypris of crustaceans, all the way to tissues which are nonliving when they fulfill their functional purpose, such as the sclerenchyma.

The change of haploid and diploid generations, the roundabouts of ontogenetic development such as different larval stages, first and second embryogeny, preservation of embryonal cell clusters, and such structures as the placentae complicate the general picture of the life span of cells and tissues in the various groups of animals and plants with true tissues. Cell replacement varies according to tissues. Table 13.8 gives a review of cell replacement, based on the data of normal wear and tear of the most important tissues of animals and plants alike. Tissues may influence the repair of other tissues as do the Schwann cells in peripheral nerve regeneration.

We can conclude from this that tissue life spans differ widely. It may also differ with regard to the life span of the cells of the same tissue but in species of different hierarchical taxonomical level. The impact of the life span of cells of different tissues and their normal renewal with regard to their behavior in the neoplastic or even malignant condition represents a neglected field of study.

In the process of possible transformation of the injured cell to the benign neoplastic, premalignant, or even malignant condition, it is important to understand the species specificity of repair or healing.

Life Span of Organisms

The picture is again complicated by the variation of the species-specific life span of different organisms which shows a characteristic relationship to the size of animals (Table 13.9 A–G).

Table 13.7

Plant Tumors with the Involvement of Meristems (a Selection) (25, 227)

Type of Meristem in Order of Magnitude	Type of Tumor Involved	Example
Succeeding meristems (*Folgemeristeme*)	Very common in galls of angiosperms, at least theoretically present in all galls containing derivatives of fully differentiated tissues	Epidermis in so-called free galls
Meristemoids	Leaf galls, especially epidermal galls	Galls of *Syndytrium* sp., *Ulmus* sp.
Phellogen	Galls of shoot and root axes	Certain epidermal galls
Cambium	Galls of shoot and root axes	Galls at roots of leguminosae
Apical meristem	Bud galls, galls on shoot axes	Proximity of primary meristem explains, at least partially, simple character of bud galls with external cecidozoa as on *Betula*

Table 13.8
Selected Species-Specific Aspects of Cellular Age (Life Span), According to Tissues and Species (An Estimate)

Tissue Group	Species	Approximate Age of Tissue	Approximate Age of Cell	Species Dependence	Remarks
Epithelia: Skin	Homo sapiens	Continued renewal from basal cell layer—holocrine secretion			Loss of embryonal potential in cells varies during life time as in meristematic tissues to total loss as in cell-invariable or nonliving tissues; life cycle (age) of cells varies from half an hour (certain bacteria) to over a hundred years as in some plant parenchymata. Tissues can be divided in those continuously renewed ones as holocrine glands, blood cells, neurons in Hydra and those lasting whole life without complete regeneration as mammalian neurons. Meristems of plants are another extreme of these cell-invariable structures with their continued cell renewal. Age of tissues and cells depends to high degree on life span of species and type of aging processes as they differ in mammals (pathologic processes) and insects (thinning of cell populations). Bulk of material is still unknown. Nutritional conditions, ability of desiccation are additional factors
Connective tissues	Variability in regenerative power concerning cell types and species, as turbellarians or mammals	Remodeling from weeks to years	From hours (lymphocytes) to 6 weeks (erythrocytes)	In its magnitude only anticipated considering developmental stages and different phyla	
Muscle tissues	Strong limitation of renewal, with exception of lowest phyla to cell invariability (cardiac musculature)	Connected with species-specific life span	Nearly as life span of species	Strong species dependence	
Nervous tissues	Hydra sp. Non-Coelenterates	Short lived Without renewal during life time	Fast renewal Without renewal during life time	Strong species dependence	
	Only limited knowledge on the life span of glia in different phyla.				
Meristematic tissues	Species-specific variation; variation by growth period; and type of meristem				
Fully differentiated tissues, e.g., parenchyma	Leaf of flower in angiosperm	1 day	1 day		
Permanent tissues	Stem of gymnosperm Gymnosperms	100 years Nonliving cell remnants exist up to 6000 years (Sequoia sp.)	100 years		

The relationship of life span and body size of the organisms is interesting. A general rule can be stated that a large body size is normally connected with a longer life span, whereas a small body size is connected with a short life span. This phenomenon of parallelism begins with a large number of offspring of the small, short living forms and a fewer number of offspring with the large, long living forms. The reason for this is that the long living, large form needs more protection against predators, more food, and must resist more environmental attacks (changes of climate, pollution). Regenerative capability and cell invariability are also more diminished in the large forms.

The heath, *Erica* sp., approximately ½ foot high, lives 3 years, whereas trees such as *Sequoia gigantea* reach a height of more than 300 feet and live up to 3000 years. Two specimens of the bristle-cone pine, *Pinus aristata*, with a proven age of 4000 and 4600 years, respectively, are considered to be the oldest presently living trees. The mouse, *Mus musculus*, lives 3 years, the descending laboratory mouse 1½ years, the elephant 50 years. The mouse weighs 20 g, the elephant 1½ tons. Also in molluscs, the largest lamellibranch, *Tridacna gigas*, has a body weight of 200 kg and a life span of approximately 85 years. In crustaceans, the small entomostraceans are short living in contrast the lobster, *Homarus* sp., that reaches a life span up to 75 years and is one of the largest of the group. In low organisms, in contrast to higher developed ones, desiccation is seen to slow down metabolism as in tardigrades. This is also the case in hibernation and related phenomena.

Capability of Healing from a Wound to DNA Repair

Healing after injury also varies greatly in vascular plants and eumetazoans. In addition, a number of variables can be found in the various subgroups of both, also with regard to granulation. In vascular plants, inflammation does not occur. Healing in plants is either bound to meristems or the repair of meristematic potential of fully differentiated adult tissues changing to succeeding meristems. Healing in eumetazoans is greatly influenced by the condition of immunity, the capability of cells deriving from the mesenchymal stem cells such as macrophages, the capability of regeneration and cell-invariability as well as other factors. The capacity of the nervous system is also important. In low organisms like platyhelminthes the network-like nervous system may have the capability of the central nervous system in higher forms, as described in Chapter 3. These factors together will not only influence the healing process but direct the possibility of neoplastic development in low organisms.

The repair of an injury of an organism therefore is a highly complicated process and shows a species-specific variation. The general comparative aspect dealing with the macroscopic appearance of wound healing down to tissue involvement in cell injury has been discussed in Chapter 12. Here it is only necessary to point out the biochemical aspects of DNA repair.

Capacity of Regeneration

Regeneration is the ordered repair of a damaged portion of the body. The phenomenon is known in both animals and plants but occurs with different intensities in the various groups. It is the ability of the organisms to replace lost parts above the level of the cellular replacement. The term regeneration is really not used in the plant kingdom. Nevertheless, especially in the plant, we are able to distinguish between easily replaceable tissues and those which are not: meristematic tissues and permanent, nonliving tissues, with the fully differentiated plant tissues in the middle. The regenerative capacity of members of the different phyla and the occurrence of the cell-invariability are reviewed in Tables 13.10 and 13.11.

Regeneration is a factor which is important in the evaluation of neoplasms or related growth processes in lower organisms and those where a very high regeneration takes place. This does not mean that regeneration will prevent neoplastic growth but it may interfere in the way that the pathologic growth process would develop in an organism with less potential regenerative capacity. Regeneration exhibits a species-specific pattern. The highest regeneration in eumetazoans is found in holothurians when evisceration occurs and total regeneration takes place. This is more remarkable as the respiratory trees in holothurians are connected with and derived from the intestinal tract.

Capacity of Cell-Invariability

Cell-invariability, with the German term *Zellkonstanz*, can be considered as contrary to high

Table 13.9A

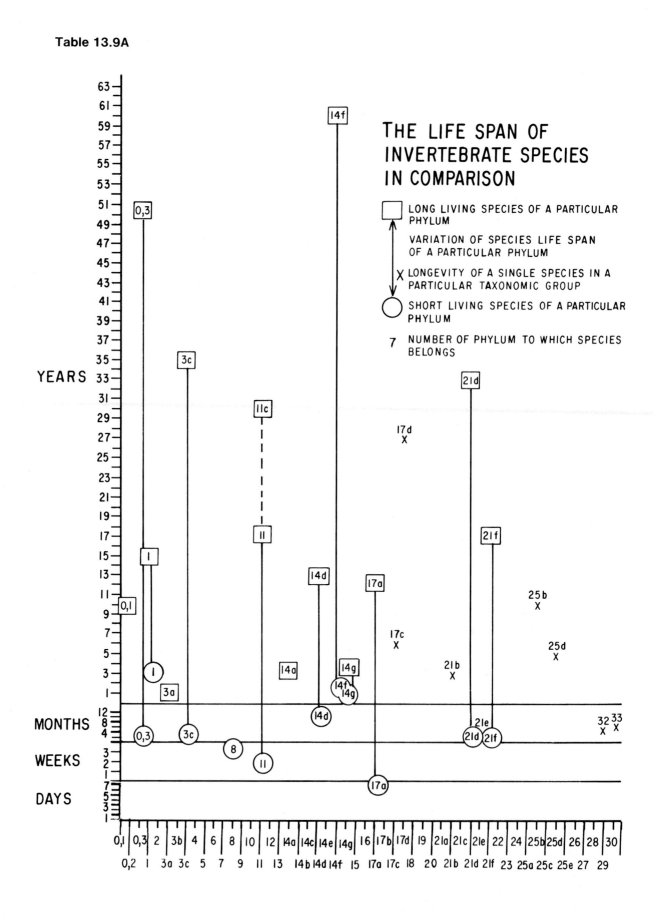

Table 13.9B

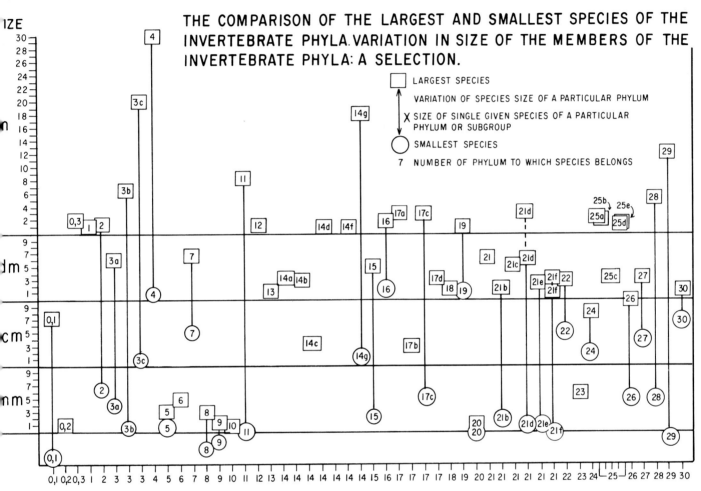

THE COMPARISON OF THE LARGEST AND SMALLEST SPECIES OF THE INVERTEBRATE PHYLA. VARIATION IN SIZE OF THE MEMBERS OF THE INVERTEBRATE PHYLA: A SELECTION.

LARGEST SPECIES
VARIATION OF SPECIES SIZE OF A PARTICULAR PHYLUM
X SIZE OF SINGLE GIVEN SPECIES OF A PARTICULAR PHYLUM OR SUBGROUP
SMALLEST SPECIES
7 NUMBER OF PHYLUM TO WHICH SPECIES BELONGS

The numbers identify the phyla (in accordance with Chapters 3, 6, and 43 and their subgroups as follows: Non-Eumetazoans: 0,1 Protozoa, 0,2 Mesozoa, 0,3 Porifera. Eumetazoans: 1 Cnidaria, 2 Ctenophora, 3 Platyhelminthes, 4 Nemertinea, 5 Gnathostomulida, 6 Entoprocta, 7 Acanthocephala, 8 Rotifera, 9 Gastrotricha, 10 Kinorhyncha, 11 Nematoda, 12 Nematomorpha, 13 Priapulida, 14 Mollusca, 14a Aplacophora, 14b Polyplacophora, 14c Gastropoda, 14d Pelecypoda, 14e Scaphopoda, 14f Cephalopoda, 15 Sipunculida, 16 Echiurida, 17 Annelida, 17a Polychaeta, 17b Oligochaeta, 17c Hirudinea, 18 Onychophora, 19 Pentastomida, 20 Tardigrada, 21 Arthropoda, 21a Merostomata, 21b Pycnogonida, 21c Arachnida, 21d Crustacea, 21e Pauropoda, 21f Symphyla, 21g Diplopoda, 21h Chilopoda, 21i Insecta, 22 Phoronida, 23 Ectoprocta, 24 Brachiopoda, 25 Echinodermata, 25a Crinoidea, 25b Asteriodea, 25c Holothuroidea, 25d Echinoidea, 25e Ophiuroidea, 26 Chaetognatha, 27 Pogonophora, 28 Hemichordata, 29 Tunicata, 30 Cephalochordata. The upper number represents the longest-living species in Table 13.9*A* and the physically largest species in Table 13.9*B*, respectively. The lower number represents the shortest-living species in Table 13.9*A* and the smallest species in Table 13.9*B*, respectively. If only one species is cited in both tables, it is marked with an × and the phylum number. For references to the particular species tabulated, see *Species-Specific Potential of Invertebrates for Toxicological Research* by H. E. Kaiser, University Park Press, Baltimore, 1980.

Table 13.9C
Life Years of Selected Vertebrates

Vertebrate	Life Span (yr)
I. Agnatha	
1. *Petromyzon marinus*	7
2. *Lampetra fluviatilis*	+1
II. Chondrichthyes	
3. *Dasyatis pastinaca*	+21
4. *Raja maculata*	+5
III. Osteichthyes	
5. *Acipenser fluvescens*	152
6. *Scomber scombrus*	3–4
IV. Dipnoi	
7. *Protopterus annectans*	18
8. *Lepidosiren paradoxa*	8
V. Amphibia	
9. *Cryptobranchus alleganiensis*	28
10. *Notophthalmus viridescens*	3
VI. Reptilia	
11. *Terrapene carolina*	88
12. *Anolis equestris*	3.5
VII. Aves	
13. *Corvus corax*	69
14. *Perdix perdix*	5
VIII. Mammalia	
15. *Balaenoptera physalus*	+80
16. *Scalopus aquaticus*	+1

Table 13.9D

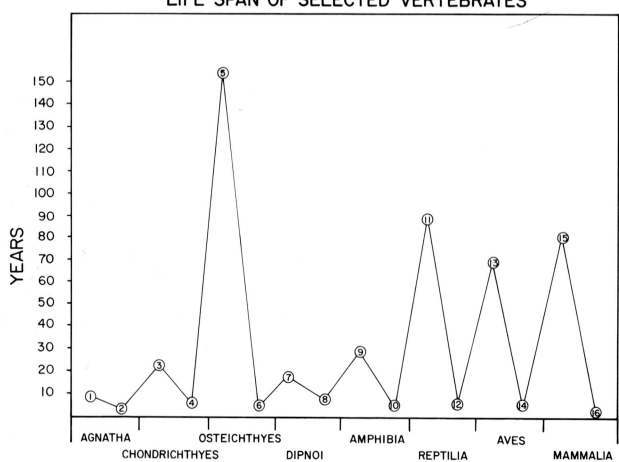

LIFE SPAN OF SELECTED VERTEBRATES

Table 13.9E
Variation in Size and Weight of Vertebrata (240a, 249a, 316a, 321a, 376a)[a]

Taxonomic Unit	Species	Size	Weight
Agnatha	*Lampetra* sp. (lamprey)	10.16 cm	85.04 g
	Petromycon sp. (lamprey)	91.44 cm	1.143 kg
Chondrichthyes	*Euprotomicrus bispinatus* or	15.24 cm	?
	Squaliolus saomenti (sharks)	?	?
	Rhincodon typus[b] (whale shark)	18.28 m	40,823.1 kg
Osteichthyes	*Pandaka pygmaea* (dwarf pygmy goby)	71–96 mm	4–5 mg
	Makaira indica (black marlin)	4.57 m	707.6 kg
	Mola mola (sunfish, headfish)	3.96 m	1496.85 kg
Amphibia			
Anura	*Phylobates limbatus* (arrow poison frog of Cuba)	1.12–1.23 cm[c]	?
	Goliath frog	33.9 cm[c], 81.48 cm	3.02 kg
Urodela	*Megalobatrachus davidianus* (Chinese giant salamander)	99.99–152.4 cm	10.541–12.972 kg[d]
Reptilia			
Squamata	*Sphaerodactylus* sp. (a gecko)	1.70–1.80 cm[c]	?
	Eunectes marinus (anaconda)	9.25 m (11.43 m)	(453.59 kg)
Crocodilia	*Crocodilus porosus* (crocodile)	3.66–4.27 m (8.23 m)	(1995.85 kg)
Aves	*Mellisuga helenae* (Helena's hummingbird)	5.79 cm (wing span 7.62 cm)	2 g
	Struthis camelus (North African ostrich)	2.43 m tall	136.08 kg
Mammalia	*Suncus etruscus* (savis whitetoothed Pygmy shrew, also called Etruscan shrew)	35–180 mm head and body 9–120 mm tail	2–35 g (usually 3–18 g)
	Giraffa camelopardalis (giraffe)	6.09 m tall	1900 kg
	Loxodonta africana africana (African bush elephant)	3.20 m tall, 3.81 m tall	5.869.67 kg (average male), 10,000 kg
	Balaenoptera musculus (blue whale)	27.43 m long, 30. m	112,500 kg, 177,800 kg

[a] The smallest species of a taxonomic unit is always given first if known. (Phylogenetic development of all groups begins with smaller forms, leading to larger forms).
[b] This shark lays also the largest eggs of any living animal.
[c] The given length is from snout to vent.
[d] Greatest weight recorded nearly 45 kg.

Table 13.9F
Life Span and Height of Selected Vascular Plants

Plant	Life Span (yr)	Height (m)
1. *Pinus aristata*	4000–4600	4
2. *Sequoiadendron giganteum*[a]	3000–3500	92
3. *Sequoia sempervirens*[b]		110
4. *Taxus baccata*	3000	7
5. *Larix decidua*	600–700	35
6. *Juniperus communis*	2000	10 (?)
7. *Eucalyptus regnans*	5000 (?)	155
8. *Ulmus sp.*	300–600	36
9. *Acer platanoides*	400–500	25
10. *Dracaena draco*	185–200	22
11. *Pirus malus*	200	18
12. *Salix alba*	150	7
13. *Erica carnea*	21	0.33

[a] The General Sherman tree has an estimated age of 2700 to 3000 years and is considered as one of the oldest redwoods.

[b] The Howard Libby tree is the tallest tree in the United States.

Table 13.9G

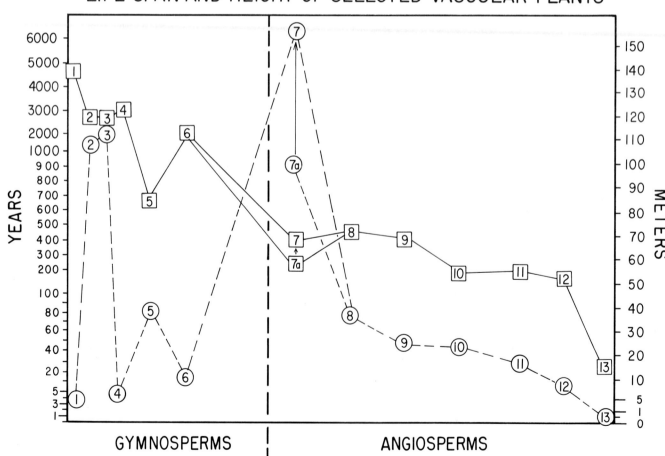

LIFE SPAN AND HEIGHT OF SELECTED VASCULAR PLANTS

Table 13.10.
Capacity of Healing or Repair from a Wound to DNA Repair (38, 41, 70, 71, 75, 76, 106, 125, 130, 137, 149–151, 298–301, 306, 312, 313, 316, 323, 324, 336, 339–341, 343, 353, 359, 360, 366, 367, 380, 381, 385)

Phylogenetic occurrence:

Practical occurrence in case of injury
ORGANISM

Molecular level

PRESENT

Eumetazoan (94, 102, 112, 127, 129)

Vascular plant (149)

MACROSCOPIC WOUND
Generally injury of body covering (2, 6, 15, 21–24, 26, 50, 53, 85, 86, 122, 328)

CELL DEATH
Varies from important to minute depending on type of wound: 1, 2, 3 grade (261, 326)
+
CELL INJURY (39, 327)
Leads to recovery of injured cells or renewed cell death

CELLULAR REACTION highly influenced by re-generative capacity and species specificity (90)	Continuation of meristems

Epithelial and muscular tis-sues depend in heavier in-jury on con-nective tis-sues for heal-ing (112, 133, 156, 160, 320, 330)

Fully differ-entiated tis-sues regain meristem ca-pacity (suc-ceeding meri-stems) in a specific man-ner. Intersti-tial tissues comparable to connective tissues in ani-mals

Permanent tissues as scleren-chymatas incapable of healing

100%
Hydra
Planarian
Echinoderm
Earthworm
Insect
Acantho-
cephalan
Rotifer
0%

Nervous tissue
Hydra 100%

Man 0%

GROWTH STIMULATION (36)
of varying degree
CHEMICAL REPAIR

GROWTH (143, 185)
HEALING

e.g. DNA repair (3, 30, 37, 42–44, 46, 48, 58, 59, 64, 67, 72, 84, 96, 99, 116, 132, 152, 159, 165, 166, 192, 204–209, 229, 237, 249, 272, 278, 282, 283, 309, 315, 347, 362, 370, 389, 393)

PRECAMBRIAN

Table 13.11
Capacity of Regeneration in Animals and Vascular Plants (5, 33, 55, 60, 68, 77, 79, 80, 82, 83, 123, 138–140, 161, 175, 180, 184–186, 189, 193, 200, 211, 217, 219, 224, 226, 228, 236, 248, 252, 259, 265, 266, 271, 291–293, 296, 303, 318, 321, 342, 345, 351, 361, 373, 387, 390, 394, 397)

Phyla and Subgroups	No Regeneration	Cellular level	Tissue level	Structural level above tissue and below organ	Organ level	Level of organ system	Level of body part	Level of whole body	Asexual reproduction
1. Protozoa		X							X
2. Mesozoa		X							
3. Porifera		X		X				X	X
4. Cnidaria		X	X					X	
5. Ctenophora		X							
6. Platyhelminthes		X	X				X	X	X
7. Nemertinea					X		X	X	X
8. Gnathostomulida		X(?)							
9. Entoprocta		X(?)							
10. Acanthocephala	X								
11. Rotifera	X								
12. Gastrotricha		X(?)							
13. Kinorhyncha		X(?)							
14. Nematoda	X								
15. Nematomorpha		X(?)							
16. Priapulida		X(?)							
17. Mollusca									
a. Monoplacophora		X							
b. Amphineura		X							
c. Gastropoda			X						
d. Pelecypoda			X						
e. Scaphopoda			X						
f. Cephalopoda			X						
18. Sipunculida		X(?)							
19. Echiurida		X(?)							
20. Annelida									
a. Polychaeta		X	X	X	X				X
b. Oligochaeta		X	X	X	X	X	X	X	X
c. Hirudinea		X(?)							
21. Onychophora		X(?)							
22. Pentastomida		X							
23. Tardigrada	X								
24. Arthropoda									
a. Merostomata		X					X		
b. Pycnogonida		X					?		
c. Arachnida		X					X		
d. Crustacea		X					X		
e. Pauropoda		X					?		
f. Symphyla		X					?		
g. Diplopoda		X					?		
h. Chilopoda		X							
i. Insecta		X					X		
25. Phoronida								X	X
26. Ectoprocta								X	X
27. Brachiopoda		X(?)							
28. Echinodermata									
a. Crinoidea		X	X						
b. Asteroidea		X					X		
c. Holothuroidea		X				X			
d. Echinoidea		X		X					
e. Ophiuroidea		X	X						
29. Chaetognatha		X	X						
30. Pogonophora		X							
31. Hemichordata		X							

Table 13.11—_continued_

Phyla and Subgroups	No Regeneration	Regeneration at							
		Cellular level	Tissue level	Structural level above tissue and below organ	Organ level	Level of organ system	Level of body part	Level of whole body	Asexual reproduction
32. Tunicata		X							
33. Cephalochordata		X							
34. Vertebrata									
a. Pisces		X	X						
b. Amphibia		X	X				X		
c. Reptilia		X	X						
d. Aves		X	X						
e. Mammalia		X	X				X(?)		
35. Tracheophyta	X	X	X				X	X	X

Table 13.12
Capacity of Cell-Invariability in Eumetazoans and Vascular Plants[a]

Phyla	Grading[b]			
	1	2	3	4
1. Protozoa	X			
2. Mesozoa	X			
3. Porifera	X			
4. Cnidaria	X			
5. Ctenophora	X			
6. Plathyhelminthes	X	X		
7. Nemertini				
8. Gnathostomulida				
9. Entoprocta				
10. Acanthocephala			X	
11. Rotifera				X
12. Gastrotricha				
13. Kinorhyncha				
14. Nematoda			X	
15. Nematomorpha			X	
16. Priapulida			X	
17. Mollusca			X	
18. Sipunculida			X	
19. Echiurida			X	
20. Annelida				
21. Onychophora				
22. Pentastomida				
23. Tardigrada				X
24. Arthropoda			X	
25. Phoronida			?	
26. Ectoprocta			?	
27. Brachiopoda			?	
28. Echinodermata			X	
29. Chaetognatha				
30. Pogonophora				
31. Hemichordata				
32. Tunicata				
33. Cephalochordata				
34. Vertebrata			X	
35. Vascular Plants		X	X	

[a] Only phyla with analogous and basic characteristics are indicated.
[b] 1, No cell invariability; 2, partial cell invariability with possibility of regaining embryonal potential; 3, partial cell invariability without regaining embryonal potential; 4, complete cell invariability without regaining embryonal potential.

regeneration. The phyla exhibiting this phenomenon are listed in Table 13.12. In both kingdoms, cell-invariability is distributed differently. Cell-invariability can be found in different groups of eumetazoans and vascular plants either with regard to certain body portions, the tissues as such, or in whole organisms with living cells such as rotifers and tardigrades. In animals, it occurs either in the whole body of a species of a particular phylum as in rotifers, in certain organs as in acanthocephalans or, as in certain tissues, for example in the nervous tissue in man. The characteristic number of cell nuclei can be seen as a special case. Another variation is introduced by those tissues of the plant kingdom which have to be nonliving to fulfill their particular task such as providing support and other functions, as for example the sclerenchyma in vascular plants.

In contrast to the only cell-invariable tissue in our body, the nerve tissue, the neurons of the coelenterate *Hydra* are highly regenerative structures (see Chapter 3).

Some pathologists consider the cardiac musculature as cell-invariable tissue. But in the case of heart hypertrophy, the enlarged cells of the cardiac musculature are able to produce tetraploid nuclei with cell enlargement and in tissue cultures the cardiac cells are able to produce DNA. Table 13.12 summarizes cell-invariability.

References

1. Abesadze, A. I., Bogvelishvili, M. V., Kvernadze, M. G., and Iosava, G. G. (1978): Role of the spleen in regulating thrombocytopoiesis. *Biull. Eksp. Biol. Med.*, 86:718–720.
2. Abolins-Krogis, A. (1976): Ultrastructural study of the shell-repair membrane in the snail, *Helix pomatia* L. *Cell Tissue Res.*, 172:455–476.
3. Ahmed, F. E., and Setlow, R. B. (1977): Different rate-limiting steps in excision repair of ultraviolet- and N-acetoxy-2-acetylaminofluorene-damaged DNA in normal human fibroblasts. *Proc. Natl. Acad. Sci. U.S.A.*, 74:1548–1552.
4. Akhtar, M., Kott, E., and Brooks, B. (1977): Extrarenal Wilms' tumor; report of a case and review of the literature. *Cancer*, 40:3087–3091.
5. Al-Barwari, S. E., and Potten, C. S. (1976): Regeneration and dose-response characteristics of irradiated mouse dorsal epidermal cells. *Int. J. Radiat. Biol.*, 30:201–216.
6. Al-Salman, A. H., Sayegh, F. S., and Chappell, R. P. (1979): Wound

healing of endosteal vitreous carbon implants in dogs. *J. Prosthet. Dent.*, 41:83–89.

7. Altman, P. L., and Dittmer, D. S. (eds.) (1964): *Biology Data Book.* FASEB, Bethesda, Md.

8. Altman, P. L., and Dittmer, D. S. (eds.) (1972): *Biology Data Book*, Ed. 2, *Vol. 1.* FASEB, Bethesda, Md.

9. Altman, P. L., and Dittmer, D. S. (eds.) (1973): *Biology Data Book*, Ed. 2, *Vol. 2.* FASEB, Bethesda, Md.

10. Altman, P. L., and Dittmer, D. S. (eds.) (1974): *Biology Data Book*, Ed. 2, *Vol. 3.* FASEB, Bethesda, Md.

11. Altman, P. L., Dittmer D. S., and Katz, D. (1979): *Biological Handbooks; III. Inbred and Genetically Defined Strains of Laboratory Animals. Part I. Mouse and Rat.* FASEB, Bethesda, Md.

12. Amarjit, S., Singh, A., and Singh, R. (1977): Nasopharyngeal teratoma. *Indian J. Cancer*, 14:367–369.

13. Amler, M. H. (1977): The age factor in human extraction wound healing. *J. Oral Surg.*, 35:193–197.

14. Andreasen, J. O., Reinholdt, J., Riis, I., Dybdahl, R., Söder, P. O., and Otteskog, P. (1978): Periodontal and pulpal healing of monkey incisors preserved in tissue culture before replantation. *Int. J. Oral Surg.*, 7:104–112.

15. Anke, T., Oberwinkler, F., Steglich, W., and Schramm, G. (1977): The strobilurins—new antifungal antibiotics from the basidiomycete *Strobilurus tenacellus*. *J. Antibiot. (Tokyo)*, 30:806–810.

16. Aristizabal, S., Davis, J. R., Miller, R. C., Moore, M. J., and Boone, M. L. (1978): Bilateral primary germ cell testicular tumors; report of four cases and review of the literature. *Cancer*, 42:591–597.

17. Arita, N., Ushio, Y., Abekura, M., Koshino, K., and Hayakawa, T. (1978): Embryonal carcinoma with teratomatous elements in the region of the pineal gland. *Surg. Neurol.*, 9:198–202.

18. Artzt, K., and Damjanov, I. (1978): Spontaneous extragonadal teratocarcinoma in a mouse. *Lab. Anim. Sci.*, 28:584–586.

19. Askenase, P. W., Hayden, B., and Gershon, R. K. (1977): Evanescent delayed-type hypersensitivity; mediation by effector cells with a short life span. *J. Immunol.*, 119:1830–1835.

20. Aubert, J., Casamayou, J., Denis, P., Hoppler, A., and Payen, J. (1978): Intrarenal teratoma in a newborn child. *Eur. Urol.*, 4:306–308.

21. Baldwin, K. M. (1977): The fine structure of healing over in mammalian cardiac muscle. *J. Mol. Cell Cardiol.*, 9:959–966.

22. Baroldi, G., and Silver, D. (1975): The healing of myocardial infarcts in man. *G. Ital. Cardiol.* 5:465–476.

23. Bazin, S., LeLous, M., and Delaunay, A. (1976): Collagen in granulation tissues. *Agents Actions*, 6:272–276.

24. Bazin, S., Bailey, A., LeLous, M., Nicolétis, C., and Delaunay, A. (1975): Collagen polymorphism in human scars. *C.R. Acad. Sci. (D) (Paris)*, 281:1447–1449.

25. Beiderbeck, R. (1977): *Pflanzentumoren.* Verlag Eugen Ulmer, Stuttgart.

26. Benfer, J., and Struck, H. (1977): Wound healing at low temperature. *Med. Welt*, 28:326–327.

27. Bengtsson, A., Grimelius, L., Johansson, H., and Ponten, J. (1977): Nuclear DNA-content of parathyroid cells in adenomas, hyperplastic and normal glands. *Acta Pathol. Microbiol. Scand (A)*, 85:455–460.

28. Bergh, N. P., Gatzinsky, P., Larsson, S., Ludin, P., and Ridell, B. (1978): Tumors of the thymus and thymic region; III. Clinicopathological studies on teratomas and tumors of germ cell type. *Ann. Thorac. Surg.*, 25:107–111.

29. Bernstine, E. G., Koyama, H., and Ephrussi, B. (1977): Enhanced expression of alkaline phosphatase in hybrids between neuroblastoma and embryonal carcinoma. *Somatic Cell Genet.*, 3:217–225.

30. Bertazzoni, U., Scovassi, A. I., Stefanini, M., Giulotto, E., Spadari, S., and Pedrini, A. M. (1978): DNA polymerases alpha beta and gamma in inherited diseases affecting DNA repair. *Nucleic Acids Res.*, 5:2189–2196.

31. Bianchi, A., and Cudmore, R. E. (1978): Salivary gland tumors in children. *J. Pediatr. Surg.*, 13:519–521.

32. Bierman, E. L. (1978): The effect of donor age on the in vitro life span of cultured human arterial smooth-muscle cells. *In Vitro*, 14:951–955.

33. Bischoff, R. (1975): Regeneration of single skeletal muscle fibers in vitro, *Anat. Rec.*, 182:215–235.

34. Bishop, L. (1978): Intracranial teratoma in a domestic rabbit. *Vet. Pathol.*, 15:525–530.

35. Bisht, J. S. (1975): Cyclic changes in the pituitary gland in correlation with the testicular cycle in a hill-stream teleost, *Schizothorax richardsonii* (Gray and Hard). *Acta Anat. (Basel)*, 92:443–453.

36. Blomgren, H., and Baral, E. (1977): Depressed responder and stimulator capacities of peripheral lymphocytes from patients with advanced breast cancer in the mixed lymphocyte culture. *Cancer Lett.*, 2:177–184.

37. Bodell, W. J., and Banerjee, M. R. (1978): DNA repair in normal and preneoplastic mammary tissues. *Cancer Res.*, 38:736–740.

38. Bohn, H. (1977): Conditioning of a glass surface for the outgrowth of insect epidermis (*Leucophaea maderae*, Blattaria). *In Vitro*, 13:100–107.

39. Bole, G. G., Jr., Jourdian, G. W., and Wright, J. E. (1975): Isolation and chemical characterization of a granuloma glycoprotein that inhibits macrophage phagocytosis, *J. Lab. Clin. Med.*, 86:1018–1031.

40. Bondarchuk, L. G., Epifantseva, M. A., Lukina, N. L., and Berezovskii,

M. E. (1977): Giant teratoma of the mediastinum in a 5-month-old infant. *Grudn. Khir.*, 6:82–83.

41. Borek, E., Baliga, B. S., Gehrke, C. W., Kuo, C. W., Belman, S., Troll, W., and Waalkes, T. P. (1977): High turnover rate of transfer RNA in tumor tissue. *Cancer Res.*, 37:3362–3366.

42. Bose, K., Karran, P., and Strauss, B. (1978): Repair of depurinated DNA in vitro by enzymes purified from human lymphoblasts. *Proc. Natl. Acad. Sci. U.S.A.*, 75:794–798.

43. Bowden, G. T., Hohneck, G., and Fusenig, N. E. (1977): DNA excision repair in ultraviolet-irradiated normal and malignantly transformed mouse epidermal cell cultures. *Cancer Res.*, 37:1611–1617.

44. Bowden, G. T., Giesselbach, B., and Fusenig, N. E. (1978): Postreplication repair of DNA in ultraviolet light-irradiated normal and malignancy transformed mouse epidermal cell cultures. *Cancer Res.*, 38:2709–2718.

45. Bradley, R. M., and Kim, Y. H. (1977): Quantitative morphological changes in epiglottal taste buds over the life span of the sheep. *Ann. Rech. Vet.*, 8:492–494.

46. Brambilla, G., Cavanna, M., Carlo, P., and Finollo, R. (1978): DNA repair synthesis in primary cultures of kidneys from BALB/c and C3H mice treated with dimethylnitrosamine. *Cancer Lett.*, 5:153–159.

47. Brasch, R. C., De Lorimier, A. A., Herzog, R. J., and Van Natta, F. C. (1978): Extragonadal endodermal sinus (yolk sac) tumor. Angiographic findings and literature review. *Pediatr. Radiol.*, 7:115–118.

48. Brash, D. E., and Hart, R. W. (1978): DNA damage and repair in vivo. *J. Environ. Pathol. Toxicol.*, 2:79–114.

49. Breining, H., Helpap, B., Cappel, S., Sturm, K. W., and Lymberopoulos, S. (1977): Morphological findings on the brain of rats after local freezing. *Acta Neuropathol. (Berl.)*, 37:137–140.

50. Bröte, L., and Stendahl, O. (1975): The function of polymorphonuclear leukocytes after surgical trauma. *Acta Chir. Scand.*, 141:565–570.

51. Brubaker, L. H., Essig, L. J., and Mengel, C. E. (1977): Neutrophil life span in paroxysmal nocturnal hemoglobinuria. *Blood*, 50:657–662.

52. Bumbic, S., Lenosavic, M., and Stefoski, M. (1977): Teratoma of the base of the tongue and neck in a newborn female infant. *Srp. Arh. Celok. Lek.*, 105:543–547.

53. Buntrock, P., Schnitzler, S., and Uerlings, I. (1974): Stimulation of experimentally induced tissue granulation by agglutinin obtained from *Helix pomatia* L. albumin glands (Anti-APH)—Part II (author's Transl.). *Exp. Pathol. (Jena)*, 9:64–72.

54. Burke, D. C., Graham, C. F., and Lehman, J. M. (1978): Appearance of interferon inducibility and sensitivity during differentiation of murine teratocarcinoma cells in vitro. *Cell*, 13:243–248.

55. Calvo, W., Fliedner, T. M., Herbst, E.; Hügl, E., and Bruch, C. (1976): Regeneration of blood-forming organs after autologous leukocyte transfusion in lethally irradiated dogs; II. Distribution and cellularity of the marrow in irradiated and transfused animals. *Blood* 47:593–601.

55a. Cantwell, G. E., Shortino, T. J., and Robbins, W. E. (1966): The histopathological effects of certain carcinogenic 2-fluorenamine derivatives on larvae of the house fly. *J. Invertebr. Path.* 8(2):167–174 (see Ref. 67, Chap. 48).

56. Canty, T. G., and Siemens, R. (1978): Malignant mediastinal teratoma in a 15-year-old girl. *Cancer*, 41:1623–1626.

57. Casciano, D. A., Farr, J. A., Oldham, J. W., and Cave, M. D. (1978): 2-Acetylaminofluorene-induced unscheduled DNA synthesis in hepatocytes isolated from 3-methylcholanthrene treated rats. *Cancer Lett.*, 5:173–178.

58. Cerutti, P., Shinohara, K., and Remsen, J. (1977): Repair of DNA damage induced by ionizing radiation and benzo(a)pyrene in mammalian cells. *J. Toxicol. Environ. Health*, 2:1375–1386.

59. Cerutti, P. A., Sessions, F., Hariharan, P. V., and Lusby, A. (1978): Repair of DNA damage induced by benzo(a)pyrene diol-epoxides I and II in human alveolar tumor cells. *Cancer Res.*, 38:2118–2124.

60. Chandebois, R. (1975): Symptoms and causation of the planarian diseases related to cancer. *Oncology*, 32:86–100.

61. Chattopadhyaya, P. K., and Chattopadhyaya, G. (1978): Dermoid cyst of the mesentery. *J. Indian Med. Assoc.*, 70:227–228.

62. Chaudhry, A. P., Lore, J. M. Jr., Fisher, J. E., and Gambrino, A. G. (1978): So called hairy polyps or teratoid tumors of the nasopharynx. *Arch. Otolaryngol.*, 104:517–525.

63. Chebanu, F. A., Kushch, A. A., and Zelenin, A. V. (1977): DNA content in dysplasias and early invasive forms of cervical cancer. *Vopr. Onkol.*, 23:64–66.

64. Chilton, M. D., Drummond, M. H., Merio, D. J., Sciaky, D., Montoya, A. L., Gordon, M. P., and Nester, E. W. (1977): Stable incorporation of plasmid DNA into plant cells; the molecular basis of crown gall tumorigenesis. *Cell*, 11:263–271.

65. Cooper, J. T., and Goldstein, S. (1977): Comparative studies on human skin fibroblasts; life span and lipid metabolism in medium containing fetal bovine or human serum. *In Vitro*, 13:473–476.

66. Corfield, V. A., and Hay, R. J. (1978): Effects of cystine or glutamine restriction on human diploid fibroblasts in culture. *In Vitro*, 14:787–794.

67. Cornelis, J. J. (1978): The influence of inhibitors on dimer removal and repair of single-strand breaks in normal and bromodeoxyuridine substituted DNA of HeLa cells. *Biochim. Biophys. Acta*, 521:134–143.

68. Craddock, V. M. (1976): Effect of a single treatment with the alkylating carcinogens dimethylnitrosamine and methyl methanesulphonate on liver regenerating after partial hepatectomy; III. Effect on DNA synthesis in vivo and on DNA polymerase activity assayed in vitro. *Chem. Biol. Interact.*, 15:247–256.

69. Curry, S. L., Smith, J. P., and Gallagher, H. S. (1978): Malignant teratoma of the ovary; prognostic factors and treatment. *Am. J. Obstet. Gynecol.*, 131:845–849.

70. Custico, W., and Cheung, C. H. (1977): Embryogenetic cell type, organ site sequence specificity in human cancers. *Cancer Res.*, 37:4166–4172.

71. Dabrowski, R., Maslinski, C., and Olczak, A. (1977): The role of histamine in wound healing; I. The effect of high doses of histamine on collagen and glycosoaminoglycan content in wounds. *Agents Actions*, 7:219–224.

72. Darwish, D. H. (1978): The effect of sex steroids on the in vitro synthesis of DNA by malignant ovarian tumours. *Br. J. Obstet. Gynaecol.*, 85:627–633.

73. Davies, I. (1977): The effect of diet on the ultrastructure of the mid-gut cells of *Nasonia vitripennis* (Walk.) (Insecta: Hymenoptera) at various ages. *Cell Tissue Res.*, 184:529–538.

74. Davis, J. T., and Blakemore, W. S. (1978): An atypical case of retroperitoneal teratoma (letter). *Arch. Surg.*, 113:1110.

75. de Bold, A. J., and Bencosme, S. A. (1975): Selective light microscopic demonstration of the specific granulation of the rat atrial myocardium by lead-hematoxylin-tartrazine. *Stain Technol.*, 50:203–205.

76. Derby, A. (1978): Wound healing in tadpole tailfin pieces in vitro. *J. Exp. Zool.* 205:277–284.

77. Desselle, J. C. (1976): [Cytochemical analysis of muscle cell histones of *Triturus cristatus* limbs a) in normal regeneration, b) in regeneration arrested by r-irradiation, and c) in regeneration restored by implants] (Fr.) *C. R. Acad. Sci. [D] (Paris)*, 282:301–304.

78. De Terra, N. (1975): Evidence for cell surface control of macronuclear DNA synthesis in *Stentor*. *Nature*, 258:300–303.

79. Deuchar, E. M. (1975): Regeneration of the tail bud in *Xenopus* embryos *J. Exp. Zool.*, 192:381–390.

80. De Vries, O. M., and Wessels, J. G. (1975): Chemical analysis of cell wall regeneration and reversion of protoplasts from *Schizophyllum commune*. *Arch. Microbiol.*, 102:209–218.

81. Dische, M. R., and Gardner, H. A. (1978): Mixed teratoid tumors of the liver and neck in trisomy 13. *Am. J. Clin. Pathol.*, 69:631–637.

82. Dmitrieva, E. V. (1975): [Reparative regeneration of muscle fibers of the skeletal type and reasons for its delay in local x-ray irradiation] (Rus.). *Arkh. Anat. Gistol. Embriol.*, 68:31–36.

83. Donaldson, D. J., and Mason, J. M. (1975): Cancer-related aspects of regeneration research: A review. *Growth*, 39:476–496.

84. Dudnikova, G. N. (1977): DNA synthesis by granulation tissue fibroblasts under conditions of stimulation of the wound process. *Biull. Eksp. Biol. Med.*, 84:352–354.

85. Dustmann, H. O., and Puhl, W. (1976): [Age dependent possibilities for healing in cartilage injuries (experimental investigations with animals)] (Ger.). *Z. Orthop.*, 114:749–764.

86. Dustmann, H. O., and Puhl, W. (1977): [Healing possibilities of cartilage lesions in dependence on age] (Ger.). *Hefte Unfallheilkd.*, 129:259–264.

87. Dyban, P. A., and Mikhailov, V. P. (1978): Comparative study of mouse teratoids developed from blastocysts and embryos at the three germ layer stage. *Arkh. Anat. Gistol. Embriol.*, 75:8–16.

88. Edwards, A. J. (1977): Lymphocyte depression by cancer. *Ann. R. Coll. Surg., Engl.*, 59:222–230.

89. Egger, H. (1977): Malignant ovarian teratoma with mature glial peritoneal metastases. *Geburtshilfe Frauenheilkd.*, 37:698–700.

90. Ehrlich, H. P., Grislis, G., and Hunt, T. K. (1977): Evidence for the involvement of microtubules in wound contraction. *Am. J. Surg.*, 133:706–709.

91. Elias, M. F., Elias, P. K., Pentz, C. A., 3rd, and Sorrentino, R. N. (1977): Heart/body weight ratios for aging high and low blood pressure mice. *Exp. Aging Res.*, 3:231–238.

92. Enerbäck, L., and Mellblom, L. (1978): Growth related changes in the content of heparin and 5-hydroxytryptamine of mast cells. *Cell Tissue Res.*, 187:367–378.

93. Eneström, S., and Von Essen, C. (1977): Spinal teratoma. *Acta Neurochir. (Wien)*, 39:121–126.

94. England, M. A., and Cowper, S. V. (1977): Wound healing in the early chick embryo studied by scanning electron microscopy. *Anat. Embryol. (Berl.)*, 152:1–14.

95. Erenpreis, Ia. G., and Erenpreisa, E. A. (1978): Current state of the problem of electron-cytochemical detection of DNA. *Arkh. Anat. Gistol. Embriol.*, 75:70–76.

96. Erickson, L. C., Osieka, R., and Kohn, K. W. (1978): Differential repair of 1-(2-chloroethyl)-3-(4-methylcyclohexyl)-1-nitrosourea-induced DNA damage in two human colon tumor cell lines. *Cancer Res.*, 38:802–808.

97. Erickson, R. P. (1977): Differentiation and Other Alloantigens of Spermatozoa, in *Immunobiology of Gametes*, edited by M. Edidin and M. H. Johnson. Cambridge University Press, Cambridge.

98. Evans, R. W. (1966): *Histological Appearances of Tumours*, Ed. 2. Williams & Wilkins, Baltimore.

99. Fanta, D., Topaloglou, A., and Altmann, H. (1978): Studies on the DNA-excision repair in lymphocytes of patients with recurrent Herpes simplex. *Bull. Cancer (Paris)*, 65:341–346.

100. Farooki, Z. Q., Hakimi, M., Arciniegas, E., and Green, E. W. (1978): Echocardiographic features in a case of intrapericardial teratoma. *J. Clin. Ultrasound*, 6:108–110.

101. Farwell, J. R., Dohrmann, G. J.; Flannery, J. T. (1978): Intracranial neoplasms in infants. *Arch. Neurol.*, 35:533–537.

102. Field, S. B., and Hornsey, S. (1977): Repair in normal tissues and the possible relevance to radiotherapy. *Strahlentherapie*, 153:371–379.

103. Finger, H., Heymer, B., Emmerling, P., and Hof, H. (1977): Antibody-forming potential of lymph nodes in aged mice, with special reference to the influence of adjuvant. *Gerontology*, 23:185–204.

104. Fliedner, T. M., and Heit, H. (1975): [Senescence in cell renewal systems[(Ger.). *Verh. Dtsch. Ges. Pathol.*, 59:71–77.

105. Fodstad, O., and Pihl, A. (1978): Effect of ricin and abrin on survival of L1210 leukemic mice and on leukemic and normal bone-marrow cells. *Int. J. Cancer*, 22:558–563.

106. Fong, T. P., Ko, S. T., Streczyn, M., and Westerman, M. P. (1976): Chronic anemia, wound healing, and red cell 2,3-diphosphoglycerate. *Surgery*, 79:218–223.

107. Foss, S. D. (1977): DNA-variations in neighbouring epithelium in patients with bladder carcinoma. *Acta Pathol. Microbiol. Scand. (A)*, 85:603–610.

108. Fox, H., and Elston, C. W. (1978): Pathology of the placenta. *Major Probl. Pathol.*, 7:1–491.

109. Frederiksen, P., Thommesen, P., Kjaer, T. B., and Bichel, P. (1978): Flow cytometric DNA analysis in fine needle aspiration biopsies from patients with prostatic lesions. Diagnostic value and relation to clinical stages. *Acta Pathol. Microbiol. Scand. (A)*, 86:461–464.

110. Frisk, C. S., Wagner, J. E., and Doyle, R. E. (1978): An ovarian teratoma in a guinea pig. *Lab. Anim. Sci.*, 28:199–201.

111. Fujisawa, K., and Shiraki, H. (1978): Study of axonal dystrophy; I. Pathology of the neuropil of the gracile and the cuneate nuclei in ageing and old rats, a stereological study. *Neuropathol. Appl. Neurobiol.*, 4:1–20.

112. Gabbiani, G., LeLous, M., Bailey, A. J., Bazin, S., and Delaunay, A. (1976): Collagen and myofibroblasts of granulation tissue. A chemical, ultrastructural and immunologic study. *Virchows Arch. Cell Pathol.*, 21:133–145.

113. Gabka, J., Harnisch, H., and Witt, H. (1977): Mixed tumors (II). *Quintessenz*, 28:197–201.

114. Gachelin, G. (1978): The cell surface antigens of mouse embryonal carcinoma cells. *Biochim. Biophys. Acta*, 516:27–60.

114a. Gateff, E. (1978): The genetics and epigenetics of neoplasms in *Drosophila*. *Biol. Rev.*, 53:123–168.

115. Gehring, W. J., and Schubiger, G. (1975): Expression of homeotic mutations in duplicated and regenerated antennae of *Drosophila melanogaster*. *J. Embryol. Exp. Morphol.*, 33:459–469.

116. Giannelli, F. (1978): Xeroderma pigmentosum and the role of DNA repair in oncogenesis. *Bull. Cancer (Paris)*, 65:323–334.

117. Giess, M. C. (1977): [Influence of sexual activity on longevity in adult male *Drosophila melanogaster*] (Fr.). *C. R. Acad. Sci. (D) (Paris)*, 285:233–235.

118. Giess, M. C., and Planel, H. (1977): Influence of sex on the radiation-induced life span modifications in *Drosophila melanogaster*. *Gerontology*, 23:325–334.

119. Gill, J. E., Wheeless, L. L., Jr., Hanna-Madden, C., Marisa, R. J., and Horan, P. K. (1978): A comparison of acridine orange and Feulgen cytochemistry of human tumor cell nuclei. *Cancer Res.*, 38:1893–1898.

120. Giustini, F. G., Sohn, S., and Khosravi, M. (1978): Pelvic abscess and perforation of the sigmoid colon by a segment of benign cystic teratoma; an unusual complication of induced abortion. *J. Reprod. Med.*, 20:291–292.

121. Goldenberg, N. J. (1978): Dermoid perforation of the colon. *Gastrointest. Radiol.*, 3:221–222.

122. Gordon, R. E., and Lane, B. P. (1977): Cytokinetics of rat tracheal epithelium stimulated by mechanical trauma. *Cell Tissue Kinet.*, 10:171–181.

123. Gottlob, R. (1977): Endothelial regeneration; The role of smooth muscle cells, blood cells and histiocytes. *Prog. Biochem. Pharmacol.*, 13:276–282.

124. Grajewski, S. (1978): Case of malignant teratoma located retroperitoneally. *Wiad. Lek.*, 31:129–130.

125. Grimes, D. W. (1978): Why some fractures don't heal. *Mod. Med. Asia*, 14:8–10.

126. Gupta, R. K., and Gupta, P. (1977): Cystic ovarian teratoma in a girl of 5 years presenting as acute intestinal obstruction. *J. Indian Med. Assoc.*, 68:235–236.

127. Gywat, L. J., Daicker, B. C., and Gloor, B. P. (1978): Wound healing in the feline retina following mechanical trauma. *Albrecht Von Graefes Arch. Klin. Ophthalmol.*, 206:269–280.

128. Hall, I. A., Lee, K. H., Starnes, C. O., Eigebaly, S. A., Ibuka, T., Wu, Y. S., Kimura, T., and Haruna, M. (1978): Antitumor agents; XXX. Evalu-

ation of alpha-methylene-gamma-lactone-containing agents for inhibition of tumor growth, respiration, and nucleic acid synthesis. *J. Pharm. Sci.*, 67:1235–1239.

129. Hall, S. M. (1978): The Schwann cell; a reappraisal of its role in the peripheral nervous system. *Neuropathol. Appl. Neurobiol.*, 4:165–176.

130. Hallmans, G. (1978): Healing of experimentally induced burn wounds. A comparative study of the healing of exposed burn wounds and burn wounds covered with adhesive zinc-tape and a scanning electron microscopic study of the microvasculature of wound healing in the rabbit ear. *Scand. J. Plast. Reconstr. Surg.*, 12:105–109.

131. Hallowes, R. C., Rudland, P. S., Hawkins, R. A., Lewis, D. J., Bennet, D., and Durbin, H. (1977): Comparison of the effects of hormones on DNA synthesis in cell cultures of nonneoplastic and neoplastic mammary epithelium from rats. *Cancer Res.*, 37:2492–2504.

132. Hanawalt, P. C. (1977): DNA repair processes: An overview, in *DNA Repair Processes*, pp. 1–19, edited by W. W. Nichols *et al.* Symposium Specialists, Miami.

133. Hansen, T. M. (1975): Collagen development in granulation tissue as compared with collagen of skin and aorta from injured and non-injured rats. *Acta Pathol. Microbiol. Scand. (A)*, 83:721–732.

134. Harper, W. F., and McNicol, E. M. (1977): A histological study of normal vulvar skin from infancy to old age. *Br. J. Dermatol.*, 96:249–253.

135. Hassenstein, E. O. (1977): An unusual regression of pulmonary metastases from embryonal carcinoma of the testis. *Br. J. Radiol.*, 50:668–670.

136. Hatzihaberis, F., Stamatis, D., and Staurinos, D. (1978): Giant epignathus. *J. Pediatr. Surg.*, 13:517–518.

137. Hayes, H., Jr. (1977): A review of modern concepts of healing of cutaneous wounds. *J. Dermatol. Surg. Oncol.*, 3:188–193.

138. Hays, E. F., Firkin, F. C., Koga, Y., and Hays, D. M. (1975): Hemopoietic colony forming cells in regenerating mouse liver. *J. Cell Physiol.*, 86:213–219.

139. Heacock, A. M., and Agranoff, B. W. (1976): Enhanced labeling of a retinal protein during regeneration of optic nerve in goldfish. *Proc. Natl. Acad. Sci. U.S.A.*, 73:828–832.

140. Hellerström, C., Andersson, A., and Gunnarsson, R. (1976): Regeneration of islet cells, *Acta Endocrinol. (Kbh.)*, 83:145–160.

141. Hendry, W. F., Tyrrell, C. J., Macdonald, J. S., McElwain, T. J., and Peckham, M. J. (1977): The detection and localization of abdominal lymph node metastases from testicular teratomas. *Br. J. Urol.*, 49:739–745.

142. Hilf, R. (1977): RNA: DNA ratios in human tumors. *J. Natl. Cancer Inst.*, 59:1053–1054.

143. Hofnung, M. J. (1978): Relations between mutagenesis and carcinogenesis. *Biochimie*, 60:1151–1171.

144. Hogan, B., Fellous, M., Avner, P., and Jacob, F. (1977): Isolation of a human teratoma cell line which expresses F9 antigen. *Nature*, 270:515–518.

145. Holden, S., Bernard, O., Artzt, K., Whitmore, W. F., Jr., and Bennett, D. (1977): Human and mouse embryonal carcinoma cells in culture share an embryonic antigen (F9). *Nature*, 270:518–520.

146. Hong, W. K., Wittes, R. E., Hajdu, S. T., Cvitkovic, E., Whitmore, W. F., and Golbey, R. B. (1977): The evolution of mature teratoma from malignant testicular tumors. *Cancer*, 40:2987–2992.

147. Horky, J., Vacha, J., and Znojil, V. (1978): Comparison of life span of erythrocytes in some inbred strains of mouse using 14C-labelled glycine. *Physiol. Bohemoslov.*, 27:209–217.

148. Hoshino, T., Nomura, K., Wilson, C. B., Knebel, K. D., and Gray, J. W. (1978): The distribution of nuclear DNA from human brain-tumor cells. *J. Neurosurg.*, 49:13–21.

149. Hotta, Y., Chandley, A. C., and Stern, H. (1977): Meiotic crossing-over in lily and mouse. *Nature*, 269:240–242.

150. Howes, R. M., and Hoopes, J. E. (1977): Current concepts of wound healing. *Clin. Plast. Surg.*, 4:173–179.

151. Huang, B., Rifkin, M. R., and Luck, D. J. (1977): Temperature-sensitive mutations affecting flagellar assembly and function in *Chlamydomonas reinhardtii*, *J. Cell Biol.*, 72:67–85.

152. Huang, P. H., and Stewart, B. W. (1978): Dimethylnitrosamine-induced structural damage to DNA results from repair of O-6-methylguanine rather than repair of 7-methylguanine. *Cancer Lett.*, 5:161–166.

153. Hug, O. (1977): Introduction in the problem of the time factor and its therapeutical significance. *Strahlentherapie*, 153:362–370.

154. Hulsey, T. K., Burnham, S. J., Neblett, W. W., O'Neill, J. A., Jr., and Meng, H. C. (1977): Delayed burn wound healing in essential fatty acid deficiency. *Surg. Forum*, 28:31–32.

155. Hundert, P., Koltin, Y., Stamberg, J., Wertzberger, R. (1978): Repair of UV-induced damage in wild-type and mutant strains of *Schizophyllum commune*. *Mutat. Res.*, 50:157–162.

156. Hunt, T. K., Conolly, W. B., Aronson, S. B., and Goldstein, P. (1978): Anaerobic metabolism and wound healing; an hypothesis for the initiation and cessation of collagen synthesis in wounds. *Am. J. Surg.*, 135:284–289.

157. Hurd, J. K., Jr. (1978): Benign cystic teratoma of the fallopian tube. *Obstet. Gynecol.*, 52:362–364.

158. Ide, C. H., Davis, W. E., and Black, S. P. (1978): Orbital teratoma. *Arch.*

159. Ikenaga, M., Takebe, H., and Ishii, Y. (1977): Excision repair of DNA base damage in human cells treated with the chemical carcinogen 4-nitroquinoline 1-oxide. *Mutat. Res.*, 43:415–427.

160. Im, M. J., Freshwater, M. F., and Hoopes, J. E. (1976): Enzyme activities in granulation tissue; energy for collagen synthesis. *J. Surg. Res.*, 20:121–125.

161. Ingoglia, N. A., Weis, P., and Mycek, J. (1975): Axonal transport of RNA during regeneration of the optic nerves of goldfish. *J. Neurobiol.*, 6:549–563.

162. Irvin, T. T. (1978): Effects of malnutrition and hyperalimentation on wound healing. *Surg. Gynecol. Obstet.*, 146:33–37.

163. Ishihara, M. (1977): Histological and histochemical study on auto-transplantation between different kinds of cartilage. *Aichi. Gakuin Daigaku Shigakkai Shi.*, 15:229–244.

164. Ishikawa, T., and Takayama, S. (1978): Ovarian neoplasia in ornamental hybrid carp (Nishikigoi) in Japan. *Ann. N.Y. Acad. Sci.*, 298:330–341.

165. Ishikawa, T., Takayama, S., and Kitagawa, T. (1978): Autoradiographic demonstration of DNA repair synthesis in ganglion cells of aquarium fish at various age in vivo. *Virchow's Arch. Cell Pathol.*, 28:235–242.

166. Ivanov, S. D., and Dzhioev, F. K. (1977): Binding of 2-acetylaminofluorene-9-^{14}C with rat liver nucleic acids during malignization and in primary hepatomas. *Biull. Eksp. Biol. Med.*, 83:332–334.

167. Izquierdo, J. N. (1977): Increased cell proliferation with persistence of circadian rhythms in hamster cheek pouch neoplasms. *Cell Tissue Kinet.*, 10:313–322.

168. Jacob, F. (1978): The Leeuwenhoek Lecture, 1977. Mouse teratocarcinoma and mouse embryo. *Proc. R. Soc. Lond. (Biol.)*, 201:249–270.

169. Jacquet, M., Affara, N., Jakob, H., Nicolas, J. F., Jacob, F., and Gros, F. (1977): Complexity of polysomal messenger RNA in mouse teratocarcinoma cell lines, in *The Organization and Expression of the Eukaryotic Genome*, edited by E. M. Bradbury and K. Javaherian. Academic Press, London.

170. Jakob, H., Buckingham, M. E., Cohen, A., Dupont, L., Fiszman, M., and Jacob, F. (1978): A skeletal muscle cell line isolated from a mouse teratocarcinoma undergoes apparently normal terminal differentiation in vitro. *Exp. Cell Res.*, 114:403–408.

171. Japundzic, I. P., Mimicoka, J. I., and Japundzic, M. M. (1978): The ontogenetic evolution of acidic phosphoprotein phosphatase activity in the lymphatic tissue and the liver of the rat. *Biochimie*, 60:489–498.

172. Joel, J. (1980): Ein Teratom auf der Arteria pulmonalis innerhalb des Herzbeutels. *Virchows Arch. Pathol. Anat.*, 122:381.

173. Jones, P. G., and Campbell, P. E. (eds.) (1976): *Tumours of Infancy and Childhood.* Blackwell Scientific Publications, London.

174. Josipovic, V. (1978): Primary cardiac tumors. *Glas. Srp. Akad. Nauka (Med.)*, 305:57–79.

175. Kantorova, V. I. (1975): [The osteogenic role of the dura mater in adult rabbits during regeneration of the skull] (Rus.). *Ontogenez*, 6:63–70.

176. Kaplan, E. (1977): Squamous cell carcinoma arising in a dermoid cyst of the ovary. A case report. *S. Afr. Med. J.*, 52:1128–1129.

177. Karnaukhov, V. K. (1978): Life span of *Fasciola* in man. *Med. Parazitol. (Mosk.)*, 47:24–25.

178. Kastendieck, H., Böcker, W., and Hüsselmann, H. (1976): [Ultrastructure and formal pathogenesis of embryonal rhabdomyosarcoma] (Ger.). *Z. Krebsforsch.*, 86:55–68.

179. Katenkamp, D., and Stiller, D. (1978): Contractile connective tissue cells and wound healing. Function of myoid fibroblasts in reparative regeneration of mesenchymal tissue. *Z. Exp. Chir.*, 11:17–26.

180. Katenkamp, D., Stiiller, D., and Schulze, E. (1976): Ultrastructural cytology of regenerating tendon—an experimental study. *Exp. Pathol. (Jena)*, 12:25–37.

181. Kaufmann, P., Gentzen, D. M., and Davidoff, M. (1977): The ultrastructure Langhans cells in pathologic human placentas. *Arch. Gynaecol.*, 222:319–332.

182. Kavkalo, D. N. (1978): Effect of dodecyl guanidine acetate on healing time of surgical wounds in animals. *Klin. Khir.*, 7:38–41.

183. Kayser, J., and Lavollay, J. (1978): [Growth and longevity of Wistar rats receiving a diet whose protein content is rapidly lowered in relation to aging] (Fr.). *C. R. Acad. Sci. (D) (Paris)*, 286(14):1109–1112.

184. Kent, S. (1978): Cell regeneration, the aging process, and cancer control. *Geriatrics*, 33:112–118.

185. Khomullo, G. V., Ivanenko, T. V., and Lotova, V. I. (1977): DNA synthesis in connective tissue elements of regenerating skin under the influence of thyrocalcitonin and hypoxia. *Biull. Eksp. Biol. Med.*, 84:618–621.

186. Kiernan, J. A. (1978): An explanation of axonal regeneration in peripheral nerves and its failure in the central nervous system. *Med. Hypotheses* 4:15–26.

187. Kimler, S. C., and Muth, W. F. (1978): Primary malignant teratoma of the thyroid; case report and literature review of cervical teratomas in adults. *Cancer*, 42:311–317.

188. Kirk, D., King, R. J., Heyes, J., Peachey, L., Hirsch, P. J., and Taylor, R. W. (1978): Normal human endometrium in cell culture; I. Separation and characterization of epithelial and stromal components in vitro. *In Vitro*, 14:651–662.

189. Kittlick, P. D., Hadhazy, C., and Olah, E. H. (1975): Studies on cartilage formation; XVIII. Changes of the composition of glycosaminoglycans in regenerating articular surface. *Acta Biol. Acad. Sci. Hung.*, 26:165–174.

190. Kivisaari, J. (1975): Oxygen and carbon dioxide tensions in healing tissue. *Acta Chir. Scand.*, 141:693–696.

191. Klass, M. R. (1977): Aging in the nematode *Caenorhabditis elegans*; major biological and environmental factors influencing life span. *Mech. Ageing Dev.*, 6:413–429.

192. Kondo, S. (1977): A test for mutation theory of cancer; carcinogenesis by misrepair of DNA damaged by 4-nitroquinoline 1-oxide. *Br. J. Cancer*, 35:595–601.

193. Koritsanszky, S., and Hartwig, H. G. (1974): The regeneration of the monoaminergic system in the cerebral ganglion of the earthworm, *Allolobophora caliginosa*. A morphological and microspectrofluorimetrical analysis. *Cell Tissue Res.*, 151:171–186.

194. Kosiakov, G. A., and Razinkov, A. G. (1978): Malignant ovarian folliculoma in an 8-year-old girl. *Pediatriia*, 1:75–76.

195. Koval, T. M., Myser, W. C., Hart, R. W., and Hink, W. F. (1978): Comparison of survival and unscheduled DNA synthesis between an insect and a mammalian cell line following X-ray treatments. *Mutat. Res.*, 49:431–435.

196. Krahenbuhl, J. L., and Remington, J. C. (1977): Inhibition of target cell mitosis as a measure of the cytostatic effects of activated macrophages on tumor target cells. *Cancer Res.*, 37:3912–3916.

197. Kranz, D. (1977): [Wound healing in old age (experimental studies on rats)] (Ger.). *Zentralbl. Chir.*, 102:1160–1170.

198. Kranz, D., Hecht, A., and Fuhrmann, I. (1975): The influence of age on the wound healing of experimental myocardial infarction in rats. *Exp. Pathol. (Jena)*, 11:107–114.

199. Kranz, D., Hecht, A., and Fuhrmann, I. (1976): The influence of hyperthyroidism and hypothyroidism on the wound healing of experimental myocardial infarction in the rat. *Exp. Pathol. (Jena)*, 12:129–136.

200. Kranz, V. D., and Richter, W. (1975): [Neurogenesis and regeneration in the brain of teleosts in relation to age (autoradiographic studies)] (Ger.). *Z. Alternsforsch.*, 30:371–382.

201. Krumerman, M. S., and Chung, A. (1977): Squamous carcinoma arising in benign cystic teratoma of the ovary; a report of four cases and review of the literature. *Cancer*, 39:1237–1242.

202. Kurman, R. J., and Norris, H. J. (1978): Germ cell tumors of the ovary. *Pathol. Annu.*, 13:291–325.

203. Kuwabara, T., Perkins, D. G., and Cogan, D. G. (1976): Sliding of the epithelium in experimental corneal wounds. *Invest. Ophthalmol.*, 15:4–14.

204. Lange, C. S., Martin, P., Ferguson, P., and Resnick, M. A. (1977): The organization and repair of DNA in the mammalian chromosome. *Biopolymers*, 16:1083–1092.

205. Lange, C. S., Liberman, D. F., Clark, R. W., and Ferguson, P. (1977): The organization and repair of DNA in the mammalian chromosome; I. Calibration procedures and errors in the determination of the molecular weight of native DNA. *Biopolymers*, 16:1063–1081.

206. Lange, C. S., Liberman, D. F., Clark, R. W., Ferguson, P., and Sheck, L. E. (1977): The organization and repair of DNA in the mammalian chromosome; III. Determination of the molecular weight of a mammalian native DNA. *Biopolymers*, 16:1093–1114.

207. Laszlo, J., Fyfe, M. J., Swedwick, D., Lee, L., and Brown, O. (1978): Comparison of metoprine (DDMP) and etoprine (DDEP) by measuring the inhibition of deoxyuridine incorporation into the DNA of human leukemic cells 1, 2, 3. *Cancer Treat. Rep.*, 62:341–344.

208. Lea, M. A. (1977): Regulation of macromolecular synthesis in Morris hepatomas. *Adv. Exp. Med. Biol.*, 92:289–305.

209. Leigh, B. (1978): The formation and recovery of two-break chromosome rearrangements from irradiated spermatozoa of *Drosophila melanogaster*. *Mutat. Res.*, 49:45–54.

210. Leith, A. (1978): Detection of limited life span in small clones. *J. Theor. Biol.*, 71:453–464.

211. Letnansky, K. (1975): The phosphorylation of nuclear proteins in the regenerating and premalignant rat liver and its significance for cell proliferation. *Cell Tissue Kinet.*, 8:423–439.

212. Levy, S. B., Rubenstein, C. B., and Tavassoli, M. (1976): The spleen in Friend leukemia; II. Nonleukemic nature of spleen stroma. *J.N.C.I.*, 56:1189–1195.

213. Lim, C., and Lovell, R. T. (1978): Pathology of the vitamin C deficiency syndrome in channel catfish (*Ictalurus punctatus*). *J. Nutr.*, 108:1137–1146.

214. Lin, R. Y., Rappoport, A. E., Deppisch, L. M., Natividad, N. S., and Katz, W. (1977): Squamous cell carcinoma of the urachus. *J. Urol.*, 118:1066–1067.

215. Linares, H. A. (1976): Granulation tissue and hypertrophic scars, in *the Ultrastructure of Collagen*, pp. 93–107, edited by J. J. Longacre. Charles C Thomas, Springfield, Ill.

216. Linthicum, D. S., Marks, D. H., Stein, E. A., and Cooper, E. L. (1977): Graft rejection in earthworms; an electron microscopic study. *Eur. J. Immunol.*, 7:871–876.

217. Liozner, L. D. (1975): Characteristics of the mammalian capacity of regeneration. *Ontogenez*, 6:450–457.

218. LiVolsi, V. A., and Perzin, K. H. (1975): Inflammatory pseudotumors (inflammatory fibrous polyps) of the esophagus. A clinicopathologic study. *Am. J. Dig. Dis.*, 20:475–481.

219. Loeb, J. N., and Yeung, L. L. (1975): Synthesis and degradation of ribosomal RNA in regenerating liver. *J. Exp. Med.*, 142:575–587.

220. Luntz, M. H., Kaufmann, J. C., and Spiller, M. (1975): Sutures and iris wound-healing in the baboon. *Adv. Ophthalmol.*, 30:171–184.

221. Lupulescu, A. (1975): Effect of prostaglandins on protein, RNA, DNA and collagen synthesis in experimental wounds. *Prostaglandins*, 10:573–579.

222. Maekawa, H., and Yamana, K. (1975): Alkaline phosphatase isoenzymes of *Xenopus laevis* embryos and tissues. *J. Exp. Zool.*, 192:155–164.

223. Maj, S., Sitarska, E., and Szczygiel, M. (1977): Free amino acids in leukemic leukocytes. *Acta Haematol. Pol.*, 8:15–20.

224. Malyshev, I. I. (1977): Regeneration of the myocardium of fetuses and newborn rabbits. *Arkh. Patol.*, 39:53–58.

225. Manabe, S., Shima, I., and Yamauchi, S. (1975): Cytokinetic analysis of osteogenic cells in the healing process after fracture. *Acta Orthop. Scand.*, 46:161–176.

226. Mandi, V., Hadhazy, C., Rethy, A., Kiss, E. K., and Glant, T. (1975): Studies on cartilage formation; XVI. Chemical and histochemical assay of lipids in the regenerating articular cartilage. *Acta Biol. Acad. Sci. Hung.*, 26:115–133.

227. Mani, M. S. (1964): *Ecology of Plant Galls*. Dr. W. Junk Publishers, The Hague.

228. Manski, W. (1975): Immunological comparison of normal, regenerating, and cultured corneal cells. *Arch. Ophthalmol. (Paris)*, 35:167–180.

229. Manthorpe, R., Garbarsch, C., and Lorenzen, I. (1975): Glucocorticoid effect on repair processes in vascular connective tissue. Morphological examination and biochemical studies on collagen RNA and DNA in rabbit aorta, *Acta Endocrinol (Copenh.)*, 80:380–397.

230. Mantovani, A. (1978): Effects on in vitro tumor growth of murine macrophages isolated from sarcoma lines differing in immunogenicity and metastasizing capacity. *Int. J. Cancer*, 22(6):741–746.

231. Mantovani, A., Polentarutti, N., Sironi, M., Vecchi, A., Spreafico, F., and Garattini, S. (1978): Macrophage-mediated cytostatic activity on tumour cells after treatment with Triton WR 1339. *Eur. J. Cancer*, 14:229–235.

232. Mareel, M. M., and Vakaet, L. C. (1977): Wound healing in the primitive deep layer of the young chick blastoderm. *Virchow's Arch. Cell Pathol.*, 26:147–157.

233. Martin, R. G., and Oppenheim, A. (1977): Initiation points for DNA replication in nontransformed and simian virus 40-transformed Chinese hamster lung cells. *Cell*, 11:859–869.

234. Massie, H. R., Baird, M. B., and Williams, T. R. (1978): Increased longevity of *Drosophila melanogaster* with diiodomethane. *Gerontology*, 24:104–110.

235. Mastropaolo, W., and Lang, C. A. (1978): DNA polymerase profile during the mosquito life span. *Exp. Gerontol.* 13:207–211.

236. Matulionis, D. H. (1976): Light and electron microscopic study of the degeneration and early regeneration of olfactory epithelium in the mouse. *Am. J. Anat.*, 145:79–99.

237. Maurice, P. A., and Lederrey, C. (1977): Increased sensitivity of chronic lymphocytic leukemia lymphocytes to alkylating agents due to a deficient DNA repair mechanism. *Eur. J. Cancer*, 13:1033–1039.

238. McCormack, T. J., Plassche, W. M., Jr., and Lin, S. R. (1978): Ruptured teratoid tumor in the pineal region. *J. Comput. Assist. Tomgr.*, 2:499–501.

239. McGinnis, J. P., Jr., and Parham, D. M. (1978): Mandible-like structure with teeth in an ovarian cystic teratoma. *Oral Surg.*, 45:104–106.

240. McManus, M. J., Dembroske, S. E., Pienkowski, M. M., Anderson, T. J., Mann, L. C., Schuster, J. S., Vollwiler, L. L., and Weisch, C. U. (1978): Successful transplantation of human benign breast tumors into the athymic nude mouse and demonstration of enhanced DNA synthesis by human placental lactogen. *Cancer Res.*, 38:2343–2349.

240a. McWhirter, N., and McWhirter, R. (1977): *Guiness Book of World Records*, pp. 44–97. Sterling Publishing Co., New York.

241. Meerovitch, E., and Bomford, R. (1977): Macrophage potentiation by *Trichinella spiralis*. *Ann. Trop. Med. Parasitol.*, 71:245–248.

242. Mendez Amezcus, G., and De la Torre Rendon, F. E. (1979): Congenital gastric teratoma in a premature newborn infant. *Bol. Med. Hosp. Infant Mex.*, 36:255–265.

243. Menezes, A. H., Bell, W. E., and Perret, G. E. (1977): Hypothalamic tumors in children. Their diagnosis and management. *Childs Brain*, 3:265–280.

244. Meyer, J. C., and Weiss, H. (1977): [Different behavior of human melanoma cells from primary tumor and metastases in vitro] (Ger.). *Dermatologica*, 155:210–217.

245. Michlmayr, G. (1978): T-lymphocytes and their function in Hodgkin's disease. *Fortschr. Med.*, 96:1928–1932.

246. Micu, D. (1977): Metabolic disturbances of the lymphoid cells and their significance for clinical pathology. *Med. Interne*, 15:3–12.

247. Miegeville, M., Morin, O., and Vermeil, C. (1977): Autoradiography of the exchanges that can occur between murine sarcoma cells (BP 8) and yeast cells (*Saccharomyces cerevisiae*, complete or protoplast). *C. R. Soc. Biol. (Paris)*, 171:879–882.

248. Militzer, K. (1976): [Quantitative histometric investigations on the epidermis and corium of rat paw after experimental inflammation] (Ger.). *Arch. Dermatol. Res.*, 256:151–166.

249. Milo, G. E., Blakeslee, J., Yohn, D. S., and DiPaolo, J. A. (1978): Biochemical activation of aryl hydrocarbon hydroxylase activity, cellular distribution of polynuclear hydrocarbon metabolites, and DNA damage by polynuclear hydrocarbon products in human cells in vitro. *Cancer Res.*, 38:1638–1644.

249a. Minton, S. A., Jr., and Minton, M. R. (1973): *Giant Reptiles*, pp. 187–206. Charles Scribner's, New York.

250. Mittal, A. K., Rai, A. K., and Banerjes, T. K. (1977): Studies on the pattern of healing of wounds in the skin of a cat-fish *Heteropneustes fossilis* (Bloch) (Heteropneustidae, Pisces). *Z. Mikrosk. Anat. Forsch.*, 91:270–286.

251. Mogilevskaia, K. A., and Loiko, E. E. (1978): Organismoid teratoma of the retroperitoneal space in a child. *Vestn. Khir.*, 120:118.

252. Molisch, H. (1938): *The Longevity of Plants*. English Ed. The Translator, New York.

252a. Moment, G. B. (1975): On the non-hormonal control of the termination of regeneration. *Growth*, 39:233–240.

253. Morello, D., Gachelin, G., Dubois, P., Tanigaki, N., Pressman, D., and Jacob, F. (1978): Absence of reaction of a xenogenic anti-H-2 serum with mouse embryonal carcinoma cells. *Transplantation*, 26:119–125.

254. Moriuchi, A., Nakayama, I., Muta, H., Taira, Y., and Takahara, O. (1977): Gastric teratoma of children—a case report with review of the literature. *Acta Pathol. Jpn.*, 27:749–758.

255. Mosely, L. H., and Finseth, F. (1977): Cigarette smoking; impairment of digital blood flow and wound healing in the hand. *Hand*, 9:97–101.

256. Movshovich, B. L., and Naddachina, T. A. (1977): Myocardial infarct repair in the light of clinico-biochemical and morphological studies. *Kardiologiia*, 17:108–114.

257. Müller, I., and Wolf, F. (1978): A correlation between shortened life span and UV-sensitivity in some strains of *Saccharomyces cerevisiae*. *Mol. Gen. Genet.*, 160:231–234.

258. Müller, W., Brämisch, R., Afra, D., and Schwenzfeger, A. (1977): Cytophotometric investigations of the nuclear DNA content in ependymomas and plexus-papillomas. *Acta Neuropathol. (Berl.)*, 39:255–259.

259. Nabeshima, Y. I., Tsurugi, K., and Ogata, K. (1975): Preferential biosynthesis of ribosomal structural proteins by free and loosely bound polysomes from regenerating rat liver. *Biochim. Biophys. Acta*, 414:30–43.

260. Nandi, S. (1978): Role of hormones in mammary neoplasia. *Cancer Res.*, 38:4046–4049.

261. Nasiell, M., Kato, H., Auer, G., Zetterberg, A., Roger, V., and Karlen, L. (1978): Cytomorphological grading and Feulgen DNA-analysis of metaplastic and neoplastic bronchial cells. *Cancer*, 41:1511–1521.

262. Nathan, P., Law, E. J., Ogle, J. D., and MacMillan, B. G. (1976): Proteolytic enzyme activity in the granulation tissue of the human burn wound. *J. Trauma*, 16:912–918.

263. Naumova, L. P., Samorodova, N. I., and Sandakhchiev, L. S. (1975): [Polar distribution of RNA in the cytoplasm of *Acetabularia mediterranea*] (Rus.). *Ontogenez*, 6:99–104.

264. Nochomovitz, L. E., and Rosai, J. (1978): Current concepts on the histogenesis, pathology, and immunochemistry of germ cell tumors of the testis. *Pathol. Annu.*, 13:327–362.

265. Nordlander, R. H., and Singer, M. (1976): Synaptoid profiles in regenerating crustacean peripheral nerves. *Cell Tissue Res.*, 166:445–460.

266. Oehmichen, M., and Huber, H. (1976): Reactive microglia with membrane features of mononuclear phagocytes. *J. Neuropathol. Exp. Neurol.*, 35:30–39.

267. Ohashi, T., Shimamura, Y., Miyake, L., Harada, L., and Namba, S. (1977): The epidermoid and dermoid cysts of the central nervous system—reported of unusual cases. *No Shinkei Geka*, 5:585–592.

268. Ohkawara, A., and Aoyagi, T. (1977): Wound healing—some biochemical aspects, in *Biochemistry of Cutaneous Epidermal Differentiation*, pp. 274–87, edited by M. Seiji and I. A. Bernstein. University Park Press, Baltimore.

269. Oi, R. H., and Dobbs, M. (1978): Lactating breast tissue in benign cystic teratoma. *Am. J. Obstet. Gynecol.*, 130:729–731.

270. Oppermann, H. C., and Willich, E. (1978): [X-ray diagnosis and differential diagnosis of mediastinal tumors in childhood] (Ger.). *Radiologe*, 18:218–227.

271. Owen, S. E., Weiss, H. A., and Prince, L. H. (1942): Carcinogens and planarian tissue regeneration.

272. Paffenholz, V. (1978): Correlation between DNA repair of embryonic fibroblasts and different life span of 3 inbred mouse strains. *Mech. Ageing Dev.*, 7:131–150.

273. Pallin, B., Ahonen, J., Rank, F., and Zederfeldt, B. (1975): Granulation tissue formation in oophorectomized rats treated with female sex hormones; I. A histological study. *Acta. Chir. Scand.*, 141:702–709.

274. Pallin, B., Ahonen, J., and Zederfeldt, B. (1975): Granulation tissue formation in oophorectomized rats treated with female sex hormones; II. Studies on the amount of collagen and on tensile strength. *Acta Chir. Scand.*, 141:710–714.

275. Papaioannou, V. E., Gardner, R. L., McBurney, M. W., Babinet, C., and Evans, M. J. (1978): Participation of cultured teratocarcinoma cells in mouse embryogenesis. *J. Embryol. Exp. Morphol.*, 44:93–104.

276. Parsons, R. W. (1977): Scar prognosis. *Clin. Plast. Surg.*, 4:181–186.

277. Pegels, C. C. (1978): Statistical effects of varying blood life span from 14 to 28 days. *Transfusion*, 18:189–192.

278. Perekalin, D. V. (1975): [DNA reproduction in the organism of planarians in postinjury recovery] (Rus.). *Tsitologiia*, 17:1084–1086.

279. Pereverzev, B. L. (1978): Quantity of RNA in the life cycle of normal and tumorous cells. *Dokl. Akad. Nauk. SSSR*, 241:946–948.

280. Peries, J., Debons-Guillemin, M. C., Canivet, M., Emanoil-Ravicovitch, R., Tavitian, A., Boiron, M. (1977): Multiplication of murine C-type viruses in mouse teratocarcinoma cell lines. *Nouv. Rev. Fr. Hematol. Blood Cells*, 18:383–390.

281. Pero, R. W., Brynglesson, C., and Brandt, L. (1977): Carcinogen-induced repair and binding in the DNA of chronic lymphocytic leukemic lymphocytes. *Cancer Lett.*, 2:311–317.

282. Pero, R. W., Bryngelsson, T., Rudduck, C., and Levan, G. (1978): Polycyclic hydrocarbon-induced rat sarcomas correlated to disturbances in the deoxyadenylate regions of the tumor DNAs. *Eur. J. Cancer*, 14:961–969.

283. Pero, R. W., Bryngelsson, C., Mitelman, F., Kornfält, R., Thulin, T., and Norden, A. (1978): Interindividual variation in the responses of cultured human lymphocytes to exposure from DNA damaging chemical agents; inter-individual variation to carcinogen exposure. *Mutat. Res.*, 53:327–341.

284. Pickart, L., Millard, M. M., Beiderman, B., and Thaler, M. M. (1978): Surface analysis and depth profiles of calcium in hepatoma cells during pyruvate-induced DNA synthesis. *Biochim. Biophys. Acta*, 544:138–143.

285. Planck, S. R., and Mueller, G. C. (1977): DNA chain growth in isolated Hela nuclei. *Biochemistry*, 17:2778–2782.

286. Platt, J. E. (1976): The effects of ergocornine on tail height, spontaneous and T4-induced metamorphosis and thyroidal uptake of radioiodide in neotenic *Ambystoma tigrinum*. *Gen. Comp. Endocrinol.*, 28:71–81.

287. Pochedly, C., and Necheles, T. F. (eds.) (1973): *Major Problems in Childhood Cancer*. Charles C Thomas, Springfield, Ill.

288. Podboronov, V. M., and Stepanchenok-Rudnik, G. I. (1977): Bactericidal factor in arthropods (review of the literature). *Med. Parazitol. (Mosk.)*, 46:92–99.

289. Ponten, J., and Westermark, B. (1978): Properties of human malignant glioma cells in vitro. *Med. Biol.*, 56:184–193.

290. Prasad, C. N., Mitra, S. K., and Pathak, I. C. (1977): Gastric teratoma in a newborn baby. *Indian Pediatr.*, 14:855–856.

291. Pressman, E. K., Razumova, V. P., Sandakhchiev, L. S. (1974): [Morphogenesis of reconstructed enucleated *Acetabularia* cells] (Rus.). *Acetabularia Ontogenez*, 5:532–535.

292. Price, C. H. (1977): Regeneration in the central nervous system of a pulmonate mollusc, *Melampus*. *Cell Tissue Res.*, 180:529–536.

293. Purves, D. (1975): Functional and structural changes in mammalian sympathetic neurones following interruption of their axons. *J. Physiol. (Lond.)*, 252:429–463.

294. Quigley, E. M., Doyle, C. T., and Brady, M. P. (1977): Thyroid teratoma in infancy. *Ir. J. Med. Sci.*, 146:298–299.

295. Raekallio, J. (1977): The synergistic effect of humoral factors, extracellular matrix and cells in wound healing. *Fortschr. Med.*, 95:1299–1304.

296. Ramos, S., and Acha, I. G. (1975): Cell wall enzymatic lysis of the yeast form of *Pullularia pullulans* and wall regeneration by protoplasts. *Arch. Microbiol.*, 104:271–277.

297. Recondo, J., and Libshitz, H. I. (1978): Mediastinal extragonadal germ cell tumors. *Urology*, 11:369–375.

298. Reidy, M. A., and Bowyer, D. E. (1977): Scanning electron microscopy of aortic endothelium following injury by endotoxin and during subsequent repair. *Prog. Biochem. Pharmacol.*, 13:175–181.

299. Reinhardt, C. A., Hodgkin, N. M., and Bryant, P. J. (1977): Wound healing in the imaginal discs of *Drosophila*; I. Scanning electron microscopy of normal and healing wing discs. *Dev. Biol.*, 60:238–257.

300. Renne, J. (1977): [Experimental contribution on the healing tendency of cartilage bone transplants after short intra-articular preservation] (Ger.). *Hefte Unfallheilkd.*, 129:360–364.

301. Repesh, L. A., and Oberpriller, J. C. (1978): Scanning electron microscopy of epidermal cell migration in wound healing during limb regeneration in the adult newt, *Notophthalmus viridescens*. *Am. J. Anat.*, 151:539–555.

302. Revich, G. G., Savina, M. I., and Toguzov, R. T., [Changes in the content of different nuclear proteins and DNA from diploid and polyploid hepatocytes in regenerating liver of mice] (Rus.). *Biokhimiia*, 40:790–794.

303. Reznikov, K. Iu. (1978): Proliferative potential of vertebrate brain cells and their role in brain regeneration. *Usp. Sovrem. Biol.*, 86:99–113.

304. Rizzino, A., Sato, G. (1978): Growth of embryonal carcinoma cells in

serum-free medium. *Proc. Natl. Acad. Sci. U.S.A.*, 75:1844–1848.

305. Rodermel, S. R., and Smith-Sonneborn, J. (1977): Age-correlated changes in expression of micronuclear damage and repair in *Paramecium tetraurelia*. *Genetics*, 87:259–274.

306. Roland, J. (1976): [Fibroblast and myofibroblast in the granulation tissue] (Fr.). *Ann. Anat. Pathol. (Paris)*, 21:37–44.

307. Rose, H. (1977): [Biological bases of aging] (Ger.). *ZFA (Dresden)*, 32:11–17.

308. Rosenbaum, T. J., Soule, E. H., and Onofrio, B. M. (1978): Teratomatous cyst of the spinal canal. Case report. *J. Neurosurg.*, 49:292–297.

309. Ross, W. E., Ewig, R. A., and Kohn, K. W. (1978): Differences between melphalan and nitrogen mustard in the formation and removal of DNA cross-links. *Cancer Res.*, 38:1502–1506.

310. Rupniewska, Z. M., Rozynkowa, D., Kowalewski, J., and Kurowska, M. (1978): Mononuclear peripheral blood cells in patients with non-Hodgkin's lymphoma synthesizing DNA in vitro. *Acta Haematol. Pol.*, 9:169–177.

311. Russo, R., Anguissola, G. B., Scalia, D., Gallucci, V., and Fasoli, G. (1978): The usefulness of the phonocardiography in the diagnosis of the extrinsic obstruction of the pulmonary artery. Report of a case. *G. Ital. Cardiol.*, 8:789–794.

312. Ruzicka, F., Pawlowsky, J., Erber, A., and Nowotny, H. (1976): [Three cases of eosinophilic leukemia with atypical granulation in the eosinophils and neutrophils] (Ger.). *Blut*, 32:337–346.

313. Ryvniak, V. V., and Vtiurin, B. V.: [The ultrastructure of the cellular elements of granulation tissue] (Rus.). *Arkh. Patol.*, 37:14–20.

314. Saleuddin, A. S. (1975): An electron microscopic study on the formation of the periostracum in *Helisoma* (Mollusca). *Calcif. Tissue Res.*, 18:297–310.

315. Sasada, M., Sawada, H., Nakamura, T., and Uchino, H. (1978): DNA repair in human leukemic leucocytes treated with neocarzinostatin. *Gan*, 69:407–412.

316. Sawada, K. (1978): Wound repair of the mouse cerebral cortex—an electron microscopic study. *Fukuoka Igaku Zasshi*, 69:298–318.

316a. Scheffer, V. B. (1979): Whales great and small, in *Wild Animals of North America*, pp. 167–207. National Geographic Society, Washington, D.C.

317. Scheidegger, S. (1977)): Maximal human life span. A pathological study. *Praxis*, 66:1138–1140.

318. Schierhölter, R., and Honegger, H. (1975): Morphology of the corneal endothelium under normal conditions and during regeneration after mechanical injury. *Adv. Ophthalmol.*, 31:34–99.

319. Schmidt, M.,.and Sperling, W. (1978): Report on 2 highly-mature, retroperitoneally located, twin teratomas in a male newborn infant; fetus in fetu. *R.O.E.F.O.*, 128:369–371.

320. Schroeder, J. J., James, J., Muller, J. H., Everts, V., and Klopper, P. J. (1977): The epithelium in healing experimental standard lesions in the gastric mucosa of the rat. A light microscopical and scanning electron microscopical study. *Digestion*, 15:397–410.

321. Schulitz, K. P. (1976): [Regeneration of the synovia] (Ger.). *Z. Orthop.*, 114:161–176.

321a. Schultz, L. P. (1948): *The Ways of Fishes*. D. Van Nostrand, New York.

322. Schwartz, A. G., and Moore, C. J. (1977): Inverse correlation between species life span and capacity of cultured fibroblasts to bind 7,12-dimethylbenz(a)anthracene to DNA. *Exp. Cell Res.*, 109:448–450.

323. Schwartz, S. M., Stemerman, M. B., and Benditt, E. P. (1975): The aortic intima; II. Repair of the aortic lining after mechanical denudation. *Am. J. Pathol.*, 81:15–42.

324. Sciubba, J. J., Waterhouse, J. P., and Meyer, J. (1978): A fine structural comparison of the healing of incisional wounds of mucosa and skin. *J. Oral Pathol.*, 7:214–227.

325. Seidel, M. V., Howard, R. J., and Balfour, H. H., Jr. (1978): A virological study of human kidney explant cultures from renal allograft recipients. *Transplantation*, 25:193–196.

326. Seitz, H. D., Köhnlein, H. E., Ocker, K., and Tonn, M. (1978): Studies on wound healing and secondary and tertiary wounds. *Z. Exp. Chir.*, 11:121–127.

327. Sevitt, S. (1978): Pathology of injury; some problems and new horizons. *Injury*, 10:22–30.

328. Shah, N. K., Kripke, B. J., Sanzone, C. F., and Cosman, E. B. (1978): Histological evaluation of cutaneous wound healing in presence of nitrous oxide in rats. *Anesth. Analg. (Cleve.)*, 57:527–533.

329. Shapot, V. S., and Likhtenshtein, A. V. (1978): Genetic nature of neoplastic transformation. *Tsitol. Genet.*, 12:73–84.

330. Shekhter, A. B., Berchenko, G. N., and Nikolaev, A. V. (1977): Macrophage-fibroblast interaction and its possible role in regulating collagen metabolism during wound healing. *Biull. Eksp. Biol. Med.*, 83:627–630.

331. Shibata, T., and Mori, W. (1978): A study on the melanin-laden dendritic cell (melanocyte) in ovarian cystic teratoma. *Acta Pathol. Jpn.*, 28:225–233.

332. Shin, K. H., Freeman, C. R., and Stachewitsch, A. (1978): Primary intracranial mixed choriocarcinoma and malignant teratoma. *J. Can. Assoc. Radiol.*, 29:129–131.

333. Shivers, R. R., and Brightman, M. W. (1976): Trans-glial channels in ventral nerve roots of crayfish, *J. Comp. Neurol.*, 167:1–26.

333a. Shortino, T. J., et al. (1963): Effect of certain carcinogenetic 2-fluorenamine derivates on larvae of the house fly, *Musca domestica* Linnaeus. *J. Insect. Pathol.*, 5:489–492.

334. Siewing, R. (1969): *Lehrbuch der vergleichenden Entwicklungsgeschichte der Tiere*. Paul Parey Verlag, Berlin.

335. Sikora, K., Stern, P., and Lennox, E. (1977): Immunoprotection by embryonal carcinoma cells for methylcholanthrene-induced murine sarcomas. *Nature*, 269:813–815.

336. Simnett, J. D., and Fisher, J. M. (1976): Cell division and tissue repair following localized damage to the mammalian lung. *J. Morphol.*, 148:177–184.

337. Sobis, H., and Vandeputte, M. (1977): Yolk sac derived teratomas and carcinomas in hamsters. *Eur. J. Cancer*, 13:1175–1181.

338. Sobis, H., Park, B., and Vandeputte, M. (1978): Immunological enhancement of hybrid teratomas derived from yolk sac. *Transplantation*, 26:178–180.

339. Sonntag, W., and Paulini, K. (1977): The vascularisation of the granulation tissue in different ages. Its importance for wound healing. *Aktuel Gerontol.*, 7:253–256.

340. Spadaro, J. A. (1977): Electrically stimulated bone growth in animals and man. Review of the literature. *Clin. Orthop.*, 122:325–332.

341. Spector, G. J. (1977): Leucine and alanine aminopeptidase activities in experimentally induced intradermal granulomas and late stages of wound healing in the rat. *Lab. Invest.*, 36:1–7.

342. Stark, M. M., Nicholson, D. J., Soelberg, K. B., Kempler, D., and Pelzner, R. B. (1977): The effects of retraction cords and electrosurgery upon blood pressure and tissue regeneration in rhesus monkeys. *J. Dent. Res.*, 56:881–888.

343. Stemerman, M. B., Spaet, T. H., Pitlick, F., Cintron, J., Lejnieks, I., and Tiell, M. L. (1977): Intimal healing. The pattern of reendothelialization and intimal thickening. *Am. J. Pathol.*, 87:125–142.

344. Swenberg, J. A. (1977): Chemical- and virus-induced brain tumors. *Natl. Cancer Inst. Monogr.*, 46:3–10.

345. Stephan-Dubois, F., and Biver, G. (1974): [Action of dactinomycin on the caudal regeneration of *Tubifex tubifex* (Annelida, Oligochaeta)] (Fr.). *C. R. Soc. Biol. (Paris)*, 168:1068–1071.

346. Strickland, S., and Mahdavi, V. (1978): The induction of differentiation in teratocarcinoma stem cells by retinoic acid. *Cell*, 15:393–403.

347. Strong, J. E., and Crooke, S. T. (1978): DNA breakage by tallysomycin. *Cancer Res.*, 38:3322–3326.

348. Suseelan, A. V., Gupta, I. M., Viswanathan, V., and Udekwu, F. A. (1977): Teratoma of the thyroid gland. *Int. Surg.*, 62:586–587.

349. Sutow, W. W., Vietti, T. J., and Fernbach, D. J. (eds.) (1977): *Clinical Pediatric Oncology*, Ed. 2. C. V. Mosby, St. Louis.

350. Svedbergh, B. (1975): Effects of artificial intraocular pressure elevation on the corneal endothelium in the vervet monkey (*Cercopithecus aethiops*). *Acta Ophthalmol., (Copenh)* 53:839–855.

351. Svendgaard, N. A., Björklund, A., and Stenevi, U. (1976): Regeneration of central cholinergic neurones in the adult rat brain. *Brain Res.*, 102:1–22.

352. Symann, M., Fontebuoni, A., Quesenberry, P., Howard, D., and Stohlman, F., Jr. (1976): Fetal hemopoiesis in diffusion chamber cultures; I. The pattern of pluripotent stem cell growth. *Cell Tissue Kinet.*, 9:41–49.

353. Takeuchi, K., Okabe, S., Takagi, K., and Umeda, N. (1977): Influence of aspirin on healing of chronic gastric ulcers in dogs. *Digestion*, 16:51–56.

354. Tarhan, S., White, R. D., and Moffitt, E. A. (1977): Anesthesia and postoperative care for cardiac operations. *Ann. Thorac. Surg.*, 23:173–193.

355. Taylor-Papadimitriou, J., Shearer, M., and Watling, D. (1978): Growth requirements of calf lens epithelium in culture. *J. Cell Physiol.*, 95:95–103.

356. Theppisai, H., Shuangshoti, S., and Amatyakul, A. (1977): Neuroblastoma arising in metastasizing ovarian teratoma. *J. Med. Assoc. Thai.*, 60:396–404.

357. Thomas, C. B., Osieka, R., and Kohn, K. W. (1978): DNA cross-linking by in vivo treatment with 1-(2-chloroethyl)-3-(4-methylcyclohexyl)-1-nitrosourea of sensitive and resistant human colon carcinoma xenografts in nude mice. *Cancer Res.*, 38:2448–2454.

358. Thomason, P. R., and Matzke, H. A. (1975): Effects of ischemia on the hind limb of the rat. *Am. J. Phys. Med.*, 54:113–131.

359. Timson, J. (1977): Caffeine. *Mutat. Res.*, 47:1–52.

360. Timur, M., Roberts, R. J., and McQueen, A. (1977): Carrageenin granuloma in the plaice (*Pleuronectes platessa*); a histopathological study of chronic inflammation in a teleost fish. *J. Comp. Pathol.*, 87:89.

361. Tjernshaugen, H., and Gautvik, K. M. (1976): Nucleotidase activity in regenerating liver and in clonal strains of hepatoma and pituitary cells in culture. *J. Cell. Physiol.*, 88:13–22.

362. Trenin, A. S. (1977): Carminomycin induction of single-stranded breaks in the DNA of tumor cells. *Antibiotiki*, 23:400–403.

363. Tumrasvin, W., Sucharit, S., and Vutikes, S. (1977): Studies on the life history of *Megaselia scalaris* (Loew) in Thailand. *Southeast Asian J. Trop. Med. Public Health*, 8:74–76.

364. Ungerleider, R. S., Donaldson, S. S., Warnke, R. A., and Wilbur, J. R.

(1978): Endodermal sinus tumor; the Stanford experience and the first reported case arising in the vulva. *Cancer*, 41:1627–1634.

365. Urrutia, J., Undurraga, A., and Aguila, P. (1978): Primary teratocarcinoma of the mediastinum. *Rev. Med. Chil.*, 1:34–38.

366. Van Bogaert, L. J., De Coninck, A., Vrebos, J., and Verheecke, G. (1977): Studies on the possible influence of the so-called wound healing reaction on DNA synthesis in organ culture. *Virchows Arch. Cell Pathol.*, 25:75–82.

367. Van Dam, R. H., Boot, R., Van der Donk, J. A., and Goudswaard, J. (1978): Skin grafting and graft rejection in goats. *Am. J. Vet. Res.*, 39:1359–1362.

368. VanDenbos, G., and Frieden, E. (1976): DNA synthesis and turnover in the bullfrog tadpole during metamorphosis. *J. Biol. Chem.*, 251:4111–4114.

369. Van Heukelem, W. F. (1977): Laboratory maintenance, breeding, rearing, and biomedical research potential of the Yucatan octopus (*Octopus maya*). *Lab. Anim. Sci.*, 27:852–859.

370. Viceps-Madore, D., and Mezger-Freed, L. (1978): Studies on DNA repair in frog and human cells exposed to an acridine half-mustard (ICR 191) and to MNNG. *Mutat. Res.*, 49:357–370.

371. Vincent, A. L., and Ash, L. R. (1978): Further observations on spontaneous neoplasms in the Mongolian gerbil, *Meriones unguiculatus. Lab. Anim. Sci.*, 28:297–300.

372. Vitello, L., Breen, M., Weinstein, H. G., Sittig, R. A., and Blacik, L. J. (1978): Keratan sulfate-like glycosaminoglycan in the cerebral cortex of the brain and its variation with age. *Biochim. Biophys. Acta*, 539:305–314.

373. Vladimirova, I. G. (1975): Growth and respiration of regenerating tissues of the axolotl tail. *Sov. J. Dev. Biol.*, 5:88–91.

374. Vogel, H. G. (1977): Strain of rat skin at constant load (creep experiments); influence of age and desmotropic agents. *Gerontology*, 23:77–86.

375. Von Albertini, A. (1974): *Histologische Geschwulstdiagnostik.* Georg Thieme Verlag, Stuttgart.

376. Von Denffer, D. (1976): In: *Strasburger's Textbook of Botany,* edited by E. Strasburger. Tischer, London.

376a. Walker, E. P. (1975): *Mammals of the World,* pp. 141–142, 155, 1137, 1319–1324, 1405–1408. Johns Hopkins University Press, Baltimore.

377. Waller, M., and Waller, H. (1978): [Diploid and aneuploid human cell lines from autopsy material in long term cultures. Investigations of growth behaviour and karyotype] (Ger.). *Zentralbl. Allg. Pathol.*, 122:236–248.

378. Walter, J. B. (1976): Wound healing. *J. Otolaryngol.*, 5:171–176.

379. Watanabe, I., Kasai, M., and Suzuki, S. (1978): True teratoma of the liver—report of a case and review of the literature. *Acta Hepatogastroenterol. (Stuttg.)*, 25:40–44.

380. Weber, G. (1977): Enzymology of cancer cells (first of two parts). *N. Engl. J. Med.*, 296:486–492.

381. Weber, G., Prajda, N., and Williams, J. C. (1975): Biochemical strategy of the cancer cell; malignant transformation-linked enzymatic imbalance. *Adv. Enzyme Regul.*, 13:3–23.

382. Weinstein, R. A., Rubinstein, A. S., and Choukas, N. C. (1976): Sequential electron microscopic healing study of grafted palatal mucosa. *J. Dent. Res.*, 55:16–21.

383. Wheeler, J. E. (1978): Extraovarian teratoma with peritoneal gliomatosis. *Hum. Pathol.*, 9:232–234.

384. Whitcomb, M. E., and Parker, R. L. (1977): Abnormal lymphocyte protein synthesis in bronchogenic carcinoma. *Cancer*, 40:3014–3018.

385. White, A. A., 3rd, Panjabi, M. M., and Southwick, W. O. (1977): The four biomechanical stages of fracture repair. *J. Bone Joint Surg.*, 59A:188–192.

386. Widdus, R., Taylor, M., Powers, L., and Danielli, J. F. (1978): Characteristics of the "life spanning" phenomenon in *Amoeba proteus.* Independent nuclear and cytoplasmic ability to impose finite "life span." *Gerontology*, 24:208–219.

387. Widmann, J. J., and Fahimi, H. D. (1975): Proliferation of mononuclear phagocytes (Kupffer cells) and endothelial cells in regenerating rat liver. A light and electron microscopic cytochemical study. *Am. J. Pathol.*, 80:349–366.

388. Williams, G. M., ter Haar, A., Krajewski, C., Parks, L. C., and Roth, J. (1975): Rejection and repair of endothelium in major vessel transplants. *Surgery*, 78:694–706.

389. Yager, J. D., Jr., and Miller, J. A., Jr. (1978): DNA repair in primary cultures of rat hepatocytes. *Cancer Res.*, 38:4385–4394.

390. Yamada, T. (1977): Control mechanisms in cell-type conversion in newt lens regeneration. *Monogr. Dev. Biol.*, 13:1–126.

391. Yanko, L., and Behar, A. (1978): Teratoid intraocular medulloepithelioma. *Am. J. Ophthalmol.*, 85:850–853.

392. Yeschua, R., Bab, I. A., Wexler, M. R., and Neuman, Z. (1977): Dermoid cyst of the floor of the mouth in an infant. Case report. *J. Maxillofac. Surg.*, 5:211–213.

393. Yew, F. H., and Johnson, R. T. (1978): Human B and T lymphocytes differ in UV-induced repair capacity. *Exp. Cell Res.*, 113:151–160.

394. Yoshida, H. (1975): [Histopathological study on degeneration and regeneration of damaged photoreceptor cells; 3. Electron histochemical study on phosphorylase activity in the photoreceptor cell of the photocoagulated rabbit retina] (Jpn.). *Acta Soc. Ophthalmol. Jpn.*, 79:1585–1593.

395. Zerner, J., Wilkis, J. L., and Fenn, M. E. (1978): Oral contraceptive therapy and benign hepatic lesions in females. *J. Maine Med. Assoc.*, 69:161–164.

396. Zetter, B. R., and Martin, G. R. (1978): Expression of a high molecular weight cell surface glycoprotein (LETS protein) by preimplantation mouse embryos and teratocarcinoma stem cells. *Proc. Natl. Acad. Sci. U.S.A.*, 75:2324–2328.

397. Znidaric, D., and Lui, A. (1974): Regeneration of proximal and distal body part in Hydra exposed to ultraviolet light (2535 Å). *Z. Mikrosk. Anat. Forsch.*, 88:637–648.

14

Chrono-Oncology

Francis Levi, Franz Halberg, Mark Nesbit, Erhard Haus, and Howard Levine

INTRODUCTION

A considerable body of cytokinetic, pharmacologic and biochemical information has served with relative success as a basis for the currently employed schedules of oncostatic therapy, both at the experimental and at the clinical level (3, 24, 77, 137). However, in 1972, Mathé (91) suggested that the expectation of further benefits from chemotherapy is limited. An explanation proposed by others for this apparent "stagnation" of therapeutic progress is that conventional methods for improving the selective toxicity ratio (135) of carcinostatic agents have reached their limit (162). Tannock (148) indicates that the major factor favorably affecting the outcome of chemotherapy is the availability of active drugs with acceptable host toxicity. In such a situation, extensively documented rhythms in immunologic, hormonal, and other variables pertinent to oncogenesis as well as to tolerance of oncostatic agents by host and tumor may well be exploited for the prevention and treatment of cancer.

FACTORS AFFECTING CARCINOGENESIS

External Agents

The major role played by bioperiodicity in chemical carcinogenesis has been repeatedly studied (27, 43, 47, 70, 100). In several studies, local skin exposure to a carcinogen such as dimethylbenzanthracene (DMBA) or 3-methylcholanthrene induced a different number of tumors (e.g., sarcomas) as a function of the circadian stage in which the agent was applied.

Such a circadian stage dependence of host susceptibility to a carcinogen evaluated after injection of DMBA into the submandibular gland of hamsters is seen in Figure 14.1. In two separate studies, carried out by Anand P. Chaudhry in Minnesota (11), six groups of animals had a fixed dose of DMBA injected into the submandibular gland, one group at each of six circadian times separated by consecutive 4-hr spans during 24 hr. Three months later the hamsters were killed and the presence of tumors (sarcomas) in excised glands were determined. Sarcoma was found in 80% of the animals injected at one time—6 hours after light onset (6 HALO)—and 35% of those injected at another time (22 HALO). In both studies, the stage of the organism at the time of injection was sufficiently important to tip the scale between sarcoma and no sarcoma 3 months after administration of the carcinogen. It overrode the effects of a multitude of factors impinging upon the organism during the 3-month span.

Similarly, a circadian rhythm in DMBA-induced mammary carcinogenesis was demonstrated in mice implanted with ectopic pituitaries or muscle isografts and orally fed with DMBA at 1 of 6 circadian stages (Figure 14.1). The highest incidence of DMBA-induced breast cancers in mice and DMBA-induced submandibular sarcomas in hamsters occurred if the carcinogenic agent was administered toward the end of the light (rest) span. It is commonly supposed that a condition for circadian susceptibility rhythms to occur is a short half-life, i.e., the rapid elimination of an agent from the body. In the case of DMBA, the host is exposed to the

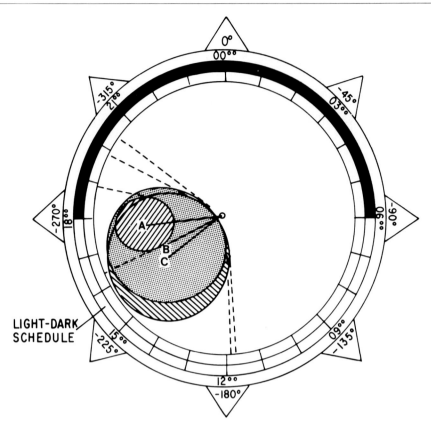

SINGLE COSINOR

KEY TO ELLIPSES	P	NO. OBS.	% RHYTHM	MESOR SE	AMPLITUDE (95% CL.)	ACROPHASE (ϕ) (95% CL)
A SERUM CORTICOSTERONE	<0.001	31	62	98 4.2	45 (27.7 62)	−265°(−246 −284)
B BREAST CANCER INCIDENCE IN MICE	0.026	12	55	100 8.0	38 (4.9 71)	−237°(−177 −298)
C SARCOMA INCIDENCE IN HAMSTERS	0.031	20	34	91 10.1	40 (3.4 77)	−242°(−173 −305)

A: IN ADULT D$_8$♀ MICE

B: ADULT D$_8$ ♀ MICE IMPLANTED WITH ECTOPIC PITUITARY OR MUSCLE ISOGRAFTS. 32 MONTHS LATER SUBGROUPS WERE FED DMBA (2mg/1.2cc OLIVE OIL/20gm BODY WEIGHT BY ESOPHAGEAL INSTILLATION) AT ONE OF SIX 4-HOURLY TIME POINTS. (HAUS et al.)

C: 21-25 HAMSTERS INJECTED WITH DMBA INTO THE SUBMANDIBULAR GLAND AT ONE OF 6 CIRCADIAN STAGES 15 WEEKS EARLIER (CHAUDHRY et al.)

Figure 14.1 Cosinor presentation of the circadian rhythm in murine susceptibility to a chemical carcinogen and its phase relationship to serum corticosterone. Dimethylbenzantracene (DMBA)-induced sarcomas in hamsters; DMBA-induced breast carcinomas and serum corticosterone in mice. The cosinor method (50, 51) consists of fitting cosine functions to the data series available. By doing so, the method yields the parameters of the best fitting cosine function for any a priori selected period (e.g. 24 hr). This method also yields a P value from an F-test in testing the zero-amplitude assumption. In the presence of a rhythm, this assumption is rejected, yielding a P value < 0.05. When the P value is > 0.05, the zero-amplitude assumption is accepted, and no rhythm can be described with the period tested for this data series. The parameters yielded by the cosinor method are: 1) the mesor: average value of the rhythm, which is close to the mean, if the data are obtained at equal intervals over an integral number of periods; 2) the amplitude: the total extent of predictable variability of the "best fitting" cosine function above *or* below the mesor; and 3) the acrophase: the timing of the maximum of the best fitting cosine function, relative to any chosen reference. The polar plot displays these last two parameters. The outer rim indicates the dominant synchronizing schedule (e.g. light-dark) for the period considered. The scale is in

agent for a considerable span following a single administration. Under such conditions, just as in the case of exposure to noise for only a very few seconds, the response of the organism is bioperiodic rather than constant (42). Thus, we can introduce the importance of rhythms to carcinogenesis by showing that the process itself is circadian-stage dependent under controlled conditions (11) as well as under ordinary conditions (100).

Hormonal Environment

The hormonal environment has also long been known to influence carcinogenesis and tumor growth, as illustrated notably by the current concept of cancer hormono-dependence. Thus the role played by the pituitary and/or the hypothalamus in breast-cancer genesis was documented in Bagg albino (C) mice (46, 54). This strain does not carry the Bittner agent—a virus that will enhance the development of breast cancer. Figure 14.2 dramatically indicates the carcinogenic effect of the pituitary isograft: 200 C mice were assigned at random to 10 groups of 20 mice each. One group received no treatment while the others received various tissue implants. All groups were observed for 800 days, shown on the horizontal scale of each rectangle.

An effect of the hypothalamus stands out clearly. Of the 60 animals receiving a hypothalamus with a pituitary, 20 received a pituitary in the axilla on one side and a hypothalamus in the axilla on the other side, i.e., the two tissues were inserted contralaterally. In this case, some breast cancers were recorded but fewer than in the other groups. Yet fewer breast cancers were recorded in a group receiving, through the same trocar but separately in succession, first one tissue and then the other. This group (represented in the second rectangle in the second column), although it received the two tissues successively, had yet fewer cancers. The decrease in the incidence of breast cancer in the latter two groups, as compared to that in the groups receiving pituitary and other tissues, has not been separately tested for statistical significance. However, the effect of the hypothalamus in the group receiving the pituitary and hypothalamus jointly, i.e., by the same trocar, as compared to groups 4–7, is statistically significant.

It seems clear than in most C mice studied in the absence of a known virus, the hypothalamus prevented the development of breast cancer. Whether a similar manipulation can also be successful when, under certain conditions, a pituitary in situ becomes carcinogenic, remains a problem for further study. Some process in the hypothalamus could be responsible for certain endocrine aspects of human breast cancer that would render the pituitary in situ similar to the ectopic pituitary. In the cited mouse studies, the pituitary had been intentionally rendered independent by relocation away from hypothalamic controls. It seems possible that some other procedures which reconstitute any lost hypothalamic controls may also be curative or even preventive via the control of a spectrum of rhythms in prolactin secretion by the pituitary. Bromoergocryptin, now applied for the treatment of cancer without considerations of timing, may be worthy of chronobiologic investigation. It is in this context that the detection of any increased breast cancer risk in terms of an altered, e.g., circannual, prolactin rhythm (149, Chapter 37) or some more readily assessed marker rhythm—conceivably an alteration of a temperature rhythm—could be useful. Such studies with chronopsies of body temperature and other variables are overdue (37, 38).

Risk factors associated with breast cancer and revealed by dyschronism in breast temperature and several hormonal variables are discussed in Chapter 37 of this volume. Such results, not only in the case of prolactin but also for thyroid-stimulating hormone (TSH), point to a spectrum of rhythms of different frequencies that may exert an influence in different ways. Thus, an alteration if not obliteration of the circannual rhythm in plasma prolactin and an increase in extent of circannual variation in TSH seem to be correlated with a high risk of breast cancer.

RECEPTOR RHYTHMS A BASIS FOR CHRONOHORMONOTHERAPY

The responsiveness of target tissues to various agents, notably hormones, undergoes variations with several frequencies. A circadian rhythm in cytoplasmic estrogen receptor content of breast tissue characterizes mice with and without pituitary isografts and demonstrated differences

degrees, with 360° ≡ the period length chosen. The vector outward from the pole indicates the acrophase by its direction and the amplitude, usually by its length. The ellipse represents the 95% confidence region for the amplitude-acrophase pair.

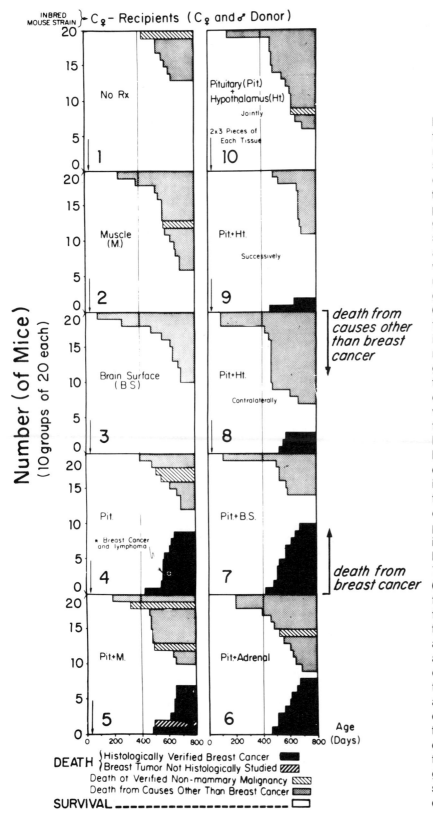

Figure 14.2 Role of the pituitary and the hypothalamus in the incidence of mouse breast cancer. Breast cancers shown as black areas are found abundantly in those subgroups of 20 mice that on two occasions received three pituitaries by trocar into the axilla. The glands have been administered as the sole tissue (see fourth rectangle from above in column 1) or in combination with muscle (see fifth rectangle in column 1) or with adrenal (see fifth rectangle in column 2) or with brain surface (see fourth rectangle in column 2). At the moment of appearance of a histologically validated breast cancer, a step is made from the bottom of a given rectangle upward, at a time corresponding on the abscissa to the appearance of the cancer, whereas if there is no histologic validation of the nature of the breast tumor, the area of the step upward is hatched. When an animal dies without a breast tumor, a descending staircase indicates the moment of its death. Hatching indicates that a malignancy other than a histologically validated breast cancer was the cause of death. A comparison of these bottom rows, summarizing the incidence of cancer in C mice bearing pituitary isografts (rectangles 4–7), with the 3 cells above in column 1 (rectangles 1–3), leaves little doubt of the efficacy of ectopic pituitary function for inducing mammary cancer in mice of the Bagg albino strain. More specifically, at 800 days of age, roughly one-half of about 800 animals receiving pituitary isografts (alone or with tissues that all turned out to be controls, *i.e.,* muscle, adrenal, or brain surface) had histologically verified cancer. By contrast, after the same interval, no single breast cancer had been observed in about 60 control C animals given no treatment or given isografts only of muscle or brain surface (see top three rectangles in left column).

in breast cancer risk (Fig. 14.3) (79). In this study 7-week-old BALB/c mice received a subcutaneous implant of (a) 3 pituitaries or (b) 3 pituitaries with 3 hypothalami or (3) 3 fragments of muscle alone. The animals were multiply housed in light from 06:00 to 18:00 alternating with darkness. Seven weeks after implantation, subgroups of animals of all 3 treatment groups were killed at 4-hr intervals during 24 hr. Breasts were removed and cytoplasmic estrogen receptors determined by the saturation method, using dextran-coated charcoal. A circadian rhythm in estrogen receptor content was quantified by cosinor analysis of data from each of the 3 treatment groups. The average receptor content (mesor) in the animals bearing a pituitary implant (which demonstrably develop breast cancer) was about twice that of the mice with a muscle implant; the latter had a breast cancer incidence of only 1%. A reduction in the rate of pituitary-induced breast cancer by addition of hypothalamic tissue, as discussed above, was not reflected in a lower receptor level.

The quantified circadian and circannual rhythms in hormone receptors from murine mammary gland (59), avian oviduct (141), and rat, calf, and pig uteri (68) can be viewed in the light of a previously demonstrated *in vivo* and *in vitro* change in the responsiveness of the murine adrenal cortex to ACTH, suggesting the broader scope of rhythmic changes in cellular responsiveness, infradian as well as circadian.

Beyond the scope of reported yearly fluctuations in estrogen receptor concentrations of human breast cancer (68), a circannual rhythm has recently been documented in this variable (65). One tumor biopsy was obtained from each of 797 patients with histologically validated primary breast cancer in Minnesota from 11/74 to 11/78. The highest levels were found in late fall

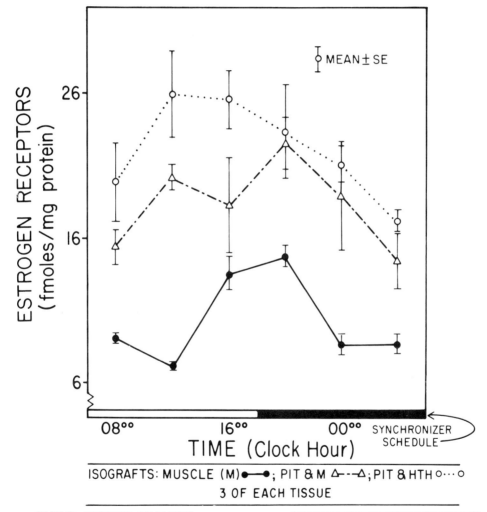

ISOGRAFTS: MUSCLE (M)●—●; PIT & M △--△; PIT & HTH ○···○
3 OF EACH TISSUE

TABLE: COSINOR ANALYSIS

ISOGRAFT	MESOR± SE	AMPLITUDE± SE	ACROPHASE(°)[†] ± 95 CI	RHYTHM DETECTION(P)
MUSCLE	10.2±0.4	3.1±0.6	-282(-259,-304)	<.001
PIT. +MUSCLE	18.8±0.9	3.4±1.3	-292(-250,-333)	.042
PIT. +HTH	22.1±0.8	4.3±1.1	-235(-205,-265)	.004

[†]REFERENCED TO MIDNIGHT (360°≡24H)

Figure 14.3 Estrogen receptor concentrations in breast of mice with low (muscle) or high (pituitary) risk of breast cancer. *PIT*, pituitary; *HTH*, hypothalamus.

and the lowest in spring. This difference was statistically significant and ranges from 30.1 ± 5.9 to 12.2 ± 2.2 fmol/mg protein. The data were fitted by a cosine function with a chosen period of 1 year ($P = 0.04$). Such findings may imply the need for a time-qualification of cancer hormono-dependence along the circadian and the circannual scales; when the choice between hormonotherapy and chemotherapy for treating a patient with advanced breast cancer is based on estrogen receptor concentration, it may not depend on when the biopsy was done but rather on the circannual stage when one or the other is expected to be more effective.

CHRONOTOLERANCE FOR SINGLE AGENTS

Host protection is unquestionably improved by programming the time when potentially toxic

single therapeutic agents are applied once or repeatedly (41, 42, 61). Thus, there is an opportunity for an immediate exploitation of information on rhythms that provides predictable or assessable times of highest host sensitivity. Laboratory experiments aimed at timing the radiotherapy or chemotherapy of cancer according to bodily rhythms are cases in point. In these instances and in others, one avoids drug administration (or restricts the dose) during a susceptible stage of the host's pertinent rhythms and administers most if not all of the drug during the stage of resistance. In principle, this shielding in time is analogous to the protection gained by shielding in space, as in radiotherapy.

Chronotolerance for Radiation

In an unpublished study on 420 mice, a predictable change of about 100 r in LD_{50} of whole-

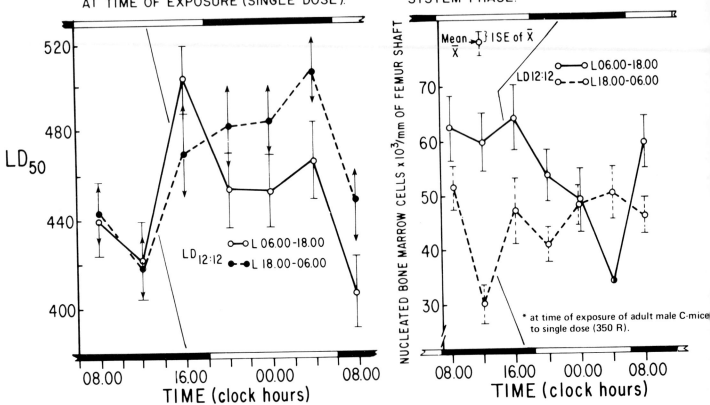

a) LD_{50} of Whole body X-ray irradiation of mice and circadian system phase at time of exposure to single dose. b) Bone marrow depression by whole body X-irradiation in relation to circadian system phase at time of exposure of adult male C-mice to single dose (350 r). Circadian radiosensitivity rhythm of mice after standardization for 14 days on 2 lighting regimens differing 180° in phase. LD_{50} in roentgens. Data obtained in 1958 in the Chronobiology Laboratories, University of Minnesota. Circadian rhythm in LD_{50} (a) and bone marrow depression (b). A remarkable circadian change in radiosensitivity also characterizes the Chinese hamster.

Figure 14.4 Mouse chronotolerance for whole-body x-irradiation as gauged by LD_{50} (a) and surviving nucleated bone marrow cells (b).

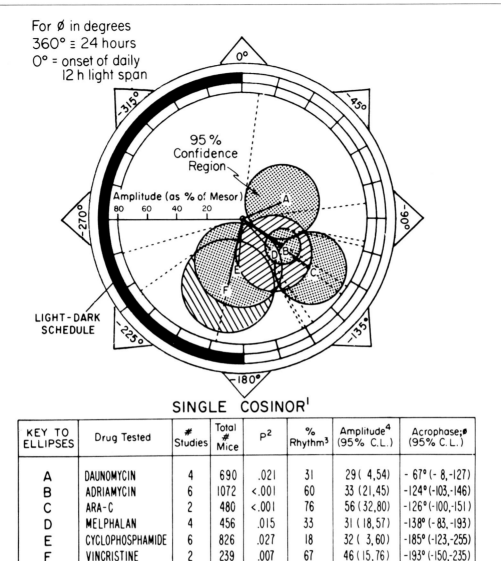

For Ø in degrees
360° ≡ 24 hours
0° = onset of daily
12 h light span

95%
Confidence
Region

Amplitude (as % of Mesor)
80   60   40   20

LIGHT-DARK
SCHEDULE

SINGLE COSINOR[1]

KEY TO ELLIPSES	Drug Tested	# Studies	Total # Mice	P[2]	% Rhythm[3]	Amplitude[4] (95% C.L.)	Acrophase;ø (95% C.L.)
A	DAUNOMYCIN	4	690	.021	31	29 (4,54)	- 67° (- 8,-127)
B	ADRIAMYCIN	6	1072	<.001	60	33 (21,45)	-124° (-103,-146)
C	ARA-C	2	480	<.001	76	56 (32,80)	-126° (-100,-151)
D	MELPHALAN	4	456	.015	33	31 (18,57)	-138° (- 83,-193)
E	CYCLOPHOSPHAMIDE	6	826	.027	18	32 (3,60)	-185° (-123,-255)
F	VINCRISTINE	2	239	.007	67	46 (15,76)	-193° (-150,-235)

1) Results from least-squares fitting of 24-h cosine curve
2) P from test of zero-amplitude hypothesis
3) % Rhythm = % of total variability attributable to fitted cosine
4) Expressed as % of Mesor

Figure 14.5. Single cosinor presentation of mouse chronotolerance for a single injection of various oncostatic drugs. Evaluated from data on percentage survival vs. treatment-timing.

body x-irradiation was shown to depend on the circadian stage of dosing (Fig. 14.4a) (41). A difference in the mortality of rats subjected to whole-body x-irradiation at two times of day was later reported (103). Subsequently Rugh *et al.* (122), studying the same problem in mice, and Straube (145), using rats, reported that rhythmic variations in radiosensitivity of rodents were not apparent. These reports were re-evaluated by Menaker (94) and by Pizzarello *et al.* (104), who again presented information supporting the occurrence of a circadian susceptibility-resistance cycle to whole-body irradiation in the mouse.

In our laboratory, Garcia Sainz *et al.* (28)

studied the loss of body weight in Fischer rats after x-irradiation of the upper half of the body only. They found that the dose of x-rays required to obtain a 20% weight loss of the animals 8 days after irradiation varied as a function of circadian system phase at the time of exposure. The highest resistance of the animals to radiation-induced weight loss occurred during the second half of the light span (LD12:12, light from 06:00 to 18:00), corresponding to the time of lowest mortality in the same animals and also in mice and rats exposed to whole-body x-irradiation (28). A circadian rhythm in host tolerance of whole-body x-irradiation was also demon-

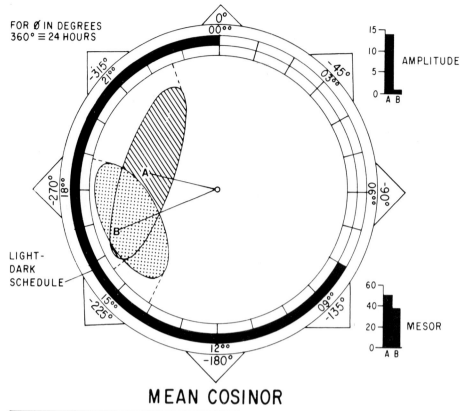

FOR Ø IN DEGREES
360° ≡ 24 HOURS

AMPLITUDE

MESOR

LIGHT-
DARK
SCHEDULE

MEAN COSINOR

KEY TO ELLIPSES	P	NO. STUDIES	MESOR	AMPLITUDE (95% CL)	ACROPHASE (θ) (95% CL)
A PERCENT SURVIVORS	<0.001	7	50	13.9 (8.7 24.1)	−283°(−233 −339)
B TEMPERATURE (°C)	0.002	5	37	0.62(0.4 0.84)	−249°(−211 −283)

P=PROBABILITY OF HYPOTHESIS "AMPLITUDE =0" ; NO. OBS.=NUMBER OF OBSERVATIONS
PR=PERCENT RHYTHM (PERCENT OF VARIABILITY ACCOUNTED FOR BY COSINE CURVE)
95% CL = CONSERVATIVE 95% CONFIDENCE LIMITS DERIVED FROM COSINOR ELLIPSE

Figure 14.6 Mean cosinor presentation of rat chronotolerance for cisplatin as evaluated from percent survivors at 50% mortality and referred to rectal temperature as a marker rhythm of the host. Summary of 7 studies (1055 rats), between March and November.

strated in the Chinese hamster by Lappenbusch (81). Furthermore, he demonstrated a circadian rhythm in the rate of mitosis (MI = mitotic index) of the white cells in the bone marrow. The highest MI was found to correspond to the lowest $LD_{50/30}$,[1] and the lowest MI corresponded to the highest $LD_{50/30}$, with a statistically significant linear correlation between $LD_{50/30}$ values and rate of mitosis. In hamsters, the number of circulating white blood cells 30 days after irradiation (800 r) at lowest MI was similar to control values, while hamsters exposed at highest MI had much lower values throughout this 30-day span. The number of peripheral white blood

cells may thus represent a marker rhythm of host sensitivity to radiations, reflecting the rate of mitosis in the bone marrow.

Vacek et al. (155), Ueno (154), and Vacek and Rotkovska (156) suggested that a higher number of surviving hematopoietic stem cells may be the cause of the differences in the mortality of mice irradiated at different circadian system phases.

In our laboratory, Haus et al. (60) delivered a single whole-body x-irradiation (350 r) to 406 adult male Bagg albino (C) mice. The animals were singly housed and standardized in two periodicity rooms with inverted lighting regimens, each consisting of 12 hr of light alternating with 12 hr of darkness. In one room light onset was at 06:00, in the other at 18:00. After 2 weeks of standardization, mice received a single dose of irradiation at 1 of 6 circadian stages, each

---

[1] Dose which kills 50% of the animals within 30 days from administration.

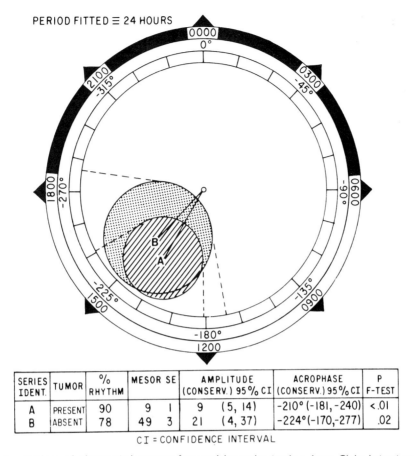

PERIOD FITTED ≡ 24 HOURS

SERIES IDENT.	TUMOR	% RHYTHM	MESOR	SE	AMPLITUDE (CONSERV.)	95% CI	ACROPHASE (CONSERV.)	95% CI	P F-TEST
A	PRESENT	90	9	1	9	(5, 14)	-210°	(-181, -240)	<.01
B	ABSENT	78	49	3	21	(4, 37)	-224°	(-170, -277)	.02

CI = CONFIDENCE INTERVAL

Figure 14.7 Similar timing of chronotolerance for arabinosylcytosine (*ara-C*) in intact and leukemic mice.

separated by 4 hr. On day 4 postirradiation, all the mice were killed and femur bone marrow cellularity examined. The highest number of surviving bone marrow cells was found in mice irradiated near the end of the light (rest) span in both rooms (Fig. 14.4b). In 1246 mice standardized in the same conditions, the circadian rhythm in the lethality of a single dose of x-irradiation was confirmed. The highest tolerance of these mice, exposed to 410 or 450 r of whole-body irradiation, occurred during the late light (rest) span (60). Thus, a circadian rhythm in host tolerance for a single dose of whole-body x-irradiation characterizes several rodent species investigated (mouse, rat, hamster). This rhythm is related to the circadian rhythm characterizing the mitotic rate of the bone marrow stem cells before any irradiation, also discussed by Pizzarello *et al.* (105). The time of highest tolerance of radiation occurs in the daily late rest span of these animals, when the rate of mitoses in the bone marrow is lowest.

Failure to follow the basic rules of controlled animal experimentation in general, including those of periodicity analysis in particular, may explain some of the seemingly "negative" and confusing results reported in the existing literature on the subject.

Chronotolerance for Oncostatic Drugs

A circadian stage dependence has been demonstrated in murine tolerance for numerous oncostatic drugs (54) (Figs. 14.5 and 14.6). Results of Haus *et al.* (61) (Fig. 14.7), Scheving *et al.* (130), and Rose *et al.* (120) indicate that the timing of such tolerance rhythms in tumor-bearing animals may be similar to that in healthy animals. Murine data of this kind allow an evaluation of the gain in tolerance achieved by proper drug timing (Fig. 14.8).

If, as a minimum, cancer chronotherapy would exploit chronotolerance, it could prove to be as successful in the clinic as it has been on laboratory rodents. If such proves to be the case, it should be introduced as broadly as scrubbing before surgery (44). To achieve this goal, much more coordinated research in both the laboratory and clinic is needed, beyond the overwhelming evidence already on record concerning the hours of changing resistance and the corresponding chronopharmacokinetics.

EXPERIMENTAL CANCER CHRONOTHERAPY

First Step in Experimental Cancer Chronotherapy: Circadian Stage Dependence in Response of Murine L1210 Leukemia to Single Drug, Arabinosylcytosine (ara-C)

The question posed for these studies of ara-C was simply: Given a recommended dose (240 mg/kg for each course) and frequency of administration (q3h × 8, q4d × 4) for the treatment of

mouse L1210 leukemia (137), is there a therapeutic advantage in varying individual doses according to the animal's circadian tolerance rhythm?

A number of studies involving over a thousand mice (54, 55, 61) demonstrated that a circadian sinusoidal modulation of the 3-hourly doses could double the cure rate (from 10 to 20%) and increase the survival time by 60% if the highest doses were given near the acrophase of tolerance for this drug; *i.e.*, near midlight for mice kept in a lighting regimen consisting of light (L) for 12 hr alternating with darkness (D) for 12 hr (LD12:

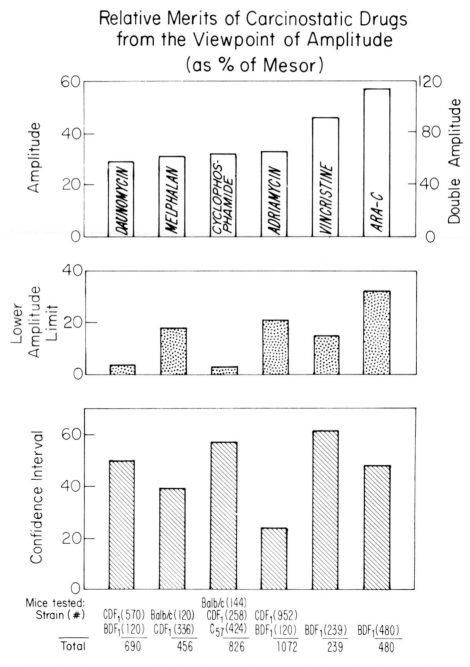

Figure 14.8 Potential gains from a proper timing of several oncostatic drugs in mice are evaluated from data on chronotolerance. (From fit of 24-hr cosine to survival data from 6 timepoints (4-hr apart) on mice in light and darkness alternating at 12-hr intervals.)

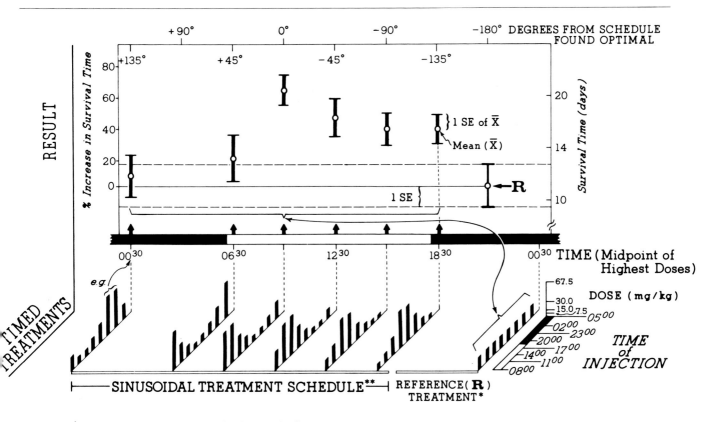

Figure 14.9. Survival of leukemic mice after the administration of arabinosylcytosine (ara-c) on different schedules. L1210 leukemia inoculated on 1-26-72. A 60% improvement in survival times of leukemic mice results from the administration of the highest doses of arabinocylcytosine (ara-C) near its acrophase of chronotolerance.

12) (Figs. 14.9 and 14.10). Recently, studies by Rose *et al.* (120) led them to question the merits of chronotherapy in the same model (murine L1210 leukemia treated with ara-C). However, critical evaluation of their data actually provides strong confirmation of the earlier findings cited above (53) (Fig. 14.11).

The advantage of chronotherapy also can be demonstrated in terms of the number of surviving leukemic cells at the end of ara-C treatment. Assuming that: (a) even one surviving L1210 cell can be lethal within 45 days after treatment; (b) there are no drug-related deaths; and (c) all leukemic cells are equally sensitive to ara-C, one can use the Poisson distribution to estimate the average (expected) number of surviving L1210 cells per mouse (136). Results from the study described above indicated a value of 1.6 cells/animal in the group treated with the optimal sinusoidal schedule and 2.3 cells/animal in the homeostatically treated group.

While such computations quantify the advantage of chronotherapy, they do not explain it. One plausible explanation requires abandon-

ment of the assumption that all L1210 cells are equally sensitive to the drug. Ara-C-induced DNA damage requires the presence of the enzyme deoxycytidine kinase. A high level of this enzyme is found in L1210 cells (63). Assuming that the activity of this enzyme varies among leukemic cells and that a higher drug concentration is required to kill cells with lower enzyme activity, one can explain the greater effectiveness of a sinusoidal dose schedule by the fact that higher doses can be administered at circadian stages of greater host tolerance.

With this explanation, cells that survive ara-C treatment can be expected to be relatively resistant to the drug by virtue of a low enzyme level. If enzyme activity is genetically based a drug-resistant strain may then be propagated. An alternative possibility is that L1210 cells may mutate to a resistant state (5). In either case, the complete elimination of tumor cells by a single agent may require the exploitation of the agents' specificity in relation to stages of the tumor's circadian cell cycle, as well as of circadian and other rhythms in host tolerance.

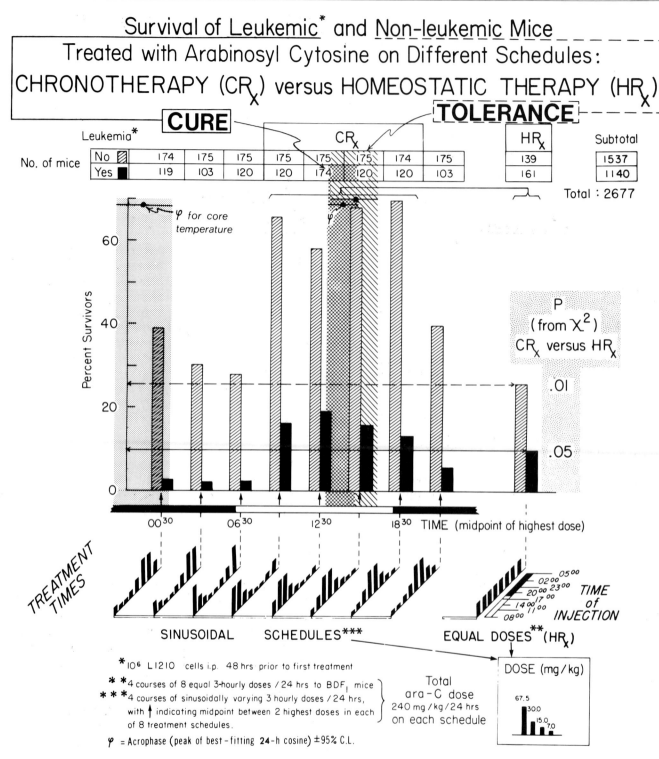

Figure 14.10 Doubling of cure rate of leukemic mice when the highest 3-hr doses of arabinosylcytosine (ara-C) (within each circadian sinusoidal treatment) are given near the acrophase of chronotolerance of ara-C.

Chronochemotherapy with Drug Combinations

The development of drug resistance can be circumvented to some extent by combining two agents (5), as has been demonstrated for L1210 leukemia using ara-C and 1-(2-chloroethyl)-3-cyclohexyl-1-nitrosourea (CCNU) (124). Such com-

binations of two or several oncostatic drugs are generally recognized to have led to an improvement in the potency of cancer chemotherapy as a consequence of therapeutic synergism (32). The latter, however, can exhibit different degrees as a function of the interval and/or the sequence of administering the drugs, as has been

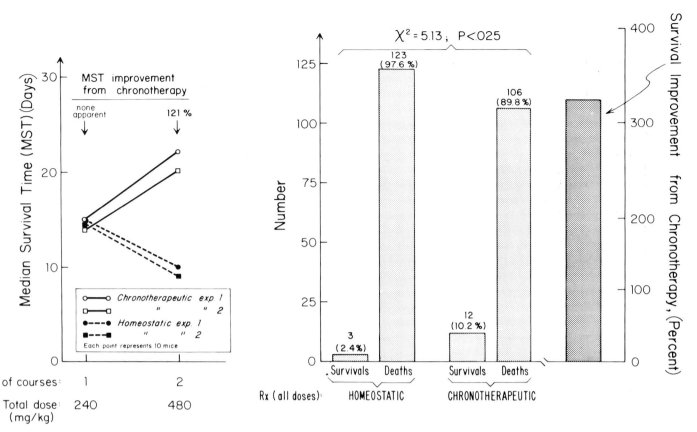

Figure 14.11 Advantage of chronotherapeutic over homeostatic treatment of murine leukemia assessed by two endpoints: median survival time (left) and percentage of long term survivors (right). The merits of chronotherapy with β-arabinosylcytosine (ara-C) against mouse L1210 leukemia become obvious when the number of courses of circadian sinusoidal treatment (q3h × 8) with ara-C increases. (Data from W. C. Rose *et al.* (120).)

shown for several drug combinations, notably methotrexate (MTX) and L-asparaginase (157), 1,3-bis(2-chloroethyl)-1-nitrosourea (BCNU) and MTX (158), ara-C and CCNU (124), vincristine (VCR) and cyclophosphamide (Cy) (115).

Unfortunately, such studies have not considered the circadian-stage dependence of the toxicity and effectiveness of several of these agents. Thus, an effect observed in relation to different sequences and/or intervals between two (or more) drugs may also reflect the relation of the timing to any temporal periodic organization of both the tumor and the host and the consequent changing sensitivity to each drug, as emphasized by the following studies with chronobiologic designs. In mouse L1210 leukemia treated with a combination of ara-C and Cy (129) (Fig. 14.12), in a rat immunocytoma treated with a combination of adriamycin (Adr) and *cis*-diamminedichloroplatinum (cisplatin, cis-P) (64, 138) (Fig. 14.13) and in a rat mammary adenocarcinoma treated with Adr and L-phenylalanine mustard (melphalan, PAM) (52) (Fig. 14.14), only one drug in the combination was tested for its circadian stage dependent antitumor effectiveness at a

therapeutic level. In each of the studies mentioned above, the best therapeutic results were obtained when the drug was given near the previously determined circadian acrophase of murine chronotolerance for it.

Data published by Tobias *et al.* (151) may also be viewed with rhythms in mind. These data reportedly reveal a synergistic effect of a combination of Adr (5 mg/kg) and Cy (100 mg/kg) on mouse L1210 leukemia. They also show that whether the second drug was given concomitantly with or 24 hr after the first, the results in terms of long term survivors were identical in the case of the Cy→Adr sequence and not very dissimilar for the Adr→Cy sequence. With time intervals ranging from zero (concomitant administration) to 8 hr for either drug sequence (Figs. 14.15 and 14.16), the percentage of long term survivors appeared to be progressively lower. The question thus arose as to a possible circadian periodicity in the antitumor effectiveness of each agent, given as a second drug. As an attempt to account for this variation in effectiveness of each drug combination, a single cosine function with a 24-hr period was fitted (50) to

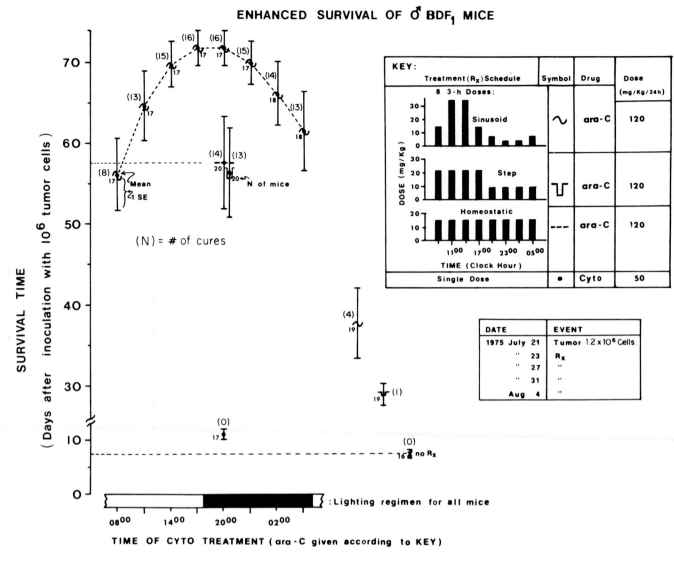

Figure 14.12. Combination of arabinosylcytosine (ara-C) and cyclophosphamide (Cyto) against mouse L1210 leukemia. A single course of treatment demonstrates a time-dependent synergistic effect of both drugs, as gauged by percentage of survivors at 75 days after inoculation of 1.2×10^6 L1210 cells. The optimal time for Cy injection is near its acrophase of mouse chronotolerance. (Ten of 10 mice without tumor but treated with ara-C sinusoid and Cyto at 20:00 alive at end of study.) (Reproduced with permission from L. E. Sheving *et al.* (129).)

the limited data of six mean values during a single 24-hr span. Regrettably no original data were available for a 16-hr span, including almost all of the dark span. This data-gap strongly biases the results; nevertheless, a test of the zero-amplitude (no rhythm) hypothesis yielded a *P* value of 0.04 for the Adr→Cy sequence, indicating the presence of a rhythm. For the Cy→Adr sequence, the *P* value was 0.16.

A log transformation also was applied to the data to evaluate the rate of mouse removal from the potentially dead population, that is, the cure rate from leukemia; analyses of these transformed data revealed a circadian rhythm in this variable for both sequences. Moreover, both ac-

rophases remained within the 95% confidence interval of the tolerance acrophase for the second drug in each sequence (Figs. 14.17 and 14.18). Such results from treatment of L1210 leukemia with the Adr→Cy and Cy→Adr sequences have recently been confirmed by appropriately designed studies (129a).

In this same model (murine L1210 leukemia) Scheving *et al.* (129) demonstrated that the potency of an observed therapeutic synergism between ara-C and Cy depended on the time of administration of Cy as above cited. In four different studies, the authors used different total doses of ara-C always given on the "best" sinusoidal schedule (55, 61). Cy was given on the same

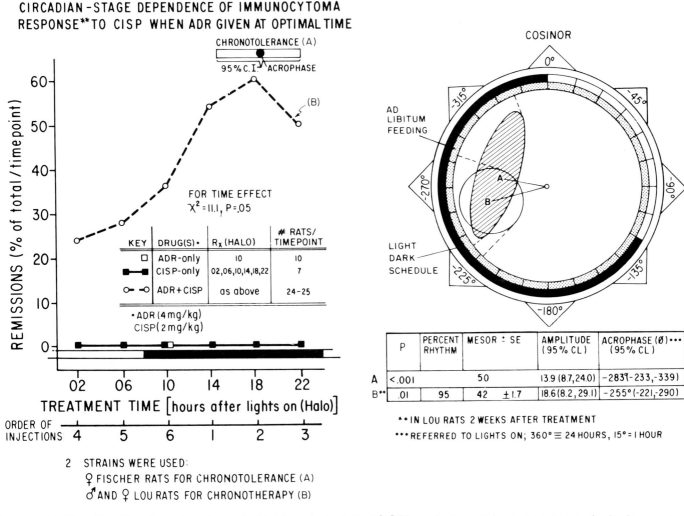

Figure 14.13. Combination of adriamycin (Adr) and cisplatin (CISP) against a rat immunocytoma. A single course of treatment induces a circadian-stage dependent synergistic effect as gauged by % complete remissions. The optimal time for CISP injection is near its acrophase of chronotolerance.

day as ara-C but at one of 8 different circadian stages to different groups of mice. The acrophase of the circadian rhythm in percent of long term survivors as a function of Cy-timing, in combination with ara-C, was at approximately 10 hr after lighting onset (10 HALO) of the daily lighting regimen (LD12:12), very close to the above-mentioned acrophase of cure rate in the Adr→Cy combination.

As an attempt to demonstrate the merits of chronotherapy with nonlethal drug combinations, the cosinor analysis of cures as shown in Figure 14.17 concerns one of these four ara-C→Cy studies. Cy chronotolerance and *therapeutic* chronosynergism with two different nonlethal two-drug combinations (Adr→Cy and ara-C→Cy) exhibit a similar timing.

In summary, various experimental tumor models have been treated with the following two-drug combinations: sequential Adr→PAM, Adr→cis-P, ara-C→Cy, Adr→Cy and Cy→Adr. In each case the acrophase of antitumor effectiveness of the second agent given at different circadian stages, as gauged by percent cures or percent complete remissions, occurred within the 95% confidence interval of that agent's tolerance acrophase. Thus, the circadian stage of drug administration seems quite clearly to be a major factor underlying the observed synergism of drug combinations used in therapy of cancer.

Chronochemotherapy with a Single Agent

It should be noted that, at least in the case of single drug administration, the optimal circadian treatment time in terms of an effect on tumor

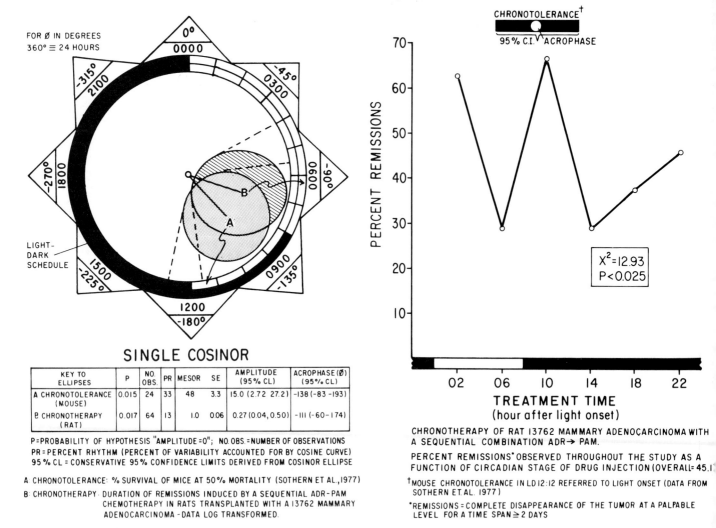

SINGLE COSINOR

KEY TO ELLIPSES	P	NO. OBS.	PR	MESOR	SE	AMPLITUDE (95% CL)	ACROPHASE (∅) (95% CL)
A CHRONOTOLERANCE (MOUSE)	0.015	24	33	48	3.3	15.0 (2.72 27.2)	-138 (-83 -193)
B CHRONOTHERAPY (RAT)	0.017	64	13	1.0	0.06	0.27 (0.04, 0.50)	-111 (-60 -174)

P=PROBABILITY OF HYPOTHESIS "AMPLITUDE=0"; NO.OBS.=NUMBER OF OBSERVATIONS
PR=PERCENT RHYTHM (PERCENT OF VARIABILITY ACCOUNTED FOR BY COSINE CURVE)
95% CL = CONSERVATIVE 95% CONFIDENCE LIMITS DERIVED FROM COSINOR ELLIPSE

A: CHRONOTOLERANCE: % SURVIVAL OF MICE AT 50% MORTALITY (SOTHERN ET AL.,1977)

B: CHRONOTHERAPY: DURATION OF REMISSIONS INDUCED BY A SEQUENTIAL ADR-PAM
CHEMOTHERAPY IN RATS TRANSPLANTED WITH A 13762 MAMMARY
ADENOCARCINOMA -DATA LOG TRANSFORMED.

CHRONOTHERAPY OF RAT 13762 MAMMARY ADENOCARCINOMA WITH
A SEQUENTIAL COMBINATION ADR→ PAM.

PERCENT REMISSIONS* OBSERVED THROUGHOUT THE STUDY AS A
FUNCTION OF CIRCADIAN STAGE OF DRUG INJECTION (OVERALL= 45.1)

†MOUSE CHRONOTOLERANCE IN LD 12:12 REFERRED TO LIGHT ONSET (DATA FROM
SOTHERN ET. AL. 1977)

*REMISSIONS = COMPLETE DISAPPEARANCE OF THE TUMOR AT A PALPABLE
LEVEL FOR A TIME SPAN ≧ 2 DAYS

Figure 14.14. Sequential combination of Adriamycin (Adr) and melphalan (L-phenylalanine mustard, PAM) against a rat mammary adenocarcinoma. Treatment consisted in 0.8 mg/kg i.p. Adr from D_{11} to D_{19} post-tumor inoculation (except on D_{16-17}), followed by 1.6 mg/kg p.o. PAM 3 times a week until death of 50% of the animals. The proportion of rats which went into complete remission (C) and the duration of these complete remissions (B) were greater when the drugs were given near the acrophase of mouse chronotolerance for both drugs. All 24 rats which were not implanted with tumor, but received the treatment, were alive at the end of the study.

size may differ appreciably from that based on survival. Thus, regression of an immunocytoma in LOU rats treated daily with methylprednisolone was most pronounced if treatment occurred near the middle of the light span. In contrast, animals treated near mid-darkness each day had the longest mean survival span (Fig. 14.19) (78).

In the same model (LOU rat-immunocytoma) a single injection of Adr induced a faster tumor regression, but also a faster regrowth, if the injection occurred near midlight (near the acrophase of Adr tolerance), as compared to other circadian stages. Consequently, animals treated at this time had a shorter mean life span (Fig. 14.20) (33). These results suggest that a rapid

reduction in tumor cell population may also increase the rate of recruitment of resting tumor cells in the "cell cycle."

Data are also available for the antitumoral effect of Cy given every 2 days to mice inoculated with a mammary cancer (2). They show that mice injected between 4 and 12 HALO—overlapping the 95% CI for mouse chronotolerance for Cy—exhibit the smallest tumor sizes. The worst effect is also found to overlap the 95% CI of tolerance (between 12 and 20 HALO). At this time the mitotic index of the tumor was found to be at the nadir of a pronounced circadian rhythm. It seems, thus, that a greater oncostatic effect results in this model from treatment taking advantage of a combination of host chronotolerance and tumor susceptibility rhythms (Fig. 14.21).

CHRONOPHARMACOKINETICS

Work on the optimization of chronotherapeutic agents depends further on temporal aspects of pharmacokinetics. These aspects include rhythmic (i.e., circadian) variation of drug bioavailability and of excretion in urine, feces, sweat, and saliva, as well as of the undesired or desired effect of the drug. Statistically significant circadian rhythms have been demonstrated for the several parameters used to characterize pharmacokinetics (44, 116, 118, 146). Differences in the pharmacokinetic parameters of urinary excretion of the anti-tumor drug cis-P were found to depend on the circadian stage of the kidney function when rats or patients receive this drug (66, 84). In both species, when cis-P was injected near the circadian stage associated with a high

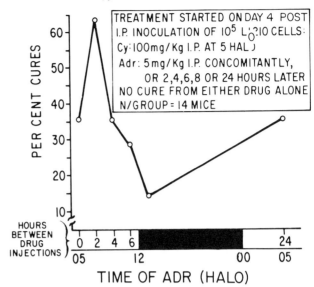

Variation in response to combination chemotherapy due to interval or to circadian rhythm?

Figure 14.16. A nonlethal combination of cyclophosphamide-Adriamycin (Cy→Adr) exhibits a time-dependent synergistic effect on mouse L1210 leukemia, as evaluated by percentage of cures. An optimal therapeutic effect results from the administration of Adr near its acrophase of chronotolerance. HALO = hours after light onset. (Data from B. S. Tobias *et al.* (151).)

urine volume (low kidney function), cisP was excreted faster, in greater amount, and in lower concentration than when injected at a circadian stage of low urine volume (high kidney function). Such differences explain the observed murine chrononephrotoxicity of this drug (83). The relevance of chronopharmacokinetics is further indicated by the claim that the bioavailability of drugs is the major factor determining the outcome of chemotherapy (148).

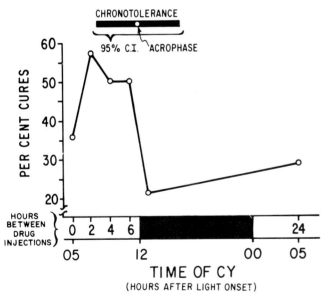

Figure 14.15. A nonlethal combination of Adriamycin-cyclophosphamide (Adr→Cy) exhibits a time-dependent synergistic effect on mouse L1210 leukemia, as evaluated by percentage of cures. An optimal therapeutic effect results from the administration of Cy near its acrophase of chronotolerance. Treatment on day 4 post i.p. inoculation of 10^5 L1210 cells. Adr (5 mg/kg) injected i.p. at 5 hr after light onset to all groups of 7–14 mice each. Cy (100 mg/kg) injected i.p. either concomitantly, 2, 4, 6, 8, or 24 hr later. No cure resulted from either drug alone. (Data from B. S. Tobias *et al.* (151), and from E. Haus *et al.* (61a).)

CHRONOCYTOKINETICS: THE CIRCADIAN CELL CYCLE

Circadian mitotic rhythms (39, 40, 48) have been reviewed and documented as ubiquitous and amenable to gradual (but not abrupt) schedule shifts. Some of these rhythms also have been explored with reference to related biochemical phenomena and underlying mechanisms: cellular, adrenocortical, pituitary, and other (39, 43, 48). Such observations occurred at about the same time as the proposal (80) and development (112, 131) of circadian time-invariant cell kinet-

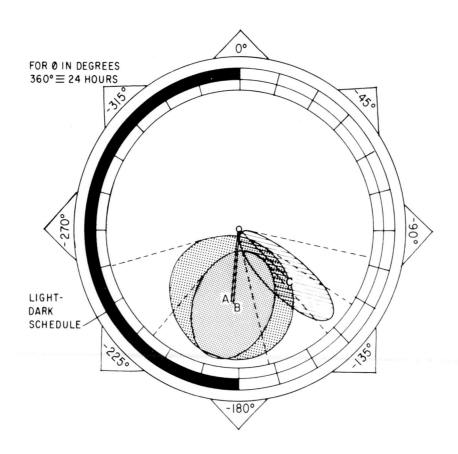

KEY TO ELLIPSES	P	PR	MESOR	SE	AMPLITUDE (95% CL)	ACROPHASE (∅) (95% CL)
A CHRONOTOLERANCE[1]	0.027	17.7	103	8.2	32 (3.1, 60)	-185° (-123, -256)
B CHRONOSYNERGISM[2]	0.014	81.4	78	3.0	21.9 (6.1, 38)	-184° (-137, -220)
C " [3]	0.037	88.9	1.1	0.11	0.7 (0.1, 1.3)	-128° (-85, -153)

(1) % SURVIVORS AT END OF 6 STUDIES (HAUS ET AL. 1974); CY ALONE.

(2) % CURES OF MOUSE L1210 LEUKEMIA (STUDY I OF SCHEVING ET AL. 1977); CY AND ARA-C.

(3) % CURES OF MOUSE L1210 LEUKEMIA (TOBIAS ET AL. 1975); DATA LOG TRANSFORMED; CY AND ADR.

Figure 14.17. Cyclophosphamide (Cy). Cosinor presentation of mouse chronotolerance for Cy and chronosynergism of Cy in combination with arabinosylcytosine (ara-C) or Adriamycin (Adr) against mouse L1210 leukemia.

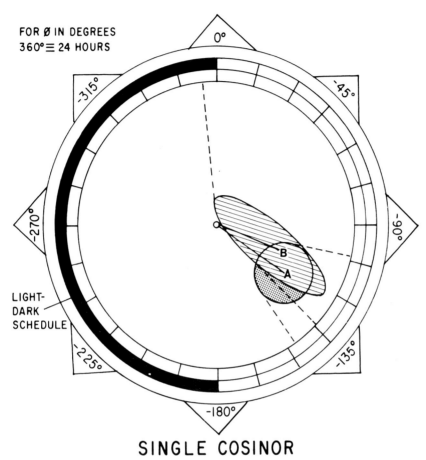

FOR Ø IN DEGREES
360° ≡ 24 HOURS

LIGHT-
DARK
SCHEDULE

SINGLE COSINOR

KEY TO ELLIPSES	P	NO. OBS.	PR	MESOR	S.E.	AMPLITUDE (95% CL)	ACROPHASE (Ø) (95% CL)
A CHRONOTOLERANCE	<0.001	36	59.8	48	1.58	15.7 (9.9 21.4)	-124°(-103-146)
B CHRONOTHERAPY (CY→ADR)	0.033	6	89.6	1.0	0.13	0.62 (0.05 1.37)	-111°(-5,-134)

P=PROBABILITY OF HYPOTHESIS "AMPLITUDE=0"; NO.OBS.=NUMBER OF OBSERVATIONS
PR=PERCENT RHYTHM (PERCENT OF VARIABILITY ACCOUNTED FOR BY COSINE CURVE)
95% CL=CONSERVATIVE 95% CONFIDENCE LIMITS DERIVED FROM COSINOR ELLIPSE

A: CHRONOTOLERANCE: % SURVIVORS AT 50% MORTALITY (SOTHERN ET.AL.,(1977)
B: CHRONOTHERAPY OF L1210 LEUKEMIA WITH CY→ADR SEQUENCE (TOBIAS ET.AL. 1975)
CURE RATE (DATA LOG TRANSFORMED)

Figure 14.18. Adriamycin (Adr). Cosinor presentation of mouse chronotolerance for Adr and chronosynergism of Adr in combination with cyclophosphamide (Cy) against mouse L1210 leukemia.

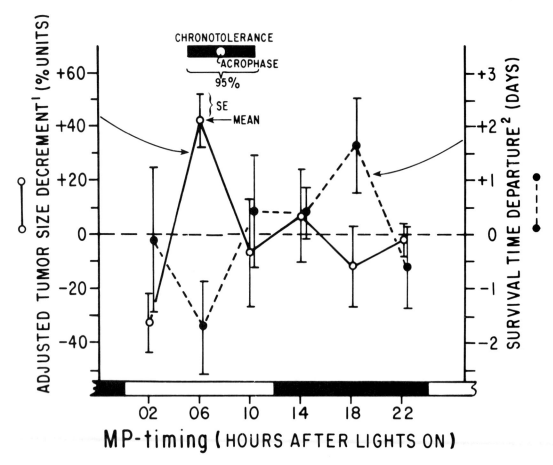

(1) DEPARTURE FROM OVERALL REGRESSION OF RAT TUMOR SIZE DECREMENT (RELATIVE TO NON-TREATED CONTROLS) ON LOG MP-DOSAGE DURING FIRST WEEK OF TREATMENT; THE HIGHER THE VALUE, THE GREATER THE RESPONSE TO TREATMENT.

(2) DEPARTURE FROM OVERALL REGRESSION OF SURVIVAL TIME ON LOG MP-DOSAGE; THE HIGHER THE VALUE, THE LONGER THE SURVIVAL TIME.

Figure 14.19 Methylprednisolone (MP). Single drug treatment of a rat immunocytoma. Immunocytoma size and survival times. The optimal antitumor effect of MP results from its administration near its acrophase of chronotolerance, but the optimal increase in life span is exhibited in rats treated 12 hours later, when MP is least tolerated. (Rat chronotolerance separately evaluated from body weight loss subsequent to daily oral MP treatment in healthy rats.)

ics. By the end of the 1950s, a combination of classical histology, radioactive tracer methods, and wet chemistry had led to the documentation of a circadian cell cycle in rodent liver (Fig. 14.22). This circadian liver cell cycle summarized contributions from a (very small) dividing subpopulation and a much larger nondividing one in the same organ. With this qualifying restriction, one obtained a first temporal map of processes in the immature growing organ leading to energy storage and release (such as glycogen deposition) and of a sequence of phenomena related to RNA, DNA, and mitosis. (This order of sequential "activation" was considered in the 1950s.)

Figure 14.23 suggests that this sequence of circadian cellular events may be similar in immature growing mouse liver, in a unicell (22, 23), in the hamster's cheek pouch epithelium (72, 73), and in human bone marrow (92).

In tetrahymena cells Scherbaum and Zeuthen (125) achieved a good degree of synchronization both of DNA replication and of mitosis by heat shocks spaced one cell generation apart. In a much smaller fraction of cells than in the case of tetrahymena, but with a host of mapped systemic and local variables, DNA metabolism and mitoses in intact immature (growing) mouse liver exhibited without shocks a light-dark synchronized or a free-running rhythm for a num-

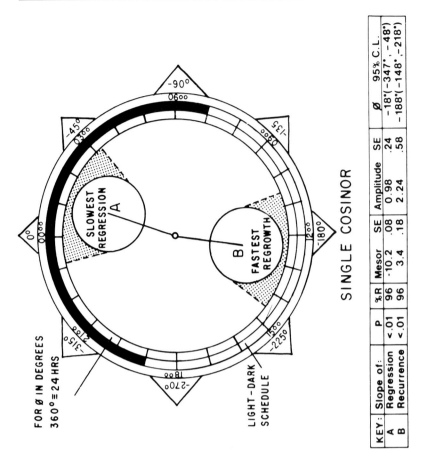

SINGLE COSINOR

KEY:	Slope of:	P	%R	Mesor	SE	Amplitude	SE	Ø	95% C.L.
A	Regression	<.01	96	-10.2	.08	0.98	.24	-18°(-347°,-48°)	
B	Recurrence	<.01	96	3.4	.18	2.24	.58	-188°(-148°,-218')	

Figure 14.20. Adriamycin (Adr). Single drug treatment of a rat immunocytoma. Slopes of tumor regression and regrowth. The optimal antitumor effect of a single i.p. injection of Adr (6 mg/kg) results from its administration near its murine acrophase of chronotolerance. However, the optimal increase in life span resulting from the slowest tumor regrowth corresponds to Adr injection at a time of worse drug chronotolerance.

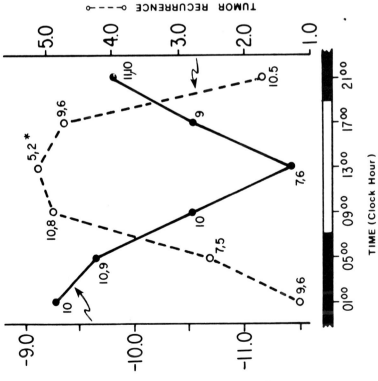

* N of rats at start and end of span covered by slope given with each point

** Tumor size determined every two days as length x width; size on day of $R_x \equiv 100\%$

ber of circadian cycles. The circadian frequency and/or acrophase synchronization for different processes in the same organ (labeling of phospholipid, RNA, and DNA, as well as mitosis in growing mouse liver) is altered in continuous light (47). Studies under constant conditions re-

vealing changes in relations of loosely coupled rhythmic webs, and the manipulation of several synchronizers (51) in attempts to separate tightly coupled circadian webs, can serve for a critical analysis, *inter alia,* of problems of chronocytokinetics, and may be complemented by a (chron-

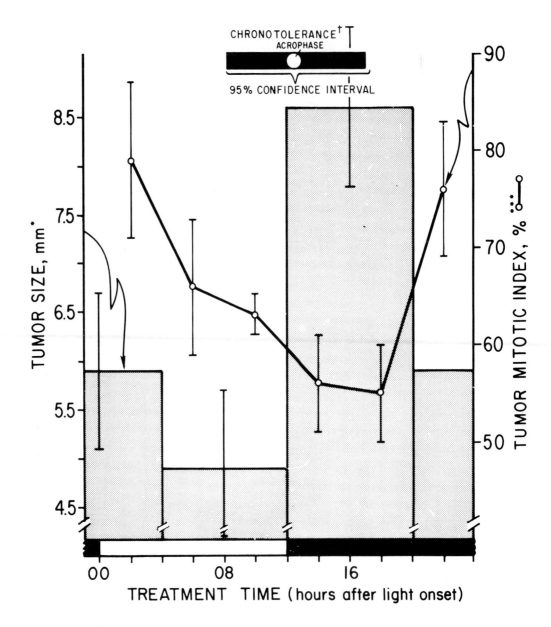

$\frac{^*D+d}{2}$ = MEAN OF TWO DIAMETERS OF TUMORS ON DAY 15 AFTER START
OF TREATMENT
TUMOR SIZE OF UNTREATED MICE 13.6±0.8mm
**Rx: 0.05 mg CYCLOPHOSPHAMIDE/gr I.P. EVERY 2 DAYS.
***% OF CELLS IN MITOSIS; TUMOR BEARING UNTREATED MICE
DATA FROM BADRAN, A.F. AND ECHAVE LLANOS, J.M.: J.NATL.CANCER INST. 35:
285-290, 1965 AND †HAUS et al: CHRONOBIOLOGIA, 1: 270-280, 1976

Figure 14.21.   Cyclophosphamide (Cy). Single drug treatment of a mouse adenocarcinoma. Cy-induced tumor shrinkage may result from interaction between circadian host chronotolerance of Cy and a pronounced circadian rhythm in tumor mitotic index. (For tumor size and mitotic index, $P = 0.05$.)

The Circadian Cell Cycle, *bottom of figure,* an Alternative to the letters G (for gaps in knowledge), *top of figure*

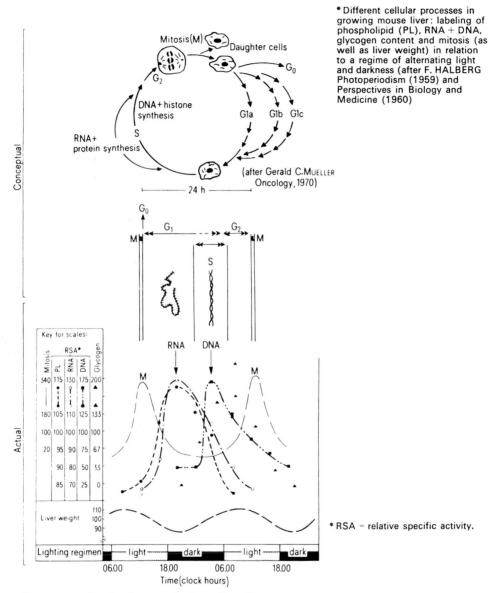

*Different cellular processes in growing mouse liver: labeling of phospholipid (PL), RNA + DNA, glycogen content and mitosis (as well as liver weight) in relation to a regime of alternating light and darkness (after F. HALBERG Photoperiodism (1959) and Perspectives in Biology and Medicine (1960)

(after Gerald C. MUELLER Oncology, 1970)

*RSA = relative specific activity.

Circadian stage of 24-h synchronized events in the cell cycle. Different cellular processes in growing mouse liver: Labeling of phospholipid (PL), RNA and DNA, glycogen content and mitosis (as well as liver weight) in relation to a regime of alternating light and darkness. RSA, relative specific activity. Sensitive stages of the cell cycle may become directly amenable to therapeutic exploitation by timing carcinostatic treatment according to rhythms.

Figure 14.22. The circadian cell cycle in immature growing mouse liver.

obiologically designed) periodic administration of growth-inhibiting (55, 121) or growth-promoting (85) agents. Circadian metabolic and mitotic bioperiodicities also stand out clearly in certain regenerative processes, e.g., when the proportion of cells participating in division is substantially enlarged by a procedure such as partial hepatectomy (48) and in certain cancers (55). Circadian variation in labeling (6, 8, 9, 12, 29, 35, 62, 69, 71–

73, 82, 95, 96, 102, 107, 112, 126–128, 132, 152–153) and cell division is the more important when it influences widely used indices of kinetics as well as responses to agents such as pituitary growth hormone (46, 85) and anticancer drugs (54, 55, 61, 129, 130).

Among several approaches tending toward chronocytokinetics (Table 14.1), Guiguet *et al.* (36) proposed a mathematical model of cellular

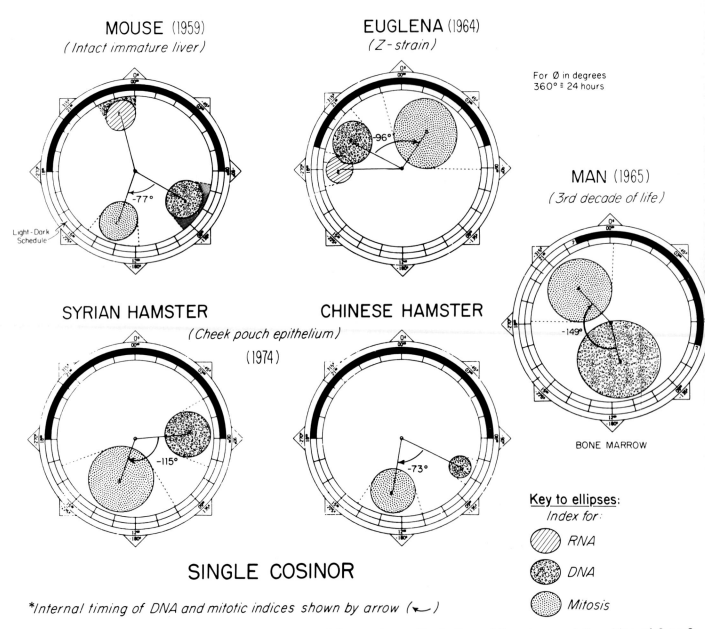

Figure 14.23. Chronocytokinetics in different living systems. Illustration of the phase relationships of 2 or 3 major events of cell division.

Table 14.1
Desirability of Wedding Different Approaches toward Chronocytokinetics

I. Some modeling by kineticists in this decade and "diurnal" (time of day) effects if not rhythms

Author(s)	Year	Reference	Kinds of Rhythmic Sources of Variation			
			None	Time of day "diurnal"	Circadian rhythm[a]	Rhythm spectrum[a]
Klein and Valleron	1975	*Biomedicine Express*, 23:214		X		
Brockwell	1975	In *Mathematical Models in Cell Kinetics*, pp. 24–25, edited by A.J. Valleron. European Press, Ghent, Belgium.		X		
Klein and Valleron	1977	*Journal of Theoretical Biology*, 64:27–42		X		
Hartmann and Møller	1978	In *Biomathematics and Cell Kinetics*, University of Paris, Feb. 27–28		X		
Rotenberg	1977	*Journal of Theoretical Biology*, 66:389–398	"Rhythm" induction			
Hopper and Brockwell	1978	*Cell and Tissue Kinetics*, 11: 205–225		X		
Hahn	1970	*Mathematical Biosciences*, 6:295–304	X			
Kim, Bahrani, and Woo	1974	*IEEE Transactions, Biomedical Engineering* BME-21:387–398	X			
Kim and Woo	1975	*Cell and Tissue Kinetics*, 8:199–200	X			

II. Localization (at least for liver) several decades ago of actual timing of S and M, with schedule manipulation for 1) synchronization, 2) shifting, and 3) free-running (rather than as mere "time of day" effect) and avoidance of gaps (G_0, G_1, G_2) by 1) mapping [with systemic and organ markers (inter alia, rectal temperature, blood eosinophils, liver weight and glycogen rhythms)], bioperiodic mitosis and labeling not only of DNA but also of RNAs and phospholipid and by 2) scrutinizing pace-making corticoid effects

Author(s)	Year	Reference	None	Time of day "diurnal"	Circadian rhythm[a]	Rhythm spectrum[a]
Halberg, Halberg, Barnum, and Bittner	1959	In *Photoperiodism and Related Phenomena in Plants and Animals*, pp. 803–878, edited by R.B. Withrow. Publ. No. 55, American Association for the Advancement of Science, Washington, D.C.			X	X
Halberg, Haus, and Scheving	1980	*Biomathematics and Cell Kinetics*, edited by A.J. Valleron, Elsevier/North-Holland, Amsterdam			X	X
Halberg, Carandente, Cornelissen, and Katinas	1977	*Chronobiologia*, 4 (Suppl. 1): 1–189			X	X

[a] In the light of inferential statistical tests.

events allowing for the circadian variations in any or all of the stages of an unidentified cell cycle. This was done by inclusion of sinusoidal variations in the probabilities of transition from any compartment of the cell cycle to the next.

However, the role that further knowledge in cytokinetics may play in improving chemotherapeutic schedules has recently been questioned (148). Thus, the acrophase of DNA synthesis in the bone marrow of rats occurs precisely at a time corresponding to highest murine tolerance of some so-called "S-phase-specific" oncostatic drugs (Fig. 14.24)[2]; such results further amplify the need for combining chronocytokinetics with chronopharmacokinetics in the study of cell damage with oncostatic agents.

[2] L. E. Sheving, unpublished data.

TOWARD CHRONOIMMUNOPOTENTIATION AND CHRONOIMMUNOTHERAPY

Immune Functions Exhibit Rhythms of Various Frequencies

Circadian rhythms have been recently documented for numerous immunologic variables including lymphocyte stimulation with mitogens (134, 150), graft vs. host reaction (16), spleen-colony-forming units (144), plaque-forming cells (25), phagocytic activity (147), and natural killer cell activity (26); and circadian rhythms have long been known in related variables, notably for serum corticosterone and blood eosinophils, leukocytes, and lymphocytes in various animal species (39).

Moreover, circadian rhythms have been demonstrated in the rejection of rat kidney allografts (114) and rat skin homografts and isografts (56) (Fig. 14.25); the high numbers of host vs. graft reactions occurred for grafts performed between 6 and 10 HALO or at 22 HALO, respectively. Such a difference in timing may be related to differences among animal species and tissue models, as well as to selective modulations of the circadian time structure by other frequencies. Skin grafts were performed in January 1971, while renal grafts were done between July and October 1971. A possible circannual modulation of circadian aspects of graft rejection needs to be considered.

Circaseptan (approximately 7-day) rhythms also have been demonstrated in the incidence of

rejections of kidney transplants by rats (114) and human beings (19). Kidney rejection occurred most frequently at multiples of 7.7 days in rats and of 8.1 days in human beings (Fig. 14.26); these periodicities were not differentiable from a 7-day period.

Circaseptan rhythms in antigenically triggered lymphocytes were also demonstrated by re-analyzing data published and kindly provided by Raine *et al.* (113). In guinea pigs with chronic relapsing experimental allergic encephalomyelitis followed for 387 days after antigenic induction of the disease, a circaseptan rhythm could be shown in B and T cells, with 3 relapses out of 4 occurring at multiples of 7 days post-antigen injection and with all 4 relapses happening when T-lymphocyte number was low (Table 14.2).

These data indicate that a circaseptan rhythm after antigenic stimulation characterizes both

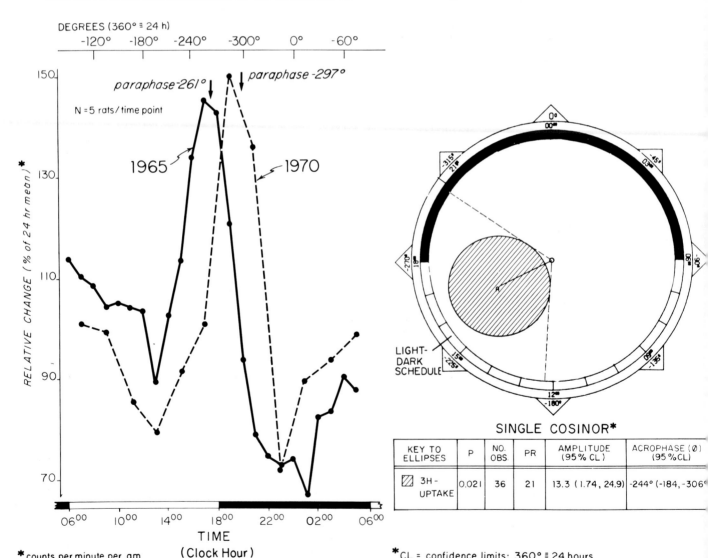

KEY TO ELLIPSES	P	NO. OBS.	PR	AMPLITUDE (95% CL)	ACROPHASE (∅) (95% CL)
▨ ³H-UPTAKE	0.021	36	21	13.3 (1.74, 24.9)	-244° (-184, -306°)

SINGLE COSINOR*

*CL = confidence limits; 360° ≡ 24 hours

Figure 14.24. [³H]Thymidine uptake in rat bone marrow (femur) shows a circadian rhythm of DNA synthesis reproducible from 1 year to the other. (Scheving *et al.*).

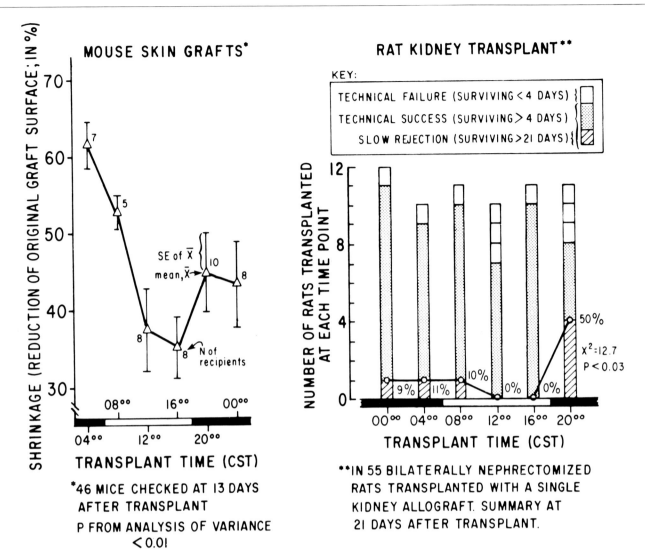

Figure 14.25. Mouse skin graft and rat kidney transplant rejections exhibit statistically significant circadian rhythms, almost in antiphase. Apparent differences in graft "take" may relate to differences in species, tissue grafted and/or modulation by other periodicities.

"arms" (T and B) of the immune system. Evidence for cyclic 7-day responses in number of IgM secreting cells and IgG secreting cells after T-independent antigen challenge also has been reported (14, 34, 119).

Chronoimmunomodulation: does a spectrum of frequencies (circadian, circaseptan, and circannual) determine immunostimulation or suppression with Lentinan? An attempt was made to exploit both circadian and circaseptan perioicities in optimizing the response of a rat immunocytoma to Lentinan. This polysaccharide was extracted from the most popular edible mushroom in Japan, *Lentinus edodes*, by Chihara et al. (15).

Lentinan has been defined as a T-oriented adjuvant or specific T-helper factor (18, 21, 86). In several studies on mice inoculated subcutaneously with sarcoma 180, treatment with Len-

tinan before or after tumor inoculation induced complete regression of the tumors (87). However, the effectiveness of this treatment depended on the strain of mice. Lentinan has also been demonstrated to be a host-mediated carcinostatic agent in several other solid tumors with high heterogeneity, and also in a mouse syngeneic methylcholanthreneinduced fibrosarcoma (161).

Against this background, a small preliminary study on LOU rats in our laboratories demonstrated that Lentinan could induce a transient inhibition of immunocytoma growth if given 6 hr after lighting onset (6 HALO) daily for 5 days prior to tumor inoculation. Two studies were then performed to examine possible circadian and circaseptan influences on the effectiveness of Lentinan against this tumor; the first study began in December 1978 and the second in May 1979. The endpoints were tumor size just before

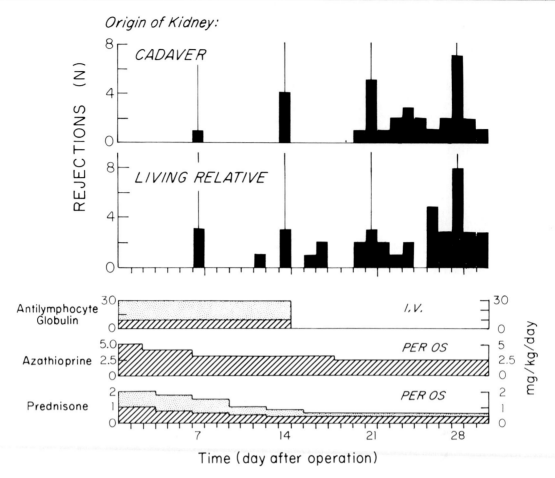

Figure 14.26. Circaseptan rhythm in the incidence of human kidney graft rejections.

Table 14.2
Circaseptan Rhythms Detected by Least-Squares Analyses (Chronobiologic window) in Different Classes of Lymphocytes after Antigenic Stimulation[a]

Lymphocyte	Best-fitting Period (days)	P	Mesor[b]	Double Amplitude[b]	Acrophase[c]
B-cell	7.4	0.02	1.43	0.80	6.3 (5.1, 7.4)
Early T-cells	7.0	0.08	1.59	1.3	2.9 —
	6.6	0.07	1.16	1.2	5.6 —
Late T-cells	7.2	0.07	2.16	1.0	3.6 —
All T-cells	7.0	0.01	1.78	1.2	3.1 (2.3, 4.1)

[a] A longitudinal survey of immunity in a guinea pig with chronic allergic encephalomyelitis. Blood samples (28) collected over 387 days after disease induction with isologous spinal cord (in complete Freund's adjuvant) in the nuchal area. (Data from C. S. Raine *et al.* (113).)
[b] Number of cells $\times 10^6$.
[c] In days from disease induction.

the first death was observed—on day 20 and day 19 after tumor inoculation in the first and second studies, respectively, percentage of survivors at 50% overall mortality, and mean survival times.

In the first study (involving 128 rats),[3] circadian and circaseptan stage dependence of Lentinan action was found in LOU rats treated prior to immunocytoma inoculation. Lentinan was injected i.p. daily at one of 6 circadian stages (2, 6, 10, 14, 18, 22 HALO) for 7 days in a total dose of 21 mg/kg. Rats at each circadian stage were assigned to 4 subgroups, two receiving sinusoidal doses of Lentinan, one with higher doses in the first several days (A), the second vice versa (B), while a third subgroup received equal doses of Lentinan each day (H), and a fourth was injected only with saline (C) (Table 14.3 and Fig. 14.27). Analyses of variance of tumor growth

[3] Lentinan was kindly provided by Dr. Goro Chihara, scientist, National Cancer Institute, Tokyo, Japan, who coauthored a first report (14a).

Table 14.3
Experimental Design of Study I

Subgroup	Group (HALO Time)[a]						Days Prior to Tumor Inoculation						
	1 (2)	2 (6)	3 (10)	4 (14)	5 (18)	6 (22)	7	6	5	4	3	2	1
A	6[b]	6	6	5	6	6	3.0[c]	5.0	5.5	4.1	1.9	0.6	1.0
B	6	6	6	6	6	6	3.0	1.0	0.6	1.9	4.1	5.5	5.0
H	6	4	6	5	5	6	3.0	3.0	3.0	3.0	3.0	3.0	3.0
C	4	3	3	4	4	4	None[d]						

[a] HALO = hours after light onset.

[b] No. of rats per group and subgroup. Total number of rats = 128 (104 given Lentinan, 22 controls given Dulbecco's medium and 2 added controls that received no injection) standardized with 8 hr of light alternating with 16 hr of darkness.

[c] Daily dose of Lentinan (mg/kg). Total cumulative Lentinan dose same (21 mg/kg) for subgroups A, B, and H.

[d] Dulbecco's medium, 1 ml/kg daily.

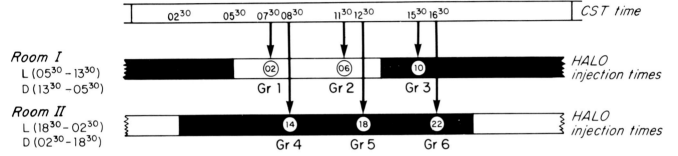

Figure 14.27. Experimental design of the first Lentinan study under conditions of synchronization with a 24-hr periodic lighting regimen. After 15 days of standardization, rats in Rooms I and II are expected to be in a similar circadian stage, when reference is made to light onset, but in an almost opposite circadian stage when referred to standard time. Such a scheme allows treatment at convenient clock hours (CST) for long term studies. (Lighting regimens in both rooms consist of light (L) for 8 hr alternating with darkness (D) for 16 hr (LD8:16); Groups 1, 2, and 3 housed from day of birth in Room I; Groups 4, 5, and 6 housed in Room II for 3 weeks prior to as well as during treatment; all animals singly housed beginning 3 weeks prior to first treatment. HALO = hours after lighting onset.)

documented the occurrence of a circaseptan and circadian stage dependence ($P \leq 0.05$). Tumor growth inhibition, survival rate and survival times were increased in rats receiving Lentinan during their daily rest span or near the daily onset of activity on schedule A and decreased in rats receiving the polysaccharide near the middle or late activity span under schedule H. While the "best" treatments slowed tumor growth and reduced the death rate as compared to data from controls, the "worst" treatments produced an opposite response (Figs. 14.28 and 14.29, Table 14.4).

The second study[4] (involving 308 rats) tested several circaseptan schedules, in addition to six circadian stages of Lentinan administration. The design was similar to that of the first study (Table 14.5) except that the lighting schedule was LD12:12 rather than LD8:16. Results from the cosinor method indicated a statistically significant circadian stage dependence of Lentinan action (irrespective of circaseptan schedule) upon tumor growth, percentage of survivors at 50% mortality and survival times (Table 14.6). Surprisingly, the acrophases of the rhythm in Lentinan effect upon tumor growth was about in antiphase with that observed in the first study (Fig. 14.30). When data at different circadian stages (irrespective of any circaseptan scheduling) were examined, it became apparent that Lentinan did not exhibit any effect at all on tumor size (compared to that of saline-injected controls) when given at 14, 18, or 22 HALO in either study. On the other hand, its administration at 2, 6, or 10 HALO yielded a favorable effect in the first study but an unfavorable one

[4] Lentinan was kindly provided by Dr. James Byram, scientist, Department of Pathology, Peter Bent Brigham Hospital, Boston, MA 02115, and Dr. M. Phillips, Department of Medicine, Allergy and Immunology, Hospital of University of Pennsylvania, Philadelphia, PA 19104.

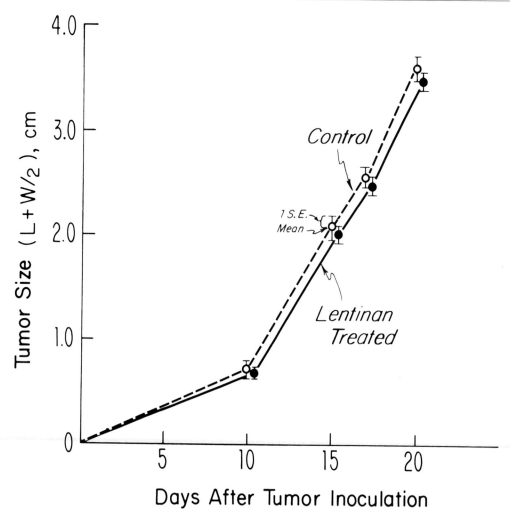

Figure 14.28. Immunocytoma growth in rats with or without Lentinan pre-treatment. Summary of pooled data from rats treated at different circadian stages and on different circaseptan schedules. Such a summary obscures time-dependent response of Lentinan-treated animals in comparison with controls. (Cumulative dose of 21 mg/kg given in 7 consecutive daily doses.)

in the second (Table 14.7). Since the only apparent difference between the two studies was the time of year when they were performed, a circannual influence upon the circadian system involved in Lentinan action should be considered. Such a circannual influence was recently documented in our laboratories for murine chronotolerance for arabinosylcytosine and cisplatin.

Two-way analyses of variance for data on tumor growth and survival time also indicated a statistically significant effect of circadian stage. In neither case could a main effect of circaseptan schedule be demonstrated. However, the presence of a statistically significant interaction term in the case of tumor growth suggests that an effect of circaseptan schedule depends on circadian stage. Further evidence of a circaseptan effect was provided by a χ^2 test of data on

percent survival at 50% overall mortality ($\chi^2 =$ 18.5; $P \sim 0.01$). Thus it appears that the optimal circadian timing for Lentinan administration may vary appreciably along the scale of a year. Furthermore, Lentinan action may be either favorable, unfavorable or absent depending on the circannual and circadian stage and possibly also on circaseptan modulation of a daily dose.

The main host factor reportedly responsible for retarding tumor growth is the generation of cytotoxic small lymphocytes (CTL) after contact with tumor antigens. CTL response has been shown to be greatly increased by Lentinan treatment after tumor inoculation and this increase was strictly schedule- and dose-dependent (57, 58). The first 3 days following tumor inoculation are critical for the mounting of such a Lentinan-induced increase in CTL response (57, 58, 87). Furthermore, a depressed CTL response could

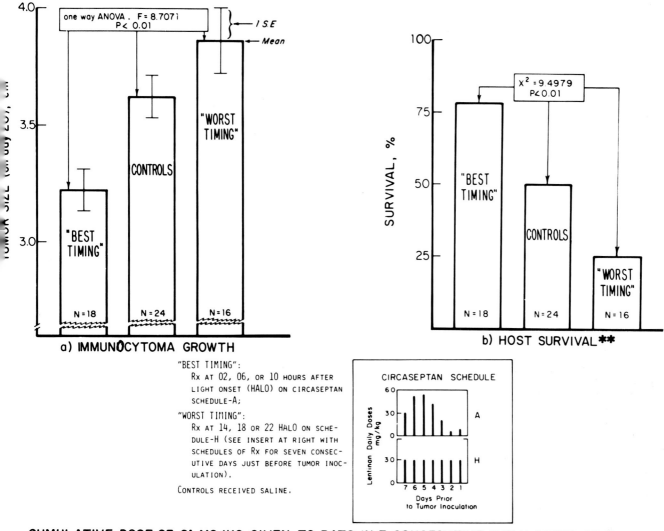

"BEST TIMING":
Rx at 02, 06, or 10 hours after light onset (HALO) on circaseptan schedule-A;

"WORST TIMING":
Rx at 14, 18 or 22 HALO on schedule-H (see insert at right with schedules of Rx for seven consecutive days just before tumor inoculation).

Controls received saline.

CUMULATIVE DOSE OF 21 MG/KG GIVEN TO RATS IN 7 CONSECUTIVE DAILY DOSES BEFORE TUMOR INOCULATION.

✸✸ % SURVIVORS AT 50% OVERALL MORTALITY.

Figure 14.29. Circadian and circaseptan dependence of immunomodulation with Lentinan (first study). (a) Bargraph of immunocytoma growth, supplemented by results of an analysis of variance, illustrates the beneficial or harmful effect of Lentinan according to its timing. (b) Bargraph of survival rate at 50% mortality, supplemented by results of a χ^2 analysis, further supports that immunopotentiation can turn to immunosuppression according to the timing of Lentinan.

Table 14.4
Effect of 7-Daily Consecutive Doses of Lentinan Prior to Inoculation of Immunocytoma to LOU Rats on Mean Survival Time[a]

	Circaspetan Lentinan Schedule[b]			ANOVA
	A	H	None (Controls)	
Circadian stage of treatment (HALO[c])	2, 6, 10	14, 18, 22	Pooled	
No. of rats	18	16	24	$F = 3.3371$
Survival time (mean ± SE)	24.8 ± 0.4	23.3 ± 0.5	23.8 ± 0.3	$P < 0.05$

[a] Results of one-way analysis of variance (ANOVA) summarize the role played by the circadian-stage of administration and the circaseptan modulation of the daily dose.

[b] Seven-daily consecutive dose of Lentinan as follows: Schedule A: 3.0, 5.0, 5.5, 4.1, 1.9, 0.6, 1.0 mg/kg; Schedule H: fixed dose of 3 mg/kg.

[c] HALO: hours after light onset (rats standardized in LD8:16).

Table 14.5
Experimental Design of Study II

Subgroup	Group (HALO Time)[a]						Days Prior to Tumor Inoculation						
	1 (2)	2 (6)	3 (10)	4 (14)	5 (18)	6 (22)	7	6	5	4	3	2	1
Lentinan:													
A	6[b]	6	6	6	6	6	5.5[c]	5.0	3.0	1.0	0.6	1.9	4.1
B	6	5	6	6	6	6	4.1	5.5	5.0	3.0	1.0	0.6	1.9
C	5	6	6	5	6	6	1.9	4.1	5.5	5.0	3.0	1.0	0.6
D	6	6	6	6	6	6	0.6	1.9	4.1	5.5	5.0	3.0	1.0
E	6	6	6	6	6	6	1.0	0.6	1.9	4.1	5.5	5.0	3.0
F	6	6	6	6	6	6	3.0	1.0	0.6	1.9	4.1	5.5	5.0
H	6	6	6	6	6	6	3.0	3.0	3.0	3.0	3.0	3.0	3.0
Saline:													
S	10	10	9	10	10	10	None						

[a] HALO = hours after light onset.
[b] Number of rats per subgroup. Total number of rats = 308 (249 given Lentinan, 59 controls given saline) standardized with 12 hr of light alternating with 12 hr of darkness.
[c] Daily dose (mg/kg). Total cumulative dose same (21 mg/kg) for all subgroups A–F and H.

Table 14.6
Results from Single Cosinor[a] Analysis of Three Indices of Lentinan Action upon Immunocytoma Growth in LOU Rats (Study II)

Variables (Units)	N	PR	Mesor	Amplitude	Acrophase (95% CL)
Tumor growth (cm)[b]	249	9.4	3.0	0.15	−68° (−38, −97)
Survivors (%)[c]	42	34.2	49	22.4	−245° (−210, −279)
Survival time (hr)	249	8.7	558	13.1	−238° (−208, −269)

[a] Period fitted = 24 hr. P = probability of zero amplitude < 0.001 for each variable. N = number of observations. PR = percent rhythm. Mesor = rhythm-adjusted mean. Amplitude = half of the variability predicted by fitted cosine. Acrophase in degrees from light onset (LD12:12) with 360° ≡ 24 hr. 95% CL = conservative 95% confidence limits derived from cosinor ellipse.
[b] Tumor size on day 19 after tumor inoculation.
[c] At 50% overall mortality.

be observed if Lentinan was given in the late part of the time span associated with an immune response (D_5 to D_9) following tumor inoculation (57). This is consistent with the present report that an undesirable effect of Lentinan also can result from a wrongly scheduled administration before tumor inoculation.

In addition, the cytotoxicity of peritoneal cells against tumor reportedly peaks at 7 days after administration of Lentinan, but is not present in the peritoneal cells collected 14, 20, and 30 days after administration (86). An algebraic immunomodulation, possibly depending on "circaseptan" timing of a single dose of 1 mg/mouse Lentinan in relation to antigenic sensitization and challenge with Schistosoma eggs in mice, was recently suggested (10) and is depicted in Figure 14.31.

Turning back to the preliminary study, anal-

ysis of the fresh spleen weights of dead animals as a function of days after tumor inoculation (regardless of whether or not they had received Lentinan) also showed a circaseptan rhythm (Fig. 14.32). Since these data cover only a 10-day span from day 19 after tumor inoculation, they must be regarded in the light of reports on the occurrence of rhythms of 7-day periodicity in the number of plaque-forming cells after a single antigenic challenge (4, 74, 119, 142, 160). It goes without saying that the role played by circadian, circaseptan, and circannual rhythms upon immunomodulation deserves further study. Furthermore, our reports suggest that chronobiological investigations considering the spectrum of frequencies appear to be necessary to understand the crucial role played by the temporal relationship between the administration of an "immunopotentiator" and tumor challenge,

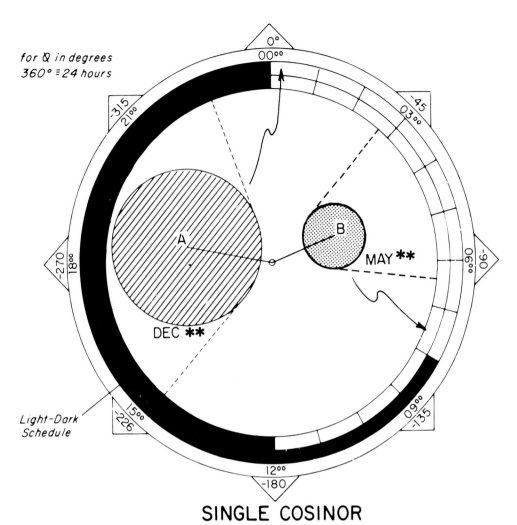

SINGLE COSINOR

Key to Ellipses	P	No. Obs.	PR	Mesor ±SE	Amplitude (95% CL)	Acrophase (95% CL)
A. Study I	0.018	108	7.4	3.5 ±0.05	0.20(0.03,0.36)	-280°(-221,-339)
B. Study II	<0.001	249	9.4	3.0 ±0.02	0.15(0.08,0.22)	- 68°(-39, -97)

DATA ON IMMUNOCYTOMA SIZE (MEAN DIAMETER, CM) IN RATS 20 DAYS (A) o OR 19 DAYS (B) AFTER TUMOR INOCULATION, AS A FUNCTION OF CIRCADIAN STAGE OF PRIOR LENTINAN TREATMENT (IRRESPECTIVE OF CIRCASEPTAN SCHEDULE), FITTED WITH 24 HOUR COSINE CURVE.

✱✱ Considering all circaseptan sub groups receiving Lentinan (N= 3 in A and N = 7 in B).

Figure 14.30. Cosinor presentation of circadian rhythm in Lentinan immunomodulation as evaluated by tumor size: Results from first and second study. The direction of the line (vector) directed outward from the center of the figure represents the rhythm's acrophase in relation to the circular scale. The circular region at the tip of the vector indicates the joint 95% confidence regions for the rhythm's amplitude and acrophase. The largest tumor sizes (indicated by the acrophases) results from Lentinan treatment at 2 opposite circadian stages according to the circannual stage of this treatment.

which sometimes results in tumor promotion rather than inhibition (Table 14.8). Our findings encourage further investigations of rhythms in the immune system and the development of multifrequency schedules in immunotherapy as well as in oncostatic chemotherapy and radiotherapy.

ADDED CIRCASEPTAN (AND OTHER) RHYTHMS OF INTEREST FOR CHRONO-ONCOLOGY

Circaseptan rhythms also have been reported in DNA synthesis and in the mitotic index of rat

Table 14.7
Comparisons between Tumor Growth as a Function of the Circadian Stages of Lentinan Administration in December and May

Month (study)	Tumor Size (cm)				
	Lentinan[a]		Saline (all)[a]	One-Way ANOVA[a]	
	2+6+10[b]	14+18+22[b]		F	P
December (I)	3.35 ± 0.07	3.63 ± 0.07	3.63 ± 0.10	4.736	~ 0.01
May (II)	3.03 ± 0.03	2.87 ± 0.03	2.89 ± 0.05	5.746	< 0.01

[a] Mean and standard error.
[b] In hours after light onset.
[c] Analysis of variance.

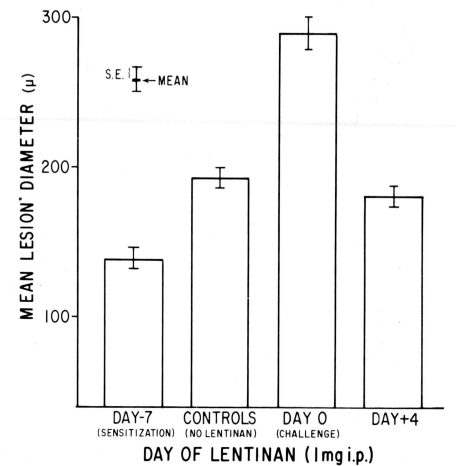

*LUNG GRANULOMAS ON DAY 8 AFTER CHALLENGE WITH EGGS OF SCHISTOSOMA MANSONI IN MICE SENSITIZED SEVEN DAYS EARLIER.

Figure 14.31. Effect of Lentinan on pulmonary granuloma evaluated 8 days after intravenous injection of *Schistosoma mansoni* eggs into sensitized CBA/J mice. The action of Lentinan is determined by the time of administration of a single 1-mg dose in relation to day of challenge. Sensitization occurred 7 days before challenge. Lentinan was given either concomitantly with sensitization, or 7 days later (concomitantly with challenge) or 4 days after challenge. Controls received an equivalent volume of saline instead of Lentinan. (Data from Byram *et al.* (10).)

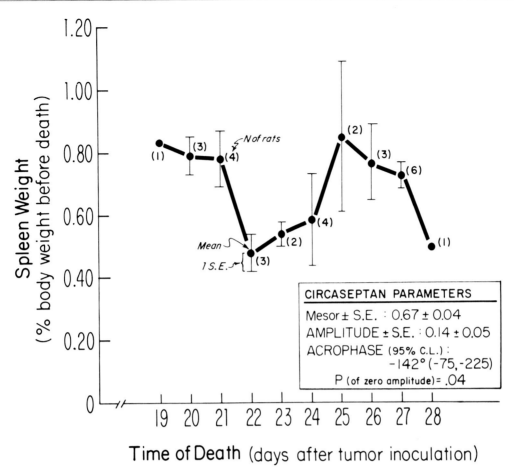

Figure 14.32. Circaseptan periodicity in spleen weight after tumor inoculation as revealed by data collected between days 19 and 28 post-tumor inoculation and analyzed by the single-cosinor method. Such results must be considered with regard to documented circaseptan periodicities in, e.g., the number of plaque-forming cells. The first acrophase (high value) of relative spleen weight is predicted to occur 2.8 days after tumor challenge, when Lentinan presence is required to show any antitumor effectiveness. (Fresh spleen weight obtained upon death of rats with or without previous Lentinan treatment. Parameter estimates based on least squares fit of 7-day cosine curve; acrophase reference = day of tumor inoculation, with $360° \equiv 7$ days $(-142° = 2.8$ days.)

kidney during compensatory hypertrophy (67). Circaseptan rhythms are not only revealed after antigenic or traumatic stimulation, but have also been demonstrated notably in urine volume and urinary 17-ketosteroid excretion (49, 140), and in oral temperature (14), collected from ("unstimulated") human beings living under usual routine. Other species also exhibit such rhythms; they have been demonstrated, e.g., for oviposition in an arthropod (13) and for the enzyme hydroxyindole-o-methyl-transferase in rat pineal gland of either sex (159). Furthermore, cyclic variations in the infradian domain (which may include circaseptan periodicity) have been reported in the response of lymphocytes to phytohemagglutinin in healthy individuals (20) and in hematologic studies of toxicity from cyclophosphamide and irradiation (89, 97, 99).

Thus, circaseptan periodicity can be regarded as a component of the spectrum of rhythms characterizing life (45, 49); it awaits further exploitation in tumor immunotherapy and in all kinds of immunosuppressive therapy. Moreover, the role played by bioperiodic phenomena on the so-called immunosurveillance system (7) seems to imply frequencies other than circadian and circaseptan, since circannual rhythms in numerous immunologic variables have been documented in human beings, notably for immunoglobulins in healthy adults (117), for surface Ig bearing B lymphocytes (1), and for complement.

In addition, a circamenstrual modulation of the circadian response to a subcutaneous injection of histamine has been demonstrated (93).

In short, a wide spectrum of rhythms of different frequencies characterizing (among others) lymphocytic function needs to be considered for cancer chronotherapy as well as for cancer chronophylaxis.

Table 14.8
Promotion as Well Inhibition of Tumor Growth by "Immunotherapeutic" Agents

Reference	Agent	Dose Range	Route	Schedule	Model	Results	Factors Deemed Responsible
D. O. Chee and A. J. Bodurtha: *International Journal of Cancer*, 14:137–143, 1974	BCG (8.10^8 organisms/mg)	0.0005–0.5 mg	s.c.	Once weekly for 6 weeks; tumor administration last day of treatment	Mouse B16 melanoma	Tumor growth promoted or reduced	Dose-dependence
G. Mathé et al.: *European Journal of Cancer*, 11:801–807, 1975	BCG (7.10^6 organisms/mg)	1 mg	s.c., i.v.	Day 3 or 7, or 14 before test	(DBA/$2\times$C57B1/6)f$_1$ mice	Macrophage activation test null or increased	Route and schedule
			s.c., i.v.	idem	idem	Hemolytic plaque-forming assay-null or increased antibody formation	Route and schedule
H. T. Wepsic et al.: *Cancer Research*, 36:1950–1953, 1976	BCG (Wall)	75–150 µg	s.c., i.v.	Day 14 before tumor inoculation	Idem + Lewis lung carcinoma	Tumor growth promoted or reduced	Route
			s.c.	Day 32, 21 or 14 before, concomitantly with, or day 12 after inoculation	Morris 3924a hepatoma in ACI rats	Tumor growth promoted, reduced or unchanged	Schedule
F. C. Sparks and J. H. Breeding: *Cancer Research*, 34:3262–3269, 1974	BCG (Tice)	0.1 ml	Intratumor	Day 15 after tumor inoculation	C$_3$H mice with BP fibrosarcoma	Tumor growth promoted	
	BCG ± neuramidinase		Site of tumor inoculation	Day 7 after tumor inoculation	C$_{57}$BL/6 mice with MCA-1 fibrosarcoma	Tumor growth promoted	Host-tumor system
	BCG ±neuramidinase		Intratumor and s.c.	Day 14 after tumor inoculation	C$_3$H mice with MCA-2 fibrosarcoma	Tumors completely regressed	
	BCG ±neuramidinase	6.9×10^5 to 6.9×10^6 Organisms	s.c., intratumor, axilla	Day 9 &/or 23 after tumor inoc.	C$_3$H mice with MC-43 fibrosarcoma	Tumor growth promoted or inhibited	Dose and schedule
N. L. Levy et al.: *Cancer*, 10:244–248, 1972	BCG (MSD)	0.1 ml	Intratumor	Once (3 weeks before lymphocyte toxicity array)	66-yr male patient with widely metastatic melanoma	Tumor growth promoted; death	Blocking activity of serum against cell-mediated cytotoxicity

Reference	Agent	Dose	Route	Schedule	Tumor model	Effect	Comments
E. G. Bliznakov: Bionedicine, 26:73–76, 1977	Summarizes BCG, levamisole, zymosan, coenzyme Q10: "immunostimulation and depression . . . are two diverse expressions of the same system;" needs consideration of dose, time, route, intervals between multiple administration						
R. Bomford: International Journal of Cancer, 19:673–679, 1977	C. parvum (Co-parvax)	7–350 µg	s.c., i.v.	Day 7 before, or concomitantly with or day 7 after inoculation	Mouse CBA T6T6 with transplanted methylcholanthrene-induced fibrosarcoma	Tumor growth promoted or reduced, or unchanged	Schedule, route and dose of tumor cells
D. A. Berd and M. S. Michell: Cancer Research, 36:4119–4124, 1976	C. parvum	0.25–1 mg	i.p., i.v.	Day 7 before tumor inoculation	Mouse C57BL/6 (H-2^b) challenged with L1210 leukemia (allogeneic mice)	Tumor promotion; in-vitro-spleen cell-mediated and antibody cytotoxicity suppressed	Dose and route dependence

MARKER RHYTHMS FOR CLINICAL CANCER CHRONOTHERAPY

In clinical practice, the best compromise in treatment-timing between that showing highest antitumor activity and that with lowest antihost activity must be explored by the use of marker rhythms. These should indicate the temporal stages of sensitivity (to the agent used) for both the host and tumor.

Host Temperature

As a marker rhythm of the host's temporal organization, the circadian rhythm in core temperature has been shown to exhibit a consistent phase relationship to the circadian rhythms of murine tolerance for several drugs, such as Adr (101), PAM, and cisP (83). For example, in the case of Adr, a 180° shift in the tolerance rhythm (Fig. 14.33) was accomplished by manipulation of the availability of food and was accompanied by a similar shift in the temperature rhythm. Whether in cancer patients core temperature also may be a reliable marker rhythm to indicate the internal time of highest host tolerance is presently under investigation. An adequate instrumentation for data collection from continuous temperature and activity monitoring is now available (TherMologs and Solicorders). These devices are small pocket-size units equipped with an electronic memory and connected to a rectal or surface temperature probe and/or to a wrist bracelet registering activity.

Such devices allow a sampling frequency as high as 1/sec. The observation span depends on the sampling frequency chosen. For example, with a sampling frequency of 1/12 min, data can be automatically collected throughout 15 days. An example of the reliability of rectal temperature monitoring by such a device is depicted in Figures 14.34 and 14.35 for a mildly hypertensive man. When analyzed by rhythmometric procedures, the circadian rhythm in core temperature remained remarkably consistent from day to day during a 9-day span, except when the subject experienced a mild laryngitis. This further documents what many previous reports have shown, the adequacy of host temperature as a consistent marker rhythm. Such data also point out the sensitivity of the temperature rhythm to an ongoing mild pathologic process, and prompts investigation of any disease- or treatment-induced alterations in temperature rhythm in cancer patients.

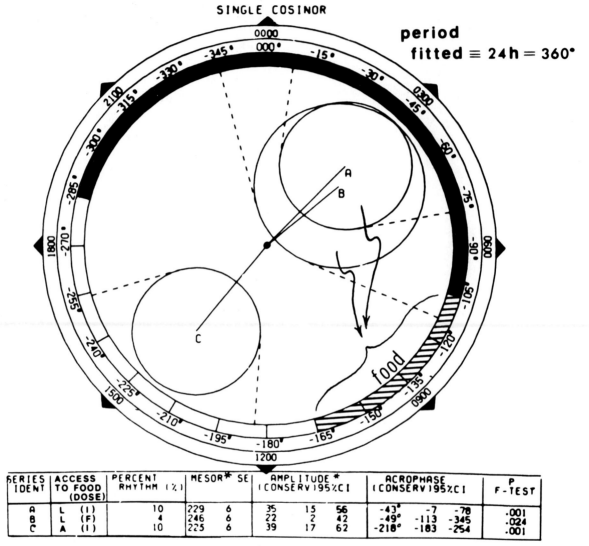

SERIES IDENT	ACCESS TO FOOD (DOSE)	PERCENT RHYTHM (%)	MESOR* SE		AMPLITUDE* (CONSERV)95%CI			ACROPHASE (CONSERV)95%CI			P F-TEST
A	L (I)	10	229	6	35	15	56	-43°	-7	-78	.001
B	L (F)	4	246	6	22	2	42	-49°	-113	-345	.024
C	A (I)	10	225	6	39	17	62	-218°	-183	-254	.001

L = Limited to first 4h in 12h light span

A = Ad lib.

I = Dose by weight at injection time

F = Dose fixed

Figure 14.33. Cosinor presentation of the shiftability of murine chronotolerance for Adriamycin by meal timing. Mean survival time in hours after LD$_{90}$. Food ad libitum or restricted to the first 4 hr of light (resting span).

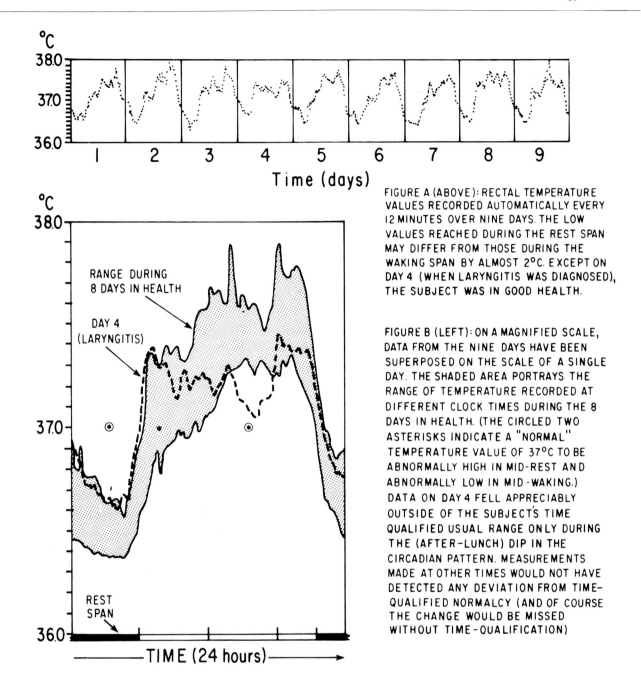

FIGURE A (ABOVE): RECTAL TEMPERATURE VALUES RECORDED AUTOMATICALLY EVERY 12 MINUTES OVER NINE DAYS. THE LOW VALUES REACHED DURING THE REST SPAN MAY DIFFER FROM THOSE DURING THE WAKING SPAN BY ALMOST 2°C. EXCEPT ON DAY 4 (WHEN LARYNGITIS WAS DIAGNOSED), THE SUBJECT WAS IN GOOD HEALTH.

FIGURE B (LEFT): ON A MAGNIFIED SCALE, DATA FROM THE NINE DAYS HAVE BEEN SUPERPOSED ON THE SCALE OF A SINGLE DAY. THE SHADED AREA PORTRAYS THE RANGE OF TEMPERATURE RECORDED AT DIFFERENT CLOCK TIMES DURING THE 8 DAYS IN HEALTH. (THE CIRCLED TWO ASTERISKS INDICATE A "NORMAL" TEMPERATURE VALUE OF 37°C TO BE ABNORMALLY HIGH IN MID-REST AND ABNORMALLY LOW IN MID-WAKING.) DATA ON DAY 4 FELL APPRECIABLY OUTSIDE OF THE SUBJECT'S TIME QUALIFIED USUAL RANGE ONLY DURING THE (AFTER-LUNCH) DIP IN THE CIRCADIAN PATTERN. MEASUREMENTS MADE AT OTHER TIMES WOULD NOT HAVE DETECTED ANY DEVIATION FROM TIME-QUALIFIED NORMALCY (AND OF COURSE THE CHANGE WOULD BE MISSED WITHOUT TIME-QUALIFICATION)

Figure 14.34. Rectal temperature values recorded automatically every 12 minutes over 9 days from 60-year-old man with controlled mesor-hypertension. Chronogram (*A*) and time-qualified range of variation (*B*), which allows detection of a pathologic process.

Urinary Variables: Host and Tumor Marker Rhythms

Other potential readily assessed marker rhythms of the host are those in urinary variables, notably urine volume (10a). The latter proved adequate for predicting rat chronotolerance for a single therapeutic dose of cisP and for following up the toxicity of this drug (83) (Fig.

14.36). In human beings, urine volume has long been known to exhibit circadian variations (106, 133). Such a circadian rhythm persisted in healthy subjects even when at rest, deprived of food and hydrated p.o. every hour for 1 or 2 days (133), and also in myeloma patients (162) (Fig. 14.37). Reproducibility throughout the year of the characteristics of the circadian urine volume rhythm in a single individual has been documented (139). However, interindividual differ-

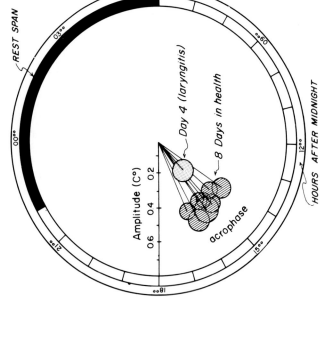

AMPLITUDES AND ACROPHASES OF 24-HOUR COSINE CURVES FITTED TO DATA FROM EACH DAY SEPARATELY ARE DISPLAYED ON THIS "COSINOR" PLOT. THE AMPLITUDES ARE REPRESENTED BY THE LENGTHS AND THE ACROPHASES BY THE ANGULAR POSITIONS OF THE "CLOCK HANDS" IN RELATION TO LINEAR AND CIRCULAR SCALES, RESPECTIVELY. THE SHADED CIRCLE AT THE TIP OF EACH "HAND" INDICATES THE 95% CONFIDENCE REGION FOR THE TRUE AMPLITUDE AND ACROPHASE ON THAT PARTICULAR DAY. THE CLEAR SEPARATION OF THE CONFIDENCE REGION FOR DAY 4 FROM THOSE OF THE OTHER DAYS ILLUSTRATES GRAPHICALLY THE STATISTICALLY HIGHLY SIGNIFICANT PERTURBATION OF THE TEMPERATURE RHYTHM ON THAT DAY OF LARYNGITIS.

EVEN IF MEASUREMENTS HAD BEEN OMITTED DURING THE MIDDAY SPAN WHEN VALUES WERE LOWER THAN "NORMAL," THE STATISTICAL **SIGNIFICANCE OF** THE RHYTHM PARAMETERS WOULD HAVE DEMONSTRATED THE PERTURBATION-- ACTUALLY BY AS RIGOROUS AND IMMEDIATE A TEST RESULT AS NON-OVER- LAPPING 95% CONFIDENCE INTERVALS (NOT SHOWN).

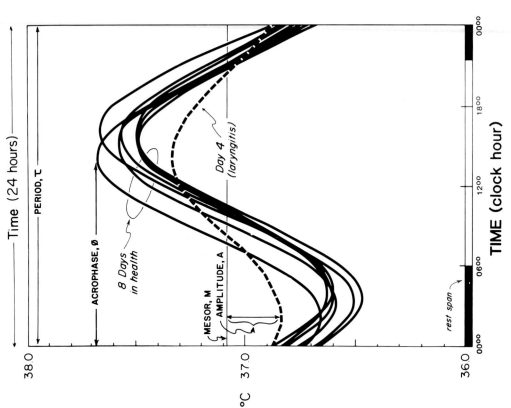

SUPERPOSED 24-HOUR COSINE CURVES FITTED SEPARATELY TO DATA FROM EACH DAY. THE SMALLER AMPLITUDE OF THE CURVE FITTED TO THE DATA OF DAY 4 (DASHED CURVE) SEEMS EVIDENT, BUT STILL REQUIRES A STAT- ISTICAL TEST OF DEVIATION FROM THE SET OF MACROSCOPICALLY SIMILAR CURVES FOR THE OTHER 8 DAYS.

Figure 14.35. Cosinor analyses of 9 consecutive days of automatic recording of rectal temperature from 60-year-old man with controlled mesor-hypertension, on his usual routine.

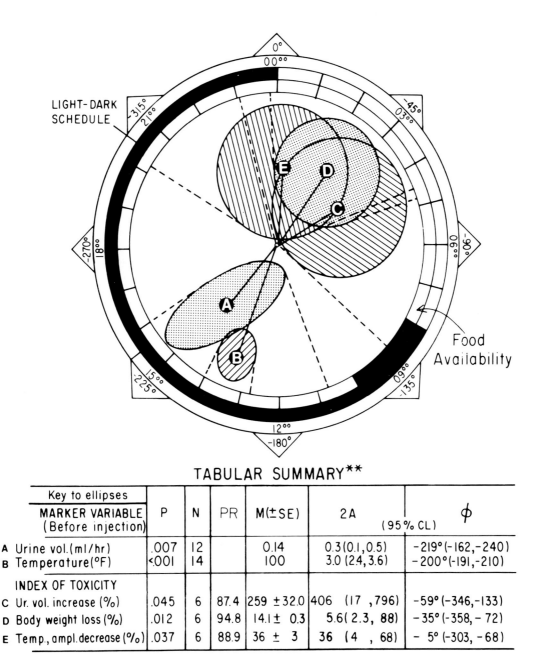

TABULAR SUMMARY**

Key to ellipses MARKER VARIABLE (Before injection)	P	N	PR	M(±SE)	2A (95% CL)	φ
A Urine vol.(ml/hr)	.007	12		0.14	0.3(0.1,0.5)	-219°(-162,-240)
B Temperature(°F)	<.001	14		100	3.0 (2.4,3.6)	-200°(-191,-210)
INDEX OF TOXICITY						
C Ur. vol. increase (%)	.045	6	87.4	259 ±32.0	406 (17 ,796)	-59°(-346,-133)
D Body weight loss (%)	.012	6	94.8	14.1± 0.3	5.6(2.3, 88)	-35°(-358,- 72)
E Temp., ampl.decrease (%)	.037	6	88.9	36 ± 3	36 (4 , 68)	- 5° (-303,- 68)

** Results from mean cosinor for marker variables (N = number of series) and from single cosinor for indices of toxicity (N = number of values fitted, each value representing rats treated at a given time point.)
P = P-value obtained from the zero amplitude test in single cosinor analysis; PR = percent rhythm or amount of variability accounted for by cosine fit; M = mesor or rhythm adjusted mean; 2A = extent of predictable variability (double amplitude); Ø = acrophase or time of maximum in fitted cosine curve with light onset = reference time and 360° ≡ 24h; C = mean daily urine volume (U) increase = (U$_2$-U$_1$)/(U$_1$); D = mean body weight (W) loss = (W$_1$-W$_2$)/(W$_1$); E = mean decrease in the amplitude (A) of the temperature circadian rhythm = (A$_1$-A$_2$)/(A$_1$); with (1) = values observed before injection and (2) = values observed during the 6 d post injection span.

Figure 14.36. Cosinor presentation of rat chronotolerance for a for single therapeutic dose of cisplatine (5 mg/ kg intraperitoneally) in relation to two host marker rhythms (urine volume and temperature). Drug tolerance is here evaluated from urine volume increase, body weight loss and reduction of the amplitude of temperature circadian rhythm, during the 6-day postinjection span.

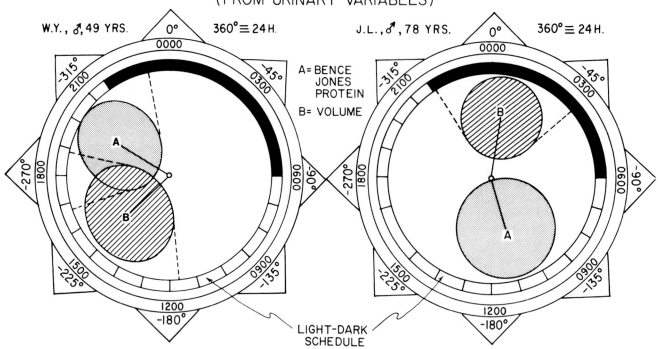

Figure 14.37. Urinary marker rhythms of the host and tumor in 2 myeloma patients.

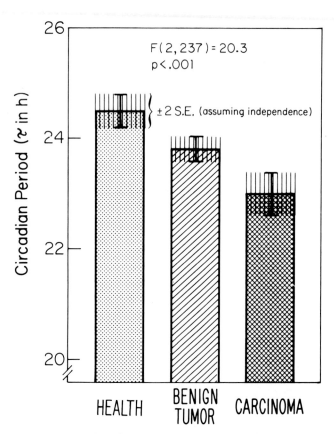

Figure 14.38. Cancer chronopathology: different candidate circadian periods in surface temperature recorded over a healthy and a cancerous breast.

ences may exist in the phase relationship of two potential marker rhythms, as reported in the case of urine volume and temperature (75) or urine volume and urinary sodium (10a). In such cases, the more adequate marker rhythm will have to be chosen as a function of the drugs used.

Tumor Temperature

Marker rhythms documented to reflect a periodic stage of tumor sensitivity to oncostatic agents include tumor surface temperature. In the case of breast cancer, symmetric location of thermal probes on both breasts allows comparisons between the healthy and the diseased breast, and shows alteration in the circadian period of the rhythm as a graded function of the severity of the pathologic process (Fig. 14.38) (31) (see Chapter 37). Resynchronization of the circadian surface temperature rhythm over the cancerous human breast with that over the healthy breast has been reported to correlate with an early detection of a clinical response to an active antitumor drug (88).

Tumor temperature has been correlated with mitosis in oral cancers (17) and with increased ^{32}P uptake (presumably an indirect measure of processes leading to mitosis) in breast cancer (143).

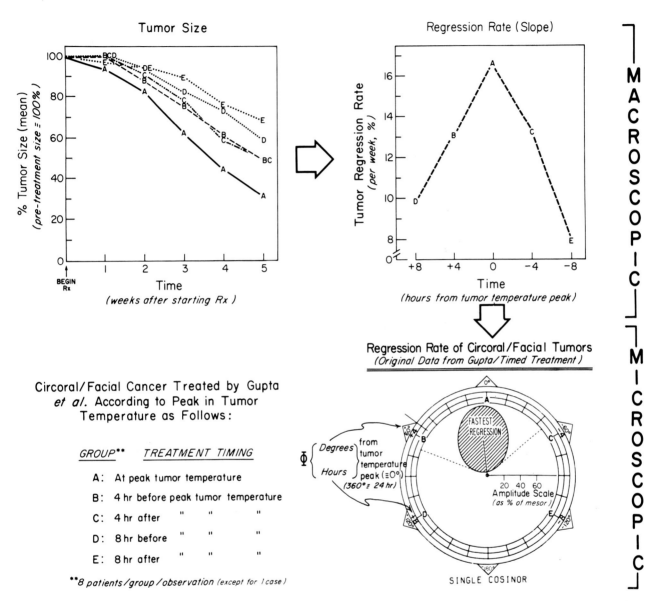

Figure 14.39. Chronoradiotherapy of oral cancers referred to tumor surface temperature as a tumor marker rhythm and evaluated by a short term therapeutic endpoint.

Table 14.9
Long-term Follow-up after Circadian Chronoradiotherapy of Oral Cancers (from Deka, 1975): Evaluation of Disease-free Patients

Treatment group	A	B	C	D	E	Controls
Treatment time[a]	0	−4	+4	−8	+8	Time-unqualified
No. of Patients	8	8	8	8	8	10
No. lost to follow-up (time of loss)	1 (12 mo)	1 (12 mo)	1 (18 mo)	2 (12 mo)	2 (3 and 18 mo)	1 (3 mo)
Time of Evaluation (month)[b]						
3	7:1[c]	4:4	4:4	4:4	4:4	5:5
6	7:1	4:4	3:5	4:4	2:6	4:6
12	6:2	3:5	3:5	3:5	2:6	4:6
18	5:3	2:6	2:6	2:6	1:7	3:7
24	5:3	2:6	2:6	2:6	1:7	3:7
Percent disease-free at 24 months	62.5	25	25	25	12.5	30

[a] In hours, from tumor temperature peak.
[b] In months, from the end of treatment course.
[c] Number disease free:number with recurrence.
[d] Peak test (Savage *et al.* (123): $P < 0.05$.

Clinical Circadian Chronoradiotherapy

With tumor temperature as a marker rhythm, chronoradiotherapy of oral cancers with external beam radiation has been investigated in two studies by Gupta, Deka *et al.* A first study included 3 groups of 19–22 patients. All patients received standard therapy of 240 r daily, 5 days each week, for 5 weeks (total tumor dose 6000 r). Patients were either treated with the usual once-a-day dose, without regard to the timing of treatment, or with fractionated doses (120 r in the morning *and* 120 r in the evening on each day of treatment), or with once-a-day doses given near the peak of tumor temperature, monitored before treatment as a marker rhythm. Patients irradiated near the peak of tumor temperature exhibited the fastest tumor regression.

In a second, double-blind study, 40 patients with oral cancers received the same total tumor dose at one of 5 different circadian stages of tumor temperature. The latter was measured every 2–4 hr during a 3–4-day span preceding treatment. Thus, 5 groups of 8 patients each were irradiated either near the peak of tumor temperature, 4 hr before or after, or 8 hr before or after the tumor temperature peak.

Tumor regression (as gauged by weekly measurements of tumor size during the 5 weeks of therapy) depended on the circadian stage of tumor temperature at the time of irradiation (Fig. 14.39) (54). The fastest tumor regression was found in patients treated near the peak of tumor temperature and was statistically validated as such by the cosinor method.

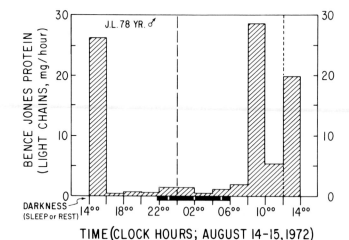

Figure 14.40. Circadian rhythm in a urinary tumor marker rhythm (light chain excretion) in a multiple myeloma patient.

Eight patients (1 or 2 per group) were lost to follow-up. However, at 24 months after treatment, the highest proportion of disease-free patients was observed in the group treated near the peak of tumor temperature. This peak in disease-free patients was statistically validated by the peak test (122) (Table 14.9).

Other Clinically Relevant Marker Rhythms of the Tumor

While tumor temperature seems to be an adequate marker rhythm for tumor sensitivity to

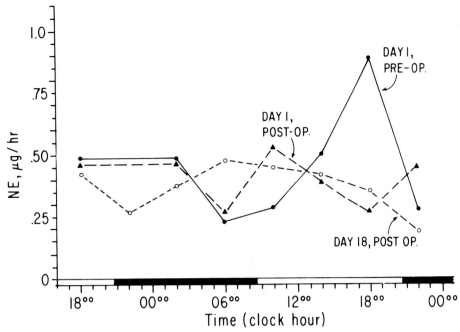

Figure 14.41. Circadian rhythm in a urinary tumor marker rhythm in a 2-year-old male patient with a retinoblastoma before and after tumor removal by surgery.

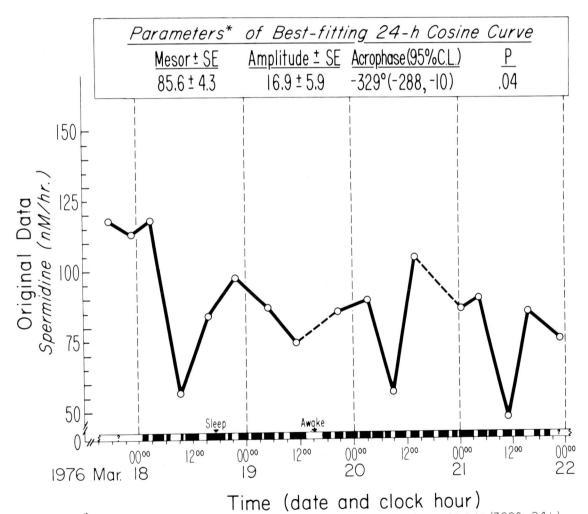

*Mesor and amplitude in nM/hr., acrophase in degrees after midnight (360° ≡ 24 h). Estimates based on least squares fitting of 24-h cosine curve; p-value from test of zero amplitude.

Figure 14.42. Circadian rhythm in urinary polyamines as markers of the host-tumor system in a male infant with neuroblastoma.

oncostatic agents, other tumor rhythms may also be amenable to monitoring by noninvasive techniques. This would be especially important for inaccessible tumors; *e.g.,* monitoring urinary light chain excretion in myeloma patients (Fig. 14.40), urinary epinephrine in retinoblastoma patients (Fig. 14.41), or urinary polyamine excretion (Fig. 14.42) in various types of cancer. Rhythms of periods longer than 24 hr have also been shown to characterize several tumors, notably chronic myelogenous leukemia, where a 72-day period was found for leukocytes and platelets either without (Fig. 14.43) or with treatment. Similar periodicities in this disease have also been reported (30, 99), even despite a constant nontoxic chemotherapeutic regimen (76, 90). Exploitation of those rhythms for therapeutic purposes deserves further investigation. Rhythms in other specific tumor markers such as carcinoembryonic antigen, α-fetoprotein, βHCG, and others are presently investigated.

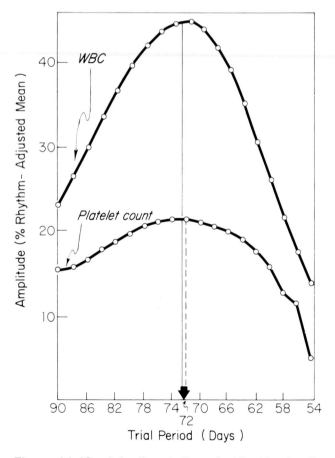

Figure 14.43. Infradian rhythm of white blood cells and platelets in a chronic myelogenous leukemia patient, resolved by rhythmometry procedures.

CONCLUSION

The existence of a temporal structure with a wide spectrum of different frequencies characterizes each living system, at each level of organization, and indicates an urgent need for a chrono-oncology.

Circadian rhythms in several variables pertinent to oncogenesis, such as lymphocytic functions, hormones, and cell division, provide a background for the observed circadian stage-dependence of chemically induced oncogenesis. These variables, however, also may be characterized by several other bioperiodicities, notably circaseptan, circatrigintan, and circannual. Thus, alteration of the circannual rhythm in prolactin may be a prominent factor contributing to increased risk of breast cancer. Such data underline the role that may be played by chronophylaxis, as a first step before chronotherapy.

Exploitation of bioperiodic phenomena for cancer chronotherapy should lead to a significant therapeutic improvement. Numerous studies document circadian rhythms in murine tolerance for several oncostatic agents, as well as circadian-stage dependence for the antitumor effectiveness of several nonlethal two-drug combinations.

These findings prompt investigations along the lines of chronokinetics of cells and drugs (chronocytokinetics and chronopharmacokinetics) coupled to chronopharmacodynamics to provide rationales for the design of optimal (chrono-)oncostatic schedules.

Optimal treatment schedules also may include consideration of circaseptan rhythms in host tolerance and in tumor sensitivity to carcinostatic modalities. For example, it was suggested that exploitation of circadian and circaseptan periodicities can tip the scale between anticancer immunostimulation or suppression with Lentinan, an immune adjuvant. A possible circannual influence upon the circadian system involved in Lentinan action also was indicated. Such results may relate to reportedly conflicting experimental and clinical results of tumor immunotherapy.

For the purpose of carrying experimental results to the clinic, host and tumor marker rhythms are needed. Automatically recorded host and/or tumor temperature seems promising in this respect. Results from circadian chronoradiotherapy of oral cancers, timed by the circadian rhythm in tumor temperature, have demonstrated the clinical pertinence of cancer chronotherapy.

Urinary variables such as volume, electrolytes, polyamines, epinephrine and Bence-Jones protein also exhibit circadian rhythms that can be considered potential marker rhythms depending on the kind of tumor and/or oncostatic agent(s) used.

Such temporal considerations should improve clinical experience with several experimentally proven synergistic drug combinations, and increase the selective toxicity ratio of combined carcinostatic modalities.

Acknowledgment. We thank Dr Walter Nelson for valuable discussions and critical reading of the manuscript. This work was supported by U.S. Public Health Service (GM-13981), National Cancer Institute (CA-14445 and CP-55702), National Institute of Occupational Safety and Health (OH-00631), National Institute of Aging (AG-00158), Environmental Protection Agency (R804512) and the St. Paul-Ramsey Medical Education and Research Foundation.

References

1. Abo, T., and Kumagai, K. (1978): Studies of surface immunoglobulins on human B lymphocytes; III. Physiological variations of SIg+ cells in peripheral blood. *J. Immunol.*, 33:441-452.
2. Badran, A. F., and Echave Llanos, J. M. (1965): Persistence of mitotic circadian rhythm of a transplantable mammary carcinoma after 35 generations: its bearing on the success of treatment with endoxan. *J.N.C.I.*, 2:285-290.
3. Baserga, R., and Wiebel, F. (1969): The cell cycle of mammalian cells. *Int. Rev. Exp. Pathol.*, 7:1-30.
4. Britton, S., and Moller, G. H. (1968): Regulation of antibody synthesis against *Escherischia coli* endotoxin I. *J. Immunol.*, 100:1326-1334.
5. Brockman, R. W. (1974): Circumvention of resistance, in *Pharmacological Basis of Cancer Chemotherapy*, pp. 691-771. Proc. 27th Symp. Fundamental Cancer Research— M.D. Anderson Hospital and Tumor Institute. Williams & Wilkins, Baltimore.
6. Brown, J. M., and Berry, R. J. (1969): Effects of x-irradiation on the cell population kinetics in a model tumour and normal tissue model. *Br. J. Radiol.*, 42:372-377.
7. Burnet, F. M. (ed.) (1970): *Immunological Surveillance*. Pergamon Press, New York.
8. Burns, E. R., and Scheving, L. E. (1975): Circadian influence on the waveform of the frequency of labeled mitoses in mouse corneal epithelium. *Cell Tissue Kinet.*, 8:61-66.
9. Burns, E. R., Scheving, L. E., Pauly, J. E., and Tsai, T. H. (1976): Effect of altered lighting regimens, time-limited feeding, and presence of Ehrlich ascites carcinoma on the circadian rhythm in DNA synthesis of mouse spleen. *Cancer Res.*, 36:1538-1544.
10. Byram, J. E., Sher, A., DiPietro, J., and Von Lichtenberg, F. (1979): Potentiation of schistosome granuloma formation by Lentinan, a T-cell adjuvant. *Am. J. Pathol.*, 94:201-222.
10a. Charyulu, K., Halberg, F., Reeker, E., Haus, E., and Buchwald, H. (1974): Autorhythmometry in relation to radiotherapy: Case report as tentative feasibility check. In: *Chronobiology*, pp. 265-272, Proc. Int. Soc. for the Study of Biological Rhythms, Little Rock, Ark. L. E. Scheving, F. Halberg and J. E. Pauly, eds. Georg Thieme Publishers, Stuttgart; Igaku Shoin, Ltd., Tokyo.
11. Chaudhry, A. P., and Halberg, F. (1960): Rhythms in blood eosinophils and mitoses of hamster pinna and pouch; phase alterations by carcinogen. *J. Dent. Res.*, 39:704.
12. Cheng, H., and Leblond, C.P. (1974): Origin, differentiation and renewal of the four main epithelial cell types in the mouse small intestine; V. Unitarian theory of the origin of the four epithelial cell types. *Am. J. Anat.*, 141:537.
13. Chiba, Y., Cutkomp, L. K., and Halberg, F. (1973): Circaseptan (7-day) oviposition rhythm and growth of spring tail, *Folsomia candida* (*Collembola: Isotomidae*). *Int. J. Cycle Res.*, 4:59-66.
14. Chiba, Y., Chiba, K., Halberg, F., and Cutkomp, L. K. (1977): Longitudinal evaluation of circadian rhythm characteristics and their circaseptan modulation in an apparently healthy couple, in *Chronobiology in Allergy and Immunology*, pp. 17-35, edited by J. McGovern, A. Reinberg

and M. Smolensky. Charles C Thomas, Springfield, Ill.
14a. Chihara, G., Carandente, F., and Halberg, F. (1979): Chronoimmunology and temporal effects of Lentinan upon LOU rat immunocytoma growth. *Proc. AACR/ASCO20*:111 (abstr. 449).
15. Chihara, G., Hamuro, J., Maeda, Y. Y., Arai, Y., and Fukuoka, F. (1970): Fractionation and purification of the polysaccharides with marked antitumor activity, especially Lentinan from *Lentinus edodes* (Berk.) Sing. (an edible mushroom). *Cancer Res.*, 30:2776-2781.
16. Cornelius, E. A., Yunis, E. J., and Martinez, C. (1969): Cyclic phenomena in the graft vs. host reaction. *Proc. Soc. Exp. Biol. Med.*, 131:680-684.
17. Deka, A. C. (1975): Application of chronobiology to radiotherapy of tumours of the oral cavity. M.D. Thesis, Post-Graduate Institute of Medical Education and Research, Chandigarh, India.
18. Dennert, D. W., and Tucker, D. (1973): Antitumor polysaccharide lentinan; a T-cell adjuvant. *J.N.C.I.*, 51:1727-1729.
19. DeVecchi, A., Halberg, F., Sothern, R. B., Cantaluppi, A., and Ponticelli, C. (1978): Circaseptan rhythmic aspects of rejection in treated patients with kidney transplant. *Proc. Intl. Symp. Clin. Chronopharmacol., Chronotherapeutics and Chronopharmacy*, Tallahassee, Florida, February 9-12, in press.
20. Dionigi, R., Zonta, A., Albertario, F., Galeazzi, R., and Bellinzona, G. (1973): Cyclic variations in the response of lymphocytes to phytohemagglutinin in healthy individuals. *Transplantation*, 16:550-557.
21. Dresser, D. W., and Phillips, J. M. (1974): The orientation of the adjuvant activities of *Salmonella typhosa* lipopolysaccharides and lentinan. *Immunology*, 27:895-902.
22. Edmunds, L. N. (1964): Replication of DNA and cell division in synchronously dividing cultures of *Euglena gracilis*. *Science*, 145:266-268.
23. Edmunds, L. N. (1977): Clocked cell cycle clocks; I. Cell cycle clocks, cell division cycles and circadian rhythms. II. Implications towards chronopharmacology and aging, in *Proc. Conf. Biological Rhythms and Aging*, St. Petersburg Beach, Florida. *Waking and Sleeping*, 1:227-252.
24. Ellison, R. R., Holland, J. F., Weil, M., Jacquillat, C., Boiron, M., Bernard, J., Sawitsky, A., Rosner, F., Gossof, B., Silver, R. T., Karanas, A., Cutter, J., Gpurr, C. L., Hayes, D. M., Blom, J., Leone, L. A., Haurani, R., Kyle, R., Hutchinson, J. L., Forcier, R. J., and Moon, J. H. (1968): Arabinosyl cytosine—a useful agent in the treatment of acute leukemia in adults. *Blood*, 32:507-523.
25. Fernandes, G., Halberg, F., Yunis, E., and Good, R. A. (1976): Circadian rhythmic plaque-forming cell response of spleens from mice immunized with SRBC. *J. Immunol.*, 117:962-966.
26. Fernandes, G., Halberg, F., Halberg, E., Miranda, M., and Good, R. A. (1978): Circadian rhythm in natural cell-mediated cytotoxicity against RLl lymphoma cells measured with ^{31}Cr releasing assay. *Proc. Intl. Symp. Clin. Chronopharmacol., Chronotherapeutics and Chronopharmacy*, Tallahassee, Florida, February 9-12, pp. 41-42.
27. Frei, J., and Ritchie, A. C. (1964): Diurnal variations in the susceptibility of mouse epidermis to carcinogen and its relationship to DNA synthesis. *J.N.C.I.*, 31:1213-1220.
28. Garcia-Sainz, M., Halberg, F., and Moore, V. (1968): Periodicidad en la respuesta biologica a la radiacion bio-ensayo en roedores. *Rev. Mex. Radiol.*, 22:131-146.
29. Gasser, R. F., Scheving, L. E., and Pauly, J. E. (1972): Circadian rhythms in the mitotic index of the basal epithelium and in the uptake rate of ^{3}H-thymidine by the tongue of the rat. *J. Cell. Physiol.*, 80:437-441.
30. Gatti, R. A., Robinson, W. A., Deinard, A. S., Nesbit, M., McCullough, J. S., Ballow, M., and Good, R. A. (1973): Cyclic leukocytosis in chronic myelogenous leukemia; new perspectives on pathogenesis and therapy. *Blood*, 41:771-782.
31. Gautherie, M., and Gros, C. (1977): Circadian rhythm alteration of skin temperature in breast cancer. *Chronobiologia*, 4:1-17.
32. Goldin, A., Venditti, J. M., and Mantel, N. (1974): Combination chemotherapy; basic considerations, in *Antineoplastic and Immunosuppressive Agents*, Part I, pp. 411-448, edited by A. C. Sartorelli and D. G. Johns. Springer Verlag, New York.
33. Good, R. A., Sothern, R. B., Stoney, P. J., Simpson, H., Halberg, E., and Halberg, F. (1977): Circadian state dependence of adriamycin-induced tumor regression and recurrence rates in immunocytoma-bearing LOU rats. *Chronobiologia*, 4:174.
34. Grossman, Z., Asofsky, R., DeLisi, C. (1980): The dynamics of antibody secreting cell production: Regulation of growth and oscillations in the response to T independent antigens (in press).
35. Grube, D. D., Auerbach, H., and Brues, A. M. (1970): Diurnal variations in the labeling index of mouse epidermis. *Cell Tissue Kinet.*, 3:363-373.
36. Guiguet, M., Klein, B., and Valleron, A. J. (1978): Diurnal Variation and the analysis of percent labelled mitoses curves, in *Biomathematics and Cell Kinetics*, pp. 191-220, edited by A. J. Valleron and P. D. M. Macdonald. Elsevier/North-Holland Biomedical Press, Amsterdam.
37. Halberg, E., Halberg, F., Haus, E., Cornélissen, G., Wallach, L. A., Smolensky, M., Garcia-Sainz, M., Halberg, H. W., and Shons, A. R. (1978): Towards a chronopsy; Part I. Chronobiologic case report and thermopsy complementing the biopsy. *Chronobiologia*, 5:241-250.
38. Halberg, E., Halberg, F., Cornélissen, G., Simpson, H. W., and Taggett-

Anderson, M. A. (1979): Towards a chronopsy; Part II. A thermopsy revealing asymmetrical circadian variation in surface temperature of human female breasts and literature review. *Chronobiologia*, 6:231–257.

39. Halberg, F. (1953): Some physiological and clinical aspects of 24-hour periodicity. *J. Lancet*, 73:20–32.

40. Halberg, F. (1959): Physiologic 24-hour periodicity: general and procedural considerations with reference to the adrenal cycle. *Z. Vitamin-Hormon- Fermentforsch.*, 10:225–296.

41. Halberg, F. (1960): Temporal coordination of physiologic function. *Cold Spring Harbor Symp. Quant. Biol.*, 25:289–310.

42. Halberg, F. (1962): Physiologic 24-hour rhythms; a determinant of response to environmental agents, in *Man's Dependence on the Earthly Atmosphere*, pp. 48–98, edited by K. E. Schaefer. Macmillan, New York.

43. Halberg, F. (1964): Organisms as circadian systems; temporal analysis of their physiologic and pathologic responses, including injury and death, in *Walter Reed Army Institute of Research Symposium, Medical Aspects of Stress in the Military Climate*, pp. 1–36.

44. Halberg, F. (1976): From aniatrotoxicosis and aniatrosepsis toward chronotherapy. Introductory remarks to the 1974 Capri Symposium on timing and toxicity: the necessity for relating treatment to bodily rhythms. *Tempus non solum dosis venenum facit.* In: *Chronobiological Aspects of Endocrinology*, pp. 1–34, edited by J. Aschoff, F. Ceresa and F. Halberg. F. K. Schattauer Verlag, Stuttgart.

45. Halberg, F., Ratte, J., Kühl, J. F. W., Najarian, J., Popovich, V., Shiotsuka, R., Chiba, Y., Cutkomp, L., and Haus, E. (1974): Rythmes circaseptidiens—environ 7 jours—synchronisés ou non avec la semaine sociale. *C. R. Acad. Sci. (Paris)*, 278:2675–2678.

46. Halberg, F., Bittner, J., and Cole, H. (1978): Endocrine implants and breast cancer in the mouse. *Physiologist*, 1:31–32.

47. Halberg, F., and Barnum, C. P. (1961): Continuous light or darkness and circadian periodic metabolism in C and D₈ mice. *Am. J. Physiol.*, 201: 227–230.

48. Halberg, F., Halberg, E., Barnum, C. P., and Bittner, J. J. (1959): Physiologic 24-hour periodicity in human beings and mice, the lighting regimen and daily routine, in *Photoperiodism and Related Phenomena in Plants and Animals*, pp. 808–878, edited by R. B. Withrow. Publ. No. 55. American Association for the Advancement of Science, Washington, D.C.

49. Halberg, F., Engeli, M., Hamburger, C., and Hillman, D. (1965): Spectral resolution of low-frequency, small-amplitude rhythms in excreted 17-ketosteroid; probable androgen-induced circaseptan desynchronization. *Acta Endocr. (Copenh.)*, 50 (Suppl. 103):5–54.

50. Halberg, F., Johnson, E. A., Nelson, W., Runge, W., and Sothern, R. (1972): Autorhythmometry procedures for physiologic self-measurements and their analysis. *Physiol. Teacher*, 1:1–11.

51. Halberg, F., Carandente, F., Cornélissen, G., and Katinas, G. S. (1977): Glossary of chronobiology. *Chronobiologia*, 4 (Suppl. 1):1–189.

52. Halberg, F., Nelson, W., Levi, F., Culley, D., Bogden, A., Taylor, D. J. (1979): Chronotherapy of 13762 mammary tumor in rats. *Int. J. Chronobiology*, in press

53. Halberg, F., Nelson, W., Cornélissen, G., Haus, E., Scheving, L. E., Good, R. A. (1979): On methods for testing and achieving cancer chronotherapy. *Cancer Treatment Reports.* 63:1428–1430

54. Halberg, F., Gupta, B. D., Haus, E., Halberg, E., Deka, A. C., Nelson, W., Sothern, R. B., Cornélissen, G., Lee, J. K., Lakatua, D. J., Scheving, L. E., Burns, E. R. (1977): Steps toward a cancer chronopolytherapy. In: Proc. XIVth International Congress of Therapeutics, Montpellier, France, L'Expansion Scientifique Francaise, Paris, pp. 151–196.

55. Halberg, F., Haus, E., Cardoso, S. S., Scheving, L. E., Kühl, J. F. W., Shiotsuka, R., Rosene, G., Pauly, J. E., Runge, W., Spalding, J. F., Lee, J. K., and Good, R. A. (1973): Toward a chronotherapy of neoplasia: tolerance of treatment depends upon host rhythms. *Experientia*, 29: 909–934.

56. Halberg, J., Halberg, E., Runge, W., Wicks, J., Cadotte, L., Yunis, E. J., Katinas, G., Stutman, O., and Halberg, F. (1974): Transplant chronobiology, in *Chronobiology*, pp. 320–328, edited by L. E. Scheving, F. Halberg, and J. E. Pauly. Igaku Shoin Ltd., Tokyo.

57. Hamuro, J., Röllinghoff, M., and Wagner, H. (1978): β(1→3)-Glucan mediated augmentation of alloreactive murine cytotoxic T lymphocytes *in vivo. Cancer Res.*, 38:3080–3085.

58. Hamuro, J., Wagner, H., and Röllinghoff, M. (1978): β(1→3)-Glucans as a probe for T-cell specific immune adjuvants; II. Enhanced *in vitro* generation of cytotoxic T lymphocytes. *Cell. Immunol.*, 38:328–335.

59. Haus, E., and Halberg, F. (1970): Circannual rhythm in level and timing of serum corticosterone in standardized inbred mature C mice. *Environ. Res.*, 3:81–106.

60. Haus, E., Halberg, F., Loken, M. K., and Kim, U. S. (1973): Circadian rhythmometry of mammalian radiosensitivity, in *Space Radiation Biology*, pp. 435–474, edited by A. Tobias and P. Todd. Academic Press, New York.

61. Haus, E., Halberg, F., Scheving, L. E., Cardoso, S. S., Kühl, J. F. W., Sothern, R., Shiotsuka, R. N., Hwang, D. S., and Pauly, J. E. (1972): Increased tolerance of leukemic mice to arabinosyl cytosine given on schedule adjusted to circadian system. *Science*, 177:80–82.

61a. Haus, E., Fernandes, G., Kühl, J. F. W., Yunis, E. J., Lee, J.-K., and Halberg, F. (1974): Murine circadian susceptibility rhythm to cyclo-

phosphamide. *Chronobiologia*, 1:270–280.

62. Hegazy, M. A. H., and Fowler, J. F. (1973): Cell population kinetics of plucked and unplucked mouse skin. *Cell Tissue Kinet.*, 6:17–33.

63. Ho, D. H. W. (1973): Distribution of kinase and deaminase of 1-β-D-arabinofuranosylcytosine in tissues of man and mouse. *Cancer Res.*, 33:2816–2820.

64. Hrushesky, W. J., Sothern, R. B., Halberg, F., Haus, E., and Kennedy, B. J. (1978): Towards an experimental circadian chronotherapy with *cis*-diamminedichloroplatinum (Pl) and adriamycin (Ad) gauged by survival prolongation in immunocytoma-bearing rats. *Clin. Res.*, 26:710A.

65. Hrushesky, W., Teslow, T., Halberg, F., Kiang, D., and Kennedy, B. J. (1979): Temporal components of predictable variability along the 1-year scale in estrogen receptor concentration of primary human breast cancer. *Proc. Am. Soc. Clin. Oncol.*, 20:C165.

66. Hrushesky, W. J., Pleasants, M., Levi, F., Halberg, F., Borch, R. F., Theologides, A., and Kennedy, B. J. (1980): Toward clinical chronotherapy: circadian chronopharmakinetics of cisdiamminedichloroplatinum in five patients with widely metastatic cancer. *Chronobiologia*, 6:113, 1979.

67. Hubner, K. (1967): Kompensatorische Hypertrophie, Wachstum und Regeneration der Rattenniere. *Ergeb. Allg. Pathol. Anat.*, 100:1–80.

68. Hughes, A., Jacobson, H. I., Wagner, R. K., and Jungblut, P. W. (1976): Ovarian-independent fluctuations of estradiol receptor levels in mammalian tissues. *Mol. Cell. Endocrinol.*, 5:379–388.

69. Hume, W. J., and Potten, C. S. (1976): The ordered columnar structure of mouse filiform papillae. *J. Cell Sci.*, 22:149–160.

70. Iversen, U. (1970): Diurnal variations in susceptibility of mouse skin to the tumorigenic action of methylcholanthrene. *J.N.C.I.*, 45:269–276.

71. Izquierdo, J. N. (1977): Increased cell proliferation with persistence of circadian rhythms in hamster cheek pouch neoplasms. *Cell Tissue Kinet.*, 10:313–322.

72. Izquierdo, J. N., and Gibbs, J. S. (1972): Circadian rhythms of DNA synthesis and mitotic activity in hamster cheek pouch epithelium. *Exp. Cell Res.*, 71:402–408.

73. Izquierdo, J. N., Gibbs, J. S. (1974): Turnover of cell-renewing populations undergoing circadian rhythms in cell proliferation. *Cell Tissue Kinet.*, 7:99–111.

74. Jehn, V., and Tannenberg, W. (1970): Characterization of 2 different types of direct plaque-forming cells. *Clin. Exp. Immunol.*, 6:913–918.

75. Kanabrocki, E. L., Scheving, L. E., Halberg, F., Brewer, R. L., and Bird, T. J. (1975): Circadian variation in presumably healthy young soldiers. Department of the Army, Document PB228437, Natl. Technical Information Service, U.S. Department of Commerce, P.O. Box 1553, Springfield, Virginia.

76. Kennedy, B. J. (1970): Cyclic leucocyte oscillations in chronic myelogenous leukemia during hydroxyurea therapy. *Blood*, 35:4751–4760.

77. Kline, I., Venditti, J. M., Tyrer, D. D., and Goldin, A. (1966): Chemotherapy of leukemia L1210 in mice with 1-β-D-arabinofuranosylcytosine hydrochloride. Influence of treatment schedules. *Cancer Res.*, 26:853–859.

78. Kuzel, M., Zinneman, H., Nelson, W., Halberg, F., Rosen, G., Scheving, L. E., and Haus, E. (1978): Competing circadian effects of methylprednisolone and rat weight, light chains, immunocytoma size and survival. *Chronobiologia*, 5:295–311.

79. Labrosse, K., Haus, E., Lakatua, D. J., and Halberg, F. (1978): Circadian rhythm in mammary cytoplasmic estrogen receptor content in mice with and without pituitary isografts and demonstrated differences in breast cancer risk. Proceedings of the Endocrinology Society 60th Annual Meeting, Abstract 661.

80. Lajtha, L. G., Oliver, R., and Ellis, F. (1954): Incorporation of ³²P and adenine ¹⁴C into DNA by human bone marrow cells *in vitro. Br. J. Cancer*, 8:367–379.

81. Lappenbusch, W. L. (1972): Effect of circadian rhythm on the radiation response of the Chinese hamster (*Cricetulus griseus*). *Radiat. Res.*, 50: 600–610.

82. Leblond, C. P., and Cheng, H. (1976): Identification of stem cells in the small intestine of the mouse, in *Stem Cells of Renewing Cell Population*, pp. 7–31, edited by A. B. Cairnie, P. K. Lala, and D. G. Osmond. Academic Press, London.

83. Levi, F., Ernsberger, P., Cornélissen, G., and Taddeini, L. (1979): Potential marker rhythms of cisplatine (cisP) chronotoxicity; urine volume and core temperature. *Proc. Am. Soc. Clin. Oncol.*, 20:C519.

84. Levi. F., Pleasants, M., Hrushesky, W., Borch, R. F., and Halberg, F. (1979): Rat urinary chronopharmacokinetics of the anti-tumor drug cisplatine (CP). *Chronobiologia*, 6:127.

85. Litman, T., Halberg, F., Ellis, S., and Bittner, J. J. (1958): Pituitary growth hormone and mitoses in immature mouse liver. *Endocrinology*, 62:361–364.

86. Maeda, Y. Y., Chihara, G. (1971): Lentinan, a new immuno-accelerator of cell-mediated responses. *Nature*, 229:634.

87. Maeda, Y. Y., Hamuro, J., Yamada, Y. O., Ishimura, K., and Chihara, G. (1973): The nature of immunopotentiation by the polysaccharide lentinan and the significance of biogenic amines in its action, in *Immunopotentiation*, pp. 259–341 (Ciba Found. Symp.), Vol. 18, edited by G. E. W. Wolstenholme and J. Knight. Elsevier/Excerpta Medica/North Holland, Amsterdam.

88. Mansfield, C. M. (1968): Use of heat-sensing device in cancer therapy. *Radiology*, 91:673–678.

89. Many, A., and Schwartz, R. S. (1971): Periodicity during recovery of immune response after cyclophosphamide treatment. *Blood*, 37:692–695.

90. Mastrangelo, R. (1976): A specific spontaneous leucocyte cycle in chronic myelogenous leukemia. *Tumori*, 62:197–204.

91. Mathe, G. (1972): La meilleure chimiothérapie du monde ne peut que ce qu' elle peut. *Nouv. Presse Med.*, 1:1753–1756.

92. Mauer, A. M. (1965): Diurnal variation of proliferative activity in the human bone marrow. *Blood*, 26:1–7.

93. McGovern, J. P., Smolensky, M. H., and Reinberg, A. (1977): Circadian and circannual rhythmicity in cutaneous reactivity to histamine and allergenic extracts, in *Chronobiology in Allergy and Immunology*, pp. 79–116, edited by J. P. McGovern, M. Smolensky, and A. Reinberg. Charles C Thomas, Springfield, Ill.

94. Menaker, M. (1964): X-rays: Are there cyclic variations in radiosensitivity? *Science*, 143:597.

95. Messier, B., and Leblond, C. P. (1960): Cell proliferation and migration as revealed by radioautography after injection of ^{3}H-thymidine into male rats and mice. *Am. J. Anat.*, 106:247–285.

96. Moller, U., Larsen, J. K., and Faber, M. (1974): The influence of injected tritiated thymidine on the mitotic circadian rhythm in the epithelium of the hamster cheek pouch. *Cell Tissue Kinet.*, 7:231–239.

97. Morley, A., and Stohlman, F., Jr. (1969): Periodicity during recovery of erythropoiesis following irradiation. *Blood*, 34:96–99.

98. Morley, A., and Stohlman, F., Jr. (1970): Cyclophosphamide-induced cyclical neutropenia. *N. Engl. J. Med.*, 282:643–646.

99. Morley, A. A., Baikie, A. G., and Galton, D. A. (1967): Cyclic leucocytosis as evidence for control in chronic granulocytic leukemia. *Lancet*, 2:1320–1323.

100. Mottram, J. C. (1965): A diurnal variation in the production of tumors. *J. Pathol. Bacteriol.*, 57:265–267.

101. Nelson, W., Halberg, F., and Scheving, L. (1974): Meal timing as an adjuvant of experimental chronotherapy; circadian rhythm in tolerance of adriamycin by mice on a 24-hour cyclic lighting regimen—the usually dominant synchronizer routine—is shifted by restricting feeding to early light span. *Chronobiologia*, 1:315–316.

102. Pilgrim, C., Erb, W., and Maurer, W. (1963): Diurnal fluctuations in the numbers of DNA synthetizing nuclei in various mouse tissues. *Nature*, 199:863.

103. Pizzarello, D. J., Witcofski, R. L., and Lyons, E. A. (1963): Variations in survival time after whole-body radiation at two times of day. *Science*, 139:349.

104. Pizzarello, D. J., Isaak, D., Chua, K. E., and Rhyne, A. L. (1964): Circadian rhythmicity in the sensitivity of two strains of mice to whole-body radiation. *Science*, 145:286–291.

105. Pizzarello, D. J., and Witcofski, R. L. (1970): A possible link between diurnal variations in radiation sensitivity and cell division in bone marrow of male mice. *Radiology*, 97:165–167.

106. Popper, H. (1938): Die physiologischen Schwankungen der Nierenarbeit. *Klin. Med. (Vienna)*, 134:196.

107. Potten, C. S. (1974): The epidermal proliferative unit: the possible role of the central basal cell. *Cell Tissue Kinet.*, 7:77–88.

108. Potten, C. S. (1975): Kinetics and possible regulation of crypt cell populations under normal and stress conditions. *Bull. Cancer*, 62:419–430.

109. Potten, C. S. (1976): Small intestine crypt stem cells, in *Stem Cells of Renewing Cell Populations*, pp. 79–84, edited by A. B. Cairnie, P. K. Lala, and D. G. Osmond. Academic Press, London.

110. Potten, C. S., and Hendry, J. H. (1975): Differential regeneration of intestinal proliferative cells and cryptogenic cells after irradiation. *Int. J. Radiat. Biol.*, 27:413–424.

111. Potten, C. S., Jessup, B. A., and Croxson, M. B. (1971): Incorporation of tritiated thymidine into the skin and hair follicles; II. Daily fluctuations in ^{3}H-TdR and ^{3}H-UR levels. *Cell Tissue Kinet.*, 4:413–421.

112. Quastler, H., and Sherman, F. G. (1959): Cell population kinetics in the intestinal epithelium of the mouse. *Exp. Cell Res.*, 14:420–438.

113. Raine, C. S., Traugott, V., and Stone, S. H. (1978): Suppression of chronic allergic encephalomyelitis: relevance to multiple sclerosis. *Science*, 201:445–448.

114. Ratte, J., Halberg, F., Kuhl, J. F. W., and Najarian, J. S. (1977): Circadian and circaseptan variations in rat kidney allograft rejection, in *Chronobiology in Allergy and Immunology*, pp. 250–257, edited by J. McGovern, A. Reinberg, and M. Smolensky. Charles C Thomas, Springfield, Ill.

115. Razek, A., Vretti, T., and Valeriote, F. (1974): Optimum time sequence for the administration of vincristine and cyclophosphamide *in vivo*. *Cancer Res.*, 34:1857–1861.

116. Reinberg, A., and Halberg, F. (1971): Circadian chronopharmacology. *Ann. Rev. Pharmacol.*, 2:455–492.

117. Reinberg, A., Schuller, E., Delasnerie, N., Clench, J., and Helary, M. (1977): Rythmes circadiens et circannuels des leucocytes, proteines totales, immunoglobuline A, G et M. Etude chez 9 adultes jeunes et sains. *Nouv. Presse Med.*, 6:3819–3823.

118. Reinberg, A., Clench, J., Ghata, J., Halberg, F., Abulker, C., Dupont, J., and Zagulla-Mally, Z. (1975): Rythmes circadiens des paramètres de l'excretion urinaire du salicylate (chronopharmacocinetique) chez l'homme adulte sain. *C. R. Acad. Sci. (Paris)*, 280:1697–1699.

119. Romball, C. G., and Weigle, W. O. (1973): Cyclical appearance of antibody-producing cells after a single injection of serum protein antigen. *J. Exp. Med.*, 138:1426–1442.

120. Rose, W. C., Trader, M. W., Russer, R., Jr., and Schabel, F. M., Jr. (1978): Chronochemotherapy of L1210 leukemia mice with cytosine arabinoside or cyclophosphamide. *Cancer Treat. Rep.*, 62:1337–1349.

121. Rotenberg, M. (1977): Selective synchrony of cells of differing cycle times. *J. Theor. Biol.*, 66:389–398.

122. Rugh, R., Castro, V., Balter, S., Kennelly, E. V., Marosden, D. S., Warmund, J., and Wollin, M. (1963): X-rays: Are there cyclic variations in radiosensitivity? *Science*, 142:53–56.

123. Savage, I. R., Rao, M. M., and Halberg, F. (1962): Test of peak values in physiopathologic time series. *Exp. Med. Surg.*, 20:309–317.

124. Schabel, F. M., Jr. (1968): *In vivo* leukemic cell kill kinetics and "curability" in experimental organisms, in *The Proliferation and Spread of Neoplastic Cells*, pp. 379–408. Williams & Wilkins, Baltimore.

125. Scherbaum, O., and Zeuthen, E. (1954): Induction of synchronous cell division in mass cultures of *Tetrahymena piriformis*. *Exp. Cell Res.*, 6:211–227.

126. Scheving, L. E., and Chiakulas, J. J. (1965): Periodicity in thymidine-H^3 uptake. *Exp. Cell Res.*, 39:161–169.

127. Scheving, L. E., and Pauly, J. E. (1967): The circadian phase relationship of thymidine ^{3}H uptake, labeled nuclei, grain counts and cell division rate in rat corneal epithelium. *J. Cell. Physiol.*, 32:677–683.

128. Scheving, L. E., Burns, E. R., and Pauly, J. E. (1977): Coincidence in timing between the synthetic and mitotic stages of the cell cycle in liver parenchymal cells in mice bearing an 8-day Ehrlich ascites tumor (EAT), in *Proceedings of the XII Conference of the International Society of Chronobiology*, pp. 427–432. Publishing House "Il Ponte," Milan.

129. Scheving, L. E., Burns, E. R., Pauly, J. E., Halberg, F., and Haus, E. (1977): Survival and cure of leukemic mice after circadian optimization of treatment with cyclophosphamide and arabinosyl cytosine. *Cancer Res.*, 37:3648–3655.

129a. Scheving, L. E., Burns, E. R., Pauly, J. E., and Halberg, F. (1980): Circadian bioperiodic response of mice bearing advanced L1210 leukemia to combination therapy with Adriamycin and cyclophosphamide. *Cancer Res.*, 40:1511–1515.

130. Scheving, L. E., Haus, E., Kuhl, J. F. W., Pauly, J. E., Halberg, F., and Cardoso, S. S. (1976): Close reproduction by different laboratories of characteristics of circadian rhythm in 1-β-D-arabinofuranosylcytosine tolerance by mice. *Cancer Res.*, 36:1133–1137.

131. Sherman, F. G., Quastler, H., and Wimber, D. R. (1961): Cell population kinetics in the ear epidermis of mice. *Exp. Cell Res.*, 25:114–119.

132. Sigdestad, C. P., Bauman, J., and Lesher, S. W. (1969): Diurnal fluctuations in the number of cells in mitosis and DNA synthesis in the jejunum of the mouse. *Exp. Cell Res.*, 58:159–162.

133. Simpson, G. E. (1926): Diurnal variations in the rate of urine excretion for 3-hour intervals. Some associated factors. *J. Biol. Chem.*, 59:107–122.

134. Simpson, H., Tavadia, H. B., Fleming, K., Hume, P., Halberg, E., and Halberg, F. (1973): A study to evaluate any circadian rhythms in the reactivity of human lymphocytes to mitogens or antigen, in Workshop 2 on Chronobiology and Allergy, Proceedings of the International Conference on Allergy, Tokyo, abstract 314.

135. Skipper, H. E. (1965): The effect of chemotherapy on the kinetics of leukemic cell behavior. *Cancer Res.*, 25:1544–1550.

136. Skipper, H. E., Schabel, F. M., and Wilcox, W. S. (1964): Experimental evaluation of potential anticancer agents; XIII. On the criteria and kinetics associated with "curability" of experimental leukemia. *Cancer Chemother. Rep.*, 35:3–111.

137. Skipper, H. E., Schabel, F. M., Jr., and Wilcox, W. S. (1967): Experimental evaluation of potential anticancer agents; XXI. Scheduling of arabinosylcytosine to take advantage of its S-phase specificity against leukemia cells. *Cancer Chemother. Rep.*, 51:125–165.

138. Sothern, R. B., Halberg, F., Hrushesky, W., and Doe, R. P. (1978): Circadian optimization of cis-diamminedichloroplatinum (Pl) and adriamycin (Ad) combination (PlAd) therapy of an immunocytoma gauged by complete remission or cure. *Clin. Res.*, 26:712A.

139. Sothern, R. B., Leach, C., Nelson, W., Halberg, F., and Rummel, J. A. (1974): Characteristics of urinary circadian rhythms in a young man evaluated on a monthly basis during the course of 21 months. *Chronobiologia*, 1 (Suppl. 1):73–82.

140. Sothern, R. B., Simpson, H. W., Leach, C., Nelson, W. L., and Halberg, F. (1980): Individually assessable human circadian, circaseptan and circannual urinary rhythms (with temporal compacting and editing procedures) (in press).

141. Spelsberg, T. C., Boyd, P., Halberg, F. (1980): Circannual rhythm in chick oviduct progesterone receptor and nuclear acceptor, in *Chronopharmacology*, Proceedings of the 7th International Congress of Pharmacology Satellite Symposium on Chronopharmacology, edited by A. Reinberg, and F. Halberg. Pergamon Press, Oxford (in press).

142. Stimpfling, J. H., and Richardson, A. (1967): Periodic variations of the hemagglutinin response in mice following immunization against sheep red blood cells and allo-antigens. *Transplantation, 5*:1496–1503.

143. Stoll, B. A., and Burch, W. (1968): Surface detection of circadian rhythm in ^{32}P content of cancer of the breast. *Cancer, 21*:193–196.

144. Stoney, P. J., Halberg, F., and Simpson, H. W. (1975): Circadian variation in colony-forming ability of presumably intact murine bone marrow cells. *Chronobiologia, 2*:319–324.

145. Straube R. L. (1963): Examination of diurnal variation in lethally irradiated rats. *Science, 142*:1062.

146. Sturtevant, F. M. (1976): Chronopharmacokinetics of ethanol; I. Review of the literature and theoretical considerations. *Chronobiologia, 3*:237–264.

147. Szabo, I., Kovats, T. G., and Halberg, F. (1978): Circadian rhythm in murine reticuloendothelial function. *Chronobiologia, 5*:137–143.

148. Tannock, I. (1978): Cell kinetics and chemotherapy: a critical review. *Cancer Treat. Rep., 62*:1117–1133.

149. Tarquini, B., Gheri, R., Romano, S., Costa, A., Cagnoni, M., Lee, J. K., and Halberg, F. (1979): Circadian mesor-hyperprolactinemia in fibrocystic mastopathy. *Am. J. Med., 66*:229–237.

150. Tavadia, H., Fleming, K. A., Hume, P., and Simpson, H. W. (1977): Circadian variations in the quantity and quality of lymphocyte traffic in human peripheral venous blood, in *Chronobiology in Allergy and Immunology*, pp. 187–203, edited by J. McGovern, A. Reinberg, and M. H. Smolensky. Charles C Thomas, Springfield, Ill.

151. Tobias, B. S., Parker, L. M., Tattersall, M. H. N., and Frei, E., III (1975): Adriamycin/cyclophosphamide and adriamycin/melphalan in advanced L1210 leukemia. *Br. J. Cancer, 32*:199–207.

152. Tvermyr, E. M. F. (1969): Circadian rhythms in epidermal mitotic activity. Diurnal variations in the mitotic index, mitotic rate and mitotic duration. *Virchows Arch. Cell Pathol., 2*:318–325.

153. Tvermyr, E. M. F. (1972): Circadian rhythms in hairless mouse epidermal DNA-synthesis as measured by double labelling with H3-thymidine. *Virchows Arch. Cell Pathol., 11*:43–54.

154. Ueno, Y. (1968): Diurnal rhythmicity in the sensitivity of haematopoietic cells to whole-body irradiation of mice. *Int. J. Radiat. Biol., 14*:307–312.

155. Vacek, A., Davidova, E., Druzhinin, Y., Hosek, B., and Chlumecky, J. (1967): Circadian rhythmicity in the effect of irradiation on the endogenous colony formation in the spleen of irradiated mice. *Int. J. Radiat. Biol., 13*:539–547.

156. Vacek, A., Rotkovska, D. (1970): Circadian variations in the effect of x-irradiation on the hematopoietic stern cells of mice. *Strahlentherapie, 140*:302–306.

157. Vadlamudi, S., Subba Reddy, W., and Goldin, A. (1972): Schedule-dependent therapeutic synergism for L-asparaginase and methotrexate in leukemic mice. *Proc. Am. Assoc. Cancer Res., 13*:31.

158. Venditti, J. M., Kline, I., Tyrer, D. D., and Goldin, A. (1965): 1,3-bis(2-Chloroethyl)-1-nitrosurea (NSC 409962) and methotrexate (NSC 740) as combination therapy for advanced mouse leukemia L1210. *Cancer Chemother. Rep., 48*:35–39.

159. Vollrath, L., Kantazjian, A., and Howe, C. (1975): Mammalian pineal gland; 7 rhythmic activity. *Experientia, 31*:458–460.

160. Weigle, W. O. (1975): Cyclical production of antibody as a regulatory mechanism in the immune response. *Adv. Immunol., 21*:87–111.

161. Zakany, J., Chihara, G., and Fachet, J. (1980): Effect of lentinan on tumor growth in murine allogenic and syngeneic hosts. *Int. J. Cancer, 25*:371–376.

162. Zinneman, H. H., Halberg, F., Haus, E., and Kaplan, N. (1974): Circadian rhythms in urinary light chains, serum iron and other variables of multiple myeloma patients. *Int. J. Chronobiol., 2*:3–16.

163. Zubrod, C. G. (1978): Selective toxicity of anticancer drugs; presidential address. *Cancer Res., 38*:4377–4384.

15

Chronobiological Aspects of Comparative Experimental Chemotherapy of Neoplasms

L. E. Scheving

INTRODUCTION

Chronobiology is the branch of science that explores mechanisms of biological time structure including the important rhythmic manifestations of life (16). Although it is a comparatively young science, the writers of ancient times, including the poets, were fascinated with rhythmic events, particularly as they pertained to leaf and petal movements. Many of the important early scientific investigations into rhythmic behavior were performed on plants; and in 1958 E. Bünning (5) summarized work done up to that time, including his own important contributions. Since then a number of review papers relative to plants have appeared (8).

The past three decades have been a period of rapid proliferation of data on rhythms in plants and animals, and it is the mammalian forms that will be considered primarily in this chapter. Rhythms of many frequencies and at all levels of animal life, as well as from all levels of biological organization, have been demonstrated. Oscillation has been firmly established as a fundamental property of all life. Because of the regularity of these rhythms, some refer to them as biological or physiological clocks. The range of frequencies that has been found in the living systems extends from cycles of less than a second to cycles of a year or more. It is noteworthy that many, but not all, clearly correspond to physical, environmental frequencies, such as the natural light-dark cycle. There is strong evidence that many rhythms are adaptive and serve to adjust the organism to periodic changes in its environment. This chapter will concentrate on the frequency corresponding to the 24-hr rotation of the earth. This Halberg (12) called "circadian" (*circa*, about; *dies*, day). The adjective "diurnal" is sometimes used synonymously with circadian, but diurnal is better used to describe animals active by day as opposed to "nocturnal" animals which are active by night.

Circadian rhythms are ubiquitous in eukaryotic unicellular and multicellular organisms. Recent data on the growth rates of bacteria suggest that circadian rhythms as well as those of higher frequencies (ultradian) also characterize the prokaryotic cell (15, 47).

AN EXAMPLE OF A CIRCADIAN RHYTHM

One of the earliest documented and most extensively studied hormonal rhythms in mammals is the serum steroid rhythm (34). This rhythm, illustrated for both rat and man in Figure 15.1, will be used to demonstrate some of the basic properties of rhythms and the special terminology used to describe their behavior. In diurnally active man, serum steroids begin to be secreted from the adrenal gland prior to awakening and reach their peak levels in the blood shortly after he arises. In the nocturnally active rat, the peak occurs shortly before his active period begins. The 4-fold or greater variation (amplitude) seen along the 24-hr time scale clearly shows that such variation is not a minor fluctuation around a 24-hr mean that could be ignored in experimental design (33). It also should be noted that rhythms with frequencies higher than circadian (ultradian) (49) and lower than circadian (infradian or circannual) (22) also characterize serum steroids as well as other variables.

SYNCHRONIZATION

An understanding of the important concept of synchronization is essential to appreciating the complexity of the circadian system (2, 13, 30). Many animals in nature are synchronized to the natural light-dark cycle, while those in the laboratory were usually synchronized to an artificial light-dark cycle. The serum steroid rhythm of the rodent illustrated in Figure 15.1 is such a synchronized rhythm. The synchronizing force is also called the *zeitgeber* (time-giver), entraining agent, clue, or cue. The best evidence that light is the dominant synchronizer of the rodent comes from inversion studies. If one shifts the light-dark cycle 180°, the circadian rhythm will eventually invert, but not immediately (42). Such is strong evidence for the influence of the light-dark cycle on animals. Man, on the other hand, seems to be less dependent on the environmental light-dark cycle; his circadian system is more strongly synchronized to his social cycle (50).

For organisms (plant or animal) in the synchronized state, rhythmic variables normally have a fixed time relationship. For example, one expects to find for both man and the rodent that body temperature is highest during the organism's active stage. Thus the temperature and activity rhythms are internally synchronized, their timing or phasing being nearly the same. For other variables in the normal synchronized state, however, the timing could be as much as 180° out of phase. If the usual time relationship among variables is altered, in that rhythms which once exhibited similar frequencies now exhibit altered frequencies with phase differences, the rhythms are described as internally desynchronized. Such internal desynchronization might occur in an organism isolated from the synchronizing force or, transiently, in an organism that is adjusting to a change in the synchronizing cycle. Examples are a laboratory animal adjusting to an inverted light-dark cycle, a man adjusting to a new social cycle required after rapid displacement by "jet" through several time zones, or a shift worker adjusting to a new activity routine.

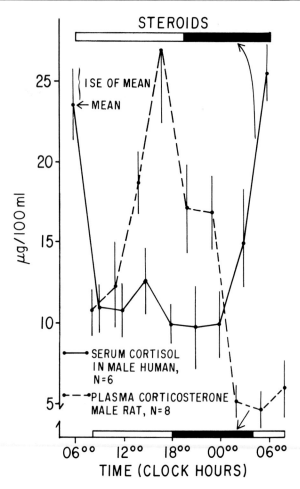

Figure 15.1. Prominent circadian fluctuation of the predominant serum steroids of rat and man. The rats were standardized to a light-dark cycle (14 hr of light alternating with 10 hr of darkness) and fed *ad libitum* for 2 weeks prior to the study. For man, the meal times were 0700, 1245, and 1645 hr; rest or sleep time was 2100–0600. The subjects were awakened, however, for sampling at 2400 and 0300 (34).

FREE-RUNNING RHYTHMS

Scientists once thought that periodic biological behavior was nothing more than a direct response to some periodicity in the physical environment, such as the light-dark cycle, temperature, feeding, etc. De Mairan, the mathematician and astronomer, was fascinated with daily periodic behavior in the movement of leaves. In 1729 (9) he found that the leaves of plants would continue their periodic behavior when kept in a darkened cave, away from sunlight and open air; this suggested that some endogenous factor in the plant was responsible for its behavior.

Interestingly, if we remove the rodent (or other animal) from the effect of the light-dark cycle mediated by their eyes (by blinding), or if we subject the animals to continuous light, the rhythms for steroids as well as for other variables will continue. Under such conditions, however, it is rare that the circadian frequencies of these rhythms will any longer be precisely 24 hr; usually they only approximate 24 hr, and consequently their timing changes predictably each day in relation to clock time. Such rhythms are described as "free-running"; the same phenomenon characterizes both plant and animal life and is strong evidence of the innate and endogenous nature of rhythms as well as for their genetic origin.

It should also be noted that recently a great deal of interest has centered around rhythmic variables that seem to free-run for no apparent reason. Such may play a role in the many well-known diseases which have a periodic component in severity; for example, patients with depression or mania might suffer from abnormalities in the internal phase relationships among different circadian systems. This hypothesis is currently being explored (3).

MECHANISMS OF RHYTHMS

The finding that the length of a free-running may be characteristic for each individual is strong evidence that rhythmicity has a genetic basis. More recent evidence from genetic studies on plants and *Drosophila* (the fruit fly) supports this view. For *Drosophila*, it was found that a

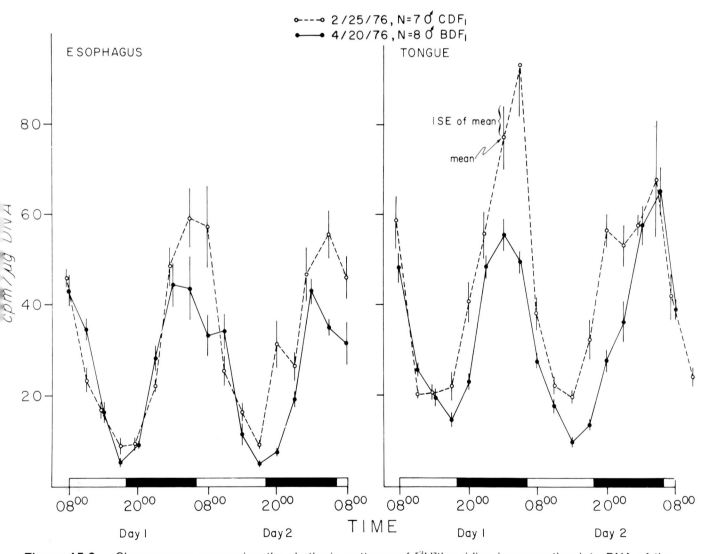

Figure 15.2. Chronograms comparing the rhythmic patterns of [³H]thymidine incorporation into DNA of the esophagus and tongue of two different strains of male mice. Note the high degree of reproducibility in the phasing of the rhythms in these similarly standardized animals (38). The abscissa represents the light-dark cycle under which the mice were standardized: light 0600–1800; dark 1800–0600.

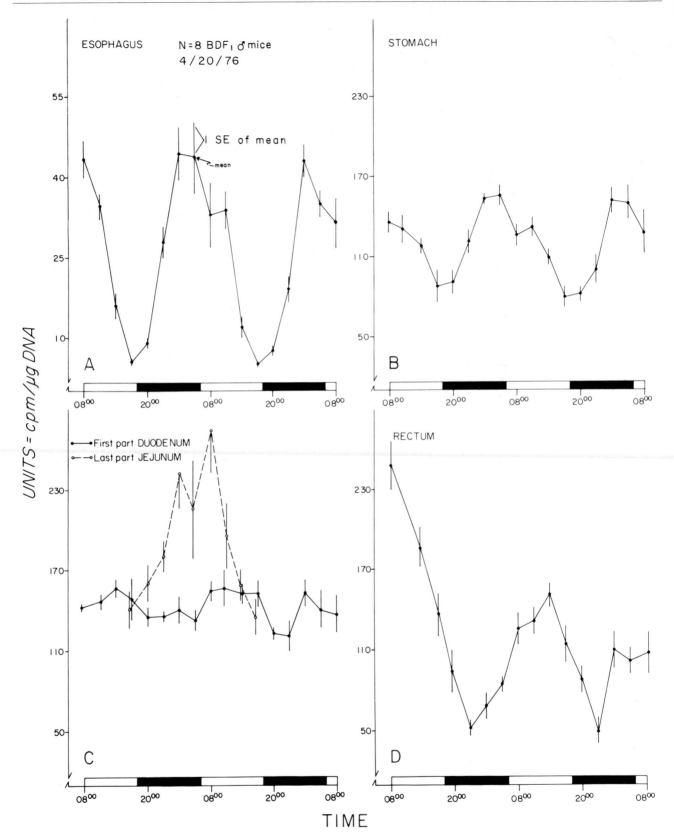

Figure 15.3. Chronograms illustrating the rhythmic patterns of [³H]thymidine incorporation into DNA in five different regions of the alimentary canal of male CD_2F_1 mice (38).

small region on the X-chromosome is responsible for the circadian rhythm in both activity and emergence, and for the length of the natural free-running period (25).

Many attempts have been made through experiments on mammals to elucidate the mechanism of rhythmicity. Among these were studies employing the classical endocrinological approaches of adrenalectomy, hypophysectomy, cerebral ablation, and pinealectomy; and, more recently, a great deal of interest has been given to the possible role of the suprachiasmatic nucleus as a rhythm generator (19, 27, 45). In spite of such studies, I believe no single regulator has been found that will account for the control of all rhythmic variables. Halberg has shown that certain aspects of 24-hr periods are controlled by the adrenal and pituitary glands, and has suggested that the adrenocortical cycle deserves serious consideration as a mechanism, possibly underlying man's adaption to his daily routine (11, 14). Incidentally, the adrenal glands will continue to secrete and respond circadianally for several cycles when grown *in vitro* (1). There also have been numerous attempts to locate the central regulator of circadian phenomenon at the unicellular level; these have been unsuccessful unless a more recent hypothesis should prove true. This hypothesis postulates that circadian oscillation is generated, and synchronization is effected, by temporal variation within membrane properties themselves (29, 48).

In spite of many models and much data, it is still being questioned whether oscillation for a given organism is driven by a master oscillator; or by a population of circadian oscillators; or by a population of noncircadian biochemical oscillators. Even though the majority of chronobiologists accept the endogenous nature of rhythms, one school postulates that circadian rhythms are generated by an interaction of several external forces—such as light, temperature, electromagnetic variation and possibly by yet unknown, subtle geophysical forces—with metabolism (4). Space does not permit discussion of this interesting and important concept.

RHYTHMS IN CELL DIVISION

The following examples are selected because they are primarily relevent to the main theme of this chapter. Figure 15.2 demonstrates the

rhythmic variation in the cell division rate of both the esophagus and tongue of the mouse. It is striking that the rate of DNA synthesis in the esophagus varies as much as 700% over the 24-hr time scale. Under the conditions of this study the lowest levels occurred about the time of transition from light to dark, and the higher levels about the time of transition from dark to light. When the highest and lowest daily means were compared with the 24-hr mean for each day, both were statistically different from the daily 24-hr mean ($P < 0.005$). The rhythmic pattern in DNA synthesis within the tip of the tongue (Fig. 15.2) similar; this is shown for two different strains of mice (38). Figure 15.3 demonstrates that a similar rhythm to that described in Figure 15.1 has been demonstrated in five different regions of the alimentary canal (38). It should be noted that the amplitude of the rhythm in the duodenum is not nearly as high as in other regions. This brings up the point that the cell-division rate in a certain tissue or region of an organ may show a low-amplitude rhythm while other tissues or even different regions of the same organ may show very high-amplitude rhythms. In our experience, the rhythms of DNA synthesis in most tissues of the body tend to be of the high-amplitude type. It should also be noted that the DNA-synthesis rhythms in many, but not all, tissues have a somewhat similar

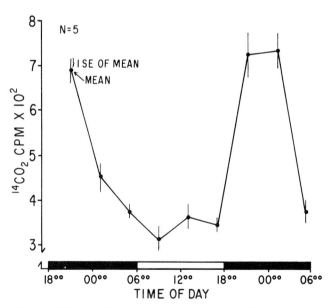

Figure 15.4. Circadian variation in ornithine decarboxylase activity of male rat liver. The activity was determined by the measurement of $^{14}CO_2$ release from L-[^{14}C]ornithine produced by incubation with supranatants (46).

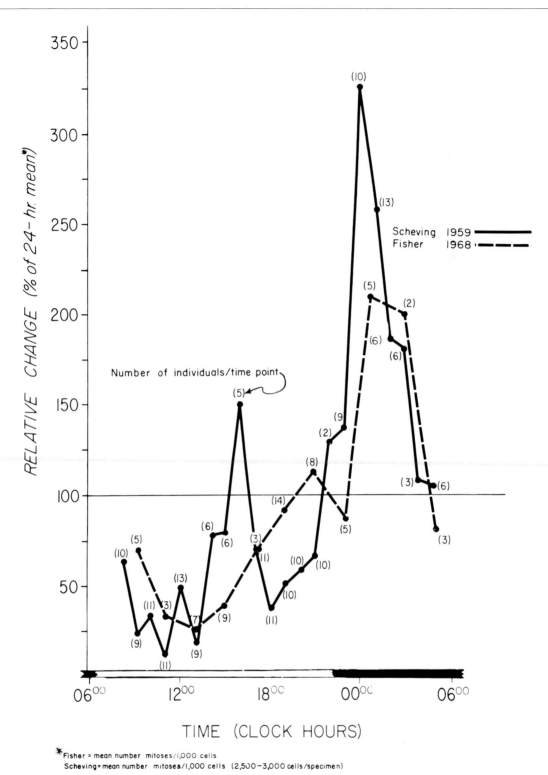

Figure 15.5. The rhythm in the mitotic index in the adult human epidermis. A majority of the cells divide at a predictable phase of the circadian system. Remarkable reproducibility has been demonstrated in studies done many miles (London, Chicago) and many years apart (10,32).

phasing to that described for the esophagus. Because of this it serves no purpose to demonstrate further examples of DNA-synthesis rhythms in other tissues. It should be noted, however, that other variables associated with growth are also rhythmic, such as polyamines (21) and ornithine decarboxylase (46) (Fig. 15.4). Figure 15.5 demonstrates the rhythmic variation

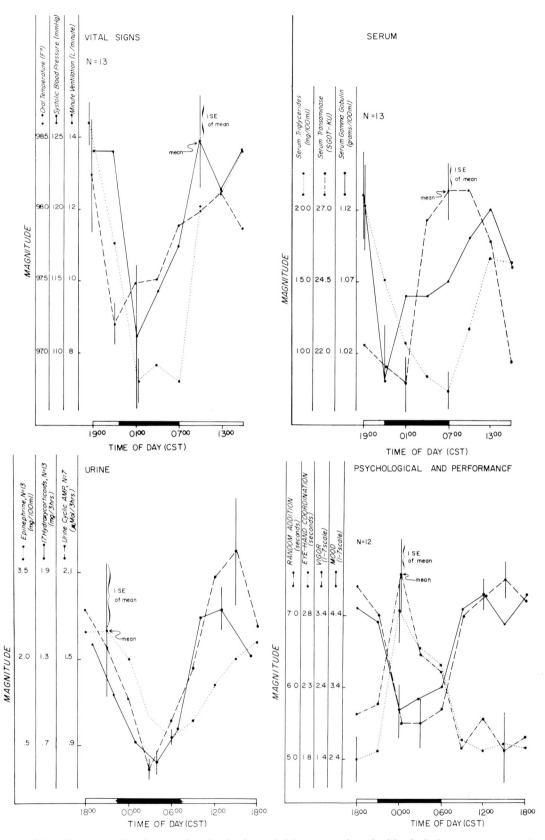

Figure 15.6. Circadian variation in man for rhythmic variables associated with vital signs, components of serum and urine as well as for psychological and performance variables in presumably healthy young men. Meal times: 0830, 1430, and 1630; rest or sleep time: 2245 to 0700 for all but the group subjected to psychological and performance testing who sleep from 2100 to 0600 with meals at 0700, 1245, and 1645. The details of this study have previously been published (24, 40).

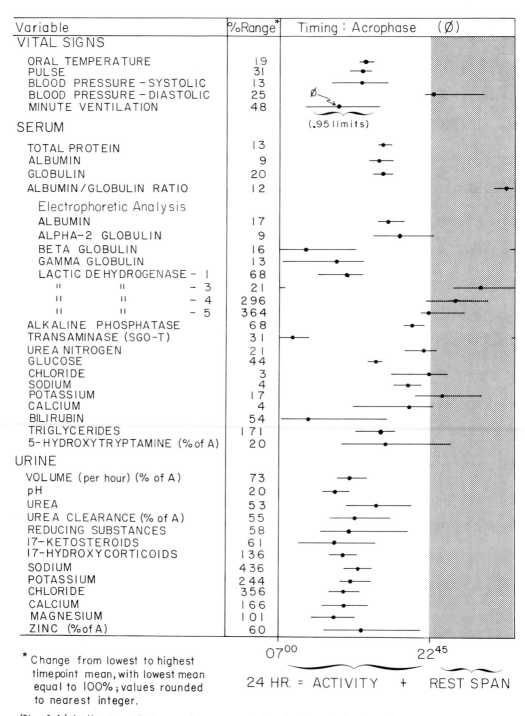

Figure 15.7. Acrophase map showing data obtained from studies on 13 young men. The map illustrates 41 different rhythmic variables in vital signs and in constituents of serum and of urine. Meal times were 0830, 1430, and 1630; rest or sleep time was 2245–0700. The *dot* represents the time when the crest of the rhythm occurs in relation to the rest-activity cycle. The *horizontal bars* represent the confidence interval. The center column gives the average 24-hr range of change for the group, that is, the percent difference between the highest recorded means.

in the cell division rate of human skin; most of the cell division in the skin takes place at night (10, 32).

RHYTHM VARIABLES OF MAN

Irrespective of whether one measures vital signs, components in serum, urine, or even mood, vigor, the ability to estimate time or perform a task, each fluctuates in a predictable manner and still each rhythm is modifiable (Fig. 15.6). The same data as shown in Figure 15.6 as well as additional data were analyzed by an inferential statistical method commonly referred to as the "cosinor" (17, 18). The cosinor technique, frequently used by us, is one of several objective methods by which time-series data can be analyzed. Essentially, the time-series data are fitted to a 24-hr cosine curve by the method of least squares and the rhythmic parameters are determined; this is readily done by computer. The rhythmic parameters include mesor (overall 24-hr mean if the data are equidistant), ampli-

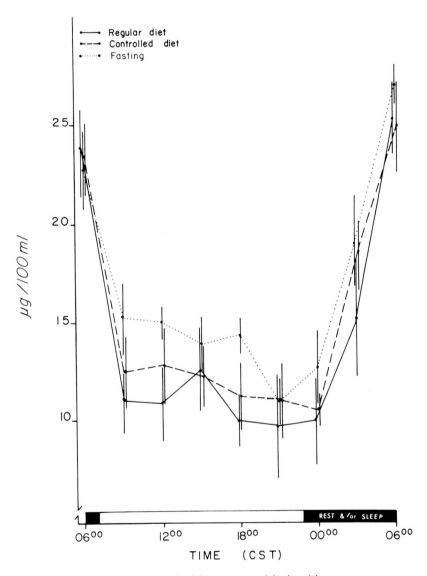

Figure 15.8. Circadian variation in serum cortisol in presumably healthy young men over a 24-hr span. The regular diet consisted of each person eating from the same menu at 0615, 1215, and 1630 (the quantity eaten was not controlled). The controlled diet means that a fixed amount and type of food was eaten by each individual at each sampling time. The fasting group received no food (only water) from 1630 of the day prior to the first sampling time (0600). The phasing of the rhythm in each case remained remarkably similar. Rest or sleep time was from 2100 to 0600; however, the subjects were awakened for sampling at 2400 and 0300. Each point represents the mean ± S.E. of six individuals.

tude, and acrophase. The computer-determined acrophase (point estimate, illustrated by a dot in Fig. 15.7) represents the time when the crest occurs in relation to the rest activity cycle, and the confidence limits are also shown (horizontal bars). Only the acrophases for each variable studied are shown in Figure 15.7. The percentage range of change, shown in Column 2, is the average difference between the lowest and highest mean values over the 3-day period; temperature, however, is an exception because the actual change is shown in degrees rather than as a percentage. Note that in this case 41 different variables were measured (18, 24). This finding in itself does not imply that all the variation shown in Figures 15.6 and 15.7 need to be anything more than responses to food intake, etc. However, we do know that many of the variables listed in this acrophase map will continue to fluctuate in individuals deprived of food during the sampling period. Among them is cortisol, illustrated in Figure 15.8, where it can be seen that the phasing of the rhythm for a group of individuals is minimally disturbed by meal timing. Moreover the same rhythm persists even if the individuals do not sleep or rest.

DRUG SUSCEPTIBILITY RHYTHMS

Because the biological system is rhythmically changing, it follows that the organism is biochemically a different entity at different circadian phases. Therefore, it reacts differently to identical stimuli at different circadian times. This variation has been documented many times using a variety of stimuli which have included carcinogens, immunizing agents, and physical agents, as well as toxic agents such as drugs, chemicals, and poisons. Several reviews of this phenomenon have appeared (28, 31, 43).

Within the past few years a series of studies, which largely have been a collaborative effort of two chronobiology laboratories (the Universities of Arkansas and Minnesota), have shown that by applying chronobiological methods and concepts to the treatment of normal and leukemic mice, host tolerance to a carcinostatic drug could be dramatically improved. Figure 15.9 illustrates the results of the first of this series of studies. These data clearly show that there is a rhythm in the susceptibility of the host to 1-β-D-arabinofuranosylcytosine (ara-C) (7, 39).

A question asked in 1971 was what could be done with such chronobiologically determined

toxicity data in the area of cancer chemotherapy. To explore such a question, it would be ideal to have some accepted reference data which had been determined without chronobiological considerations with which to compare. Fortunately the excellent work of Skipper et al. (44) involving the treatment of L1210 leukemic mice with ara-C seemed to offer such a reference. Skipper and his co-workers consistently were able to eradicate 1 × 10⁵ leukemic cells (sometimes 10⁶) without animal deaths due to toxicity; this was accomplished by giving 4 courses of 120 mg of ara-C per kg body weight in equal doses spaced at 3-hr intervals over a 24-hr span. Between each course was a 3-day rest span. Courses of 240 mg per kg of ara-C given on the same schedule were so toxic that they killed all the animals.

An experiment was designed to determine if the host tolerance to BD_2F_1 mice to the 240 mg/kg dose could be improved by applying chrono-

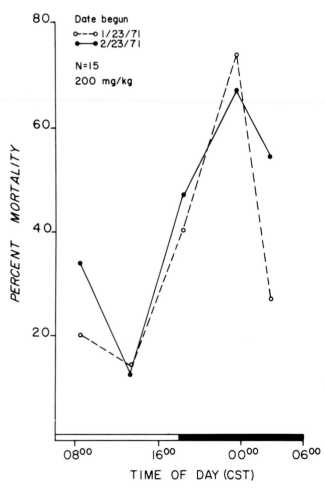

Figure 15.9. Circadian susceptibility rhythm of BD_2F_1 mice to 1-β-D-arabinofuranosylcytosine (ara-C) given once to each group daily on five consecutive days at single, defined, circadian system phases (37a, 39).

biological methods and concepts (23). This was done by inoculating BD_2F_1 mice with L1210 leukemic cells and administering the 240 mg per kg of the ara-C in a special manner. The special manner involved giving the drug in 8 equal doses at 3-hr intervals; it was given thus in a sinusoidally increasing and decreasing amount over the 24-hr span. A number of different sinusoidal treatment schedules were designed and some of

these are illustrated in Figure 15.10. The "best" (most effective) sinusoidal treatment schedules resulted when the largest amount of the drug was given at the times of peak host resistance to the drug and the smallest dose was administered when the animals were more susceptible (41).

Since this drug is cell-cycle specific in that it specifically inhibits DNA synthesis, it was of interest to compare its susceptibility (mortality)

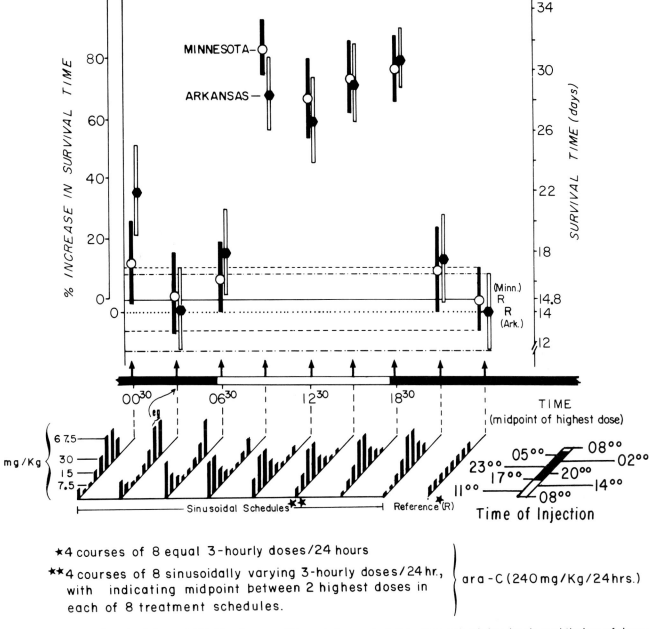

Figure 15.10. Survival time of CD_2F_1 mice on different drug administration schedules (*top*); and timing of doses of ara-C (*bottom*) in sinusoidal and reference (*R*) schedules. All treatment schedules comprise four courses, each consisting of a total of 240 mg/kg/24 hr. When the same total dose of ara-C is given, certain sinusoidal drug-administration schedules are definitely better tolerated by mice than are other sinusoids or than is a currently conventional reference treatment schedule of 8 equal doses over a 24-hr span. Also note unequivocal reproducibility of chronotoxicity to ara-C in experiments done on the same days in different laboratories in different geographic locations (45).

rhythm to the rhythm characterizing DNA synthesis in the duodenum (Fig. 15.11). In this case the peak of mortality is associated with that phase of the circadian system when DNA synthesis is lowest. This would imply that ara-C is having its greatest effect at the time of conversion of the cells from G_1 to S. It has been claimed that this is the most vulnerable part of the cell cycle to many inhibitors of DNA. The application of such an approach, as described above, in a number of different studies ultimately led to a report of an increase not only in host tolerance to the drug but also in the numbers of cures

when compared to the reference schedule that could be obtained using the single drug, ara-C, alone against an inoculum of 1×10^6 L1210 leukemic cells (26). A comprehensive review of these studies and their implications to chronotherapy has been published (47). It should be pointed out that Figure 15.10 demonstrates clearly the remarkable reproducibility relative to host toxicity data that can be achieved from one laboratory to another (41).

The doubled cure rate alluded to in the paragraph above was at best only about 28% of all mice bearing an inoculum of 1×10^6 leukemic

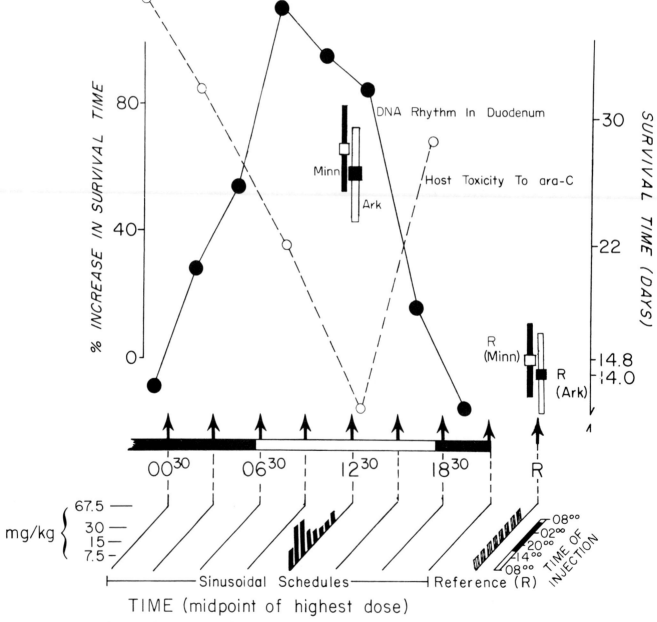

Figure 15.11. Comparison of the ara-C toxicity rhythm to the rhythm in DNA synthesis in the duodenum (see text, also Ref. 28).

cell with treatment started 44 hr after tumor implant (26). Obviously, if one was to achieve a better than 28% cure rate it would be necessary to give more than one drug. Cure in this case involved animals alive and apparently healthy at 60 days after tumor inoculation.

Our objective in the next series of studies was to cure as many mice as possible who had been previously inoculated with about 1×10^6 tumor cells. Such was accomplished by administering 4 courses of the best ara-C sinusoidal schedule (see Figure 15.11) and also by administering in combination the drug cyclophosphamide once

per course but at different circadian times for different groups of mice. Cyclophosphamide, like ara-C, also was found to vary in its toxicity when administered at different circadian times. The end result of these studies was that one could, at certain circadian phases with the ara-C sinusoidal approach plus cyclophosphamide, cure close to 100% of all mice bearing an inoculum of 1.2×10^6 L1210 leukemic cells (Fig. 15.12) (37a). As indicated above, nothing comparable could be accomplished using either drug alone. Moreover, using the two drugs in combination without chronobiological consideration, too

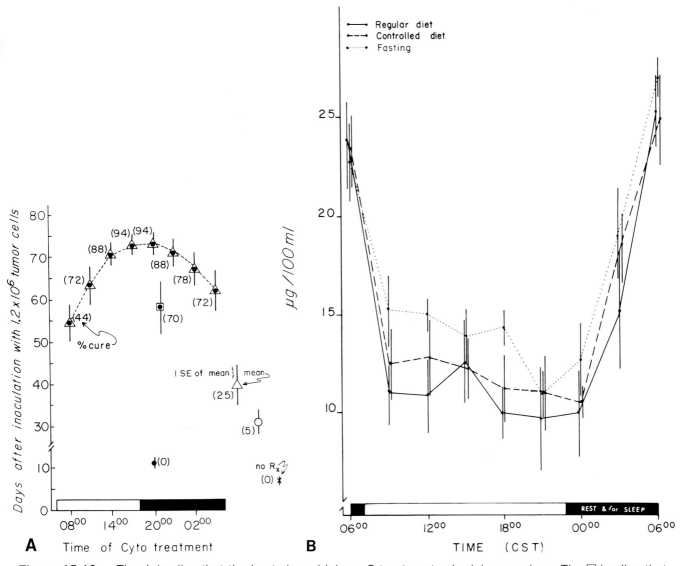

Figure 15.12. The △ implies that the best sinusoidal ara-C treatment schedule was given. The □ implies that the reference schedule of treatment was administered; for review of both modes of treatment, refer to Figure 12.11. The ● implies that cyclophosphamide (*Cyto*) was administered to combination with ara-C once/course to each mouse; however, different groups received it at different circadian phases, △. The percentages of cures (percentage alive at 75 days after tumor inoculation) are shown in parentheses. Horizontal scale, time when cyclophosphamide was administered. The groups that did not receive cyclophosphamide are shown just to the right of the time scale. *N* for each group was 20.

many animals died from acute drug toxicity (15%); thus the same high rate of cure could not be achieved.

The next series of studies had as their objective to determine with the same approach whether or not an inoculum of 5×10^6 cells could be cured with treatment started 44 hr after inoculation. It was found that such an inoculum was too high to achieve anywhere near what had been achieved with the less advanced disease stage described above. Even in this situation, however, the chronobiological approach demonstrated better therapeutic efficacy when compared to the nonchronobiological approach.

In succeeding studies a combination of three drugs, ara-C, cyclophosphamide, and vincristine, were employed with limited degrees of success in curing an inoculum of 5×10^6 L1210 tumor cells. This was followed by a series of studies involving a fourth drug, methylprednisolone. Finally, a combination of the above four drugs as well as the fifth drug, diaminetrichloroplatinum (*cis*-platinum) was found to be remarkably effective (6, 35).

Ultimately we were able, by manipulating the dosages of the above five drugs in a chronobiological manner, to increase significantly the cure rate in mice that had received an inoculum of 5×10^6 tumor cells with treatment initiated 44 hr after inoculation. In fact, at certain circadian

phases as many as 88% of the mice were cured (in this case, those mice alive 75 days after tumor inoculation). In this situation as before, however, the conventional or nonchronobiological approach resulted in an overwhelming number of deaths due to drug toxicity (6a, 35, 36, 50).

More recently, cyclophosphamide, 100 mg/kg, and Adriamycin, 5 mg/kg, were found to be synergistic in treating L1210 leukemic mice that were inoculated with 1×10^5 L1210 cells 4 days prior to treatment. In this case only one course of treatment was given. There was a dramatic circadian variation in response as monitored by mean survival time and cure rate (Figs. 15.13 and 15.14). The variation in cure rate (mice alive and apparently free of disease 75 days post-tumor inoculation) as a function of treatment timing ranged from 8 to 68% in male animals standardized to 12 hr of light alternating with 12 hr of darkness. Similarly, in female mice standardized to 8 hr of light alternating with 16 hr of darkness, the cure rate ranged from 0 to 56% depending on when the drugs were injected during the 24-hr span. No cures were obtained with either drug alone (37).

The maximum cure rate was recorded when the two drugs were administered in the early part of the dark portion of the light-dark cycle (whether 12 hr of light and 12 hr of darkness or 8 hr light and 16 hr darkness), whereas maxi-

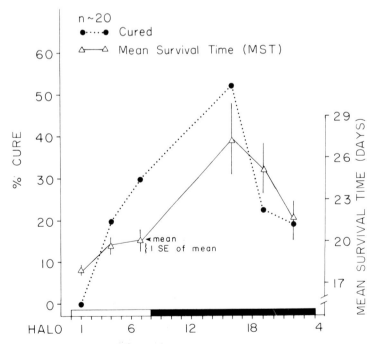

Figure 15.13. Variation in cure rate of leukemic mice depending on timing of concomitant treatment with cyclophosphamide and Adriamycin. One study was done on male mice in LD 12:12; another was done on female mice in LD 8:16. HALO—hours after lights on. (The details of this study have been published; see Ref. 37.)

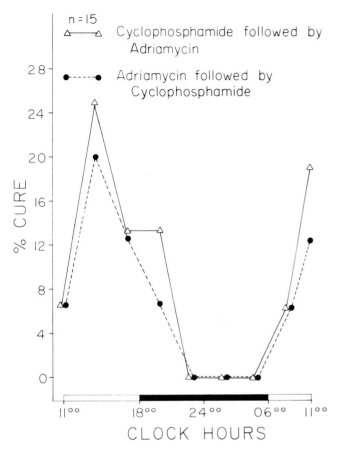

Figure 15.14. Effects of drug sequence and interval (probably confounded by circadian variation) on responsive leukemic mice to cyclophosphamide and Adriamycin. First drug given at 1100 (5 hr after onset of lights) and second drug given either concomitantly or 3, 6, 9, 12, 15, 18, 21, or 24 hr later. (The details of this study have been published; see Ref. 37.)

mum mortality occurred following treatment early in the light span.

Extensive evidence also documents that maximal therapeutic advantage as obtained when the two drugs were separated by 2- or 3-hr intervals and that this effect of drug sequencing was strongly circadian-stage dependent (37).

The results at present demonstrate clearly in the experimental model that one should not ignore the circadian variation in tolerance when dealing with chemotherapy or sequencing studies. The evidence is compelling that the temporal organization in general carries with it significant implications not only for cancer chemotherapy but equally importantly for basic cancer research. Perhaps we can come to better grips with the mechanism of cancer if we consider the rhythmic nature of cell division in the first place. It seems quite safe to predict that in any future edition of this book more dramatic results of experimental chronotherapy will be reported.

Even more important, it is hoped that successful results will be forthcoming from studies on humans; we know of at least one study now getting underway that is designed to test the feasibility of the clinical application of chronotherapy. This latter task presents many problems, and among them will be the identification of appropriate marker rhythms to gauge therapeutic efficacy.

References

1. Andrews, R. V., and Folk, G. E. (1963): Circadian metabolic patterns in cultured hamster adrenals. *J. Comp. Biochem. Physiol.*, 11:393.
2. Aschoff, J. (1960): Exogenous and endogenous components in circadian rhythms. *Cold Spring Harbor Symp. Quant. Biol.*, 25:11.
3. Atkinson, M., Kripke, D. F., and Wolf, S. R. (1975): Autorhythmometry in manic-depressives. *Chronobiologia*, 2:325.
4. Brown, F. A. (1965): A unified theory for biological rhythms, in *Circadian Clocks*, p. 231, edited by J. Aschoff. North-Holland Publ. Co., Amsterdam.
5. Bünning, E. (1958): *The Physiological Clock*. Springer-Verlag, New York.
6. Burns, E. R., and Scheving, L. E. (1980): *Chronobiologia*, 7:41.
6a. Burns, E. R., Scheving, L. E., and Pauly, J. E. (1977): Chronochemotherapy of L1210 leukemia with cytosine arabinoside (ara-C) in combination with cyclophosphamide (C) or C + vincristine (V). *Proc. Am. Assoc. Cancer Res.*, 18:197.
7. Cardoso, S. S., Scheving, L. E., and Halberg, F. (1970): Mortality of mice as influenced by the hour of day of drug (ara-C) administration. *Pharmacologist*, 12:302.
8. Cummings, B. G., and Wagner, E. (1968): Rhythmic processes in plants. *Ann. Rev. Plant Physiol.*, 19:381.
9. De Mairan, M. (1729): *Observations Botaniques*, p. 35. Hist. Acad. Roy. Sci., Paris.
10. Fisher, L. B. (1968): The diurnal mitotic rhythm in the human epidermis. *Br. J. Dermatol.*, 80:75–80.
11. Halberg, F. (1953): Some physiological and clinical aspects of 24-hour periodicity. *J. Lancet*, 73:20.
12. Halberg, F. (1959): Physiologic 24-hour periodicity; general and procedural considerations with reference to the adrenal cycle. *Vitam. Horm. Fermentforsch.*, 10:225.
13. Halberg, F. (1960): Temporal organization in physiological function. *Cold Spring Harbor Symp. Quant. Biol.*, 25:289.
14. Halberg, F. (1969): Chronobiology. *Ann. Rev. Physiol.*, 31:675.
15. Halberg, F., and Connor, R. L. (1961): Circadian organization and microbiology; variance spectra and periodogram on behavior of *Escherichia coli* growing in fluid cultures. *Proc. Minn. Acad. Sci.*, 29:226.
16. Halberg, F., and Katinas, G. (1973): Chronobiologic glossary. *Int. J. Chronobiol.* 1:31.
17. Halberg, F., Tong, Y. L., and Johnson, E. A. (1967): Circadian system phase—an aspect of temporal morphology; procedures and illustrative examples, in *Cellular Aspects of Biorhythms*, p. 20, edited by H. v. Mayersbach. Springer-Verlag, Berlin.
18. Halberg, F., Johnson, E. A., Nelson, W., and Sothern R. (1972): Autorhythmometry procedures for physiological self-measurement and their analysis. *Physiol. Teacher*, 1:1.
19. Halberg, F., Powell, E. W., Lubanovic, W., Sothern, R. B., Brockway, B., Pasley, R. N., and Scheving, L. E. (1977): Glossary of chronobiology. *Chronobiologia, Suppl. IV*, p. 190.
20. Halberg, F., Haus, E., Cardoso, S. S., Scheving, L. E., Kühl, J. F. W., Shiotsuka, R., Rosene, G., Pauly, J. E., Runge, W., Spalding, J. E., Lee, J. K., and Good, R. A. (1973): Toward a chronotherapy of neoplasia; tolerance of treatment depends on host rhythms. *Experientia*, 29:909.
21. Halberg, F., et al. (1976): Circadian rhythms in polyamine excretion by rats bearing an immunocytoma. *Chronobiologia*, 4:309.
22. Haus, E., and Halberg, F. (1970): Circannual rhythms in level and timing of serum corticosterone in standardized inbred mature C-mice. *Environ. Res.*, 3:31.
23. Haus, E., Halberg, F., Scheving, L. E., Cardoso, S. S., Kühl, J. F. W., Sothern, R., Shiotsuka, R., Hwang, D. S., and Pauly, J. E. (1972): Increased tolerance of leukemic mice to arabinosyl cytosine with schedule adjusted to circadian system. *Science*, 177:80.
24. Kanabrocki, E. L., Scheving, L. E., Halberg, F., Brewer, R. L., and Bird, T. J. (1973): Circadian variation in presumably healthy men under conditions of peace-time army reserve training. *Space Life Sci.*, 4:258.
25. Konopka, R. J., and Benzer, S. (1971): Clock mutants of *Drosophila melanogaster*. *Proc. Natl. Acad. Sci. U.S.A.*, 68:2112.
26. Kühl, J. F. W., Haus, E., Halberg, F., Scheving, L. E., Pauly, J. E., Cardoso, S. S., and Rosene, G. (1974): Experimental chronotherapy with ara-C;

comparison of murine ara-C tolerance on differently timed treatment schedules. *Chronobiologia, 1*:316.

27. Moore, R. Y., and Eichler, V. B. (1972): Loss of a circadian adrenal corticosterone rhythm following suprachiasmatic lesions in the rat. *Brain Res., 42*:201.

28. Moore-Ede, M. C. (1973): Circadian rhythms of drug effectiveness and toxicity. *Clin. Pharmacol. Ther., 14*:925.

29. Njus, D., Sulzman, F., and Hastings, J. W. (1974): Membrane model for the circadian clock. *Nature (Lond.), 248*:116.

30. Pittendrigh, C. S. (1960): Circadian rhythms and circadian organization of living systems. *Cold Spring Harbor Symp. Quant. Biol., 25*:1959.

31. Reinberg, A., and Halberg, F. (1971): Circadian pharmacology. *Ann. Rev. Pharmacol., 11*:455.

32. Scheving, L. E. (1959): Mitotic activity in the human epidermis. *Anat. Rec., 135*:7.

33. Scheving, L. E. (1974): Chronobiology, in *Chronobiology*, p. 221, edited by L. E. Scheving, F. Halberg, and J. E. Pauly. Igaku Shoin Ltd., Tokyo.

34. Scheving, L. E., and Pauly, J. E. (1974): Circadian rhythms; some examples and comments on clinical application. *Chronobiologia, 1*:3.

35. Scheving, L. E., Burns, E. R., Halberg, F., and Pauly, J. E.: (1980): *Chronobiologia, 7*:33.

35a. Scheving, L. E., Burns, E. R. and Pauly, J. E. (1977): Can chronobiology be ignored when considering the cancer problem? In *Prevention and Detection of Cancer, Pt. 1, Prevention, Vol. 1: Etiology*, p. 1081, edited by H. E. Neiburgs. Marcel Dekker, New York.

36. Scheving, L. E., Burns, E. R., and Pauly, J. E. (1978): Failure to synchronize the mitotic index rhythm of mouse corneal epithelium to a controlled feeding schedule. *Anat. Rec., 190*:553.

37. Scheving, L. E., Burns, E. R., Pauly, J. E., and Halberg, F.: (1980): *Cancer Res., 40*:1511.

37a. Scheving, L. E., Burns, E. R., Pauly, J. E., and Halberg, F., and Haus, E. (1977): Survival and cure of leukemic mice after circadian optimization of treatment with cyclophosphamide and 1-β-D-arabinofuranosylcytosine. *Cancer Res, 37*:3648.

38. Scheving, L. E., Burns, E. R., Tsai, T. H., and Pauly, J. E. (1978): Circadian variation in cell division in the mouse alimentary tract, bone marrow and corneal epithelium. *Anat. Rec., 191*:479.

39. Scheving, L. E., Cardoso, S. S., Pauly, J. E., Halberg, F., and Haus, E. (1974): Variation in susceptibility of mice to the carcinostatic agent arabinosyl cytosine, in *Chronobiologia*, p. 213, edited by L. E. Scheving, F. Halberg, and J. E. Pauly, Igaku Shoin Ltd., Tokyo.

40. Scheving, L. E., Halberg, F., and Kanabrocki, E. L. (1977): Circadian rhythmometry on 42 variables of 13 presumably healthy young men, in *Proceedings of the XII International Conference, Washington, D.C., August 10–13, 1975*, p. 47. Publishing House "Il Ponte," Milano.

41. Scheving, L. E., Haus, E., Kühl, J. F. W., Pauly, J. E., Halberg, F., and Cardoso, S. S. (1976): Close reproduction by different laboratories of characteristics of circadian rhythms in 1-β-D-arabinofuranosyl cytosine tolerance by mice. *Cancer Res., 36*:1133.

42. Scheving, L. E., Pauly, J. E., Von Mayersbach, H., and Dunn, J. (1974): The effect of continuous light or darkness on the rhythm of the mitotic index in the corneal epithelium of the rat. *Acta Anat., 88*:411.

43. Scheving, L. E., Von Mayersbach, H., and Pauly, J. E. (1974): An overview of chronopharmacology. *J. Eur. Toxicol., 7*:203.

44. Skipper, H. E., Schabel, F. M., and Wilcox, W. S. (1967): Experimental evaluation of potental anticancer agents; XXI. Scheduling of arabinosyl cytosine to take advantage of its S-phase specificity against leukemia cells. *Cancer Chemother. Rep., 51*:125.

45. Stephan, F. K., and Zucker, I. (1972): Rat drinking rhythms; central visual pathways and endocrine factors mediating responsiveness to environmental illumination. *Physiol. Behav., 8*:315.

46. Stone, J. E., Scheving, L. E., Burns, E. R., and Graham, M. (1974): Circadian rhythm of ornithine decarboxylase activity in mouse liver; the effect of isoproterenol and Clelland's aqueous reagent, in *Chronobiologia*, p. 33, edited by L. E. Scheving, F. Halberg, and J. E. Pauly, Igaku Shoin Ltd., Tokyo.

47. Sturtevant, R. P. (1973): Circadian variability in *Klebsiella* demonstrated by cosinor analysis. *Int. J. Chronobiol., 1*:141.

48. Sweeney, B. M. (1974): A physiological model for circadian rhythms derived from *Acetabularia* rhythm paradoxes. *Int. J. Chronobiol., 2*:25.

49. Weitzman, E. D., and Hellman, L. (1974): Temporal organization of the 24-hour pattern of hypothalamic-pituitary axis, in *Biorhythms and Human Reproduction*, p. 371, edited by M. Ferin, F. Halberg, and R. L. Vande Weile. John Wiley & Sons, New York.

50. Wever, R. (1969): Untersuchungen zur Circadianen Periodik des Menschen mit besonderer Berücksichtigung des Einflusses schwacher elektrischer Wechselfelder. *Bundesminist. Wiss. Forsch. Forschungsber., 61*:212.

16

Species Specificity of Normal Biochemical Pathways as Platform for Pathologic Pathways

Hans E. Kaiser

It is not only the morphology of the organism that shows a species-specific aspect, but also its biochemistry in the broadest sense of the word. Thus it is possible to consider normal growth and abnormal growth, since the latter is derived from the first, from these various points of view. The pathological aspect is a derivative of the normal one. In the case of morphology, the ultrastructure of the cell can be used as the common basis of comparison: the distribution of generally occurring biochemical intermediates and their metabolism are basic features. The occurrence in different specialized tissues, on the other hand, may vary. These variations may be considered differently depending on their occurrence in the number of species or the number of types; this, again, is dependent on the various phyla. Therefore with respect to morphology, developmental potential, as well as biochemically and biophysically, those characteristics that appear generally and those which appear specifically have to be recognized and differentiated. In comparative oncology, these variations in the combination of generally and specifically occurring processes will greatly influence the possible development of neoplasms in the various species. From a phylogenetic standpoint, the general phenomena are the older ones, although it is also possible that they have developed convergently. Development resulting in specific processes in lower organisms, as in bacteria, must have passed through a longer period of geological history or a longer period of evolution than the process in a more highly developed organism such as a mammal.

What are the processes that are so important for the biochemical development of neoplasms? Without a doubt, the normal biochemical pathways influence quite decisively the possible path of a specific tumor development in a specific organism due to a specific compound. On the other hand, these normal pathways may also prevent tumor development or may direct it along the diverse routes, due to the variations in the distribution of the biochemical intermediates in the organisms. Also to be considered is the action of an initiator or promoter on normal metabolism. Furthermore, blocking the entrance of carcinogens into a pathway by otherwise harmless or anticarcinogenic compounds should be considered.

A more or less uniform-appearing cell injury occurs at the beginning of each neoplastic transformation. The interrelated processes, as described in Chapter 12, form one of the uniform bases of neoplastic growth. Certain ontogenetic factors such as the definite growth processes are capable of modifying the general character to some extent. As shown in Chapter 12, the problem of cell injury and neoplastic growth can also be considered from a morphological and biochemical viewpoint. The connection between these two modes of observation is the cell ultrastructure. It is one of the essential characteristics of living organisms to break down nonspecific nutrients into low molecular building blocks which are then rebuilt into high molecular, species-specific compounds which are then utilized in the organism for normal growth. The various organisms either follow synthetic pathways which are, species-specifically widely distributed, or biosynthetic pathways for certain compounds may occur in only a small group of organisms of one or more particular species. The biosynthesis of the same type of substances, or even of a definite intermediate, may follow species-specific pathways.

The stimulants effecting the neoplastic transformation of a cell can act only through the insertion of the chemical carcinogen into the biochemical structure of the organism itself. The metabolic processes are chain reactions between different intermediates; they may lead to changes in the metabolic conditions in the organism, but not necessarily so. The stimulating factor leading to neoplastic transformation acts like a key to a lock with respect to the metabolism of the organism. If one or several steps of a definite synthetic pathway in normal metabolic synthesis is lacking, then a neoplastic transformation by a definite chemical carcinogen may not occur. Thus, the normal pathways with their specificity, as far as species, organs, and tissues are concerned, are of extreme importance. They determine whether a neoplastic transformation

due to a certain carcinogen may or may not occur; namely, why certain compounds are carcinogenic for one group of organisms while they are harmless for another. They constitute a framework for the discussions on the species-specific biochemical pathways of malignant growth (Chapter 17) as well as for an understanding of the biochemistry of neoplastic cells (Chapter 18).

For a detailed discussion of the subject, consult the following references.

References

1. Beutler, R. (1951): Vergleichende Physiologische Chemie der Tiere, in *Physiologische Chemie*, pp. 659–970, edited by Flaschenträger-Lehnartz, Springer-Verlag, Berlin.
2. Dagley, S., and Nicholson, D. E. (1970): *An Introduction to Metabolic Pathways.* Blackwell Scientific Publications, Oxford and Edinburgh.
3. Flaschenträger-Lehnartz, (1951–66): *Physiologische Chemie.* Springer-Verlag, Berlin.
4. Florkin, M., and Scheer, B. T. (1967–78): *Chemical Zoology*, Vols. *1–10.* Academic Press, New York.
5. Greenberg, D. M. (1967–75): *Metabolic Pathways*, Vols. *I–VIII.* Academic Press, New York.
6. Luckner, M. (1972): *Secondary Metabolism in Plants and Animals.* Chapman & Hall, London.
7. Mothes, K. (1966): Vergleichende Betrachtung des pflanzlichen Stoffwechsels, in *Physiologische Chemie, Vol. II*, edited by Flaschenträger-Lehnartz. Springer-Verlag, Berlin.

17

Species-Specific Biochemical Pathways of Malignant Growth

Elizabeth K. Weisburger

INTRODUCTION

Although there are easily as many as 400 well-documented experimental carcinogens and about 30 human carcinogens, studies on the biochemical basis for differences in species and strain response to carcinogens have been performed with only a few of these chemicals. This situation has occurred even though it was noted relatively early, with the first individually identified chemical carcinogens, that there were sizable differences in the response of different species to the agents (cf. 130). For example, mice were quite susceptible to tumor formation when painted with the ubiquitous carcinogen benzo[a]pyrene (BP) while rats, fowl, guinea pigs, and monkeys did not respond within a useful time period.

Despite these differences, there have been no systematic *in vivo* experiments with BP to determine the reasons for the variation in response. Furthermore, research with BP has moved into the area of metabolism by isolated cells (126) or liver microsomes (53) to identify the mutagenic and presumably activated metabolites. Currently a 7,8-diol-9,10-epoxide is the major mutagenic intermediate from BP metabolism (54). Recent advancements in the separation and identification of BP and its metabolites have facilitated studies in this area (110). Further work has indicated the very stereospecific nature of the 7,8-diol-9,10-epoxide of BP in its interactions (61, 145, 146). A BP-nucleic acid derivative has been identified as the epoxide-guanosine adduct (60).

In this review, two carcinogenic substances will be discussed in detail. The first, aflatoxin B$_1$, is a widespread environmental problem, while the second, N-2-fluorenylacetamide, is a model experimental carcinogen.

In addition, extensive tables are presented demonstrating the species-specific response to a different type of experimental carcinogen, N-nitroso-N-methylurea, and to a widely used cancer chemotherapeutic agent, melphalan.

AFLATOXIN B$_1$

Aflatoxin B$_1$, a naturally occurring carcinogen, is a toxin produced by the food spoilage fungus, *Aspergillus flavus*. Although peanuts were the original food crop found to be contaminated, many other types of foods, especially in tropical countries, harbor the fungus. Of several compounds produced by *A. flavus*, aflatoxin B$_1$ is usually the most prevalent and is certainly the most toxic of all (24, 143) (Fig. 17.1). Allcroft (3) has summarized the data on the toxicity of aflatoxins in farm animals. There were some marked differences in response to both the acute and chronic effects with no correlation between them.

With regard to experimental animals, aflatoxin B$_1$ is chiefly a hepatocarcinogen in rats, ferrets, guinea pigs, ducks (15), monkeys (1, 125), tree shrews (101), guppies (105), and rainbow trout (47). Some tumors were induced in other organs such as the kidney and gastrointestinal tract, especially in rats. The strain of rat influenced the tumor response to an appreciable extent.

In mice, a significant carcinogenic effect on the liver was obtained only if the animals received repeated doses of aflatoxin B$_1$ at the neonatal stage (127); adult mice seemed resistant to the hepatocarcinogenicity of aflatoxin B$_1$. In contrast, rainbow trout are extremely suscepti-

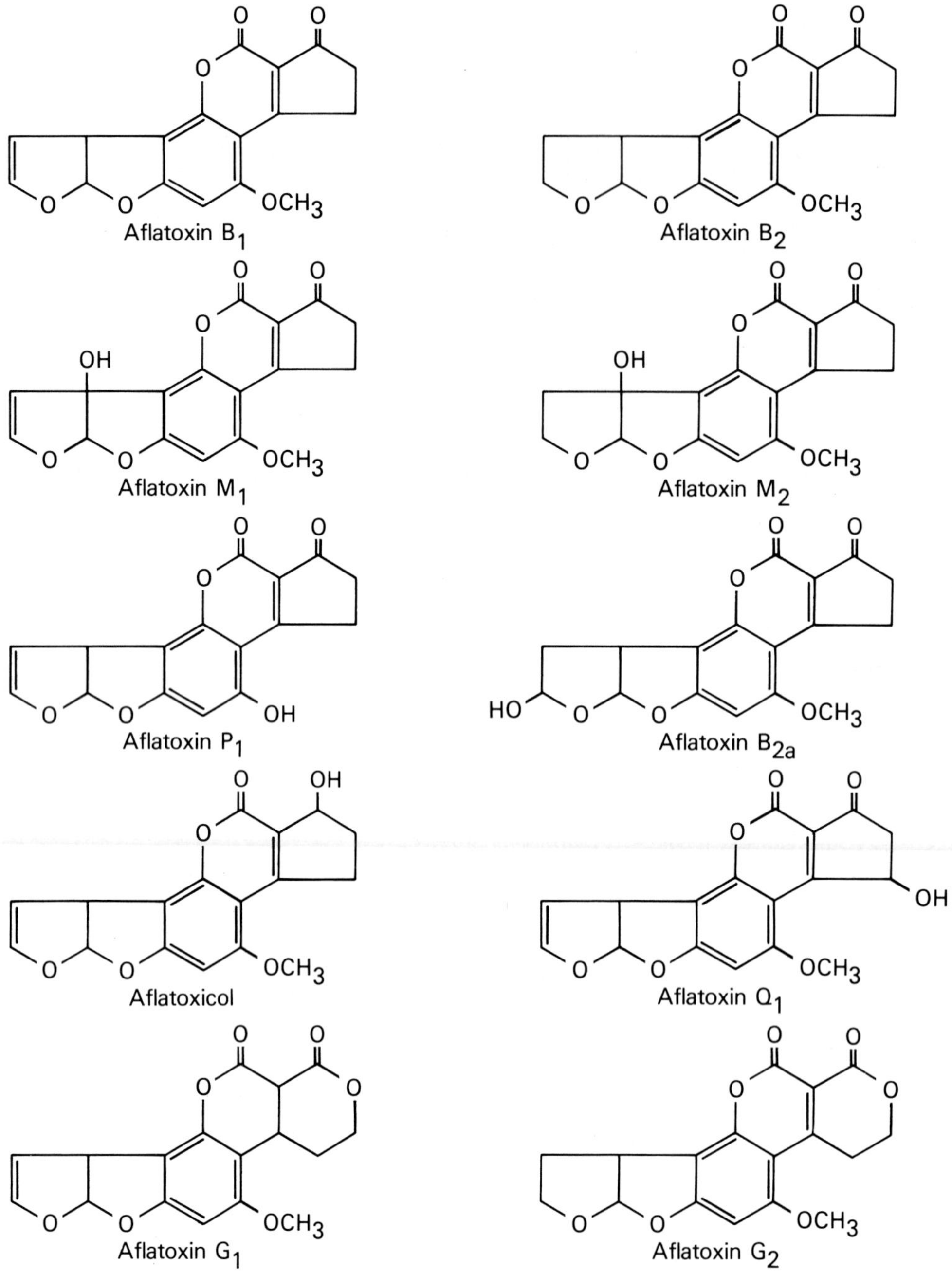

Figure 17.1. Principal aflatoxins and metabolites.

ble to both the toxicity and the hepatocarcinogenicity of aflatoxin (47). Some other types of fish, including the coho salmon and the channel catfish, are more resistant to both the acute and chronic action (47). Peculiarly, a closely related salmonid fish, the sockeye salmon (*Oncorhynchus nerka*) did develop hepatomas when fed a diet containing aflatoxin B_1 and cyclopropenoid fatty acids (128).

In vivo Studies

Definitive metabolism studies have been performed using labeled aflatoxin B_1 in rats, mice,

and monkeys (19, 20, 142). Other qualitative investigations in sheep, cattle, pigs, guinea pigs, and chickens have employed unlabeled aflatoxin B_1, relying upon fluorescence as an indicator for aflatoxin B_1 or its metabolites (68, 94).

Rats

Two different labeled forms of aflatoxin B_1 were employed, one labeled in the ring, the other in the methoxy carbon (142). When methoxy-labeled aflatoxin was injected intraperitoneally (i.p.), over 30% of the radioactivity appeared in the expired CO_2 within 24 hr. Sizable amounts were excreted in the urine and feces (approximately 40% total). Of all the organs, the liver carried the most activity. On the other hand, when ring-labeled ^{14}C-aflatoxin was injected, the feces carried 60–70% of the label, the urine about 20%. As with methoxy-labeled aflatoxin, the liver had the highest activity of the organs examined. Biliary excretion apparently was the primary pathway for the radioactivity finally appearing in the feces. The difference in excretion pattern showed that 0-demethylation of aflatoxin B_1 represents a major metabolic pathway. Nevertheless, an 0-demethylated product could not be positively identified in rat urine, only aflatoxin M_1 in which hydroxylation had occurred on the furan moiety of the aflatoxin B_1 molecule (Fig. 17.1).

Mice

Mice injected i.p. with ring-labeled aflatoxin B_1 excreted somewhat more radioactivity in the urine within 24 hr than did the susceptible rat. However, the difference was not outstanding, i.e., approximately 90% in the mouse versus 80% in the rat. More significant, perhaps, was the much lower percentage of activity from the labeled aflatoxin B_1 in the liver of the mouse, compared with the rat. On the average, the proportion in rat liver was 5-fold greater than that in the mouse. Thus, a much lower level of administered aflatoxin was retained in the liver of the mouse than in the rat.

Monkeys

The metabolism of ^{14}C-labeled aflatoxin B was investigated after both i.p. and oral administration to rhesus monkeys (19, 20). Comparing the two modes of administration, urinary excretion of radioactivity was somewhat more rapid after oral dosing. However, by 96 hr, the cumulative urinary excretion was the same after either route. An even greater proportion of a dose remained in the livers of monkeys for a much longer time when compared with mice and rats (Table 17.1).

There were differences in the relative levels of the identified urinary metabolites. Aflatoxin M_1 was the major metabolite after oral dosing while i.p. administration led to high levels of aflatoxin P_1, excreted mostly as the glucuronide conjugate (Table 17.2). At least four other minor metabolites which were not identified were also present.

Table 17.1

Excretion and Distribution of Radioactivity from Ring-labeled ^{14}C-Aflatoxin B_1 in Mice, Monkeys, and Rats[a]

	Mice 24 Hr i.p.	Rats 24 Hr i.p.	Monkeys (i.p.)			Monkeys Oral		
			24 hr	48 hr	96 hr	24 hr	48 hr	96 hr
	% of Dose							
Total excreted	89.9	80.1						
CO_2	0.3	0.4						
Urine	34.5	22.6	27	29	35	33	34	35
Feces	55.7	57.1				1	14	41
Liver	1.5	7.6	8.3	5.8	5.6			6.8

[a] Data from Wogan (142), Dalezios and Wogan (19), Dalezios et al. (20).

Table 17.2

Urinary Metabolites of Aflatoxin B_1 in Monkeys[a]

	% of Dose	
Dosing Method	i.p.	Oral
Aflatoxin P_1 glucuronide	17	3.3
Aflatoxin P_1 sulfate	3	1.2
Aflatoxin P_1		
M_1	2.3	19
B_1	0.01–0.1	0.05–0.2

[a] Data from Wogan (142), Dalezios and Wogan (19), Dalezios et al. (20).

Qualitative studies

Qualitative studies on the excretion of aflatoxin B_1 metabolites have been performed in various susceptible and resistant domestic and laboratory animals including cows, sheep, goats, ducks, chicks, rats, mice, and guinea pigs (68, 94). Rats, guinea pigs, goats, sheep, and cows converted aflatoxin B_1 to M_1 (for milk toxin), or its conjugate, but the excretion of M_1 was doubtful in mice and ducklings.

The urine of children who had eaten peanut butter contaminated with aflatoxin B_1 contained aflatoxin M_1, as determined by chemical methods and a bioassay in rainbow trout (16, 17).

To summarize these efforts, the in vivo studies of aflatoxin B_1 metabolism indicate that the toxin was generally converted to aflatoxin M_1 in most species. The demethylated metabolite, aflatoxin P_1, was positively identified only in the urine of monkeys administered B_1. Experiments with ^{14}C-labeled aflatoxin B_1 showed that the least susceptible species, the mouse, retained much less of a dose in the liver than did the rat, a susceptible animal. In turn, the primate liver retained even more of a dose and for a longer time than did the rat. If it can be assumed that humans exposed to aflatoxin might react similarly to the nonhuman primate, the implication is that human liver would also retain some ingested aflatoxin or metabolites for a long time. The adduct of aflatoxin with DNA has been isolated and identified (33, 73). Since analytical studies on urines of populations exposed to aflatoxin have not been very definitive in identifying persons at risk, a radioimmunological assay for aflatoxin has been developed (71). This technique should facilitate epidemiological studies on the possible relationship between aflatoxin ingestion and cancer.

In vitro Studies

In vitro work has been focused largely on metabolism of aflatoxin B_1 by liver preparations from a number of mammalian and avian species (103). An advantage of in vitro systems is that the metabolites formed can be isolated without the complication of additional alteration either from bacteria in the intestinal tract or other tissues reached through systemic circulation.

Using crude liver microsomal preparations from calf, chick, duckling, goat, guinea pig, mouse, pig, rat, and sheep, Patterson and Allcroft (94) found that aflatoxin B_1 was metabolized most extensively by the mouse liver preparation and least by that from the rat. In sheep, goat, or rat liver preparations, aflatoxin M_1 could be identified to a minor extent; the major metabolite, though, was an unidentified substance. Further efforts showed the unknown probably was related to or was aflatoxin B_{2a}, a hemiacetal (95). The hemiacetal was relatively unstable; addition of cysteine to the incubation mixture inhibited its breakdown so that under these conditions half the aflatoxin B_1 could be identified as B_{2a}.

The oxidative enzyme system forming M_1 was inducible by phenobarbital or aflatoxin B_1, at least in rat liver (106). An extensive study by

Bassir and Emafo (5) with both liver slices and liver microsomes from eight mammalian species (goat, sheep, rat, mouse, guinea pig, rabbit, dog, and golden hamster) showed some sizable differences in both demethylation and hydroxylation of aflatoxin B_1. Both liver slices and microsomes from dogs did not demethylate B_1, while sheep liver slices had low demethylating activity. Microsomes from guinea pigs also lacked the demethylase. As for hydroxylation to M_1, mouse liver slices and microsomes had no activity even though the mouse liver microsomes metabolized almost all the added B_1 (Table 17.3).

Another enzyme system which reduced the cyclopentenone ring of aflatoxin to an alcohol was discovered in the livers of most avian species (96). The product, called aflatoxicol, was readily formed by a soluble fraction from chicken, duck, turkey, and rabbit liver; little or no activity was present in guinea pig, mouse, or rat liver. Tissues from older birds had greater activity than those from young ones, a finding which correlated with the greater resistance of older birds to aflatoxin poisoning.

Further investigations have concentrated largely on the alteration of aflatoxin B_1 by liver preparations from primates. Büchi et al. (14) identified a hydroxylated aflatoxin B_1 (aflatoxin Q_1) as a major metabolite from either human or monkey liver in 39 or 18% yields, respectively. The hydroxy group was on the carbon atom beta to the carbonyl on the cyclopentenone ring. Steyn et al. (115) obtained a compound of similar structure with microsomes from vervet monkey (*Cereopithecus aethiops*) or baboon (*Papio ursinus*) liver. However, the physical properties of the two compounds isolated by Büchi et al. and Steyn et al. did not agree, possibly due to differences in stereochemical configuration. Steyn et al. could not detect aflatoxin P_1 even though this is a major urinary metabolite in monkeys. How-

Table 17.3
Species Differences in Metabolism of Aflatoxin B_1 by Liver Slices or Microsomes[a]

Species	Goat	Sheep	Rat	Mouse	Guinea Pig	Rabbit	Dog	Hamster
Formaldehyde (mμmol) produced per gram liver								
Slices (2 hr)	23.0 ± 1.3	6.4 ± 0.9	37.2 ± 1.9	17.8 ± 1.8	30.4 ± 1.3	36.5 ± 3.2	0	29.3 ± 2.7
Microsomes (1 hr)	61.6 ± 2.0	43.4 ± 2.5	75.1 ± 13.0	68.3 ± 7.5	0	56.3 ± 10.5	0	89.0 ± 9.0
% of B_1 metabolized								
Slices (2 hr)	91.3 ± 3.7	48.1 ± 7.4	83.8 ± 5.3	88.8 ± 5.5	83.8 ± 2.9	92.5 ± 4.8	82.8 ± 3.0	95.6 ± 2.7
Microsomes (1 hr)	98.0 ± 1.3	75.5 ± 1.5	88.8 ± 2.0	99.8 ± 0.4	94.4 ± 2.6	98.7 ± 0.5	85.6 ± 3.6	99.4 ± 0.06
% of M_1 produced								
Slices (2 hr)	1.8 ± 0.3	4.3 ± 0.6	1.6 ± 0.6	0	0.88 ± 0.1	1.1 ± 0.3	5.3 ± 1.4	5.4 ± 1.1
Microsomes (1 hr)	1.9 ± 0.5	4.8 ± 1.0	1.7 ± 0.13	0	0.9 ± 0.07	1.0 ± 0.12	5.4 ± 1.2	1.3 ± 0.3

[a] The concentration of substrate (B_1) added was 160 mμmol in all cases. Data from Bassir and Emafo (5).

ever, in the similar incubation system used by Merrill and Campbell (85) with human liver, the presence of free aflatoxin P_1, in addition to unchanged B_1, M_1, and two other unknown metabolites, was detected.

Krieger et al. (69) investigated further the conditions for the metabolism of aflatoxin B_1 in rhesus monkey liver. The hydroxylation was catalyzed by microsomal mixed function oxidases requiring NADPH and oxygen for maximum effect. Interestingly, the pH optimum for formation of aflatoxin Q_1 was 7.4 while for M_1 the optimum was 8.4.

Unfortunately, it is highly probable that the various hydroxylated aflatoxin B_1 metabolites mentioned thus far are the products of detoxification reactions as shown by the greatly reduced carcinogenic effect of those tested (144). They are less likely to point out the pathway to the activated intermediate, capable of attaching to proteins or nucleic acids or other important cellular macromolecules.

However, additional studies involving metabolism of aflatoxin B_1 by hamster, rat, and human liver microsomes, trapping the active metabolite through reaction with nucleic acids, followed by mild hydrolysis of the adduct, have yielded evidence for a new type of metabolite (34, 117, 118). In this case, what was isolated was a 2,3-dihydrodiol aflatoxin B_1 in which the olefinic double bond of the furan ring had been oxidized and

hydrolyzed (Fig. 17.2). Presumably, the active intermediate was the epoxide of aflatoxin B_1, analogous to the situation during the metabolism of polycyclic aromatic hydrocarbons. Such epoxides are fairly reactive, mutagenic, cause transformation of cells in culture, and have many attributes of the proximal carcinogen.

To summarize, there is no evidence at present that aflatoxins M_1, Q_1, P_1, and aflatoxicol detected from the in vitro studies represent an activation mechanism for aflatoxin B_1. They are probably also products of detoxification reactions. There is a greater likelihood that certain dihydrodiols, which have been identified only through trapping the intermediate, typify the actual activation pathway of aflatoxin B_1. Further investigations on the species specificity of this reaction are needed.

N-2-FLUORENYLACETAMIDE

N-2-Fluorenylacetamide (FAA) (2-acetylaminofluorene) was first proposed for use as a pesticide on tobacco, beans, and other crops instead of lead and arsenic compounds. When a thorough long-term toxicological study by Wilson et al. (141) revealed the presence of diverse types of tumors in the test animals, the use of FAA as

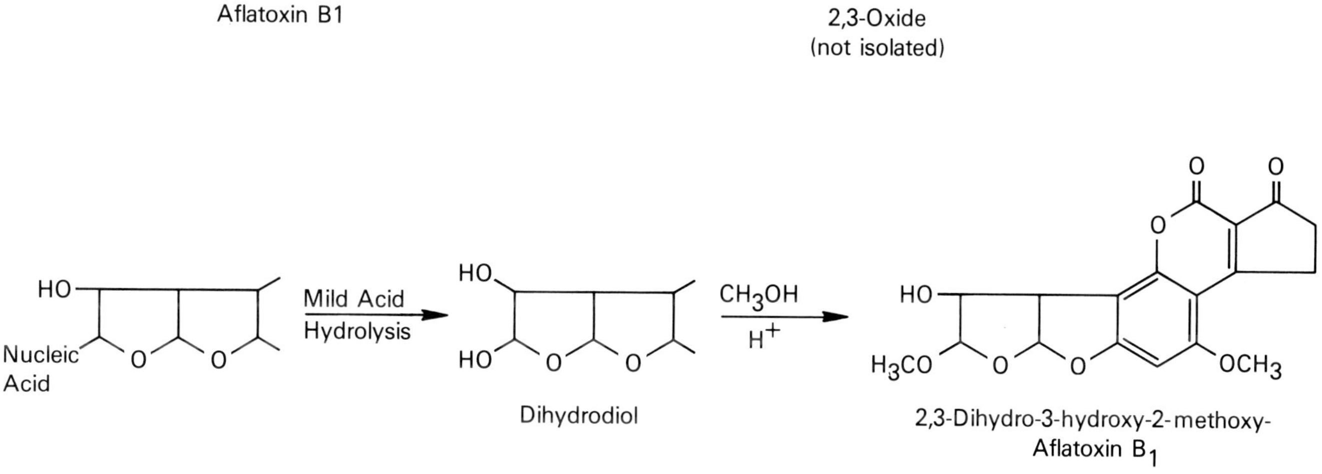

Figure 17.2. Metabolism of aflatoxin B_1 to form nucleic acid-bound derivatives.

a pesticide never came to pass (131). However, the early reports on FAA opened a new vista in cancer research. Unlike the polycyclic aromatic hydrocarbons which caused tumors at the site of application, FAA induced many types of tumors, in different organs, all remote from the point of entry. Various species of laboratory animals—mice, rats, hamsters, rabbits, cats, and dogs—were susceptible to the carcinogenic effects of FAA. Among other species, a carcinogenic action was noted in bats (48), chickens, and guppies (105), but rainbow trout, so susceptible to aflatoxin B_1, showed a minimal response (46). Bacteria were affected to some extent since FAA inhibited their growth, (8, 78). Cockroaches (*Periplanata americana*) were resistant to any carcinogenic action (116). However, FAA induced neoplastic growth or nodules in tobacco (*Nicotiana tabacum*) callus cultures, an *in vitro* system (6).

Later, it was found also that guinea pigs were resistant to the carcinogenic effect of FAA (12, 87); steppe lemmings (9), the X/Gf strain of mouse (35), and monkeys (29) were further recognized as belonging to the resistant group.

In vivo Studies

Initial efforts to study the metabolism of FAA, using isolation of metabolites from urine (7) and colorimetric techniques (90), indicated hydroxylation on the 7-position and deacetylation had occurred. However, definitive investigations were not possible until a good deal of background work on the synthesis of various hydroxylated derivatives of FAA and chromatographic methods to separate them had been developed (131, 136).

Examination of the chemical structure of FAA

(Fig. 17.3) shows that the ring positions most likely to be oxidized or hydroxylated would be the 7-, 5-, 3-, and 1-positions. Syntheses of these various hydroxy compounds and comparison with the metabolites of FAA excreted showed that 7-hydroxy-2-fluorenylacetamide (7-OH-FAA) and 5-OH-FAA were major metabolic products while 3-OH- and 1-OH-FAA were formed to a much lesser extent. In addition, at least in the rat, there were very small amounts of 8-OH-FAA and 6-OH-FAA. The corresponding deacetylated products were also excreted. However, the lower toxicity and lack of carcinogenic effect indicated that the ring hydroxylated derivatives of FAA were the result of detoxification reactions. The diversity of these products implied that several enzyme systems were probably involved (84). This premise was strengthened by the differences in the relative amounts of the detoxification products excreted in various species. Guinea pigs excreted largely 7-OH-FAA conjugates and only a trace of 5-OH-FAA. In rats, 5-OH-FAA often was more abundant than the 7-hydroxylated derivative. Small variations occurred in other species examined (Table 17.4).

However, a different type of hydroxylation, namely on the nitrogen atom, led to a substance, N-hydroxy-N-2-fluorenylacetamide (N-OH-FAA), which was both more toxic and carcinogenic than the parent FAA (88). In addition, N-OH-FAA could be activated by esterification to yield a strong electrophile (86). This moiety, in turn, reacted with model cellular constituents such as methionine, cysteine, guanosine, or deoxyguanosine, affording arylamidated products analogous to the material obtained from *in vivo* studies (86).

With techniques available for determining the

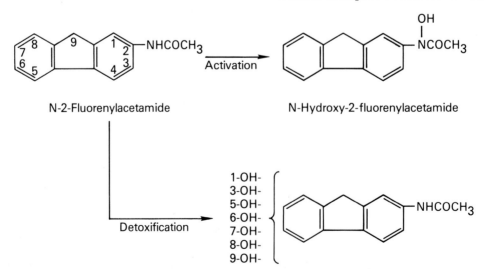

Figure 17.3. *N*-2-Fluorenylacetamide and metabolites.

Table 17.4
Hydroxylation of FAA by Various Species

Species	Carcinogenic Effect of FAA	N-Hydroxylation by Liver in vitro	Urinary Excretion of Major Metabolites (% of Dose)		
			N-OH-FAA	7-OH-FAA	5-OH-FAA
Cat	+	+	1.5	38	2.1
Chicken	+	+			
Dog	+	+	5.2	0.7	
Guinea pig	−	−		90	trace
Hamster	+	+	5–6	28–35	4–5
Human	?	+	4–14	25–30	1.5
Mastomys			2.3	8.7	3–7
Monkey	?	+	0.6–2.7	7.2–18	
Mouse	+	+	1.8–3.5	20	3.4
X/Gf strain mouse	−	?	1.5	25	2.0
Rabbit	+	+	13[a]	28[a]	0[a]
Rainbow trout	−	−		3.0	0.21
Rat	+	+	0.3–15[b]	12	7
Steppe lemming	−		0.8	22	0.9

[a] After one dose.
[b] After repeated administration.

metabolites of FAA, it became apparent that one reason for the resistance of guinea pigs to FAA was that they either did not form N-OH-FAA, or else rapidly converted any that was formed to a less effective substance (Table 17.4). Kiese and Wiedemann (65) reported that guinea pigs injected with large doses of FAA excreted 0.03% of the deacetylated form of N-OH-FAA, 2-fluorenylhydroxylamine, in the urine. In the rats, the hydroxylamine itself was largely excreted as 7-OH-FAA, 5-OH-FAA, and N-OH-FAA (135). However, when synthetic N-OH-FAA was administered to guinea pigs orally or subcutaneously, they developed tumors (87). In general, there was a fair correlation between N-hydroxylation in a given species and the susceptibility to tumor induction by FAA. One exception has been the X/Gf mouse, recently found to form and excrete N-OH-FAA, despite its resistance to the carcinogenicity of FAA (39). Another point of interest was that humans were also capable of N-hydroxylating FAA, although to a fairly variable extent (137).

The N-hydroxylation of FAA could be inhibited appreciably in rats by administration of other compounds such as 3-methylcholanthrene which induced the enzymes increasing detoxification of FAA, thereby decreasing the carcinogenic effect. However, in the hamster 3-methylcholanthrene along with FAA increased the amount of N-OH-FAA, with a subsequent heightened carcinogenic action (32). The mechanism of this difference between rats and hamsters is unknown at present. Nevertheless, N-hydroxylation itself did not provide an expla-

nation to some of the differences in carcinogenicity of FAA. Male rats, for example, were more susceptible to liver cancer than females even though female rats excreted more of the glucuronide of N-OH-FAA and the actual amount of circulating N-OH-FAA was similar. When studies were made on the further activation of N-OH-FAA by esterification with endogenous anions such as sulfate, phosphate, glucuronic acid, or acetate, it was found that sulfotransferase levels were higher in the livers of male rats than in females. Other species, i.e., hamsters, mice, rabbits, and guinea pigs, had lower levels than the rat, in rough agreement with the biological effect of FAA in the liver of each species (21, 22, 44, 58). (Table 17.5).

However, the sulfotransferase enzyme was lacking in certain tissues which were highly susceptible to the carcinogenicity of FAA, namely, mammary tissue and the sebaceous gland of the ear (Zymbal's gland) (57). Therefore, production of the 0-sulfate ester of N-OH-FAA through the sulfotransferase system may be important in rat liver. For other tissues, other mechanisms may hold.

Further investigation indicated phosphorylation of the N-hydroxy group yields a reactive intermediate (74, 77). Also, activation by acylation (75) or by N-0 acyltransfer (67) has been studied. The latter enzyme (arylhydroxamic acid acyltransferase) was present in many tissues of rats, hamsters, rabbits, guinea pigs, and monkeys, which is more akin to the effect of the parent carcinogen. The enzyme levels were very low or immeasurable, however, in dogs, mice,

Table 17.5
Species Variation in Enzymes Activating N-OH-FAA

Species	Acyltransferase[a] in Tissue			Liver Sulfotransferase[b]
	Liver	Small intestine	Colon	
Rat	1.13–2.12	0.26–0.39	0.27–0.42	56–59 male
(Sprague-Dawley male)				9–10 female
Mouse	0.02–0.05	0.02–0.03	0.01–0.02	1
Guinea pig	0.08–0.10	0.07–0.19	0.07–0.14	1
Hamster	2.13–3.40	0.96–1.31	0.26–0.38	1–2
Rabbit	2.08–5.21	0.16–1.61	0.02–0.11	5–6
Dog	0.01–0.02	0.01	0.01	
Monkey	0.51–0.61	<0.01–0.10	<0.01–0.01	
Goat	0.02	0.02		

[a] Measured as 2-fluorenamine bound to tRNA (nmol/20 mg tissue/20 min). Data from King and Olive (67).

[b] Expressed as μg of o-methylthio-FAA formed from N-OH-FAA. Data from DeBaun et al. (22).

and goats, even though mice and dogs do yield tumors on feeding FAA (Table 17.5).

Current separation techniques have enabled the isolation and identification of deoxyguanosine adducts of N-OH-FAA (36). As with other potent carcinogens, a radioimmunological assay for the adduct has been developed (99).

Summarizing the results of many experiments, it appears that N-hydroxylation is a necessary, but not sufficient, first step for the expression of the carcinogenicity of FAA. However, this reaction is not by itself the only one involved in the carcinogenic process. Further reactions, controlled by various enzyme systems, appear necessary.

In vitro Metabolism

The main reactions of FAA which have been studied using in vitro techniques include deacetylation-acetylation, hydroxylation, both on the nitrogen and ring carbons, and reduction of N-OH-FAA to FAA.

Deacetylation-Acetylation

Rat or mouse liver slices or homogenates converted FAA to the free amine in an air or oxygen atmosphere (42, 132). Peters and Gutmann (97) observed that the reverse reaction or acetylation of 2-fluorenamine to FAA or the diacetyl derivative also occurred in rat liver slices, probably involving acetyl coenzyme A. Deacylase activity was present in many rat tissues. An enzyme present in guinea pig liver microsomes was quite active in deacetylation of FAA to the free amine (59, 64). In liver cytosols from various species there was no correlation between rate of acetylation of 2-fluorenamine, in the presence of ace-

tyl coenzyme A, and susceptibility to the carcinogenicity of FAA (82). Hamster had the highest activity, followed by guinea pig, mouse, and rat while no acetylation occurred in dog liver cytosol.

More emphasis has been placed recently on deacetylation of N-OH-FAA; in this case, deacetylation has been accomplished by a soluble deacylase and also by a microsomal enzyme which was very high in guinea pig and hamster, lower in the rabbit, and least in the rat (55). Liver cytosols from the rabbit and then the hamster, in the presence of acetylcoenzyme A, were most active in N-acetylation of fluorenylhydroxylamine or 2-fluorenamine to the corresponding amides. Rat or mouse cytosol had much lower activity (76).

Hydroxylation

Hydroxylation of FAA by liver slices, or fortified liver homogenates from rats was investigated by Gutmann et al. (43), Peters and Gutmann (98), and Booth and Boyland (10). However, the chromatographic systems did not allow separation of the metabolites produced, and N-hydroxylation of FAA had not been discovered at that time. Liver cell fractions were investigated further by Seal and Gutmann (109) who found that liver from the hamster yielded the most active fractions, followed by the guinea pig, rat, rabbit, and fowl. The main ring hydroxylated metabolites of FAA were identified from the incubation mixtures.

After the discovery of N-hydroxylation of FAA in vivo, this observation was extended to in vitro systems. There have been several reviews covering this topic (56, 133, 134). Irving (55) reported that liver microsomes from ham-

Table 17.6
Varied Effects of *N*-Nitrosomethylurea in Different Species

Order	Species and Strain	Route	Dose Single	Dose Total	Tumor Sites	Reference
Primates:	Genus *Macaca* African green monkey	Oral	10–40 mg/kg	2.4–134 g	Squamous cell carcinomas of mouth, pharynx, esophagus, tongue	Adamson et al. (2)
	Cynomolgus Rhesus (*Macaca mulatta Rhesus*)					
Lagomorpha	Rabbit (*Oryctolagus cuniculus*)	Intravenous, monthly or biweekly	10–20 mg/kg body wt		Gliomas of brain, spinal cord tumors, intestinal carcinomas, hemangiosarcomas	Schreiber et al. (108)
	Rabbit	Intravenous, biweekly	10 mg/kg	660 mg	Brain, spinal cord, nerves	Stavrou (113)
Rodentia	Hamster, Chinese	Subcutaneous injection	2.5–9.7 mg/kg body wt	31.6–174.6 mg/kg	Injection site, fibrosarcomas	Reznik et al. (102)
	Hamster, European (*Cricetus cricetus*)	Subcutaneous, weekly	5.65–22.6 mg/kg		Fibrosarcomas, carcinomas, carcinosarcomas at injection site, forestomach papillomas	Mohr et al. (89)
	" "	Intravenous, weekly for 18 weeks	2.5–10 mg/kg	45–180 mg/kg	Heart, stomach, oral and nasal cavities, lymphatic system	Ketkar et al. (63)
	Hamster, Syrian (*Mesocricetus auratus*)	Intravenous	2.5–5 mg	7.5–12.5 mg	Odontogenic tumors, carcinomas of oral cavity	Herrold (50)
	" "	Intragastric, 2 times weekly for 4 months		32 mg	Odontogenic tumors, carcinomas of oral cavity	
	Hamster, Syrian (*Mesocricetus auratus*)	Cutaneous, 3 times weekly	0.35 mg	12.6 mg	Skin, papillomas, carcinomas at application site	Graffi & Hoffmann (37)
	" "	Subcutaneous, weekly	1.4–3.5 mg/kg		Injection site sarcomas, forestomach papillomas	Hass et al. (45)
	" "	Subcutaneous, weekly	0.5–1 mg	5–9 mg	Injection site sarcomas, forestomach, vagina, ovary	Herrold (49)
	" "	1% solution applied to tracheal epithelium 10 to 30 times	5 mg	50–150 mg	Carcinomas, papillomas and polyps of tachea and larynx	Yarita et al. (147)
	Rat, BD (*Rattus norvegicus*)	Intravenous injection	70–100 mg/kg (single dose)		Forestomach papillomas, sarcomas of kidney, carcinomas along digestive tract	Druckrey et al. (26)
	Rat, BD II	Intravenous injection, weekly	5 mg/kg	232 mg/kg	Brain tumors, nephroblastoma, uterine sarcoma, spinal cord	Druckrey et al (25)
	Rat BD	Oral, daily	4–8 mg/kg		Forestomach	Druckrey et al. (27)
	Rat, BUF/N	Intravenous, 3 month injections	50 mg/kg	150 mg/kg	Mammary (89% in 77 days)	Gullino et al. (41)
	Rat, F344	" "	"	"	Mammary (89% in 94 days)	"
	Rat, Sprague-Dawley	" "	"	"	Mammary (73% in 86 days)	"
	Rat, CD-Fischer	Intrarectal, 3 times weekly for 10 weeks	1–2.5 mg	30–75 mg	Large intestine, thymic lymphoma	Narisawa et al. (93)

Table 17.6—*continued*

Order	Species and Strain	Route	Dose Single	Dose Total	Tumor Sites	Reference
	Rat, Lewis	Intravenous, monthly	25 mg/kg		Mammary tumors (65% of females), brain (males)	Bots and Willigh (11)
	Rat, Sprague-Dawley, newborn	Intracerebral, single dose	0.05–1.6 mg		Fibrosarcoma of kidney, breast carcinoma	Kelly et al. (62)
	Rat, Wistar	Oral	90 mg/kg (at pH 4)		Odontoma in periodontal membrane	Ebling et al. (30)
	Rat, Wistar	Oral, to pregnant rat	5 mg/kg		Neuroblastoma on spinal cord (in offspring)	Brucher and Ermel (13)
	Rat, Wistar	Oral, 5 times weekly	4–8 mg/kg	758 mg/kg	Brain	Thomas and Sierra (121)
	Rat, Wistar (Porton)	Oral	90 mg/kg 7.2 mg single dose		Kidney, forestomach, small & large intestine, skin	Leaver et al. (72)
	Rat, Wistar/Lewis	Bladder instillation, 3 doses at biweekly intervals	1.5 mg	4.5 mg	Bladder carcinomas	Sporn et al. (112)
	Rat, Wistar	Bladder instillation, 4 doses on alternate weeks	1.5 mg	6 mg	Bladder carcinomas	Hicks and Wakefield (51)
	Rat, Wistar newborn	Intraperitoneal, single dose	50 mg/kg		Kidney, forestomach, small intestine, breast	Terracini and Testa (120)
	Rat, Wistar 5 weeks old	Intraperitoneal, single dose	50 mg/kg		Kidney, lymphoma, breast, intestine	Terracini and Testa (120)
	Rat, Wistar	Intraperitoneal injection, weekly	10 mg/kg	230 mg/kg	Local tumors, neurinoma	Thomas et al. (122)
	Rat, Wistar	Intravenous, single dose	70 mg/kg		Kidney, breast, lymphoma, lung, colon	Murthy et al. (91)
	Rat, Wistar	Cutaneous, 3 times weekly	1.75 mg	87.5 mg	Skin papillomas, basal cell & squamous cell carcinomas	Graffi and Hoffmann (37)
	Rat	Intraperitoneal injection after partial hepatectomy	45–90 mg/kg (single dose)		LIver, breast, lymphoma, kidney, intestine, injection site sarcomas	Craddock and Frei (18)
	Mouse BC3f F₁ newborn (*Mus musculus*)	Intraperitoneal, single dose	50 mg/kg		Lung, lymphoma, forestomach, liver	Terracini and Testa (120)
	Mouse BC3f F₁, 5 weeks old	Intraperitoneal, single dose	50 mg/kg		Forestomach, lymphoma, lung	
	Mouse XVII Bln and AB (*Mus musculus*)	Cutaneous	0.35 mg	12.6 mg	Skin papillomas,	Hoffmann and Graffi (52)
	Mouse XVII Bln, newborn	Cutaneous	50–100 mg/kg		Leukemia	Graffi and Hoffmann (38)
	Mouse, Ha/ICR Swiss (*Mus musculus*)	Intrarectal, single to 30 doses	0.06–1.5 mg	1.8–22.5 mg	Large intestine,	Narisawa et al. (93)
	Mouse, Swiss, newborn (*Mus musculus*)	Subcutaneous, single dose	50 mcg		Lymphoma	Terracini and Stramignoni (119)
	Mouse, randombred albino, newborn (*Mus musculus*)	Intracerebral Subcutaneous single dose	0.05–0.8 mg 0.05–0.2 mg		Leukemia, lung Leukemia, lung	Kelly et al. (62)
	Mouse, CDF₁ newborn	Intracerebral, single dose	0.1–0.5 mg		Leukemia, lung	Kelly et al. (62)
		Subcutaneous, single dose	0.1–0.2 mg		Leukemia, lung	
	Guinea pig (*Cavia porcellus*)	Oral (drinking water) 5 days weekly	0.4 g/kg body wt		Stomach, pancreas, ear duct	Druckrey et al. (28)
	Guinea pig, Strain 13	Intragastric	10 mg/kg body wt	135 mg (average)	Pancreas	Reddy et al. (100)
	Guinea pig, Strain 2 (*Cavia porcellus* 1976)	Intrarectal	79–89 mg		Large intestine	Narisawa et al. (92)

Table 17.6—*continued*

Order	Species and Strain	Route	Dose Single	Dose Total	Tumor Sites	Reference
Carnivora	Dog, mongrel (*Canis familiaris*)	Intravenous	20 mg/kg	3.3–4.3 g	Brain, spleen, lungs, heart	Warzok *et al.* (129)
	Dog, boxer (*Canis familiaris*)	5 mg/kg weekly for 36 weeks, intravenous	5 mg/kg	180 mg/kg	Malignant neurinoma (small intestine, heart, stomach, colon), sarcoma (small intestine), hemangiosarcoma (spleen, heart), hemangioma (skin), malignant lymphoma (liver, spleen)	Denlinger *et al.* (23)
Artiodactyla Suidae	Pig, miniature, Hanford strain (*Sus scrofa*)	Oral	10 mg/kg	55–117 g	Stomach, mostly multiple	Stavrou *et al.* (114)

sters, dogs, rabbits, chickens, and cats, in decreasing order, formed N-OH-FAA from FAA in the presence of a NADPH generating system. When NADPH was added, N-OH-FAA was also formed by microsomes from rat and mouse liver. Guinea pig or human liver microsomes did not produce N-OH-FAA from FAA in either system (Table 17.4). However, Enomoto and Sato (31) later found variable responses in human liver microsomes; those from patients with liver disease had undetectable levels of N-OH-FAA while relatively high amounts were formed by other samples. Species variations in the ring- and N-hydroxylation of FAA *in vitro* were confirmed by Lotlikar *et al.* (81). Enzyme induction by pretreatment with 3-methylcholanthrene was studied concomitantly.

N-Hydroxylation of FAA with guinea pig liver microsomes was not detected in either of these experiments. However, Kiese *et al.* (66) reported that 2-fluorenamine was converted to fluorenylhydroxylamine by guinea pig liver microsomes. The hydroxylamine was not detected as such but was oxidized to 2-nitrosofluorene which could be determined spectrophotometrically. The discrepancy between these reports has not been resolved.

Baetcke *et al.* (4) recently claimed that modifications in the amount of microsomal protein used and the buffer system enhanced the metabolism of FAA *in vitro*. As much as 30% of added FAA was converted to N-OH-FAA by mouse liver microsomes, a much higher level than in any previous studies.

The question of what enzyme systems are involved in hydroxylation of FAA *in vitro* has been investigated through differential induction and inhibition by compounds such as 3-methyl-cholanthrene, phenobarbital, 3-aminotriazole, and carbon monoxide.

On the basis of such experiments, it was concluded that hydroxylation of FAA was accomplished by a family of microsomal enzymes (83, 84). Because carbon monoxide treatment had the least effect on N-hydroxylation in hamster or rat liver microsomes, it was decided that cytochrome P-450 was not involved in the N-hydroxylation reaction. However, later work using higher levels of CO indicated that a cytochrome P-450 dependent mixed function oxidase may be responsible (123, 124). In any event, the enzyme apparently was not a mixed-function amine oxidase such as catalyzes the oxidation of primary, secondary, and tertiary amines (79). Further studies in this area with purification of the enzymes may help to elucidate some of the differences in species specificity.

Reduction

A soluble fraction of liver reduced N-OH-FAA to FAA with activity decreasing from hamster, rabbit, rat, mouse, and guinea pig in that order (80). Deacetylation of part of the FAA produced to 2-fluorenamine also occurred (40, 80). Of interest is the fact that the bacteria found in the lower intestinal tract of mammals also reduce N-OH-FAA to FAA (140).

VARIED EFFECTS OF N-NITROSOMETHYLUREA IN DIFFERENT SPECIES

N-Nitroso-N-methylurea was selected as an example of a carcinogen which has been tested

Table 17.7
Species-dependent toxicity and carcinogenicity of melphalan (NSC-8806)

Species	Toxicity		Carcinogenicity	Reference
	Level	Route		
Man (*Homo sapiens*)	$TD_{10} = 67$ mg/kg	Oral	+ (Myeloma; leukemia)	Kyle *et al.* (70)
Rhesus monkey (*Macaca mulatta*)	Fatal = 0.43 mg/kg (daily)	i.v.		Schmidt *et al.* (107)
	$\dfrac{Fatal}{4} = 0.11$ mg/kg (daily)	i.v.		
Dog (*Canis familiaris*)	Fatal = 0.43 mg /kg (daily)	i.v.		Schmidt *et al.* (107)
	$\dfrac{Fatal}{4} = 0.11$ mg/kg (daily)	i.v.		
Cat (*Felis catus*)	$LD_{10} = 33.3$ $\mu M/kg$ (10.4 mg/kg)	i.v.		White (139)
Rabbit (*Ochotona* sp.) (Family: Leporidae)	$LD_{10} = 33.3$ $\mu M/kg$ (10.4 mg/kg)	i.v.		White (139)
Guinea pig (*Cavia porcellus*)	$LD_{10} = 52.9$–66.3 $\mu M/kg$	Oral		White (139)
Rat (*Rattus norvegicus*) Holtzman	$LD_{10} = 7.8$ $\mu M/kg$	i.p.		Schmidt *et al.* (107)
	$LD_{10} = 7.6$ $\mu M/kg$	i.v.		Schmidt *et al.* (107)
	$LD_{10} = 13$ $\mu M/kg$	Oral		Schmidt *et al.* (107)
Fischer	$LD_{10} = 4.4$ $\mu M/kg$	i.p.		Schmidt *et al.* (107)
	$LD_{10} = 9.8$ $\mu M/kg$	Oral		
Sprague-Dawley (CD)		i.p.	+ Peritoneal sarcomas	Weisburger *et al.* (138)
Mouse (*Mus musculus*) Rolfsmeyer	$LD_{10} = 15$ $\mu M/kg$	i.p.		Schmidt *et al.* (107)
	$LD_{10} = 21$ $\mu M/kg$	Oral		Schmidt *et al.* (107)
LAF$_1$ (male)	15 $\mu M/kg$	i.p.		Schmidt (107)
(female)	25 $\mu M/kg$	i.p.		Schmidt (107)
BDF (male)	15 $\mu M/kg$	i.p.		Schmidt (107)
(female)	15 $\mu M/kg$	i.p.		Schmidt (107)
(female)	21 $\mu M/kg$	oral		Schmidt (107)
S Strain		Skin painting + croton oil	+ Skin tumors	Salaman and Roe (104)
A/J		i.p.	+ Lung adenomas	Shimkin *et al.* (111)
Swiss		i.p.	+ Lung tumors, lymphosarcomas	Weisburger *et al.* (138)

in many species and by different routes of administration. This compound has a multifaceted effect; it induces tumors at the site of application as well as at many remote sites. By proper selection of the animal model, dosage, and route of administration, one can induce many types of tumors which serve as excellent models for human cancers. Thus, intravenous injection in female rats can yield a high percentage of mammary tumors which are better models of human breast cancer than those induced by 7,12-dimethylbenz[a]anthracene. Similarly, instillation into the bladder or colon leads to tumors of these tissues in a relatively short period. In addition, nitrosomethylurea has a definite transplacental effect and induces tumors of the nervous system in the offspring of exposed pregnant animals. Many N-nitroso compounds are not effective carcinogens when painted on the skin of rodents, but nitrosomethylurea is a potent carcinogen in this respect. The propensity of this compound and its analogs or derivatives to affect the nervous system indicates that nitrosoureas can pass through the blood-brain barrier. Thus, besides its utility in research on chemical carcinogenesis, nitrosomethylurea serves as a model for many effective drugs employed for treatment of brain neoplasms (Table 17.6).

CARCINOSTATIC COMPOUNDS FROM A SPECIES-SPECIFIC POINT OF VIEW SHOWN IN THE CASE OF MELPHALAN

Carcinostatic compounds, or antineoplastic agents, are chemical compounds of different molecular structure which show an inhibitory effect on the growth of tumors. They are, therefore, the basic tool of chemotherapy. It is the purpose of this section to show species-specific variations to selected compounds (Table 17.7).

These compounds have been found naturally in unicellular procaryotic organisms (bacteria), in unicellular eucaryotic organisms as protozoa, in fungi, plants, and invertebrate animals (eumetazoa) if occurring naturally; they also have been prepared synthetically.

Antineoplastic drugs may act as a factor, lowering the risk of malignant growth after the onset of premalignant stages, such as papillomas. This is understandable if it is realized that very rarely a regression or self-healing, even of malignant neoplasms, has been observed. Such a group of compounds, working in this manner, at least in the rat, are the synthetic retinoids, and especially 13-cis-retinoic acid. The majority of antineoplastic drugs work by an inhibition of the growth of malignant cells and tissues.

Antineoplastic drugs have been tested on the malignant neoplasms of different sites, different histogenesis, in various species. The groups of organisms tested have included viruses, bacteria, protozoans, invertebrates, and especially vertebrates. The main groups of tested vertebrates have been the fishes, amphibia, birds, and the

mammals, of which especially the primates, carnivora, lagomorpha, rodentia, perissodactyla, and artiodactyla have been tested or treated with chemotherapeutic agents. Concerning primates, human tissues in organ and/or tissue culture, implanted human tumors, cell cultures of human neoplasms, as the HeLa cells, or as treatment in patients on one hand or nonhuman primates, monkeys and apes, have been investigated.

Concerning carnivora, main emphasis has been given to the investigation and treatment of cat and dog, largely from the point of view of pet treatment; some investigations on zoo species, such as lions, may exist. With regard to lagomorpha, the rabbit is the species of focus, especially as an experimental animal.

The most important order of mammals for research with carcinostatic compounds have been and are the rodents, with the following sequence of genera—mouse, rat, hamster, and guinea pig.

In perissodactyla, the horse is the focal point as a domesticated animal and in the artiodactyla the miniature pig as research animal together with cattle, goats, sheep, and pigs as domesticated animals.

Acknowledgment. The author appreciates the dedicated secretarial assistance of Mrs. Frances M. Williams.

References

1. Adamson, R., Correa, P., and Dalgard, D. (1973): Occurrence of a primary liver carcinoma in a rhesus monkey fed aflatoxin B₁. *J. Natl. Cancer Inst.*, 50:549–553.
2. Adamson, R. H., Krolikowski, F. J., Correa, P., Sieber, S. M., and Dalgard, D. W. (1977): Carcinogenicity of 1-methyl-1-nitrosourea (NMU) in nonhuman primates. *J. Natl. Cancer Inst.*, 59:415–422.
3. Allcroft, R. (1969): Aflatoxicosis in farm animals. In *Aflatoxin, Scientific Background, Control and Implications* pp. 237–264, edited by L. A. Goldblatt. Academic Press, New York.
4. Baetcke, K. P., Gough, B. J., and Shellenberger, T. E. (1974): Modified system *in vitro* for the metabolism of 2-acetylaminofluorene. *Biochem. Pharmacol.*, 23:1745–1752.
5. Bassir, O., and Emafo, P. O. (1970): Oxidative metabolism of aflatoxin B₁ by mammalian liver slices and microsomes. *Biochem. Pharmacol.*, 19:1681–1687.
6. Bednar, T. W., and Linsmaier-Bednar, E. M. (1972): Induction of plant tissue neoplasms *in vitro* by substituted fluorenes. *Chem. Biol. Interact.*, 4:233–238.
7. Bielschowsky, F. (1945): A metabolite of 2-acetamidofluorene. *Biochem. J.*, 39:287–289.
8. Bielschowsky, F., and Green, H. N. (1942): 2-Aminofluorene as growth inhibitor for bacteria and rats. *Nature*, 149:526–527.
9. Bolonina, N. I. (1965): On resistance of the steppe lemming to some chemical carcinogenic agents and tumorigenic viruses. *Vopr. Onkol.*, 11:80–83.
10. Booth, J., and Boyland, E. (1957): The biochemistry of aromatic amines. 3. Enzymic hydroxylation by rat-liver microsomes. *Biochem. J.*, 66:73–78.
11. Bots, G. T. A., and Willighagen, R. G. J. (1975): Tumours in the mammary gland induced in Lewis rats by intravenous methylnitrosourea. *Br. J. Cancer*, 31:372–374.
12. Breidenbach, A. W., and Argus, M. F. (1956): Attempted tumor induction in guinea pigs. *Q. J. Florida Acad. Sci.*, 19:68–70.
13. Brucher, J. M., and Ermel, A. E. (1974): Central neuroblastoma induced by transplacental administration of methylnitrosourea in Wistar-R rats. *J. Neurol.*, 208:1–16.
14. Büchi, G. H., Müller, P. M., Roebuck, B. D., and Wogan, G. N. (1974): Aflatoxin Q₁: A major metabolite of aflatoxin B₁ produced by human liver. *Res. Commun. Chem. Pathol. Pharmacol.*, 8:585–592.
15. Butler, W. H. (1969): Aflatoxicosis in laboratory animals. In *Aflatoxin.*

Scientific Background, Control and Implications, pp. 223–236, edited by L. A. Goldblatt. Academic Press, New York.

16. Campbell, T. C., Caedo, J. P., Jr., Bulatao-Jayme, L., Salamat, L., and Engel, R. W. (1970): Aflatoxin M₁ in human urine. *Nature*, 227:403–404.

17. Campbell, T. C., Sinnhuber, R. O., Lee, D. J., Wales, J. H., and Salamat, L. (1974): Hepatocarcinogenic material in urine specimens from humans consuming aflatoxin. *J. Natl. Cancer Inst.*, 52:1647–1649.

18. Craddock, V. M., and Frei, J. V. (1974): Induction of liver cell adenomata in the rat by a single treatment with N-methyl-nitrosourea given at various times after partial hepatectomy. *Br. J. Cancer*, 30:503–511.

19. Dalezios, J. I., and Wogan, G. N. (1972): Metabolism of aflatoxin B₁ in rhesus monkeys. *Cancer Res.*, 32:2297–2303.

20. Dalezios, J. I., Hsieh, D. P. H., and Wogan, G. N. (1973): Excretion and metabolism of orally administered aflatoxin B₁ by rhesus monkeys. *Food Cosmet. Toxicol.*, 11:605–616.

21. DeBaun, J. R., Miller, E. C., and Miller, J. A. (1970): N-Hydroxy-2-acetylaminofluorene sulfotransferase: its probable role in carcinogenesis and in protein-(methion-S-yl) binding in rat liver. *Cancer Res.*, 30:577–595.

22. DeBaun, J. R., Rowley, J. Y., Miller, E. C., and Miller, J. A. (1968): Sulfotransferase activation of N-hydroxy-2-acetylaminofluorene in rodent livers susceptible and resistant to this carcinogen. *Proc. Soc. Exp. Biol. Med.*, 129:268–273.

23. Denlinger, R. H., Koestner, A., and Swenberg, J. A. (1978): Neoplasms in purebred boxer dogs following long-term administration of N-methyl-N-nitrosourea. *Cancer Res.*, 38:1711–1717.

24. Detroy, R. W., Lillehoj, E. B., and Ciegler, A. (1971): Aflatoxin and related compounds. In *Microbial Toxins. Fungal Toxins*, Vol. VI, pp. 3–178, edited by A. Ciegler, S. Kadis, and S. J. Ajl, Academic Press, New York.

25. Druckrey, H., Ivankovic, S., and Preussmann, R. (1964): Selektive Erzeugung von Hirntumoren bei Ratten durch Methylnitrosoharnstoff. *Naturwissenschaften*, 51:144.

26. Druckrey, H., Steinhoff, D., Preussmann, R., and Ivankovic, S. (1964): Erzeugung von Krebs durch eine einmalige Dosis von Methylnitroso-Harnstoff und verschiedenen Dialkylnitrosaminen an Ratten. *Z. Krebsforsch.*, 66:1–10.

27. Druckrey, H., Preussmann, R., Ivankovic, S., and Schmähl, D. (1967): Organotrope carcinogene Wirkungen bei 65 verschiedenen N-Nitroso-Verbindungen an BD-Ratten. *Z. Krebsforsch.*, 69:103–201.

28. Druckrey, H., Ivankovic, S., Bücheler, J., Preussmann, R., and Thomas, C. (1968): Erzeugung von Magen- und Pankreas-Krebs beim Meerschweinchen durch Methylnitroso-Harnstoff und -urethan. *Z. Krebsforsch.*, 72:162–182.

29. Dyer, H. M., Kelly, M. G., and O'Gara, R. W. (1966): Lack of carcinogenic activity and metabolic fate of fluorenylacetamide in monkeys. *J. Natl. Cancer Inst.*, 36:305–322.

30. Ebling, H., Barbachan, J. J. D., do Valle, J. G. C., and De Oliveira, L. Y. (1973): N-Methyl-N-nitrosourea-induced odontogenic neoplasms in rats. *J. Dental Res.*, 52:177.

31. Enomoto, M., and Sato, K. (1967): N-Hydroxylation of the carcinogen 2-acetylaminofluorene by human liver tissue *in vitro*. *Life Sci.*, 6:881–887.

32. Enomoto, M., Miyake, M., and Sato, K. (1968): Carcinogenicity in the hamster of simultaneously administered 2-acetamidofluorene and 3-methylcholanthrene. *Gann*, 59:177–186.

33. Essigmann, J. M., Croy, R. G., Nadzan, A. M., Busby, W. F., Jr., Reinhold, V. N., Büchi, G. H., and Wogan, G. N. (1977): Structural identification of the major DNA adduct formed by aflatoxin B₁ *in vitro*. *Proc. Natl. Acad. Sci.*, 74:1870–1874.

34. Garner, R. C. (1973): Chemical evidence for the formation of a reactive aflatoxin B₁ metabolite, by hamster liver microsomes. *F.E.B.S. Lett.*, 36:261–264.

35. Goldfeder, A. (1974): Characterization of X/Gf mice with respect to their resistance to oncogenesis. *Trans. N. Y. Acad. Sci.*, 36:59–77.

36. Goodman, J. I. (1976): Separation of the products of the reaction of deoxyguanosine with N-acetoxy-2-acetylaminofluorene by high pressure liquid chromatography. *Anal. Biochem.*, 70:203–207.

37. Graffi, A. and Hoffmann, F. (1966): Starke kanzerogene Wirkung von N-Methyl-N-Nitroso-Harnstoff auf die Hamster- und Rattenhaut im Tropfungsversuch. *Arch. Geschwulstforsch.*, 28:234–248.

38. Graffi, A., and Hoffmann, F. (1966): Starke leukämogene Wirkung von N-Methyl-nitroso-Harnstoff bei der Maus nach einmaliger Applikation an neugeborenen Tieren. *Acta Biol. Med. Ger.*, 17:K33–K35.

39. Grantham, P. H., Mohan, L. C., and Weisburger, E. K. (1976): Metabolism of N-2-fluorenylacetamide in X/Gf strain mice: Lack of a correlation between biochemical interaction and carcinogenicity. *J. Natl. Cancer Inst.*, 56:649–651.

40. Grantham, P. H., Weisburger, E. K., and Weisburger, J. H. (1965): Dehydroxylation and deacetylation of N-hydroxy-N-2-fluorenylacetamide by rat liver and brain homogenates. *Biochim. Biophys. Acta*, 107:414–424.

41. Gullino, P. M., Pettigrew, H. M., and Grantham, F. H. (1975): N-Nitrosomethylurea as mammary gland carcinogen in rats. *J. Natl. Cancer Inst.*, 54:401–414.

42. Gutmann, H. R., and Peters, J. H. (1954): Studies on the action of rat liver on 2-acetylaminofluorene. *J. Biol. Chem.*, 211:63–74.

43. Gutmann, H. R., Peters, J. H., and Burtle, J. G. (1956): The metabolism *in vitro* of fluorene derivatives by rat liver: hydroxylation and protein binding. *J. Biol. Chem.*, 222:373–386.

44. Gutmann, H. R., Malejka-Giganti, D., Barry, E. J., and Rydell, R. E. (1972): On the correlation between the hepatocarcinogenicity of the carcinogen, N-2-fluorenylacetamide, and its metabolic activation by the rat. *Cancer Res.*, 32:1554–1561.

45. Haas, H., Mohr, U., and Krüger, F. W. (1973): Comparative studies with different doses of N-nitrosomorpholine, N-nitrosopiperidine, N-nitrosomethylurea, and dimethylnitrosamine in Syrian golden hamsters. *J. Natl. Cancer Inst.*, 51:1295–1301.

46. Halver, J. (1965): Hepatomas in fish. In *Primary Hepatoma*, pp. 103–112, edited by W. J. Burdette. University of Utah Press, Salt Lake City, Utah.

47. Halver, J. E. (1969): Aflatoxicosis and trout hepatoma. In *Aflatoxin. Scientific Background, Control and Implications.* pp. 265–306, edited by L. A. Goldblatt. Academic Press, New York.

48. Heldt, L. W., Rowe, N. H., and Spain, J. D. (1974): Response at fifteen weeks of the big brown bat (*Eptesicus fuscus*) to intraperitoneal injections of N-2-acetylaminofluorene. *Cancer Res.*, 34:2807–2809.

49. Herrold, K. M. (1966): Carcinogenic effect of N-methyl-N-nitrosourea administered subcutaneously to Syrian hamsters. *J. Pathol. Bacteriol.*, 92:35–41.

50. Herrold, K. M. (1968): Odontogenic tumors and epidermoid carcinomas of the oral cavity. An experimental study in Syrian hamsters. *Oral Surg.*, 25:262–272.

51. Hicks, R. M., and Wakefield, J. S. J. (1972): Rapid induction of bladder cancer in rats with N-methyl-N-nitrosourea. I. Histology. *Chem. Biol. Interact.*, 5:139–152.

52. Hoffmann, F., and Graffi, A. (1966): Histologische Veränderungen an der Mausehaut während der kanzerogenen Einwirkung von N-Methyl-N-nitroso-Harnstoff. *Arch. Geschwulstforsch.*, 28:89–102.

53. Holder, G., Yagi, H., Dansette, P., Jerina, D. M., Levin, W., Lu, A. Y. H., and Conney, A. H. (1974): Effects of inducers and epoxide hydrase on the metabolism of benzo[a]pyrene by liver microsomes and a reconstituted system: Analysis by high pressure liquid chromatography. *Proc. Natl. Acad. Sci. U.S.A.*, 71:4356–4360.

54. Huberman, E., Sachs, L., Yang, S. K., and Gelboin, H. V. (1976): Identification of mutagenic metabolites of benzo[a]pyrene in mammalian cells. *Proc. Natl. Acad. Sci. U.S.A.*, 73:607–611.

55. Irving, C. C. (1964): Enzymatic N-hydroxylation of the carcinogen 2-acetylaminofluorene and the metabolism of N-hydroxy-2-acetylaminofluorene-9-¹⁴C *in vitro*. *J. Biol. Chem.*, 239:1589–1591.

56. Irving, C. C. (1970): Conjugates of N-hydroxy compounds. In *Metabolic Conjugation and Metabolic Hydrolysis*, Vol. I, pp. 53–119, edited by W. H. Fishman. Academic Press, New York.

57. Irving, C. C., Janss, D. H., and Russell, L. T. (1971): Lack of N-hydroxy-2-acetylaminofluorene sulfotransferase activity in the mammary gland and Zymbal's gland of the rat. *Cancer Res.*, 31:387–391.

58. Jackson, C. D., and Irving, C. C. (1972): Sex differences in cell proliferation and N-hydroxy-2-acetylaminofluorene sulfotransferase levels in rat liver during 2-acetylaminofluorene administration. *Cancer Res.*, 32:1590–1594.

59. Järvinen, M., Santti, R. S. S., and Hopsu-Havu, V. K. (1971): Partial purification and characterization of two enzymes from guinea-pig liver microsomes that hydrolyze carcinogenic amides 2-acetylaminofluorene and N-hydroxy-2-acetylaminofluorene. *Biochem. Pharmacol.*, 20:2971–2982.

60. Jeffrey, A. M., Jennette, K. W., Blobstein, S. H., Weinstein, I. B., Beland, F. A., Harvey, R. G., Kasai, H., Miura, I., and Nakanishi, K. (1976): Benzo[a]pyrene-nucleic acid derivative found *in vivo*: structure of a benzo[a]pyrenetetrahydrodiol epoxide-guanosine adduct. *J. Am. Chem. Soc.*, 98:5714–5715.

61. Kapitulnik, J., Wislocki, P. G., Levin, W., Yagi, H., Jerina, D. M., and Conney, A. H. (1978): Tumorigenicity studies with diol-epoxides of benzo[a]pyrene which indicate that (±)-trans-7, 8-dihydroxy-9,10-epoxy-7,8,9,10-tetrahydrobenzo[a]pyrene is an ultimate carcinogen in newborn mice. *Cancer Res.*, 38:354–358.

62. Kelly, M. G., O'Gara, R. W., Yancey, S. T., and Botkin, C. (1968): Carcinogenicity of 1-methyl-1-nitrosourea in newborn mice and rats. *J. Natl. Cancer Inst.*, 41:619–626.

63. Ketkar, M., Reznik, G., Haas, H., Hilfrich, J., and Mohr, U. (1977): Tumors of the heart and stomach induced in European hamsters by intravenous administration of N-methyl-N-nitrosourea. *J. Natl. Cancer Inst.*, 58:1695–1699.

64. Kiese, M., and Renner, G. (1966): The hydrolysis of acetanilide and some of its derivatives by enzymes in the microsomal and soluble fraction prepared from livers of various species. *Arch. Exp. Pathol. Pharmak.*, 252:480–500.

65. Kiese, M., and Wiedemann, I. (1966): Excretion of N-hydroxy-2-aminofluorene by guinea pigs injected with 2-acetylaminofluorene. *Biochem. Pharmacol.*, 15:1882–1885.

66. Kiese, M., Renner, G., and Wiedemann, I. (1966): N-hydroxylation of 2-aminofluorene in the guinea pig and by guinea pig liver microsomes *in vitro*. *Arch. Exp. Pathol. Pharmak.*, 252:418–423.

67. King, C. M., and Olive, C. W. (1975): Comparative effects of strain, species, and sex on the acyltransferase- and sulfotransferase-catalyzed activations of N-hydroxy-N-2-fluorenylacetamide. *Cancer Res.*, 35:906–912.

68. Koes, M. T., Forrester, L. J., and Brown, H. D. 81973): Metabolism of aflatoxin B₁ by the guinea pig. *Food Cosmet. Toxiol.*, 11:463–466.

69. Krieger, R. I., Salhab, A. S., Dalezios, J. I., and Hsieh, D. P. H. (1975): Aflatoxin B₁ hydroxylation by hepatic microsomal preparations from the rhesus monkey. *Food Cosmet. Toxicol.*, 13:211–219.

70. Kyle, R. A., Pierre, R. V., and Bayrd, E. D. (1975): Multiple myeloma and acute leukemia associated with alkylating agents. *Arch. Intern. Med.*, 135:185–192.

71. Langone, J. J., and Van Vunakis, H. (1976): Aflatoxin B₁ specific antibodies and their use in radioimmunoassay. *J. Natl. Cancer Inst.*, 56:591–595.

72. Leaver, D. D., Swann, P. F., and Magee, P. N. (1969): The induction of tumours in the rat by a single oral dose of N-nitrosomethylurea. *Br. J. Cancer*, 23:177–187.

73. Lin, J.-K., Miller, J. A., and Miller, E. C. (1977): 2,3-Dihydro-2-(guan-7-yl)-3-hydroxy-aflatoxin B₁, a major acid hydrolysis product of aflatoxin B₁-DNA or -ribosomal RNA adducts formed in hepatic microsome-mediated reactions and in rat liver *in vivo*. *Cancer Res.*, 37:4430–4438.

74. Lotlikar, P. D., and Luha, L. (1971): Acetylation of carcinogenic hydroxamic acids by carbamoyl phosphate to form reactive esters. *Biochem. J.*, 124:69–74.

75. Lotlikar, P. D., and Luha, L. (1971): Acetylation of the carcinogen N-hydroxy-2-acetylaminofluorene by acetyl coenzyme A to form a reactive ester. *Mol. Pharmacol.*, 7:381–388.

76. Lotlikar, P. D., and Luha, L. (1971): Enzymic N-acetylation of N-hydroxy-2-aminofluorene by liver cytosol from various species. *Biochem. J.*, 123:287–289.

77. Lotlikar, P. D., and Wasserman, M. B. (1970): Reactive phosphate ester of the carcinogen 2-(N-hydroxy) acetamidofluorene. *Biochem. J.*, 120:661–665.

78. Lotlikar, P. D., Fukuda, S., and Yamamoto, N. (1972): Effects of the carcinogen 2-acetylaminofluorene and its derivatives on bacteria and bacteriophages. *Mol. Pharmacol.*, 8:645–650.

79. Lotlikar, P. D., Wertman, K., and Luha, L. (1973): Role of mixed-function amine oxidase in N-hydroxylation of 2-acetamidofluorene by hamster liver microsomal preparations. *Biochem. J.*, 136:1137–1140.

80. Lotlikar, P. D., Miller, E. C., Miller, J. A., and Margreth, A. (1965): The enzymatic reduction of the N-hydroxy derivative of 2-acetylaminofluorene and related carcinogens by tissue preparations. *Cancer Res.*, 25:1743–1752.

81. Lotlikar, P. D., Enomoto, M., Miller, J. A., and Miller, E. C. (1967): Species variations in the N- and ring-hydroxylation of 2-acetylaminofluorene and effects of 3-methylcholanthrene pretreatment. *Proc. Soc. Exp. Biol. Med.*, 125:341–346.

82. Lower, G. M., Jr., and Bryan, G. T. (1973): Enzymatic N-acetylation of carcinogenic aromatic amines by liver cytosol of species displaying different organ susceptibilities. *Biochem. Pharmacol.*, 22:1581–1588.

83. Matsushima, T., and Weisburger, J. H. (1972): Effect of carbon monoxide or of 3-aminotriazole on C- and N-hydroxylation of the carcinogen N-2-fluorenylacetamide by liver microsomes of hamsters pretreated with 3-methylcholanthrene. *Xenobiotica*, 2:423–430.

84. Matsushima, T. Grantham, P. H., Weisburger, E. K., and Weisburger, J. H. (1972): Phenobarbital-mediated increase in ring- and N-hydroxylation of the carcinogen N-2-fluorenylacetamide and decrease in amounts bound to liver deoxyribonucleic acid. *Biochem. Pharmacol.*, 21:2043–2051.

85. Merrill, A. H., Jr., and Campbell, T. C. (1974): Preliminary study of *in vitro* aflatoxin B₁ metabolism by human liver. *Toxicol. Appl. Pharmacol.*, 27:210–213.

86. Miller, J. A., and Miller, E. C. (1969): The metabolic activation of carcinogenic aromatic amines and amides. *Prog. Exp. Tumor Res.*, 11:273–301.

87. Miller, E. C., Miller, J. A., and Enomoto, M. (1964): The comparative carcinogenicities of 2-acetylaminofluorene and its N-hydroxy metabolite in mice, hamsters, and guinea pigs. *Cancer Res.*, 24:2018–2032.

88. Miller, E. C., Miller, J. A., and Hartmann, H. A. (1961): N-Hydroxy-2-acetylaminofluorene: a metabolite of 2-acetylaminofluorene with increased activity in the rat. *Cancer. Res.*, 21:815–824.

89. Mohr, U., Haas, H., and Hilfrich, J. (1974): The carcinogenic effects of dimethylnitrosamine and nitrosomethylurea in European hamsters (*Cricetus cricetus* L.). *Br. J. Cancer*, 29:359–364.

90. Morris, H. P., and Westfall, B. B. (1950): Some studies of the excretion of diazotizable material after feeding 2-acetylaminofluorene to rats. *Cancer Res.*, 10:506–509.

91. Murthy, A. S. K., Vawter, G. F., and Bhaktaviziam, A. (1973): Neoplasms in Wistar rats after an N-methyl-N-nitrosourea injection. *Arch. Pathol.*, 96:53–57.

92. Narisawa, T., Wong, C.-Q. and Weisburger, J. H. (1975): Induction of carcinoma of the large intestine in guinea pigs by intrarectal instillation of N-methyl-N-nitrosourea. *J. Natl. Cancer Inst.*, 54:785–787.

93. Narisawa, T., Wong, C.-Q., Maronpot, R. R., and Weisburger, J. H. (1976): Large bowel carcinogenesis in mice and rats by several intrarectal doses of methylnitrosourea and negative effect of nitrite plus methylurea. *Cancer Res.*, 36:505–510.

94. Patterson, D. S. P., and Allcroft, R. (1970): Metabolism of aflatoxin in susceptible and resistant animal species. *Food Cosmet. Toxicol.*, 8:43–53.

95. Patterson, D. S. P., and Roberts, B. A. (1970): The formation of aflatoxins B₂ₐ and G₂ₐ and their degradation products during the *in vitro* detoxification of aflatoxin by livers of certain avian and mammalian species. *Food Cosmet. Toxicol.*, 8:527–538.

96. Patterson, D. S. P., and Roberts, B. A. (1971): The *in vitro* reduction of aflatoxins B₁ and B₂ by soluble avian liver enzymes. *Food Cosmet. Toxicol.*, 9:829–837.

97. Peters, J. H., and Gutmann, H. R. (1955): The acetylation of 2-aminofluorene and the deacetylation and concurrent reacetylation of 2-acetylaminofluorene by rat liver slices. *J. Biol. Chem.*, 216:713–726.

98. Peters, J. H., and Gutmann, H. R. (1956): Stimulation of hydroxylation and protein binding of the carcinogen 2-acetylaminofluorene in rat liver homogenates. *Arch. Biochem. Biophys.*, 62:234–236.

99. Poirier, M. C., Yuspa, S. H., Weinstein, I. B., and Blobstein, S. (1977): Detection of carcinogen-DNA adducts by radioimmunoassay. *Nature*, 270:186–188.

100. Reddy, J. K., Svoboda, D. J., and Rao, M. S. (1974): Susceptibility of an inbred strain of guinea pigs to the induction of pancreatic adenocarcinoma by N-methyl-N-nitrosourea. *J. Natl. Cancer Inst.*, 52:991–993.

101. Reddy, J. K., Svoboda, D. J., and Rao, M. S. (1976): Induction of liver tumors by aflatoxin B₁ in the tree shrew (*Tripaia glis*), a nonhuman primate. *Cancer Res.*, 36:151–160.

102. Reznik, G., Mohr, U., and Kmoch, N. (1976): Carcinogenic effects of different nitroso compounds in Chinese hamsters: N-dibutylnitrosamine and N-nitrosomethylurea. *Cancer Letters*, 1:183–188.

103. Roebuck, B. D., and Wogan, G. N. (1977): Species comparison of *in vitro* metabolism of aflatoxin B₁. *Cancer Res.*, 37:1649–1656.

104. Salaman, M. H., and Roe, F. J. C. (1956): Further tests for tumour-initiating activity: N,N-di-(2-chloroethyl)-p-aminophenylbutyric acid (CB 1348) as an initiator of skin tumour formation in the mouse. *Br. J. Cancer*, 10:363–377.

105. Sato, S., Matsushima, T., Tanaka, N., Sugimura, T., and Takashima, F. (1973): Hepatic tumors in the guppy (*Lebistes reticulatus*) induced by aflatoxin B₁, dimethylnitrosamine, and 2-acetylaminofluorene. *J. Natl. Cancer Inst.*, 50:765–778.

106. Schabort, J. C., and Steyn, M. (1969): Substrate and phenobarbital inducible aflatoxin-4-hydroxylation and aflatoxin metabolism by rat liver microsomes. *Biochem. Pharmacol.*, 18:2241–2252.

107. Schmidt, L. H., Fradkin, R., Sullivan, R., and Flowers, A. (1965): Comparative pharmacology of alkylating agents. Part I. *Cancer Chemother. Rep. (Suppl.)*, 2:1–401.

108. Schreiber, D., Jänisch, W., Warzok, R., and Tausch, H. (1969): Die Induktion von Hirn- und Rückenmarktumoren bei Kaninchen mit N-Methyl-N-nitrosoharnstoff. *Z. Ges. Exp. Med.*, 150:76–86.

109. Seal, U. S., and Gutmann, H. R. (1959): The metabolism of the carcinogen N-(2-fluorenyl)acetamide by liver cell fractions. *J. Biol. Chem.*, 234:648–654.

110. Selkirk, J. K., Croy, R. G., and Gelboin, H. V.. (1974): Benzo[a]pyrene metabolites: efficient and rapid separation by high-pressure liquid chromatography. *Science*, 184:169–171.

111. Shimkin, M. B., Weisburger, J. H., Weisburger, E. K., Gubareff, N., and Suntzeff, V. (1966): Bioassay of 29 alkylating chemicals by the pulmonary-tumor response in strain A mice. *J. Natl. Cancer Inst.*, 36:915–935.

112. Sporn, M. B., Squire, R. A., Brown, C. C., Smith, J. M., Wenk, M. L., and Springer, S. (1977): 13-cis-retinoic acid: inhibition of bladder carcinogenesis in the rat. *Science*, 195:487–489.

113. Stavrou, D. (1969): Zur Morphologie und Histochemie experimentell induzierten Hirntumoren beim Kaninchen. *Z. Krebsforsch.*, 73:98–109.

114. Stavrou, D., Dahme, E., and Kalich, J. (1976): Gastroonkogene Wirkung von Methylnitrosoharnstoff beim Miniaturschwein. *Res. Exp. Med.*, 169:33–43.

115. Steyn, P. S., Vieggaar, R., Pitout, M. J., Steyn, M., and Thiel, P. G. (1974): 3-Hydroxyaflatoxin B₁: a new metabolite of *in vitro* aflatoxin B₁ metabolism by vervet monkey (*Cercopithecus aethiops*) liver. *J. Chem. Soc. (Perkin I)*, 1:2551–2552.

116. Sutherland, D. J. (1969): Effects of certain carcinogens on *Periplanata americana*. In *Neoplasms and Related Disorders of Invertebrate and Lower Vertebrate Animals*, National Cancer Institute Monograph 31 pp. 433–445.

117. Swenson, D. H., Miller, J. A., and Miller, E. C. (1973): 2,3-Dihydro-2,3-dihydroxy-aflatoxin B₁: an acid hydrolysis product of an RNA-aflatoxin B₁ adduct formed by hamster and rat liver microsomes *in vitro*. *Biochem. Biophys. Res. Commun.*, 53:1260–1267.

118. Swenson, D. H., Miller, E. C., and Miller, J. A. (1974): Aflatoxin B₁-2,3-

oxide: evidence for its formation in rat liver *in vivo* and by human liver microsomes *in vitro*. *Biochem. Biophys. Res. Commun.*, 60:1036–1043.

119. Terracini, B., and Stramignoni, A. (1967): Malignant lymphomas and renal changes in Swiss mice given nitrosomethylurea. *Eur. J. Cancer, 3:* 435–436.

120. Terracini, B. and Testa, M. C. (1970): Carcinogenicity of a single administration of N-nitrosomethylurea: a comparison between new-born and 5-week-old mice and rats. *Br. J. Cancer, 24:*588–598.

121. Thomas, C., and Sierra, J. L. (1967): Hirntumoren bei Ratten nach oraler Gabe von N-Nitroso-N-ethyl-Harnstoff. *Naturwissenschaften, 54:*228.

122. Thomas, C., Sierra, J. L., and Kersting, G. (1968): Neurogene Tumoren bei Ratten nach intraperitonealer Applikation von N-Nitroso-N-Methyl-Harnstoff. *Naturwissenschaften, 55:*183.

123. Thorgeirsson, S. S., Felton, J. S., and Nebert, D. W. (1975): Genetic differences in the aromatic hydrocarbon-inducible N-hydroxylation of 2-acetylaminofluorene and acetaminophen-produced hepatotoxicity in mice. *Mol. Pharmacol., 11:*159–165.

124. Thorgeirsson, S. S., Jollow, D. J., Sasame, H. A., Green, I., and Mitchell, J. R. (1973): The role of cytochrome P-450 in N-hydroxylation of 2-acetylaminofluorene. *Mol. Pharmacol., 9:*398–404.

125. Tilak, T. B. G. (1975): Induction of cholangiocarcinoma following treatment of a rhesus monkey with aflatoxin. *Food Cosmet. Toxicol., 13:* 247–249.

126. Vadi, H., Moldeus, P., Capdevila, J., and Orrenius, S. (1975): The metabolism of benzo[a]pyrene in isolated rat liver cells. *Cancer Res.,* 35:2083–2091.

127. Vesselinovitch, S. D., Mihailovich, N., Wogan, G. N., Lombard, L. S., and Rao, K. V. N. (1972): Aflatoxin B₁, a hepatocarcinogen in the infant mouse. *Cancer Res., 32:*2289–91.

128. Wales, J. H., and Sinnhuber, R. O. (1972): Hepatomas induced by aflatoxin in the sockeye salmon (*Oncorhynchus nerka*). *J. Natl. Cancer Inst., 48:*1529–1530.

129. Warzok, R., Schneider, J., Schreiber, D., and Jänisch, W. (1970): Experimental brain tumors in dogs. *Experientia, 26:*303–304.

130. Weisburger, E. K. (1971): Testing of new compounds for long-term toxicity. *J. Soc. Cosmet. Chem., 22:*825–838.

131. Weisburger, E. K., and Weisburger, J. H. (1958): Chemistry, carcinogenicity and metabolism of 2-fluorenamine and related compounds. *Adv. Cancer Res., 5:*331–431.

132. Weisburger, J. H. (1955): The enzymic deacetylation of the carcinogen 2-acetylaminofluorene and related compounds. *Biochim. Biophys. Acta,* 16:382–390.

133. Weisburger, J. H. and Weisburger, E. K. (1971): N-oxidation enzymes. In *Handbook of Experimental Pharmacology*, Vol. XXVIII, Pt. 2, pp. 312–333, edited by B. B. Brodie and J. R. Gillette. Springer-Verlag, New York.

134. Weisburger, J. H., and Weisburger, E. K. (1973): Biochemical formation and pharmacological, toxicological, and pathological properties of hydroxylamines and hydroxamic acids. *Pharmacol. Rev., 25:*1–66.

135. Weisburger, J. H., Grantham, P. H., and Weisburger, E. K. (1966): The metabolism of N-2-fluorenylhydroxylamine in male and female rats. *Biochem. Pharmacol., 15:*833–839.

136. Weisburger, J. H., Weisburger, E. K., Morris, H. P., and Sober, H. A. (1956): Chromatographic separation of some metabolites of the carcinogen N-2-fluorenylacetamide. *J. Natl. Cancer Inst., 17:*363–374.

137. Weisburger, J. H., Grantham, P. H., VanHorn, E., Steigbigel, N. H., Rall, D. P., and Weisburger, E. K. (1964): Activation and detoxification of N-2-fluorenylacetamide in man. *Cancer Res., 24:*475–479.

138. Weisburger, J. H., Griswold, D. P., Jr., Prejean, J. D., Casey, A. E., Wood, H. B., Jr., and Weisburger, E. K. (1975): The carcinogenic properties of some of the principal drugs used in clinical cancer chemotherapy. *Recent Results Cancer Res., 52:*1–17.

139. White, F. R. (1960): New agent data summaries. Sarcolysin and related compounds. *Cancer Chemother. Rep., 6:*61–93.

140. Williams, J. R., Jr., Grantham, P. H., Marsh, H. H., III, Weisburger, J. H., and Weisburger, E. K., (1970): The participation of liver fractions and of intestinal bacteria in the metabolism of N-hydroxy-N-2-fluorenylacetamide in the rat. *Biochem. Pharmacol., 19:*173–188.

141. Wilson, R. H., De Eds, F., and Cox, A. J., Jr. (1941): The toxicity and carcinogenic activity of 2-acetaminofluorene. *Cancer Res., 1:*595–608.

142. Wogan, G. N. (1969): Metabolism and biochemical effects of aflatoxins. In *Aflatoxin. Scientific Background, Control and Implications*, pp. 151–186, edited by L. A. Goldblatt. Academic Press, New York.

143. Wogan, G. N. (1974): Naturally occurring carcinogens. In *The Physiopathology of Cancer: Biology and Biochemistry*, Vol. I, pp. 64–109, edited by F. Homburger. Karger, Basel.

144. Wogan, G. N., and Paglialunga, S. (1974): Carcinogenicity of synthetic aflatoxin M₁ in rats. *Food Cosmet. Toxicol., 12:*381–384.

145. Yagi, H., Akagi, H., Thakker, D. R., Mah, H. D., Koreeda, J., and Jerina, D. M. (1977): Absolute stereochemistry of the highly mutagenic 7,8-diol-9,10-epoxide derived from the potent carcinogen trans-7,8-dihydroxy-7,8-dihydrobenzo[a]pyrene. *J. Am. Chem. Soc., 99:*2358–2359.

146. Yang, S. K., McCourt, D. W., Roller, P. P., and Gelboin, H. V. (1976): Enzymatic conversion of benzo[a]pyrene leading predominantly to the diol-epoxide r-7, t-8-dihydroxy-t-9,10-oxy-7,8,9,10-tetra-hydrobenzo[a]pyrene through a single enantiomer of r-7, t-8-dihydroxy-7,8-dihydrobenzo[a]pyrene. *Proc. Natl. Acad. Sci. U.S.A., 73:*2594–2598.

147. Yarita, T., Nettesheim, P., and Williams, M. l. (1978): Tumor induction in the trachea of hamsters with N-nitroso-N-methylurea. *Cancer Res.,* 38:1667–76.

18

Biochemistry of the Neoplastic Cell

Henry C. Pitot

THE BIOCHEMISTRY OF NEOPLASIA *IN VIVO*

Although the discoveries of chemical, physical, and biological carcinogenic agents have been perhaps the most exciting and significant in our understanding of the causation of cancer and of many aspects of its prevention, nothing has intrigued the biological scientist more than the biochemistry of the cancer cell in relation to that of normal cells.

Glycolysis of Cancer Cells—the Warburg Theory

During the early part of this century and extending into the 1920's, the predominant investigations of the biochemistry of cancer centered around the monumental studies of Otto Warburg. In 1930 Warburg published his book (49) on the metabolism of tumors, in which he demonstrated that a wide variety of neoplasms investigated, including benign and malignant, both human and lower animal, exhibited a significant, if not very high, rate of glycolysis. Warburg's hypothesis, which was reiterated in 1956 (50), states that cancer cells originate from normal cells as a result of an irreversible injury to their respiration, said injury to the normal cell being compensated for in the cancer cell by increased fermentation of glucose (glycolysis). Until 15 years ago there were very few, if any, exceptions to this generalization, although many normal tissues exhibited equally high and, in some instances, even higher rates of glycolysis than the vast majority of tumors studied; examples are embryonic tissue, the retina, and the renal papilla (2). In view of this fact, two questions have

arisen that have never been answered satisfactorily by proponents of the Warburg hypothesis. The first is the association of glycolysis with growth rate. A number of studies carried out in various laboratories demonstrate a reasonable degree of correlation of glycolytic rate with growth rate of tumors in many systems. We shall come back to this point in more detail later, but it is clear that glycolysis in most neoplasms may be a secondary event possibly resulting from the loss of control of cellular replication. The second unanswered question is the validity of many comparisons between neoplastic tissues and the cells from which they arose. This takes us back to the definition of neoplasia, which involved *relative autonomy, i.e.,* relative to the tissue from which the neoplasm arose (26). Unfortunately, Warburg (50) and also Greenstein (8, 9) attempted to generalize their results to all neoplasms. Today it is clear that comparisons of normal liver with highly differentiated hepatocellular carcinomas reveal little, if any, differences in the glycolytic capacities of the two tissues, although, as these neoplasms continue to be transplanted, they tend to increase their glycolytic activity. Earlier investigations in the 1950's demonstrated the existence of primary hepatomas with little or no increased glycolytic rate as compared with liver (7). Malignant lymphoblasts glycolyze at essentially the same rate as their normal counterparts, and it is likely that malignant teratomas do not exhibit a degree of glycolysis in excess of that found in embryonic tissues. Thus, in support of Warburg's original hypothesis, most neoplasms do have relatively high rates of glycolysis, but, just as normal karyotypes occur in early neoplasia, normal glycolytic rates do exist in many neoplasms. Increased glycolysis may, therefore, be a characteristic of tumor progression, similar to the occurrence of many karyotypic changes in neoplasms.

The Convergence Hypothesis of Greenstein (9)

Approximately two decades ago, the late Jesse Greenstein, author of "The Biochemistry of Cancer" (7), the next major text after Warburg's work on the biochemical characterization of neoplasia (49), proposed that the biochemical constitution of tumors tended to converge to a relatively common enzymatic pattern. Several authors, including V. R. Potter of the McArdle Laboratory (31), pointed out that the Greenstein hypothesis had not challenged that of Warburg but actually extended it. Warburg's ideas of convergence of tumors were limited to the area of glycolysis and respiration, whereas those of Greenstein extended to a number of enzymatic functions in the cell (9). Greenstein understood and realized the importance of using valid tissue comparisons: he was among the first biochemists to realize the importance of comparing liver with hepatomas, since each is a relatively homogeneous cellular population. In stating the hypothesis of convergence, Greenstein recognized its limitations, although perhaps not the importance of such limitations in an understanding of the cancer problem in general. As we shall see later, exceptions to the Greenstein hypothesis have become more numerous, especially in early neoplasia. Like the Warburg hypothesis, the Greenstein idea of the convergence of neoplasms to a biochemically uniform cell type is untenable as a unique characteristic of neoplasia in the light of modern-day studies. A number of neoplasms may be maintained by multiple transplantations *in vivo* in a phenotypically highly differentiated state (28). This has been shown both with experimental hepatomas and mammary adenocarcinomas. Thus, the differentiated characteristics of many neoplasms may be retained, and such cells do not converge to a universally uniform malignant phenotype. Also, however, in the same manner as the effect of the Warburg concept on cancer research, Greenstein's experiments and ideas have served to open new areas of fruitful investigation.

The Deletion Hypothesis

Unlike the two hypotheses mentioned above, the deletion hypothesis, first advanced by the Millers more than 25 years ago (19, 20), was not based on studies with many different neoplasms, but rather evolved from investigations on the production of hepatic cancer by the feeding of aminoazo dyes. The basic experimental observation was that the dye became bound in a covalent fashion to protein(s) of the liver of the dye-fed animal, whereas little or no dye binding occurred in the protein of the tumors ultimately produced. The Millers thus postulated that carcinogenesis resulted from "a permanent alteration or loss of protein essential for the control of growth..." (19). Later studies by Sorof and others (43) indicated that the proteins to which the dyes were bound in the greatest amounts comprised an electrophoretically slow-moving class termed the h_2 proteins. These proteins were found to be missing from the neoplasms that were produced by dye feeding. More recent investigations with highly differentiated neoplasms have shown the presence of the h_2 protein in these tumors, although still little or no dye binding occurred in this fraction (22). Furthermore, it is now clear that, for the covalent linkage between amine carcinogens and liver macromolecules to occur, aromatic amine carcinogens must be "activated" by N-hydroxylation and subsequent esterification. Thus, the absence of the dye binding in the neoplasms may be the result of a difference in blood supply, an absence of N-hydroxylase, or both, or of some other factors. Later studies by Miller and by Heidelberger (*cf.* 13) showed that a completely analogous situation took place in skin carcinogenesis by hydrocarbons. A protein has been isolated from mouse skin that binds hydrocarbons in a direct relationship to their carcinogenic activity for the skin. Electrophoretically this protein has many of the characteristics of the h proteins of liver. More recent studies by Levin et al. (18), Thakker et al. (46) and Yang et al. (54), have demonstrated that the most "active" form of the hydrocarbons is in all likelihood a diolepoxide in which the epoxidation is not in the "K" region.

After the original proposal of the deletion hypothesis, Potter (31) suggested that the protein deletions occurring during carcinogenesis may be associated with enzymes involved in catabolic reactions, a view compatible with the Greenstein hypothesis as well as with some of the biological aspects of neoplasia, such as rapid growth. Furthermore, several experimental hepatomas demonstrated a complete lack of many catabolic reactions characteristic of liver. However, not long after the initial proposal of the catabolic deletion hypothesis, a series of highly differentiated hepatocellular carcinomas were produced in the laboratory of Dr. Harold Morris, and their chemical characteristics were studied by numerous investigators (22). These studies demonstrated that these neoplasms exhibited nearly all of the normal hepatic enzymatic functions investigated and, in several instances, lacked any abnormal glycolytic capacity. These neoplasms also showed an extreme divergence in their biochemical phenotype, so it is apparent that no two of these highly differentiated neoplasms are phenotypically identical. In fact, extensions of these investigations to primary hepatomas, mammary carcinomas, and even preneoplastic lesions have confirmed the ubiquitousness of this phenotypic heterogeneity.

The Minimal Deviation Concept

As a result of investigations with the highly differentiated Morris hepatomas, Potter proposed the concept of the "minimal deviation" tumor (31) at the opposite end of the spectrum from those neoplasms conforming to the original Greenstein convergence hypothesis (9). Potter's concept was that some neoplasms were probably very closely related to or virtually identical with the initiated cell and deviated only slightly from normal with respect to the growth characteristics or some other necessary function for neoplasia. As these cells progressed, the deviation from the cells of origin increased in the moderately or maximally deviated neoplasm. Thus, the term "minimal deviation hepatoma" appeared to apply to a number of the Morris neoplasms. While there has been some discussion of this concept in the literature, its correlation with both morphology and karyotype appears to present a reasonable distinction among the degrees of differentiation of various neoplasms.

The Molecular Correlation Concept

Shortly after the demonstration of the existence of the minimal deviation hepatomas, Weber and his associates embarked on an extensive biochemical analysis of the enzymatic patterns of these neoplasms. These workers attempted to assemble the data into a modification of the Greenstein hypothesis but in direct relation to cell replication and the growth rate of the neoplasm (51). Thus, by the molecular correlation concept, certain enzymatic abnormalities seen in a class of neoplasms as compared with their cells of origin may be closely correlated with the growth rate of the tumor. Other functions, usually those more closely associated with the degree of differentiation of the organ, show little or no relation to the growth rate of the neoplasm. Weber's investigations have now been extended to include several different types of experimental neoplasms, numerous enzymatic functions, and specific metabolic pathways (51). A compilation of much of this information may be seen in Table 18.1. However, the relation of these data to the process of initiation or to the initial transformation of the neoplastic cell is open to some question. Just as in the case of the Warburg concept and of convergence, it is much more likely that the molecular correlation concept is a function of the progression of the neoplasm and that the metabolic changes seen may be related to this process, to the karyotypic abnormalities that occur, and to other changes secondary to the initial neoplastic transformation. Nevertheless, these data are quite useful for our understanding of the overall metabolism of many malignant neoplasms in relation to the ultimate therapy directed at the metabolic changes seen in the metabolism of the cancer.

CONTROL MECHANISMS IN CANCER

With the advances in recent years in our knowledge of normal cells, it has been possible to study the biological characteristics of the relative autonomy of tumors from a chemical viewpoint. The hormonal control of enzyme activity and enzyme synthesis has now been well studied in many laboratories and is quite applicable to our understanding of the biochemistry of the neoplastic cell. A significant number of studies on the regulation of enzyme levels during hepatocarcinogenesis have been published (26), although no generalization can be made. With some carcinogens, the induction of certain enzymes by hormones is deleted or modified, whereas other hepatocarcinogens have no effect on the same system. Clearly, the acute administration of a number of hepatocarcinogens markedly inhibits most hormonal effects on enzyme synthesis, but the relationship of these phenomena to the neoplastic transformation is as yet unclear.

Within the fully developed neoplastic cell, the feed-back regulation of enzyme activity by metabolic effectors has in general displayed no dissimilarities between normal and neoplastic tissues. On the other hand, the environmental con-

Table 18.1
Biochemical Functions Correlated with Growth Rate in Hepatomas[a]

Carbohydrate Metabolism	Nucleic Acid Metabolism	Protein and Amino Acid Metabolism	Other Metabolic Areas

Glucose synthesis: Decreased
  Glucose-6-phosphatase
  Fructose-1,6-diphosphatase
  Phosphoenolpyruvate carboxykinase
  Pyruvate carboxylase
Glucose catabolism: Increased
  Glycolysis
  Heoxkinase
  Phosphofrunctokinase
  Pyruvate kinase
Pentose phosphate pathway: Increased
  C-1/C-6 oxidation of glucose
Specific phosphorylating enzymes: Decreased
  Fructokinase and glucokinase
Fructose metabolism: Decreased
  Thiokinase
  Aldolase
Resposiveness to glucocorticoid stimulation: Decreased
  Response of gluconeogenic enzymes
Isozyme shift
  High K_m Isozymes: Decreased
  Low K_m Isozymes: Increased
	DNA synthesis: Increased
	  Thymidine Incorporation into DNA
	  Thymidine kinase
	  DNA polymerase
	  Thymidylate synthetase
	  Deoxycytidylate deaminase
	  DNA nucleotidyltransferases ribonucleotide reductase
	DNA catabolism: Decreased
	  Thymidine degradation to CO_2
	RNA synthesis: Increased
	  Aspartate carbamyltransferase tRNA methylase
	RNA catabolism: Decreased
	  Xanthine oxidase
	  Uricase
	RNA metabolic response to glucocorticoid stimulation: Decreased
		Protein synthesis: Increased
		  Amino acid incorporation into protein (alanine, aspartate, glycine, serine, Isoleucine valine)
		Decrease: S-adenosylmethionine synthetase
		Enzymes catabolizing amino acids:
		  Decreased
		  Tryptophan pyrrolase
		  Serotonin deaminase
		  5-Hydroxytryptophan decarboxylase
		  Glutamate dehydrogenase
			Polyamine synthesis: Increased
			  Ornithine decarboxylase
			Urea cycle: Decreased
			  Ornithine carbamyltransferase
			Lipid metabolism: Decreased
			  Lipid content
			  Glycerophosphate dehydrogenase
			  Butyrate to acetoacetate
			Respiratory activity: decreased
			  Oxygen consumption
			  Mitochondrial protein content respiratory ATP production

[a] From Weber (51).

trol of enzyme synthesis and degradation is significantly different when normal and neoplastic cells are compared in appropriate systems. Many of these examples have been demonstrated with the highly differentiated minimal deviation hepatomas and include deletion or modification of the regulation of the synthesis of a number of gluconeogenic enzymes as well as the dietary regulation of fatty acid synthesis and carbohydrate degradation (28). The one abnormality in control mechanisms that appears to be a characteristic of all hepatomas and is possibly applicable to other types of neoplasms is the loss of feedback control of cholesterol synthesis. This effect, which centers around the regulation of the synthesis of the key enzyme HMG-CoA reductase, a microsomal enzyme, has been described in both experimental and human neoplasms of the liver as well as in leukemic cells (41). Recently, Sabine (37) has raised some questions concerning the significance of this generalization on the basis of the inability of neoplastic cells to accumulate and metabolize cholesterol (10), and at least one report indicat-

ing that not all spontaneous hepatomas had lost feedback control (17). The regulation of drug-metabolizing enzymes is also defective in hepatomas, although not ubiquitously (11). It is of interest that, despite the abnormal or deleted mechanisms for the regulation of specific enzyme synthesis in neoplasms, the *in vitro* model for studies of the regulation of enzyme synthesis has been with an inducible enzyme, tyrosine aminotransferase, in a hepatoma cell line in culture (29).

BIOCHEMICAL THEORIES OF CANCER IN RELATION TO ABNORMAL CONTROL MECHANISMS

With the advent of the minimal deviation hepatomas as exceptions to the Warburg, Greenstein, and deletion hypotheses, theories concerned with abnormalities in cellular regulation or "relative autonomy" became significant. Potter proposed the feedback deletion hypothesis (31), suggesting that "in the minimal deviation hepatomas there has been a break in feedback control of cell division." Clearly other feedback controls were abnormal in such neoplasms, but in order to define the neoplasm operationally, growth regulation became most significant. On the other hand, it is not unlikely that the abnormality of the environmental control of growth in the neoplastic cell is basically the same as the abnormality(s) evident in the regulation of enzymes not involved in growth.

Within the last 5 years, the abnormalities in enzyme regulation as well as in growth control seen in neoplasms have been compared with the biochemistry of late fetal and early neonatal tissues, especially in liver. Such a correlation has been related to the isozymic profile of a number of enzymes by Weinhouse and Ono (52) as well as Dunaway et al. (6), Sato et al. (38), and others (24). Potter (31, 32) and others have emphasized the potential importance of the analogy between neoplastic and fetal tissue. Their contentions are enhanced by the demonstration in a wide variety of neoplasms of the appearance of fetal antigens, a clear demonstration of major abnormalities in the regulation of genetic expression in the neoplastic tissues. Furthermore, in most instances the fetal antigens appearing in the neoplastic cell are not directly related to cell replication.

DIFFERENTIATION AND ALTERED TEMPLATE STABILITY OF NEOPLASIA

A number of investigators have now demonstrated that messenger RNA molecules are stabilized for extended periods of time in the cytoplasm of mammalian cells. Furthermore, such stabilization of messenger RNA templates is an integral part of the process of cellular differentiation occurring in the development of the fetus. More than a decade ago Pitot (26) proposed that an alteration in template stability of neoplastic cells could be the basis of the initial transformation event in neoplasia, resulting in a "molecular mask" in the form of the neoplastic phenotype but with the normal genotype.

The details of the concept of altered template stability have given rise to a hypothetical cytoplasmic structure, termed the membron (27). This model proposed that the stabilization of messenger RNA templates occurs within differentiated mammalian cells through an associa-

tion of the messenger RNA molecule with intracellular membranes, especially those of the endoplasmic reticulum. Studies by Pitot and his associates have documented differences in the messenger RNA template lifetime for four different enzymes in liver and in three separate hepatomas. Furthermore, the lifetime of the messenger RNAs for any one enzyme in each of the hepatomas appears to be distinct. Thus, the content of altered template stability may explain the extreme diversity and phenotypic heterogeneity that is so characteristic not only of hepatomas but also of many other types of neoplasms including mammary adenocarcinomas, myelomas, and thyroid carcinomas (27).

On the basis of the concept of altered template stability, the neoplastic transformation may be equated with an abnormal differentiation, resulting in a new phenotype. In this instance, however, the differentiation occurs in adult somatic tissues and is the result of the reprogramming of the expression of genetic information as a consequence of the interaction of the biologic, chemical, and/or physical environment with the genome itself. Furthermore, the concept implies that the neoplastic transformation need not be solely the direct result of changes in cellular gene populations and chromosomal structure but can also result from heritable cytoplasmic changes comparable to the phenomenon of differentiation.

RESOLUTION OF THE SOMATIC MUTATION AND ALTERED TEMPLATE STABILITY HYPOTHESES IN LIGHT OF THE NATURAL HISTORY OF NEOPLASIA

It is obvious to any investigator in the field of oncology that the evidence for a genetic basis for the neoplastic transformation is almost overwhelming, although almost entirely indirect. The fact that chemical carcinogens are mutagenic or may be converted to mutagens is important but not direct evidence for the genetic origin of neoplasia. The only direct evidence that neoplasms are genetically abnormal is that most malignant neoplasms exhibit karyotypic abnormalities in their later stages of development. On the other hand, the evidence for an epigenetic basis of neoplasia comes principally from studies of nuclear transplantation and the recent investigations demonstrating that teratoma cells inoculated into blastulas may exhibit complete reversion to the normal phenotype on development of the organism to the adult (see below).

Pitot (27) has attempted to reconcile these two apparently discrepant concepts by relating them to the natural history of the development of neoplasms *in vivo*. This concept is seen in Table 18.2. The process of initiation, originally proposed by Berenblum, Boutwell, and others, is seen here to be the result of an altered differentiation resulting in a transformed cell with a perfectly normal genome but a heritably altered phenotype. In most neoplasms, however, this neoplastic phenotype tends to render the genotype relatively unstable in that the natural history and tendency of such well-differentiated neoplasms, if allowed to continue their growth, is to develop chromosomal abnormalities and thus truly genetic alterations as compared with their cell of origin. This development may be related to a basic membrane change that can affect the nuclear membrane such that the association of chromosome or chromosomal components with this structure leads to abnormal mitotic activity. Obviously, cells may be transformed directly into the promoted or progressed state without ever passing through the initiated state.

Although this thesis is clearly far from proven, the recent studies of Mintz and Illmensee (21) and those of Gardner and his associates (25) bear on this thesis. As mentioned above, teratoma cells placed into blastulas develop as normal cells. However, Gardner and his associates extended these studies and showed that only those teratoma cells exhibiting normal karyotypes developed in this manner. Aneuploid teratoma cells inoculated into blastulas developed into normal-appearing mice at birth, but these animals developed numerous teratomas and died shortly after birth. These two studies indicate that neoplastic cells do exist with perfectly normal genomes, whereas those with obvious genomic abnormalities appear to have irreversibly fixed the neoplastic state. It is of interest that, whereas Berenblum's original concept proposed that the phenomenon of tumor initiation was irreversible but tumor promotion was reversible, the above proposal indicates that initiation may not always result from a genetic change and that promotion or progression of a neoplasm to the point of karyotypic abnormalities results in an irreversible change.

THE BIOCHEMISTRY OF TRANSFORMED CELLS *IN VITRO*

Perhaps the best model in which to study the biochemistry of neoplastic cells compared with their normal counterparts may be found in systems of normal and transformed cells *in vitro*, when both are derived from the same tissue or cellular source. The first of such systems to be described, and still one of the best examples, was that of normal embryonic chick fibroblasts compared with fibroblasts transformed by Rous virus *in vitro* (45).

This system, as well as a number of other *in vitro* systems in which normal and transformed cells can be readily compared, has exhibited a number of interesting and relatively uniform biochemical characteristics. However, virtually all of the systems studied have been mesenchymal in origin. Thus, any generalizations that have been proposed would be restricted to mesenchymal neoplasms, although, as we will see, certain conclusions reached with the Rous sarcoma virus and the chemical transformation of fibroblasts are applicable to some epithelial cultures.

Table 18.2
Pathogenesis or Natural History of Neoplasia

Initiation		Promotion
	Biology	
Highly differentiated neoplasms with normal karyotype	Tumor progression	Biologically malignant neoplasms exhibiting known or morphologically abnormal karyotypes
	Molecular Biology	
Heritable membrane alterations associated with altered stabilities of mRNA, resulting in stable new phenotype	Alterations in membrane-genome interaction	Gene multiplicities and/or deletions. Karyotypic changes

MEMBRANE TRANSPORT OF CELLS TRANSFORMED *IN VITRO* AND OF THEIR NORMAL COUNTERPARTS

One of the earliest investigations of the biochemical changes accompanying transformation *in vitro* concerned various membrane functions (12, 30). In particular, the transport of small molecules across the plasma membrane of transformed cultured cells was compared with this process in their cells of origin. In RNA virus-transformed cells there was an increase in the rate of glucose uptake concomitant with the first appearance of morphologic changes in the virus-infected cells (12). Furthermore, the available evidence indicated that this increase was dependent on the transformation process; e.g., hexokinase activity did not change at the time of transformation by the RNA oncogenic virus, but the transformed morphology occurring in the cells after virus infection correlated with increased sugar transport, whereas the rate of sugar uptake in "revertant" cells was identical to that seen in the nontransformed cells. Perhaps the most conclusive evidence in support of this contention was carried out with temperature-sensitive mutants of Rous sarcoma virus. In these experiments, transformation of the cells occurred at 36°C but not at 41.5°C. Similarly, the enhanced sugar transport was observed only at the permissive temperature (36°C); by shifting the temperature of the culture to 41.5°C, one could decrease sugar transport to the level seen in the nontransformed cell. This change appears to be related to an increase in the V_{max} of the transport system and not to the affinity of the sugar for the transport system. More recent studies indicated that the bound forms of hexokinase and of several other glycolytic and shunt enzymes increased significantly in Rous sarcoma virus-transformed cells. On the other hand, a recent study by Venuta and Rubin (48) demonstrated that normal chick fibroblasts increased their rate of glucose transport up to 10-fold when the cells were starved with respect to glucose, although fast-growing normal cells doubled their rate of uptake of the sugar after starvation. Cells transformed with Rous sarcoma virus do not show any change in the rate of glucose uptake during starvation. Unlike cells transformed with RNA oncogenic viruses, SV40 virus transformation of mouse cells does not specifically enhance sugar transport (12). Transport mechanisms following chemical carcinogenesis in vitro have not as yet been studied in detail.

CHARACTERISTICS OF THE SURFACE MEMBRANE OF NORMAL AND TRANSFORMED CELLS *IN VITRO*

The phenomenon of contact inhibition, which may be related to tumor invasion and possibly tumor metastases, was first described in cell culture and probably involves some alteration in the surface of the neoplastic cell. Attempts to study such alterations biochemically were rather unsuccessful until the demonstration by Rapin and Burger of the agglutination of virally transformed cells in vitro (33); the source of the agglutinin was from wheat germ. In contrast, the parent cells from which they were derived did not agglutinate when specific plant materials were added to the medium. The purified material was found to be a glycoprotein having a molecular weight of approximately 18,000. This material was found to react with a number of neoplastic cells obtained from tumors growing in vivo as well as cells transformed in culture by chemicals, x-rays or viruses, or "spontaneously" transformed. In many instances revertant cells in vitro lost their agglutinability.

Since these earlier experiments, several other plant agglutinins have been found to affect neoplastic cells in a similar manner. In addition, some nontransformed cells also exhibited agglutinability, thus making the original generalization invalid (42). Burger and others (33, 34) demonstrated that treatment of normal cells with trypsin for very short periods of time rendered them agglutinable by the lectin. This last experiment indicated that normal cells contained receptor sites for the plant agglutinins (lectins) but that these sites were normally protected or covered over by some peptide components of the surface membrane. Some variants of polyoma-transformed cells showed varying degrees of agglutination by another material, concanavalin A (34). Sachs' laboratory (14) has demonstrated that normal fibroblasts in mitosis are agglutinated by concanavalin A as well as by the wheat germ lectin, whereas transformed fibroblasts in mitosis are not agglutinated by these lectins. These studies, together with those mentioned above concerning the enzymatic treatment of membranes, would argue for a certain degree of mobility of the sites that bind the agglutinins of plant lectins. Such a phenomenon has been demonstrated in lymphocytes, in which fluorescent concanavalin A is localized at one pole of the cell. Neoplastic lymphocytes did not exhibit this phenomenon, which has been termed "capping." Furthermore, the capping induced by concanavalin A did not affect the binding of the wheat germ agglutinin over the surface of the normal cell; this indicates a differential mobility of the receptor sites for the two lectins. Using the electron microscope, Nicolson (23) demonstrated that, in the case of cells agglutinable with concanavalin A, the lectin was associated with patches of the plasma membrane, whereas in nonagglutinable cells it was found randomly dispersed. This patchy distribution of concanavalin A receptor sites on the surface of many transformed cells is probably the result of an increased mobility of concanavalin A receptors in these cells.

Becker (1) has also demonstrated a differential lectin agglutination of fetal and malignant hepatocytes as compared with adult hepatocytes. The latter, even after treatment with protease, were not agglutinated by concanavalin A, whereas fetal liver cells and hepatoma cells were agglutinated by this lectin. Thus, these epithelial cells appear to have different numbers of concanavalin A binding sites; this is not the case with the mesenchymal cells studied thus far.

In accord with the changes in lectin binding sites described above, biochemical studies of the surface membranes of normal and transformed cells *in vitro* have shown interesting differences. Inbar and Schinitzky (15) have recently demonstrated that the increased fluidity of the surface membranes of malignant lymphoma cells from mice can be correlated with a marked decrease in cholesterol content of these membranes. Surface glycoproteins and gangliosides of cells transformed by viruses, chemicals, and x-rays *in vitro* showed significant but not necessarily common differences when compared with nontransformed cells cultured *in vitro* (5). In agreement with these findings is the demonstration by several investigators (35) of lowered levels in transformed cells of glycosyl transferase involved in the synthesis of glycoproteins and gangliosides in the surface membrane. These findings, coupled with the suggestion that surface galactosyl transferase activity may be related to cell-to-cell interaction, offer the possibility that in the near future we may be able to understand the mechanisms of contact inhibition, cell adhesiveness, and lectin effects on cells in relation to plasma membrane structure and enzymology.

CYCLIC NUCLEOTIDES AND TRANSFORMATION *IN VITRO*

Although it is more than 20 years since the discovery by Sutherland and Rall (44) of cyclic AMP, the possible role of this "second messenger" in the neoplastic transformation has been suggested only within the last decade. The studies by Pastan and his associates (16, 53), who demonstrated that the addition of cyclic AMP to transformed cell cultures resulted in an alteration in their morphology to that of normal, contact-inhibited cells with a lower growth rate, represented the initial findings in this now very rapidly moving area. It appears that the concentration of cyclic AMP in cells transformed *in vitro* is generally about half that of the concentration seen in corresponding nontransformed cells. Furthermore, in Rous sarcoma virus-transformed chick embryo fibroblasts, plasma membrane adenylate cyclase activity is reduced, and the K_m for ATP is significantly lower in normal cells than in the transformed cells.

More recently another cyclic nucleotide, cyclic GMP, has been shown by Goldberg and Haddox (7) and others (39) to vary with cell replication in a manner opposite to that seen with cyclic AMP—that is, cyclic GMP levels increase when cells are stimulated to replicate, whereas the levels of this cyclic nucleotide are decreased in starved cells, in which cyclic AMP levels increase. These changes in cyclic nucleotides have even led to the initial utilization of cyclic AMP in attempts to treat neoplasms *in vivo* as well as regulating the replication of their cells *in vitro*.

Perhaps one of the more interesting aspects of the cyclic nucleotides and transformation *in vitro* is the recent demonstration of a correlation between cyclic nucleotide concentrations and their effects on changes seen in the surface membrane. Willingham and Pastan (53) have demonstrated that, in at least one strain of cultured cells, low levels of intracellular cyclic AMP may be correlated with increased agglutinability by concanavalin A, whereas high levels of the cyclic nucleotide are seen in those cells exhibiting decreased agglutinability. Cyclic AMP also appears to affect the glycopeptide composition of the surface membranes of cultured cells, and the morphologic changes seen in cultured neoplastic cells after the addition of cyclic nucleotides are also associated with a reappearance of contact inhibition of growth in these cells.

In somewhat more differentiated cells, such as those of the neuroblastoma in culture, cyclic AMP addition to the culture actually regulates the morphologic differentiation of these cells in culture in that the addition of the cyclic nucleotide enhances differentiation of the neuroblastoma cells to differentiated neurons; this is accompanied by a decrease in cellular proliferation. In contrast to the effects of cyclic AMP, the addition of a nucleic acid base analog, 5-bromodeoxyuridine, to cultures of differentiating tissues (whether normal or transformed) inhibits morphologic differentiation of these cells. In certain neoplastic cells, especially melanomas, differentiated characteristics are lost when these cells are cultured in the presence of this analog (4). Furthermore, the tumorigenicity of mouse melanoma cells treated with the analog is markedly inhibited (40). However, after return of the cultured cells to a medium that does not contain the analog, normal differentiated characteristics and tumorigenicity reappear rather rapidly. One of the most interesting effects of this analog is its ability to "rescue" viruses from cells that are not producing the virus but that contain viral information within their genome. In this instance it would appear that the analog tends to enhance "differentiation" of the expression of the viral genome (36).

PLASMINOGEN ACTIVATOR(S) IN TRANSFORMED CELLS

Over three decades ago, investigators using tissue culture techniques were aware of the fact that certain neoplastic cells grown in vitro had the ability to lyse plasma clots rapidly. This observation has recently been re-evaluated, and Reich and his associates (47) have demonstrated that many cells transformed in vitro release into the culture medium a proteolytic factor that has the ability to activate plasminogen, an inactive precursor of the proteolytic enzyme plasmin. The plasminogen activator of SV40-transformed cells growing in vitro has been characterized as a protein of molecular weight 50,000 (3). The production of this activator can be correlated in many transformed cells with the other characteristics that we have described above, agglutinability and the suppression of tumorigenicity by 5-bromodeoxyuridine. Again, however, we are faced with the fact that the plasminogen activator is not produced by all cells transformed in vitro or in vivo. Thus, although activator production may be an important characteristic of specific transformants, it does not appear to be a ubiquitous characteristic of the neoplastic transformation. Unfortunately, at our present state of knowledge it is impossible to define the malignant transformation biochemically either in vivo or in vitro. Clearly the phenotypic heterogeneity characteristic of highly differentiated

neoplasms in vivo is a property of neoplasia that was predicted by the morphologic variation in cancers described by pathologists during the past century. Although cultured cells offer the best possible delineation of critical differences between normal and neoplastic cells, as yet no generalizations applicable to all neoplasms have come from these studies.

References

1. Becker, F. F. (1974): Differential lectin agglutination of fetal, dividing-postnatal, and malignant hepatocytes. *Proc. Natl. Acad. Sci. U.S.A.*, 71: 4307.
2. Burk, D., Woods, M., and Hunter, J. (1967): On the significance of glycolysis for cancer growth with special reference to Morris rat hepatomas. *J. Natl. Cancer Inst.*, 38:839.
3. Christman, J. K., and Acs, G. (1974): Purification and characterization of a cellular fibrinolytic factor associated with oncogenic transformation: the plasminogen activator from SV40-transformed hamster cells. *Biochim. Biophys. Acta*, 340:339.
4. Christman, J. K., Silagi, S., Newcomb, E. W., Silverstein, S. C., and Acs, G. (1975): Correlation suppression by 5-bromodeoxyuridine of tumorigenicity and plasminogen activator in mouse melanoma cells. *Proc. Natl. Acad. Sci. U.S.A.*, 72:47.
5. Coleman, P. L., Fishman, P. H., Brady, R. O., and Todaro, G. J. (1975): Altered ganglioside biosynthesis in mouse cell cultures following transformation with chemical carcinogens and X-irradiation. *J. Biol. Chem.*, 250:55.
6. Dunaway, G. A. Jr., Morris, H. P., and Weber, G. (1974): A comparative study of rat liver, muscle and hepatoma 3924A phosphofructokinase isozymes. *Cancer Res.*, 34:2209.
7. Goldberg, N. B., and Haddox, M. K. (1977): Cyclic GMP metabolism and involvement in biological regulation. *Ann. Rev. Biochem.*, 46:823.
8. Greenstein, J. P. (1954): *Biochemistry of Cancer*, 2nd Ed. Academic Press, New York.
9. Greenstein, J. P. (1956): Some biochemical characteristics of morphologically separable cancers. *Cancer Res.*, 16:641.
10. Harry, D. S., Morris, H. P., and McIntyre, N. (1971): Cholesterol biosynthesis in transplantable hepatomas: evidence for impairment of uptake and storage of dietary cholesterol. *J. Lipid Res.*, 12:313.
11. Hart, L. G., Adamson, R. H., Morris, H. P., and Fouts, J. R. (1965): The stimulation of drug metabolism in various rat hepatomas. *J. Pharmacol. Exp. Ther.*, 149:7.
12. Hatanaka, M. (1974): Transport of sugars in tumor cell membrane. *Biochim. Biophys. Acta*, 355:77.
13. Heidelberger, C. (1970): Chemical carcinogenesis, chemotherapy: cancer's continuing core challenge. *Cancer Res.*, 30:1549.
14. Inbar, M., Rabinowitz, Z., and Sachs, L. (1969): The formation of variants with a reversion of properties of transformed cells. III. Reversion of the structure of the cell surface membrane. *Int. J. Cancer*, 4:690.
15. Inbar, M., and Schinitzky, M. (1974): Increase of cholesterol level in the surface membrane of lymphoma cells and its inhibitory effect of ascites tumor development. *Proc. Natl. Acad. Sci. U.S.A.*, 71:2128.
16. Johnson, G. S., Friedman, R. M., and Pastan, I. (1971): Cyclic AMP-treated sarcoma cells acquire several morphological characteristics of normal fibroblasts. *Ann. N. Y. Acad. Sci.*, 185:413.
17. Kandutsch, A. A., and Hancock, R. L. (1971): Regulation of the rate of sterol synthesis and the level of β-hydroxy-β-methylglutaryl coenzymes A reductase activity in mouse, liver and hepatomas. *Cancer Res.* 31:1396.
18. Levin, W., Wood, A. W., Yagi, H., Dansette, P. M., Jerina, D. M., and Conney, A. H. (1976): Carcinogenicity of benzo[a]pyrene 4,5-, 7,8-, and 9,10-oxides on mouse skin. *Proc. Natl. Acad. Sci. U.S.A.*, 73:243.
19. Miller, E. C., and Miller, J. A. (1947): The presence and significance of bound aminoazo dyes in the livers of rats fed p-dimethylaminoazobenzene. *Cancer Res.*, 7:468.
20. Miller, J. A., and Miller, E. C. (1971): Chemical carcinogenesis: mechanisms and approaches to its control. *J. Natl. Cancer Inst.* 47:V.
21. Mintz, B., and Illmensee, K. (1975): Normal genetically mosaic mice produced from malignant teratoma cells. *Proc. Natl. Acad. Sci. U.S.A.*, 72:3585.
22. Morris, H. P. (1965): Studies on the development, biochemistry, and biology of experimental hepatomas. *Adv. Cancer Res.*, 9:227.
23. Nicolson, G. L. (1976): Trans-membron control of the receptors on normal and tumor cells. II. Surface changes associated with transformation and malignancy. *Biochim. Biophys. Acta*, 458:1.
24. Nordmann, Y., and Shapira, F. (1967): Muscle type isoenzyme of liver aldolase in hepatomas. *Eur. J. Cancer*, 3:247.
25. Papaionnou, V. E., McBurney, M. W., Gardner, R. L., and Evans, M. J.

(1975): Fate of teratocarcinoma cells injected into early mouse embryos. *Nature, 258:*70.

26. Pitot, H. C. (1964): Altered template stability: the molecular mask of malignancy. *Perspect. Biol. Med., 8:*50.

27. Pitot, H. C. (1974): Neoplasia: a somatic mutation or a heritable change in cytoplasmic membranes? *J. Natl. Cancer Inst., 53:*905.

28. Pitot, H. C. (1975): Metabolic controls and neoplasia. In *Cancer—A Comprehensive Treatise*, pp. 121–154, edited by F. F. Becker. Plenum Press, New York.

29. Pitot, H. C., Peraino, C., Morse, P. A., and Potter, V. R. (1964): Hepatoma in tissue culture compared with adapting liver *in vivo*. *Natl. Cancer Inst. Monogr., 13:*229.

30. Pollack, R. E., and Hough, P. V. C. (1975): The cell surface and malignant transformation. *Ann. Rev. Med., 25:*431.

31. Potter, V. R. (1964): Biochemical perspectives in cancer research. *Cancer Res., 24:*1085.

32. Potter, V. R. (1969): Recent trends in cancer biochemistry: The importance of studies on fetal tissue. *Can. Cancer Conf., 8:*9.

33. Rapin, A. M. C., and Burger, M. M. (1974): Tumor cell surfaces: general alterations detected by agglutinins. *Adv. Cancer Res., 20:*1.

34. Rosenblith, J. Z., Ukena, T. E., Yin, H. H., Berlin, R. D., and Karnovsky, M. J. (1973): A comparative evaluation of the distribution of concanavalin A-binding sites on the surface of normal, virally-transformed, and protease-treated fibroblasts. *Proc. Natl. Acad. Sci. U.S.A., 70:*1625.

35. Roth, S., Patterson, A., and White, D. (1974): Surface glycosyltransferases on cultured mouse fibroblasts. *J. Supramol. Struct., 2:*1.

36. Rowe, W. P., Lowy, D. R., Teich, N., and Hartley, J. W. (1972): Some implications of the activation of murine leukemia virus by halogenated pyrimidines. *Proc. Natl. Acad. Sci. U.S.A., 69:*1033.

37. Sabine, J. R. (1975): Defective control of lipid biosynthesis in cancerous and precancerous liver. *Progr. Biochem. Pharmacol., 10:*269.

38. Sato, S., Matsushima, T., and Sugimura, T. (1969): Hexokinase isozyme patterns of experimental hepatomas of rats. *Cancer Res., 29:*1437.

39. Seifert, W., and Rudland, P. S. (1974): Cyclic nucleotides and growth control in cultured mouse cells: correlation of changes in intracellular 3′:5′ cGMP concentration with a specific phase of the cell cycle. *Proc. Natl. Acad. Sci. U.S.A., 71:*4920.

40. Silagi, S. (1971): Modification of malignancy of 5-bromodeoxyuridine. *In Vitro, 7:*105.

41. Siperstein, M. D., Grude, A. M., and Morris, H. P. (1971): Loss of feedback control of hydroxymethylglutaryl coenzyme A reductase in hepatomas. *Proc. Natl. Acad. Sci. U.S.A., 86:*315.

42. Sivak, A., and Wolman, S. R. (1972): Classification of cell types: agglutination and chromosomal properties. *In Vitro, 8:*1.

43. Sorof, S., Young, E. M., and Ott, M. G. (1958): Soluble liver h proteins during hepatocarcinogenesis by aminoazo dyes and 2-acetylaminofluorene in the rat. *Cancer Res., 18:*33.

44. Sutherland, E. W., and Rall, T. W. (1960): Relation of adenosine-3′,5′-phosphate and phosphorylase to the actions of catacholamines and other hormones. *Pharmacol. Rev., 12:*265.

45. Temin, H. (1963): Further evidence for a converted, non-virus producing state of Rous sarcoma virus-infected cells. *Virology, 20:*235.

46. Thakker, D. R., Yagi, H., Lu, A. Y. H., Levin, W., Conney, A. H., and Jerina, D. M. (1976): Metabolism of benzo[a]pyrene: Conversion of (±)-trans-7,8-dihydroxy-7,8-dihydrobenzo[a]pyrene to highly mutagenic 7,8-diol-9,10 epoxides. *Proc. Natl. Acad. Sci. U.S.A., 73:*3381.

47. Unkeless, J. C., Tobia, A., Ossowski, L., Quigley, J. P., Rifkin, D. D., and Reich, E. (1973): An enzymatic function associated with transformation transformed by avian RNA tumor viruses. *J. Exp. Med., 137:*85.

48. Venuta, S., and Rubin, H. (1975): Effects of glucose starvation on normal and Rous sarcoma virus-transformed chick cells. *J. Natl. Cancer Inst., 54:*395.

49. Warburg, O. (1930): *Metabolism of Tumors.* Arnold Constable, London.

50. Warburg, O. (1956): On the origin of cancer cells. *Science, 123:*309.

51. Weber, G. (1974): Molecular correlation concept. In *The Molecular Biology of Cancer*, pp. 487–521, edited by H. Busch. Academic Press, New York.

52. Weinhouse, S., and Ono, T. (1972): *Isozymes and Enzyme Regulation in Cancer.* Gann Monograph 13. Univ. of Tokyo Press, Tokyo.

53. Willingham, M. C., and Pastan, I. (1974): Cyclic AMP mediates the concanavalin A agglutinability of mouse fibroblasts. *J. Cell Biol., 63:*288.

54. Yang, S. K., McCourt, D. W., Roller, P. P., and Gelboin, H. V. (1976): Enzymatic conversion of benzo[a]pyrene leading predominantly to the diol-epoxide r-7,t-8-dihydroxy-5-9,10-oxy-7,8,9,10-tetrahydroxybenzo[a]pyrene through a single centiomer of r-8,t-8-dihydroxy-7,8-dihydrobenzo[a]pyrene. *Proc. Natl. Acad. Sci. U.S.A., 73:*2594.

19

In Vitro Metabolism of Polynuclear Aromatic Hydrocarbons in Deep-Sea Fishes

John J. Stegeman

The world's oceans can serve as sinks for many toxic chemicals which are regionally or globally distributed. Foreign compounds, such as polychlorinated biphenyls, can be found in all segments of the water column and in animals living there (5). Atmospheric transport seems to be a prominent route of introduction of such compounds in many regions (4), yet whatever the mechanism of introduction or of transport through the water column, foreign organic compounds accumulate in recent marine sediments.

Carcinogenic polynuclear aromatic hydrocarbons are among those compounds found in sediments from rivers, lakes, near-shore marine waters and from the deep ocean. Levels in sediments near industrial areas are in general much higher than those in more remote regions. There are some exceptions. An example may be taken from Laflamme and Hites (6). $C_{20}H_{12}$ polynuclear aromatic hydrocarbons, including benzofluoranthenes, benzopyrenes and perylene, were found at concentrations of 33 ppm in Charles River sediments, 1.7 ppm in New York Bight sediments and 0.034 ppm in the Nares Abyssal Plain (6). These 3 samples were mostly benzofluoranthene and benzopyrenes. A fourth site, the Cariaco Trench, contained 1.66 ppm $C_{20}H_{12}$, but in this case perylene was the dominant component. A diagenetic source is postulated for this compound suggesting a complex geochemistry in some regions, as yet not well understood.

Not only the geochemistry but also the biochemistry of such compounds is poorly understood for the deep sea. This is not surprising when one considers the difficulties in obtaining suitable samples from ocean depths. However, some information is available on hydrocarbon biotransformation in deep sea fishes.

It is now known that submammalian vertebrates including fishes can metabolize polynuclear aromatic hydrocarbons via cyctochrome P-450 (3, 8). As in mammals aromatic hydrocarbons can induce increased levels of aryl hydrocarbon (benzo[a]pyrene) hydroxylase in fishes and apparently such increased rates of metabolism identified *in vitro* correspond to increased rates of metabolism of compounds *in vivo* as well, (9). In fishes from coastal and nearshore waters the levels of benzo[a]pyrene hydroxylase can be quite high, and in some cases these high levels can be correlated with hydrocarbon contamination (7, 11). In general, however, we have noticed that coastal fishes living or feeding in association with the bottom have higher levels of benzo[a]pyrene hydroxylase than those active animals which inhabit the water column.

By comparison, benthic fishes living in the deeper waters, from the continental shelf to the continental rise, have lower levels of benzo[a] pyrene hydroxylase than do animals living closer to shore. Table 19.1 gives values for hepatic benzo[a]pyrene hydroxylase in a closely related group of benthic species, commonly called rattails, taken from depths of 400–3000 meters in the western North Atlantic. While these values are much lower than in nearshore species, the strong inhibition of benzo[a]pyrene hydroxylase by 7,8-benzoflavone may indicate the animals are being affected by compounds similar to 3-methylcholanthrene, known to in-

Table 19.1 Hepatic Benzo[a]pyrene Hydroxylase in Benthic Fishes[a]

Species (N)	Sampling Depth (meters)	Benzo[a]pyrene Hydroxylase (units/g liver)[b, c]	Influence of 10^{-4} M 7,8-Benzoflavone (% inhibition)
Flounder			
Pseudopleuronectes americanus (3)	10	4895 ± 450	91.6 ± 2
Rattails			
Nezumia (6)	420	750 ± 293	40.6
Coryphaenoides carapinus (2)[d]	1375	1814 ± 750	99.0
Coryphaenoides armatus (8)	2705–2970	806 ± 358	94.6
Coryphaenoides leptolepis (1)	2970	246	94.4

[a] Deep benthic fishes collected and assayed on cruise 43 of R/V OCEANUS, Woods Hole Oceanographic Institution, April 11–18, 1978.
[b] Units are expressed as picomoles 3-OH-benzo[a]pyrene equivalents produced per minute in a 20-min incubation using a postmitochondrial supernatant preparation. Activity is normalized to liver weight.
[c] Assays were carried out according to Stegeman (11) at 20°C for flounder and 20°C for rattails.
[d] These fish were juveniles. All others were nongravid adults.

Table 19.2 Bioactivation of benzo[a]pyrene to Toxic and Mutagenic Derivatives by Scup (Stenotomus versicolor) Liver Mixed-Function Oxygenases[a]

Incubation Conditions	Bacterial Survival (%)	Mutant Fraction[b] ($\times 10^{-8}$)
Complete (12.5 μg benzo[a]pyrene/ml)	5	47.2
Minus benzo[a]pyrene	100	0.55
Minus NADPH	91	0.21

[a] Incubation of Salmonella typhimurium strain TA-98 with untreated scup liver microsomes and appropriate cofactors.
[b] Mutant fraction refers to the number of His$^+$ revertants per number of survivors.
Data taken from Stegeman (10).

duce a cytochrome P-450 (cytochrome P-448) sensitive to 7,8-benzoflavone in mammals (13). This possibility is not inconsistent with the predominantly benthic habitat and feeding patterns of these animals and the presence of polynuclear aromatics in oceanic sediments.

The metabolism of aromatic hydrocarbons in fish can proceed via glutathione transferases and conjugating enzymes to detoxified products (1). However, strong evidence obtained with mammals links metabolism to certain electrophilic metabolites with formation of active car-

cinogenic forms of some polynuclear aromatic hydrocarbons. Recent evidence indicates that metabolism of compounds such as benzo[a]pyrene by fish also results in formation of metabolites which are both toxic and mutagenic (Table 19.2).

It would seem carcinogenic hydrocarbons in freshwater systems and in coastal marine sediments may contribute to the appearance of tumors in fishes and other aquatic animals (2, 12). There are virtually no studies of tumors in animals from the deep sea. Yet, the presence of environmental hydrocarbons and the ability of deep-sea fishes to metabolize these compounds suggests that activation of chemical carcinogens there is possible. Surveys of pathology in deep-sea samples may indicate whether this presumed remote environment is in fact at risk from environmental carcinogens and mutagens.

Acknowledgments: This work was supported by the National Science Foundation grant No. OCE76-84415. I thank Albert Sherman and Heidi Kaplan for technical assistance.

References

1. Bend, J. R., James, M. O., and Dansette, P. M. (1977): *In vitro* metabolism of xenobiotics in some marine animals. *Ann. N.Y. Acad. Sci,* 298:505.
2. Brown, E. R., Hazdra, J. J., Keith, L. Greenspan, I. Kwapinski, J. B. G., and Beamer, P. 1973. Frequency of fish tumors found in a polluted watershed as compared to nonpolluted Canadian waters. *Cancer Res.,* 33:189.
3. Chevion, M., Stegeman, J. J., Peisach, J., and Blumberg, W. E. (1977): Electron paramagnetic resonance studies on hepatic microsomal cytochrome P-450 from a marine teleost fish. *Life Sci.,* 20:895.
4. Harvey, G. R. and Steinhauer, W. G. 1976. Transport pathways of polychlorinated biphenyls in Atlantic water. *J. Mar. Res.,* 34:561.
5. Harvey, G. R., Miklas, H. P., Bowen, V. T., and Steinhauer, W. G. (1974): Observations on the distribution of chlorinated hydrocarbons in Atlantic Ocean organisms. *Sears Found. J. Marine Res.,* 32:103.
6. Laflamme, R. E., and Hites, R. A. (1980): The global distribution of polycyclic aromatic hydrocarbons in recent sediments. *Geochim. Cosmochim. Acta,* 42:289.
7. Payne, J. F. (1976): Field evaluation of benzo[a]pyrene hydroxylase induction as a monitor for marine pollution. *Science,* 191:945.
8. Pohl, R. J., Bend, J. R., Guarino, A. M., and Fouts, J. R. (1974): Hepatic microsomal mixed-function oxidase activity of several marine species from coastal Maine. *Drug Metab. Dispos.,* 2:545.
9. Statham, C. N., Elcombe, C. R., Szyjka, S. P., and Lech, J. J. (1978): Effect of polycyclic aromatic hydrocarbons on hepatic microsomal enzymes and disposition of methylnaphthalene in rainbow trout *in vitro. Zenobiotica,* 8:65.
10. Stegeman, J. J. (1977): Fate and effects of oil in marine animals. *Oceanus,* 20:59.
11. Stegeman, J. J. (1978): Influence of environmental contamination on cytochrome P-450 mixed-function oxygenases in fish; implications for recovery in the Wild Harbor Marsh. *J. Fish. Res. Bd. Can.* 35:668.
12. Stich, H. F., Acton, A. B., and Forrester, C. R. (1976): Fish tumors and sublethal effects of pollutants. *J. Fish. Res. Bd. Can.,* 33:1993.
13. Weibel, F. J., Leutz, J. C., Diamond, L., and Gelboin, H. V. (1971): Hydrocarbon (benzo[a]pyrene) hydroxylase in microsomes from rat tissues; differential inhibition and stimulation by benzoflavones and organic solvents. *Arch. Biochem. Biophys.,* 144:78.

20

Ultrastructural Aspects of Neoplasia and Preneoplastic Lesions

Benjamin F. Trump and Raymond T. Jones

Introduction

The subject of the ultrastructure of neoplastic cells is one which is undergoing a rapid evolution at the present time. This is the result of intensive studies on the ultrastructure of experimental neoplasms as well as an equally intensive development of electron microscopy (EM) in the diagnosis of cancer (5, 34). All of these studies are beginning to reveal extensive information about neoplastic cells at the ultrastructural level which is fundamental not only to an understanding of tumor cell biology but also is badly needed to improve methods for diagnosis of tumors at the time of resection, biopsy, autopsy, and cytopathology. The diagnostic application of EM is relatively new but promises to be of material assistance in future tumor classification.

It is still fair to state that there is no single morphological feature of neoplastic cells at the light or EM level which permits them to be separated with certainty from normal cells. The patterns of the ultrastructural features are, however, quite significant and often diagnostic. There is probably no single organelle found in tumor cells which is not found in normal cells nor is the converse true.

And yet there is asolutely no doubt that the pathologist can, with morphology alone, diagnose cancer with a very high degree of precision and even recognize the site of origin in metastases in many cases. Using EM in addition, this precision will undoubtedly go higher.

The use of EM with cytochemistry has been of material assistance in assessing differentiation at the cellular and subcellular levels. This is of great importance in neoplasia because it is at this level that key features of differentiation are often expressed and, frequently, classification at the light microscopical level is difficult or impossible. The field of diagnostic EM has been rapidly expanding in recent years, see series by Trump and Jones (43, 44). It may be that in the future increasing use of EM will provide improved quality control for diagnostic surgical pathology. In addition to application in the area of tissue examination, EM is also currently being applied to the study of cytopathologic specimens.

Another important feature of relevance in considering the ultrastructure of neoplasia is that many of the ultrastructural features in neoplastic cells represent reactions of the tumor cells to various types of injury including anoxia, ischemia, chemotherapeutic agents, radiation, etc., and it is important not to confuse such reactions with features which are characteristic or specific of the neoplastic cell. Many other features in neoplasms represent more chronic injury or reactions to injury, as discussed in Chapter 12, including repair and healing, hyperplasia, metaplasia, etc. Many more experiments in the future will be needed to completely separate these features from those which represent the alterations implicit in the neoplastic process.

NUCLEUS

Many features of the cancer cell nucleus have, of course, been described by light microscopy especially in cytopathologic literature (19). At the ultrastructural level it is frequent that irregularities of the nuclear envelope occur (Fig. 20.1). Such irregularities of the nuclear envelope occur (Fig. 20.1). Such irregularities can be extremely deep, sometimes forming large pseudoinclusions (Fig. 20.2) which can be identified by their nuclear envelope lining (42). Such irregularities are extrinsic in the cerebriform nuclei of mycosis fungoides. Entrapment of cytoplasm, probably by the pinching off of such invaginations, has also been shown to lead to the development of true intranuclear inclusions of lipid and sometimes membranous debris. Nuclear "bodies" are

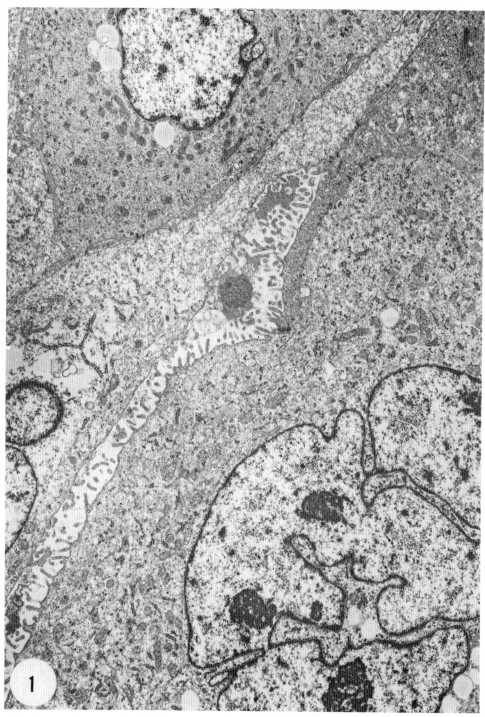

Figure 20.1. Electron micrograph of apocrine carcinoma of the human breast. Note the very irregular and indented nuclei which are characteristic of neoplastic cells. Note also that the cells join with junctional complexes surrounding typical lumens which are characteristic of adenocarcinomas. Secretory material is present within the lumen. (Courtesy of Dr. A. Shamsuddin.)

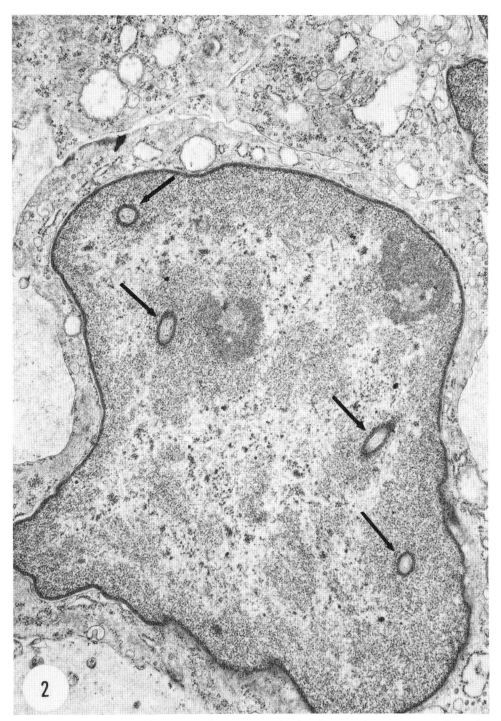

Figure 20.2. Electron micrograph of osteogenic sarcoma in the femur of a human patient showing a typical neoplastic cell nucleus with marked irregularities of contour, clumping of chromatin, and numerous pseudoinclusions (*arrows*). (Courtesy of Dr. A. Shamsuddin.)

often seen in different cells but can be seen in normal cells as well. These have been classified by Bouteille et al. (6). The nuclear chromatin pattern often shows numerous chromatin centers although these can be difficult to visualize in thin section studies. The nucleoli are large and often, of course, multiple nucleoli are pres-

ent. The alterations of the chromatin patterns that are so easily seen by light microscopy and especially in Pap smears are difficult to visualize in thin sections. Sometimes, however, one can appreciate these changes. Especially one can commonly recognize attachment of the nucleolus to the nuclear envelope—a finding also common in regenerating cells. The nucleolonema is frequently widely dispersed with many large areas of pars amorpha. Many nucleolar changes have been described even in premalignant cells including the so-called stratification which also occurs following treatment of cells with several inhibitors of RNA synthesis; many of these inhibitors are carcinogens. Other changes include dispersion and formation of intranuclear bodies seen after other carcinogens such as ethionine (27). Whether or not these are in any way specific for inducers of neoplasia has not been determined; however, it is clear that many carcinogenic agents show nucleolar changes at an early stage.

The presence of numerous mitotic figures, sometimes abnormal, typifies malignant neoplasia. These can often be recognized in electron micrographs. It is important to keep in mind that such increased numbers of mitoses do not necessarily reflect increased cell division; recent studies indicate that they frequently imply mitotic arrest.

THE CELL MEMBRANE

The cell or plasma membrane is currently visualized as a complex of macromolecules which also interacts with elements within the cell including cytoskeletal contractile and tubular macromolecules and which consists of a lipid bilayer in which a variety of proteins, some of them transmembrane, are embedded (37). Many of these proteins exhibit lateral mobility and the lipid components are of a variable fluidity. Proteins on the exterior aspect of the membrane are decorated with polysaccharide or glycoprotein complexes which form the glycocalyx and which contain a number of important cell surfaces including tumor antigens. In the cancer cell there are numerous modifications in the macromolecular composition of the cell surface (36). These include alterations in the components such as glycoproteins, glycolipids and proteins, changes in surface enzymes especially increase in proteases and glycosidases, changes in membrane transport systems, often increases in the transport systems of sugars and amino acids, and changes in receptor mobility especially the mobility of lectin binding sites such as those which bind concanavalin A (29). These latter seem to involve alterations in membrane protein interactions with elements of the cytoskeleton

and are further discussed under that section below.

The use of freeze etching, which splits the membrane and reveals the patterns of the intramembranous proteins, promises to be of great utility in the further study of membrane changes in neoplasia (31). This will probably be especially effective when combined with correlative studies of immunoreactive materials in the cell membrane, *i.e.*, surface tumor and embryonic antigens, etc.

Cilia are very uncommonly seen in neoplasms. In fact, absence of cilia is a classic cytopathologic criterion of a malignant cell (19). Actually very few neoplasms in experimental animals have been described to have cilia. In our experience this is rare in the extreme.

Alterations of the cell membrane are numerous and probably very important in neoplastic cells (Figs. 20.3 and 20.4). Some of these changes may be, in fact, crucial to the process of transformation as well as to the biology of metastasis. Cell membrane changes also appear to be closely related to cytoskeletal and contractile elements of the cell including microtubules and microfilaments (50). Changes of cell junctions may relate to the invasive growth of cells and to altered cell to cell communication. In many epithelial tumors the membrane specializations found in the cell of origin are lost and replaced by a different pattern. A good example is adenocarcinomas of the kidney originating from the pars recta of the proximal tubules which has a very well-developed microvillus brush border (8, 13). Following neoplastic transformation the well-developed long microvilli which form the brush border are completely lost and replaced by short stubby villi which are much more widely spaced (Fig. 20.5). In adenocarcinomas of the colon, similar simplification of the cell surface is seen. This is especially prominent in scanning EM (31). Changes of the membrane associated filaments are also characteristics and sometimes represent markers of neoplastic cells. In tumors derived from the gastrointestinal tract and lung for example, the terminal web is characteristically seen beneath the microvillus surface. This can be of assistance in establishing the origin of such a tumor and is apparently retained as a counterpart of the endodermal epithelium. It has recently been observed that, in invasive versus noninvasive carcinomas of the skin, the arrangement of microfilaments and their number nearer the cell membrane is markedly different (25). This could conceivably relate to altered cell motility which in turn could be related to the pro-

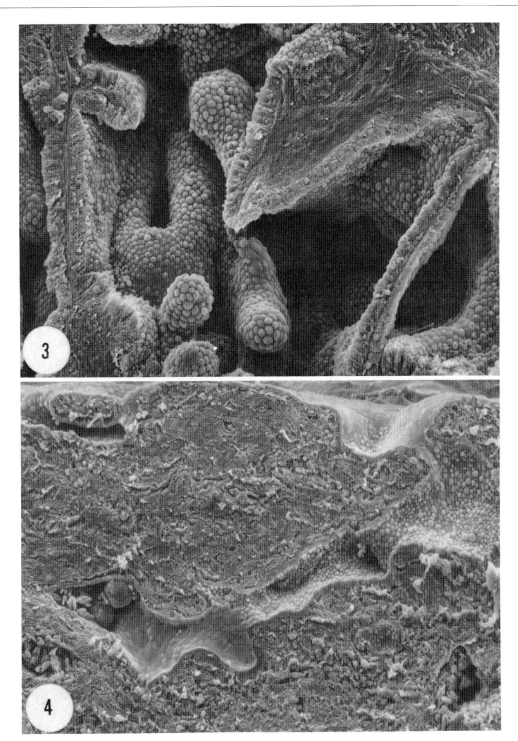

Figure 20.3.   Scanning electron micrograph of human prostate showing the typical acinar pattern with multiple infoldings covered with epithelial cells disposed in a regular pattern. Note the stratified nature of the epithelium and the very irregular shape of the epithelium on the papillae extending into the acinar lumens. (Courtesy of Dr. H. Sanefuji.)

Figure 20.4.   Human prostate derived from an immediate autopsy cultured *in vitro* for 2 weeks after 2 doses of MNNG at a dose of 5 μg/ml each dose. This is the cut service of the explant. At the top of the picture the outgrowth of epithelium over the surface is noted and growth down into the gland can also be seen. Note that in contrast to the normal there is an irregular growth pattern, piling up of cells and irregularity of cell shape and size. (Courtesy of Dr. H. Sanefuji.)

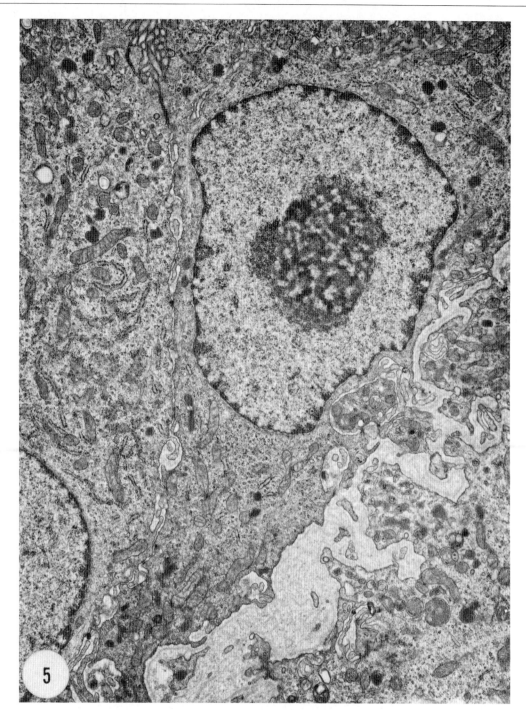

Figure 20.5. Electron micrograph of experimentally induced adenocarcinoma in the rat kidney following 36 weeks of exposure to fluorobiphenylacedimide. Many of the features of neoplastic cells are shown. Note the poorly developed microvilli at the surface in marked contrast to those of the normal pars recta from which this neoplasma originates. Note also the small irregular mitochondria, the numerous ribosomes, the large irregular nucleus with large nucleolus and the very irregular basal lamina interspersed with cell processes. (Courtesy of Dr. J. H. Dees.)

cess of invasion. Studies using immunologic identification of actin in a series of normal and neoplastic tissues suggest markedly altered patterns and increased numbers of actin filaments in neoplastic cells (11).

Changes in cell surface antigenic markers need further study; however it seems evident that changes in surface antigens (1) can identify and characterize transformed cells, α-fetoprotein and carcinoembryonic antigens (CEA) being examples. In the neoplasms of the bronchus, adenocarcinomas and epidermoid carcinomas may show different amounts of CEA (Fig. 20.6) (16).

Many features of the cell surface are of importance in diagnostic EM. These include the formation of cell junctions along intra- and intercellular alveoli in adenocarcinomas. Such differentiation features do not occur in epidermoid carcinomas (Fig. 20.7). The types of cell junctions in neoplasia vary but need much more study. Along these alveoli, intermediate junctions, and sometimes desmosomes are seen, possibly tight junctions occur also. These form a terminal bar similar to those seen in normal secreting epithelia.

The large vacuoles commonly used as a criterion of adenocarcinoma in pap smears usually represent the so-called intracellular alveoli (14) referred to above. These invaginations of the cell membrane show the usual surface membrane specializations along their surface and typically contain secretory products such as mucus. Often they appear to have pinched off from the cell surface.

The presence of a well-developed terminal web beneath the surface epithelium commonly occurs in tumors of the gastrointestinal tract and to a lesser extent in lung tumors. Whether or not this typifies these tumors needs further study as it may be of diagnostic significance. The terminal web is composed of filaments growing in several directions, including up into the microvilli. Such filaments may be related to actin and result in changes in cell shape.

Whether or not the quantity and quality of cell junctions differ in neoplasia in any consistent pattern needs much more study as it could be important in cell-cell communications, cell movement, contact inhibition, invasiveness, and propensity to metastasis. Cell junction alterations have been described by Loewenstein (21) in culture of malignant epithelium and in hepatomas. Cell-to-cell communication appeared to be impaired as measured by injection of fluorescein and electrical pulses. In epidermoid carcinomas of several organs numerous desmosomes are typically seen. The thickening of the inner leaflet of the cell membrane that typifies the lining transitional epithelium of the bladder persists in at least the well-differentiated tumors of this organ (15).

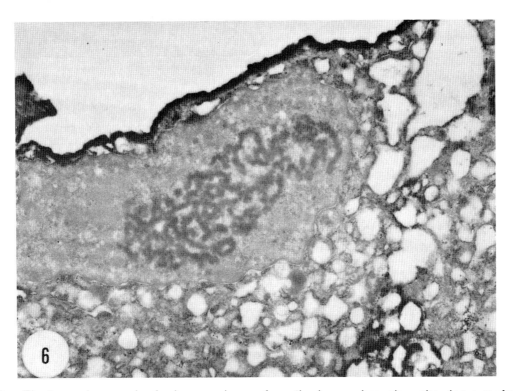

Figure 20.6.   Electron micrograph of adenocarcinoma from the human bronchus showing a surface epithelial cell with prominent reaction product for carcinoembryonic antigen (CEA) over the cell surface and within membrane elements in the cell interior. Experiments in our laboratory reveal that beginning with epidermoid metaplasia there is a marked increase in the amount of immunoperoxidase staining for CEA which ultimately is much greater in adenocarcinomas and epidermoid carcinomas. CEA was demonstrated using the Sternberger technique. (Courtesy of P. Phelps.)

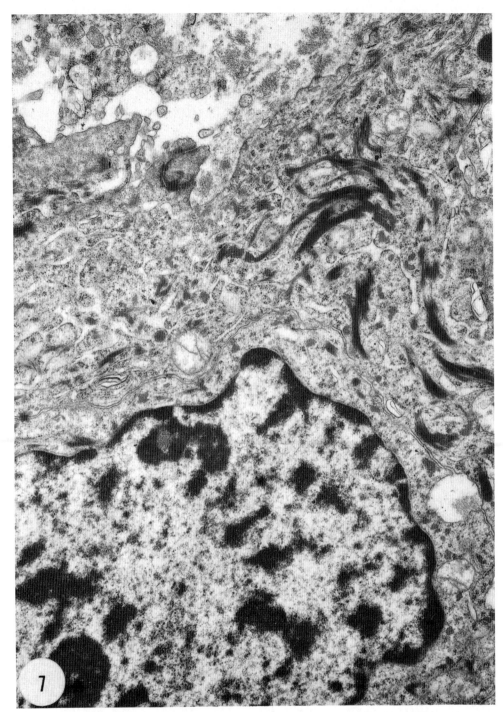

Figure 20.7. Electron micrograph of epidermoid carcinoma of the lung in a human patient. Note the characteristic features of this type of neoplasm including a paucity of organelles, inconspicuous mitochondria, and large bundles of tonofilaments beginning to form keratohyalin. The nucleus shows clumped irregular chromatin and a very irregular boundry. (Courtesy of Dr. A. Shamsuddin.)

THE ENDOPLASMIC RETICULUM

Numerous alterations in the endoplasmic reticulum (ER) have been described in neoplastic cells and in experimental neoplasia where histogenesis and comparisons with cell of origin can be determined (2). There are always changes in this important organelle. In some studies of transplantable tumors characteristic changes occur in a given cell type. The changes include alterations of shape, size and distribution including whorls in fingerprint formations, meandering cisternae, extensive proliferation of rough and often smooth ER, branching cisternae, irregular spacing of ribosomes and rough ER, and budding of the walls of cisternae into the lumens. Again, these changes are difficult to distinguish from the proliferative changes often induced by chemical carcinogens and, indeed, all of these may be related. During the preneoplastic stages following treatment with a number of carcinogens including halogenated hydrocarbons in saffrole, the endoplasmic reticulum in hepatic parenchymal cells undergoes massive hypertrophy associated with changes in the mixed function oxidase system. These changes seem to persist into the transformed cell and may well be indicators of the etiologic chemical agent. Other changes characteristic of rapidly dividing cells include the so-called peared cisternae and annulate lamellae. Marked enzyme changes typically occur in the endoplasmic reticulum of neoplastic cells, for example, the prominent deficiency of glucose-6-phosphatase (Figs. 20.8 and 20.9) in the ER of both renal (13) and hepatic adenocarcinomas in rat (also see Chapter 18 by Pitot in this volume). The dispo-

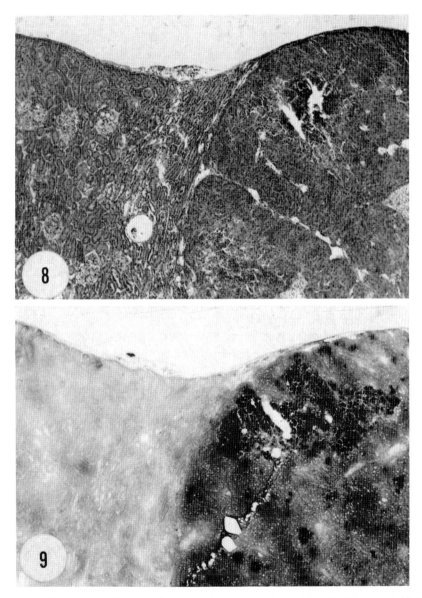

Figure 20.8. Section of kidney containing adenocarcinoma produced by *N*-4-fluoro-4-biphenylacedimine. The large neoplasm on the right is elevating the capsule and compressing adjacent tissue. These neoplasms arise from the pars recta of the proximal tubule over a period of months following continuous feeding of the carcinogen. (Reproduced with permission from B. M. Heatfield *et al.: Journal of the National Cancer Institute, 57:* 795, 1976.)

Figure 20.9. Same neoplasm showing a stain for glucose-6-phosphate dehydrogenase which is markedly increased in the tumor. (Courtesy of Dr. B. M. Heatfield.)

sition in differentiation of the ER can also be of diagnostic assistance in surgical pathology. For example, those adenocarcinomas which are devoid of well-developed alveoli, possess well-developed and smooth ER. Tumors of steroid producing cells including the adrenal and the sex organs typically show an abundance of smooth endoplasmic reticulum (3, 4).

PEROXISOMES

Peroxisomes are recently described ubiquitous organelles containing a variety of oxidative enzymes readily demonstrated with the diaminobenzidine reaction for catalase (17, 33, 40). Though peroxisomes occur in virtually all cell types examined, they are particularly well developed in the form of large microbodies in hepatic parenchymal cells and in the cells of the renal proximal convoluted tubules. Changes in peroxisomes also seemingly occur in tumors as composed with the cell of origin. There may be a degree of parallelism between the growth rate of the tumor and the degree of development of the peroxisomes. For example, relatively well-differentiated slow growing hepatomas have large microbodies resembling those seen in normal cells; the opposite is true in fast growing hepatomas (28). Their role in normal as well as abnormal cell function remains to be completely determined; however, they seem to be involved in fatty acid oxidation (20) and possibly in gluconeogenesis (7).

GOLGI APPARATUS AND SECRETORY GRANULES

The degree of development of the Golgi apparatus varies in different neoplasms and probably again differs from the cell of origin and is probably roughly proportional to the secretory activity of the tumor cell, that is, secretory derived cells including exocrine and endocrine adenocarcinomas. Both have well-developed Golgi apparatuses as well as appropriate secretory granules. Cells showing an epidermoid differentiation as well as many sarcomas and other poorly differentiated neoplasms have very poorly developed Golgi apparatus commensu-

rate with their probable lack of secretory activity.

In association with the Golgi apparatus are secretory granules of various types which persist as features of cell differentiation in neoplastic cells. For example, tumors derived from mucus-producing epithelia commonly still produce mucus and often this is only visualized at the EM level especially when combined with EM cytochemistry (23, 24, 46).Tumors of endocrine glands commonly still retain the small dense core granules characteristic of such differentiation (Fig. 20.10). Compared combined EM and cytochemical studies of such tumors have given rise to the so-called APUD concept (30) and the concept of so-called APUDOMAS. Morphological characterization, however, is relatively crude in separating various types of endocrine granules though differences do occur even in routinely fixed embedded tissues. Currently increasing application of immunocytochemistry at the light and EM levels especially using immunoperoxidase methods promises to be of material assistance in assessing these types of granules in the future (39). Other important granules in surgical pathological diagnosis are the melanin and premelanin granules which persist even in amelonotic melanomas and can sometimes only be recognized by the use of EM.

LYSOSOMES

All neoplastic cells possess lysosomes and it is usually only when comparisons are carefully made with the cell of origin that the marked changes in these organelles can be visualized. In general, tumors appear to have fewer and smaller lysosomes than the cell of origin and these tend to have less enzyme activity such as acid phosphatase. This is particularly true in tumors derived from the liver and kidney. On the other hand, tumor cells often possess numerous residual bodies and autophagic vacuoles some of which may represent sublethal reactions to injury of the cells as a result of hormone stimulation, chemotherapeutic or radiation treatment or normal blood supplies. One tumor, the granular cell myoblastoma is eosinophilic and granular at the light microscopic level simply because of large numbers of debris-filled residual bodies which fill the cytoplasm (38). An interesting current finding is that hemosiderin

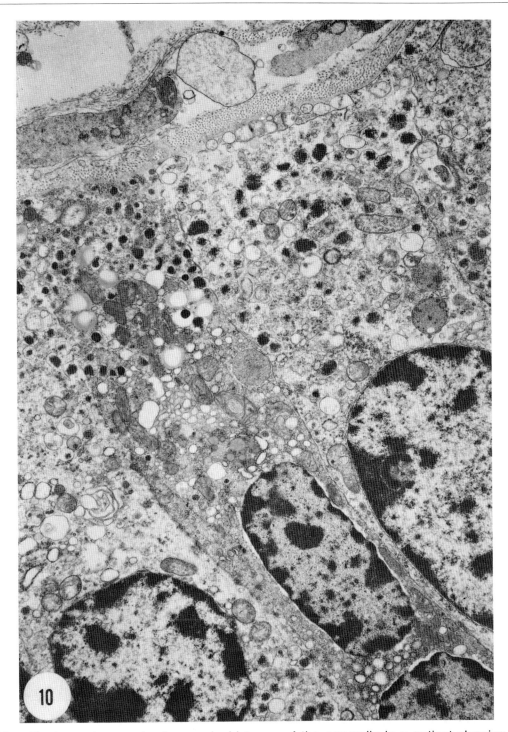

Figure 20.10.   Electron micrograph of a carcinoid tumor of the appendix in a patient showing the basalar aspects of the neoplastic cells which contain numerous dense core granules surrounded by a single membrane. This is an example of a neoplastic cell which preserves secretory activities related to the cell of origin. (Courtesy of Dr. A. Shamsuddin.)

and ferritin storage within hepatoma cell lysosomes is greatly diminished (51). This has been useful as a marker of preneoplastic and neoplastic change in the hepatic parenchyma. This reduction in the amount of stored iron, following

systemic loading, may relate to abnormal uptake and/or synthesis and transport of iron including its macromolecular derivatives, ferritin and hemosiderin. The other finding concerning lysosomes is that protease activities including fibrinolysin are often high in tumor cells; some of these may be membrane associated (18). Whether or not the lysosomes play a role in the initiation of neoplasia has often been debated and reviewed but still remains unknown.

MITOCHONDRIA

Mitochondria show numerous changes in neoplastic cells as compared with the cell of origin. It is a well-known generalization that from the biochemical point of view tumor cells are relatively deficient in oxidative enzyme activity and more active in glycolytic systems, an observation first made and developed by Otto Warburg (49). Electron microscopy reveals that tumor mitochondria are, in the case of malignant neoplasms, generally smaller and more irregular than their normal counterparts. This is especially obvious in tumors of epithelia such as the kidney proximal tubule which have extremely well-developed mitochondria (8, 13). Histochemical activities of oxidative enzymes (*i.e.*, succinic dehydrogenase) are typically reduced in the neoplastic cell and, when isolated, the mitochondria often show loose coupling and poor respiratory control. In addition to their small size and irregular shape, the mitochondria are often bizzare in configuration with branching, dumbbell, and doughnut-shaped forms. Megamitochondria are sometimes observed. Cristae are sometimes unusual and in lamellar configurations.

The morphology of the mitochondria can also be of diagnostic help in the so-called oncocytic tumors or oncocytomas which are characterized by eosinophilic granular cytoplasms. The mitochondria are prominent and closely packed, occupying much of the available cytoplasm. Peculiarities of cisternal differentiation characteristic of the cell of origin can also be of significance. The best example is the tubular cristae of the renal cortical epithelial cells which is maintained in adrenal cortical adenomas and carcinomas (3, 4).

CELL SAP OR CYTOSOL

The cell sap or cytosol representing the continuous phase of the cytoplasm has not received significant attention until recently. Apart from muscle cells with their well-developed myofila-

ments, and various cells with glycogen and lipid deposits, little attention has been directed toward this compartment. Recently with the realization of the important role of the cytoskeletal and contractile elements of the cytoplasm and the interactions of these with the cell membrane and other intracellular organelles, much attention is being directed toward this compartment and many important answers appear to be forthcoming (10, 35). It appears that many vital cell activities, including those mediated by hormones or other mediators, involve changes in this compartment, some of which are in connection with the cytoskeletal and contractile filaments. Some of these are mediated by rapid ion shifts including calcium. Wotosewick and Porter (52) using high voltage EM have placed great attention on three-dimensional organization in the cytosol, especially as it involves the clustering of materials around meandering cisternae and other formed elements.

General

Deposits of glycogen and lipid are seen in tumor cells and these give a clear appearance by light microscopy. So-called clear cell carcinomas often are the mere light microscopic representations of epidermoid or adenocarcinomas containing abundant glycogen and/or lipid. Some tumors such as renal cortical carcinomas are typically characterized by large amounts of glycogen and lipid. Characteristic aggregates of glycogen are also of diagnostic help in Ewing's sarcoma (41). Many of these reactions, however, are results of cell injury occurring in the neoplasm and of metabolic alterations, for example, in the process of glycogenolysis.

Microtubules

Microtubules exist in a dynamic equilibrium between the polymerized form recognizable by EM and the subunits which can polymerize or depolymerize rapidly and under hormonal-ionic control. It is currently evident that microtubules interact closely with elements of the cell membrane (see above) and in transformed cells these membrane attachments may be altered. The use of immunofluorescence and immunoperoxidase methods coupled with conventional and high voltage EM promises to yield much more information about these elements. The role in mitosis has been clear for some time, however, recently the role and a variety of other cell movements including absorption, secretion, and motility have been elucidated. It is evident also that several important cancer chemotherapeutic agents including the Vinca alkaloids and some additional compounds exert a primary effect by depolymerizing or pushing the equilibrium toward the subunits of these systems (47).

Microfilaments

Microfilaments which apparently are contractile include actin, myosin, and related proteins. They are seen in all cells including muscle. Again they can be demonstrated by immunofluorescence or immunoperoxidase, and interact both with microtubules and with the cell surface proteins. Changes in microfilaments inducible by hormones may relate to changes in cyclic AMP, cyclic GMP, and cytosol calcium. Concentrations of filaments are often seen near the plasma membrane and their state of contraction is apparently related to cell shape. One recent study implicates correlation between aggregates of contractile filaments near the cell surface and invasiveness (25). Changes in these filaments in their membrane attachments could relate to shape, motility, metastasis, and invasion.

Other Filaments

Other larger filaments in the order of 100 nm in diameter are seen in all cell types, often referred to as tonofilaments (Fig. 20.11) and exhibiting intimate relationships with cell junctions especially the so-called desmosome. These large filaments need much more characterization. Some of them appear to relate to keratin and keratinization. Many large filaments are characteristic of certain neoplasms such as astrocytomas where they are typical of epidermoid differentiation and are sometimes not evident by light microscopy (12). Again, the use of more advanced techniques including immunofluorescence and immunoperoxidase will be necessary to further characterize these structures and their significance.

EXTRACELLULAR MATERIALS

A variety of extracellular components occur in neoplasms including what is often called the stroma with its connective tissues, support blood vessels, and connective tissue fibers. These are often host-derived while structures, such as basal laminae, appear to be the products of tumor cell secretion. Basal laminas and their orientation relative to tumor cell groups can be of diagnostic significance as adenocarcinomas show a characteristic polarity of lumens, cells, and basal lamina. Surrounding of individual cells by basal lamina material is of help in the diagnosis of liposarcomas (Fig. 20.12) (45). Endothelial stromal interactions are of evident importance in the process of invasion and metastasis. In some organs such as the breast and prostate hormonal influences may modify not only the epithelium but also the stromal and stromal-epithelial interchanges. Much more study on both normal and abnormal differentiation is needed on these relationships. Abnormal polymerization of fibrillar proteins in the form of so-called amyloid appears in certain tumors of the thyroid (48). Calcification of extracellular debris possibly phospholipid can result in the lamellar concretions known as psammoma bodies which are very numerous in certain tumors, for example, serous cystadenocarcinomas of the ovary (9).

ULTRASTRUCTURAL FEATURES RELATED TO TUMOR ETIOLOGY

Actual visualization of ultrastructural features which specifically relate to etiology is a very difficult and poorly understood area both with viral and chemical carcinogens. A few features relevant to this area will be discussed.

Viral

In most tumors definitely shown to be produced by viruses, EM has not revealed virus particles in most cases. In some instances, however, viral antigens can be demonstrated and sometimes a true virus can be demonstrated following reexamination by EM. A tumor-like lesion molluscum contagiosum does reveal pox virus particles (32) as some papillomas and other proliferative lesions including benign warts in several mammals. Viral particles can also be demonstrated in the kidney tumor cells during certain stages of the Lucké virus-induced adenocarcinoma of the kidney of frogs (22).

Chemical

In the case of chemical carcinogens, again, there is no specific morphologic change which also identifies the nature of the chemical or even the fact that chemical agents did indeed induce

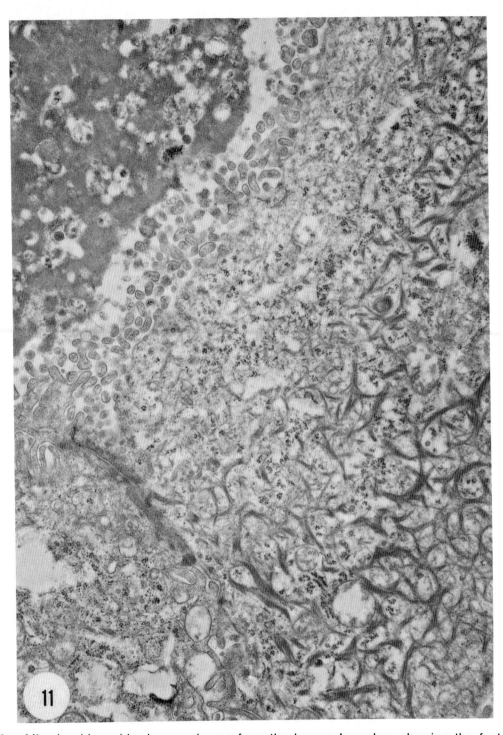

Figure 20.11. Mixed epidermoid adenocarcinoma from the human bronchus showing the features of both adeno- and epidermoid carcinomas. Note the lumen at the upper right where the cells join with junctional complexes with numerous microvilli along the apical surface. Beneath the surface the organelles include numerous bundles of tonofilaments characteristic of epidermoid carcinoma. (Reproduced with permission from E. M. McDowell *et al.: Journal of the National Cancer Institute, 61:* 587, 1978.)

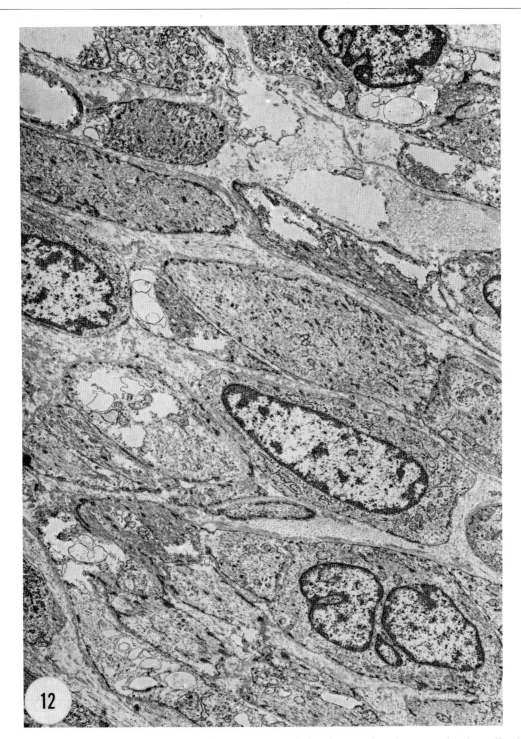

Figure 20.12. Electron micrograph of a leiomyosarcoma of the femur showing neoplastic cells derived from smooth muscle. Note the spindle shape of the cells each of which is surrounded by a basal lamina and the characteristic clusters of filaments in dense plaques along membrane which characterize smooth muscle. (Courtesy of Dr. A. Shamsuddin.)

the neoplasms. Perhaps the nearest tumor so far identified is the change described in the endoplasmic reticulum resulting from chemical stimulation of liver cells by carcinogens (26), the response of the ER of the tumor being initially adaptive but relating to changes in mixed function oxidase systems in modification of carcinogen metabolism. These changes can be sometimes observed to persist into the neoplastic stage.

References

1. Abeley, G. I., Assecritova, I. V., Kraeusky, N. D., Perova, S. D., and Perevodchikova, N. I. (1967): Embryonal serum α-globulin in cancer patients; diagnostic value. *Int. J. Cancer*, 2:551–558.

2. Apffel, C. A. (1978): The endoplasmic reticulum membrane system and malignant neoplasia. *Prog. Exp. Tumor Res.*, 22:317-362.

3. Bloodworth, J. M. B., Jr. (1975): The adrenal, in *Endocrine Pathology Decannial 1966-1975*, pp. 391-421, edited by S.S. Sommers. Appleton-Century-Crofts, New York.

4. Bloodworth, J. M. B., Jr., Horvath, E., and Kovacs, K. (1980): Fine structural pathology of the endocrine system, in *Diagnostic Electron Microscopy, Vol. 3*, pp. 359-527, edited by B.F. Trump and R.T. Jones. John Wiley & Sons, New York.

5. Bonikos, D. S., Bensch, K. G., and Kempson, R. L. (1976) The contribution of electron microscopy to the differential diagnosis of tumors. *Beitr. Pathol.*, 158:417-444.

6. Bouteille, M., Kalifat, S. R., and Delarue, J. (1967): Ultrastructural variations of nuclear bodies in human diseases. *J. Ultrastruct. Res.*, 19:474-486.

7. De Duve, C. (1975): Exploring cells with a centrifuge, in *Les Prix Nobel EN 1974*, p. 142, Norstedt and Son, Stockholm.

8. Dees, J. H., Reuber, M. D., and Trump, B. F. (1976): Adenocarcinoma of the kidney; I. Ultrastructure of renal adenocarcinomas induced in rats by N-(4'-fluoro-4-biphenylyl)acetamide. *J. Natl. Cancer Inst.*, 57:779-794.

9. Ferenczy, A., and Richart, R. M. (1974): *Female Reproductive System: Dynamics of Scan and Transmission Electron Microscopy*, pp. 288-290. John Wiley & Sons, New York.

10. Fuller, G. M., and Brinkley, B. R. (1976): Structure and control of assembly of cytoplasmic microtubules in normal and transformed cells. *J. Supramol. Struct.*, 5:497-514.

11. Gabbiani, G., Csank-Brassert, J., Schneeberger, J.-C., Kapanci, Y., Trenchev, P., and Holborow, J. (1976): Contractile proteins in human cancer cells; immunofluorescent and electron microscopic study. *Am. J. Physiol.*, 83:457-474.

12. Garcia, J. H., and Mena, H. (1978): The diagnosis of central nervous system disorders by transmission electron microscopy, in *Diagnostic Electron Microscopy, Vol. 2*, pp. 351-394, edited by B. F. Trump, and R. T. Jones. John Wiley & Sons, New York.

13. Heatfield, B. M., Hinton, D. E., and Trump, B. F. (1976): Adenocarcinoma of the kidney; II. Enzyme histochemistry of renal adenocarcinomas induced in rats by N-(4'-fluoro-4-biphenylyl)acetamide. *J. Natl. Cancer Inst.*, 57:795-808.

14. Hess, F. G., McDowell, E. M., and Trump, B. F. (1978): Intracellular alveoli (IA)—important cytologic criteria of adeno differentiation in bronchogenic carcinomas. *Acta Cytol.*, 22:596-597.

15. Hicks, R. M., and St. John Wakefield, J. (1976): Membrane changes during urothelial hyperplasia and neoplasia. *Cancer Res.*, 36:2502-2507.

16. Hill, T. A., Anthony, R. L., Sutherland, J. S., and Trump, B. F. (1980): Carcinoembryonic antigen in the lung; a review of localization in normal and neoplastic human lung. *Arch. Pathol. Lab. Med.* (in press).

17. Hruban, Z., and Rechzigel, M. (1969): Microbodies and related particles. *Int. Rev. Cytol.* [Suppl]:1-89.

18. Jones, P., Benedict, W., Strickland, S., and Reich, E. (1975): Fibrin overlay methods for the detection of single transformed cells and colonies of transformed cells. *Cell*, 5:323-329.

19. Koss, L. G. (1968): *Diagnostc Cytology and its Histopathologic Bases*, J. B. Lippincott, Philadelphia.

20. Lazarow, P. B., and de Duve, C. (1976): A fatty acyl-CaD oxidizing system in rat liver peroxisomes; enhancement by clofibrate, a hypolipidemic drug. *Proc. Natl. Acad. Sci. U.S.A.*, 73:2043-2046.

21. Loewenstein, W. R. (1975): Cellular communication by permeable membrane junctions, in *Cell Membranes Biochemistry Cell Body and Pathology*, p. 105, edited by G. Weissmann, and R. Clarborne. H. P. Publishing Co., New York.

22. Lunger, P. D. (1964): The isolation and morphology of the Lucké frog kidney tumor virus. *Virology*, 24:138-145.

23. McDowell, E. M., Barrett, L. A., Glavin, F., Harris, C. C., and Trump, B. F.: (1978): The respiratory epithelium; I. Human bronchus. *J. Natl. Cancer Inst.*, 61:539-549.

24. McDowell, E. M., McLaughlin, J. S., Merenyi, D. K., Kieffer, R. F., Harris, C. C., and Trump, B. F. (1978): The respiratory epithelium; V. Histogenesis of lung carcinomas in the human. *J. Natl. Cancer Inst.*, 61:587-606.

25. McNutt, N. S. (1976): Ultrastructural comparison of the interface between epithelium and stroma in basal cell carcinoma and control human skin. *Lab. Invest.*, 35:132-142.

26. Merkow, L. P., Epstein, S. M., Farber, E., Pardo, M., and Bartus, B. (1969): Cellular analysis of liver carcinogenesis; III. Comparison of the ultra-structure of hyperplastic liver nodules and hepatocellular carcinomas induced in rat liver by 2-fluorenylacetamide. *J. Natl. Cancer Inst.*, 43:33-63.

27. Miya, K., and Steiner, J. W. (1967): Fine structure of interphase liver cell nuclei in acute ethionine intoxication. *Lab. Invest.*,16:677-692.

28. Mochizuki, Y., Hruban, Z., Morris, H. R., Slesers, D., and Vigil, E. L. (1971): Microbodies of Morris hepatomas. *Cancer Res.*, 31:763-773.

29. Nicholson, G.L., and Poste, G. (1976): The cancer cell; dynamic aspects and modifications in cell-surface organization. *N. Engl. J. Med.*, 295:197.

30. Pearse, A. G. E. (1969): The cytochemistry and ultrastructure of polypeptide hormone-producing cells of the APUD series and embryologic, physiologic and pathologic implications of the concept. *J. Histochem.*, 17:303-313.

31. Phelps, P. C., Toker, C., and Trump, B. F. (1979): Surface ultrastructure of normal, adenomatous, and malignant epithelium from human colon. SEM/79/III: 169-175.

32. Postlethwaite, R. (1970): Molluscum contagiosum; a review. *Arch. Environ. Health*, 21:432-452.

33. Riede, U. N., Moore, G. W. and Sandritter, W. (1980): Peroxisomes in cellular injury and disease, in *Pathobiology of Human Disease*, edited by B. F. Trump, R. T. Jones, and A. Laufer. Gustav Fisher, New York (in press).

34. Rosai, S., and Rodriquez, H. A. (1968): Application of electron microscopy to the differential diagnosis of tumors. *Am. J. Clin. Pathol.*, 50:555.

35. Schenk, P. (1974): Microfilaments in human epithelial cancer cells. *Z. Krebsforsch.*, 84:241-256.

36. Scott, R. E., and Furcht, L. T. (1976): Membrane pathology of normal and malignant cells; a review. *Human Pathol.*, 7:519.

37. Singer, S. J. (1975): Architecture and topography of biologic membranes, in *Cell Membranes, Cell Biology, and Pathology*, edited by G. Weissman and R. Clarborne. H. P. Publishing Co., New York.

38. Sobel, H. J., Schnarz, R. and Marquat, E. (1973): Light and electron microscope study of the origin of granular cell myoblastoma. *J. Pathol.*, 109:101-111.

39. Sternberger, L. A. (974): *Immunocytochemistry*. Prentice-Hall, Englewood Cliffs, N. J.

40. Svoboda, D. J., and Reddy, J. K. (1974): Some biologic properties of microbodies (peroxisomes). *Pathobiol. Ann.*, 1974:1-32.

41. Tanayama, S., and Sugawa, I. (1970): Electron microscopic observation of Ewing's sarcoma—a case report. *Acta Pathol. Jpn.*, 20:87-101.

42. Trump, B. F., McDowell, E. M., and Arstila, A. U. (1980): Cellular reaction to injury, in *Principals of Pathobiology*, Ed. 3, pp. 20-111, edited by R. B. Hill and M. F. La Via, Oxford University Press, New York.

43. Trump, B. F., and Jones, R. T. (eds.) (1978): *Diagnostic Electron Microscopy, Vol. I*. John Wiley & Sons, New York.

44. Trump, B. F., and Jones, R. T. (Eds.) (1978): *Diagnostic Electron Microscopy, Vol. II*. John Wiley & Sons, New York.

45. Trump, B. F., Jesudason, M. L., and Jones, R. T. (1978): Ultrastructural features of diseased cells, in *Diagnostic Electron Microscopy, Vol. I*, pp. 1-88, edited by B. F. Trump and R. T. Jones. John Wiley & Sons, New York.

46. Trump, B. F. McDowell, E. M., Glavin, F., Barrett, L. A., Becci, P. J., Schürch, W., Kaiser, H. E., and Harris, C. C (1978): The respiratory epithelium; III. Histogenesis of epidermoid metaplasia and carcinoma in situ in the human. *J. Natl. Cancer Inst.*, 61:563-575.

47. Tyson, G. E., and Bulger, R. E. (1972): Endothelial detachment sites in glomerular capillaries of vinblastine-treated rats. *Anat. Rec.*, 172:669-674.

48. Valenta, L. J., Michel-Bechet, M., Mattson, J. C., and Singer, F. R. (1977): Microfollicular thyroid carcinoma with amyloid rich stroma resembling the medullary carcinoma of the thyroid [MCT]. *Cancer*, 39:1573-1586.

49. Warburg, O. (1926): *Über den Stoffwechsel der Tumoren*. Springer, Berlin. (English Translation by F. Dickens (1930), Constable, London.)

50. Weinstein, R. S., Alroy, J., and Pavli, B. U. (1980): Pathobiology of cell junctions, in *Pathobiology of Human Disease*, edited by B. F. Trump, R. T. Jones, and A. Laufer. Gustav Fisher, New York (in press).

51. Williams, G. M., Klaiber, M., Parker, S. E., and Farber, E. (1976): Nature of early appearing carcinogen-induced liver lesions resistant to iron accumulation. *J. Natl. Cancer Inst.*, 57:157-165.

52. Wotosewick, J. J., and Porter, K. R. (1976): Stereo high voltage electron microscopy of whole cells of the high diploid line, W1-38. *Am. J. Anat.*, 147:303-323.

21

Selected Biophysical Aspects of Neoplastic Growth

Donald F. H. Wallach

GENERAL INTRODUCTION

Wide and intensive investigation over several decades indicates that tumorigenesis and malignancy do not derive from unique, simple, biochemical, or molecular biological defects. On the contrary, it now appears that each tumor, malignant or not, is an entity *sui generis*, due to crucial deviations in the *state* of certain cellular components from the normal situation. This possibility has led to some intensive explorations into the state of (a) *water* and of (b) the *membranous compartments* in normal vs. tumor cells. The latter topic has been the focus of extremely active investigation and is continuing to receive the most vigorous attention. It has been reviewed *in extenso* by Wallach (35). The state of cellular water in normal vs. neoplastic cells has also been examined intensively of late and experimentation in this area has recently been combined with investigations into the possible states of major ionic solutes in the intracellular water of normal vs. neoplastic tissues.

This brief review deals primarily with physical approaches to the above ideas about water, or membrane, state and neoplastic transformation. It is not intended to be a comprehensive review of the literature and does not deal with a number of aspects of neoplasia which have been studied by techniques that are essentially physical, such as ultrastructure (electron microscopy) cellular communication (electrophysiological methods), and surface charge (electrokinetic techniques), all of which focus on different functional aspects of the neoplastic (malignant) condition. The emphasis here is rather on questions of state in the physical sense and on methods of approaching this by physical techniques.

STATE OF WATER IN NORMAL AND NEOPLASTIC TISSUES

Introduction

Possible differences between the states of water within normal and neoplastic cells have been explored by nuclear magnetic resonance (NMR). When placed in a magnetic field, the field experienced by a given atomic nucleus within a molecule depends not only on the applied magnetic field but also on the magnetic microenvironment of the nucleus. Because a nuclear magnetic moment slightly polarizes the bonding electrons of a molecule magnetically, and this polarization can transmit the instantaneous spin state of one nucleus to another, one tends to obtain a distribution of resonant frequencies about the mean resonant frequency of the isolated nucleus. However, the above process is usually countered by *spin lattice relaxation*, whereby energy of excited nuclear spins is transferred by a radiationless mechanism into the lattice of total nuclei in a time, T_1, describing the lifetime of the spin states (10^{-5}–10^{-4} sec). Spin lattice relaxation depends primarily on transition between spin states induced by dipoles fluctuating near the resonance frequency of the nuclei under study.

A second relaxation process that provides important information is "*spin-spin relaxation.*"

Spin-coupled nuclei, with unhindered mobility, tumble rapidly and the field of dipoles imposed upon one nucleus by its neighbors is time-averaged. However, when the motion of coupled nuclei is constrained in some fashion, e.g., by high local viscosity, the field experienced by one nucleus varies with the motions of the surrounding nuclei. The nuclei will then precess out of phase with one another, leading to band broadening. This dipole interaction is described by the relaxation time, T_2, which is the time constant for the rate at which precessing nuclei get out of phase.

Water Proton NMR (PMR)

Numerous research groups (Damadian (6), Damadian et al. (7–9), Hazelwood et al. (16, 17), Hollis et al. (18–21), Frey et al. (13), Weisman et al. (36), Kiricuta et al.(26, 27), Block (2) block and Maxwell (3), Economou et al. (11), Inch et al. 24), Saryan et al. (32), Coles (5) have shown that PMR spin lattice relaxation time (e.g., T_1) of experimental tumors (mostly in rodents) are generally longer than those from normal tissues. These findings have led to the suggestion that PMR might be useful in the diagnosis of human cancer.

Damadian (6) was the first to use PMR techniques as possible means to discriminate between normal and tumor tissues. He observed differences between the relaxation times of normal tissues and tumor tissues, and interpreted these in terms of a significant decrease in the degree of ordering of intercellular water in malignant tissues. Subsequently Hazlewood et al. (16) measured the relaxation times and diffusion coefficients of water protons in normal and tumor tissues and attributed the increase in the relaxation times for tumor tissues to a change in the interaction of water with the macromolecular structures of the cell. Moreover, the same group (Hazelwood et al. (17)) argued that the genotype of the host influences the relaxation times. However, Kiricuta and associates (26–28) have argued all along that the relationship between the relaxation times, T_1 and T_2 of neoplastic vs. normal tissues, are derived from the relative hydrations of these tissues. Their conclusions concerning T_1 were confirmed by Inch et al. (24) and Saryan et al. (32). In addition Block (2), Block and Maxwell (3), and Coles (5) have demonstrated the correlation between water content and the T_2 times in rat tissues. Clearly,

if proton relaxation time measurements are to be used for cancer diagnosis, it must be shown definitively that elevation of such relaxation times are sufficiently characteristic of the malignant state and specific to malignant tissues. This does not appear to be the case.

Thus, Hollis et al. (20) have shown that Morris hepatoma 7800, chemically induced, transplantable malignant rat hepatoma, with an intermediate growth rate, has a T_1 value identical to that of skeletal muscle. For this reason, this group (Hollis et al. (21)) studied a series of six other Morris hepatomas and determined T_1 values, growth rates, and water contents of these hepatomas as well as a mouse fibrosarcoma and two mouse lymphosarcomas. They also examined a variety of other tissues such as brain, heart, spleen, skeletal muscle, kidney, and liver. Their data show rather clearly that the T_1 values of the malignant hepatomas are not invariably longer than those of normal tissues. Indeed there is a considerable overlap, with the values for brain, heart, skeletal muscle, and spleen falling in the middle. The data also show that the T_1 valves depend primarily on the hydration of the tissues, correlating well with direct determinations of water content. Moreover, there was a rough correlation of T_1 and water content with tumor growth rate. *Importantly*, the degree of overlap revealed was such that normal and malignant tissues could not be adequately distinguished by the method.

Also, Kiricuta and Simplaceanu (28) have demonstrated that the main cause of observed differences between the relaxation times, T_1 and T_2, of normal vs. neoplastic tissues is due to the generally higher hydration of the latter. These investigators used pulsed PMR to differentiate between normal and malignant tissues. Their data document a good correlation between the spin lattice (T_1) and spin lattice spin (T_2) relaxation times and tissue water content in all normal tissues as well as neoplastic tissues, with T_1 more sensitive than T_2 to tissue hydration. Because of their findings, they argue that pulse PMR techniques are not likely to produce meaningful results as long as water content is the principal cause of differences in the relaxation values.

Coles (5) performed measurements of pulse PMR relaxation times, T_1 and T_2 at 2.7 MHz and 15 MHz on water protons in isolated fragments of liver, kidney, spleen, muscle, and brain from normal mice and in the same tissues as well as tumors of mice developing a solid ascites sarcoma (following subcutaneous implantation of tumor fragments). An improved spectrometer design made it possible to show that T_1 and T_2 of all tissues, except brain, were increased by the presence of the tumor in the animal. The T_1 and T_2 responses of liver and kidney were proportional to the size of the tumor. The smaller responses shown by T_1 in spleen (15 MHz) and T_1 and T_2 in muscle (2.7 MHz) also showed a significant correlation with tumor size. The relaxation times for the tumors showed a significant negative correlation with tumor size, *i.e.*, the times decreased as tumor size increased. A detailed analysis of the results showed a pattern consistent with the effects expected if tissue water content increased and tumor water content decreased as tumor sizes increased. The analysis further indicated that the effects arose primarily through changes in the fraction of water bound to fast-exchange sites on protein.

The combination of the natural variation of relaxation times between different individuals and the proportionality of the relaxations time response and tumor size indicate that measurements of tissues would not be very useful to indicate the presence of a tumor somewhere in the animal. Indeed, in the case of the tumor studied, the tumor would have to reach 5% of body weight before the relaxation times in sensitive tissues would be sufficiently outside the normal range to give a significant result. Conceivably, successive measurements of a single individual by an *in vivo* technique might be more useful and might permit a monitoring of growth or regression of a tumor.

A number of publications have dealt with the NMR of nuclei other than the hydrogen of cell water in terms of the diagnosis and possible treatment of cancer. The logic of these studies, as stated by Damadian and Cope (8) is that such studies might provide "chemical profiles" of various cancers and that these could lead to a more rational application of chemotherapy.[1]

Damadian and Cope (8) have examined the potassium (^{39}K) NMR of various normal and malignant tissues in rats and mice. They measured the NMR relaxation times (T_1) of potassium in brain, liver, spleen, muscle, kidney, small intestine, and testis and compared these with six types of cancer in rats and mice. They found that the T_1 differences between cancerous and corresponding normal tissues were rather small (perhaps 24% longer for the neoplastic tissues) but that the increase was statistically significant at the 2% level. The authors argue that in general, the NMR "spin-signature" appeared to be distinctive for a given type of tumor, and suggest that (^{39}K) NMR measurements might be useful for diagnosis of cancer in surgical biopsy specimens.

Chemical measurements of water and sodium concentrations showed that the tumors appeared enriched in these substances, without differing in the potassium concentration. This finding is attributed to a "marked reduction of selectivity for potassium vs. sodium in cancers," surely a somewhat extended interpretation.

In another study, Goldsmith and Damadian (15) have compared the ^{23}Na NMR of normal and cancerous tissues. They compared the spin lattice relaxation times (T_1) of muscle, liver, kidney, intestine, and testis with those of Walker 256 carcinosarcoma, Novikoff hepatoma, Ehrlich-ascites carcinoma (grown in solid form), and Sarcoma 180. They report that the T_1 values for the tumors were generally longer than those for the normal tissues with the greatest difference occurring between rat liver ($T_1 = 6.5$ msec) and Novikoff hepatoma ($T_1 = 23.7$ msec). No differences validly distinctive of neoplasia were ob-

---

[1] Such elemental analyses can now be rapidly achieved by electron microscopic x-ray analysis and this method has been tested in comparsions of normal and neoplastic leukocytes. X-rays are produced when any electrically charged particle with sufficient kinetic energy is rapidly decelerated. When this process involves multiple collision and a successive loss of fractions of the total kinetic energy a continued x-ray spectrum is obtained. These considerations apply to electron microscopy, because the primary electrons which constitute the electron beam in electron microscopy are rapidly decelerated when they impinge on the sample. The x-rays that are generated by the deceleration of the beam electrons can be collected and analyzed by either a wavelength dispersive or energy dispersive system. Since characteristic x-rays of the various elements vary in a systematic and predictable manner according to their atomic number, the elemental compo-

sition of the sample volume subjected to the electron beam can be determined. This technique of x-ray microanalysis is particularly useful in studying nonhomogeneous samples such as tumors or cells. Very small amounts of many elements can be measured and localized within the cell with ultrastructural accuracy and under direct electron microscopic control. Yarom *et al.* (37) have applied electron microscopic x-ray analysis to compare the elemental contents of normal and leukemic lymphocytes. The lymphocytes were purified, buffered, and fixed with glutaraldehyde, thin sections (120 nm) cut, and these examined unstained with an electronic microscopic x-ray analyzer. Despite the relatively poor contrast and resolution, due to lack of staining, different cells and some of their organelles could easily be recognized and it was possible to focus the electron beam onto areas of interest with relative ease. It took about 50 sec to develop a reasonable elemental spectrum. It was possible to get strong signals for phosphorus, sulfur, chlorine, calcium, cooper, and zinc and the concentration of some of these elements appeared to be disease-related. In this feasibility study, leukemic lymphocytes showed considerably lower levels of nuclear zinc than normal lymphocytes, whereas phosphorus was only moderately decreased.

served. Estimation of the tissues sodium from the signal intensity of the reasonances indicated that all four tumor types contained more sodium than any of the normal tissues. This observation was partly confirmed by conventional chemical analyses. The authors argue that, as a method of quantitation, NMR compares "favorably with other commonly used techniques such as flame photometry or atomic absorption spectra photometry in that it avoids time consuming and destructive sample digestion required by the latter." However, flame photometry is certainly a very inexpensive, clinically widely used method and NMR is expensive and not acessible to most hospitals. Also analyses of heterogeneous cell samples are of questionable value in any case.

Zaner and Damadian (39, 40) have studied phosphorus NMR in normal vs. neoplastic cells. Their experimentation had two aims. The first was to isolate "cancer-specific" NMR absorption frequencies that might aid in the *diagnosis* of cancer. The second was to utilize such frequencies—if they existed—in cancer *therapy*.

The logic for the *diagnostic* application is that a frequency scanning approach would avoid the difficulties that arise with pulse NMR, namely that the tumor signal is diluted out by signals from normal tissues including stroma.[2] Frequency-dependent NMR might avoid the problem since "specific" cancer lines would appear regardless of lines originating from normal tissues—which would lie elsewhere in the radiofrequency spectrum.

Concerning *therapy* the authors present a somewhat euphoric idea: if cancer-specific lines exist one could employ radiofrequency (rf)-radiation at frequencies that would damage only neoplastic tissues and leave normal tissues unharmed. The frequencies for treatment would be selected from high resolution scans of the malignant tumor. It is argued that these frequencies should also hold for metastatic foci, allowing treatment without localizing these foci. The therapeutic effect would then be due to tumor hyperthermia by rf-radiation, a modality that is now being actively explored by more direct approaches (e.g., Overgaard and Overgaard (30)).

The results presented by Zaner and Damadian (39, 40) are marginal. They show no clear evidence for any "cancer specific" rf-frequency. Moreover, the authors' calculations indicate that

the energies that can be absorbed by use of NMR are much too small to lead thermic tissues destruction. Despite this they retain the concept, arguing that it might be possible to use nuclear resonance to "trigger a tumor destruction even though the energies are too small to heat."

STUDIES ON THE MEMBRANE STATE

Spin Label Studies

Barnett *et al.* (1) have attempted to estimate the "fluidity" of membrane lipids in normal and neoplastically converted fibroblasts by use of spin label measurements. They exposed the various cell types to a nitroxide derivative of the tadecanoic acid and then recorded the electron spin resonance (ESR) spectra of the nitroxide groups after washing the cells. They interpreted their results to mean that the molecular motions of the lipid probes were somewhat less "ordered" in the neoplastic cells than in the normal fibroblasts, and attributed this to a greater "fluidity" of the lipids in the plasma membrane of neoplastic cells.

Gaffney (14) used a similar approach in an attempt to evaluate the "inherent flexibility of the lipid acyl chains in intact membranes" of normal mouse 3T3 fibroblasts and several virally transformed variants thereof (SV40, polyoma, and Rous sarcoma virus) by means of several fatty acid spin labels. The fatty acid spin labels were chosen to have the reporter group, the nitroxide residue, at varying distances from the carboxyl terminal of the label. The label was transferred to intact, cultured cells as in the experiments of Barnett *et al.* (1).

The results (Gaffney (14)) show *no* significant difference in inherent "lipid flexibility" in normal vs. transformed mouse fibroblasts, as measured by the behavior of the various spin label probes. Also, it was found important, for reliable comparisons, to adequately control temperature, since differences in water content or sample positioning could lead to very considerable extents of microwave sample heating. Conceivably this technicality might have been the basis for the differences between normal and neoplastic cells reported by Barnett *et al.* (1).

Unfortunately, serious flaws in these spin label experiments prevent meaningful interpretation of differences, or lack of such, observed between normal and transformed cells and prevent conclusions about plasma membrane "fluidity." *First*, no measurements of label up-

---

[2] The authors argue that a solution to this problem could be obtained by using appropriate "focussing methods." This is improbable, however, because all tumor cells have normal cells associated with them, for example fibroblasts, endothelium, and lymphocytes.

take were made, an essential requirement for comparisons of multimembrane, multicompartment systems, such as different intact cells. *Second*, nitroxide lipid analogs tend to perturb and "fluidize" their microenvironment; they also partition preferentially into fluid domains. *Third*, nitroxide spin labels are inactivated (reduced) to different degrees by different cells. *Fourth*, and most important, nitroxide-labeled fatty acids bind to all kinds of biomembranes, liposomes, oil droplets, as well as diverse proteins. Some membranes give "fluid" signals, others do not. Fatty acid spin probes in oil droplets give "fluid" signals, but the same probes bound to hydrophobic domains in proteins indicate "immobilization."

The experiments can thus give no information as to the location(s) of the probes and there is certainly no reason to assume that they are restricted to plasma membranes. A slightly greater amount of adsorbed albumin (from medium) in the normal cells would give the appearance of greater "fluidity" in the transformed cells. An increased oil droplet content (common in many neoplastic cells) would also give the appearance of greater membrane "fluidity." Differential uptake of the spin probes by the two cell categories together with different reduction rates of nitroxide free radicals (e.g., secondary to enhanced aerobic glycolysis in neoplastic cells) may further confuse the issue.

NMR Studies

Nicolau *et al* (29) have measured the ^{1}H and ^{13}C NMR of lipids in normal and SV40 virus-transformed hamster embryo fibroblast "membranes." For this the two cell types were sonicated and inside the material pelleted by centrifugation at 6×10^6 g· min. The pellets were then washed once with water, repelleted, lyophilized, washed twice in D_2O, and resuspended to a concentration of 15% w/w for NMR.

The authors obtained well resolved ^{1}H and ^{13}C NMR spectra with material from both normal and transformed cells. Measurements of the ratios of the ^{13}C T_2 values [normal/transformed] suggested increased intermolecular motion in the membranes from the transformed cells. The authors carried out a study of the temperature dependence of the (CH$_2$) line in the ^{1}H spectra in the temperature range 25–70°C and discovered a sloping Arrhenius plot for the normal material but not in the case of the material from

transformed cells. They argue on this basis that the "fluidity" of the phospholipid region in the transformed cell membrane seemed to be significantly higher than that observed in the normal cell material. The basis for this interpretation of the rather unusual Arrhenius plot (Raison (31)) is quite unclear.

This study is not very informative, because the particulate mixture studied is totally uncharacterized. Certainly some tumor cells differ from normal in terms of lipid content, and even composition, the proportion of various intercellular membranes etc. (Wallach (35)) but there is tremendous variability—between various membranes of a given cell and between given membranes of diverse normal and neoplastic cells. Therefore, even approximate conclusions require careful membrane fraction and characterization. The authors' conclusions that their data indicate a change in tumor plasma membranes are not justified.

Fluorescence Studies

Lipid Probes

Inbar *et al.* (23) describe the use of the aromatic fluorophore 1,6-diphenyl-1,3,5-hexatriene (DPH) as a probe of the "fluidity" of the plasma membranes of normal and neoplastic lymphocytes. They exposed intact normal rat or mouse lymph node cells, normal human peripheral blood lymphocytes, leukemic human blood lymphocytes (chronic lymphocytic leukemia) and cells of a Moloney virus-induced mouse T-cell lymphoma, to aqueous dispersions of DPH and thereafter measured polarization, p, and made estimates of membrane microviscosity, by reference to the variation of DPH polarization with medium viscosity for unbound DPH. Their data show that the polarization of DPH taken up by leukemic mouse and human lymphocytes was 84% and 92%, respectively, of that found in normal rodent or human lymphoid cells. The viscosities in the DPH microenvironment would therefore be 43% and 25% lower in neoplastic rodent and human lymphoid cells than in the normal cells at 4°C. The authors conclude that the plasma membrane lipids of the neoplastic cells are more "fluid" than those of normal lymphoid cells.

Shinitzky and Inbar (34) reported further on their attempts to measure "microviscosity" differences between normal and neoplastic cells by use of DPH. In these experiments they tested the behavior of the probe, in liposomes and biological membranes of different cholesterol/phospholipid molar ratio and at different temperatures. They also examined normal and malignant (SV40-transformed) hamster fibroblasts grown *in vitro*, as well as normal rat or mouse lymphocytes, compared with the Moloney virus-transformed mouse T-type lymphoma cells. As before, the DPH was added to intact cells.

It appears from the results that, in the case of the fibroblasts, the neoplastic conversion produces a higher lipid "microviscosity," whereas in the case of lymphocytes, malignant transformation causes a lower lipid "microviscosity." The authors' attempt to correlate these data with their finding that in model systems the "microviscosity" correlates with cholesterol/phospholipid ratio, *i.e.*, that an increase in this ratio produces an increase in microviscosity.

The authors argue that there is "a marked reduction of the molar ratio of cholesterol to phospholipids in the membranes of leukemic cells" and that this "induces the significant reduction in the membrane microviscosity as compared to normal lymphocytes." However, they have not measured plasma membrane cholesterol and their claims are totally contradictory to the findings of very high rates of cholesterol biosynthesis and cholesterol levels in a variety of leukemic lymphocytes (*cf.* Wallach (35)).

The experiments of Inbar *et al.* (23) and Shinitzky and Inbar (34) also contain more basic defects which preclude secure interpretation. *First*, the binding measurements, needed for comparisons between cells, are lacking. *Second*, fluorescent probes such as DPH like other probes may alter their microenvironment and tend to localize in preexisting fluid domains. *Third*, the cell types used are not comparable, particularly rodent lymph node cells and a T-cell population. *Fourth*, and most crucial, the experiments provide no clue as to the location(s) of the DPH. The fact that DPH fluorescence intensifies after addition of the cells does not mean penetration "into the surface membrane," but partition into various sites within the cell.

The authors argue vigorously, but not convincingly, that their label is located predominantly in the surface membrane. However, the evidence presented in support of this contention consists primarily of the undocumented statement that fluorescent microscopy shows fluorescent cell periphery after addition of the label. It is acknowledged that the labeled cells bleach very rapidly, preventing photography of the peripheral fluorescence, and no studies on isolated membranes have apparently been carried out. It is argued, nevertheless, that "unless otherwise proven, we will continue to relate the DPH signal to the cell surface membrane, even though conclusive evidence for it are not yet in hand."

In my view, the authors' contentions not withstanding, the observed differences in polarization could reflect different proportions of the neutral fat, altered membrane proportions, and many other uncontrolled variables.

Dionisi *et al.* (10) have studied the fluorescent probe, 1-analinonaphthalene-8-sulfonate (ANS) for its reaction with "plasma membranes" isolated from liver and from a Morris hepatoma. Unfortunately, their fractionation techniques do not take into account the fact that an entirely different product is produced by applying almost identical fractionation methods, two cell types of very different surface characteristics. They find that both membrane types cause an intensification of ANS fluorescence and a blue shift of the emission maximum. The blue shift was 20 nm in the case of the normal liver membranes and 35 nm in the tumor membranes.

Unfortunately, the study does not take into account the extensive information, now available, concerning ANS binding, nor does it utilize the established phenomenon that membrane-bound ANS can be localized much better by its capacity to act as an acceptor for the excitation energy of membrane-protein tryptophan. The data thus merely indicate that ANS goes into fairly hydrophobic domains and that the membrane preparation from the Morris hepatoma seems to exhibit a somewhat larger binding capacity for ANS to sites of lower polarity.

Edwards *et al.* (12) have carried out investigations on the baby hamster kidney cells, BHK21, and Rous sarcoma virus-transformed lines derived from BHK21, BHKT1, and BHKT2 in order to establish some correlation between membrane structure of the transformed cells with that of normal cells. They employed normal spectrofluorimetric techniques to investigate the fluorescence of N-phenyl-1-naphthylamine in the cell membranes and also laser photolysis to excite pyrene and derivatives of pyrene in the cell membrane. All the studies were carried out on intact cells. Incorporation of the probes was rather empirical. Thus pyrenebutyric acid and N-phenyl-1-naphthylamine were incorporated into the cells by incubating these with the probes, coated on the walls of the container, in the ratio 20 μl of pyrenebutyric acid per 10^6 cells and 10 μl of N-phenyl-1-naphthylamine per 10^6

cells. Pyrene was prepared as an acetone stock solution (10^{-2} M) and 40 μl of this combined with 10 ml of phosphate-buffered saline to produce a fine suspension to 4 parts of cells. After incubation at 37°C the cells were removed and resuspended in phosphate-buffered saline.

N-Phenyl-1-naphthylamine gave the following results. The two transformed lines had a red shifted emission spectrum compared with the BHK21 line. Moreover, the microviscosity calculated at 23°C and 37°C showed that the environment experienced by the probe was most rigid in BHK21, less so in BHKT1, and still less so than in BHKT2. It is considered therefore that the environment of N-phenyl-1-naphthylamine is more polar in the transformed cells, but that its microviscosity is lower than that of normal cells.

The fluorescent lifetimes of pyrene and pyrenebutyric acid were similar in all cell types. Excimer fluorescence was observed at high pyrene concentrations and at two different temperatures. The data showed a greater yield of excimer in BHK21 at 23°C than in BHKT1 and BHKT2 at this temperature. However, at 37°C there was no significant differences between BHK21 and BHKT2. This might be taken to indicate a possibly decreased mobility of the pyrene probe in the membranes of the transformed cells at least at 23°C—that is, if the probe is only in the membranes.

The authors also studied the quenching of pyrene and pyrenebutyric acid by O_2, Na^+, I^-, Tl^+, NO_3^- and nitromethane. The data show that the quenchers can move into the membrane to deactivate the pyrene singlet excited state. The rate constant for quenching was generally lower in the BHKT1 and BHKT2 cells than in BHK21 cells with the exception of iodide quenching of pyrene in BHKT2. Also, quencher penetration into BHKT1 is slower than into BHKT2 and BHK21, but BHKT2 is similar to BHK21 in this respect. O_2 behaves identically in all three cells.

Ideally this kind of study might provide some meaningful information if one can correctly exclude the perturbing effects of the probes on the membranes. N-Phenyl-1-naphthylamine probably lies at polar-apolar interfaces, with the aromatic moiety located in more apolar regions. Pyrene is less polar and is expected to lie in a more apolar environment. Also, its life time is much longer and the probe can consequently diffuse considerable distances during an experimental measurement. Consequently pyrene gives "a summary of the rigidity of the environment visited by the excited" molecules. This

volume would be much larger than what is seen by the probe N-phenyl-1-naphthylamine, which would report only about restricted microdomains.

Taken at face value the results suggest that the transformed cells allow greater localized mobility—monitored by the N-phenyl-1-naphthylamine—but also exhibit *reduced* long range mobility of molecules such as pyrene.

Unfortunately this study also contains the flaws already discussed in connection with previous probe studies on intact cells. There is absolutely no information as to the location of the probes, the relative volume of the various membrane compartments in the different cell types, the accessibility of the probes in the different compartments, and the possibility of artificial compartments such as lipid droplets, etc. This study, therefore, does not provide reliable or interpretable information as to membrane alterations in neoplasia.

Fluorescent Lectins

Inbar *et al.* (22) and Shinitzky and Inbar (34) have attempted to probe the "mobility" of plasma membrane proteins by use of fluorescein-labeled concanavalin A (F-Con A), wheat germ agglutinin (F-WGA), and soybean agglutinin (F-SBA).

These experiments were designed to compare the decay rates of fluorescence polarization of free and cell-bound fluorescein-lectin conjugates. Since the relaxation rate, τ, of fluorescein ($\sim 4\ \mu sec$) is vastly less than that of the proteins, these workers constructed plots of $1/\tau$ vs. $\eta_0\tau/\eta$ where η_0 is the viscosity of aqueous buffer and η that of a buffer solution containing sucrose (up to 70%). At high values of $\eta_0\tau/\eta$ $1/\tau$ reflects predominantly the mobility of the protein rather than that of the fluorophore, thereby allowing evaluation of ρ_0, the relaxation rate of the coupled proteins, as well as the anisotropies, r_0, of the coupled proteins. The ρ_0 and r_0 values were then compared with the corresponding values, ρ and r, or the F-lectins absorbed by diverse cells. Unfortunately, the effects of medium viscosity on the fluorescence polarization of cell-bound lectins was not evaluated.

The authors argue that the ρ values reflect those of the membrane lectin receptors and that differences in ρ indicate alterations in receptor mobility. They further contend that the receptor mobility is greater in neoplastic fibroblasts than in normal cells and lower in neoplastic lymphocytes than in normal lymphoid cells. They interpret the data to indicate major changes of membrane "fluidity" with neoplastic conversion! This conclusion is not justified for the following reasons. (a) The relaxation times lie almost two orders of magnitude below that of the 20 μ sec for rhodopsin which is a small protein with a proven high rotational mobility; many membrane proteins show much lower mobility than rhodopsin. (b) The ρ values for concanavalin A "bound" to normal lymphocytes and SV40 transformed fibroblasts do not differ significantly from the solution value (in contrast to F-WGA and F-SBA). (c) There is no information on the effect of fluorescein coupling on the subunit association of the lectins; a change could modify binding. (d) The cells are not comparable: rat lymph node cells are not appropriate controls for mouse T-cells. Cultured fibroblasts should be compared with neoplastic variants derived therefrom. (e) The measurements were carried out at 24°C, where concanavalin A is rapidly interiorized into cells. (f) There were no binding studies. These are essential for comparisons since one cannot, a priori, assume a single type of binding site for each cell. (g) At the concanavalin A levels used (20 μg/ml) concanavalin A receptors of transformed fibroblasts aggregate. This should restrict diffusional rotation. But the authors argue for greater mobility in F-concanavalin A treated transformed fibroblasts than in normal cells.

It appears that the concanavalin A experiments considered here do not give any insight into "receptor mobility." Indeed, there might be trivial reasons for the observed differences, for example: (a) Under the conditions employed, part of the lectin is no longer membrane bound, but on the way to intracellular digestion; this process can vary from one cell to the next. (b) Membrane-bound lectins rotate independently about sites of attachment to receptors, but this rotation varies from cell to cell depending on receptor distribution. (d) Receptors are bound to membranes with varying affinities (Schmidt-Ullrich and Wallach (33), Bornens et al. (4)). Whatever the interpretation of the data, the authors' conclusion that the observed relaxation rates reflect membrane "fluidity" appears premature and certainly cannot be generalized.

Recently there have been several attempts to measure the lateral mobility of the receptors for concanavalin A by use of *photobleaching approaches*. In these studies, concanavalin A and/ or its succinylated derivative labeled with fluo-rescein-isothiocyanate and the labeled lectin were allowed to react with the cells to be tested. After washing, geometrically defined areas on the surface of individual cells are photobleached by laser pulses and the rate of fluorescence return to the bleached spots used to evaluate the apparent mobility of the receptors. Zagyanski and Edidin (38) applied this technique to a comparison of embryonic mouse fibroblasts composed of cells C1 1D (probably neoplastic). In the case of the embryonic fibroblasts, slow recovery was detected with concanavalin A and more rapid recovery of fluorescence with the succinylated derivative. In the case of the C1 1D cells, no recovery of fluorescence was observed.

In another study, Jacobson et al. (25) compared normal and SV40-transformed fibroblasts using essentially the same technique. Their data indicated that a considerable proportion of the bound, fluorescein-labeled, concanavalin A molecules do not move appreciably and also that one could not detect any significant difference between the normal and neoplastic cells by this method. These results are basically similar to those obtained by Zagyanski and Edidin (38).

Neither of the photobleaching studies can be related to the polarization studies using fluorescent lectins (Inbar et al. (22), Shinitzky and Inbar (34)). Also, laser-photobleaching experiments are flawed by the fact that part of the energy in the laser illumination used to produce irreversible bleaching is converted into heat, conceivably leading to elevations of the temperature in the microenvironment fluorophores, a fact that cannot be prevented by controlling bulk temperature. The laser pulses might thus (a) artificially heat, coagulate, or inactivate membrane protein: (b) artificially fluidize or even chemically alter membrane lipids; and (c) both. It would therefore appear that experiments of this type cannot, in their present form, provide unambiguous information about membrane structure.

CONCLUSIONS

A variety of physical techniques of proven potency in other areas have been applied to differentiate between normal and neoplastic cells, with emphasis on the states of water and of membranes. The results to date have been disappointing and inconclusive largely because the physical approaches have been applied in relative isolation from biological and biochemical concepts. Progress in this area will require concentratedly interdisciplinary efforts on tested, relevant biological systems.

References

1. Barnett, R. E., Furcht, L. T., and Scott, R. E. (1974): Differences in membrane fluidity and structure in contact-inhibited and transformed cells. *Proc. Natl. Acad. Sci. U.S.A.*, 71:1992–1994.
2. Block, R. E. (1973): Factors effecting proton magnetic resonance linewidths of water in cellular rat tissues. *FEBS Lett.*, 34:109–112.
3. Block, R. E., and Maxwell, G. P. (1974): Proton magnetic resonance studies of water in normal and tumor rat tissues. *J. Magnet. Reson.*, 14:329.
4. Bornens, M., Karsenti, E., and Avrameas, S. (1976): Cooperative binding of concanavalin A at 4°C and microredistribution of concanavalin A receptors. *Eur. J. Biochem.*, 65:61–69.
5. Coles, P. A. (1976): Dual-frequency proton spin relaxation measurements on tissues from normal and tumor-bearing mice. *J. Natl. Cancer Inst.*, 57:389–393.
6. Damadian, R. (1972): Tumor detection by nuclear magnetic resonance. *Science*, 171:1151–1153.
7. Damadian, R. Zaner, K., Hor, D., and Dimaio, T. (1973): Human tumors detected by NMR. *Physiol. Chem. Physi.*, 5:381–402.
8. Damadian, R., and Cope, F. W. (1974): NMR in cancer; V. Electronic diagnosis of cancer by potassium (^{39}K) nuclear magnetic resonance; spin signatures and T_1 beat patterns. *Physiol. Chem. Phys.*, 6:309–322.
9. Damadian, R., Zaner, K., Hor, K. and DiMaio, T. (1974): Human tumors detected by NMR. *Proc. Natl. Acad. Sci. U.S.A.*, 71:1471–1473.
10. Dionisi, O., Galeotti, T., Terranova, T., Arflan, P., and Azzi, A. (1975): Interaction of fluorescent probes with plasma membranes from rat liver and Morris hepatoma 3924A. *FEBS Lett.*, 49:346–349.
11. Economou, J. S., Parks, L. C., Saryan, L. A., Hollis, D. P., Czeisler, J. L., and Eggleston, J. C. (1973): Detection of malignancy by nuclear magnetic resonance. *Surg. Forum*, 24:127–129.
12. Edwards, H. E., Thomas, K. J., Burleson, G. R., and Kulpa, C. F. (1976): The study of Rous sarcoma virus-transformed baby hamster kidney cells using fluorescent probes. *Biochim. Biophys. Acta*, 448:451–459.
13. Frey, H. E., Knispel, R. R., Kruuv, J., Sharp, R. T., Thompson, R. T., and Pintar, M. M. (1972): Proton spin lattice relaxation studies of non-malignant tissues of tumorous mice. *J. Natl. Cancer Inst.*, 49:903–906.
14. Gaffney, D. J. (1975): Fatty acid chain flexibility in the membranes of normal and transformed fibroblasts. *Proc. Natl. Acad. Sci. U.S.A.*, 72:664–668.
15. Goldsmith, N., and Damadian, L. (1975): NMR in cancer; VII. Sodium-23 magnetic resonance of normal and cancerous tissues. *Physiol. Chem. Phys.*, 7:263–269.
16. Hazlewood, C. F., Chang, D. C., Medina, D., Cleveland, G., and Nichols, B. L. (1972): Distinction between the pre-neoplastic and neoplastic states of murine mammary glands. *Proc. Natl. Acad. Sci. U.S.A.*, 69:1478–1480.
17. Hazlewood, C. F., Cleveland, G., and Medina, D. (1974): Relationship between hydration and proton nuclear magnetic resonance relaxation times in tissues of tumor-bearing and non-tumor bearing mice. Implications for cancer detection. *J. Natl. Cancer Inst.*, 52:1849–1853.
18. Hollis, D. P., Saryan, L. A., and Morris, H. P. (1972): A nuclear magnetic resonance study of water in two Morris hepatomas. *Johns Hopkins Med. J.*, 131:441–444.
19. Hollis, D. P., Economou, J. S., Parks, L. C., Eggleston, L. A., Saryan, L. A., and Czeisler, J. L. (1973): Nuclear magnetic resonance studies of several experimental and human malignant tumors. *Cancer Res.*, 33:2156–2160.
20. Hollis, D. P., Saryan, L. A., Economou, J. S., Eggleston, J. C., Czeisler, J. L., and Morris, H. P. (1974): Nuclear magnetic resonance studies of cancer; V. Appearance and development of tumor systemic effect in serum and tissues. *J. Natl. Cancer Inst.*, 53:807–815.
21. Hollis, D. P., Saryan, L. A., Eggleston, J. C. and Morris, H. P. (1975): Nuclear magnetic resonance studies of cancer; VI. Relationship among spin lattice relaxation times; growth rate and water content of Morris hepatomas. *J. Natl. Cancer Inst.*, 54:1469–1472.
22. Inbar, N., Shinitzky, M., and Sachs, L. (1973): Rotational relaxation times of concanavalin A bound to surface membrane of normal and malignant transformed cells. *J. Mol. Biol.*, 81:245–253.
23. Inbar, N., Shinitzky, M., and Sachs, L. (1974): Microviscosity in the surface membrane lipid layer of intact normal lymphocytes and leukemic cells. *FEBS Lett.*, 38:268–270.
24. Inch, W. R., McCredie, J. A., Knispel, R. R., Thompson, R. P., and Pintar, M. N. (1974): Water content and proton spin relaxation time for malignant and non-malignant tissues from mice and humans. *J. Natl. Cancer Inst.*, 52:353–356.
25. Jacobson, K., Wu, E., and Post, G. (1976): Measurement of the translational mobility of concanavalin A in glycerol-saline solutions and on the cell surface by fluorescence recovery after photobleaching. *Biochim. Biophys. Acta*, 433:215–222.
26. Kiricuta, I. C., Demco, D., and Simplaceanu, V. (1972): Spin echo study of the proton transfer of water in malignant tumor tissue, in *Proceedings of the 8th National Symposium of Biophysics, Timisoara, Romania*, pp. 55–61.
27. Kiricuta, I. C., Demco, D., and Simplaceanu, V. (1973): State of water in normal and tumor tissue. *Arch. Geschwulstforsch.*, 42:226–228.
28. Kiricuta, I. C., and Simplaceanu, V. (1975): Tissue water content and nuclear magnetic resonance in normal and tumor tissues. *Cancer Res.*, 35:1164–1167.
29. Nicolau, Cl., Dietrich, W., Steiner, N. R., Steiner, S., and Melnick, J. L. (1975): ^{1}H and ^{13}C nuclear magnetic resonance spectra of the lipids in normal and SV40 virus—transformed hamster embryo fibroblast membranes. *Biochim. Biophys. Acta*, 382:311–321.
30. Overgaard, K., and Overgaard, J. (1972): Investigation on the possibility of a thermic tumor therapy; I. Shortwave treatment of a transplanted ascites mouse memory carcinoma. *Eur. J. Cancer*, 8:65–78.
31. Raison, J. K. (1973): The influence of temperature-induced phase changes on the kinetics of respiratory and other membrane-associated enzyme systems. *Bioenergetics*, 4:285–309.
32. Saryan, L. A., Hollis, D. P., Economou, J. L., and Eggleston, J. C. (1974): Nuclear magetic resonance studies of cancer; IV. Correlation of water content with tissue relaxation times. *J. Natl. Cancer Inst.*, 52:599–602.
33. Schmidt-Ullrich, R., and Wallach, D. F. H. (1975): Cooperativity in concanavalin A binding to thymocyte membranes; correlation with polymerization of a receptor glycoprotein. *Biochem. Biophys. Res. Commun.*, 69:1011–1018.
34. Shinitzky, M., and Inbar, M. (1976): Microviscosity parameters and protein mobility in biological membranes. *Biochim. Biophys. Acta*, 433:133–149.
35. Wallach, D. F. H. (1975): *Membrane Molecular Biology of Neoplastic Cells*. Elsevier-North Holland, New York.
36. Weisman, I. D., Bennett, L. H., Maxwell, L. R., Sr., Woods, M. W., and Burk, D. (1972): Recognition of cancer *in vivo* by NMR. *Science*, 178:1288–1290.
37. Yarom, R., Hall, T. A., and Polliack, A. (1976): Electron microscopic x-ray microanalysis of normal and leukemic human lymphocytes. *Proc. Natl. Acad. Sci. U.S.A.*, 73:3690–3694.
38. Zagyansky, Y., and Edidin, M. (1976): Lateral diffusion of concanavalin A receptors in the plasma membrane of mouse fibroblasts. *Biochim. Biophys. Acta*, 733:209–214.
39. Zaner, K., and Damadian, R. (1975): ^{31}P as a nuclear probe for malignant tumors. *Science*, 189:729–731.
40. Zaner, K. S., and Damadian, R. (1975): NMR in cancer; IX. The concept of cancer treatment by NMR: A preliminary report of high resolution NMR of phosphorous in normal and malignant tissues. *Physiol. Chem. Phys.*, 7:437–451.

22

The Control Theory as a Mathematical-Regulatory Method (Tool) for Better Understanding of Normal and Malignant Cellular Growth

Werner Düchting

INTRODUCTION

Comparative oncology is a science in its own right, which is as diversified as the umbrella science comparative pathology. In the different sections of Chapter 7 it was attempted to show this multiplicity of problems by selected examples. The preceding chapters by Trump and Wallach deal with ultrastructural and biophysical aspects of the problem. It is appropriate to show in this chapter which contributions the regulatory circuits can make to the tracing of cellular transformation using the science of control theory. The material is arranged to show how this is accomplished. The second question of interest is how it applies to comparative oncology. The tracing of neoplastic transformation and of cell transformed to malignancy on one hand and the regression of neoplasms on the other hand can be better understood from a species-specific point of view. But in cellular transformation, as well as in metastatic spread and reaction (even in tumors of the same histologic type), occur species-specific similarities as well as dissimilarities. The relatively new methods may be able to contribute new insight in the transformation of the cellular and subcellular pattern during histogenesis in different species. The section is included here because it is an extension of the biophysical aspects of the problem in methods of biophysics to applied physics or engineering, especially systems analysis.

The rapid advances in the field of control and system theory have given the impetus to investigate the regulation of the growth process of cells by means of model building and computer simulation. In recent years numerous biomathematical and biophysical models of the cell cycle kinetics and cell renewal systems have been developed. Some of them deal with stochastic theory of cell proliferation (14) using difference equations (12) or following the theory of branching processes (10).

In addition to this line of research this contribution tries to explain cell renewal processes as closed loop negative feedback circuits. By applying the control theory to cell renewal systems, an attempt is made here to interpret malignant neoplastic growth as unstable control loops.

BASIC CONTROL LOOP

The very first model (3) developed for this purpose was based on a simple block diagram of a single-loop control circuit (Fig. 22.1). Starting from this control process with rather simplified assumptions the criterion for the stability of the regulator gene has been developed when disturbances have caused irreversible changes in the DNA of the regulator gene. The DNA defect leads to a monotonic or oscillatory increase of the cells if the system has become structurally unstable.

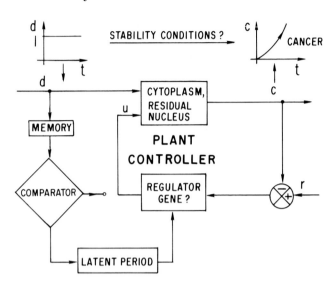

Figure 22.1. Block diagram of a control process of cell proliferation. Controlled variable *c*, deviation of the number of cells from the steady state; reference input *r*, *e.g.*, hormones; disturbances *d*, carcinogens, *e.g.*, damps of tar, mechanical stimuli, radiological rays, viruses, chronic inflammations, environmental perturbations; control signal *u*, production of specific regulation substances, *e.g.*, enzymes.

MACROMODEL OF THE BLOOD-FORMING PROCESS

There are two reasons for specifying the overall model of Figure 22.1 for the process of forming red blood cells: (a) the field of erythropoiesis offers the best and most numerous sets of data gained by experiments (2), (b) the reticulocyte counts of patients with special leukemia show an oscillatory behavior (1), and (c) the dynamic balance between cell gain and cell loss in a normal case itself calls for an interpretation by control theory. Therefore, a deterministic model of the blood-forming process has been developed in which it is possible to change disturbances, parameters, and structures (Fig. 22.2). The aim is to find out the transient response curves of erythrocytes by using digital simulation. With this model at hand it is most interesting to study diseases of the blood-forming processes and to interpret them by means of control theory (5–7).

In the simplified block diagram of Figure 22.2 the reference variable *R* represents the required tissue oxygen symbolized by an equivalent number of erythrocytes. If a deviation $E = R - C$ arises between the reference input signal *R* and the controlled variable *C* (momentary number of red cells), the hormone erythropoietin produced mainly in the kidney affects the determined stem cell compartment in the bone marrow to feed the proliferation pool with a certain number Y32 of the determined stem cells. The

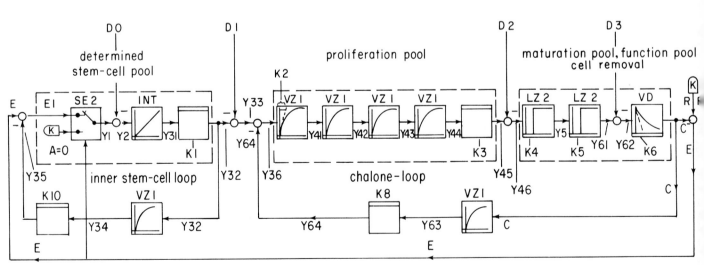

Figure 22.2. Multiloop erythropoietic feedback control block diagram. Y1, determined stem cells = quantity of erythropoietin; Y32, committed stem cells; Y41, proerythroblasts; Y42, macroblasts; Y43, basophilic erythroblasts; Y44, polychromatic erythroblasts; Y5, onchochromatic erythroblasts; Y61, Y62, erythrocytes/reticulocytes; *C*, controlled variable = red blood cells; *R*, reference input = desired number of erythrocytes = required tissue oxygen; *E*, error, deviation = erythrocytes = quantity of erythropoietin; *D*, disturbances, *e.g.*, viruses, rays, vitamin and iron deficiency, bleeding, sudden hypoxia.

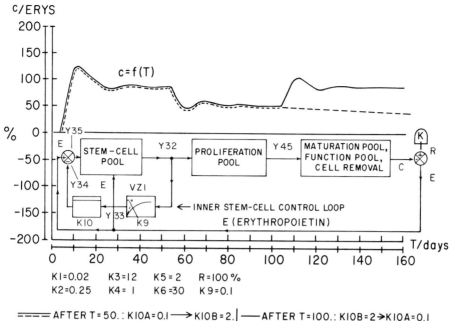

Figure 22.3. Red cell response $C = f(T)$ to changes of the gain K10 of the inner stem cell control loop.

switching function operator SE2 symbolizes the switching activities of the genes. Step by step the determined stem cells pass different pools in which the cell division and cell differentiation take place, then as reticulocytes or erythrocytes C they enter the peripheral blood and after a mean life span of about 120 days they are finally removed.

Interacting subsystems have led to two additional internal control loops. The chalone hypothesis (13) with tissue-specific unspecified mitotic inhibitors is represented by the right inner loop and the produced committed stem cells (15) have a direct negative feedback on their own compartment along the left inner stem cell loop of Figure 22.2.

The time behavior of the single-control-loop elements is described in Figure 22.2 by the respective time responses. Their notations were chosen corresponding to the terminology of the block-oriented programming language ASIM (*Analog SIMulation*) of the firm AEG-Telefunken, which was used for the computer simulation.

In addition to the symbolic first-order transfer function elements VZ1 in the proliferation pool there are delay elements LZ2 in the maturation pool and—for the removal of cells—the delayed derivative element VD. The output response to the stem-cell pool is symbolized by an integrator INT and by the switching-function operator SE2 (comparator). The switching mechanism repre-

sents the activity of genes which initiate the dividing process from resting stem cells to daughter cells. The proportional standard block symbols K1 and K3 indicate the gains of the corresponding phases. In Figures 22.2 the points can also be made out at which the disturbances D0, D1, D2, and D3 act on the control loop. These disturbances cause a sudden reduction of cells in the respective pool, the disturbances being viruses, rays, vitamin- or iron-deficiency, sudden haemorrhage, or environmental perturbations.

For different cases the system can be stimulated by disturbances, parametrical or structural changes and subsequently the time response of the erythrocytes $C = (f(T)$ can be determined by computer simulation.

The first example describes the case of an aplastic anemia and results in a curve of erythrocyte response $C = f(T)$ shown in Figure 22.3. It represents the situation that at the time $T = 50$ days a sudden change of the parameter K10 of the inner stem cell control loop takes place. The increased feedback factor K10 leads to a conspicuously decreasing response of red blood cells (dashed line in Fig. 22.3) which is similar to clinical observations of aplastic anemia. On the other hand it can be shown in a second example (7) that structural changes, *e.g.*, a defect of the comparator (SE2) of the stem cell pool of Figure 22.2 can cause the control loop to become unstable. Then the simulation run leads to a rising

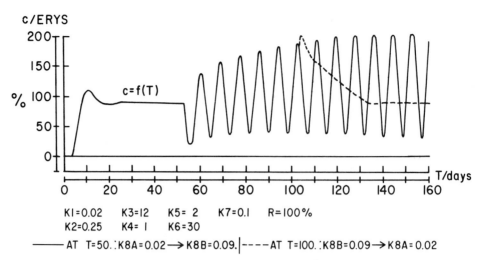

Figure 22.4. Red blood cell responses $C = f(T)$ to changes of the gain K8 of the inner feedback Chalone-loop (see Fig. 22.2).

oscillation course of the red cell response symbolizing certain forms of polycythemia (Fig. 22.4).

GENERALIZED MODEL OF PROLIFERATING CELLS

The erythropoiesis control system configuration described in Figure 22.2 is, however, unsuitable for studying the behavior of a single cell in the different compartments. Therefore, a generalized multiloop and multicompartmental model has been developed (Fig. 22.5) which fulfills the following additional requirements:

1. The existence and location of a cell in a pool can be ascertained at any moment,
2. The mean life span of each cell can be variably fixed and controlled,
3. Every single cell can be eradicated at any desired moment by disturbances from outside.

According to the compartment hypothesis (8, 11) the process of cell division and differentiation takes its course from an undetermined stem cell in the bone marrow (symbolized by signal AO3 of Fig. 22.5) through various stages of development until they finally become mature cells. An example of these mature cells are the erythrocytes S3 which are sent into the peripheral blood.

Each of the single compartments in the model has an identical structure and they are all connected in series but they contain a limited number of viable cells—the maximal number varying from compartment to compartment. The strict arrangement of the cells in the outlined blocks

has been made for reasons of clarity. It is not a statement of the real local position of cells in a pool in which the cells, e.g., Z1.5, Z2.12, and Z3.4, could be arranged next to each other.

Compartment 2 gets the impulses for forming new cells from the previous compartment 1. In this model special subroutines produce the input signals C21, when a cell is being divided and is advancing into the adjacent compartment. A digital logic device ascertains and registers the presence of each cell in the specific compartment. The total number of cells present in compartment 2 is symbolized by S2. S2 is compared in the control loop II with the desired number of cells S22 which represents for instance the required tissue oxygen. If the controlled variable S2 sinks below the reference signal S22 by a certain fixed value the pulser SIØL sends an output signal (S23)—symbolizing a humoral agent—to the stem cell pool. The resulting feedback signal is called S00. The fictive switch SE1 in the stem cell pool, which symbolizes the gene activities, is temporarily closed and delivers a stem cell for the erythrocytic track.

The subsystem of an "artificial cell" (Fig. 22.6) with multi-input and multi-output signals contains analog transfer elements as integrators INT, elements (LZ) with variable delay times, switching components SE, and digital transfer elements as, for instance, logical elements MEMR (memory elements). A detailed description of the subsystem of a single cell is given in Düchting (8).

Important fixed input signals are: the dividing impulses C, the disturbance signals ZA or ZB, the mean life span TA or TB and the input channels UA, VA, NA, etc., to alter the life span

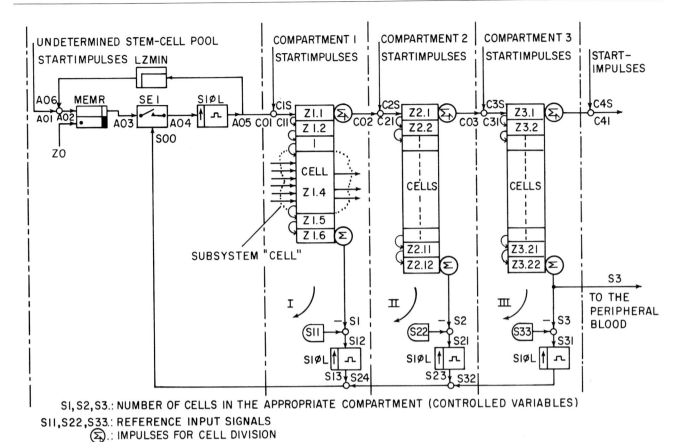

Figure 22.5. Simplified block diagram of a generalized cell renewal feedback-control system.

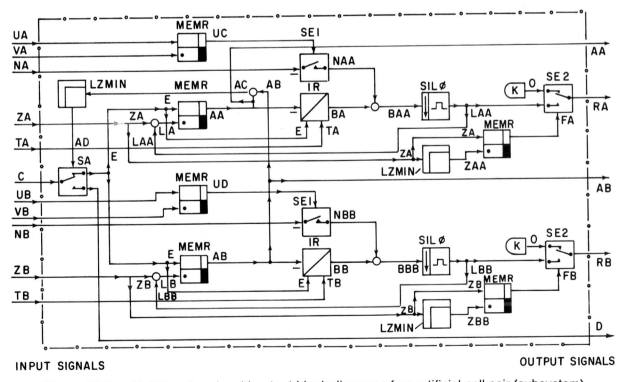

INPUT SIGNALS

OUTPUT SIGNALS

Figure 22.6. Multi-input and multi-output block diagram of an artificial cell pair (subsystem).

of the single cell externally. The most important output signals are AA or AB which prove the existence of cells by the variables logic "1." The newly formed daughter cells enter the following compartments via the outlets RA and RB.

As the design of the generalized model is very flexible, it is possible to carry out case studies which would be impossible in a practical experiment.

In the following computer simulations the reference signals S11, S22, and S33 were programmed in such a manner that the average number of cells is two in compartment 1, four in compartment 2, and eight in compartment 3. The mean value of the fictive life span of cells in the single departments varies between 0.967 and 1.05 days and the standard deviation shows values between 0.197 and 0.333.

The most frequent case in reality is that single

cells of different compartments, being in the DNA-phase, are destroyed directly or indirectly by external disturbances (Fig. 22.7). The arising deviations from the norm are compensated by several internal control loops. If the disturbances of Figure 22.7 are assumed and the reference signal S11 in the control loop I is doubled as a result of the disturbances, Figure 22.7 shows the dynamic behavior of the cells in each compartment. The plot IMP = $f(T)$ illustrates that only loop I of Figure 22.7 is an active control loop while there is no feedback impulse to the stem cell pool generated in the loops II and III. The loops II and III are always present and serve as redundant backup circuits.

Advancing to a further stage of development the time behavior, as outlined in Figure 22.8, is obtained when, from $T = 8.5$ days onward, a programmed perturbation occurs in all cells of

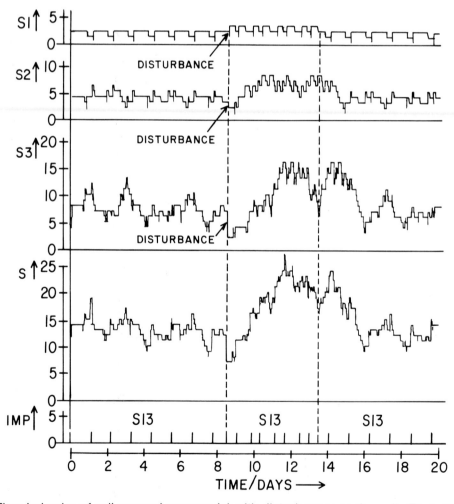

Figure 22.7. Time behavior of cell renewal process (a) with disturbances to the cells Z1.1, Z2.3, Z3.1 till Z3.5 at $T = 8.5$ days and (b) with doubled reference signal S11 in loop I until $E = 13.5$ days. S1, S2, S3, number of cells in the appropriate compartment; S, number of total cells (S = S1 + S2 + S3); and IMP, feedback impulses (S13, S23, S32).

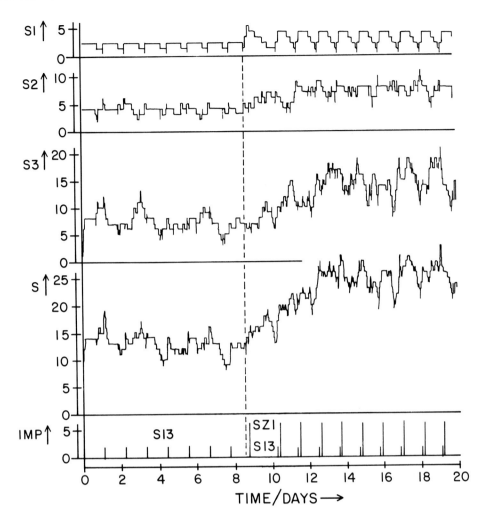

Figure 22.8. Time behavior of cell renewal process without disturbances but with a permanent additional impulse in the feedback loop after T = 8.5 days. S1, S2, S3, number of cells in the appropriate compartment; S, number of total cells (S = S1 + S2 + S3); and IMP, feedback impulses (S13, S23, S32).

compartment 1. Each cell which is being divided in the first compartment affects the stem cell pool—in addition to the normal control impulses S13—to deliver a further cell to the erythrocytic track. Without changing the reference signals of the system, the above oscillating behavior of cells with an increased mean value in some compartments represents a stage of transition to malignant disorders of cell renewal processes. Thus the structural alteration which causes one additional impulse SZ1 leads to a time course which is similar to a tumor-like behavior.

GROWTH PATTERN OF NORMAL AND TRANSFORMED CELLS

The models developed so far disregarded the local position of cells in an array and the cell-to-

cell interactions of adjacent cells in a tissue. This shortcoming is compensated by a new approach constructing a model which allows computer predictions about the organization, local arrangements and cell kinetics of a self-renewal system using microcomputer systems. Additional conditions enable the introduction of the study of the proliferation of two cell systems growing in competition with different speed.

Basic questions concerning the structure of cell renewal systems with regard to information and automata theory have been answered in the papers of Gardner (9) and Lindenmayer (16).

The starting point of the new approach of constructing a cell renewal model is a small homogenous two-dimensional grid section of a larger tissue (Fig. 22.9). The model is to be organized in a way to satisfy the following conditions:

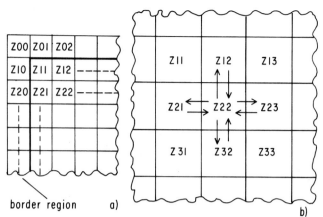

border region   a)   b)

Figure 22.9.   Grid configuration of cells.

1. To start the growing process of each single cell by an initial signal at any desired discrete moment,
2. To assign the mean life span of each cell to a life span matrix element deliberately or to change it within a limited region,
3. To destroy each single cell at any desired discrete moment by external disturbances, e.g., by irradiation which can be simulated by a "reset signal" in the computer program,
4. To grow two competitive cell systems which differ in the life span of their clones, and
5. To display on a plotter the local position of the single cells and also the total number of all living cells at any arbitrary discrete moment.

Further on a set of formation rules is given assuming an intercellular communication between a cell and its adjacent cells in a row and a column, but not with cells diagonally arranged (Fig. 22.9b). The exchange of information includes the mutual message about the actual state of cells and also the sending of and receiving of dividing and resetting instructions. In detail the given formation rules are:

1. A cell can come to life only if there is at least one living neighbor cell in each row or column,
2. If a living cell is surrounded by dead or destroyed horizontal or vertical cells only, this cell is isolated and dies at once.
3. A cell division happens only if a dividing cell finds an empty space next to itself. Otherwise, no cell division take place and the cell dies,
4. If there are several "vacancies" in the direct neighborhood of a cell, a pseudo-binary random generator decides which empty space is to be occupied by the daughter cell,
5. The cells in the border lines (Fig. 22.9a) follow additional conditions. The state of a boundary cell is registrated by all neighbor cells and is enclosed in the data processing mechanism, but division and reset signals are exchanged between this cell and its inner neighbor cell only.

From the viewpoint of automata theory a self-reproducing cell system can be considered as an asynchronous state-controlled sequential cir-

cuit. In this model the outputs are not only dependent on the input signals, but also on the momentary interior states of the cells. Therefore it is reasonable to study the dynamics of a self-reproducing cell system by means of a computer model of a state-controlled circuit, e.g., with the help of a microcomputer system, e.g., of the firm INTEL.

For this purpose, numerous subprograms (Fig. 22.10) have been set up for the listed specifications, for instance "the entering of data of the life span into a storage device," the treatment of borderline cells," "the pseudo-binary random generator," "the control of a run along the elements of the cell matrix," "the entering of marker data of competing cells into an intermediate storage."

Assuming different initial and boundary conditions it is possible to study the space and time behavior of disturbed self-reproducing cell systems by raising deliberated disturbances, e.g., reset instructions which are equivalent to a biological removal either by rays or by surgical operations. First each cell of a 10 × 10 matrix is given a constant life span deliberately fixed according to an equipartition (Fig. 22.10) with two cell systems (○ and ▲) growing with different speed. Then there are written in, the initial and

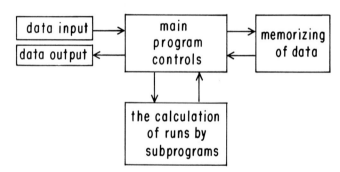

Figure 22.10.   Organization of the program.

3	6	4	3	6	4	5	3	6	3
6	3	5	7	4	6	3	5	7	4
5	7	3	4	7	3	4	6	5	3
3	7	4	5	6	4	7	5	3	6
7	5	3	4	5	7	4	3	4	7
6	3	6	5	3	4	7	5	6	5
3	7	4	3	4	7	5	4	3	7
3	5	7	4	5	3	6	3	7	6
4	6	7	3	5	3	4	6	3	6
3	5	6	7	3	4	6	7	4	7

cell system ○
(fast growing)

7	10	8	7	10	8	9	7	10	7
10	7	9	11	8	10	7	9	11	8
9	11	7	8	11	7	8	10	9	7
7	11	8	9	10	8	11	9	7	10
11	9	7	8	9	11	8	7	8	11
10	7	10	9	7	8	11	9	10	9
7	11	8	7	8	11	9	8	7	11
7	9	11	8	9	7	10	7	11	10
8	10	11	7	9	7	8	10	7	10
7	9	10	11	7	8	10	11	8	11

cell system △
(slowly growing)

Figure 22.11.   Life span matrices of two different cell systems.

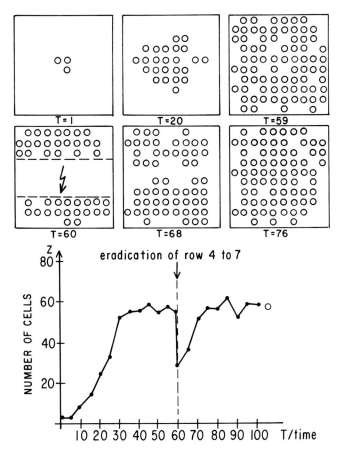

Figure 22.12. Disturbed cell renewal process of the fast growing cell system (○).

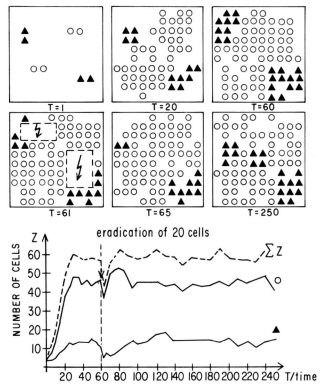

Figure 22.13. Disturbed cell renewal process of two mixed cell systems with different life spans.

reset instructions, the number of sequential runs and the time step of the output signals. Controlled by the master program (Fig. 22.11) the cell matrix is treated, one element after the other, row by row. As a result the local distribution of the living cells and their total number (without the border cells) are put out on a graphic display or a high speed plotter after the pass time of $T = 1$ time unit. The next step is to reduce the life spans in the cell matrix (Fig. 22.10) by the value 1 and to start the second run. When the life span of a cell gets to "zero," the cell is being divided provided that all boundary conditions regarding the adjacent cells are given. The same values of life span as fixed in Figure 22.10 are assigned to the newly formed daughter cells. Starting from three initial cells which at $T = 1$ time unit are rapidly growing in the center of the matrix, it can be observed that the cell renewal process (Fig. 22.12) following the given formation rules reaches the stationary state at $T = 45$ time units. When interpreting the curve $Z = f(T)$ attention has to be paid to the fact that Z represents the total number of living cells *without* the borderline cells. A disturbance at the time of

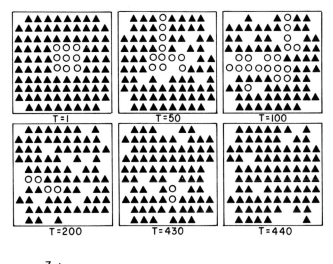

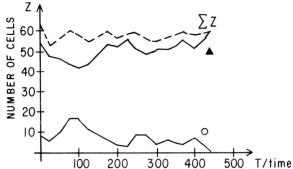

Figure 22.14. Cell renewal process of two competing cell systems with special initial conditions.

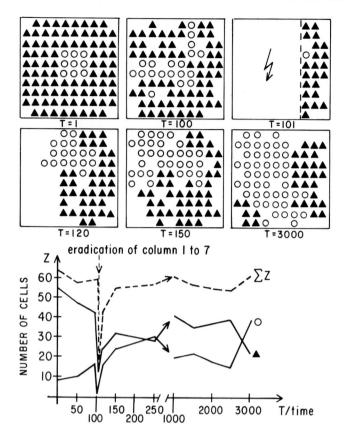

Figure 22.15. Cell renewal process of two competing cell systems with a partial surgical removal of the neoplastic tissue.

$T = 60$ killing all the cells of the rows 1 to 4 Figure 22.12 is already leveled at $T = 75$ time units.

The next assumption in Figure 22.13 is a mixed cell system growing with two different speeds. The origin of the cells is marked by different signs. Here it can be noticed that in the stationary state the ratio of the rapidly proliferating cells to the slowly growing ones is about 3:1 after $T = 40$ time units. After a deliberate disturbance at $T = 61$ the number of cells swings back to the previous steady state after a short overshoot or transition reaction.

When starting from a completely occupied matrix at $T = 1$ according to Figure 22.14 and when assuming a core of 3×3 matrix with rapidly growing cells which could be interpreted as malignant neoplastic tissue, the normal (benign) cells have occupied all spaces of the cell matrix at $T = 440$. If, however, the number of the malignant cells is increased by enlarging the core of the matrix from 3×3 to 6×6, an oscillating time course of both cell systems of almost about the same mean value can be ob-

served after a long term run after $T = 500$ time units.

Returning to the malignant 3×3 core matrix of Figure 22.14 and assuming a surgical removal of the cell columns 1–7 at $T = 101$, it can be made out in Figure 22.15 that the only malignant cell which was not removed by this operation is able to increase rapidly to the value of about 40 cells after $T = 3000$ time units.

If there are several malignant cell clones distributed over the total system of the cell renewal process, an oscillation of the cell population around an almost constant mean value of $Z = 30$ cells can be observed (Fig. 22.16). This oscillation process had not been reduced even after a period of $T = 10,000$ time units as could be demonstrated by a long term run.

Figure 22.17 shows the change of the cell configuration of a neoplastic tissue which is placed

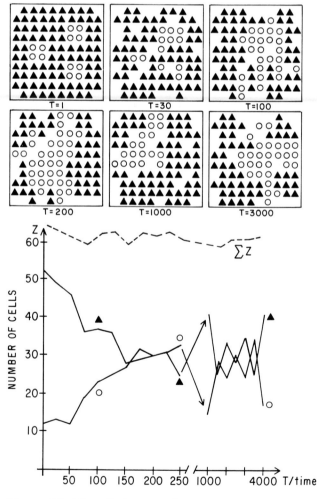

Figure 22.16. Cell renewal process of two competing cell systems with special initial conditions.

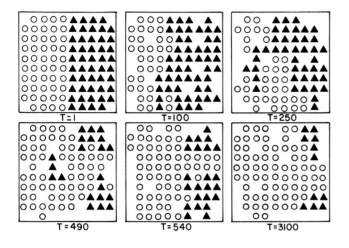

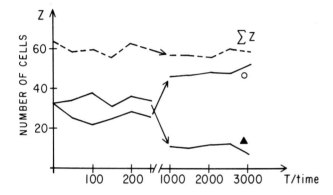

Figure 22.17. Cell renewal process of normal and neoplastic tissue touching each other.

CONCLUSIONS

Resuming the results one can say that

1. The control models developed in this contribution make it possible to describe the dynamics of different blood diseases with the same model,
2. Special forms of disorders or hemopoietic regulation can be interpreted as unstable feedback control loops,
3. An enlarged model has been developed step by step taking into acount the cell-to-cell communication and the local arrangement of cells in a tissue.

The hypothesis proposed should stimulate physicians to look for further deliberated tests with cell cultures.

References

1. Chikkappa, G., Borner, G., Burlington, H., Chanana, A. D., Cronkite, E. P., Öhl, S. Pavelec, M., and Robertson, J. S. (1976): Periodic oscillations of blood leukocytes, platelets, and reticulocytes in a patient with chronic myelocytic leukemia. *Blood*, 47:1023–1030.
2. Dörmer, P. (1973): *Kinetics of Erythropoietic Cell Proliferation in Normal and Anaemic Man. A New Approach Using Quantitative* ^{14}*C-Autoradiography.* Gustav-Fischer Verlag, Stuttgart.
3. Düchting, W. (1968): Krebs, ein instabiler Regelkreis, Versuch einer Systemanalyse. *Kybernetik*, 5:70–77.
4. Düchting, W. (1970): Spezifische Immunitätsbildung—ein kybernetisches Denkmodell. *Messen Steuern Regeln*, 6:216–222.
5. Düchting, W. (1973): Entwicklung eines Erythropoiese-Regelkreismodells zur Computersimulation. *Blut*, 27:342–350.
6. Düchting, W. (1975): Computersimulationen von Zellerneuerungssystemen. *Blut*, 31:371–388.
7. Düchting, W. (1976): Computer simulation of abnormal erythropoiesis—an example of cell renewal regulating systems. *Biomed. Tech.*, 21:34–43.
8. Düchting, W. (1976): A cell kinetic study on the cancer problem based on the automatic control theory using digitla simulation, *J. Cybernet.*, 6:139–172.
9. Gardner, M. (1971): On cellular automata, self-reproduction, the Garden of Eden and the game life. *Sci. Am.*, 224:112–117.
10. Jagers, P. (1975): *Branching Processes with Biological Applications.* John Wiley & Sons, New York.
11. Jansson, B. (1975): Simulation of cell-cycle kinetics based on a multicompartmental model. *Simulation*, pp. 99–108.
12. Kim, M., Bahrami, K., and Woo, K. B. (1975): Mathematical description and analysis of cell cycle kinetics and the application to Ehrlich ascites tumor. *J. Theor. Biol.* 50:437–459.
13. Kivilaakso, E., and Rytömaa, T. (1971): Erythrocytic chalone, a tissue-specific inhibitor of cell proliferation in the erythron. *Cell Tissue Kinet.*, 4:1–9.
14. Korn, A. P., Henkelman, R. M., Ottensmeyer, F. P., and Till, J. E. (1973): Investigations of stochastic model of haemopoiesis. *Exp. Hematol.*, 1:362–375.
15. Lajtha, L. G. (1975): Haematopoietic stem cells. *Br. J. Haematol.*, 29:529–535.
16. Lindenmayer, A. (1975): Developmental algorithms for multicellular organisms; a survey of L-systems. *J. Theor. Biol.*, 54:3–22.

side by side to a normal one. After a long term run of $T = 3000$ it can be seen that the malignant cells for the most part have infiltrated into the "normal" region and that neoplastic tissue is already dominant.

These results show a great similarity to morphological cuts and to cell kinetic curves both gained by experiments. They are to stimulate further deliberated tests with cell cultures.

23

Selected Aspects of Species-Specific Viral Action: Introduction

Hans E. Kaiser

Viruses comprise one group of initiators or promoters which are able to cause neoplastic development in different organisms. They are not only able to react with the host cell, initiating neoplastic development, but they are also able to participate in a chain reaction of transformation with a chemical, physical, or other type of initiator or promoter acting on a host cell. They are highly complicated molecular compounds with the ability to multiply in the cell. They have certain characteristics in common with genes, a fact which warrants placing the sections on selected aspects of species-specific viral action in this part of the study. Certain viruses may be split by a chemical or physical carcinogen in the form of a mutation from a gene of the host.[1] This assumption may be made by the fact that viruses share the following three main characteristics with genes:

1. Identical reproduction in the host cells

2. Imprint imposition ("Merkmalsauslösung")
3. Ability to undergo mutation

For details see "Lack of Species Specific Restoration of Oncornavirus Transforming Genes" in Chapter 25, "Viral Genes Involved in Tumorigenesis" in Chapter 26, and "The Possible Role of a Virus in Genetic Tumor Formation" in Chapter 33.

The subchapter on species-specific viral action is hence followed by the section on genetics in relation to tumorigenesis. Very little data exist on oncogenetic viruses in invertebrates and further studies are urgently needed. In vertebrates, the oncornaviruses (oncogenic RNA viruses) have been selected. Tumorigenic viruses also play an important role in plants; of these, the best known is the wound tumor virus. The species-specific biology of the tumor viruses is thus the linkage. It is my opinion that in tumorigenesis the viruses perform as chemical compounds with a special form of action.

---

[1] H. E. Kaiser, unpublished data.

24

Invertebrates and Oncogenic Viruses

Hans E. Kaiser

If we consider the number of species of invertebrates in relation to the spontaneous neoplasms described and the investigations conducted in invertebrates, we cannot fail to note that a tremendous discrepancy exists. In other words, a wide field is open for study. The few data available suggest that investigation of oncogenic viruses in invertebrates would be highly rewarding, if performed against a background of the variations in normal growth, ontogeny, histology, and distribution of chemical compounds that are found (Table 24.1). Dawe (15) also called for investigations of the causal genetic relationship of invertebrate neoplasms and viruses. The older literature was discussed by Krieg (31) and a brief review was provided by Vago (60) summarizing the problem of oncogenesis in invertebrates. In particular, a comparison of oncogenic invertebrate viruses (which are at least involved in such events as cell proliferations) with oncogenic vertebrate viruses has yet to be made (63). These viruses include the baculoviruses and iridoviruses (18), tumor-inducing-factor, and western X-disease virus. Analogies between vertebrates and invertebrates appear to exist (46).

Studies by Matz and co-workers (42–45) seem to be the most convincing. The cell-free transmission to the epithelial neoplasms of intestinal tumors in the migratory locust (*Locusta migratoria*) was found to be possible by studies of tissue suspensions, the hemolymph, cell-free filtrates, as well as extracted tumor RNA. Biochemical and electron microscopical investigations point to an oncornavirus (32, 58, 59, 61, 63–68).

An epidemic disease known as "curly tail disease" of the planarian platyhelminth (*Dugesia dorotocephala*) was described by Dawe (16). In-

clusion bodies have been found but no virus isolation was achieved. The disease is characterized by a bending at a certain point of its development.

As far as oncogenic viruses of invertebrates are concerned, most of our knowledge is derived from the study of insects. Infection of the leafhopper (*Colladomus montanus*) with the western X-disease virus resulted among other findings with cell proliferation in the esophagus that resembled polyp formation (62).

In the European spruce saw fly (*Gilpinia herzyaeniae*), Bird (7) observed proliferations of the intestinal regenerating crypts of the midintestine caused by the polyhedrosis virus. In an advanced larval stage, these proliferations resulted in large growth processes, up to metamorphosis, composed of a necrotic pigmented center surrounded by large, virus-infected epithelial cells and enclosed within spindle cells, all without signs of malignancies. The studies were repeated, confirmed, and expanded by Neilson and Elgee (47).

Studies of the fruit fly (*Drosophila melanogaster*) with respect to melanized hemocytic aggregations are of special interest because they point to relationships between an oncogenic virus and the genetic properties of the host (26). These relationships are also known in vertebrates.

The oncological nature of the aggregations has yet to be demonstrated. Burdette (9) showed that oncogenic viruses, such as RSV and SV40, exhibit characteristics which vary in different strains. Occurrences of lethality, interaction with genes, and chromosome aberrations have been reported.

Many attempts have been made to isolate the

Table 24.1
Review of the Possible Role of Viruses in Oncogenic and Related Processes in Invertebrates

Phylum and Species	Spontaneous	Experimental Application	Type of Viruses	Action	Reference
Protozoa					
Paramecium sp.	Yes	Cytoplasmic particles	Comparable to Bittner factor		51, 55–57
Platyhelminthes					
Class: Planaria					
Dugesia dorotocephala	Yes		?	Bending of tail	16
Arthropoda					
Class: Insecta					
Order: Orthoptera					
Locusta migratoria	Yes		Oncornavirus	Intestinal "tumors"	32, 58, 59, 61, 63–68
Locusta migratoria, Periplaneta americana		Yes, nerve severance	?	Freeing of latent virus	54
Leucophaea maderae _Callodomus montanus_		Yes	Western X-disease virus	Cell proliferation in esophagus	62
Order: Diptera					
Gilpinia hercyniae	Yes		Polyhedrosis	Proliferations at midintestinal epithelium	47
Drosophilia melanogaster	Yes		RSV, SV40	Melanotic changes	9
Pieris brassicae	Yes		DNA factor		33–41
Order: Lepidoptera					
Bombyx mori		Yes	Tipula virus	Epidermal proliferations	29
Agrotis segetum		Yes	Granulosis virus 1 and 2	Proliferations	48, 49

virus from _Drosophila_ tissues and melanotic tumors (14, 17, 19, 20, 27, 28, 53).

Gene dependent cytoplasmic factors have been made plausible in a number of investigations (4–6, 30). Burton and co-workers (10, 12, 13) as well as Friedman _et al._ (21–24) isolated a tumor inducing factor (TIF) from larval tissues. The studies of Barigozzi (4), Jainchill (30), Burton and Friedman (11), Friedman et al. (24), and Ghelelovitch (25) also belong in this category. Virus particles have been observed in the especially affected strains by Akai et al. (1), Bairati (2, 3), Perott et al. (50), and Rae and Green (52).

A factor containing DNA was isolated from the "cabbage butterfly" (_Pieris brassicae_) after infection with derivatives of folic acid by L'Helias (33–41). This factor was also active in _Drosophila_ (39). L'Helias, the author of these investigations, developed a hypothesis which points toward a split of a changed DNA which appears in the cytoplasm (39).

Tumor-like epidermal proliferations were produced by Hukuhara (29) in the silk moth (_Bombyx mori_) by inoculation of larvae with _Tipula iridescent_ virus.

Proliferations in the dark moth (_Agrotis segetum_) (48) were seen by Paillot after infection with granulosis virus Type 1 and 2 (49). He reported proliferations only of the fat body in contrast to the epidermal changes induced by Type 2. According to Scharrer (54) nerve severance may lead through nullification of innervation to the freeing and activation of a latent virus. These studies have been done with _Periplaneta americana_, _Leucophaea maderae_, and _Locusta migratoria_.

It was stated earlier that the phenomenon of neoplastic growth also exhibits a gradual phylogenetic development. In particular, a species-specific review of the countless variations of neoplastic (and even more abnormal) growth reveals a phylogenetic parallel reflected in recent appearance and pattern of neoplastic growth and related phenomena (see also (8).)

Questionable in this respect and in this context are the cytoplasmic killer particles described by Sonneborn (55–57) and detected in _Paramecium_ sp., a ciliated protozoan, which have been compared to oncogenic viruses, especially the Bittner factor in vertebrates. Prier (51) associated these particles, called kappa particles, with bacteria.

The few facts available to us regarding possible viral oncogenesis in invertebrates indicate that a very wide field of research awaits us; these few data fit well into the overall comparative and phylogenetic picture of neoplastic development.

References

1. Akai, H., Gateff, E., Davis, L. E., and Schneiderman, H. A. (1967): Virus-like particles in normal and tumorous tissue of *Drosophila*. *Science*, 157: 810.
2. Bairati, A., Jr. (1962): Preliminary observations on the ultrastructure of the lymph gland cells of *Drosophila melanogaster*. *J. Electr. Microsc. (Tokyo)*, 2:1–13.
3. Bairati, A., Jr. (1963): L'organo dell'emolinfa nella larva di *Drosophila melanogaster* in ceppi portatori di tumori melanotici. *Fourth Atti Congr. Ital. Microsc. Elettronica (Padua)*, pp. 114–118.
4. Barigozzi, C. (1963): Relationship between cytoplasm and chromosome in the transmission of melanotic tumors in *Drosophila*, in *Biological Organization at the Cellular and Supercellular Level. A Symposium*, edited by R. J. C. Harris. Academic Press, New York.
5. Barigozzi, C., and Dravina, A. M. (1963): Cold Spring Harbor, Long Island, N.Y. Dept. of Genetics, Carnegie Institute of Washington. *Drosophila Inform. Serv.*, 37:64.
6. Barigozzi, C., Halfer, C., and Scorbati, G. (1962): Melanotic tumors of *Drosophila*; a partially Mendelian character. *Heredity*, 17:561–575.
7. Bird, F. T. (1949): Tumors associated with virus infection in insects. *Nature*, 163:777–778.
8. Black, I. B., and Axelrod, J. (1970): The regulation of some biochemical circadian rhythms, in *Biochemical Action of Hormones*, pp. 135–155, edited by G. Litwack. Academic Press, New York.
9. Burdette, W. J. (1969): Tumors, hormones and viruses in *Drosophila*. *Natl. Cancer Inst. Monogr.*, 31:303.
10. Burton, L. (1955): Carcinogenic effects of an extractable larval tumor agent. *Trans. N.Y. Acad. Sci.*, 17:301–308.
11. Burton, L., and Friedman, F. (1957): A tumor inducing factor in *Drosophila melanogaster*; II. Its characteristics and biological nature. *Ann. N.Y. Acad. Sci.*, 68:356.
12. Burton, L., Friedman, F., and Mitchell, H. K. (1956): Purification of an inherited tumor-inducing factor in *Drosophila melanogaster*. *Cancer Res.*, 16:880–884.
13. Burton, L., Harnly, M. H., and Kopac, M. J. (1956): Activity of a tumor factor in *Drosophila* development. *Cancer Res.*, 16:402–407.
14. Castiglioni, M. C., and Beati, S. (1954): Production of pseudotumors in *Drosophila* after injection of haemolymph. *Experientia*, 10:501–502.
15. Dawe, C. J. (1965): (cited from E. A. Steinhaus) Symposium on microbial insecticides; IV. Diseases of invertebrates other than insects. *Bacteriol. Rev.*, 29:388–396.
16. Dawe, C. J. (1969): Phylogeny and oncogeny. *Natl. Cancer Inst. Monogr.*, 31:1–40.
17. Erk, F. C., and Nevole, N. A. (1962): The occurrence of heritable melanotic tumors in *Drosophila* after larval feeding on extracts of tumorous flies. *Genetics*, 47:951–952.
18. Fenner, F. (1976): *Classification and Nomenclature of Viruses*. Second Report of the International Committee on Taxonomy of Viruses. S. Karger, Basel.
19. Friedman, F., and Burton, L. (1956): Benign and invasive tumors induced in *Drosophila* by an inherited tumor-inducing factor. *Cancer Res.*, 16: 1059–60.
20. Friedman, F., Harnly, M. H., and Burton, L. (1954): The effects of TU[6] larval fluid and vitamins on tumor production in *Drosophila melanogaster*. *Proc. Am. Assoc. Cancer Res.*, 1:15.
21. Friedman, F., Burton, L., and Mitchell, H. K. (1957): Characteristics of an inherited tumor-inducing factor in *Drosophila melanogaster*. *Cancer Res.*, 17:208–214.
22. Friedman, L., Burton, L., and Mitchell, H. K. (1957): A tumor-inducing factor in *Drosophila melanogaster*; I. Purification and action. *Ann. N.Y. Acad. Sci.*, 68:349–356.
23. Friedman, F., Burton, L., Kaplan, M. L., Kopac, M. J., and Harnly, M. H. (1959): The etiology and development of a melanotic tumor in *Drosophila*, in *Pigment Cell Biology*, pp. 279–299 edited by M. Gordon. Academic Press, New York.
24. Friedman, F., Kassel, R., Burton, L., Kaplan, M. L., and Rottino, A. (1960): A rapid (24-hour) bioassay for detection of human and mouse tumor factor. *Proc. Soc. Exp. Biol. Med.*, 103:16–19.
25. Ghelelovitch, S. (1963): Le déterminisme physiologique de la formation des tumeurs mélanique chez la Drosophile (*D. melanogaster*). *Bull. Cancer*, 50:399–411.
26. Ghelelovitch, S. (1975): Tumeurs mélaniques héréditaires de la Droso-

27. Harker, J. E. (1963): Tumors. In: *Insect Pathology*, Vol. I, pp. 191–213, edited by E. A. Steinhaus. Academic Press, New York.
28. Harshbarger, J. C., and Taylor, R. L. (1968): Neoplasms of insects. *Annu. Rev. Entomol.*, 13:159.
29. Hukuhara, T. (1964): Induction of epidermal tumor in *Bombyx mori* Linnaeus with tipula iridescent virus. *J. Insect. Pathol.*, 6:246.
30. Jainchill, J. L. (1963): A cytoplasmic factor and tumor genes for the melanotic tumor in the tu y² vg *Drosophila melanogaster*. Doctoral thesis, New York University, New York.
31. Krieg, K. (1973): *Invertebrates in Tumour Research*. Theodor Steinkopff, Dresden.
32. Krieg, K. and Wittmann, W. (1969): Adenopapillome der Riechschleimhaut beim Schaf, in *Handbuch der Virusinfektionskrankheiten bei Tieren*, Vol. V, Pt. 2, pp. 769–777, edited by H. Rohrer. Gustav Fischer Verlag, Jena.
33. L'Helias, C. (1957): Tumeurs d'insectes provoquées par l'acide folique. *C. R. Acad. Sci. (Paris)*, 244:1678–1680.
34. L'Helias, C. (1959): Purification partielle du facteur viral induisant les tumeurs provoquées artificiellement chez, *C. R. Acad. Sci. (Paris)*, 248: 3646–3648.
35. L'Helias, C. (1959): Facteur inducteur de tumeurs provoqué par l'acid folique chez Pieris en diapause. *Ann. Biol.*, 35:232–249.
36. L'Helias, C. (1960): Tumor induction factor provoked by folic acid in *Pieris brassicae* during the diapause. *Folia Biol. (Praha)*, 6:310–318.
37. L'Helias, C. (1961): Transmission génétique du facteur inducteur de tumeur à la *Drosophila*. *C. R. Acad. Sci. (Paris)*, 252:2015–2016.
38. L'Helias, C. (1962): On the role of pterins photolabile and thermolabile intermediates in the synthesis of the endocrine complex hormone of insects. *Gen. Comp. Endocrinol.*, 2:612–613.
39. L'Helias, C. (1964): Étude du facteur inducteur de tumeurs (ADN) induit par les déséquilibre de croissance. *Bull. Biol. Fr. Belg.*, 98:511–542.
40. L'Helias, C. (1964): Côntrole chez les insectes de la synthése des hormones de croissance par les ptérines agissant par induction ou par repression en fonction de la température et de la photopériode. *Ann. Endocrinol. (Paris)*, 25:66–71.
41. L'Helias, C. (1966): Induction de désordres tissulaire chez les insectes par altération de l'equilibre entre facteurs de croissance ptérinique et hormones de croissance et mécanisme de cette induction. *Ann. Endocrinol. (Paris)*, 27:343–352.
42. Matz, G. (1964): Transmission de tumeurs chez les insectes par l'hemolymphe et par filtrats acellulaire du tumeurs broyees. *J. Insect Physiol.*, 10:141–145.
43. Matz, G. (1969): Histology and transmission of *Locusta migratoria* (L.) tumors insecta orthoptera. *Natl. Cancer Inst. Monogr.*, 31:465.
44. Matz, G. (1975): Les tumeurs chez les insectes. *C. R. Soc. Biol. (Paris)*, 169:784–787.
45. Matz, G., Weil, J. H., Joly, P., and Ebel, J.-P. (1964): Transmission de tumeurs chez les insectes par un acide nucleique extrait des tumeurs. *C. R. Acad. Sci. (Paris)*, 258:4366.
46. Messow, C. (1960): *Regeneration und Entzündung vom Standpunkt der vergleichenden Pathologie*. Schaper Publisher, Hanover.
47. Neilson, M. M., and Elgee, D. E. (1968): Tumorlike bodies in virus-infected and non-infected adults of the spruce sawfly, *Diprion hercyniae*. *J. Invertebr. Pathol.*, 10:70–75.
48. Paillot, A. (1935): Nouvel ultravirus parasite d'*Agrotis segetum* provoquant une proliferation de tissus infectes. *C. R. Acad. Sci. (Paris)*, 201: 1062.
49. Paillot, A. (1936): Contribution à l'étude des maladies à ultravirus des insectes. *Ann. Epiphyt. Phytogenet.*, 2:341–379.
50. Perott, M., Bairati, E., and Bairati, A., Jr. (1968): Ultrastructure of the melanotic masses in two tumorous strains of *Drosophila melanogaster* (tuB₃ and freckled). *J. Invertebr. Pathol.*, 10:122–38.
51. Prier Cytologia (Leningrad), 12:137.
52. Rae, P. M. M., and Green, M. M. (1968): Virus-like particles in adult *Drosophila melanogaster*. *Virology*, 34:187.
53. Rohrborn, G. (1957): Versuche zur Induktion melanotischer Bildungen durch zellfreie Gewebsextracte bei *Drosophila melanogaster*. *Wilhelm Roux' Arch. Entwicklungsmech. Org.*, 150:115.
54. Scharrer, B. (1959). Remarks in the discussion: Histolysis and tumors, in *Physiology of Insect Development*, edited by G. L. Campbell. University of Chicago Press, Chicago.
55. Sonneborn, T. M. (1939): *Paramecium aurelia*; mating types and groups, lethal interactions, determination and inheritance. *Am. Nat.*, 73:390–413.
56. Sonneborn, T. M. (1943): Gene and cytoplasm; I. The determination and inheritance of the killer character in variety 4 of the *P. aurelia*; II. The bearing of determination and inheritance of characters in *P. aurelia* on problems of cytoplasmic inheritance, pneumococcus transformation, mutations and development. *Proc. Natl. Acad. Sci. U.S.A.*, 29:329–343.
57. Sonneborn, T. M. (1945): The dependence of the physiological action of a gene on a primer and the relation of primer to gene. *Am. Nat.*, 79:318–

339.

58. Urbaneck, D. (1969): Leukose bei anderen Haussäugetieren (Hund, Katze, Schwein, Schaf, Pferd), in *Handbuch der Virusinfektionskrankheiten bei Tieren, Vol. V*, Pt. 1, pp. 175–212, edited by H. Rohrer. Gustav Fischer Verlag, Jena.

59. Urbaneck, D., and Wittmann, W. (1969): Leukosen der Mäuse, in *Handbuch der Virusinfektionskrankheiten bei Tieren, Vol. V*, Pt. 1, pp. 213–298, edited by H. Rohrer. Gustav Fischer Verlag, Jena.

60. Vago, C. (1975): Formations tumorales et proliferations cellulaires chez les invertebres. *C. R. Soc. Biol. (Paris),* 169:778–784.

61. Vogel, K., Wittmann, W., and Krieg, K. (1969): Virusbedingte Neoplasmen der Vögel (virusbedingte aviare Tumoren), in *Handbuch der Virusinfektionskrankheiten bei Tieren, Vol. V*, Pt. 1, pp. 331–673, edited by H. Rohrer. Gustav Fischer Verlag, Jena.

62. Whitcomb, R. F., and Jensen, D. D. (1968): Proliferative symptoms in leafhoppers infected with western x-disease virus. *Virology,* 35:174.

63. Wittmann, W. (1969): Allgemeines zur Virusätiologie von Tumoren, in *Handbuch der Virusinfektionskrankheiten bei Tieren, Vol. V*, Pt. 1, pp. 13–40, edited by H. Rohrer. Gustav Fischer Verlag, Jena.

64. Wittmann, W. (1969): Tumoren der Kaltblüter, in *Handbuch der Virusinfektionskrankheiten bei Tieren, Vol. V*, Pt. 2, pp. 805–820, edited by H. Rohrer. Gustav Fischer Verlag, Jena.

65. Wittmann, W., and Krieg, K. (1969): Fibromatosen, in *Handbuch der Virusinfektionskrankheiten bei Tieren, Vol. V*, Pt. 1, pp. 299–320, edited by H. Rohrer. Gustav Fischer Verlag, Jena.

66. Wittmann, W., and Krieg, K. (1969): Durch Adenoviren bedingte Tumoren, in *Handbuch der Virusinfektionskrankheiten bei Tieren, Vol. V*, Pt. 1, pp. 321–332, edited by H. Rohrer. Gustav Fischer Verlag, Jena.

67. Wittmann, W., and Krieg, K. (1969): Durch Papovaviren bedingte Tumoren, in *Handbuch der Virusinfektionskrankheiten bei Tieren, Vol. V*, Pt. 2, pp. 687–767. Gustav Fischer Verlag, Jena.

68. Wittmann, W., and Krieg, K. (1969): Das Mammakarzinom der Mäuse, in *Handbuch der Virusinfectionskrankheiten bei Tieren, Vol. V*, Pt. 2, pp. 779–804, edited by H. Rohrer. Gustav Fischer Verlag, Jena.

25

Species-Specific Actions of Vertebrate Oncornaviruses: Origins, Interactions, and Oncogenesis

Peter J. Fischinger and Arthur E. Frankel

INTRODUCTION

In considering comparative aspects of tumor virus interaction with vertebrate host cells, no group of known animal tumor viruses is better suited for this purpose than the single-stranded RNA tumor viruses (oncornavirus, oncovirus, retrovirus). More is known about the evolution, life cycle, specific enzymes, structural proteins, specific nucleotide sequences, comparative evolution, and infectious potential than of any other virus group. Oncornaviruses are very richly represented in all species, not only as horizontally transmitted infectious agents but also as an integral part of normal cellular genetic content of a given species (2, 8, 10, 19, 31, 81, 82). They exemplify a unique concept in life strategy: a duality of form so that the genes replicate both on an RNA and a DNA level. Although the common mode of extracellular presentation is that of single-stranded RNA, the exact double-stranded DNA counterpart (the provirus) is the genetically stable and probably the more important alternative form (37, 40, 81, 82). Thus oncornaviruses can be strictly considered as DNA viruses with an extracellular life cycle in an RNA version of the same nucleotide sequences. Oncornaviruses are essentially ubiquitous in vertebrate species (Table 25.1). Intense examination of many species has given a clear understanding that even within the DNA of single species, multiple varieties of retroviruses exist which share no nucleotide sequences with each other, as well as retroviruses of related groups which do contain common and related information. Generally oncornaviruses exist as multiple copies (2–10/haploid genome) within the cell DNA and strictly obey the laws of Mendelian segregation in appropriate intraspecies crosses (2, 14, 19, 42, 46, 57). The wealth of varieties and the multiple DNA copies of retroviruses in cells has given estimates which show that at least in the thoroughly studied mouse species ~0.01% of total cellular genetic information is that of retrovirus DNA (5). What the natural role of oncornavirus may be is still under speculation, and various aspects of gene variation, gene amplification, and differentiation have been considered (20, 40, 82).

A very clear function, however, is the capacity of some oncornaviruses to cause or provoke neoplastic disease *in vivo* and to be able to transform appropriate cells in culture, which, when inoculated into appropriate hosts, produce progressive metastatic tumors. Direct involvement of viral genes is implied by the existence of temperature-sensitive mutants of oncornaviruses which show that a viral gene function is needed to maintain the phenotype of the transformed state (74, 84). From a pragmatic point of view three functional groups of oncornaviruses of vertebrates, limited at present to the "C" type morphological criteria, will be considered (15).

Table 25.1
Isolation of C-Type Oncornaviruses from Vertebrate Species: A Selected Sprectrum[a]

Species	Varieties and Relatedness	Oncogenic Spectrum	Molecular Origins	References (Selected)
Teleosts	Several	Unknown	Unknown	87
Reptilian	Several vipers	Unknown	Unknown	31
Avian				
(Chicken)	Mostly eco-, some xeno-, rare amphotropic, all related	Leukosis, sarcomas, epithelial tumors. Some not documented as oncogenic	Chicken mostly	81
(Pheasant	Ecotropic	Unknown	Pheasant mostly	29
(Duck, turkey)	Ecotropic	Avian sp.	Duck, turkey	61, 66
Murine sp.				
(Mouse)	Eco-, xeno-, and amphotropic; all at least partially related	Leukemias, sarcomas, some not documented as oncogenic	M. musculus	2, 8, 46, 48, 52, 56
(Mouse)	Xenotropic	Not documented.	M. caroli	53
(Mouse)	Eco- and xenotropic	Not documented.	M. cervicolor	5
(Rat)	Eco- and xenotropic	Sarcomas	Rat	48, 69, 70
Feline	Eco- and xenotropic	Lymphomas, sarcomas	Cat (rat related)	53
	Xeno-, not related to ecotropic	Xeno, unknown	Cat (baboon related)	24
Porcine	Xenotropic	Unknown	Pig (mouse related)	12
Primate				
(Woolly monkey)	Ecotropic (one isolate)	Unknown, sarcomas	Asian mice	90
(Gibbon)	Ecotropic, related	Lymphomas	Asian mice	47
(Baboon)	Xenotropic, all	Unknown	Papio sp.	7

[a] "C" type viruses have also been reported in many other vertebrate species. These have not as yet been well characterized, or are in the process of being examined. Some of the species include hamster, guinea pig, horse, sheep, deer, rhesus, and marmoset. Several reports of "C" type particle detection and isolation from man have also been reported.

The first group consists of truly endogenous oncornaviruses which can be elicited by various means from normal cells of a species; whose total genetic information is within the DNA of that species, and which can be controlled by various normal repressive mechanisms by cells of the species of origin (54). The second functional group consists of leukemia-leukosis inducing oncornaviruses. This is a widely prevalent group which is involved in disease under both laboratory and field conditions. Examples of this group include commercially important avian leukosis viruses which can regularly decimate chicken flocks, and the feline leukemia virus group which is the causative agent of feline lymphoma, the most common and prevalent neoplasm of domestic cats (4, 32, 61, 63, 64, 81). The leukemia type of oncornavirus which are capable of in vitro growth do not overtly transform cells in tissue culture. This may be due to a lack of appropriate white blood stem cell precursors in culture rather than a lack of transforming potential. Both tissue culture derived and tumor derived leukemia viruses are capable of inducing disease in new hosts. The third group consists of oncornaviruses which cause solid tumors—generally but not exclusively sarcomas—in animals and produce discrete foci of transformed cells in tissue culture. Sarcoma type oncornaviruses are much more scarce and have a complex genetic makeup. All known sarcoma viruses can be considered as accretions of leukemia type oncornavirus specific nucleotide sequences and additional genetic information which because of its species specific relevance will be discussed in detail (20, 28, 58, 71–73, 78).

Because of the unique origins of vertebrate oncornaviruses, species-specific effects will be considered in a dual mode. First, we will consider the replication of oncornaviruses in the cells of species of origin as well as in cells of other species whether or not these viruses transform cells or cause tumors. Second we will consider transforming effects of specific viral genes apart from viral replication. The potential life cycles of these oncornaviruses can be considered in various modes so that replication of virus and its oncogenic or transforming effects can be clearly dissociated. As seen below the cellular species specific constraints or oncornavirus replication may have little or no effect on individual viral genes capable of inducing and maintaining the neoplastic state.

LIFE CYCLE OF ONCORNAVIRUSES

A brief replicative life cycle of a standard leukemia "C" type viral RNA is as follows. The mature virion is composed of a diploid genome—two identical RNA strands of about 10^4 nucleotides (~35 S value) each. The two strands are connected to each without covalent bonds around the 5' termini (43–45, 88). Like cellular messenger RNAs each viral 3' end terminates in a polyadenylic acid sequence (50–200 nucleotides). The total viral RNA genome sediments with a 70 S value (41, 43, 81). Each 35 S strand is also the messenger, "sense" strand which can be directly translated into viral proteins (3, 30). Associated with viral genomic RNA are three critical structures: (a) the reverse transcriptase, that unique enzyme that will eventually copy single-stranded RNA into a double-stranded DNA circle (4, 80); (b) two small viral proteins, one a basic p10 (p = protein 10 (10×10^3 dalton)) RNA associated protein, and a p12, an acidic phospoprotein displaying RNA binding specificity (4, 67, 68); and (c) transfer RNAs which vary with virus type (18, 43). These structures are enclosed in a quasi-icosahedral core shell composed primarily of the major viral protein (p27–31) (4, 67). The next layer appears to resemble the sugars and lipids of cell membranes. In that outer envelope layer lies the major viral surface glycoprotein (gp70–85) which specifies viral surface properties such as attachment, species host range, interference, and major protective immunogenic determinants (4, 16, 41). Several additional minor proteins are also found on the envelope subsurface.

The infectious virion attaches itself to the surface of the cell to a gp71 receptor site and the virion is taken in by pinocytosis. After several hours the virion becomes uncoated and the formation of provirus begins. No "early" virion proteins are known to be made prior to DNA synthesis. Reverse transcriptase initiates DNA synthesis from the RNA template at a specific site 100–150 nucleotides from the 5' end (17, 43). The initiation site is at the attachment of a specific transfer RNA whose ~16 nucleotides of the fourth loop appear to be attached to viral RNA. Synthesis of a single-stranded DNA begins in a 3'→5' direction (17). As the 100–150 RNA nucleotides have been transcribed into complementary ss DNA the 5' end of the molecule has been reached. The solution to the remainder of viral RNA transcription is that the 5' and the 3' ends of viral RNA are identical and the final ss DNA at the 5' end is complementary to the RNA of the 3' terminus (36, 45). This allows a looping over and circularization of viral RNA and thus the entire DNA copy of viral RNA can be made. At the same time two functions of the reverse transcriptase enzyme are noted, one of which is

an RNAse "H" a "hybridase" which destroys the viral RNA and the second which synthesizes the complementary DNA strand (4, 81). The final product is a double-stranded (ds) DNA circular copy of the initial single-stranded RNA. It is probably the circular viral ds DNA "provirus" which integrates into cellular DNA as a linear molecule, presumably by the same classical mechanisms employed by bacteriophages and plasmid circular structures (76). The provirus can now simply replicate as a normal cellular DNA constituent (37) (*cf.* addendum).

The afferent leg of the replicative cycle consists of proviral negative strand transcription by cellular RNA polymerase to yield a ss RNA which is later polyadenylated by cellular enzymes and enters the cell cytoplasm. Some of this viral RNA serves as template for translation and some of it ends up in the virions. Translation begins from the 5' end as a large precursor polyprotein(s) (59, 88). The precursor(s) are specifically cleaved, the individual viral proteins aggregate in a structured manner about the cell surface and budding of the virion occurs as a specific membrane evagination at the budding site. Viral RNA strands coalesce at that time into a 70 S diploid structure (88).

A special and important variant of this cycle is the defective form of oncornaviruses best exemplified by some sarcoma viruses. In a simple way a defective variant can be a deletion mutant which has lost part of its RNA specifically in the reverse transcriptase and the major envelope glycoprotein regions (28, 60). Such a defective virion contains a reverse transcriptase and/or envelope borrowed from an intact replicating, e.g., leukemia "helper" virus (23, 39, 60). Intracellular entry is regulated by the helper virus envelope glycoprotein, and DNA synthesis by the reverse transcriptase of helper virus. A circular DNA copy of sarcoma virus is made and integrates into host cell DNA presumably in the same manner as leukemia virus DNA. It should be noted that at this point that deletion mutants must conserve the identical terminal sequences, otherwise looping over and total DNA transcription could not occur. The integrated sarcoma proviral DNA does transcribe its RNA which is later polyadenylated (18, 36, 45). In sarcoma viruses the RNA is translated at least as those genes responsible for the maintenance of transformation. Some sarcoma viruses translate additional viral proteins or their precursors positioned near the 5' end of sarcoma virion RNA (59). Because the mammalian sarcoma virus RNA is apparently incapable of coding for functional envelope or reverse transcriptase proteins, virion formation and maturation do not occur and no infectious virus is produced. This is considered as a "nonproductive" state in the sarcoma virus transformed cells (39).

Should the "nonproductive" cell be infected with a autonomously replicating leukemia helper virus, then the sarcoma virus RNA can use helper virus specified proteins and become a hybrid virion, i.e., with sarcoma virus RNA on the inside and a helper virus envelope on the outside. Such forms of sarcoma virus are common and have been named as "pseudotypes" (39).

SPECIES-SPECIFIC ORIGINS OF NUCLEOTIDE SEQUENCES COMPRISING LEUKEMIA TYPE OF ONCORNAVIRUSES

Historically chicken leukosis viruses were isolated from chickens, mouse leukemia viruses from various strains of mice, feline leukemia viruses from lymphomatous cats, etc. (1, 2, 32, 55, 56, 60, 61, 63, 81). However, that precedent does not apply at this time, namely, that the DNA of the species with disease from which the virus was isolated was also the origin of that oncornavirus (9, 11, 12, 42, 53, 90). Several sets of evidence unequivocally demonstrate that some leukosis-leukemia viruses are part of normal species genomic DNA information. Although initially the normal cloned cells of some species could release infectious oncornavirus spontaneously, elegant experiments dealing with inductive processes demonstrated that each cell in a number of species tested could derepress endogenous oncornavirus (1, 2, 7, 52, 53). Favorite and still the most efficient agents were found to be halogenated pyrimidines which had to incorporate into cellular DNA in order to create control perturbations which resulted in release of virus (54). The converse line of evidence consisted of using such an "endogenous" virus isolate in asking whether it indeed comes from the DNA of that species. This was accomplished by making radioactively labeled complementary DNA (cDNA) from viral RNA by the endogenous reverse transcriptase reaction and by reacting this cDNA with cellular DNA in great excess under conditions of liquid hybridization (5, 13, 26, 79). A positive reaction is driven by the presence of complementary sequences in cell DNA and denotes not only a qualitative presence or absence but also the number of copies found in cellular DNA. A complete reaction of viral cDNA with cellular DNA denotes that indeed the virus isolated was derived from proviral sequences in the DNA of that species. An additional benefit derives from the fact that the DNA·DNA hybrids obtained will have a high affinity for each other under conditions such as high temperature which would tend to dissociate them. Thus the temperature of strand separation ("melting") is contingent among other factors on the degree of similarity or relationship of the two DNA strands (49). In this manner the degree of relationship among viruses and cellular DNA can be readily established by "melting" temperature properties of DNA·DNA hybrids (5, 6, 10, 27, 72, 73).

Two general classes of "endogenous," autonomously replicating viruses can be derepressed from normal or tumor cells of a species. First, there were viruses which could replicate in the cells of the species from which they were isolated and these were generally relatively specific. These were termed "ecotropic" and a number of these were shown to be leukemogenic when tested in the same species (1, 47, 51, 63). The second group could not replicate in the cells of the species of origin but otherwise had a very extensive host range in many vertebrate species. These were named as "xenotropic," and with some exceptions are well repressed from replication in cells of the species from which they originated (8, 51). The xenotropic viruses extensively tested for oncogenicity were those of chickens, mice, and cats.

None of these were found to be oncogenic up to this time in either homologous or heterologous hosts. The murine xenotropic viruses have been implicated in some strains of mice as potentially causative or contributory factors in autoimmune disease (51). Germane features of xenotropic viruses of all species tested so far are that they are inducible from normal cells of the species, and that they exist in multiple copies in the DNA of the species. A critical property is that as determined by molecular hybridization, using either viral high molecular weight RNA or complementary ssDNA of the xenotropic virus, the entire genome is represented in the parental cellular DNA (5, 7, 53, 61). As seen below, the parental cell can and does effectively deal with repression of the xenotropic endogenous virus group. A subset of truly endogenous viruses is best exemplified by some common ecotropic viruses from the high leukemia incidence strains, such as the AKR mouse leukemia virus. This virus is easily inducible by various agents and is often spontaneously released (54). The AKR ecotropic virus appears in the "normal" weanling mouse and is present in high titers during leukemogenesis. The AKR mouse is programmed for early death of leukemia and the AKR virus is the presumptive causative agent because it can induce identical disease as a replicating virus in low leukemia incidence mice as well as rats. From a molecular point of view, it has been determined that every AKR mouse cell has several copies of the entire AKR genome in its DNA. However, other mouse strains do not contain the AKR-specific information although these do contain various sets of murine xenotropic virus nucleotide sequences. Crosses of AKR mice and mice without these sequences have clearly determined that the AKR genes segregate according to Mendelian laws. Thus the AKR mouse, and many related mouse strains, clearly contain a totally endogenous, ecotropic and leukemogenic virus (19).

The second major group of leukemia type oncornaviruses is that which appears to contain most but not all of the nucleotide sequences in host DNA. This group represents most of the classical leukemogenic vertebrate leukemia type viruses. Typically the chicken leukosis virus group, such as avian myeloblastosis virus, lymphoid leukosis viruses, and related neoplastic disease causative agents have the majority of information encoded in chicken cell DNA (57, 81, 86). The majority of these nucleotide sequences are very closely related to the information found in chicken cells. However, a segment of the virus genome (~15%) is not found in normal chicken cells although more remotely related sequences may be present (57, 86). In the mouse an exactly analogous situation is present in those mouse strains which do not contain AKR virus-specific sequences (19). The feline leukemia virus group is also analogous to the above (61). The majority of feline leukemia virus nucleotide sequences are found as reasonably related multiple copies in normal cat cells but there also seems to be additional leukemia virus-specific information which is not present in normal cat cells. An interesting point of digression is found in cat cells. The prototype systems of chickens and mice show that the majority of sequences of avian and murine xenotropic viruses are closely related and that many group-specific antigenic determinants are found in proteins of either set of viruses. In contrast, as an exception, easily isolated feline xenotropic virus is very different and appears to share essentially no sequences in common with feline leukemia virus (13, 24).

Another well-studied group of viruses also falls into the category of oncogenic retroviruses whose sequences are not found in the normal DNA of the affected species. These viruses are the so-called gibbon ape lymphoma virus and the wooly monkey sarcoma and its associated helper virus (47, 90). The gibbon virus can be horizontally transmitted and cause leukemia in other gibbons, whereas the wooly monkey isolate has not been shown to be leukemogenic. The two viruses are very closely related to each other by nucleic acid hybridization and share group-specific antigens as well (5, 13, 53, 68). When cellular DNA of gibbon and wooly monkey was examined for viral nucleotide sequences essentially no relationship was found. DNA of various related primates was also quite negative for the virus group. After the examination of a large number of species the host with the most compatible DNA was found to be an Asian mouse (5, 53). A final group of oncornaviruses associated with mammalian leukemia is represented by the presumptive bovine leukemia virus (54). This virus does not seem to be related to other mammalian leukemia viruses antigenically. No cross-reactive interspecies antigens have been as yet found on the major viral proteins. The present evidence seems to causally associate this virus with bovine leukemia. The virus genomic information does not appear to be at all found in normal bovine DNA. However, as expected the proviral nucleotide sequences are found in virus-infected cells and in tumor cells. It is not known whether the bovine leukemia virus sequences are found in the DNA of some other species.

FOURTH DIMENSION OF SPECIES SPECIFICITY

The general schema of oncornavirus success is to be able to integrate as proviral DNA into its host and from then on replicate as normal cellular DNA. This successful strategy has an important ramification: can an oncornavirus integrate so successfully that it can become part of the germ plasm of the species, and could this have occurred as some recent or past event. There is an impressive amount of evidence which leads to the interpretation that some oncornaviruses present at this time as truly endogenous viruses of one species must have been transferred from another species in its past evolutionary history (6, 8, 14). The most thoroughly studied example is the domestic cat. The true endogenous xenotropic virus of the cat is the

RD-CCC virus (24). Multiple proviral copies are found in the DNA of all domestic cats and related cats of the Mediterranean basin (14, 61). The virus can be easily induced from cat cells derived from many organs. The feline family represents by taxonomy a number of quite closely related species. Nucleic acid hybridization of the so-called unique sequences (found as one copy/haploid genome) nicely confirms this close relationship (61, 75). The relatedness is specifically determined as the lowering of melting temperature of the interspecies DNA·DNA hybrids which is in turn based on the increase of mismatching of bases in the hybrid (49). The progression of nucleic acid relatedness is comensurate with the accepted taxonomical schema. When the RD-CCC viral complementary DNA was used as a probe to follow this relationship, a profound difference was noted. All domestic cats and all wild cats of the Mediterranean area were highly positive for viral sequences which were quite identical among various species. In contrast all other wild cats including the larger cats were uniformly negative. There was no progression from positive to negative, and the positives were very localized in terms of paleogeography (14). Shortly after the isolation of RD-CCC virus and the determination of its origins, an endogenous oncornavirus of baboons was isolated from various baboon species (7). A remarkable degree of both immunologic similarity of the major antigenic determinants was found between the RD-CCC and the baboon virus groups. Nucleic acid homology confirmed that a very close relationship existed (13, 67). The baboon provirus DNA was found to be completely present in baboon DNA as multiple proviral copies. Related primate species showed a proportion of the viral genome in this DNA proportional to their evolutionary distance (10). The melting of the DNA hybrids between baboon oncornavirus complementary DNA and cellular DNA of various primate species also has a reduced melting temperature exactly as expected from the evolutionary degree of relationship. Thus the baboon proviral DNA sequences evolved as the species evolved from a common progenitor. The expected evolutionary radiation of the proviral sequences of the baboon provirus among related old world monkeys contrasts sharply with the pattern of detection of the baboon-like RD-CCC proviral sequences among various cat species. The most reasonable interpretation is that about 50–60 million years ago a progenitor of the baboon virus derived from the baboon ancestors was transferred into the germ plasm of the ancestor small cat genus which eventually gave rise to domestic cats (10, 11). The nucleotide sequences of the respective germinal proviruses in cats and baboons since that event appear to have undergone significant changes; however, the degree of similarity is still remarkable.

A second such transfer was documented when a porcine "C" type virus was isolated. This virus was present in the DNA of the pig and closely related species. It was totally absent from other related artiodactyls. The virus, however, was quite related to murine viruses. Accordingly a transfer of ancestral endogenous mouse virus to pigs was postulated (12).

Based on the above probable event two pertinent questions can be raised: (a) Are such radical gene transfers going on? and (b) Can one reproduce in the laboratory the insertion of a previously absent provirus into the germ line of the species? The answer to both questions is positive.

The first example can be illustrated with the so-called primate leukemia and sarcoma virus isolates. The gibbon ape leukemia virus and the wooly monkey sarcoma virus were each isolated from neoplasms in the respective species (47, 90). The two viruses are remarkably similar to each other and share many antigens as well as nucleotide homology. Their major antigenic determinants differ from other oncornavirus groups (67). All of the above isolates occurred within the last few years. Several of the gibbon virus isolates were recently derived from lymphomas of gibbons occurring as small clusters in animal colonies in South East Asia. The neoplasm has been experimentally transmitted by the virus to other gibbons. The critical question was whether this is a virus of gibbons or related species as determined by homology of viral nucleotide sequences to primate cellular DNA. The answer was surprising in that no DNA of any primate tested had any significant homology to the gibbon or wooly monkey oncornavirus isolates. Of all the species tested, the mouse had a slight degree of homology yet the virus was clearly not derived from the common *Mus musculus* species. After some search, an Asian wild mouse, *Mus caroli*, was found to contain a provirus which matched very closely the above primate isolates (5, 53). When *M. caroli* cells were induced by standard methods, an intact, replicating oncornavirus was isolated. This virus, although not known to be as yet oncogenic, was very closely related to the two "primate" viruses. Its nucleotide sequences were entirely present in *M. caroli* DNA; and proportionally lower, and less closely matched sets of sequences were found in the DNA of related mouse species. Accordingly a primate oncogenic virus appeared to be very similar to rodent endogenous oncornavirus(es) (53). It should be noted that the *M. caroli*-like sequences have as yet not integrated into the germ line of higher primates (10). An example where this might have occurred in part and possibly fairly recently is again the domestic cat. This species has the well-known feline leukemia virus, a classical horizontally spread oncornavirus causative of the majority of neoplastic disease in the cat. When cat cell DNA was examined, feline leukemia virus specific sequences were in large part present in cat cell DNA (61, 62). Some part of feline leukemia virus-specific sequences may be missing. Related cats did not appear to contain these sequences in their cellular DNA. Again this was suggestive that feline leukemia virus did not originate in cats. When other species were probed for related nucleotide sequences the common rat and its relatives had the closest degree of homology (9). This putative relationship is also strengthened immunologically, because there is a greater degree of relationship of the shared viral protein antigens between the common oncornaviruses of rodents and feline leukemia virus than for example with antigens found in the baboon oncornavirus (68).

In line with suggestive epidemiological and nucleic acid hybridization evidence, laboratory experiments have clearly shown that *de novo* germ line integration of an oncornavirus could be achieved (42). The Moloney isolate of murine leukemia virus is oncogenic in mice. Although multiple copies of sequences related to Moloney leukemia virus are found in normal mouse DNA, a subset of complementary DNA sequences of Moloney leukemia virus can be isolated which does not appear to be significantly homologous to normal mouse DNA. Experiments with blastula stage mouse embryos have shown that these primordial cells are capable of infection with Moloney leukemia virus. As these cells differentiate and give rise to different organ groups, those organs in adult mice derived from virus-infected cells contain Moloney leukemia virus-specific sequences in their DNA, whereas other organs in the same mouse not derived from infected cells do not contain homologous sequences. In some mice infected primordial cells differentiated into germ line cells. Thus male mice exist which can transfer Moloney leukemia virus as part of their sperm DNA. Their progeny then have Moloney leukemia virus-specific sequences in all cells. Further segregation of the provirus follows simple Mendelian laws. Thus unequivocal evidence indicates that germ line integration of an oncorna provirus can be achieved *de novo* (42).

SPECIES-SPECIFIC ORIGINS OF NUCLEOTIDE SEQUENCES UNIQUE TO SARCOMA VIRUSES

It has become amply clear within recent years that sarcomagenic oncornaviruses are recombinants formed from leukemia-type virus information and additional nucleotide sequences. It was of interest to determine the nature and species-specific distribution of nucleotide sequences unique to sarcoma viruses. The basic questions to be asked were: (a) are these viral or cellular in origin; (b) do they originate from the virus/cell of the species afflicted with the tumor from which they were isolated; (c) what is the distribution, i.e., conservation of sequences in species evolution? A summary of the origins and properties of the better studies of sarcoma virus isolates is presented in Table 25.2.

Three systems have been well characterized up to now. The avian Rous sarcoma virus contains a large molecular weight subunit RNA ($\sim 10^4$ nucleotides) (58, 81, 88). Rous sarcoma virus as a single infectious unit is typically capable both of transformation and replication. Focus purified Rous sarcoma virus causes the transformation of fibroblasts *in vitro*. The transformation defective (td) mutants have lost a small portion of their RNA (1500–2000 nucleotides) (78). The td mutants can replicate and resemble standard avian leukosis viruses. Because of this special relationship, Rous sarcoma virus complementary DNA made with the endogenous reverse transcriptase reaction could be absorbed with viral RNA from the td mutant. The residual complementary DNA was shown to represent only Rous sarcoma specific sequences and was called: "cDNA$_{src}$" (78). Sequences homologous to cDNA$_{src}$ were not found in other nontransforming avian viruses, nor in mammalian transforming viruses. When the DNA of several avian species was tested for the presence of sequences hybridizing with cDNA$_{src}$, normal chicken cellular DNA had the closest copy. The DNA$_{sarc}$ copy in chicken cells occurred about once per haploid genome and showed

Table 25.2
Representative Sarcomagenic Oncornaviruses: Anatomy and Origins of Nucleotide Sequences

Isolate	Functions: Transforms (T) Replicates (R)	Sarcoma Specific Region: "src"			Transforming host range	Region Shared with Leukemia Virus: "Common"				Leukemia virus type
		Size (nucleotides)	DNA origin	Copy frequency[a]		Size (nucleotides)	DNA origin	Copy frequency	Expression of antigen(s)[b]	
Avian sarcoma (AS) virus	T+R+ / T+R−	~1600	Chicken	1	Avian and mammalian	~8500	Chicken mostly	2-4	All or none gp85 or no polymerase	Avian leukosis virus
Murine sarcoma virus	T+R−	~1600–2000	Mouse	1	Mammalian (Some avian)	~4000–6000	Mouse mostly	5–10	polyprotein of "gag" region p30, p15, p12 or none at all	Moloney murine leukemia virus
Kirsten sarcoma virus	T+R−	3500–4500	Rat	5–10	Mammalian (possibly avian)	~2000–4500, variable results	Mouse mostly	5–10	None	Gross-AKR murine leukemia virus
Harvey sarcoma virus	T+R−	3500–4500	Rat	5–10	Mammalian	3500–4500	Mouse mostly	5–10	None	Moloney murine leukemia virus
Feline sarcoma virus	T+R−	1500	Cat[d]	1	Mammalian	3500	Cat	5–10	Polyprotein FOCMA[c], p12, p15	Feline leukemia virus
Simian sarcoma virus	T+R−	Unknown			Mammalian	Unknown			Variable, some none, some "gag" region	Simian sarcoma associated virus

[a] Relative to "unique" sequence cellular DNA, having one copy per haploid genome.
[b] p30 etc., protein M.W. 30,000, "gp" glycoprotein, "gap" group-specific antigen.
[c] Feline oncornavirus cell surface membrane antigen.
[d] There appear to be two molecularly different FeSV "src" necleotide sequences which do not hybridize with each other. Nonetheless each is represented at about one copy in normal cat DNA.

slight differences in relationship based on melting temperatures (70). The degree of presence and the exactitude of Rous cDNA$_{src}$ diminished in related avian species and was essentially not detectable in mammals. The relationships followed the predictable evolutionary taxonomic schema. In contrast the presence of cDNA of the td mutant was shown to be found only in the chickens and their closest relatives, and species such as *Coturnix* were already bereft of td virus analogous sequences (58). It was clear that the sequences of Rous cDNA$_{src}$ and those of the td mutant evolved at different rates.

An analogous analysis was carried out in the mammalian Moloney murine sarcoma virus (MSV) system. Here the sarcoma virus was defective for replication but could transform (39). Moloney sarcoma virus required a leukemia helper virus for replication; specifically for functions such as the reverse transcriptase and the envelope glycoprotein (19, 60). Helper viruses of different species could be used to donate the necessary functions to MSV. The subunit RNA of MSV was somewhat smaller than for example the typical helper virus (~7000 vs. 9000 nucleotides) (28). Complementary DNA could be again prepared to MSV and by appropriate absorptions with helper virus RNA a set of "cDNA$_{src}$" sequences could be isolated which represented only the MSV specific region (28). By examining how much of MSV RNA was protected by cDNA$_{src}$ from ribonuclease digestion it was established that about 25% of MSV contained "cDNA$_{src}$" and that 75% was composed of Moloney leukemia virus-specific nucleotide sequence. This latter subset of Moloney leukemia-like specific sequences can be considered as MSV sequences in "common" with these sequences normally a part of autonomous Moloney leukemia virus. These "common" sequences represent about one half of the Moloney leukemia virus, are located near the 5′ end, and can be translated to yield proteins of the internal group specific antigen region (25, 59). The "common" sequences are related to analogous counterparts found in other ecotropic and xenotropic murine leukemia viruses. The search for homology with cDNA$_{src}$ among other oncornaviruses showed that no viruses other than MSV contained such sequences.

DNA of various mammalian species was analyzed for sequences hybridizing with Moloney sarcoma virus cDNA$_{src}$. About one, essentially intact copy was found in mouse cells per each haploid genome (26). Related rodent cells had similar sequences, but these showed some

digression which was proportional to taxonomic distance. Other mammalian orders had extensive mismatching of their "sarc" nucleotide sequences. The degree of divergence was compared to the evolutionary rate of unique sequences in DNA and to hemoglobin DNA copies (27). It was established that cDNA$_{src}$ was about as conserved as hemoglobin and better preserved than the average copy DNA. On the other hand experiments performed with "cDNA$_{common}$" showed very different results. The cDNA$_{common}$ sequences were found with some mismatching in normal *Mus musculus* cells but essentially were already lost from *Mus caroli* or rat cells. It appeared that the sequences coding for leukemia type oncornaviruses were rapidly lost (27). It should be remembered that this is not really a loss but a replacement with different oncornaviruses which did not hybridize with standard murine ecotropic leukemia viruses. Thus the mammalian prototype sarcoma virus system had a close analogy to the avian sarcoma virus system. In both cases sarcoma viruses appeared to be recombinants involving a part or a whole ecotropic oncornavirus and cellular unique DNA information (27, 69, 79). It can be established inferentially that the "src" sequences are directly involved in the initiation and maintenance of cellular transformation (78, 84).

The recombinant status of the above prototypes is still relatively simple compared to the following variants. In several sarcoma virus isolates such as the Harvey and Kirsten, species-specific origins derive from more than one species (69–73). Both of the above viruses have a complex genealogical origin in that they were passed as both leukemia and sarcomagenic viruses in both mice and rats (69–73). Evidently recombination between mouse and rat specific genetic information occurred in the following manner. Both sarcoma viruses derive about a half or less of their informational content from ecotropic murine leukemia viruses. The murine leukemia-specific genes do not seem to be translated into any identifiable proteins (69). Both sarcoma viruses can transform cells of various species but cannot replicate unless an intact helper leukemia virus is present. The other half of their genome is quite interesting and essentially the same in both cases. Its properties are as follows: all of it is found in normal rat DNA in multiple copies. The information can be induced as RNA by halogenated pyrimidines in normal cells. Further the RNA information can be enveloped by other endogenous rat leukemia type helper virus. When enveloped, the sarcoma virus like RNA consists of large molecular weight RNA. Accordingly the genes which constitute the transforming half of the Harvey and Kirsten sarcoma virus genomes show a remarkable resemblance to an endogenous rat oncornavirus which by itself is incapable of appearing as an intact virion. What is not known at this time is whether all of the rat cell derived information is oncornavirus-like or whether some part may be composed of rat unique sequence information. In any case the following critical observation was made: because the Moloney MSV "cDNA$_{src}$" shares no sequences in common with any part of either Harvey or Kirsten sarcoma viruses a very different strategy of sarcoma virus formation was used. As shown clearly, rat cells do have closely related homolog of Moloney cDNA$_{src}$ but these sequences were not used in the formation of two typical rat-mouse hybrid sarcoma viruses. Recent information on feline oncornavirus nucleotide sequences indicates that similar joining of information resulted in the structure of feline sarcoma virus (FeSV). FeSV is composed of "common" sequences shared with FeLV and sequences which are distinct from FeLV. The distinct, or "src" subsets of sequences are actually two types found in two different isolates of FeSV. Although the two "src" sets of sequences are distinct from each other, each is found in single copy DNA in normal cat cells. The FeSV "src" sequences are about as conserved as the chicken or mouse "srcs."[1] The origins of genes comprising other mammalian sarcomagenic viruses are still under study.

SPECIES TROPISMS OF ONCORNAVIRUSES

Tropism can be considered as the capability of an oncornavirus to infect but not necessarily to replicate in the cells of a given species. Because of the complexity of possible restrictive mechanisms only the entry step will be considered at present under tropism. Entry type tropism can be described as characteristic of virus groups and can be considered in three general categories. "Ecotropic" viruses are those which can infect the cells of the species from which they were isolated regardless of the presence or

---

[1] P. J. Fischinger and A. E. Frankel, unpublished data.

absence of proviral DNA. "Xenotropic" viruses are those oncornaviruses which are capable of infecting a wide range of species but not the cells of the species from which they were originally obtained and whose DNA contain the provirus (8, 51, 52). The species of origin can repress the endogenous xenotropic virus expression (21, 51). In a general sense the term "xenotropic" has been applied in a broader meaning which encompasses also the inability of xenotropic oncornavirus to replicate in the species of origin. The "amphotropic" viruses have the capability to enter and replicate in a wide variety of hosts including the one from which they originated (33). These viruses include several genetically stable recombinant oncornaviruses which share relevant nucleotide sequences of both eco- and xenotropic viruses (22, 89). Thus the definition of "eco-", "xeno-", and "ampho-" applies to functions of structural elements of a given type of oncornavirus. Two additional levels of complexity apply. First, oncornaviruses can as many other virus groups undergo phenotypic mixing which involves the sharing of surface-entry molecules of two different viruses (89). Second, a common phenomenon of oncornaviruses is the existence of "pseudotypes" (39). These can be considered under the category of genomic masking so that the genetic information of a totally unrelated virus can be efficiently coated and enveloped by entry type molecules of another oncornavirus. It is clear that the entry tropism depends on the surface molecules, but further events are determined by the nature and competence of the incoming viral genome.

It is of interest that the species most thoroughly studied each have been found to contain eco-, xeno-, and amphotropic viruses. It is not surprising to find a variety of oncornaviruses in any one species because of the evidence that in general all species contain multiple proviral copies of oncornavirus-like sequences in their genomes. In the avian system the majority of oncornaviruses are ecotropic in both entry and replication. There is a complex genetic control system relative to the major groups of ecotropic viruses and the specific strains of chickens they are capable of infecting (4, 64, 81). Some types of chicken ecotropic viruses have coats which allow, with a much reduced efficiency, the entry of pseudotype sarcoma viruses into heterologous mammalian cells (81). Generally, however, avian ecotropic viruses are restricted to chickens and very closely related birds. Chicken ecotropic viruses are the group of viruses responsible for the majority of commercially important avian leukosis problem. These viruses are generally ubiquitous in chicken flocks and selective care must be exercised to prevent horizontal infection to neighboring flocks. The genetic information of these avian ecotropic viruses, which are closely related to each other, is generally found in normal chicken cells. However, about 15% of avian leukosis virus genomes are not found in chicken cell DNA and the species-specific origins, if any, are not as yet defined. The typical xenotropic virus of chicken is present in its entirety in chicken DNA and can be induced from normal chicken cells in a variety of ways (57, 86, 89). Typical representatives have a wide host range: they can infect cells of birds such as quail, pheasants, etc., and are less efficient in terms of entry into various mammalian cells. It is of interest that avian xenotropic virus does have the capacity of infecting and replicating certain genetically defined chicken strains (29, 81). Most other chicken cells will rigidly exclude chicken xenotropic oncornaviruses. Amphotropic type viruses have also been found, of these Rous associated virus (RAV− 60) has been demonstrated to be a stable genetic recombinant possessing informational sequences of both eco- and xenotropic avian oncornaviruses (81).

In the murine system the widely studied ecotropic leukemia viruses have a rigidly defined host range. These viruses can infect mouse cells and rat cells both *in vivo* and in culture. No other less related mammalian cells are known to be susceptible to murine ecotropic viruses. In contrast several genetically distinct types of murine xenotropic viruses exist which cannot replicate in mouse cells at all, although these are inducible from mouse cells which contain the entire xenotropic provirus (2, 50). Murine xenotropic viruses have a very wide host range including some other rodents and essentially all orders of mammals including all higher primates. Entry into some avian cells is also possible (51). Murine amphotropic viruses have been found both in nature and in the laboratory (24, 32). Some of these are now known to be recombinants in the major glycoprotein responsible for attachment to receptors of cells of various species.[2]

In the feline species the situation is quite different. Feline leukemia virus is the ecotropic representative and the major neoplastic disease-inducing agent in domestic cats (32, 63). This virus in contrast to chicken and mouse ecotropic viruses has a very wide host range, including other carnivores and many other orders of mammals including man (23). However, feline leukemia virus will not infect rodent cells of any kind. The feline xenotropic virus, whose proviral sequences are in normal cat cells DNA, is also rather unusual (21, 61). It may or may not enter cat cells but in either case will not be able to replicate in cat cells (22, 24). It is capable of growth in many primate cells; however, it appears to be restricted in baboon cells which represent the presumptive proto-origin of the xenotropic virus of cats. Again the feline xenotropic virus will not enter and replicate in rodent cells. Thus it should be noted that the wide spectrum of cells susceptible to xenotropic virus of one mammalian species is not the same spectrum of susceptibility to a xenotropic virus of another mammalian species. Second, despite a common wide host range, xenotropic viruses of various species, with some exceptions, do not share any significant common nucleotide sequences (13). In keeping with the above descriptions the eco- and xenotropic viruses of other species generally behave in a similar manner.

SOME KNOWN MECHANISMS OF RESTRICTION OF REPLICATING ONCORNAVIRUSES

Cells of different species can exert various modes of restriction on replicating oncornaviruses. As mentioned above, generally xenotropic viruses have a very broad host range while ecotropic viruses are generally limited. The first level of restriction that can be considered is the problem of entry of the virus into the cells. Essentially, all viruses have specific envelope structures that are designed for attachment to cells. Cells in turn have specific, matching surface receptor molecules. Effective combination of corresponding structures allow the entry of virus. It can be seen that blockage to entry could be exerted from both viral and cellular levels. The specific attachment molecule for oncornaviruses is the major viral structural glycoprotein (M.W. 70–85,000 gp70–85) (4, 38, 41, 67). It is necessary for attachment of virus to cell receptors because gentle removal of gp70–85 by enzymes such as bromelain will abolish infectivity. The specific digestion of the saccharide portion of the molecule by endoglycosidases demonstrates that the specificity of recognition resides

---

[2]P. J. Fischinger and A. E. Frankel, unpublished data.

in the protein part of the gp70–85 molecules (16). Accordingly, virus attaches to cells by the gp70–85 envelope structure, and feasibility of compatible receptor molecules ensures infection. Studies with purified gp70–85 have shown there is a good correlation with binding of a radiolabeled gp70–85 to a cell of a specific and its susceptibility to initiation of infection. Additionally the exposure of cell receptors to gp71–85 of a given virus will effectively block cell receptors so that intact virus cannot penetrate (41). One of the classical phenomena dealing with prevention of oncornavirus entry is specific viral interference. As now well recognized, interference can be mediated from without or from within (64, 65). The addition of inactivated virus or the exposure of cells to purified gp71–85 will effectively abolish the attachment of gp71–85 or the virus of the homologous virus interference group. A preinfection with a potentially interfering virus will establish an internal production of gp71–85 which will effectively saturate all surface cell receptors (41). This is known to be a surface phenomenon rather than an internal block because sarcoma virus pseudotypes coated with appropriate gp71–85 being interfered with also cannot exert their effect. If the same sarcoma virus were coated with a different gp71–85 envelope it is able both to get in and transform a cell (23).

The presence or absence of pre-existing major glycoprotein on cell surface is of special importance and may be the critical factor relative to entry of xenotropic viruses into their homologous species cells. Both chicken and mouse cells have been known for a long time to contain on their cell surfaces gp71–85 molecules closely related if not identical to xenotropic oncornavirus major glycoproteins (4, 38, 67). The expression of gp71–85 can and does occur generally in the abence of total xenotropic virus production (38, 81). It should be noted that in all known systems ecotropic and xenotropic viruses from the same species do not cross-interfere (4, 22, 29, 81). An additional complication arises from data which unequivocally demonstrate that in the mouse at least there is an enormous production of free gp71–85 by various cells in the body, so that mouse sera are actually virus glycoproteinemic in nature (50). Accordingly it is difficult to establish *in vivo* whether all cells are capable of expressing gp71–85 or whether specific receptors are usually saturated by exogenously produced glycoprotein. Most continuous mouse cell cultures are clearly resistant to entry of xenotropic murine oncornaviruses (22, 51).

The question whether restriction of endogenous xenotropic oncornavirus is mediated solely by surface interference exerted by the expression of corresponding gp71–85 molecule was answered both in the mouse and cat cell systems by the use of defective sarcoma virus pseudotypes coated with respective xenotropic viruses. Thus two levels of restriction could exist: (a) the pseudotype could be blocked at the surface and (b) the pseudotype could enter the cell and transform it. Because the pseudotype was defective, it could not replicate if the xenotropic helper virus was internally repressed. The defective pseudotype sarcoma virus could be shown to replicate if another nonrestricted helper type virus was added. In mouse cells it was shown that murine xenotropic oncornavirus pseudotypes were restricted in all mouse cell lines save one derived from wild mouse cells (SC-1). Entry, transformation, and appropriate sarcoma virus rescue were very efficient in SC-1 cells. However, replication of xenotropic oncornavirus was quickly stopped presumably by secondary internal restrictive mechanisms. A somewhat similar phenomenon was found in cat cells. Because of a paucity of cat cell lines a single cat cell strain was studied. When the cat cell strain was diploid prior to crisis, the cells were susceptible to the entry of defective sarcoma virus enveloped with feline xenotropic virus. However, essentially no replication of feline xenotropic virus could occur indicating internal restrictive mechanisms. When the same cat cells were carried through a crisis and developed into a continuous cell line the level of restriction also shifted to the surface. Although no whole feline xenotropic virus was produced the cells did make feline xenotropic gp70–85 and prevented the entry of sarcoma virus coated with feline xenotropic oncornavirus (21). Although further studies are needed, it appears that cells of at least two species can restrict replication of endogenous xenotropic viruses at two levels; one of which is using the production of xenotropic gp71–85 which leads to an immediate form of interference with virus entry.

The nature of intracellular restriction of oncornaviruses has not been thoroughly elucidated. The best known system of restriction occurs in the mouse ecotropic virus Fv-1 system (34). Apparently there are two alleles making cells either susceptible or resistant to N or B tropic murine leukemia viruses. F_1 generations display resistance to both N and B viruses. Sarcoma virus pseudotypes coated with N or B get in but are restricted in appropriate cells. The leukemia viruses also get into a nonpermissive cell but are stopped somewhere on the afferent leg of the replication cycle which leads to provirus integration. The probable site of action is the following. The virus gets in and is uncoated. Virus-specific complementary and double-stranded DNA get made. In the nonpermissive system the DNA does not appear to integrate and therefore no further transcription and translation and virus replication occur (44). Recent evidence indicates that N-B restriction can be overcome with large multiplicity of infection and by a transient product normally supplied by one of the nonpermitted virus infectious units very early in infection. Thus a preinfection of a nonpermissive cell by one restricted virus allows a second restricted virus to function normally. Aparently the first restricted virus makes a product which inactivates the normal cellular restrictive mechanism and the second superinfecting restricted virus can then function in an unimpaired fashion.[3]

LACK OF SPECIES-SPECIFIC RESTRICTION OF ONCORNAVIRUS TRANSFORMING GENES

Although various classes, orders, and genera of cells have specific mechanisms restricting both entry and replication of leukemia viruses, some oncogenic viruses apparently easily circumvent these obstructions. Specifically, one has to differentiate between infection and replication of an intact virus, and the infection and transformation by the transforming genes of an oncornavirus. Cell transformation by specific oncornavirus genes does not require virus replication (40, 80, 85). The best examples which demonstrate the oncogenic effects of transforming viruses are the various sarcoma viruses of birds and mammals. A general claim can be made: that competent or defective sarcoma viruses transform the cells of many species *in vitro* and induce solid tumors *in vivo* in a large variety of species.

Avian sarcoma viruses which are transforming in tissue culture are generally nondefective, so that each infectious particle can both transform and replicate. The replicating moiety appears to be essentially an intact leukosis virus, and the transforming genes are the added on portion as outlined above (58, 78). By deleting a part of the leukosis genome, avian sarcoma viruses can become transforming but defective for replication. It is clear that many avian sarcoma virus isolates induce sarcomas in chickens and closely related species. Birds do have the avian sarcoma virus-specific sequences in their normal DNA. However, it was surprising that the same avian sarcoma viruses, especially when enveloped as pseudotypes of several special avian leukosis subgroups (C, D), could induce sarcomas in mice, rats, hamsters, and also primates such as marmosets and baboons (37, 81, 85). None of the above mammals has the avian sarcoma specific sequences in its DNA. The avian sarcoma virus infected the above mammalian cells and integrated its DNA proviral form, but the infection was nonproductive (85). Although intact avian sarcoma virus could be rescued by various techniques, no mammalian transformed cells produced any infectious avian sarcoma virus. Thus the provirus was not defective in its genes but the environment rendered the virus defective. Avian sarcoma virus could also transform various cells *in vitro* in an analogous fashion: avian permissive cells were transformed and yielded virus while various mammalian cells became nonproductively transformed. Cells of many mammalian species could be transformed including human cells (81). Thus the host range spectrum of avian sarcoma virus transforming genes was much broader than the host range specified by its normal attending leukosis virus.

In the extensively studied murine sarcoma virus system rather similar principles apply. The Moloney isolate of murine sarcoma virus is defective and contains murine leukemia virus-like sequences, as well as sequences unique to sarcoma virus and normal mouse cells (28). Again murine sarcoma virus was able to transform and cause solid tumors not only in mice but also in several other species as well (39). Induction of tumors and transformation of various nonmurine mammalian cells could be readily accomplished by the formation of various pseudotypes of murine sarcoma virus (23, 39). The range of cultured cells of various species which could be transformed encompassed essentially all fibroblast cells tested including human cells. Related sarcoma viruses such as the Kirsten and Harvey isolates are composed partially of murine leukemia virus-specific sequences and rat cell derived information which at least in part resembles rat endogenous oncornavirus-like sequences. These two latter isolates cause sarcomas in several rodent species as well as in some

---

[3]R. Bassin, personal communication.

carnivores and primates when assayed as pseudotypes with appropriate envelopes (35). Tissue culture host range of transformation is quite broad. Again the spectrum of transforming ability is much wider than anticipated by the degree of relationship of viral nucleotide sequences compared to cellular DNA of many unrelated species.

Two additional sarcoma virus isolates whose nucleotide sequence and origins are not entirely clear are the feline sarcoma virus[4] and the simian sarcoma virus. Both of these are capable of causing tumors in several mammalian species and can transform a wide variety of cells in culture (77, 83). An interesting fact observed is that both sarcoma viruses may be capable of replicating in cells of some species without readily visible transformation. Further studies are required. From the above examples it is abundantly clear that, once the transforming genes of sarcoma viruses are introduced into a wide variety of molecularly related or unrelated cells, these genes can function in a way that the affected cell is rendered to behave as tumor cell. Second, cells can be virally transformed to be recognized histopathologically as sarcoma type cells with quite different genes composed of sets of nucleotide sequence unrelated to each other. Apparently there is a multiplicity of unrelated viral genes capable of provoking sarcomas.

The question whether the above observations are only a quirk of the special class of sarcomagenic oncornavirus has been in part answered by studies on several lymphoma-erythroleukemia inducing agents. Two viruses under consideration are the Abelson murine leukemia virus and the Friend murine leukemia virus (71).

Both viruses appear to be structured in a manner analogous to sarcoma viruses. Namely they contain murine leukemia-like sequences and additional nucleotide sequences whose origin is as yet unknown (73).[5] In both cases sequences implicated in transformation are those which are unrelated to murine leukemia viruses. At the time the existing pseudotypes of the above viruses are still fairly species specific for oncogenesis. Further studies are needed to determine whether other pseudotypes will extend the neoplastic host range of Abelson and Friend leukemia viruses.

Further thorough studies are needed to understand the complexity of transforming oncorna-

viruses. Specifically the presence and role of recombinant oncornaviruses is under intense investigation. Although it is clear that a multitude of different nucleotide sequences can each transform the cells of a single species it will be of great importance to understand how these sequences interact with the program of the cell genome.

REFERENCES

1. Aaronson, S. A., Hartley, J. W., and Todaro. G. (1969): Mouse leukemia virus; "spontaneous" release by mouse embryo cells after long term *in vitro* cultivation. *Proc. Natl. Acad. Sci. U.S.A.*, 64:87–94.
2. Aaronson, S. A., and Stephenson, J. R. (1973): Independent segregation of loci for activation of biologically distinguishable RNA C-type viruses in mouse cells. *Proc. Natl. Acad. Sci. U.S.A.*, 70:2055–2058.
3. Arcement, L. J., Karshin, W. L., Naso, R. B., Jamjoon, G., and Arlinghaus, R. B. (1976): Biosynthesis of Rauscher leukemia viral proteins; presence of p30 and envelope p15 sequences in precursor polypetides. *Virology*, 69:763–774.
4. Baltimore, D. (1974): Tumor viruses. *Cold Spring Harbor Symp. Quant. Biol.*, 39:1187–1200.
5. Benveniste, R. E., Callahan, R., Sherr, C. J., Chapman, V., and Todaro, G. J. (1977): Two distinct endogenous type C viruses isolated from the Asian rodent *Mus cervicolor*; conservation of virogene sequences in related rodent species. *J. Virol.*, 21:849–862.
6. Benveniste, R. E., Heinemann, R., Wilson, G. L., Callahan, R., and Todaro, G. J. (1974): Detection of baboon type C viral sequences in various primate tissues by molecular hybridization. *J. Virol.*, 14:56–67.
7. Benveniste, R. E., Lieber, M. M., Livingston, D. M., Sherr, C. J., Todaro, G. J., and Kalter, S. S. (1974): Infectious C-type virus isolated from a baboon placenta. *Nature*, 248:1720–1725.
8. Benveniste, R. E., Lieber, M. M., and Todaro, G. J. (1974): A distinct class of inducible murine type-C viruses that replicates in the rabbit SIRC cell line. *Proc. Natl. Acad. Sci. U.S.A.*, 71:602–606.
9. Benveniste, R. E., Sherr, C. J., and Todaro, G. J. (1975): Evolution of type C viral genes; origin of feline leukemia virus. *Science*, 190:886–888.
10. Benveniste, R. E., and Todaro, G. J. (1974): Evolution of C-type viral genes; inheritance of exogenously acquired viral genes. *Nature*, 252:456–459.
11. Benveniste, R. E., and Todaro, G. J. (1974): Evolution of type C viral genes; 1. Nucleic acid from baboon type-C virus as a measure of divergence among primate species. *Proc. Natl. Acad. Sci. U.S.A.*, 71:4513–4518.
12. Benveniste, R. E., and Todaro, G. J. (1975): Evolution of type C viral genes; III. Preservation of ancestral murine type C viral sequences in pig cellular DNA. *Proc. Natl. Acad. Sci. U.S.A.*, 72:4090–4094.
13. Benveniste, R. E., and Todaro, G. J. (1973): Homology between type-C viruses of various species as determined by molecular hybridization. *Proc. Natl. Acad. Sci. U.S.A.*, 70:3316–3320.
14. Benveniste, R. E., and Todaro, G. J. (1974): Multiple divergent copies of endogenous C-type virogenes in mammalian cells. *Nature*, 252:170–173.
15. Bernhard, W. (1960): The detection and study of tumor viruses with the electron microscope. *Cancer Res.*, 20:712–721.
16. Bolognesi, D. P., Collins, J. J., Leis, J. P., Moennig, V., Schäfer, W., and Atkinson, P. H. (1975): Role of carbohydrate in determining the immunological properties of the major glycoprotein (gp71) of Friend murine leukemia virus. *J. Virol.*, 16:1453–1463.
17. Callahan, R., Lieber, M. M., and Todaro, G. J. (1975): Nucleic acid homology of murine xenotropic type C viruses. *J. Virol.*, 15:1378–1384.
18. Cashion, L. M., Joho, R. H., Planitz, M. A., Billeter, M. A., and Weissmann, C. (1976): Initiation sites of Rous sarcoma virus RNA-directed synthesis *in vitro*. *Nature*, 262:186–190.
19. Chattopadhyay, S. K., Lowy, D. R., Teich, N. M., Levine, A. S., and Rowe, W. P. (1974): Qualitative and quantitative studies of AKR-type murine leukemia virus sequences in mouse DNA. *Cold Spring Harbor Symp. Quant. Biol.*, 39:1085–1101.
20. Fischinger, P. J., and Haapala, D. K. (1974): Oncoduction; a unifying hypothesis of viral carcinogenesis. *Prog. Exp. Tumor Res.*, 19:1–22.
21. Fischinger, P. J., Nomura, S., Blevins, C. S., and Bolognesi, D. P. (1975): Two levels of restriction by mouse or cat cells of murine sarcoma virus coated by endogenous xenotropic oncornavirus. *J. Gen. Virol.*, 29:51–62.
22. Fischinger, P. J., Nomura, S., and Bolognesi. D. P. (1975): A novel murine oncornavirus with dual eco- and xenotropic properties. *Proc. Natl. Acad. Sci. U.S.A.*, 72:5150–5155.
23. Fischinger, P. J., and O'Connor, T. E. (1969): Viral infection across species barriers; reversible alteration of murine sarcoma virus for growth in cat cells. *Science*, 165:714–716.

---

[4] New data obtained from C. Sherr are included in Table 25.2.
[5] D. Troxler *et al.*, unpublished data.

24. Fischinger, P. J., Peebles, P. T., Nomura, S., and Haapala, D. K. (1973): Isolation of an RD-114-like oncornavirus from a cat cell line. *J. Virol.*, 11: 978–985.
25. Fischinger, P. J., Schäfer, W., and Seifert, E. (1972): Detection of some murine leukemia virus antigens in virus particles derived from 3T3 cells transformed only by murine sarcoma virus. *Virology*, 47:229–235.
26. Frankel, A. E., and Fischinger, P. J. (1976): Moloney sarcoma virus-specific nucleotide sequences in mouse DNA and RNA. *Proc. Natl. Acad. Sci. U.S.A.*, 73:3705–3709.
27. Frankel, A. E., and Fischinger, P. J. (1977): Rate of divergence of cellular sequences homologous to segments of Moloney sarcoma virus. *J. Virol.*, 21:153–160.
28. Frankel, A. E., Neubauer, R. L., and Fischinger, P. J. (1976): Fractionation of DNA nucleotide transcripts from Moloney sarcoma virus and isolation of sarcoma virus-specific complementary DNA. *J. Virol.*, 18:481–490.
29. Fujita, D. J., Chen, Y. C., Friis, R. R., and Vogt, P. K. (1974): RNA tumor viruses of pheasants; characterization of avian leukosis subgroups. *Virology*, 60:558.
30. Gielkens, A. L. J., Van Zaane, D., Bloemers, H. P. J., and Bloemendal, H. (1976): Synthesis of Rauscher murine leukemia virus-specific polypeptides *in vitro. Proc. Natl. Acad. Sci. U.S.A.*, 73:356–360.
31. Gilden, R. V., and Oroszlan, S. (1972): Group specific antigens of RNA tumor viruses as markers for subinfections expression of the RNA tumor virus genome. *Proc. Natl. Acad. Sci. U.S.A.*, 69:1021–1025.
32. Hardy, W. D., Jr, Old, L. J., Hess, P. W., Essex, M., and Cotter, S. (1973): Horizontal transmission of feline leukemia virus. *Nature*, 244:266–269.
33. Hartley, J. W., and Rowe, W. P. (1976): Naturally occurring murine leukemia viruses in wild mice; characterization of a new "amphotropic" class. *J. Virol.*, 19:19–25.
34. Hartley, J. W., Rowe, W. P., and Huebner, J. J. (1970): Host range restrictions of murine leukemia viruses in mouse embryo cell cultures. *J. Virol.*, 5:221–225.
35. Harvey, J. J. (1964): An unidentified virus which causes the rapid production of tumors in mice. *Nature*, 204:1104–1105.
36. Hazeltine, W. A., Kleid, D. G., Panet, A., Rothenberg, E., and Baltimore, D. (1976): Ordered transcription of RNA virus genomes. *J. Mol. Biol.*, 106:109–131.
37. Hill, M., and Hillova, J. (1972): Virus recovery in chicken cells tested with Rous sarcoma cell DNA. *Nature (New Biol.)*, 237:35–39.
38. Hino, S. Stephenson, J. R., and Aaronson, S. A. (1976): Radioimmunoassays for the 70000-molecular-weight glycoproteins of endogenous mouse type C viruses; viral antigen expression in normal mouse tissues and sera. *J. Virol.*, 18:933–941.
39. Huebner, R. J., Hartley, J. W., Rowe, W. P. Lane, W. T., and Capps, W. J. (1966): Rescue of the defective genome of Moloney sarcoma virus from a non-infectious hamster tumor and the production of pseudotype sarcoma viruses with various murine leukemia viruses. *Proc. Natl. Acad. Sci. U.S.A.*, 56:1164–1169.
40. Huebner, R. J., and Todaro, G. J. (1969): Onconogenes of RNA tumor viruses as determinants of cancer. *Proc. Natl. Acad. Sci. U.S.A.*, 64:1087–1094.
41. Hunsmann, G., Moennig, V., Pister, L., Seifert, E., and Schäfer, W. (1974): Properties of mouse leukemia viruses; VIII. The major viral glycoprotein of Friend leukemia virus. Seroimmunological, interfering, and hemagglutinating capacities. *Virology*, 62: 307–318.
42. Jaenisch, R., Fan, H., and Croker, B. (1975): Infection of preimplantation mouse embryos and of newborn mice with leukemia virus; tissue distribution of viral DNA and RNA and leukemogenesis in the adult animal. *Proc. Natl. Acad. Sci. U.S.A.*, 72:4008–4012.
43. Joho, R. H., Stoll, E., Friis, R. R., Billeter, M. A., and Weissmann, C. (1975): A partial genetic map of Rous sarcoma virus RNA; location of polymerase, envelope and transformation markers, in *Animal Virology, ICN-UCLA Symposium on Molecular and Cellular Biology*, edited by D. Baltimore. W. A. Benjamin, Inc., Menlo Park, Calif.
44. Jolicouer, P., and Baltimore, D. (1976): Effect of Fv-1 gene product on proviral DNA formation and integration into cells infected with murine leukemia viruses. *Proc. Natl. Acad. Sci. U.S.A.*, 73:2236–2240.
45. Junghans, R. P., Hu, S., Knight, A., and Davidson, N. (1977): Heteroduplex analysis of avian RNA tumor viruses. *Proc. Natl. Acad. Sci. U.S.A.*, 74: 477–481.
46. Kang, C. Y., and Temin, H. M. (1974): Reticuloendotheliosis virus nucleic acid sequences in cellular DNA. *J. Virol.*, 14:1179–1188.
47. Kawakami, T. G., Huff, S. D., Buckley, P. M., Dungworth, D. L., Snyder, S. P., and Gilden, R. V. (1972): C-type virus associated with gibbon lymphosarcoma. *Nature (New Biol.)*, 235:170–171.
48. Kirsten, W. H., and Meyer, L. A. (1967): Morphologic responses to a murine erythroblastosis virus. *J.N.C.I.*, 39:311–316.
49. Laird, C. D., McConaughy, B. L., and McCarthy, B. J. (1969): Rate of fixation of nucleotide substitutions in evolution. *Nature*, 224:149–154.
50. Lerner, R. A., Wilson, C. B., Del Villano, B. C., McConahey, P. J., and Dixon, F. J. (1975): Endogenous oncornaviral gene expression in adult and fetal mice; quantitative, histologic and physiologic studies on the major viral glycoprotein, gp70. *J. Exp. Med.*, 143:151–166.
51. Levy, J. A. (1976): Endogenous C-type viruses; double agents in natural life processes. *Biomedicine*, 24:84–93.
52. Levy, J. A. (1973): Xenotropic viruses; murine leukemia viruses associated with NIH Swiss mice. *Science*, 182:1151–1153.
53. Lieber, M. M., Sherr, C. J., Todaro, G. J., Benveniste, R. E., Callahan, R., and Coon, H. G. (1975): Isolation from the Asian mouse *Mus caroli* of an endogenous type C virus related to infections primate type C viruses. *Proc. Natl. Acad. Sci. U.S.A.*, 72:2315–2319.
54. Lowy, D. R., Rowe, W. P., Teich, N., and Hartley, J. W. (1971): Murine leukemia virus; high frequency activation *in vitro* by 5-iododeoxyuridine and 5-bromodeoxyuridine. *Science*, 174:155–156.
55. Miller, J. M., Miller, L. D., Olson, C., and Gillette, K. G. (1969): Virus-like particles in phytohemagglutin-stimulated lymphocute cultures with reference to bovine lymphosarcoma. *J.N.C.I.*, 43:1297.
56. Moloney, J. B. (1966): Biological studies on a lymphoid leukemia virus extracted from sarcoma S 37; I. Origin and introductory investigations. *Natl. Cancer Inst. Monggr.*, 22:139–142.
57. Neiman, P. E. (1973): Measurement of endogenous leukosis virus nucleotide sequences in the DNA of normal avian embryos by RNA-DNA hybridization. *Virology*, 53:196–204.
58. Neiman, P. E., Wright, J. E., McMillin, C., and MacDonnel, D. (1974): Nucleotide sequences relationships of avian RNA tumor viruses: measurement of the deletion on a transformation-defective mutant of Rous sarcoma virus. *J. Virol.*, 13:837–846.
59. Oskarsson, M. K., Robbey, W. G., Harris, C. L., Fischinger, P. J., Haapala, D. K., and Vande Woude, G. J. (1975): A p60 polypeptide in the feline leukemia virus pseudotype of Moloney sarcoma virus with murine leukemia virus p30 antigenic determinants. *Proc. Natl. Acad. Sci. U.S.A.*, 72:2380–2384.
60. Peebles, P. T., Gerwin, B. I., and Scolnick, E. M. (1976): Murine sarcoma virus defectiveness; serological detection of only helper virus reverse transcriptase in sarcoma virus rescued from nonmurine S+L− cells. *Virology*, 9:488–493.
61. Purchase, H. G., Ludford, C., Nazerian, K., and Cox, H. W. (1973): A new group of oncogenic viruses; reticuloendotheliosis, chick sycytial, duck infectious anemia, and spleen necrosis viruses. *J.N.C.I.*, 51:1973.
62. Quintrell, N., Varmus, H. E., Bishop, J. M., Nicholson, M. D., and McAllister, R. M. (1974): Homologies among the nucleotide sequences of the genomes of C-type viruses. *Virology*, 58:568–575.
63. Rickard, C. G. (1969). Feline leukemia. Lymphosarcoma symposium. *J. Small Anim. Pract.*, 10:615.
64. Rubin, H., Cornelius, A., and Fanshier, L. (1961). The pattern of congenital transmission of an avian leukosis virus. *Proc. Natl. Acad. Sci. U.S.A.*, 47:1058.
65. Sarma, P. S., Cheong, M., Hartley, J. W., and Huebner, R. J. (1967): A viral interference test for mouse leukemia viruses. *Virology*, 33:180–183.
66. Sarma, P. S., Jain, D. K., Mishra, N. K., Lee, M., Vernon, M. L., Paul, P. S., and Pomeroy, B. S. (1975): Isolation and characterization of viruses from natural outbreaks of reticuloendotheliosis in turkeys. *J.N.C.I.*, 54:1355–1359.
67. Schäfer, W., Bauer, H., Bolognesi, D. P., Fischinger, P. J., Frank, H., Gelderblom, H., Lange, J., and Nermut, M. V. (1975): Studies on structural and antigenic properties of C-type viruses, in *Molecular Studies in Viral Neoplasia*, pp. 115–140. Williams & Wilkins, Baltimore.
68. Schäfer, W., de Noronha, F., Lange, J., and Bolognesi, D. P. (1971): Comparative studies on group specific antigens of RNA leukemia viruses, in *The Biology of Oncogenic Viruses*, pp. 116–123. North-Holland, Amsterdam/London.
69. Scolnick, E. M., Goldberg, R. J., and Parks, W. P. (1974): A biochemical and genetic analysis of mammalian RNA-containing sarcoma vurises. *Cold Spring Harbor Symp. Quant. Biol.*, 39:885–895.
70. Scolnick, E. M., Goldberg, R. J., and Williams, D. (1976): Characteristics of rat genetic sequences of Kirsten sarcoma virus distinct class of endogenous sequences. *J. Virol.*, 18:559–566.
71. Scolnick, E. M., Howk, K. S., Anisowicz, A., Peebles, P. T., Scher, C. D., and Parks, W. P. (1975): Separation of sarcoma-specific and leukemia virus-specific genetic sequences of Moloney sarcoma virus. *Proc. Natl. Acad. Sci. U.S.A.*, 72:4650–4654.
72. Scolnick, E. M., and Parks, W. P. (1974): Harvey sarcoma virus: a second murine type C sarcoma virus with rat genetic information. *J. Virol.*, 13: 1211–1219.
73. Scolnick, E. M., Rands, E., Williams, D., and Parks, W. P. (1973): Studies on the nucleic acid sequences of Kirsten sarcoma virus; a model for formation of a mammalian RNA-containing sarcoma virus. *J. Virol.*, 12: 458–463.
74. Scolnick, E. M., Stephenson, J. R., and Aaronson, S. A. (1972): Isolation of temperature-sensitive mutants of murine sarcoma virus. *J. Virol.*, 10: 653–657.
75. Simpson, G. G. (1959): The nature and origin of supraspecific taxa. *Cold Spring Harbor Symp. Quant. Biol.*, 24:255–271.
76. Smotkin, D., Gianni, A. M., Rozenblatt, S., and Weinberg, R. A. (1975): Infectious viral DNA of murine leukemia virus. *Proc. Natl. Acad. Sci.*

U.S.A., 72:4910–4913.

77. Snyder, S. P. (1971): Spontaneous feline fibrosarcomas; transmissibility and ultra-structure of associated virus-like particles. *J.N.C.I.,* 47:1079–1084.

78. Stehelin, D., Guntaka, R. V., Varmus, H. E., and Bishop, J. M. (1976): Purification of DNA complementary to nucleotide sequences required for neoplastic transformation of fibroblasts by avian sarcoma viruses. *J. Mol. Biol.,* 101:349–365.

79. Stehelin, D., Varmus, H. E., Bishop, J., and Vogt, P. K. (1976): DNA related to the transforming gene(s) of avian sarcoma viruses is present in normal avian DNA. *Nature,* 260:170–173.

80. Temin, H. M. (1971): Mechanism of transformation by RNA tumor viruses. *Annu. Rev. Microbiol.,* 25:609–648.

81. Temin, H. M. (1974): Cellular and molecular biology of RNA tumor viruses, especially avian leukosis-sarcoma viruses and their relatives. *Adv. Virus Res.,* 19:47–104.

82. Temin, H. M. (1974): On the origin of the genes for neoplasia: G. H. A. Clowes Memorial Lecture. *Cancer Res.,* 34:2835–2841.

83. Theilen, G. H., Gould, D., Fowler, M., and Dungworth, D. L. (1971): C-type virus in tumor tissue of wooly monkey (*Lagothris* spp.) with fibrosarcoma. *J.N.C.I.,* 47:881–888.

84. Toyashima, K., and Vogt, Pp K. (1969): Temperature sensitive mutants of an avian sarcoma virus. *Virology,* 39:930–931.

85. Varmus, H. E., Bishop, J. M., and Vogt, P. K. (1973): Appearance of virus-specific DNA in mammalian cells following transformation by Rous sarcoma virus. *J. Mol. Biol.,* 74:613–626.

86. Varmus, H. E., Heasley, S., and Bishop, J. M. (1973): Use of DNA-DNA annealing to detect new virus-specific DNA sequences in chicken embryo fibroblasts after infection by avian sarcoma virus. *J. Biol.,* 14:895–903.

87. Walker, R. (1969): Virus associated with epidermal hyperplasia in fish. *Natl. Cancer Inst. Mongr.,* 31:195–207.

88. Wang, L. H., Duesberg, P. H., Kawai, S., and Hanafusa, H. (1976): Location of envelope-specific and sarcoma-specific oligonucliotides on RNA of Schmidt-Ruppin Rous Sarcoma virus. *Proc. Natl. Acad. Sci. U.S.A.,* 73:447–451.

89. Weiss, R. A., Mason, W. S., and Vogt, P. K. (1973): Genetic recombinants and heterozygotes derived from endogenous and exogenous avian RNA tumor viruses. *Virology,* 52:535–552.

90. Wolfe, L. G., Deinhardt, F., Theilen, G. H., Rabin, H., Kawakami, T., and Bustad, L. K. (1971): Induction of tumors in marmoset monkeys by simian sarcoma virus type 1 (*Lagothrix*): a preliminary report. *J.N.C.I.,* 47:1115–1120.

Addendum. Within the last year considerable new data have shown that the formation and integration of double-stranded proviral DNA from single-stranded viral DNA is much more complex than indicated above. Molecular cloning of proviral DNA in λ bacteriophage and advanced methods of DNA sequencing have yielded new insights into molecular structure. The reader is referred to two most recent analyses of DNA structure and integration models of Moloney leukemia and sarcoma viruses (*cf.* C. Shoemaker et al.: *Proc. Natl. Acad. Sci. U.S.A.,* 77:3932, and R. Dhar et al.: *ibid.,* p. 3937, both 1980). Briefly, the critical elements consist of short terminal repeated sequences, within long terminal repeated sequences (588 base pairs). In the latter are inverted terminal sequences, sequence duplications, the transcription initiation signal, the poly-adenylylation signal, the promoter signal, the tRNA binding site and the 5′ end of viral RNA. This sequence pattern has significant analogy on a comparative basis with prokaryote insertion elements and transposable elements in eukaryotes which are flanked by inverted or directly repeated sequences and which within themselves have terminal inverted repeats. The proposed integration model based on insertion element integration suggests that circularization occurs by blunt end ligation of an 8.8 kilobase pair linear DNA. Integration could take place after specific recognition of long terminal repeats and host DNA and a formation of staggered cuts in both DNAs followed by joining of ends and the replication of the repeated sequences. In the integrated form there would be viral genes flanked by long terminal repeats that have two bases missing, and the proviral DNA will be flanked by host cell DNA four base repeats. Direct sequencing of the DNA at the host DNA-viral DNA junctions has demonstrated the validity of the model.

26

Tumors Induced by Plant Viruses*

D. V. R. Reddy

INTRODUCTION

This chapter will be concerned with tumors produced in plants by plant viruses. Infection by a very few plant viruses leads directly to the production of tumors (Table 26.1). However, there are a number of virus diseases in which overgrowths of one kind or another are produced only on certain special hosts or under certain special conditions. It is interesting that the macroscopic symptoms produced by plant viruses containing double stranded RNA (grouped under "phytoreoviruses")[1] are, with the exception of rice dwarf virus, almost exclusively hyperplastic. Unfortunately, very little work has been done on tumorigenesis by plant viruses. Wound tumor disease is the best known and most studied of any plant virus tumor disease and almost all research on it was done by L. M. Black and his associates. Thus, this chapter will almost exclusively be restricted to wound tumor disease upon which the following excellent reviews by L. M. Black (6, 7, 9) have been published.

ORIGIN, DEVELOPMENT AND CELL STRUCTURE OF TUMORS PRODUCED BY WOUND TUMOR VIRUS (WTV)

The characteristic symptoms of wound tumor disease are vein-enlargement on the leaves and tumors on the roots (Figs. 26.1 and 26.2). The origin and development of tumors were studied mostly in sweet clover (*Melilotus officinalis* and *Melilotus alba*) (Fig. 26.3) because they produce many vigorously growing root tumors of various sizes. The tumor formation was initiated at the fourth or fifth incipient lateral root behind the tip of the mother root at about the time the lateral root was emerging (24). The first sign of tumor development was noticed in the pericycle opposite the primary phloem and there was no indication that the neighboring cells of the cortex, endodermis, xylem, and cambium were affected. However, with the proliferation of the pericycle some of the endodermal and cortical cells were stretched and crushed. The first tissue to become differentiated in the tumor was an abnormal phloem which lacked sieve plates. Xylem was the next tissue to become differentiated in young tumors and it developed as radiating finger-like extensions. The xylem tissue consisted of tracheids of irregular shape and dimensions. Proliferation of cells of the meristematic tissue between the xylem and phloem and between the xylem extensions was noticed in young tumors (23). Well developed tumor tissue (Fig. 26.4) contained an outermost zone of abnormal tracheids, a middle zone of parenchymatous or meristematic cells and an inner region of pseudophloem. However, this arrangement was not invariable and sometimes meristematic tumor cells were located near the surface of the tumor and tracheids occurred intermixed with parenchymatous tumor cells and pseudophloem. No distinct layers of different tissues were observed in old tumors. Groups of abnormal tracheids encircled by parenchymatous tumor cells and a few necrotic cells were seen. The meristematic tumor cells and pseudophloem were not formed as definite layers but occurred as masses of tissue around the periphery of the groups of tracheids. Meristematic tumor cells at the periphery retained their capacity for cell division

* Dedicated to Dr. L. M. Black, Emeritus Professor, University of Illinois and Dr. L. D. Swindale, Director General, International Crops Research Institute for the Semi-Arid Tropics.
[1] Name proposed for consideration to the Reovirus Study Group of the Vertebrate Virus Subcommittee of the International Committee on Taxonomy of Viruses.

TABLE 26.1
List of Viruses which are Known to Produce Hyperplastic Symptoms

S. No.	Name of the Virus	References
1	Wound tumor virus[a]	Black (4, 8)
2	Cereal tillering disease virus[a]	Lindsten et al. (26), Milne et al. (31)
3	Arrhenatherum blue dwarf virus[a]	Mühle and Kempiak (33); Milne et al. (32)
4	Maize rough dwarf virus[a]	Lovisolo (29)
5	Rice black-streaked dwarf virus[a]	Shikata (41)
6	Fiji disease virus[a]	Hutchinson and Francki (21)
7	Maize wallaby ear virus[a]	Tyron (44), Schindler (42), Grylls (19), Reddy et al. (39)
8	Citrus vein-enation[b]	Hooper and Schneider (20)
9	Clover enation virus[b]	Bos and Grancini (14)
10	Clubroot of tobacco[b]	Valleau (45)

[a] Grouped under phytoreoviruses.
[b] Detailed studies on the characterization of the virus are lacking.

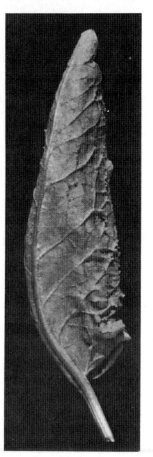

Figure 26.2. Underside of sorrel leaf, infected by wound tumor virus, showing enlarged veins. (Reproduced with permission from L. M. Black: *Progress in Experimental Tumor Research*, *15*:110–137, 1972 (10).)

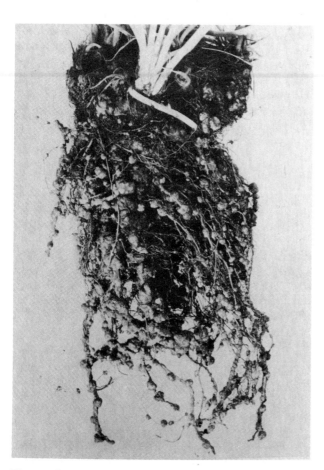

Figure 26.1. Sorrel root infected by wound tumor virus. (Reproduced with permission from L. M. Black: *Progress in Experimental Tumor Research*, *15*:110–137, 1972 (10).)

and differentiation. Occasionally cambium-like layers occurred in the tumors (24).

It is apparent that it was abnormal cell multiplication and not cell enlargement that resulted in the development of tumor tissue.

On the stems of sweet clover, tumors were produced at the point of origin of branches, at graft unions, and at the cut surface of cuttings. They originated from primary phloem fibers, phloem-parenchyma cells and from phloem procambium. Young tumors possessed regularly arranged layers of tissues comprising an inner zone of abnormal tracheids, a middle zone of meristematic tumor cells, and an outer zone of abnormal phloem. However, in older tumors, the tissues were arranged irregularly. Occasionally, slight intrusion of tumor tissue into xylem occurred during tumor development (25).

It must be mentioned that not all of the overgrowths incited by WTV originate in the pericycle or phloem. Small tumors developing from cork cambium in roots of *Rumex acetosa* were

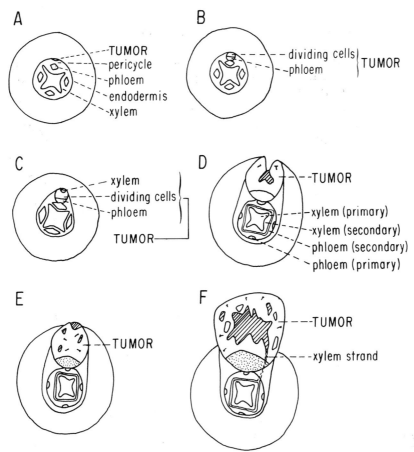

Figure 26.3. Diagramatic representation of the origin and development of root tumors in *M. alba. A*, Initiation of tumors in the pericycle opposite the primary phloem; *B*, Tumor tissue comprising approximately 30–40 cells; the innermost cells comprising abnormal phloem (stippled area); *C*, Tumor tissue comprising approximately 90–100 cells, outermost tissue differentiated into xylem (cross-lined area); *D*, Representation of overgrowth of xylem; *E*, Representation of the location of xylem at the periphery as a result of internal growth of the tumor tissue; *F*, Tumor tissue comprising approximately 1000 cells; showing central mass of xylem, basal phloem, xylem and phloem intermixed in the outer zone. (Reproduced with permission from S. M. Kelly and L. M. Black: *American Journal of Botany*, 36:65–73, 1949 (23).)

observed by Kelly and Black (23) and in certain other plants they observed overgrowths from cambium tissues.

It was shown that in many species tumor cells, especially those of pseudophloem, contained spherical cytoplasmic inclusions, called spherules (27) which were rich in arginine. The size of the spherules ranged from 4–10 μ in diameter. It is not known whether or not the spherules contained virus particles.

FACTORS INFLUENCING THE INITIATION, DEVELOPMENT, AND SIZE OF TUMORS

Hereditary Differences in Individual Plants

It was shown that sweet clover plants varied greatly in their hereditary response to infection

with the virus, some produced many prominent root tumors and others very inconspicuous ones (6). Of the various clones studied, the clone C_{10} of *M. officinalis* consistently produced excellent tumors. Since it was possible to maintain a clone by vegetative propagation of its cuttings indefinitely, clone C_{10} was used for nearly three decades to maintain WTV with consistently good results.

Role Played by Wounds in the Tumor Development

Wounds were shown to play an important role in initiating tumors in virus-infected plants (9). Lateral roots originate from the pericycle and grow out through endodermis, cortex, and epidermis. More than 80% of the root tumors originate above, below, or at the side but not opposite the emerging points of lateral roots (24).

Thus, tumors occurred on roots more frequently than on any other part of the plant. The number of tumors on stems were less because the lateral appendages of the stem are formed from superficial meristems and develop without causing wounds to the overlying tissue. Abundant production of tumors at graft unions and at the base of infected stem cuttings confirm that wounds play an important role in initiating tumors in virus-infected plants.

Role of Hormones in Tumor Production

The relationship between wounds and tumor production led to the assumption on the possible role of hypothetical hormones released from injured or killed cells (8, 10). Till now the existence of wound hormones inducing healing in plant species has not been experimentally demonstrated. However, Black and Lee (12) have shown that a number of synthetic plant growth regulating substances, including indole acetic acid and naphthalene acetic acid acted synergistically with the virus to stimulate tumor initiation. Thus, it is reasonable to assume that hormones, which are probably released from wounded cells, are playing an important role in the initiation and development of tumors.

STRUCTURE AND CHEMISTRY OF WOUND TUMOR VIRUS

WTV was shown to be icosahedral (1) 73 nm in diameter (38) and composed of 32 capsomeres, each 18 nm in diameter and consisting of 5 or 6 structural units approximately 7.5 nm in diameter (I. Kimura, personal communication). The virion possesses an amorphous outer layer consisting of 131,000 and 96,000 dalton polypeptides. The underlying capsomeres, which were visible after chymotrypsin treatment (Fig. 26.5), are composed of 36,000 and 35,000 dalton polypeptides. An inner core which resulted from the shearing effect of centrifugation of the virus through a cesium chloride gradient was found to contain the 160,000; 118,000 and 58,000 dalton polypeptides (38).

WTV contains a segmented double-stranded (ds) RNA genome and the wild isolate was reported to have 12 segments (22) which can be separated electrophoretically (34) (Fig. 26.6). WTV displays a transcriptase activity (12) which catalyzes the transcription of all 12 genome RNA segments into single stranded RNA in vitro (40).

VIRAL GENES INVOLVED IN TUMORIGENESIS

WTV was transmitted by certain agallian leafhoppers (Black, 1944) in which it multiplies (10). The virus was usually maintained in the wild (vectorial) form by continuous alternating passages in the leafhopper and in crimson clover, Trifolium incarnatum L. After inoculation of sweet clover plants by means of leafhoppers carrying the virus, it was possible to maintain WTV in cuttings of sweet clover that developed root tumors for periods of years without passage through the leafhopper vector. Virus maintained by this process for various numbers of years led to the production of WTV isolates which lost their ability to be transmitted by the vector, either partially or completely (13) with corresponding losses in specific infectivity on vector cell monolayers (28, 35). When genomes of the virus from these various isolates were examined, a single isolate contained a lower relative concentration of one or another segment than did the wild-type virus. This was attributed to a deletion mutation in the affected segment and the subsequent development of a mixed population of wild and mutant virions. Segments 1, 2, 5, and 7 showed such mutations (36). Wound tumor virion populations with the ability to replicate in sweet clover in the absence of segment 2 and segment 5 were obtained by selection. Selection for the elimination of intact segment 7 was successful but resulted in the retention of a fragment of segment 7 in quantity equimolar to the other segments. Selection aimed at eliminating segment 1 never reduced the proportion of virions carrying it below 10% (37). As illustrated in Fig. 26.7 all these various mutants have retained the ability to produce excellent tumors. Results of this study clearly indicate that WTV can multiply in sweet clover clone C_{10} and produce tumors in the absence of segments 2 and 5. It is likely that the hypothetical tumorigenic gene (10) does not occur in segments 2 and 5.

A good correlation was found between the molecular weights of segments 1, 2, 3, 4, 6, or 7, 9, 10, or 11 and those of the WTV polypeptides 160,000; 131,000; 118,000; 96,000, 58,000 and 36,000 and 35,000 daltons, respectively, suggesting a direct coding relationship between them (36). Although experimental evidence is lacking, it is likely that the segments involved in coding for structural polypeptides as well as RNA transcriptase are probably not involved in tumorigenesis. Thus, in the case of WTV, probably one of the segments of 9, 10, and 11 or segment 12 is

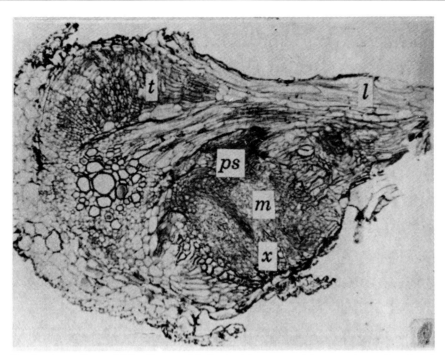

Figure 26.4. Longitudinal section of *M. alba* root infected by wound tumor virus showing later stage of tumor development. l = lateral root; m = meristematic tumor cells; Ps = Pseudophloem; x = abnormal tracheids. (Reproduced with permission from C. L. Lee: *Virology, 1:*152–164, 1955 (24).)

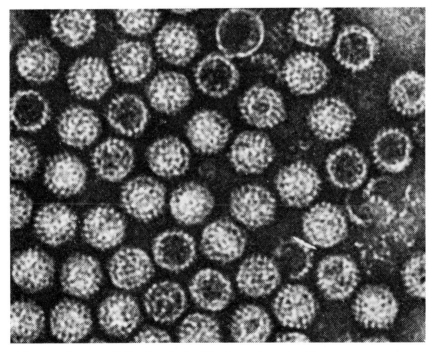

Figure 26.5. Wound tumor virus particles treated with chymotrypsin. The caposomeres are clearly discernible. The diameter of the particles is 63 nm.

playing a vital role in tumor production. This conclusion is further strengthened by the observation that the first eight segments of the genomes of WTV and rice dwarf virus which constitute about 88% of each genome, form a remarkably similar electropherogram pattern (39). Since rice dwarf virus does not produce tumors in plants, segments 9 to 12 of WTV are particularly suspected as being etiologically involved in tumor production.

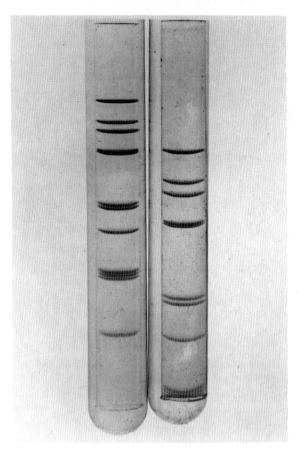

Figure 26.6. Acrylamide gels after electrophoresis of double-stranded (ds) RNA from wild wound tumor virus. Gels were stained in toluidine blue O. Movement was from top to bottom. Left side gel showing all 12 ds RNA segments and the right side one showing clear resolution of segments 4 and 5.

CONCLUSIONS

It is of special interest that seven of the eight plant viruses possessing double-stranded RNA produce tumors, whereas only three viruses are tumorigenic among the more than 200 plant viruses that do not belong to this group. Tumor tissue derived from each of more than 1,000 individual plants of different WTV isolates (36), some of which were maintained in sweet clover for nearly 25 years by continuous vegetative propagation, contained viral double-stranded RNA (D. V. R. Reddy, unpublished). Thus, tumorigenesis may be closely linked to the continuous viral replication in the case of WTV. The report of Streissle et al. (43) that after about 5 to 7 months of culturing of tumor tissue *in vitro* the virus could not be detected was not well substantiated. The particle counts in the electron microscope employed by the authors could probably only detect virus particles if the tumor tissue examined contained more than 10^9 virions per gram (18).

It is not known at the present time whether the "unique proclivity" in the WTV group for the production of tumors is related to the double-stranded nature of their RNA. Among the double-stranded RNA viruses both rice dwarf and rice black streaked-dwarf viruses multiply in rice but only the latter can produce tumors. It is probable that tumor production is not dependent on the physical property of double-strandedness of the RNA.

Since our initial attempts to detect RNA dependent DNA polymerase (reverse transcriptase) in purified WTV have failed, (D. V. R. Reddy, unpublished) it is likely that WTV-RNA is not integrated into the chromosomal DNA of a target cell. Alternatively, new and specific products, derived as a result of WTV infection, may possess the ability to incite tumors persistently activating that segment of the host cell genome which regulates continued cell growth and division. However, no bioassay exists for testing the tumorigenic capabilities of such substances. In addition, the requirement for the wound reaction, for the initiation of tumors may further complicate the development of a successful bioassay system.

Experiments performed on topophysis or phase change involving young and adult forms of certain higher plant species and crown gall (15, 16) and other plant tumor systems (for example Kostoff genetic tumors (2, 17, 30)) have demonstrated that persistent but potentially reversible changes in the phenotype without corresponding changes in the integrity of the cellular genome occur commonly in normal plant development. Thus, a deletion or permanent rearrangement of the genetic information may not be essential for attaining the neoplastic state. A persistent but potentially reverisble activation or repression of a select biosynthetic system of host cells, such as auxin-synthesizing system (16) plays a vital role in the expression of the tumor phenotype. Thus, we arrive at the most important conclusion stated first by Black (9) that one or more of the proteins coded by the genome would seem to provide the most likely agents which might inactivate a repressor gene and thereby activate an operon gene controlling cell multiplication. There is good evidence that each segment of double-stranded RNA, in the case of reoviruses, carries a monocistronic message. It is likely that one or more of the proteins coded by the lower molecular weight RNA segments of WTV may inactivate the repressor gene. Since the wounding of cells aids tumor

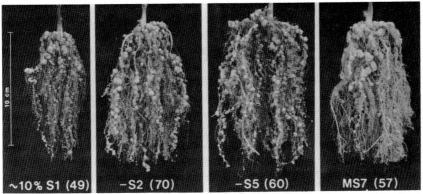

Figure 26.7. Abundant root tumors in sweet clover produced by four wound tumor virus isolates ~10% S1 (49): virion populations retained approximately 10% of segment 1; −S2(70): virions lacking segment 2; −S5(60): virions lacking segment 5; MS 7 (57): virion populations lacking segment 7 but retaining a mutant of segment 7. (Reproduced with permission from D. V. R. Reddy and L. M. Black: *Virology, 80*:336–346, 1977 (37).)

initiation, the initial repression of a select bio-synthetic system may be carried out by normal host responses to wounding.

Acknowledgment. I am grateful to Dr. L. M. Black for his many valuable comments.

References

1. Bils, R. F., and Hall, C. E. (1962): Electron microscopy of wound tumor virus. *Virology,* 1:123–130.
2. Binns, A., and Meins, F. (1973): Habituation of tobacco pith cells for factors promoting cell division is heritable and potentially reversible. *Proc. Natl. Acad. Sci.,* 70:2660–2662.
3. Black, D. R., and Knight, C. A. (1970): Ribonucleic acid transcriptase activity in purified wound tumor virus. *Virology,* 6:194–198.
4. Black, L. M. (1944): Some viruses transmitted by agallian leafhoppers. *Proc. Am. Philos. Soc.,* 88:132–144.
5. Black, L. M. (1945): A virus tumor disease of plants. *Am. J. Bot.,* 32:408–415.
6. Black, L. M. (1951): Hereditary variation in the reaction of sweet clover to the wound tumor virus. *Am. J. Bot.,* 38:256–267.
7. Black, L. M. (1958): Wound-tumor. *Proc. Natl. Acad. Sci.,* 44:364–367.
8. Black, L. M. (1965): Physiology of virus-induced tumors in plants. In *Encyclopedia of Plant Physiology,* pp. 236–266, edited by Ruhland and Lang. Springer, New York.
9. Black, L. M. (1970): Wound tumor virus. Descriptions of plant viruses No. 34. Commonwealth Mycological Institute, Kew, England.
10. Black, L. M. (1972): Plant tumors of viral origin. *Prog. Exp. Tumor Res.,* 15:110–137.
11. Black, L. M., and Brakke, M. K. (1952): Multiplication of wound-tumor virus in an insect vector. *Phytopathology,* 42:269–273.
12. Black, L. M., and Lee, C. L. (1957): Interaction of growth-regulating chemicals and tumefacient virus on plant cells. *Virology,* 3:146–159.
13. Black, L. M., Wolcyrz, S., and Whitcomb, R. F. (1958): A vectorless strain of wound-tumor virus, p. 255. 7th International Congress for Microbiology, Stockholm.
14. Bos, L., and Grancini, P. (1968): Peculiar histoid enations in white clover and their relationship to virus diseases and toxic effects of leafhopper feeding. *Phytopath. Z.,* 61:253–272.
15. Braun, A. C. (1974): *The Biology of Cancer.* Addison-Wesley, Reading, Mass.
16. Braun, A. C., and Wood, H. N. (1976): Suppression of the neoplastic state with the acquisition of specialized functions in cells, tissues and organs of crown gall teratomas of tobacco. *Proc. Natl. Acad. Sci.,* 73:496–500.
17. Carlson, P. S., Smith, H. H., and Dearing, R. D. (1972): Parasexual interspecific plant hybridization. *Proc. Natl. Acad. Sci.,* 69:2292–2294.
18. Gamez, R., and Black, L. M. (1968): Particle counts of wound-tumor virus during its peak concentration in leafhoppers. *Virology,* 34:444–451.
19. Grylls, N. E. (1975): Leafhopper transmission of a virus causing maize wallaby ear disease. *Ann. Appl. Biol.,* 79:283–296.
20. Hooper, G., and Schneider, H. (1969): The vein-enation and woody gall disease of citrus. *California Citrogr.,* 54:416, 423–424.
21. Hutchinson, P. B., and Francki, R. I. B. (1973): Fiji Disease Virus. Descriptions of plant viruses No. 119, 3 pp. Commonwealth Mycological Institute, Kew.
22. Kalmakoff, J., Lewandowski, L. J., and Black, D. R. (1969): Comparison of the ribonucleic acid sub-units of reovirus, cytoplasmic polyhedrosis virus, and wound tumor virus. *Virology,* 4:851–856.
23. Kelly, S. M., and Black, L. M. (1949): The origin, development and cell structure of a virus tumor in plants. *Am. J. Bot.,* 36:65–73.
24. Lee, C. L. (1955a): Virus-tumor development in relation to lateral-root and bacterial-nodule formation in *Melilotus alba. Virology,* 1:152–164.
25. Lee, C. L. (1955b): Anatomical changes in sweet clover shoots infected with wound-tumor virus. *Am. J. Bot.,* 42:693–698.
26. Lindsten, K., Gerhardson, B., and Pettersson, J. (1973): Cereal tillering disease in Sweden and some comparisons with oat sterile dwarf and maize rough dwarf. *National Swedish Institute for Plant Protection Contribution,* 15:151, 375–397.
27. Littau, V. C., and Black, L. M. (1952): Spherical inclusions in plant tumors caused by a virus. *Am. J. Bot.,* 39:87–95.
28. Liu, H. Y., Kimura, I., and Black, L. M. (1973): Specific infectivity of different wound tumor virus isolates. *Virology,* 51:320–326.
29. Lovisolo, O. (1971): Maize rough dwarf virus. Descriptions of plant viruses No. 72, 4 pp. Commonwealth Mycological Institute, Kew.
30. Lutz, A. (1971): Morphogenetic aptitudes of tissue cultures of unicellular origin. In "Colloq. Internat. Centre Nat. Recherche Sci. (Paris). No. 193, Les Cultures de Tissus de Plantes; (Proc. 2nd Internat. Conf. Plant Tissue Culture, Strassbourg, France, 1970). Paris: Centre Nat'l de la Recherche Scientifique, pp. 163–168.
31. Milne, R. G., Lindsten, K., and Conti, M. (1975): Electron microscopy of the particles of cereal tillering disease virus and oat sterile dwarf virus. *Ann. Appl. Biol.,* 79:371–373.
32. Milne, R. G., Kempiak, G., Lovisolo, O., and Mühle, E. (1974): Viral nature of *Arrhenatherum* blue dwarf. *Phytopath. Z.,* 79:315–319.
33. Mühle, E., and Kempiak, G. (1971): Zur Geschichte Ätiologie und Symptomatologie der Blauverzwergung des Glasshafers *Arrhenatherum elatius. Phytopath. Z.,* 72:269–278.
34. Reddy, D. V. R., and Black, L. M. (1973): Electrophoretic separation of all components of the double-stranded RNA of wound tumor virus. *Virology,* 54:557–562.
35. Reddy, D. V. R., and Black, L. M. (1974): Deletion mutations of the genome segments of wound tumor virus. *Virology,* 61:458–473.
36. Reddy, D. V. R., and MacLeod, R. (1976): Polypeptide components of wound tumor virus. *Virology,* 70:274–282.
37. Reddy, D. V. R., and Black, L. M. (1977): Isolation and replication of mutant populations of wound tumor virions lacking certain genome segments. *Virology,* 80:336–346.
38. Reddy, D. V. R., Kimura, I., and Black, L. M. (1974): Co-electrophoresis of ds RNA from wound tumor and rice dwarf viruses. *Virology,* 60:293–296.
39. Reddy, D. V. R., Grylls, N. E., and Black, L. M. (1976): Electrophoretic separation of ds RNA genome segments from maize wallaby ear virus and its relationship to other phytoreoviruses. *Virology,* 73:36–42.
40. Reddy, D. V. R., Rhodes, D. P., Lesnaw, J. A., MacLeod, R., Banerjee, A. K., and Black, L. M. (1977): *In vitro* transcription of wound tumor virus RNA by virion-associated RNA transcriptase. *Virology,* 80:356–361.
41. Shikata, E. (1974): Rice black-streaked dwarf virus. Descriptions of plant viruses No. 135, 4 pp. Commonwealth Mycological Institute, Kew.
42. Schindler, A. J. (1942): Insect transmission of "wallaby ear" of maize. *J. Australian Inst. Agricultural Sci.,* 8:35–37.
43. Streissle, G., Rizza, J. J., and Granados, R. R. (1969): Number of virus particles in wound tumor cells cultivated *in vivo* and *in vitro.* Proceedings 20th Annual Meeting. Tissue Culture Association, p. 58.
44. Tyron, H. (1910): *Report of the Department of Agriculture and Stock, Queensland for 1909–10,* pp. 81–82.
45. Valleau, W. D. (1947): Clubroot of tobacco. A wound tumor-like graft-transmitted disease of tobacco. *Phytopathology,* 37:580–582.

27

Species-Specific Molecular Biology of Tumor Viruses in Different Hosts

James B. Lewis

A number of very different kinds of viruses have now been shown to be oncogenic in that they produce cancer in animals and also can cause cells in culture to undergo transformation to growth properties characteristic of tumor cells (for a review, see ref. 89). The mechanism by which these viruses replicate, and the nature of their interaction with host cells, have been studied intensively in recent years. Many molecular biology studies have focused on the papova and adenovirus classes of DNA tumor viruses. A particularly arresting feature of the biology of these viruses is the very different ways in which a given virus will interact with different cell types. For example, simian virus 40 (SV40) has not been associated with any disease in its natural host, the adult rhesus monkey, but will induce tumors when injected into newborn hamsters (14, 31).

The behavior of SV40 in animals is paralleled by its interactions with cells in culture. Upon infection of monkey cells, SV40 will replicate, produce progeny virus, and kill the cells (84). Thus, monkey cells are "permissive" for SV40 infection. In contrast, upon infection of hamster cells with SV40, no viral DNA or virus progeny will be produced, and the cells will become "transformed" in that, like tumor cells, they no longer respond to the normal factors regulating cell growth so that they continue to divide in cultures too crowded to permit further division of the parent cells (88). Transformed permissive cells can also be isolated, either by use of stocks of defective virus (81) or as a rare event with normal virus stocks (50, 51). Cells transformed by SV40 contain copies of the viral DNA integrated into their chromosomes (8, 29, 79, 94) and express a virus-specific "T" antigen (7). T antigen is a protein of apparent molecular weight

100,000 on sodium dodecyl sulfate polyacrylamide gels induced by the SV40 A gene (68, 85, 87). The SV40 A gene product is essential both to initiate and to maintain transformation by SV40 (10, 43, 62, 69, 86). Cell-free translation studies have further shown the T antigen to be SV40 coded (72, 83). More recently, an additional A gene product of about 17,000 apparent molecular weight has been reported (73), and is referred to as "small t" to distinguish it from the above "large T" antigen. The two proteins share a common amino terminus, but have different carboxy termini (70). Each protein is involved in the process of transformation, but the two proteins seem to perform different functions, although exactly which property of transformed cells can be correlated with which protein appears to depend upon the cells used for the transformation assay (9, 26, 63, 82). It is too early to discern the mechanism of interaction of either tumor antigen with the host cell. However, the fact that mutation in the two antigens affect transformation in some cells, but not others, suggests that this area should be a rich one for future exploration of the different interactions of a tumor virus with different host cells.

The range of virus-cell interaction with human adenoviruses is even more complicated, owing in part to the existence of 31 serological types of human adenoviruses. The viruses are associated with respiratory diseases in humans, their natural host. Human cells in culture are permissive for growth of adenovirus; progeny virus is produced and the cells are killed. (For recent reviews of adenoviruses, see refs. 71 and 96.)

These adenovirus serotypes can be divided into three classes (A, B, C) which are, respectively, highly oncogenic, weakly oncogenic, and nononcogenic when injected into newborn hamsters or rats (33, 40). The nonocogenic class, which includes adenovirus type 2 (Ad2) and adenovirus type 5 (Ad5), the two serotypes that have been most extensively characterized biochemically and genetically will, however, transform rodent cells *in vitro*. Infection of rat embryo cell cultures with group C adenovirus will yield cytopathic effects from which the cultures eventually recover, leaving a small fraction of the cells transformed (24, 61). Unlike most virally transformed cells, however, these group C-transformed cells are not oncogenic in newborn rats, unless the rats are imunosuppressed (27). Further, these rat cells are not completely nonpermissive upon infection with Ad2, since a substantial fraction of the cells replicate the Ad2 DNA and produce a small amount of virus (28).

The virus-cell interaction depends not only on the cell type but also on the serotype of the virus. Hamster cells are nonpermissive for the group A serotype Ad12 but are permissive for Ad2 and Ad5. Thus, transformation of hamster cells by Ad2 and Ad5 is not ordinarily detected because of extensive cell killing. However, transformants can be isolated if hamster cells are infected by temperature-sensitive mutants of Ad5 at the restrictive temperature so that viral replication cannot occur (95).

Thus, the outcome of an infection of a given cell by a given virus is controlled by factors intrinsic to both the cell and the virus. At the moment nothing is known about the nature of these factors, nor is there in general any clear idea of where to look in the cell metabolic machinery or in the virus genome for leads to understanding these factors. A partial exception to this general ignorance is provided by the case of the semipermissive infection of monkey cells by human adenovirus. Infection of African green monkey kidney cells by adenovirus results in very low levels (about 0.1%) of virus production compared to infection of human cells. However, coinfection with SV40 enhances the level of adenovirus production from monkey cells to the same level as from human cells (74). Adenovirus infection of monkey cells can also be enhanced by use of SV40-transformed monkey cells instead of coinfection with SV40 (75, 81). A third method of obtaining enhanced infection in monkey cells is to insert into the adenovirus genome a segment of the SV40 genome. A series of nondefective adeno-SV40 hybrid viruses has been described (54, 55) in which various size fragments of SV40 DNA have been inserted into the Ad2 genome, enabling several of the hybrid viruses (Ad2$^+$ND1, Ad2$^+$ND2, and Ad2$^+$ND4) to grow on monkey cells as well as human cells.

Ad2$^+$ND1, Ad2$^+$ND2, and Ad2$^+$ND4 have in common SV40 sequences encoding the 3′ end of the early region (C-terminal end of the *A* gene protein or SV40 T antigen) and also sequences encoding the 3′ end of the late region. The enhancement function is known to be an early SV40 product, both by genetic analysis using SV40 mutants for coinfection (42) and through metabolic studies showing that protein synthesis, but not DNA synthesis, is necessary after SV40 infection for enhancement of Ad replication to occur (25).

Thus, the phenomenon of enhanced infection provides an opportunity to study the factors regulating virus-cell interactions in a case in which one particular molecule, the SV40 *A* gene product or T antigen, is known to be responsible for the difference between semipermissive and fully permissive infection. (As will be seen below, this function is located toward the carboxyterminus of the molecule, eliminating the possibility of involvement of small t antigen.) Further, one might hope that since this molecule is the product of the SV40 transforming gene, study of the mechanism of enhancement might provide a clue to the mechanism of virus-induced oncogenic transformation.

Much has been learned about the macromolecular events during the semipermissive (unenhanced) infection of monkey cells by human adenovirus. Adenovirus absorbs and enters monkey cells normally (19), and at least two early adenovirus proteins, the adenovirus T antigen and the single strand-specific DNA binding protein, are synthesized normally (19, 25, 90). Normal amounts of at least most species of virus-specific mRNA appear to be synthesized during unenhanced infection (22, 60) and viral DNA synthesis proceeds as during the infection of human cells (25, 37, 77). However, the amount of late virus-coded proteins, particularly virion components, is greatly reduced in unenhanced compared to enhanced infections (5, 18, 19, 34, 37, 46, 60). The extent of the reduction of Adenovirion protein synthesis in unenhanced infection seems to vary somewhat according to the particular line of African green monkey cells used. For example, Klessig and Anderson (46) reported that some sublines of BSC-1 cells synthesize very little of any of the virion components, whereas other BSC-1 sublines, and also CV-1 cells, show only a moderate reduction in the synthesis of most virion proteins and severe reduction only in the amount of the "fiber" virion component, which is not made in detectable amounts in unenhanced infection.

Because the most apparent difference between enhanced and unenhanced infection is at the level of virion protein synthesis, much work has focused on the hypothesis that the block to adenovirus replication in monkey cells is at the posttranscriptional level. Hybridization competition experiments have established that all the Ad sequences present late in infection of permissive cells are also present late in unenhanced infection, and that the total amount of Ad mRNA present late in unenhanced infection is comparable to that present late in permissive infection (23, 37, 60). However, since excess RNA is used for this competition, these experiments do not eliminate the possibility that substantial differences might exist between enhanced and unenhanced infections with respect to a particular species of late mRNA. To estimate the concentration of individual Ad mRNAs, (46) measured the relative rates by which RNA from enhanced and from unenhanced infections increased the rate of hybridization of specific fragments of Ad DNA. Since it is known which DNA fragments are complementary to the mRNA for each Ad-coded protein (56, 58), such methodology permits measurement of the concentration of individual Ad mRNAs. Indeed, the mRNAs for most of the viral structural proteins were present in lower concentration in the unenhanced infections, the largest difference being fiber mRNA. However, the approximately sevenfold decrease in the concentration of fiber mRNA does not seem sufficient to explain the approximately 200-fold decrease in the amount of fiber protein in unenhanced infection (D.F. Klessig, personal communication). It is possible, however, that in unenhanced infections not all of the RNA molecules containing sequences complementary to fiber are active as mRNAs. For example, adenovirus messenger RNAs, like other eucaryotic mRNAs, are formed by "splicing" together noncontiguous regions of a precursor RNA, with the deletion of intervening sequences, to form a mRNA molecule that is not colinear with the DNA sequence in which it is encoded (6, 12, 45). Consequently, differences between the "splicing" systems in different cells could result in RNA molecules not being processed into mature mRNAs. Indeed, a much higher percentage of incompletely spliced fiber mRNA is found in the cytoplasm of monkey cells with unenhanced infections compared to cells with enhanced infections (47).

A simple and direct test of whether active mRNAs are present in unenhanced infections would be to use RNA extracted from monkey cells to program cell-free protein synthesis in one of several systems which have been shown to translate Ad mRNAs efficiently, without use of specific factors from human cells (2, 4, 17, 67, 78). The polypeptides synthesized in vitro could be compared, to see if they reflected the deficiency in virion protein synthesis (especially fiber protein) seen in unenhanced infections in vivo, or whether the mRNAs from enhanced and unenhanced infections were equally active in vitro. Such an experiment has been reported twice in the literature (18, 46). Although the two experiments were done in slightly different fashions, each paper seems self-consistent and well controlled. Unfortunately, the two papers report opposite conclusions. Eron et al. (18) find that mRNA from the unenhanced infection of monkey cells yields, upon cell-free translation, the complete range of virion structural polypeptides in amounts equal to the product when mRNA from enhanced infection is used, implying that the defect in unenhanced infections is at the level of translation. Klessig and Anderson (46), on the other hand, find the same restriction in vitro and in vivo, i.e., no discernible synthesis of fiber protein and reduced synthesis of other virion proteins using mRNA from the unenhanced infection of monkey cells, consistent with the defect being at the level of mRNA production. The same result was obtained if, instead of coinfection with SV40, they used Ad2$^+$ND1 and HR140, a host-range mutant of Ad2$^+$ND1 that does not grow on monkey cells any better that does Ad2 (35), for the enhanced and unenhanced infections, respectively (D. Klessig, personal communication).

The studies of Eron et al. (18) and Klessig and Anderson (46) were made with different cell lines, infection protocols, and cell-free translation systems. However, an attempt by Klessig and Anderson (46) to use the same cell line, infection protocol, and translation system did not permit them to repeat the observation of Eron et al. (18). It is unfortunate that Eron and colleagues are no longer working on this problem, since a clear answer to this important question is prevented by the conflict in the literature.

Those authors who detected no difference in the total amount of adenovirus late mRNA present in enhanced versus unenhanced infections have reported that less adenovirus mRNA is associated with polyribosomes in unenhanced than in enhanced infection (23, 37). Such an observation is consistent with both the hypothess of a defect in the monkey cell translation machinery for adenovirus mRNA and the hypothesis of an abnormality in mRNA metabolism which makes some sequences incapable of functioning efficiently as mRNAs. However,

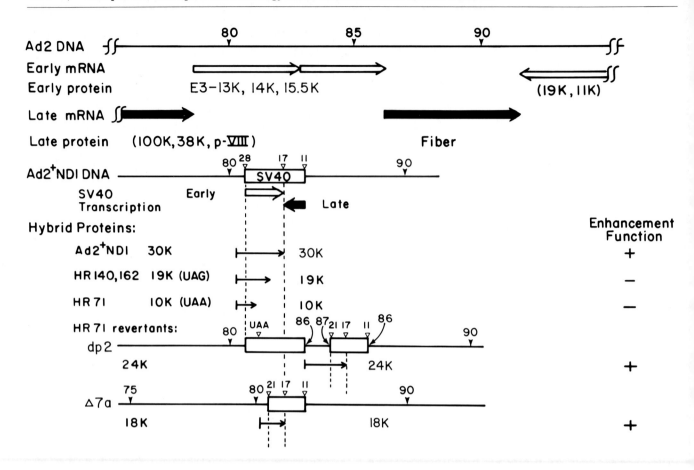

Figure 27.1. Molecules coded by the adeno-SV40 hybrid virus Ad2⁺ND1 and its mutants that enhance the replication of Ad in monkey cells. The righthand quarter of the Ad2 genome is represented diagrammatically at the top of the figure, with the map positions of the early (⇨) and late (⬛➤) mRNAs indicated. The mRNa coordinates are from Chow *et al.* (11, 13) and earlier references contained there in. The proteins encoded by these mRNAs have been identified by Lewis *et al.* (56, 57) and by Harter and Lewis (36). The hybrid virus Ad2⁺ND1 contains a deletion of 5% of Ad2 (0.80 to 0.85 map units) and an insertion of 17% of SV40 (0.11 to 0.28 map units) (38). The Ad2⁺ND1 30K protein mRNA is encoded by both Ad2 and SV40 sequences (3). The SV40 early region contained within Ad2⁺ND1 (0.17 to 0.28) could code for as much as 22,000 molecular weight of protein, so that perhaps 8000 molecular weight of this polypeptide would seem necessarily encoded by the Ad2 sequences to the left of the SV40 insertion (*i.e.*, from the region of Ad2 containing the 3' ends of the genes for the 100K, 38K, pVIII, and early E3-13K, 14K, and 15.5K proteins). It is perhaps misleading, however, to estimate the size of the Ad2⁺ND1 30K protein from mobility in sodium dodecyl sulfate (SDS) polyacrylamide gel electrophoresis. The large T antigen has an apparent molecular weight of 100,000 by electrophoretic mobility (86), yet the coding capacity of the *A* gene used for large T antigen appears to be only 87,000 MW (21, 70, 76). The chemistry of this anomaly is not understood, but it is quite possible that the proteins containing the carboxyl terminal of the large T antigen will also have anomalously high apparent molecular weights on SDS gels. Consequently, the amount of the Ad2⁺ND1-30K protein encoded by Ad2 sequences could be less than 8000 molecular weight. In any case, the host-range mutants HR140, HR162, and HR71, which have lost the ability to grow on monkey cells (*i.e.*, no enhancement function) make fragments of the 30K protein of 19,000 MW (HR140, HR162) and 10,000 molecular weight (HR71) (35). These two fragments are produced by amber (*UAG*) and ochre (*UAA*) mutations, respectively (30), which terminate protein synthesis left of the usual termination point of the large T antigen (0.17 SV40 map position) (20). Many revertants of the amber mutants produce wild-type 30K protein, presumably by reversion at the site of the original mutation. Quite possibly the amber mutation lies close enough to 0.17 SV40 map position to be within the region essential for enhancement function, and thus this mutation must be reverted. However, the ochre mutation lies farther to the left and is possibly outside the region essential for enhancement function, so that a revertant phenotype may be obtained by deletion of the region of the DNA containing this mutation (somewhere between 0.28 and 0.21 SV40 map units) so long as the reading frame was not changed beyond the deletion. Thus, ribosomes could translate the distal end of the mRNA and synthesize the carboxyl-terminal end of the large T antigen required for enhancement function. Indeed, the revertants of HR71 so far isolated (20; T. Grodzicker, E. Lukanidin, J. Lewis, and J. Sambrook, unpublished)

there is no evidence that it is the message for the most deficient proteins that is blocked in binding to polysomes.

If the defect in unenhanced infection is at the level of the monkey cells' translational machinery, it should be possible to demonstrate that a cell-free protein synthesis system prepared from permissive cells is much more efficient in translating Ad2 mRNA than is a similar system prepared from semi-permissive cells. Such a result has been reported (65, 66). A preincubated S-30 cell-free protein synthesis system prepared from SV40-transformed monkey cells or from monkey cells 16 or more hours after infection with SV40 was able to incorporate amino acid in the presence of Ad2 mRNA prepared from human cells three to five times better than was a similarly prepared S-30 from nontransformed or noninfected monkey cells. Both S-30's incorporated phenylalanine equally well in the presence of poly(U), suggesting that both S-30's were competent for translation in general, but that a specific SV40-induced factor was necessary for the efficient translation of Ad2 mRNA. Furthermore, the formation of 80S initiation complexes could be demonstrated with the use of ribosomes from monkey cells and Ad2 RNA from either permissive (human) or semipermissive (monkey) cells, if a ribosomal wash fraction from permissive cells was added. A similar fraction from semipermissvie cells was inactive.

The S-30 incorporation experiments should be interpreted cautiously. Translation of poly(U) is not an appropriate control for the proper functioning of a cell-free system in initiating translation of a natural mRNA. A more convincing control would have been the use of mRNA from uninfected or SV40-infected monkey cells, to prove that the S-30 prepared from semipermissive cells was functioning well so that the SV40-induced factor was necessary only for Ad2 mRNA. This criticism does not apply to the 80S initiation complex formation experiment, since it was shown that with SV40 mRNA the complex

formed equally well regardless of the source of the ribosome wash fraction.

A further difficulty with the S-30 experiment is the low activity of the extracts used. Assuming a counting efficiency for tritium of 10%, the S-30 extract that gave the best incorporation with Ad2 mRNA incorporated 0.5 pmol of leucine into trichloroacetic acid-insoluble radioactivity per 50 minutes per 0.15 ml reaction mixture. This system is less than $\frac{1}{1000}$ as active as a very active mammalian cell-free system (4, 78) and about $\frac{1}{50}$ as active as an average preincubated S-30 system. Comparisons made using such an inactive system might not necessarily reflect the translation ability of these cells, in that what is limiting *in vitro* might not be limiting *in vivo*.

Although fundamental questions remain about the mechanism by which SV40 enhances the replication of adenovirus in monkey cells, much progress has been made in identifying the portion of SV40 responsible. A series of nondefective adenovirus-SV40 hybrid viruses have been described (54, 55). These hybrid viruses are nondefective in that no helper Ad2 is required for growth on human cells. Further, several of these hybrids (Ad2+ND1, Ad2+ND2, and Ad2+ND4) grow as well on monkey cells as on human cells. Coinfection with SV40 is not necessary nor does it enhance the growth of these viruses on monkey cells. In these hybrids, a small, and apparently unessential, portion of the Ad genome has been deleted and a segment of the SV40 genome (the region from 0.11 to 0.28 map units in Ad2+ND1 and 0.11 to 0.59 map units in Ad2+ND4) has been inserted (52). Thus, the entire SV40 *A* gene protein is not necessary for enhancement of Ad2 growth, but rather only the portion coded for by Ad2+ND1, *i.e.*, the 30% carboxy terminal portion of the SV40 *A* gene. As expected, a protein of 28,000 to 30,000 MW not found in Ad2-infected cells is synthesized in cells infected by Ad2+ND1 (34, 59), and is encoded at least in part by SV40 since the mRNA for this Ad2+ND1 30K protein contains both

---

have lost the segment of DNA thought to contain the ochre mutation, either by outright deletion of this segment (revertants △3b, △4a, △6a, and △7a) or (in the case of revertants dp 1 and dp 2) by duplication of the region of the Ad2+ND1 genome containing the right-hand part of the SV40 sequences and the portion of the Ad2 genome immediately right of the insertion, creating a second insertion of SV40 genetic information in which the ochre mutation has been deleted. Thus, none of these revertants recreates the Ad2+ND1 30K protein. Two of these revertants (△7a and dp 2) are diagrammed above. The dp2 24K protein embodies the C-terminal end of the SV40 large T antigen and the N-terminal end of the Ad2 fiber protein. This conclusion has been confirmed by peptide analysis (20). The △7a protein presumably also has the carboxy terminal end of the SV40 large T antigen, but has as its N-terminal end the same Ad2 sequences present in the Ad2+ND1 30K protein, with only the middle (0.28 to 0.21) sequences deleted. These mutants and revertants illustrate that only the C-terminal 8000 MW of the SV40 large T antigen is necessary for enhancement function and the N-terminal identity of the protein is inconsequential.

SV40 and Ad2 sequences (3). Strong evidence that this virus-coded protein is indeed necessary for enhancement of Ad2 growth in monkey cells comes from the characterization of host-range mutants of Ad2⁺ND1 which have lost the ability to grow on monkey cells although they grow normally on human cells, and their growth on monkey cells can be enhanced by coinfection with SV40 (34, 35). Thus, these mutants have lost the enhancement function conferred upon AD2⁺ND1 by the insertion of SV40 genetic information. Two classes of these host-range mutants can be distinguished phenotypically. The first class is somewhat leaky, growing on monkey cells slightly (10-fold) better than does Ad2, but much less well (100-fold) than does Ad2⁺ND1. These mutants still synthesize a 30K protein which cannot be distinguished from wild type electrophoretically. The second class of mutants is very tight, growing no better than Ad2 on monkey cells (1000-fold less well than Ad2⁺ND1). These mutants do not make a 30K protein; instead, cell-free translation of SV40-specific mRNA from cells infected with these mutants gives rise to smaller proteins (19,000 MW for mutants HR140 and HR162 and 10,000 MW for mutant HR71). A revertant of mutant HR162 again synthesizes the 30K protein. Gesteland *et al.* (30) have demonstrated by cell-free transalation of these mutant mRNAs in the presence of yeast suppressor tRNAs that mutants HR140 and HR162 are amber nonsense mutants and that HR71 is an ochre nonsense mutant. Thus, the correlation between the absence of Ad2⁺ND1 30K protein and the absence of enhancement function in these absolute defective mutants is strong evidence for the functional role of this protein in enhancement.

The part of the SV40 *A* gene required for function in enhancement can be narrowed down even further than the 0.28 to 0.17 interval of SV40 provided by study of Ad2⁺ND1. Studies of revertants of HR71 (20; and T. Grodzicker, E. Lukanidin, J. Lewis, and J. Sambrook, unpublished results) suggest that HR71 does not give rise to revertants that synthesize the 30K protein, as does HR162. Instead, the studies whose results are summarized in Figure 27.1 show that these revertants appear to be the result of unequal recombination such that the ochre mutation has been eliminated, permitting translation of the distal (carboxyl-terminal) portion of the 30K gene. The resultant protein may be of various sizes and composed of both SV40 and Ad2 information. Further, the Ad2 component (the N terminus of the chimeric protein) is probably not the same in the different revertants. The various molecules that appear to provide the enhancement function are summarized in Figure 27.1. These proteins have in common only the C-terminal 0.04 map units (about 8000 MW of protein) of the SV40 *A* gene. Thus, only a small fraction (about 11%) of the SV40 *A* gene seems to be required for enhancement, and further, this small fragment doesn't seem to care what protein sequences are at the N-terminus of the protein, whether they be SV40 sequences or Ad2 sequences from either of two different Ad2 genes. Such conclusions are very difficult to understand in terms of any enzyme function, in which case one would expect the three-dimensional structure of the molecule to be critical for the function of the active site. Thus, the way in which this protein fragment enhances adenovirus replication in monkey cells is still obscure, but perhaps further characterization of these molecules will shed light on this mystery.

Further complicating analysis of the enhancement phenomenon is the possibility that more than one mechanism for enhancement may exist. Ad2 replication in monkey cells can be enhanced not only by the action of SV40 genetic information but also by coinfection with simian adenoviruses (1, 41, 64). The mechanism of this enhancement has not been characterized.

Klessig (44) has recently demonstrated that an Ad2 variant (HR400) can be isolated that grows as efficiently on monkey as on human cells, *i.e.*, with growth properties identical to Ad2⁺ND1 or Ad2 coinfected with SV40, even though the variant contains no SV40 genetic information (48). Apparently some Ad2 gene can be mutated to perform the function(s) filled by SV40 genetic information during enhanced infection. This mutation maps between Ad2 map positions 0.629 and 0.656 (49), entirely within the region of the Ad2 genome encoding early protein E2-72K (11, 57). This protein binds to single-strand DNA (53) and is required for DNA replication (39). Thus, if the mechanism of enhancement of adenovirus replication in monkey cells is the same in HR400 as in coinfection with SV40 genetic information, then the Ad2 E2-72K-DNA binding protein gene must, in HR400, be supplying the same function as does the SV40 *A* gene during enhancement. Significantly, the region of Ad2 responsible for transformation of rodent cells (map positions 0.01 to 0.08) (32, 80). is not at all near the region that has been altered in HR400. This may mean that the transforming function of the SV40 *A* gene is quite distinct from its function in enhancing Ad2 growth in monkey cells. Alternatively, the enhancing function in HR400 may be mechanistically different from the enhancing function of SV40 information, or transformation of cells by Ad2 and by SV40 might proceed by different mechanisms. Clearly, efforts to understand the phenomena of both restricted host range and transformation are still at an early stage.

The phenomenon of restriction of virus growth on different host cells has not been extensively studied in many other eucaryotic systems. A particularly intriguing case that should be mentioned, however, is the transformation for mammalian cells by avian RNA tumor viruses (avian retroviruses). Because the RNA tumor viruses can replicate in their host cells without killing the cells, they interact with cells in a variety of ways (see Tooze (89) for a review). The virus can replicate in a cell without transforming the cell morphologically; the virus can both replicate and transform the host cell simultaneously; or the virus can transform the host cell but not replicate. An example of this latter mode of interaction is the infection of mammalian cells by avian RNA tumor viruses. In addition to maintaining the transformed phenotype, these cells produce viral nucleic acids and antigens but no infectious virus or virus particles. Infectious virus can be produced, however, upon fusion of the transformed mammalian cells with permissive chick cells. In at least one case the block to replication in the nonpermissive cell is related to the inability of the cell to cleave a viral precursor protein. The internal virion proteins of the avian tumor viruses are synthesized as one large precursor protein, which is successively cleaved to yield three virion proteins (91). In a particular line of hamster cells transformed by the Bryan high-titer strain of Rous sarcoma virus, the larger precursor polypeptide was synthesized, but not cleaved, to form the virion proteins (15). Fusion of these cells with permissive chicken cells leads to cleavage of the precursor proteins and to formation of infectious virus. These results and others (16, 92) suggest that in this case the block to replication is the absence in the nonpermissive cell of the specific protease needed to cleave the precursor protein. A detailed elucidation of the biochemistry of virus-cell interactions in several different systems will be needed before a general picture emerges of why some cells are pemissive for a given virus and others are not.

References

1. Alstein, A. D., and Dodonova, N. N. (1968): Interaction between human and simian adenoviruses in simian cells: Complementation, phenotypic mixing and formation of monkey cell "adapted" virions. *Virology, 35:* 248–254.
2. Anderson, C. W., Lewis, J. B., Atkins, J.F., and Gesteland, R. F. (1974): Cell-free synthesis of adenovirus 2 proteins programmed by fractionated messenger RNA: A comparison of polypeptide products and messenger RNA lengths. *Proc. Natl. Acad. Sci.,* 71:2756–2760.
3. Anderson, C. W., Lewis, J. B., Baum, P. R., and Gesteland, R. F. (1976): Simian virus 40-specific polypeptides in Ad2⁺Nd1 and Ad2⁺ND4 infected cells. *J. Virol.,* 18:685–692.
4. Atkins, J. R., Lewis, J. B., Anderson, C. W., and Gesteland, R. F. (1975): Enhanced differential synthesis of proteins in a mammalian cell-free system by addition of polyamines. *J. Biol. Chem.,* 250:5688–5695.
5. Baum, S. G., Horwitz, M. S., and Maizel, J. V. (1972): Studies of the mechanisms of enhancement of adenovirus 7 infection in African green monkey cells by simian virus 40. *J. Virol.,* 10:211–219.
6. Berget, S. M., Moore, C., and Sharp, P. A. (1977): Spliced segments at the 5′ terminus of adenovirus-2 late mRNA. *Proc. Natl. Acad. Sci.,* 74:3171–3175.
7. Black, P. H., Rowe, W. P., Turner, H. C., and Huebner, R. J. (1963): A specific complement-fixing antigen present in SV40 tumor and transformed cells. *Proc. Natl. Acad. Sci.,* 50:1148–1156.
8. Botchan, M., Ozanne, B., Sugden, B., Sharp, P., and Sambrook, J. (1974): Viral DNA in transformed cells. III. The amounts of different regions of the SV40 genome present in a line of transformed mouse cells. *Proc. Natl. Acad. Sci.,* 71:4183–4187.
9. Bouck, N., Beales, N., Shenk, T., Berg P., and di Mayorca, G. (1978): New region of the simian virus 40 genome required for efficient viral transformation. *Proc. Natl. Acad. Sci.,* 75:2473–2477.
10. Brugge, J. S., and Butel, J. S. (1975): Involvement of the simian virus 40 gene A function in the maintenance of transformation. *J. Virol.,* 15:619–635.
11. Chow, L. T., Roberts, J. M., Lewis, J. B., and Broker, T. R. (1977): A cytoplasmic RNA transcript map of lytic adenovirus type 2 determined by electron microscopy of RNA:DNA hybrids. *Cell,* 11:819–836.
12. Chow, L. T., Gelinas, R. E., Broker, T. R., and Roberts, R. J. (1977): An amazing sequence arrangement at the 5′ ends of adenovirus 2 messenger RNA. *Cell,* 12:1–8.
13. Chow, L. T., Broker, T. R., and Lewis, J. B. (1979): Complex splicing patterns of RNAs from the early regions of adenovirus-2. *J. Mol. Biol.,* 134:265–304.
14. Eddy, B. E., Borman, G. S., Grubbe, G. E., and Young, R. D. (1962): Identification of the oncogenic substance in Rhesus monkey kidney cell cultures as Simian Virus 40. *Virology,* 17:65–75.
15. Eisenman, R., Vogt, V. M., and Diggleman, H. (1974): Synthesis of avian RNA tumor virus structural proteins. *Cold Spring Harbor Symp. Quant. Biol.,* 39:1067–1075.
16. Eisenman, R., and Vogt, V. M. (1978): The biosynthesis of oncovirus proteins. *Biochem. Biophys. Acta.,* 473:187–239.
17. Eron, L., Callahan, R., and Westphal, H. (1974): Cell-free synthesis of adenovirus coat proteins. *J. Biol. Chem.,* 249:6331–6338.
18. Eron, L., Westphal, H., and Khoury, G. (1975): Posttranscriptional restriction of human adenovirus expression in monkey cells. *J. Virol.,* 15:1256–1261.
19. Feldman, L. A., Butel, J. S., and Rapp, F. (1966): Interaction of a simian papovavirus and adenovirus. I. Induction of adenovirus tumor antigen during abortive infection of simian cells. *J. Bacteriol.,* 91:813–818.
20. Fey, G., Lewis, J. B., Grodzicker, T., and Bothwell, A. (1979): Characterization of a fused protein specified by the adenovirus type 2-simian virus 40 hybrid Ad2⁺ND1 dp2. *J. Virol.,* 30:201–217.
21. Fiers, W., Contreras, R., Haegeman, G., Rogiers, R., Van de Voorde, A., Van Heuverswyn, H., Van Herreweghe, J., Volckaert, G., and Ysebaert, M. (1978): Complete nucleotide sequence of SV40 DNA. *Nature (Lond.),* 273:113–120.
22. Fox, R. I., and Baum, S. G. (1972): Synthesis of viral ribonucleic acid during restriction adenovirus infection. *J. Virol.,* 10:220–227.
23. Fox, R. I., and Baum, S. G. (1974): Posttranscriptional block to adenovirus replication in non-permissive monkey cells. *Virology,* 60:45–53.
24. Freeman, A. E., Black, P. H., Vanderpool, E. A., Henry, P. H., Austin, J. B., and Huebner, R. J. (1967): Transformation of primary rat embryo cells by adenovirus type 2. *Proc. Natl. Acad. Sci.,* 58:1205–1212.
25. Friedman, M. P., Lyons, M. J., and Ginsberg, H. S. (1970): Biochemical consequences of type 2 adenovirus and simian virus 40 double infections of African green monkey kidney cells. *J. Virol.,* 5:586–597.
26. Frisque, R. J., Rifkin, D. B., and Topp, W. C. (1979): Requirements for the large T and small t proteins of SV40 in the maintenance of the transformed state. *Cold Spring Harbor Symp. Quant. Biol.,* 44:325–332.
27. Gallimore, P. H. (1972): Tumor production in immunosuppressed rats with cells transformed in vitro by adenovirus type 2. *J. Gen. Virol.,* 16:99–102.
28. Gallimore, P. H. (1974): Interactions of adenovirus type 2 with rat embryo cells. Permissiveness, transformation and *in vitro* characteristics of adenovirus transformed rat embryo cells. *J. Gen. Virol.,* 25:263–273.
29. Gelb, L. D., Kohne, D. E., and Martin, M. A. (1971): Quantitation of SV40

sequences in African green monkey, mouse and virus-transformed cell genomes. *J. Mol. Biol.*, 57:129–145.

30. Gesteland, R. F., Wills, N., Lewis, J. B., and Grodzicker, T. (1977): Identification of amber and ochre mutants of the human virus Ad2⁺ND1. *Proc. Natl. Acad. Sci.*, 74:4567–4571.

31. Girardi, A. J., Sweet, B. H., Slotnick, V. B., and Hilleman, M. R. (1962): Development of tumors in hamsters inoculated in the neo-natal period with vacuating virus, SV40. *Proc. Soc. Exp. Biol. Med.*, 109:569–660.

32. Graham, F. L., Abrahams, P. J., Mulder, C., Heijneker, H. L., Warnaar, S. O., deVrie, F. A., Fiers, W., and van der Eb, A. J. (1974): Studies on *in vitro* transformation by DNA and DNA fragments of human adenoviruses and simian virus 40. *Cold Spring Harbor Symp. Quant. Biol.*, 39:637–650.

33. Green, M. (1970). Oncogenic viruses in *Annu. Rev. Biochem.*, 39:701–756.

34. Grodzicker, T., Anderson, C., Sharp, P. A., and Sambrook, J. (1974): Conditional lethal mutants of adenovirus 2-simian virus 40 hybrids. I. Host range mutants of Ad2⁺ND1. *J. Virol.* 13:1237–1244.

35. Grodzicker, T., Lewis, J. B. and Anderson, C. W. (1976): Conditional lethal mutants of adenovirus type 2-simian virus 40 hybrids. II. AD2⁺ND1 host-range mutants that synthesize fragments of the Ad2⁺ND1 30K protein. *J. Virol.*, 19:559–571.

36. Harter, M. L., and Lewis, J. B. (1978): Adenovirus type 2 early proteins synthesized in vitro and in vivo: identification in infected cells of the 38,000- to 50,000-molecular-weight protein encoded by the left end of the adenovirus type 2 genome. *J. Virol.*, 26:736–749.

37. Hashimoto, K., Nakajima, K., Oda, K., and Shimojo, H. (1973): Complementation of translational defect for growth of human adenovirus type 2 in simian cells by a simian virus 40-induced factor. *J. Mol. Biol.*, 81:207–223.

38. Henry, P. H., Schipper, L. E., Samaha, R. J., Crumpacker, C. S., Lewis, A. M., Jr., and Levine, A. S. (1973): Studies of nondefective adenovirus 2-simian virus 40 hybrid viruses. VI. Characterization of the DNA from five nondefective hybrid viruses. *J. Virol.* 11:665–671.

39. Horwitz, M. S., Kaplan, L. M., Abboud, M., Maritato, J., Chow, L. T., and Broker, T. R. (1978): Adenovirus DNA replication in soluble extracts of infected cell nuclei. *Cold Spring Harbor Symp. Quant. Biol.*, 43:769–780.

40. Huebner, R. J. (1967): Adenovirus-directed tumor and T antigens. In *Perspectives in Virology*, Vol. V, pp. 147–166, edited by M. Pollard. Academic Press, New York.

41. Kaplan, P. M., Melnick, J. L., and Tevethis, S. (1971): Development of noncarcinogenic SA7-adenovirus 2 populations that immunize against SA7-transformed cells. *J. Natl. Cancer Inst.*, 46:565–576.

42. Kimura, G. (1974): Genetic evidence for SV40 gene function in enhancement of replication of human adenoviruses in simian cells. *Nature*, 248:590–592.

43. Kimura, G., and Itagaki, A. (1975): Initiation and maintenance of cell transformation by simian virus 40: A viral gentic property. *Proc. Natl. Acad. Sci.*, 72:673–677.

44. Klessig, D. F. (1977): Isolation of a variant of human adenovirus serotype 2 that multiplies efficiently on monkey cells. *J. Virol.*, 21:1243–1246.

45. Klessig, D. F. (1977): Two adenovirus mRNAs have a common 5′ terminal leader sequence encoded at least 10 kb upstream from their main coding sequences. *Cell*, 12:9–21.

46. Klessig, D. F., and Anderson, C. W. (1975): Block to multiplication of adenovirus serotype 2 in monkey cells. *J. Virol.*, 16:1650–1668.

47. Klessig, D. F., and Chow, L. T. (1980): Incomplete splicing of several late viral mRNAs in monkey cells infected by human adenovirus type 2. *J. Mol. Biol.*, 139:221–242.

48. Klessig, D. F., and Hassell, J. A. (1978): Characterization of a variant of human adenovirus type 2 which multiplies efficiently in simian cells. *J. Virol.*, 28:945–956.

49. Klessig, D. F., and Grodzicker, T. (1979): Mutations that allow human Ad2 and Ad5 to express late genes in monkey cells map in the viral gene encoding the 72K DNA binding protein. *Cell*, 17:957–966.

50. Knowles, B. B., Jensen, F. C., Steplweski, Z. S., and Kopsowski, H. (1968): Rescue of infectious SV40 after fusion between different SV40-transformed cells. *Proc. Natl. Acad. Sci.*, 61:42–45.

51. Koprowski, H., Jensen, F. C., and Steplewski, Z. S. (1967): Activation of production of infectious tumor virus SV40 in heterokaryon cultures. *Proc. Natl. Acad. Sci.*, 58:127–133.

52. Lebowitz, P., Kelly, T. J., Jr., Nathans, D., Lee, T. N. H., and Lewis, A. M., Jr. (1974): A colinear map relating the simian virus 40 (SV40) DNA segments of six adenovirus-SV40 hybrids to the DNA fragments produced by restriction endonuclease cleavage of SV40 DNA. *Proc. Natl. Acad. Sci.*, 71:441–445.

53. Levine, A. J., van der Vliet, P. C., Rosenwirth, B., Rabek, J., Frenkel, G., and Ensinger, M. (1974): Adenovirus-infected cell-specific DNA-binding proteins. *Cold Spring Harbor Symp. Quant. Biol.*, 39:559–566.

54. Lewis, A. M., Jr., Levin, M. J., Wiese, W. H., Crumpacker, C. S., and Henry, P. H. (1969): A nondefective (competent) adenvirus-SV40 hybrid isolated from the Ad2-SV40 hybrid population. *Proc. Natl. Acad. Sci.*, 63:1128–1135.

55. Lewis, A. M., Jr., Levine, A. S., Crumpacker, C. S., Levin, M. J., Samaha, R. J., and Henry, P. H. (1973): Studies of nondefective adenovirus 2-simian virus 40 hybrid viruses. V. Isolation of additional hybrids which

differ in their simian virus 40-specific biological properties. *J. Virol.*, 11:655–664.

56. Lewis, J. B., Atkins, J. F., Anderson, C. W., Baum, P. R., and Gestsland, R. F. (1975): Mapping of late adenovirus genes by cell-free translation of RNA selected by hybridization to specific DNA fragments. *Proc. Natl. Acad. Sci.*, 72:1344–1348.

57. Lewis, J. B., Atkins, J. F., Baum, P. R., Solem, R., Gesteland, R. F., and Anderson, C. W. (1976): Location and identification of the genes for adenovirus type 2 early polypeptides. *Cell*, 7:141–151.

58. Lewis, J. B., Anderson, C. W., and Atkins, J. F. (1977): Further mapping of later adenovirus genes by cell-free translation of RNA selected by hybridization to specific DNA fragments. *Cell*, 12:37–44.

59. Lopez-Revilla, R., and Walter, G. (1973): Polypeptide specific for cells with adenovirus 2-SV40 hybrid Ad2⁺ND1. *Nature (New Biol.)*, 244:165–167.

60. Lucas, J. J., and Ginsberg, H. S. (1972): Transcription and transport of virus-specific ribonucleic acids in African green monkey cells abortively infected with type 2 adenovirus. *J.Virol.*, 10:1109–1117.

61. McAllister, R. M., Nicolson, M. O., Lewis, A. M., MacPherson, J., and Huebner, R. J. (1969): Transformation of rat embryo cells by adenovirus type 1. *J. Gen. Virol.*, 4:29–36.

62. Martin, R. G., and Chou, J. Y. (1975): Simian virus 40 functions required for the establishment and maintenance of malignant transformation. *J. Virol.*, 15:599–612.

63. Martin, R. G., Setlow, V. P., Chepelinsky, A. B., Seif, R., Lewis, A. M., Jr., Scher, C. D., Stiles, C. D., and Avila, J. (1979): Roles of the tumor antigens in transformation by SV40. *Cold Spring Harbor Symp. Quant. Biol.*, 44:311–324.

64. Naegele, R. F., and Rapp, F. (1967): Enhancement of the replication of human adenoviruses in simian cells by simian adenovirus SV15. *J. Virol.*, 1:838–840.

65. Nakajima, K., Ishitsuka, H., and Oda, K. (1974): An SV40-induced initiation factor for protein synthesis concerned with the regulation of permissiveness. *Nature*, 252:649–653.

66. Nakajima, K., and Oda, K. (1975): The alteration ribosomes for mRNA selection concerned with adenovirus growth in SV40-infected simian cells.*Virology*, 67:85–93.

67. Oberg, B., Saborio, J., Persson, T., Everitt, E., and Philipson, L. (1975): Identification of the *in vitro* translation products of adenovirus messenger RNA immunoprecipitation. *J. Virol.*, 15:199–207.

68. Osborn, M., and Weber, K. (1974): SV40: T-antigen, the A function and transformation. *Cold Spring Harbor Symp. Quant. Biol.*, 39:267–276.

69. Osborn, M., and Weber, K. (1975): Simian virus 40 gene A function and maintenance of transformation. *J. Virol.*, 15:636–644.

70. Paucha, E., Mellor, A., Harvey, R., Smith, A. E., Hewick, R. M., and Waterfield, M. D. (1978): Large and small tumor antigens from simian virus 40 have identical amino termini mapping at 0.65 map units. *Proc. Natl. Acad. Sci.*, 75:2165–2169.

71. Philipson, L., Pettersson, U., and Lindberg, U. (1975): *Molecular Biology of Adenovirus*, pp. 1–115. Springer-Verlag, New York.

72. Prives, C., Aviv, H., Gilboa, E., Winocour, E., and Revel, M. (1975): *The Cell-Free Translation of Early and Late Classes of SV40 Messenger RNA*, pp. 305–312, edited by A.-L. Haenni and G. Beard. INSERM Symposium 47, INSERM, Paris.

73. Prives, C., Gilboa, E., Revel, M., and Winocour, E. (1977): Cell-free translation of simian virus 40 early messenger RNA coding for viral T-antigen. *Proc. Natl. Acad. Sci.* 74:457–461.

74. Rabson, A. S., O'Conor, G. T., Berezesky, I. K., and Paul, F. J. (1964): Enhancement of adenovirus growth in African green monkey kidney cell cultures by SV40. *Proc. Soc. Exp. Biol. Med.*, 116:187–190.

75. Rapp, F., and Trulock, S. C. (1970): Susceptibility to superinfection of simian cells transformed by SV40. *Virology*, 40:961–970.

76. Reddy, V. B., Thimmappaya, B., Dhar, R., Subramanian, K.N., Zain, B. S., Pan, J., Ghosh, P. K., Celma, M. L., and Weissman, S. M. (1978): The genome of SV40. *Science*, 200:494–502.

77. Reich, P. R., Baum, S. G., Rose, J. A., Rowe, W. P., and Weissman, S. M. (1966): Nucleic acid homology studies of adenovirus type 7-SV40 interactions. *Proc. Natl. Acad. Sci.*, 55:336–341.

78. Ricciardi, R., Miller, J. S., and Roberts, B. E. (1979): Purification and mapping of specific mRNAs by hybridization selection and cell-free translation. *Proc. Natl. Acad. Sci.*, 76:4927–4936.

79. Sambrook, J., Westphal, H., Srinivasan, P. R., and Dulbecco, R. (1968): The integrated state of DNA in SV40-transformed cells. *Proc. Natl. Acad. Sci.*, 60:1288–1295.

80. Sambrook, J., Botchan, M., Gallimore, P., Ozanne, B., Petterson, U., Williams, J., and Sharp, P. A. (1974): Viral DNA sequences in cells transformed by simian virus 40, adenovirus type 2 and adenovirus type 5. *Cold Spring Harbor Symp. Quant. Biol.*, 39:615–632.

81. Shiroki, K., and Shimojo, H. (1971): Transformation of green monkey kidney cells by SV40 genome: The establishment of transformed cell lines and the replication of human adenoviruses and SV40 in transformed cells. *Virology*, 45:163–171.

82. Sleigh, M. J., Topp, W. C., Hanich, R., Sambrook, J. R. (1978): Mutants of SV40 with an altered small t protein are reduced in their ability to transform cells. *Cell*, 14:79–88.

83. Smith, A. E., Bayley, S. T., Wheeler, T., and Mangel, W. F. (1975): *Cell Free Synthesis of Polyoma and SV40 Viral Proteins*, pp. 331–338, edited by A. L. Haenni and G. Beard. INSERM Symposium 47, INSERM, Paris.

84. Sweet, B. H., and Hilleman M. R. (1960): The vacuolating virus, SV40. *Proc. Soc. Exp. Biol. Med., 105*:420–427.

85. Tegtmeyer, P. (1974): Altered patterns of protein synthesis in infection by SV40 mutants. *Cold Spring Harbor Symp. Quant. Biol., 39*:9–15.

86. Tegtmeyer, P. (1975): Function of simian virus 40 gene A in transforming infection. *J. Virol., 15*:613–618.

87. Tegtmeyer, P., Schwartz, M., Collins, J. K., and Rundell, K. (1975): Regulation of tumor antigen synthesis by simian virus 40 gene A. *J. Virol., 16*:168–178.

88. Todaro, G. J., and Green H. (1964): An assay for cellular transformation by SV40. *Virology, 23*:117–119.

89. Tooze, J., ed. (1973): *The Molecular Biology of Tumor Viruses.* pp. 1–743. Cold Spring Harbor Laboratory.

90. van der Vliet, P. C., and Levine, A. J. (1973): DNA-binding proteins specific for cells infected by adenovirus. *Nature (New Biol.), 246*:170–174.

91. Vogt, V. M., and Eisenman, R. (1973): Identification of a large polypeptide precursor of avian oncornovirus proteins. *Proc. Natl. Acad. Sci., 70*: 1734–1738.

92. Vogt, V. M., Wight, A., and Eisenman, R. (1979): *In vitro* cleavage of avian retrovirus *gag* proteins by viral protease p15. *Virology, 90*:154–167.

93. Walter, G., and Martin, H. (1975): Simian virus 40-specific proteins in HeLa cells infected with nondefective adenovirus 2-simian virus 40 hybrid viruses. *J. Virol., 16*:1236–1247.

94. Westphal, H., and Dulbecco, R. (1968): Viral DNA in polyoma and SV40 transformed cell lines. *Proc. Natl. Acad. Sci., 59*:1158–1165.

95. Williams, J. F. (1973): Oncogenic transformation of hamster embryo cells *in vitro* by adenovirus type 5. *Nature, 243*:162–163.

96. Wold, W. S. M., Green, M., and Buttner, W. (1977): *Adenoviruses: The Molecular Biology of Animal Viruses*, edited by D. P. Nayak. Marcel Dekker, Inc., New York.

28

Fusion of Human Cells with Plant Protoplasts and Its Implications for Cell Differentiation

A. Lima-de-Faria

INTRODUCTION

The cellular processes that lead to the production of cancer are at present supposed to involve disturbances associated with cell function and cell differentiation. For this reason, knowledge of chromosome organization and of cell differentiation may help to understand the mechanisms which result in the appearance of cancer.

In this chapter we will summarize information that we have obtained on the following topics.

1. The evidence supporting the concept of the chromosome field and its implications for the understanding of the organization of the eukaryotic chromosome.

2. The results from the chromosome field which show that specific genes have the same location in the chromosomes of algae, higher plants, mammals, and humans.

3. This last result led to the prediction that it should be possible to fuse human cells with plant protoplasts.

4. The fusion of human cells with plant protoplasts occurred without difficulty and demonstrated that the human nucleus and the human chromosomes can survive for several days in a mixed human-plant cytoplasm surrounded by a plant cell wall.

5. Single plant cells are totipotent, *i.e.*, a whole plant can be obtained from a single plant cell growing under tissue culture conditions. The same phenomenon does not occur, however, in human cells. A human organism cannot be produced from a single cell developing under artificial conditions. The question arises whether in

human-plant heterokaryons the totipotency of the plant cell can be transferred to the human cell. We have at present no information on this question, but the fusion process is a first step in this direction.

THE ORGANIZATION OF THE EUKARYOTIC CHROMOSOME AND THE CONCEPT OF CHROMOSOME FIELD

Chromomeres vary in size and number from tissue to tissue within one organism. Similarly, the gene is a poorly defined unit as it has now become evident that it is a spliced structure in which the components may not even be located in the same chromosome. The only genetic unit that is well defined is the chromosome, since it has sharp physical limits imposed by the location of telomeres and centromeres (when the latter are terminal).

The current view of the chromosome is that it is a chaotic structure in which genes, mutations and structural rearrangements occur at random (*e.g.*, (26). In opposition to this view, I have proposed the concept of the chromosome field (12, 15). The concept is based on experimental and structural evidence which shows that the chromosome is a highly organized element. The chromosome appears to be a hierarchic structure in which centromeres and telomeres are the main organizers. Each gene has an optimal position within the centromere-telomere field. This position is called the *gene territory*. It is postu-

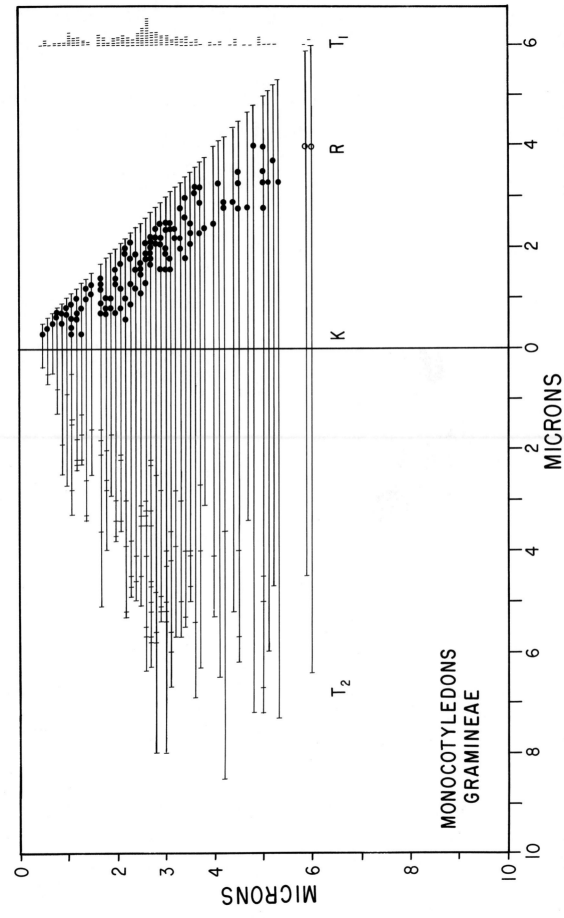

Figure 28.1. Metaphase of mitosis. Location of the nucleolar constriction (*solid circle*) where the ribosomal cistrons *R* are found) in the chromosomes of the family Gramineae. The central axis marks the position of the kinetochore *K* or centromere. By construction the telomere *T₁* of the arm containing the nucleolar organizer is located at 45° in relation to the kinetochore axis. This arm decides the position of the arm without organizer, which is on the other side of the kinetochore. The position of the telomere *T₂* is marked by a *short vertical dash*. *Small vertical dashes* in the right corner of the figure represent the number of chromosomes. The graph shows 149 chromosomes from 97 species. (Reproduced with permission from A. Lima-de-Faria: *Nature (New Biol.), 241:*136–139, 1973.)

lated that the gene has sensors that recognize messages from the centromere and the telomere regions.

The location of the genes for 28S and 18S ribosomal RNA (the nucleolus organizer region) has now been checked in more than 100 species from algae to humans (including worms, higher plants, and various mammals) and has been found to be wholly dependent on the centromere-telomere relationship (Figs. 28.1–28.8). The distribution of these genes is so regular that it can be predicted by means of a straight-line equation (13).

Other genes also have distributions in the centromere-telomere field which are the same in widely different organisms, but which differ from ribosomal genes (16–19). Such a specific gene territory allows us to classify genes as *centrons*, *medons*, and *telons* according to whether they happen to have their territory near the centromeres, in the median regions of the arms, or near the telomeres, respectively.

The DNA sequences which form the chromomere gradients are located on both sides of the centromeres. These sequences are typical centrons. They have so far been found in over 70 species of plants.

The chiasmata localized near the centromeres in *Allium* and other plant and animal species are also centrons. The regions of delayed separation in B chromosomes of plants have a location very close to the centromere. They are also centrons.

DNA sequences with their territory located in the median regions of the arms (medons) are the cold-induced regions of *Trillium* and *Fritillaria*. Other medons are the regions of human chromosomes which exhibit structural changes after UV and chemical treatment.

Typical examples of telons are the genes for 28S and 18S ribosomal RNA as they are located near the telomeres. The "knobs" (large chromomeres) of maize and many other plant species, which are located at the telomeres, or in their immediate vicinity, are also telons.

Structural rearrangements can also be classified according to their relation to the field. They may maintain the order previously established or they may disturb it. Rearrangements can accordingly be classified as *conservative*, *discordant*, *disruptive*, *destructive*, and *incompatible*. The rearrangements that least disturb the field are those that most often occur under natural conditions, such as the Robertsonian translocations which involve whole arms and thus do not alter the centromere-telomere relationship.

The concept of the chromosome field allows us to make predictions concerning gene location

and gene behavior which are difficult to conceive in terms of a chaotic view of the chromosome. For this reason, the field concept will lead to a better understanding of the problems of cell differentiation.

The field concept has also led us to postulate that a fusion between human cells and plant protoplasts should be feasible since the organization of the chromosome seems to be essentially the same in algae, higher plants, and humans.

FUSION OF HUMAN CELLS WITH PLANT PROTOPLASTS

In a first series of experiments, HeLa cells were fused with carrot protoplasts by means of polyethylene glycol and by culturing the fused components in a plant medium at 20°C. Heterokaryons were formed containing human and carrot nuclei which were surrounded by a cell wall. Nuclear contact also occurred and the percentage of heterokaryon formation ranged from 0.3 to 0.6% (3).

A similar experiment was carried out, independently of ours, involving the fusion of human cells with tobacco hybrid protoplasts by means of polyethylene glycol. It produced essentially the same results (11).

A second series of experiments carried out at our laboratory was planned with a concept to favoring the human cells. The fusion agent was inactivated Sendai virus and the plant species was *Haplopappus gracilis* which is known to tolerate high temperatures (7). The culture medium used after fusion was a modified MEM medium employed in culturing human cells and the temperature was 37°C. The fusion of the human cells with the plant protoplasts has led to the formation of heterokaryons containing one human nucleus and one *Haplopappus* nucleus. These appeared with a frequency of circa 12%. In the heterokaryons, a cell wall had formed which surrounded the two types of cytoplasms that had mixed. Human chromosomes were also present in the fused cells which had been in culture for three days (20).

SIMILAR GENES IN PLANTS AND HUMANS

The development of molecular biology and, in particular, the rapid expansion in the field of

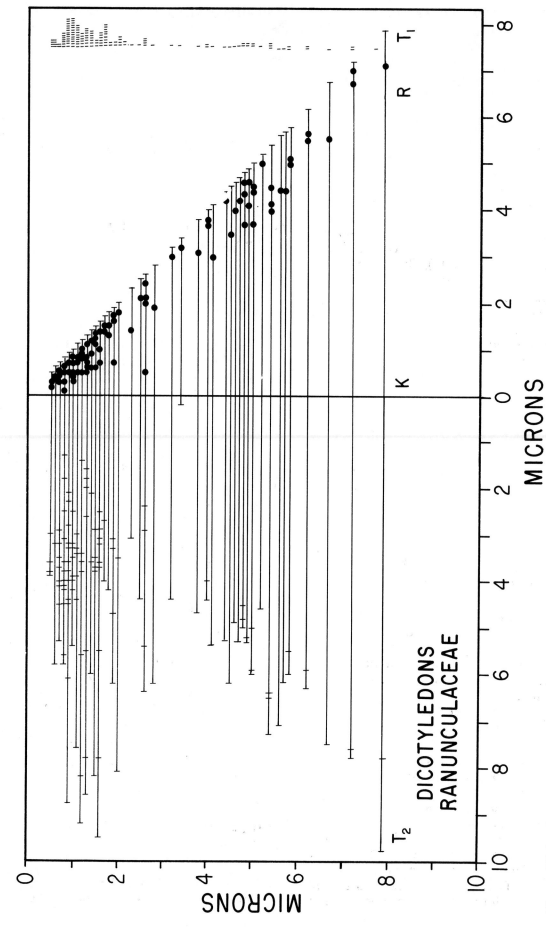

Figure 28.2. Location of the nucleolar constriction in Ranunculaceae. There are 139 chromosomes represented on the graph from 92 species. Note the occurrence of the nucleolus organizer close to telomere T_1 independent of arm length (14).

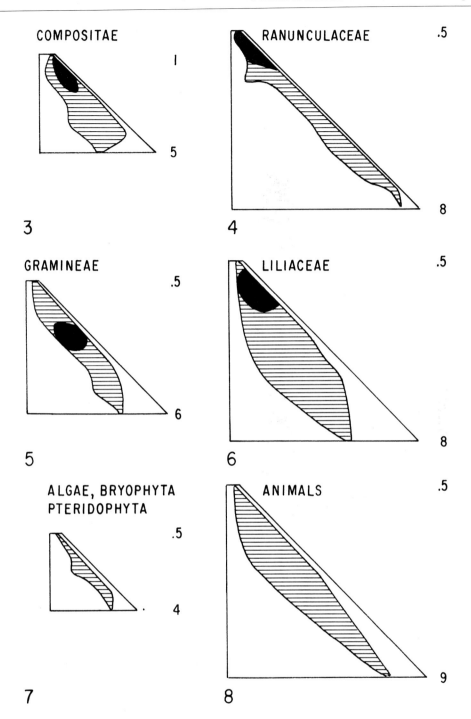

Figures 28.3–28.8. Schematic representation of the areas occupied by the nucleolar constrictions in the Compositae, Ranunculaceae, Gramineae, Liliaceae, Algae, Bryophyta, Pteridophyta, and animals (15). All locations in the animal chromosomes are from species in which the nucleoli were seen attached to the chromosomes (34 chromosomes from 19 species including man). The *black areas* represent regions of maximum frequency. The figures on the right side of each graph represent the chromosome length in μm.

molecular cytogenetics has made it possible to isolate biochemically some specific genes in eukaryotes.

Two types of genes have proved to be the easiest to isolate and analyze: the cistrons for 18S and 28S ribosomal RNA and the histone genes.

The ribosomal genes are present in humans, other animals, plants, and bacteria (review in ref. 1). The genes are so similar in the different

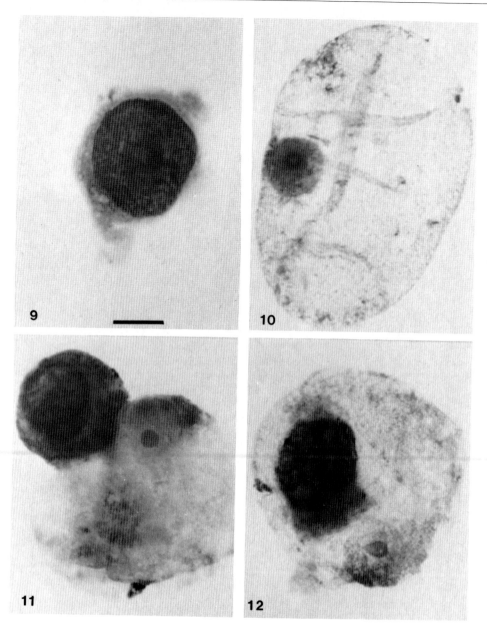

Figures 28.9–28.12. *Figure 28.9.* Human HeLa cell showing the heavily stained nucleus and deeply coloured cytoplasm. The nucleus is large and contains a large amount of heterochromatin, the cytoplasm builds a narrow band around the nucleus. *Figure 28.10. Haplopappus gracilis* protoplast that has rebuilt its cell wall (note the darker strips caused by the folds of the wall) and has acquired the bean-shaped appearance in the human medium and at 37°C. The *Haplopappus* cell is virtually indistinguishable from the controls. The cytoplasm is almost unstained and the nucleus, with only a little heterochromatin, is faintly stained but contains a distinct nucleolus. *Figure 28.11.* Beginning of cell fusion: the deeply stained human nucleus and cytoplasm (*upper left*) and the *Haplopappus* nucleus (with its distinct nucleolus) and the almost unstained plant cytoplasm (*right*). *Figure 28.12.* Heterokaryon containing a human nucleus with some cytoplasm (both darkly stained) in the center of the cell and a *Haplopappus* nucleus (*lower right*). Note the cell wall, with its folds, that surrounds the heterokaryon. The *Haplopappus* cytoplasm which is nearly unstained occupies most of the cell and involves the human nucleus.

groups of species that hybridization of RNA with DNA can be carried out by using, for instance, hamster 18S and 28S RNA and DNA of *Haplopappus*. This hybridization is most efficient mainly because of the large number of

ribosomal genes found in flowering plants Ståhle *et al.* (25) and Sinclair and Brown (24) have also obtained a high degree of hybridization between frog ribosomal RNA and barley and wheat DNA.

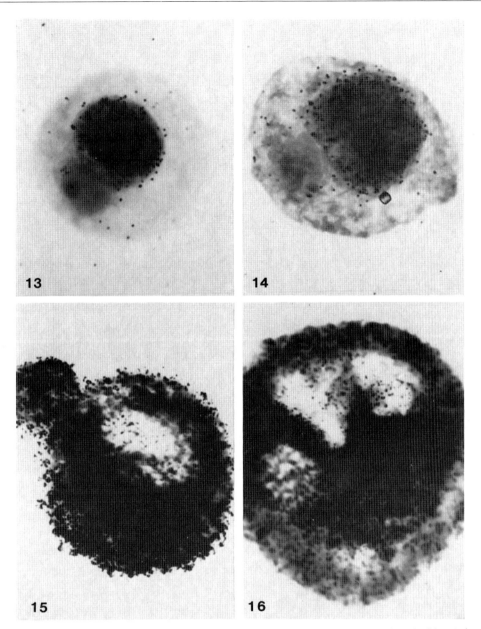

Figures 28.13–28.16. *Figures 28.13 and 28.14.* Two heterokaryons in which the darkly stained and tritium-labeled human nuclei and cytoplasms are located centrally. The *Haplopappus* nucleus in both figures is located at 8 o'clock and the plant cytoplasm is almost unstained. In Figure 28.14 the cell wall around the whole heterokaryon is particularly distinct. *Figures 28.15 and 28.16.* The reverse situation to the one depicted in the previous figures. One and two unlabeled *Haplopappus* nuclei and cytoplasms are surrounded by strongly labelled human nuclei and cytoplasms (several human nuclei are present in these heterokaryons).

The histone genes have recently been analyzed biochemically in detail (8, 9). These genes are also present in plants and humans. The histone fractions H3 and H4 have characteristic electrophoretic mobilities even when obtained from organisms as diverse as peas and cows. The amino acid sequences of H3 and H4 in these two species are very similar. H4 shows only two substitutions out of 102 amino acids and H3 four substitutions out of 135 amino acids (4).

Cytochrome *c* is another protein which is present in prokaryotes and eukaryotes and has changed little throughout millions of years of evolution. Cytochrome *c* is a protein of vital importance which functions in mitochondrial electron transfer. The amino acid sequence analysis discloses that about 60% of the total number of amino acids at corresponding positions are identical in wheat and human chains (2).

Plants also produce hemoglobin, a well-defined protein. This protein which has been studied in detail occurs mainly in leguminous plants and is called leghemoglobin (6). The amino acid sequence of the leghemoglobin of soybean has been established and, when compared with the gamma chain of human hemoglobin, shows many points of similarity. A comparison between the regions surrounding the haem-binding histidines of leghemoglobin and the human gamma chain (globin) has been made based on the genetic code. This showed that the differences in most cases involve only a single base pair giving a mutation frequency of 1.06. This means that mainly point mutations must have taken place in this part of the global chain during its evolution (5).

The fact that plants have hemoglobin genes but do not have red blood cells is of significance for understanding the organization of the eukaryotic chromosome. In our opinion the eukaryotic chromosome has such a rigid organization, established by the chromosome field, that it cannot evolve except in the direction dictated by its own molecular architecture. A gene, such as the hemoglobin gene, is formed independently of any function that it may have in the plant. The chromosome simply cannot produce anything else. The gene remains there with no obvious function. Later in the course of evolution, as other genes are produced by a process dictated by the molecular architecture, their combination may lead to a meaningful function. This may have happened, for instance, in the vertebrates when the genes for hemoglobin together with other genes led to the formation of red blood cells.

This rigid organization of the eukaryotic chromosome is supported by the finding that the ribosomal genes occupy the same position relative to kinetochores and telomeres in the eukaryotic chromosome, irrespective of whether a given chromosome belongs to the complement of an alga or of a human (15).

DNA sequence organization has been extensively carried out in animals. The genome of *Nicotiana tabacum* (one of the species used in human/plant cell fusions) was investigated by DNA/DNA reassociation for its spectrum of DNA repetition components and pattern of DNA sequence organization. Zimmerman and Goldberg (28), made this study, came to the conclusion that "the tobacco genome bears remarkable similarity to that found in the genomes of most animal species investigated to date". The animal species mentioned include man.

Not only specific genes but the overall organization of the DNA are similar in certain higher plants and in humans.

SIMILAR BIOCHEMICAL PROCESSES IN PLANTS AND HUMANS

Plants, although they do not have such highly evolved organs as animals, possess very similar chemicals and some almost identical biochemical pathways.

To start with, although plants do not have a nervous system they harbor in their cells the neurotransmitters dopamine, noradrenaline (norepinephrine), and serotonin. The nerve cells of humans and other animals communicate with one another by secreting neurotransmitters which traverse the tiny gap between two nerve cells and produce a change in the electrical activity of the receiving cell. These are messenger molecules which are released from one cell, travel a certain distance, and interact with the surface of a second cell. Among these messenger molecules are dopamine, noradrenaline, and serotonin which have a basic role in the communication between the nerve cells of animals, including humans (22). Serotonin is also a potent animal vasoconstrictor found particularly in the brain, intestinal tissue, blood platelets, and mast cells. Moreover, it stimulates uterine contraction (27).

In plants, dopamine and noradrenaline are found as derivatives of phenylpropan—amino acids. Noradrenaline is abundant in *Citrus* plants such as *Citrus aurantium* and is also present in *Portulaca oleracea*.

Serotonin is a derivative of the amino acid tryptophan. Oxidation of tryptophan leads to the formation of 5-hydroxytryptophan which results in the formation of serotonin. An intermediate compound in this chemical process, 5-hydroxytryptamine, is present in large quantities in bananas (21). Hence, although plants do not have a nervous system, they have three of the main neurotransmitters.

Some steroids are known to have androgenic and estrogenic activity in the animal kingdom, *i.e.*, they function as sex hormones which are secreted chiefly by the testis and ovary. Both androgens and estrogens have been isolated from testis and ovarian tissue. Among the sex hormones which influence the female sex cycles are estrone and estriol, two estrogenically active compounds which are found in particularly high concentrations in the urine of pregnant women. A third estrogen, β-estradiol, also present in the urine of pregnant women, is the normally secreted ovarian hormone (27).

Both estrone and estriol are found in plants. Three steroids with sexual hormone action have been described in flowering plants: the first is androstanetriol which is present in *Haplopappus heterophyllus* (Compositae). This species happens to belong to the same genus that we used in our human/plant cell fusions. The second is estrone which has been extracted from palm fruits, and the third is estriol present in willows (*Salix*) (21).

The function of these three steroids with sexual hormone action is not yet understood in plants, but we should not forget that flowering plants also have ovaries and that although these ovaries are not identical with those of mammals they have, however, the same basic function.

Ecdysone is an insect molting hormone which was first isolated from the silkworm, *Bombyx mori*. Six additional molting hormones have been isolated from a variety of insects and crustaceans.

As Hikino and Takemoto (10) point out "until five years ago who would imagine that a plant might contain an insect-molting hormone? Had there been someone with such a fantastic idea, he would have been able to discover immediately that a number of botanical extracts showed insect-molting hormone activity." In the last few years β-ecdysone has been isolated from ferns and from flowering plants. The molting hormone is present in plant species which have no close taxonomic relationship and is widely distributed since it has been found in some 80 families.

The function of ecdysone in plants is unknown. Again we have a situation where a plant produces a substance which may not necessarily have any function. The function only develops later in the course of evolution when other genes become available, which in combination produce a coordinated effect. A gene or a series of genes arise along the DNA as a consequence of its chemical properties and independently of any possible function in the plant or animal.

A corollary of such a postulate is that humans may possess a series of genes with no obvious function but that in the future, as man evolves, these nonfunctional genes may become integrated into larger gene constellations with a resulting meaningful function.

The fusion of human cells with plant protoplasts is therefore not as dramatic as it appears at first sight. The differences between the two groups of organisms may not be as profound as we have imagined.

Eukaryotic plant-like organisms may have existed approximately one billion years ago in the Protozoic era (Schopf) (23). Plants and animals must have diverged prior to this time. This seems to imply parallel lines of evolution characterized by the maintenance and acquisition of similar genes and similar biochemical pathways.

THE TOTIPOTENCY OF PLANT CELLS

A well established phenomenon in plant physiology is that a whole plant can be obtained from a single cell growing in tissue culture. The totipotency of plant cells is a most important property since it is absent in human and other animal cells.

So far it is not possible to obtain a human being from a single cell growing under artificial conditions. A fertilized human egg has this ability but not a single somatic cell.

Hence, the question arises. Can the chemical processes that lead to the totipotency in plants be transmitted to a human cell? A fusion between human cells and plant protoplasts is a first step in the investigation of such a process. However, it should be emphasized that it is only a preliminary approach to such a problem. At present the question can only be asked but no answer is available.

Acknowledgments. This work was supported by research grants from the Swedish Natural Science Research Council.

References

1. Birnstiel, M. L., Chipchase, M., Speirs, J. (1971): The ribosomal RNA cistrons. In *Progress in Nucleic Acid Research and Molecular Biology*, Vol. 11, pp. 351–389, edited by J. N. Davidson and W. E. Cohn. Academic Press, New York.
2. Dayhoff, M. O. (1971): Evolution of proteins. In *Chemical Evolution and the Origin of Life*, pp. 392–419, edited by R. Buvet and C. Ponnamperuma. North-Holland, Amsterdam.
3. Dudits, D., Rasko, I., Hadlaczky, G., and Lima-de-Faria, A. (1976): Fusion of human cells with carrot protoplasts induced by polyethylene glycol. *Hereditas, 82*:121–123.
4. Elgin, S. C. R., and Weintraub, H. (1975): Chromosomal proteins and chromatin structure. In *Annual Review of Biochemistry*, Vol. 44, pp. 725–774, edited by E. E. Snell, Annual Review, Inc., Palo Alto, Calif.
5. Ellsfolk, N. (1972): Leghaemoglobin, a plant haemoglobin, soybean. *Endeavour, 31*:139–142.
6. Ellsfolk, N., and Sievers, G. (1971): The primary structure of soybean leghemoglobin. *Acta Chem. Scand., 25*:3532–3548.
7. Eriksson, T. (1965): Studies on the growth requirements and growth measurements of cell cultures of *Haplopappus gracilis*. *Physiol. Plant.*
8. Gross, K., Probst, E., Schaffner, W., and Birnstiel, M. (1976): Molecular analysis of histone gene cluster of *Psammechinus miliaris*. 1. Fractionation and identification of 5 individual histone-messenger RNAs. *Cell, 8*:455–469.
9. Gross, K., Schaffner, W., Telford, J., and Birnstiel, M. (1976): Molecular analysis of histone gene cluster of *Psammechinus miliaris*. 3. Polarity and asymmetry of histone coding sequences. *Cell, 8*:479–484.

10. Hikino, H., and Takemoto, T. (1974): Ecdysones of plant origin. In *Invertebrate Endocrinology and Hormonal Heterophylly*, pp. 185–203, edited by W. J. Burdette. Springer-Verlag, Berlin.

11. Jones, C. W., Mastrangelo, I. A., Smith, H. H., Liu, H. Z., and Meck, R. A. (1976): Interkingdom fusion between human (Hela) cells and tobacco hybrid (GGLL) protoplasts. *Science, 193*:401–403.

12. Lima-de-Faria, A. (1954): Chromosome field in Agapanthus. *Chromosoma, 6*:330–370.

13. Lima-de-Faria, A. (1973): Equations defining position of ribosomal cistrons in eukaryotic chromosome. *Nature (New Biol.) 241*:136–139.

14. Lima-de-Faria, A. (1973): In *Modern Aspects of Cytogenetics: Constitutive Heterochromatin in Man*. Symposia Medica Hoechst 6:39–44.

15. Lima-de-Faria, A. (1976): The chromosome field. I. Prediction of the location of ribosomal cistrons. *Hereditas, 83*:1–22.

16. Lima-de-Faria, A. (1976): The chromosome field. II. The location of "knobs" in relation to telomeres. *Hereditas, 83*:23–34.

17. Lima-de-Faria, A. (1976): The chromosome field. III. The regularity of distribution of cold-induced regions. Includes the plants *Trillium* and *Fritillaria*. *Hereditas 83*:139–51.

18. Lima-de-Faria, A. (1976): The chromosome field. IV. The distribution of non-disjunction, chismata and other properties, includes plants. *Hereditas 83*:175–190.

19. Lima-de-Faria, A. (1976): Chromosome field. 5. Distribution of chromere gradients in relation to kinetochore and telomeres. *Hereditas, 84*:19–34.

20. Lima-de-Faria, A., Eriksson, T., and Kjellen, L. (1977):

21. Metzner, H. (1973): *Biochemie der Pflanzen*, pp. 1–376. Ferdinand Enke Verlag, Stuttgart.

22. Nathanson, J. A., and Greengard, P. (1977): Second messengers in brain. *Sci. Am., 237*:108–119.

23. Schopf, J. W. (1968): Microflora of the Bitter Springs Formation, late Precambrian, Central Australia. *J. Paleontol., 42*:651–688.

24. Sinclair, J. H., and Brown, D. D. (1971): Retention of common nucleotide sequences in ribosomal deoxyribonucleic acid of eukaryotes and some of their physical characteristics. *Biochemistry, 10*:2761–2769.

25. Ståhle, U., Lima-de-Faria, A., Ghatnekar, R., Jaworska, H., and Manley, M. (1975): Satellite DNA, localization of ribosomal cistrons and heterochromatin in *Haplopappus gracilis*, chromosomes. *Hereditas, 79*:21–28.

26. White, M. J. D. (1973): *Animal Cytology and Evolution*. Third Edition, Cambridge University Press, Cambridge, pp. 1–961.

27. White, A., Handler, P., and Smith, E. L. (1964): *Principles of Biochemistry*, pp. 1–1106. McGraw-Hill, New York.

28. Zimmerman, J. L., and Goldberg, R. B. (1977): DNA sequence organization in the genome of *Nicotiana tabacum*, tobacco. *Chromosoma, 59*:227–252.

29

Carcinogenesis in *Xiphophorus* and the Role of the Genotype in Tumor Susceptibility

M. Schwab and A. Anders

INTRODUCTION

About 50 years ago Myron Gordon (14), Curt Kosswig (28), and Georg Haeussler (16) discovered that certain hybrids between the platyfish (*Xiphophorus maculatus*) and the swordtail (*Xiphophorus helleri*) spontaneously develop melanomas. Since then the genetic basis for the development of the "spontaneous" melanoma has been largely elucidated (for more details, see Refs. 1–6, 15, 39).

In the last years it was shown that the melanoma as well as a large number of other types of neoplasms can be induced in *Xiphophorus* by carcinogens (36, 37). In any case the genotype appears to play an important role in determining the sensitivity or the resistance, respectively. The susceptibility for several neoplasms can be assigned to genetically defined chromosomes (35, 38) (for the most recent review on the system, see Ref. 3).

This report aims to present both the major results of the carcinogenesis studies in *Xiphophorus* and a model explaining on the basis of gene regulation the sensitivity and resistance of individuals to carcinogens.

APPROACH

The approach was to treat a large number of genetically defined genotypes (Table 29.1; see legend) including nonhybrids, their F_1 as well as backcross hybrids (*BC*) resulting from selective backcrosses, with carcinogens, and to analyze sensitivity and resistance according to the genotype.

The so-called direct acting carcinogens appear for this purpose particularly suitable. They directly interfere with the genetic material of the cell without being subjected to modification by physiological or enzymatic factors of the host (for detailed discussion, see Ref. 35). In the investigation to be presented here the nitrosamide N-methyl-N-nitrosourea (MNU), which spontaneously hydrolyzes under physiological conditions (30) to yield reactive radicals in any cell type (23), and x-rays, also generating such radicals in the cell, were applied (for details, see Refs. 33 and 38).The results obtained by using these agents should provide an understanding of the relation of the specificity of the genetic material to the resistance or sensitivity, respectively, to carcinogens (for comparison of the two agents, see Ref. 29).

CHEMICAL AND RADIATION-INDUCED NEOPLASMS

The neoplasms induced by MNU and by x-rays are of neurogenic, epithelial, and mesenchymal origin (36, 37). Neurogenic neoplasms include: melanoma, pterinophoroma, neuroblastoma, retinoblastoma, neurilemmoma; epithelial neoplasms include: papilloma, squamous cell carcinoma, solid carcinoma, and carcinoma of thyroid, kidney, liver, and gallbladder; mesenchymal neoplasms include: fibroma, fibrosar-

Table 29.1
Genotypes of *Xiphophorus* Species Treated with *N*-Methyl-*N*-nitrosourea (MNU) and X-rays[a]

Species, Populations, and Hybrids	Melanophore Spot Pattern Marker for Different Chromosomes[b]
NONHYBRIDS	
X. *maculatus* (Rio Jamapa)	$Sd, Sd', Sp, Sr, Sr', Dt, Cr, Sh, Os, Sd^{del}, Sr^{del}$
X. *maculatus* (Rio St. Pedro, Usumacinta-system)	Sh, Os; without marker
X. *xiphidium* (Rio Purification, Rio Soto la Marina)	$Fl, Ct; Fl^{del}$
X. *variatus* (Rio Panuco)	Li, Pu
X. *montezumae cortezi* (Rio Axtla, Rio Panuco-system	Sc
X. *helleri guentheri* (Belize River)	Db_1; without marker
X. *helleri guentheri* (Rio Lancetilla)	Db_2; without marker
HYBRIDS	
X. *maculatus (Rio Jamapa)* × X. *helleri* Rio Lancetilla) without marker	
F_1	$Sd, Sd', Sp, Sr, Sr', Dt, Cr, Sh, Os; Sd^{del}, Sr^{del}$
BC_n (n = 1, 3, 5, 7); BC-parent X. *helleri*	50% segregants with marker as in F_1, 50% without marker
X. *maculatus* (Rio Jamapa) × X. *montezumae*	
F_1	Sd, Sr, Sc
BC_n (n = 2, 3, 5); BC-parent X. *montezumae*	50% segregants with marker as in F_1, 50% without marker
X. *maculatus* (Rio Jamapa) × X. *xiphidium* Fl^{del}	
F_1	Sr, Sd, Sp, Sd, Sd
X. *variatus* × X. *helleri* (Rio Lancetilla) without marker	
F_1	Li
BC_n (n = 1, 4, 15); BC-parent X. *helleri*	50% segregants with marker as in F_1, 50% without marker

[a] Abbreviations: *Cr*, crescent; *Ct*, cut crescent; *Db*, dabbed; *Dt*, dot; *Fl*, flecked; Fl^{del}, deletion of flecked; *Li*, lineatus; *Os*, one spot; *Pu*, punctatus; *Sc*, spotted caudal; *Sd*, spotted dorsal; Sd^{del}, deletion of spotted dorsal; *Sd'*, spotted dorsal mutation; *Sh*, shoulder spot; *Sp*, spotted; *Sr*, striped; *Sr'*, striped mutation. (For further details, see Refs. 21 and 22.)

[b] The melanophore spot patterns are due to the expression of specific genes, each of which is located on a particular chromosome. All these genes are in any genotype coexpressed (codominant). This makes it possible to recognize the presence or absence of specific chromosomes in any genotype.

coma, rhabdomyosarcoma, leimyosarcoma, and lymphosarcoma. The MNU- and x-ray-induced neoplasms, with respect to their morphology, their structure as well as their ultrastructure, appear to be identical.

By far the most frequent lesions are melanomas (in 261 out of the 7000 fishes treated; Fig. 29.1), neuroblastomas (in 66 fishes, Fig. 29.2), solid carcinomas (in 12 fishes; Fig. 29.3), and fibrosarcomas (in 50 fishes; Fig. 29.4). They represent more than 90% of the total number of neoplasms induced.

The relative incidences of the various MNU- and x-ray-induced neoplasms are similar, suggesting that the two carcinogens trigger tumor development through the same mechanism.

ROLE OF THE GENOTYPE

Sensitivity and Resistance in Relation to the Genotype

The neoplasms induced by MNU and by x-rays are not distributed at random throughout the fishes of the different genotypes, but are confined to few of them. Nonhybrids (Table 29.1) proved to be completely resistant (Table 29.2). In contrast, F_1 and backcross hybrids were sensitive, although at considerably different degrees. While in the F_1 only the melanoma occurred (0.6% of fishes developed a neoplasm;

Figure 29.1 (a) Sd^{del}-carrying backcross segregant [(*Xiphophorus maculatus* Sd^{del}/Sd^{del} × *Xiphophorus helleri* $-/-$, F_1 × X. *helleri*, BC_1] exhibiting an induced melanoma in the upper part of the tail fin (×3). (b) Outer region of the melanoma, exhibiting relatively light pigmentation. The epidermis is hyperblastic (H&E, ×250). (c) Central area of the melanoma exhibiting dense pigmentation. Invasion of the tumor into the underlaying muscular tissue is apparent (H&E, ×250). (From thesis of S. Abdo.)

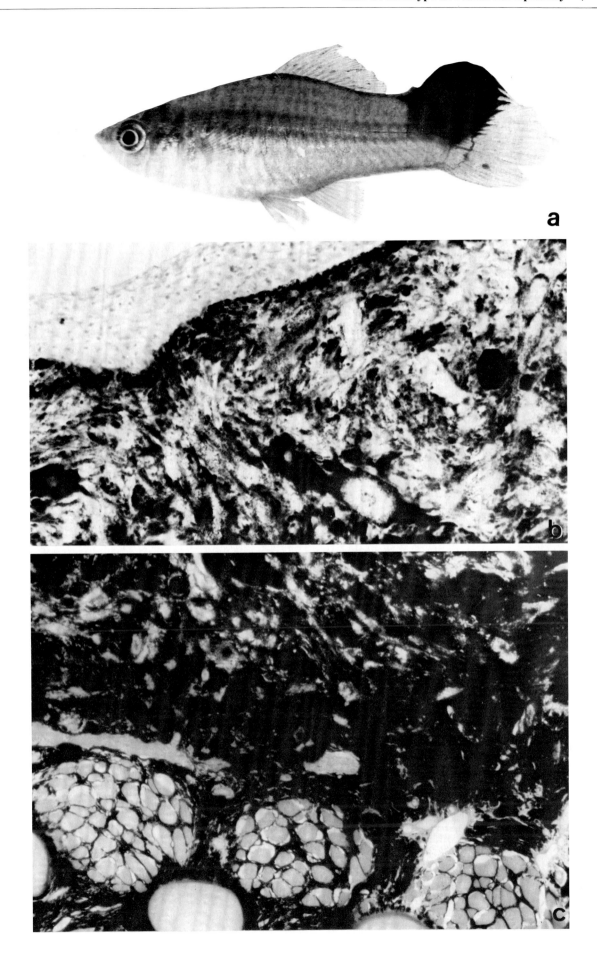

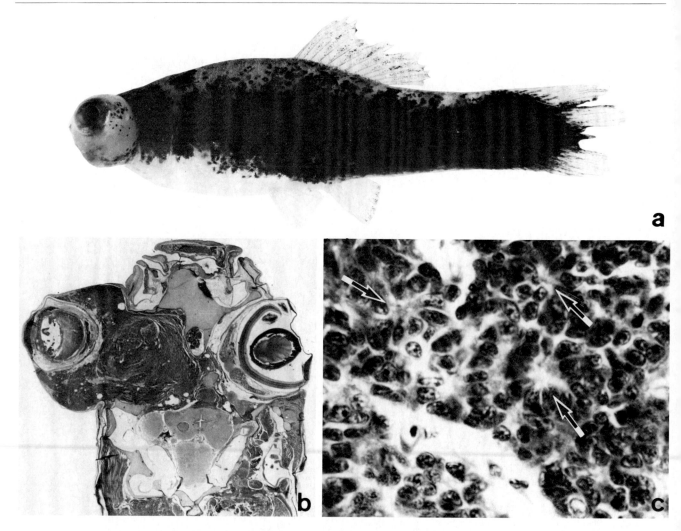

Figure 29.2 *(a)* *Li*-carrying backcross segregant [(*Xiphophorus variatus Li/Li* × *Xiphophorus helleri* −/−, *F₁*) × *X. helleri*, *BC₁*] exhibiting an induced neuroblastoma in the region of the eye (×3). *(b)* Section through the head region (H&E, ×6). *(c)* Neuroblastoma cells; note rosette-like arrangement of the tumor cells *(arrows)* (H&E, × 1000). (From thesis of G. Kollinger.)

Table 29.2), in the backcross hybrids in addition to the melanoma all the remaining neoplasms developed (7.1% of the backcross hybrids exhibited a neoplasm).

The susceptibility for the four major neoplasms, melanoma, neuroblastoma, epithelioma and fibrosarcoma can be assigned to genetically defined chromosomes; for the other neoplasms the incidences are too low in order to establish such a relation. In particular, the melanoma developed exclusively in fishes carrying any one of the chromosomes marked by the spot pattern *Li* (derived from *Xiphophorus variatus*; Table 29.1) (37), or *Sd^{del}* or *Sr* (both derived from X. *maculatus*). Furthermore, the neuroblastoma (38) and the carcinoma can be assigned to the *Li*-chromosome. The fibrosarcoma depends on the presence of another chromosome of X. *var-*

iatus (35), for which, however, we have not identified a phenotypic marker so far.

Interpretation

There is good evidence that most of the known chemical and physical carcinogens are also mutagens (31). In addition, it has been shown likely that carcinogens may cause the change of a normal cell into a neoplastically transformed cell *via* a genomic change, *i.e.*, a mutation in its broadest sense (7–11, 17, 40). In *Xiphophorus* the correlation between the chemical and radiation-induced carcinogenesis, along with the fact that most of the neoplasms most likely have a unicellular origin (see also Ref. 3), would point to a somatic mutation as the primary event triggering

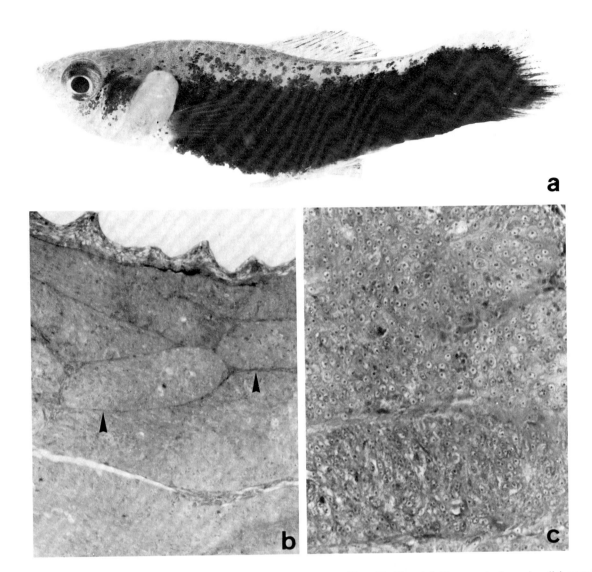

Figure 29.3. *(a)* *Li*-carrying backcross segregant (cross as in Fig. 29.2) exhibiting an induced solid carcinoma protruding from the operculum (×3). *(b)* Masses of tumor cells are surrounded by a thin rim of vascular stroma (*arrows*) (H&E, ×100). *(c)* The tumor consists of masses of round epithelial cells having round nuclei with distinct nucleoli (H&E, ×400). (From thesis of S. Abdo.)

the tumor development. This idea is further supported by the fact that a mutation in apparently the same genes located on the same chromosomes (e.g., *Li*, *Sr*, see above) can also be induced in the germ line (1, 2). In this case, germ line mutation conditioned neoplasms develop in the offspring of the treated fish. This trait is further inherited according to Mendelian prediction (for details, see Ref. 3).

On this basis it is likely that the susceptibility in the backcross hybrids, which exhibit the highest sensitivity, is controlled by a single gene; if more genes would be involved, the sensitivity would be much lower (for the relation between mutation rate, tumor incidence, and number of

genes controlling the susceptibility, see Ref. 3). In the F_1 hybrids, which have a considerably lower sensitivity, the control should be based on at the most two genes. Consequently, in the nonhybrids, which are resistant, the susceptibility is presumably controlled by several genes. One might formally interpret the differential sensitivity of the nonhybrids, the F_1 and backcross hybrids as follows (Fig. 29.5).

From any pair of parental nonhybrids, of which the hybrids and their backcross derivatives are sensitive, one parent (P_1) carries a genetic factor that favors neoplastic transformation (tentatively called "tumor gene" *Tu*). In addition, P_1 carries genetic factors controlling

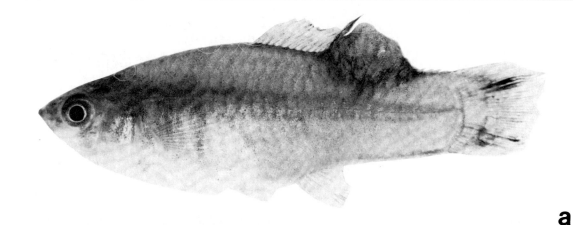

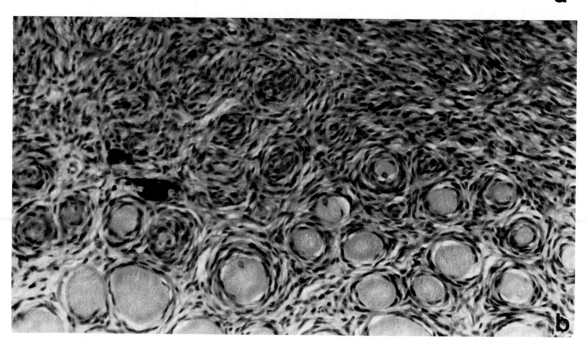

Figure 29.4. *(a)* *Li*-lacking backcross segregant (cross as in Fig. 29.2) exhibiting an induced fibrosarcoma in the region of the dorsal fin (×3). *(b)* Section through the tumor; note spindle cells irregularly arranged and invading the muscular tissue (H&E, ×250) (From thesis of S. Abdo).

Table 29.2
Sensitivity and Resistance, Respectively, of Nonhybrids, F_1 and Backcross Hybrids to the Carcinogens *N*-Methyl-nitrosourea (MNU) and X-rays

Genotype	No. of Fishes Treated[a]	Neoplasm Induced in Fishes Treated (%)	No. of Types of Neoplasms
Nonhybrid	3500	0	0
F_1	1200	0.6	1[b]
Backcross-hybrid	3300	7.1	17

[a] Approximate number.
[b] Melanoma.

Tu (tentatively called "repressing genes" *R*), one of which is linked to *Tu* on the same chromosome while others are nonlinked. Because an impairment of several *R* genes by a carcinogen in the same cell is extremely unlikely, the fish is, in effect, resistant. In the other parent (P_2) both the *Tu* and *R* are not detectable in this experiment, and are therefore not shown in Figure 29.5. The F_1 is hemizygous for both *Tu* and the linked and the nonlinked *R* genes. This situation, in which the simultaneous mutation of both *R* genes is also rather unlikely, although not impossible, may account for the low sensitivity. In the backcross generations, resulting from backcrossing of the F_1 to P_2, *Tu* is transmitted along with its linked *R* gene, while the nonlinked *R* genes, due to new combination of chromosomes, are eliminated. Fishes of this genotype have a high sensitivity, because one somatic mutation is sufficient for triggering tumor development.

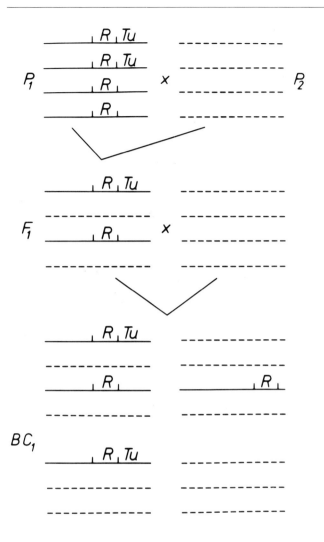

Figure 29.5. Schema displaying a genetic interpretation for the resistance of nonhybrids (P_1 and P_2) to carcinogens, the low sensitivity of the F_1, and high sensitivity of the backcross hybrids (*BC*). *Tu*, tumor gene; *R*, regulating gene repressing *Tu*; *P*, parent. (———) Chromosome of P_1; (- - - - -) chromosome of P_2. Elimination by crossings, or impairment by carcinogen-induced mutation, respectively, of all the *R* genes leads to expression of *Tu* and to subsequent neoplastic transformation. The sensitivity to carcinogens increases with decreasing number of the *R* genes. For further details see text.

DISCUSSION

Species or strain differences in the sensitivity to carcinogens have been reported for several vertebrates, such as fishes (compare Refs. 32 and 34; 35–38), the dog (12), and the mouse (13). This shows that the carcinogenicity of a physical or chemical agent is not exclusively determined by the agent itself, but depends also on the genetic makeup of the individual.

For the analysis of the genetic basis underlying the sensitivity or resistance, respectively, to carcinogens, *Xiphophorus* appears to be particularly suitable. This is mainly because a large number of chromosomes, which are marked by specific spot patterns of the skin, can easily be identified.

The results so far obtained would suggest that the resistance of the nonhybrids, which represent wild-type animals, might be due to an interaction between a gene favoring neoplastic transformation (*Tu*), and other genes repressing *Tu* (*R*). Without too much speculation, it is conceivable that *Tu* is a foreign gene of the gene pool, possibly a viral genome, that has been acquired during evolution and has been brought under genetic control exerted through the *R* genes. This idea is supported by the fact that virus particles can be induced in *Tu*-carrying fishes that are normally free of such viruses (27). Apparently there has been no selection against *Tu* in spite of its potentially deleterious effects. This would indicate, that *Tu* may perform normal functions; it could, for instance, be involved in the stimulation of cell division during the development of the embryo or during regeneration processes. At present, however, one cannot exclude that *Tu* is not a foreign gene, but is part of the natural gene pool of *Xiphophorus*.

In the course of crossing and subsequent backcrossing a part of the *R* genes becomes eliminated, while others remain. This process will result in a sensitive genotype, which upon further carcinogen-induced impairment of the remaining repressing gene(s) will develop a neoplasm. This impairment may also occur "spontaneously," although at a much lower incidence, giving rise to a "spontaneous" neoplasm. It may not be excluded that similar mechanisms as those analyzed in *Xiphophorus* account for the differential sensitivity of species or strains of other vertebrates. They may also account for the different incidences of "spontaneous" tumors observed in various strains or breeds of domesticated animals, such as the horse, dog, mouse, rat, and others (42).

From the results of the carcinogenesis studies in *Xiphorphorus*, the idea that in the origin of cancer one or several genetic changes are involved is further supported. In *Xiphophorus* several genetic changes are involved including new combination of chromosomes, which leads to a sensitive genotype, and apparently mutation, which triggers the development of the neoplasm.

This situation is, in principle, similar to that in various neoplasms in man. For instance, in retinoblastoma (24), Wilms' tumor of kidney (25), or pheochromocytoma (26) apparently two genetic events are involved, the first being on the level of the germ line leading to a sensitive genotype. The nature of this first event is still unclear, although it is felt that it might consist in a germ line mutation (18, 41). In *Xiphophorus* the first event consists in a new combination of chromosomes. The second genetic event in the above tumors in man, and in the tumors of *Xiphophorus*, appears to consist of a somatic mutation. These experiments in *Xiphophorus* would suggest that models for the etiology of cancer in general do not necessarily require two mutational events, as has been proposed by other authors (18, 41).

In our opinion, future studies with *Xiphophorus* will provide a further understanding on the interaction of the genotype and environmental factors capable of inducing abnormal growth. Furthermore, the sensitive genotypes of *Xiphophorus* should be suitable indicators for the presence of carcinogens in the environment.

SUMMARY

In *Xiphophorus* nonhybrids proved to be resistant for tumor induction by N-methyl-N-nitrosourea and by x-rays, while F_1 and backcross hybrids are sensitive, although at considerably different degrees. F_1 hybrids possess a low, backcross hybrids a high sensitivity. The results are interpreted as to imply that the resistance of the nonhybrids is due to an interaction between a certain gene favoring neoplastic transformation and a system of other genes repressing neoplastic transformation. During crossing and subsequent backcrossing the major part of the repressing genes is eliminated, and a minor part remains. This process leads to a sensitive genotype which, following further carcinogen-induced impairment of the remaining repressing gene(s), develops a neoplasm.

Acknowledgments. This work was supported by the Deutsche Forschungsgemeinschaft through Sonderforschungsbereich 103 "Zellenergetik and Zelldifferenzierung," Marburg (projects C11 and C12). It contains parts of the dissertations of S. Abdo, J. Haas, and G. Kollinger, and of the habilitation of M. Schwab.

References

1. Anders, A., Anders, F., and Klinke, K. (1973): Regulation of gene expression in the Gordon-Kosswig melanoma system; I. The distribution of the controlling genes in the genome of the xiphophorin fish, *Platypoecilus maculatus* and *Platypoecilus variatus*, in *Genetics and Mutagenesis of Fish*, pp. 33–52, edited by J. H. Schröder. Springer-Verlag, New York.

2. Anders, A., Anders, F., and Klinke, K. (1973): Regulation of gene expression in the Gordon-Kosswig melanoma system; II. The arrangement of chromatophore determining loci and regulating elements in the sex chromosomes of xiphophorin fish, *Platypoecilus maculatus* and *Platypoecilus variatus*, in *Genetics and Mutagenesis of Fish*, pp. 53–63, edited by J. H. Schröder. Springer-Verlag, New York.
3. Anders, A., and Anders, F. (1978): Etiology of cancer as studied in the platyfish-swordtail sytem. *Biochim. Biophys. Acta*, 516:61–95.
4. Anders, F. (1967): Tumour formation in platyfish-swordtail hybrids as a problem of gene regulation. *Experientia*, 23:1–10.
5. Anders, F. (1968): Genetische Faktoren bei der Entstehung von Neoplasmen. *Zentralbl. Veterinaermed.*, B15:29–46.
6. Anders, F., Kollinger, G., and Schwab, M. (1978): Tumor gene mediated hereditary and non-hereditary melanoma in the skin of xiphophorine fish, in *Skin Cancer and Virus*, edited by B. R. Balda. Springer-Verlag, New York (in press).
7. Barret, J. C., and Ts'o P. O. P. (1978): Relationship between somatic mutation and neoplastic transformation. *Proc. Natl. Acad. Sci. U.S.A.*, 75:3297–3301.
8. Barret, C. J., Tsutsui, and Ts'o, P. O. P. (1978): Neoplastic transformation induced by a direct perturbation of DNA. *Nature*, 274:229–232.
9. Benedict, W. F. (1972): Early changes in chromosomal number and structure after treatment of fetal hamster cultures with transforming doses of polycyclic hydrocarbones. *J.N.C.I.*, 49:585–590.
10. Benedict, W. F., Rucker, N., Mark, C., and Kouri, R. (1975): Correlation between the balance of specific chromosomes and the expression of malignancy in hamster cells. *J.N.C.I.*, 54:157–162.
11. Bouck, N., and diMayorca, G. (1976): Somatic mutation as the basis for malignant transformation of BHK cells by chemical carcinogens. *Nature*, 264:722–727.
12. Denlinger, R. H., Koestner, A., and Swenberg, J. A. (1978): Neoplasms in purebred boxer dogs following long-term administration on N-methyl-N-nitrosourea. *Cancer Res.*, 38:1711–1717.
13. Evans, J. T., Shows, T. B., Sproul, E. E., Paolini, N. S., Mittelman, A., and Hauschka, T. S. (1971): Genetics of colon carcinogenesis in mice treated with 1,2-dimethylhydrazine. *Cancer Res.*, 37:134–136.
14. Gordon, M. (1927): The genetics of a viviparous top-minnow *Platypoecilus*—the inheritance of two kinds of melanophores. *Genetics*, 12:253–283.
15. Gordon, M. (1959): The melanoma cell as an incompletely differentiated pigment cell, in *Pigment Cell Biology*. pp. 215–239, edited by M. Gordon. Academic Press, New York.
16. Haeussler, G. (1928): Über Melanombildung bei Bastarden von *Xiphophorus helleri* und *Platypoecilus maculatus* var. *Rubra*. *Klin. Wochenschr.*, 7:1561–1562.
17. Hart, R.W., Setlow, R. B., and Woodhead, A. D. (1977): Evidence that pyrimidine dimers in DNA can give rise to tumors. *Proc. Natl. Acad. Sci. U.S.A.*, 74:5574–5579.
18. Hethcote, H. W., and Knudson, A. G. (1978): Model for the incidence of embryonal cancers; application to retinoblastoma. *Proc. Natl. Acad. Sci. U.S.A.*, 75:2453–2457.
19. Hitotsumachi, S., Rabinowitz, Z., and Sachs, L. (1972): Chromosomal control of chemical carcinogenesis. *Int. J. Cancer*, 9:305–315.
20. Huberman, E., Mager, R., and Sachs, L. (1976): Mutagenesis and transformation of normal cells by chemical carcinogens. *Nature*, 264:360–361.
21. Kallman, K. D. (1975): The platyfish, *Xiphophorus maculatus*, in *Handbook of Genetics*, Vol. 4, pp. 81–132, edited by R. C. King. Plenum Press, New York.
22. Kallman, K., and Atz, J. W. (1967): Gene and chromosome homology in fishes of the genus *Xiphophorus*. *Zoologica*, 51:107–135.
23. Kleihues, P., and Patschke, K. (1971): Verteilung von N-(^{14}C)Methyl-N-Nitrosoharnstoff in der Ratte nach systemischer Applikation. *Z. Krebsforsch.*, 75:193–200.
24. Knudson, A. G. (1971): Mutation and cancer; statistical study of retinoblastoma. *Proc. Natl. Acad. Sci. U.S.A.*, 68:820–823.
25. Knudson, A. G., and Strong, L. C. (1972): Mutation and cancer: A model for Wilms tumor of the kidney. *J.N.C.I.*, 38:313–324.
26. Knudson, A. G., and Strong, L. C. (1972): Mutation and cancer; neuroblastoma and pheochromocytoma. *Am. J. Hum.Genet.*, 24:514–532.
27. Kollinger, G., Schwab, M., and Anders, F. (1979): Virus-like particles induced by bromodeoxyuridine in melanoma and neuroblastoma of *Xiphophorus*. *J. Cancer Res. Clin. Oncol.*, 95:239–246.
28. Kosswig C. (1927): Über Bastarde der Teleostier *Platypoecilus* und *Xiphophorus*. *Z. Indukt. Abstamm. Vererbsgsl.*, 44:253.
29. Lawley, P. D. (1976): Comparison of alkylating agent and radiation carcinogenesis. Some aspects of the possible involvement of effects on DNA, in *Biology of Radiation Carcinogenesis*, pp. 165–174, edited by J. M. Yuhan, R. R. W. Tennant, and J. Regan. Raven Press, New York.
30. Magee, P. N., Pegg, A. E., and Swann, P. F. (1975): Molecular mechanisms of chemical carcinogenesis, in *Handbuch der allgemeinen Pathologie VI/6*, pp. 329–419, edited by E. Grundmann. Springer-Verlag, New York.
31. McCann, J., Choi, E., Yamasaki, E., and Ames, B. N. (1975): Detection of carcinogens as mutagens in the *Salmonella*/microsome test; assay of 300 chemicals. *Proc. Natl. Acad. Sci. U.S.A.*, 72:5135–5139.
32. Pliss, G. B., and Khudoley, V. V. (1975): Tumor induction by carcinogenic

agents in aquarium fish. *J.N.C.I., 55*:129–136.

33. Pursglove, D., Anders, A., Doell, G., and Anders, F. (1971): Effects of x-irradiation on the genetically determined melanoma system of xiphophorin fish. *Experientia, 27*:695–697.

34. Scherf, R. H. (1976): Toxikologische Wirkungen von Diaethylnitrosamin (DÄNA) beim Guppy (*Lebistes reticulatus*). *Z. Krebsforsch., 86*:155–163.

35. Schwab, M., Abdo, S., Ahuja, M. R., Kollinger, G., Anders, A., Anders, F. and Frese, K. (1978): Genetics of susceptibility in the platyfish/swordtail tumor system to develop fibrosarcoma and rhabdomyosarcoma following treatment with N-methyl-N-nitrosourea (MNU). *Z. Krebsforsch., 91*:301–315.

36. Schwab, M., Ahuja, M. R., and Anders, F. (1976): Genetically conditioned susceptibility of specific cell types to neoplastic transformation in the xiphophorine fish. *Heredity, 34*:454–455.

37. Schwab, M., Haas, J., Abdo,S., Ahuja, M. R., Kollinger, G., Anders, A., and Anders, F. (1978): Genetic basis of susceptibility for development of neoplasms following treatment with N-methyl-N-nitrosourea (MNU)

and x-rays in the platyfish/swordtail system. *Experientia, 34*:780–782.

38. Schwab, M., Kollinger, G., Haas, J., Ahuja, M. R., Abdo, S., Anders, A., and Anders, F. (1979): Genetic basis of susceptibility for neuroblastoma following treatment with N-methyl-N-nitrosourea (MNU) and x-rays. *Cancer Res., 39*:519–526.

39. Sobel, H. J., Marquet, E., Kallman, K. D., and Corley, G. J. (1975): Melanomas in platy/swordtail hybrids, in *The Pathology of Fishes*, pp. 945–981, edited by W. E. Ribelin, and G. Migaki. University of Wisconsin Press, Madison.

40. Stich, H. F., San, R. H., and Kawazoe, Y. (1971): DNA repair synthesis in mammalian cells exposed to a series of oncogenic and non-oncogenic derivatives of 4-nitroquinoline 1-oxide. *Nature, 229*:416–419.

41. Strong, L. C. (1977): Theories of pathogenesis; mutation and cancer, in *Genetics of Human Cancer*, pp. 401–416, edited by J. J. Mulvihill, R. W. Miller, and J. F. Fraumeni. Raven Press, New York.

42. Weiss, E. (1972): Geschwuelste, in *Allgemeine Pathologie*, pp. 124–201, edited by A. Frei. Parey-Verlag, Hamburg.

30

Aberrant Tissue in *Drosophila*

Walter J. Burdette

INTRODUCTION

Melanotic tumors were first described by Bridges (3) who isolated a recessive lethal mutant, l(1)7, on the first chromosome of *Drosophila melanogaster* that caused the appearance of melanotic aggregates which were easily visible. Many years later Russell (37) was able to demonstrate that death was caused by occlusion of the gut and not because the pigmented cells were malignant. Questions have been raised about the propriety of labeling these melanotic mutants in *Drosophila*, "tumors." Since the etymology of the term from the Latin, *tumere*, has no connotation of invasion or malignancy, the designation of these mutants (11) in *Drosophila* as tumors has persisted and likely will continue merely as a means of identification. Additionally, it is unwise to discard *Drosophila* as a means for oncologic study since some tissues from larvae transplanted into adults invade adjacent tissue and kill the host (24, 39), thus fulfilling the requirements for calling these tumors malignant neoplasms. Many mutants (26, 34, 40, 41) in addition to l(1)7 have been found in various populations of *Drosophila* in the wild and in the laboratory as fortuitous observations or as the result of experimental treatments. In order to examine them in a proper setting, brief attention will be given to the life cycle in invertebrates. Its progression is controlled by hormones (15), and metamorphosis is coordinated with the puffing pattern of the giant salivary polytene chromosomes in insects.

GENETIC AND HORMONAL CONTROL OF METAMORPHOSIS

At first, genes were localized on the chromosomes of *Drosophila* by crossover mapping of mutants. Later it was possible to compare the position of genes on these maps to localization of the same genes on giant prophase salivary chromosomes which have divided in the absence of cellular division producing a convenient polytene banding pattern. It was soon noted that the puffs which appear at specific loci on these chromosomes changed their size at different times during the life cycle, and a puffing pattern correlated with metamorphosis was soon documented (1, 2). Later not only were the puffs found to contain RNA predominantly but also to respond to synthetic and naturally occurring ecdysones and juvenile hormones (12, 14, 17, 18). Also it has been found that these puffs respond *in vitro* to changing levels of the invertebrate hormones. The pattern of responsiveness is programmed in the chromosomal mechanism which somehow both provides the patterns for sequential and quantitative production of hormones and responded to a feedback mechanism poorly understood.

Insects, unlike vertebrates, have an exoskeleton. Therefore, in order to grow and differentiate, it is necessary for this chitinous armor to be replaced periodically with a larger sheath by means of the process of molting. This complex process of growth and differentiation is under the hormonal control described. The egg hatches into a mobile larva which is specialized for feeding. Then the immobile pupal stage bridges the larval and adult or imaginal stages of development. The adult emerges as an individual specialized for reproduction. Many larval structures are replaced as development proceeds by organs such as eyes, wings, and legs which develop from undifferentiated imaginal discs present in the earlier stages of development. The secretory cells of the brain respond to external stimuli, producing brain hormone which is tropic for the

461

prothoracic gland which in turn is involved in producing molting hormones (ecdysones). The corpora allata are innervated and provide juvenile hormone (in insects the ring gland consists of combined corpora allata and of combined corpora cardiaca). Balanced interaction between these hormones brings about the orderly process of development.

MELANOTIC TUMORS

Melanotic tumor strains studied in *Drosophila* are carried in inbred or isogenic cultures and each is associated with a mutant gene or genes (5, 11). Of the several principal types of tumors in *Drosophila*, they are the most numerous and begin as cellular aggregates (7) in the larval stage. With metamorphosis, these cells undergo dissolution, leaving a detritus of melanin which is usually visible in the late larval instars, pupal, and imaginal stages (26, 34). We found that antibacterial immunity may be altered in tumor strains suggesting that the cellular elements seen may be a part of the immunodefensive mechanism (16). The tumor cells attract a stroma of fusiform cells which are probably normal hemocytes also found in nontumorous strains (20). This along with melanization is similar morphologically to the reaction to injury in insects (31, 36), and therefore tumor induction by carcinogens or other noxious agents is open to more questions than their appearance as a result of genic action alone. Genes for melanotic tumors may alter viability of the strains bearing them, and at least one strain (20) (no longer in existence) was thought to be malignant. However, they are considered to be benign by investigators who work with them extensively. Early investigators (40, 41) compared them to vertebrate lymphomas and leukemias, but circulating cells in insects are not really comparable to vertebrate blood cells and identification of the origin and precursors of given cells present considerable difficulties. The *freckled* mutant produces melanization (35) of fat and pericardial cells and strains bearing it or not generally accepted as tumor stocks. Circulating cells are responsible for the disposition of those tissues confined to the larval stage. Since cells comprising the melanotic tumors can be phagocytic, this has been pointed out as additional support for hemocytic involvement in the formation of these melanotic tumors (26). Admonitions about unjustified con-

clusions concerning the nature and origin of these cellular aggregates abound (31, 36). Nevertheless, they provide an interesting system of atypical growth presenting many advantages for experimental manipulations.

The mutants in *Drosophila* which produce melanotic tumors (11) are chiefly on the second chromosome. Very few of them are allelomorphic (19), all are recessive, and principal genes are known to reside on one or more chromosomes. In addition, there are suppressor as well as enhancer genes present on the same or other chromosome(s) in some strains. Some of the primary genes and modifiers have been localized precisely, whereas the chromosomal loci of others have not been determined. Penetrance (10) is usually not complete and most of them are sensitive to temperature. When homozygous, the percentage with tumors varies from less than 1% to more than 99%, depending on the strain and the environment in which flies are raised. The same gene may bring about tumors in 9 out of 10 individuals at one temperature, whereas this may be reduced to less than 1 in 10 when the cultures are maintained at another. We found that careful experiments to produce isogenic strains (5) using inversions to prevent crossing over have not necessarily resulted in increasing penetrance. The genes themselves are apparently true mutations and not deletions, since we were able (11) to bring about reverse mutation in the $tu^{48a}vg$ bw strain by means of irradiation. Also we found that mutagens such as nitrogen mustard and carcinogens such as 20-methylcholanthrene may increase the number of tumors in tumor strains exposed to these agents (8, 13). Crowding diminishes the number of tumors, perhaps in relation to the nutritional state of the population (30).

The effect of invertebrate hormones on melanotic tumors in *Drosophila* was tested in a series of our early studies. After larvae at appropriate age were ligated posterior to the ring gland, we found (7) that the number of tumors was increased when the flow of hormone was impeded in this manner. In addition, the number of tumors increased in tumor strains into which we crossed the *l(2)gl* gene (6) which brings about a genetic reduction in the production of growth and metamorphosis hormone. It has also been demonstrated that juvenile hormone will increase the number of these tumors (33), whereas administration of both naturally occurring ecdysones and phytoecdysones will diminish the number (14, 15, 38).

When the size of representative puffs and number with tumors were determined after exposure to ecdysones and oncogenic virus both together and separately, it was found that each index puff exhibited an individual pattern of alteration in size and content of RNA and each tumor strain responded uniquely in terms of altered incidence of tumors (14, 15, 17, 18). Exposure to RNA and DNA virus tended to increase the number of tumors and inhibit puffing. Both phytoecdysones and synthetic hormones were tested and each produced its own pattern on puffing at five index loci. Inhibition of the effect of viruses on puffing was also demonstrated when concentration of ecdysones was increased in salivary glands of individuals exposed to oncogenic Rous virus. Maximal effects of hormone on puffing did not necessarily correlate with high dosages. No evidence of incorporation of oncogenic virus into chromosome(s) or passage to subsequent generations was detected. Variants of the virion for CO_2 sensitivity, both *forte* and *faible*, were introduced into tumor strains and tended to reduce the number with tumors. Subtraction or addition of heterochromatin by introducing or removing Y chromosomes in appropriate crosses of special strains did not consistently raise or lower the incidence of tumors when data for aneuploids was compared to diploids (98). We found (8) no consistent correlation between incidence of tumors and fluctuations in mutation rate when genic mutators from Florida stocks were introduced into tumor strains.

TUMOROUS HEAD

The tumorous head strain of *Drosophila* (21) exhibits curious abnormal cephalic growths. Two homozygous genes are responsible for the condition, a semidominant gene, *tu-3*, on the third chromosome and a recessive gene, *tu-1*, on the X chromosome. The latter (*tu-1*) mediates a maternal effect. Many of the males are sterile, but the entire mechanism for this feature remains unexplained since only about 20% of males are aspermic (42). The phenotype represents a striking and variable anomaly which has no features of malignancy. About three-fourths of individuals with the genotype are affected, and both genetic modifiers and environmental conditions such as temperature can alter penetrance.

OVARIAN TUMORS

Two recessive mutants in *Drosophila*, *fused(fu)* and *female sterile (fes)* cause increased numbers of divisions of ovarian cystocytes (32), and the ovarian chambers containing them can amount to as many as 10,000 cells. The rather slow process of mitosis, usually but not always yielding diploid cells, continues with transplantation. However, the cells do not invade the tissues of the host although they may invade the adjacent normal complex of egg-nurse cells in *fused* ovaries. The *fused* gene is pleiotropic, producing abnormality of wing veins as well as ovarian tumors. The *fes* gene acts earlier in ovarian development and when present in the heterozygous condition in *fu/fu* flies, the incidence of tumors is higher than in homozygous *fused* individuals without the *fes* mutant.

The late larval *lethal mutant, lethal tumorous larvae (ltl)*, results in a bloated caudal structure, but this is not associated with a cellular tumor. Zhimulev and Lytchev (43) report this anomaly to be related to abnormality of the sexual apparatus.

BLASTEMA CULTURES

Hadorn and colleagues (28, 29) have performed extensive experiments on blastema cultures transplanted into imaginal abdomens. One culture established from a 6-hr embryo of normal genotype behaved very much like a malignant mammalian neoplasm, invading ovarian follicles and surrounding the gut and malpighian tubules, resulting in death of the host in 10–12 days. These cells were carried in serial cultures *in vivo* in the adult but exhibited no imaginal differentiation when implanted into metamorphosing larva. They usually killed the larval host or disappeared during the pupal stage, although occasionally they could be identified by recovering them from the emerged adult. Bryant and Schubiger (4) reported giant and duplicated imaginal discs in the spontaneous recessive lethal mutant, *lethal (2) giant discs (l(2)gd)*. The increase in size is apparently the result of the usual rate of growth over a prolonged larval period, possibly the result of a primary endocrine defect.

TRANSPLANTABLE TUMORS

Types of tumors which are unquestionably invasive are the groups derived from giant larvae and imaginal discs. These are transplantable and malignant. A series of recessive alleles on the second chromosome cause a defect in the ring gland, alteration in hormonal production, and arrested development (23). The presence of one of these alleles is an obligatory antecedent for the malignant behavior of neuroblastomas derived from the larval brain, but these alleles are not always necessary for this behavior of imaginal discs.

Since Bridges first reported the recessive mutant, l(2)gl, causing a defect in the ring gland resulting in giant larvae and arrested development, more than 50 alleles have been described. Fifteen have been studied in detail by Gateff et al. (23). In two of the alleles, l(2)gl and l(2)gl, Gateff and Schneiderman (24, 25) isolated a transplantable malignant neuroblastoma and neoplastic imaginal discs from the presumptive adult optic center of the larval brain (22). With the exception of l(2)gl^{558} the brain and imaginal discs of these alleles vary in size and shape from the normal pattern (22). The divergence seems roughly correlated with capacity for neoplastic proliferation in situ and when transplanted into the abdomen of adult hosts. The recipients succumb as early as one week after transplantation of some tumor strains, but others are associated with longer survival of the host (25). Some imaginal discs behave in a manner similar to cells from larval brain, also killing the adult recipient. Other discs are smaller or do not grow. Golubovsky and Sokolovsky (27) suggest that mutation rather than diffusion is responsible for the frequency of l(2)gl alleles in natural populations. The viability of heterozygotes is diminished at some temperatures.

SUMMARY

A large number of mutant genes in Drosophila regularly produce cellular aggregates most of which are probably derivatives of hemocytes. These are benign and regress at various times, subsequently leaving melanotic debris as visible evidence of their prior existence. These tumors occur as a result of one or more genes acting from loci on one or more chromosomes. Each strain has characteristic penetrance which is responsive to carcinogens, viruses, hormones, and environmental conditions such as temperature and nutrition. The fes and fu genes produce an excess of ovarian cystocytes in Drosophila and lead to ovarian tumors which may be transplanted but do not invade tissues of the host. Head tumors occur as cephalic malformations which are the result of a somewhat complex system of genetic action. Imaginal discs from which adult organs develop may be abnormal in size, shape, and number in mutant stocks. When blastema cultures have been transplanted serially into the adult abdomen, invasion of host tissues leading to death of the recipient has been reported. A series of mutants on the second chromosome, which alter the normal development of the ring gland with concomitant arrested development in the form of giant larvae, yield tissue from optic center and brain that is invasive when transplanted into adults. These neoplasms, labeled neuroblastomas, have characteristics of malignancies and are frequently capable of killing the host.

Drosophila thus provides interesting biological systems of tumors, benign and malignant, often controlled by genes localized in chromosomes that show some visible evidence of genic action and are responsive to hormones that bring about differentiation and sometimes are involved in the origin and behavior of the tumors. Like most biological systems, the broad outline may appear straightforward, but closer examination can reveal puzzling complexities and leave much to be discovered. Nevertheless, it is intriguing to examine what has been disclosed so far. Even in such a relatively simple genetic system as that in Drosophila, the tumors present a complex picture but do exhibit some parallel responses when compared to those in certain human tumors. It offers biological information of interest in itself and represents an exploitable system for rapid screening of agents and mechanisms possibly related to clinical oncogenesis and therapy. At times a system such as this offers an additional means of selection between various possibilities for subsequent mammalian testing. Although the value of the results obtained in these tumors found in Drosophila in relation to etiology and management of human cancer is unknown and often debatable, the information presented suggests that periodic reexamination of current information about these invertebrate tumor strains and what they may offer in the way of better understanding of atypical growth is worthwhile.

REFERENCES

1. Becker, H. J. (1962): Die Puffs der Speicheldrüsenchromosomen von *Drosophila melanogaster*; II. Die Auslösung der Puffbildung, Ihre Spezifität und Ihre Beziehung zur Funktion der Ringdrüse. *Chromosoma*, 13:341.
2. Beerman, W. (1956): Nuclear differentiation and functional morphology of chromosomes. *Cold Spring Harbor Symp. Quant. Biol.*, 21:217.
3. Bridges, C. G. (1916): Non-disjunction as proof of the chromosome theory of heredity. *Genetics*, 1:107.
4. Bryant, P. J., and Schubiger, G. (1970): Giant and duplicated imaginal discs in a new mutant of *Drosophila melanogaster*. *Dev. Biol.*, 24:233.
5. Burdette, W. J, (1952): Incidence of tumors in isogenic strains. *J. N. C. I.*, 12:709.
6. Burdette, W. J. (1954): Effect of defective ring gland on incidence of tumors in *Drosophila*. *J. N. C. I.*, 15:367.
7. Burdette, W. J. (1954): Effect of ligation of *Drosophila* larvae on tumor incidence. *Cancer Res.*, 14:780.
8. Burdette, W. J. (1954): Effect of the mutator, *high*, on tumor incidence in *Drosophila*, *Cancer Res.*, 14:149.
9. Burdette, W. J. (1954): Heterochromatin and tumor incidence. *Drosophila Information Service*, 28:110.
10. Burdette, W. J. (1954): Penetrance of Tumors in *Drosophila*. *Drosophila Information Service*, 28:109.
11. Burdette, W. J. (1959): Tumors in *Drosophila*. *Biol. Contrib. Univ. Texas. Pub.*, 5914:57.
12. Burdette, W. J. (1964): The significance of invertebrate hormones in relation to differentiation. *Cancer Res.*, 24:521.
13. Burdette, W. J. (1965):P The significance of mutation in relation to the origin of tumors; a review. *Cancer Res.*, 15:201.
14. Burdette, W. J. (1969): Tumors, hormones, and viruses in *Drosophila*. *Natl. Cancer Inst. Monogr.*, 31:303.
15. Burdette, W. J. (1974): *Invertebrate Endocrinology and Hormonal heterophylly*. Springer, New York.
16. Burdette, W. J. (1974): Tumors in *Drosophila* and antibacterial immunity. *Contemp. Prog. Immunobiol.*, 4:283.
17. Burdette, W. J., and Anderson, R. (1965): Conditioned response of salivary-gland chromosomes of *Drosophila melanogaster* to ecdysones. *Genetics*, 51:625.
18. Burdette, W. J., and Kobayashi, M (1969): Response of chromosomal puffs to crystalline hormones *in vivo*. *Proc. Soc. Exp. Biol. Med.*, 131:209.
19. Burdette, w. J., and Olivier, H. R. (1952): Tumor incidence in F$_1$ progeny of tumor strains. *Drosophila Information Service*, 26:94.
20. El Shatoury, H. H. (1955): A genetically controlled malignant tumor in *Drosophila*. *Roux' Arch.*, 147:496.
21. Gardner, E. J. (1970): Tumorous head in *Drosophila*. *Adv. Genet.*, 15:115.
22. Gateff, E., Akai, H., and Schneiderman, H. A. (1974): Correlations between developmental capacity and structure of tissue sublines derived from the eye-antennal imaginal disc of *Drosophila melanogaster*. *Roux' Arch.*, 176:89.
23. Gateff, E., Golubovsky, M. D., and Sokdova, K. S. (1977): Lethal phase, morphology, and developmental capacities of the presumptive adult optic centers in the larval brain and the imaginal discs of fifteen *l(2)gl* alleles and a net *l(2)gl* deficiency. *Drosophila Information Service*, 52: 128.
24. Gateff, E., and Schneiderman, H. A. (1969): Neoplasms in mutant and cultured wild-type tissues of *Drosophila*. *Natl. Cancer Inst. Monogr.*, 31: 365.
25. Gateff, E., and Schneiderman, H. A. (1976): Development capacities of benign and malignant neoplasms of *Drosophila*. *Roux' Arch.*, 176:23.
26. Ghelelovitch, S. (1972): Melanotic tumors in *Drosophila melanogaster*. *Natl. Cancer Inst. Mongr.*, 31:263.
27. Golubovsky, M. D., and Sokolova, K. B. (1973): The expression and interaction of different alleles at the *l(2)gl* locus. *Drosophila Information Service*, 50:124.
28. Hadorn, E. (1969): Proliferation and dynamics of cell heredity in blastema cultures of *Drosophila*. *Natl. Cancer Inst. Monogr.*, 31:363.
29. Hadorn, E., and Schubiger, G. (196): An invasive neoplasm for embryonic cells of *Drosophila melanogaster*. *Drosophila Information Service*, 44: 190.
30. Herskowitz, H., and Burdette, W. J. (1951): Some genetic and environmental influences on the incidence of a melanotic tumor in *Drosophila*. *J. Exp. Zool.*, 117:499.
31. Jones, J. C. (1969): Hemocytes and the problem of tumors in insects. *Natl. Cancer Inst. Monogr.*, 31:481.
32. King, R. C. (1969): Hereditary ovarian tumors of *Drosophila melanogaster*. *Natl. Cancer Inst. Monogr.*, 31:323.
33. Madhaven, K. (1969): Induction of melanotic pseudotumors in *Drosophila melanogaster* by juvenile hormone. *Roux' Archiv.*, 169:323.
34. Oftedal, P. (1953): The histogenesis of a new tumor in *Drosophila melanogaster*, and a comparison with tumors in five other stocks. *Z. Indukt. Abst. Vbgl.*, 85:408.
35. Perotti, M. D., and Bairati, A., Jr. (1968): Ultrastructure of the melanotic masses in two tumorous strains of *Drosophila melanogaster* (*tuB$_3$* and *freckled*). *J. Invertebr. Pathol.*, 10:122.
36. Rotino, A., and Kopac, M. J. (1956): Pathogenesis of spontaneously-occurring and induced melanotic granuloma in *Drosophila melanogaster*. *Prog. Exp. Tumor Res.*, 8:66.
37. Russell, E. J. (1940): A comparison of benign and "malignant" tumors in *Drosophila melanogaster*. *J. Exp. Zool.*, 31:363.
38. Sang, J. H. (1969): Biochemical basis of hereditary melanotic tumors in *Drosophila*. *Natl. Cancer Inst. Monogr.*, 31:291.
39. Schneiderman, H. A. (1969): Control systems in insect development, in *Biology and the Physical Sciences*, p. 187, edited by S. Devons. Columbia University Press, New York.
40. Stark, M. B. (1935): An hereditary lymphosarcoma in *Drosophila*. *Collected Papers N.Y. Med. Coll. Flower Hosp.*, 1:379.
41. Strunge, T., Gigante, D., and Bernhard, W. (1952): Leukemia type hemopathy in Drosophila larvae, studied under the ordinary microscope and the phase contrast microscope, in *Proceedings of the Third International Society of Hematology, Rome*.
42. Woolf, C. M., Knowles, B. B., and Jarvis, M. A. (1964): Genetic analysis of fitness traits in tumorous-head strains of *Drosophila melanogaster*. *Genetics*, 50:597.
43. Zhimulev, I. F., and Lytchev, V. A. (1972): Lethal tumorous larvae. *Drosophila Information Service*, 48:49.

31

Genetic Influences on the Development of Gonadal Tumors in Mice with Emphasis on Teratomas

Leroy C. Stevens

Spontaneous tumors of the gonads of mice are rare. Slye *et al.* (24) found 28 testicular tumors in 9500 mice examined. We have examined tens of thousands of mice for testicular tumors and, except for teratomas, have never encountered one. Other workers at the Jackson Laboratory have been aware of my interest in testicular tumors for the past 23 years and, except for one possible interstitial cell tumor, only 3 or 4 teratomas have been brought to my attention.

Mice of the strains A and BALB/c are particularly susceptible to interstitial cell tumors of the testis after prolonged treatment with estrogens (1, 4, 11), but only a few spontaneous tumors have been observed in these strains (12, 13). Franks (10) found two spontaneous tumors in the same testis of a C3H/He mouse. One was an interstitial cell tumor, and the other resembled a typical Sertoli cell tumor.

Ovarian tumors occur only sporadically in most inbred strains (16, 20). Incidences of 34% and 47% have been reported for strains CE and C3HeB/De females (5, 7). Bielschowsky and D'Ath (3) and Whitten (personal communication) have found spontaneous ovarian tumors in other strains. The most common types are granulosa cell tumors and tubular adenomas, and these occur in only a few inbred strains (16). Granulosa cell tumors may be induced in sensitive strains of mice by a variety of methods including X-irradiation, transplantation of ovaries to the spleen and other sites, by remotely or directly applied chemical carcinogens (16, 17)

and by genetic deletion of ova (21, 23). Disappearance of the oocytes precedes the development of tumors by all of these methods.

Inbreeding is a genetic process and variation in tumor incidence between inbred strains constitutes evidence that genetic factors are involved.

Susceptibility to most kinds of tumors in mice is known to be determined by multiple genetic factors. There are a few cases where the effects of single genes have been identified in gonadal tumorigenesis.

A particularly striking example of the role of single genes in ovarian tumorigenesis is described by Russell and Fekete (23) and Murphy (21). All mice homozygous for viable alleles of dominant spotting (*W*) have granulosa cell tumors and complex tubular adenomas at an early age. These tumors are associated with complete oocyte deficiency, and homozygotes are born with very few or no oocytes. This system of ovarian tumor development emphasizes the dominant role played by the presence of viable oocytes, and of normal follicular development and function in the orderly differentiation of the ovary. This genetic model has the great advantage that neither the host mouse nor the tissue itself is subjected to any experimental agent, such as X-irradiation or chemical carcinogens.

Another striking example of the role of genes on gonadal tumorigenesis is the influence of several genes on the development of the spontaneous testicular teratomas that occur with pre-

467

dictable frequencies in sublines of strain 129. One-third of the males of strain 129/Sv-ter have spontaneous congenital teratomas (27).

Only three cases of testicular teratoma have been reported except in inbred strain 129 (18). This indicates that strain 129 has a combination of genes that is unique in determining susceptibility to teratocarcinogenesis. Some of the genes have been identified, and they have been useful in gaining an understanding of teratocarcinogenesis in the testes of mice.

Teratomas are different from other kinds of tumors in that they are composed of many kinds of well differentiated immature and mature tissues as well as the undifferentiated stem cells that are responsible for their growth (8, 22). The teratomas may contain neural tissue, muscle, cartilage, bone with functioning marrow, many kinds of epithelia including skin with hair and sebaceous glands and gut with muscularis, pigment and other kinds of cells (Figs. 31.1–31.7). These cells and tissues are chaotically arranged, but there are some frequently observed tissue associations. Skeletal muscle is frequently attached to cartilage or bone (Fig. 31.7). In freshly killed animals, muscular movement may be observed in teratomas. Ciliary movement may be observed in cysts. In all respects except for their disorganization, mature teratomatous tissues are normal and benign yet they are derived from potentially malignant cells (Fig. 31.8).*

Most teratomas in mice become benign and stop growing in animals at about 1 month of age. All of the stem cells differentiate and proliferation ceases. Occasionally the teratomas are malignant. They may metastasize, usually to the left renal lymph node. Several have been maintained indefinitely as progressively growing serially transplantable tumors (see below).

Usually all of the cells of teratomas in adults are differentiated. In 10-day-old males, however, they contain immature neural and other types of tissues. In mice 2 or 3 days of age the teratomas all appear to be in about the same stage of development and their composition is simple. They are composed of disorganized ectodermal and endodermal epithelial cysts with mesodermal cells between them.

When teratomas were first observed in strain 129 mice, only about 1.0% of the males were affected (28). The tumors in neonatal mice are microscopic and it was necessary to examine many serially sectioned testes to find a tumor. We attempted to increase the incidence of tera-

---

* *Editor's note:* See the last paragraph on page 837 for a comparison of the same principle in plants.

tomas to make a developmental investigation of these tumors feasible. One approach was to introduce mutant genes onto the strain 129 genetic background. The gene A^Y was selected because it had been shown to increase the incidence of other kinds of tumors (6, 32). A strain 129 mouse was mated to a C57BL/6 mouse carrying the A^Y (yellow) allele. The A^Y progeny were backcrossed to strain 129 and the A^Y progeny in the next generation were again backcrossed to strain 129. This sequence was continued for eight backcross generations. The incidence of teratomas in the A^Y mice (4/420) was only about $\frac{1}{10}$ of that in their normal littermates (35/437), indicating that the agouti locus or a very closely linked locus was involved in the susceptibility to teratocarcinogenesis of the testis.

Another gene, steel (Sl^J), was introduced onto the strain 129 genetic background. One of the most plausible explanations for the origin of teratomas was that they arose from germ cells, and the Sl^J/Sl^J genotype profoundly affects their development. $Sl^J/+$ animals are fertile, and twice as many of them had teratomas as their $+/+$ littermates (29). We do not yet understand how a single dose of Sl^J affects tumor incidence.

After the discovery that Sl^J increases the incidence of teratomas it became feasible to perform a developmental study of the microscopic prenatal tumors. They were easily identified in fetuses as young as 15 days of gestation but not younger. All of the tumors were located within the seminiferous tubules which indicated that they were derived from a component of the tubules; either the primordial germ cells or cells that would differentiate into Sertoli cells. The earliest recognizable teratomas were composed of clumps of undifferentiated embryonal cells (Fig. 31.9). Usually a cavity developed in the clump and the surrounding cells were oriented around it. They resembled the ectoderm surrounding the proamniotic cavity of normal 5-day embryos.

All of the teratomas in fetal mice of a given day of gestation were at about the same stage of development. In order to pinpoint the day of gestation when these tumors initiated development, we measured the size of the tumors in newborns, 18-, 17-, 16-, and 15-day fetuses. This made it possible for us to estimate that the tumors originated in the genital ridge at about the 12th day of gestation (Fig. 31.6).

We grafted 12-day strain 129 genital ridges to the liver, spleen, and testes of adults to see whether they would develop into testes with teratomas. Male genital ridges grafted to the liver

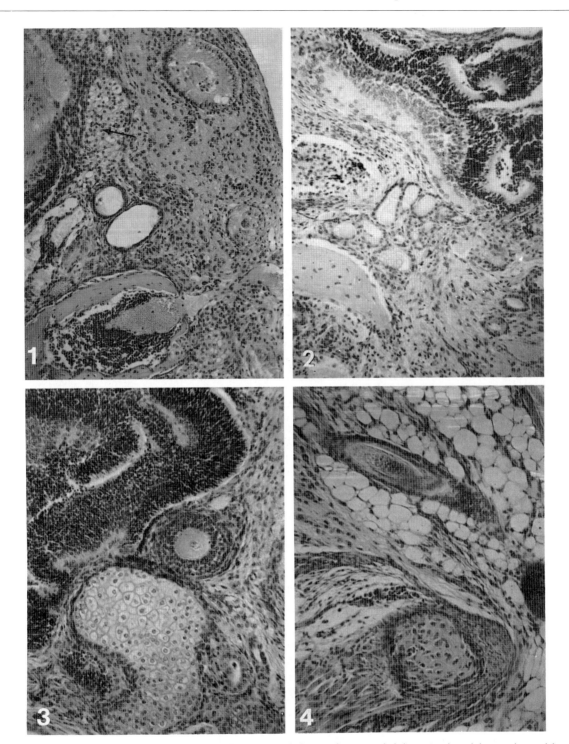

Figure 31.1. Seminiferous tubule surrounded by neural tissue (*upper right*), notochord (*arrow*), and bone with marrow (*lower left*).

Figure 31.2. Thyroid (*center*), neural tissue (*upper right*), and bone (*lower left*).

Figure 31.3. Neural tissue and cartilage.

Figure 31.4. Adipose tissue (*upper right*), hair follicle, and muscle attached to cartilage (*lower left*).

and spleen developed into testes and few of them had teratomas. In contrast, when genital ridges were grafted to the testis, most of them developed into testes with teratomas. We then had a method of experimentally inducing tera-

tomas in the mouse, and we were able to use it to find out more about the nature of teratocarcinogenesis.

When 13-day and older strain 129 genital ridges were grafted to the testis, they developed

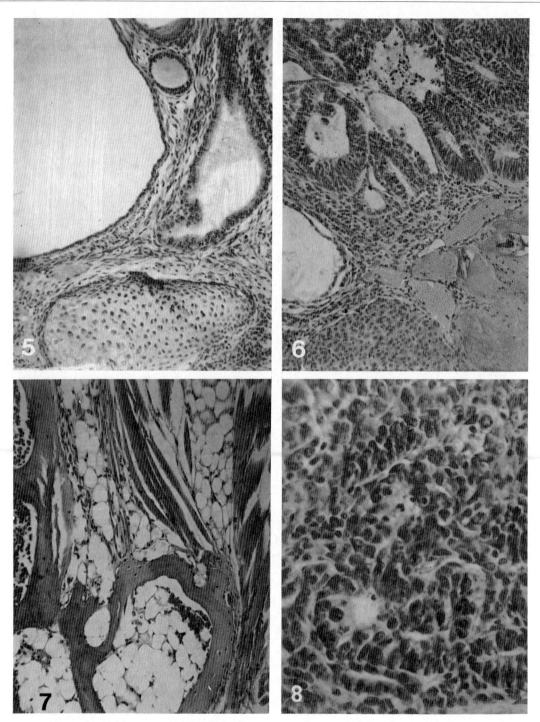

Figure 31.5. Ciliated/epithelium and cartilage.
Figure 31.6. Immature neuroepithelium (*upper*) and trophoblastic giant cells (*lower right*) in an ovarian teratoma.
Figure 31.7. Skeletal muscle attached to bone.
Figure 31.8. Undifferentiated embryonal cells. Note incipient epithelium formation (*lower left*).

into normal looking testes but only a few had teratomas. By the 14th day of gestation, a developmental change occurs in the genital ridge that makes it resistant to the formation of teratomas.

When 12-day genital ridges of other strains of mice were grafted to the testis, some developed into testes with high incidence of teratomas, some were intermediate, some low, and others were refractory to the process of teratocarcinogenesis.

The incidence of induced teratomas in strains 129 and A/He was high. However, when genital

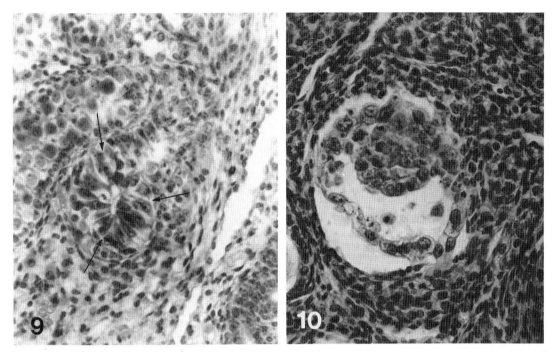

Figure 31.9. Early stage in development of a testicular teratoma. Embryonal cells (*arrows*) oriented around a central lumen within a seminiferous tubule of a 16-day fetus.

Figure 31.10. Early stage in development of an ovarian teratoma. Note similarity to normal blastocyst with outer layer of trophectoderm and, inner cell mass with endoderm formation facing segmentation cavity.

ridges from F_1 hybrid fetuses were grafted to the testis, the incidence was higher than either parental strain (26). This is interesting in view of the fact that we have examined testes of tens of thousands of F_1 hybrid adults and we have never observed a spontaneous teratoma.

When genital ridges of susceptible strains were grafted to nonscrotal sites, the incidence of teratomas was low compared to that in grafts to scrotal sites. When one of a pair of genital ridges was grafted to a scrotal testis and the other was grafted to a testis made cryptorchid surgically, there was a marked difference in the incidence of tumor formation. For strain A/He, 43% of the testes that developed in the scrotal testis had teratomas compared with 3% of those grafted to the cryptorchid testis in the same host (26). This indicated that the temperature of the graft site might be involved in the teratocarcinogenetic process. To examine this, we grafted genital ridges to the testes of adults which were housed in an incubator maintained at 37°C. This made it impossible for the scrotal testis to be cooler than body temperature. A low proportion of the testes developed with teratomas, again indicating that temperature was involved in experimentally induced teratocarcinogenesis.

The discovery of an easy experimental method of inducing teratomas enabled us to use

the gene steel to reinvestigate the cell of origin of teratomas. Homozygous *Sl/Sl* animals have very few or no primordial germ cells. If teratomas originate from primordial germ cells, *Sl/Sl* animals should be free of teratomas. *Sl/Sl* fetuses die at about 15 days of gestation. However, when 12-day *Sl/Sl* genital ridges were grafted to adult testes, they survived and developed into sterile testes. None of 75 *Sl/Sl* testes had teratomas compared to 70% (75/194) of their normal *Sl/+* or *+/+* littermates. This genetic evidence supports the morphologic evidence (i.e., all tumors are enclosed within the seminiferous tubules) that teratomas are derived from primordial germ cells (25).

Like steel, alleles at the dominant spotting locus (*W*) also affect the development of germ cells and in the homozygous state results in a phenotype similar to *Sl/Sl*. When *W* was introduced onto the strain 129 genetic background, the incidence of teratomas in *W/+* mice was the same as in their normal littermates. However, at the 8th backcross generation, one pair of mice produced 38 offspring and 8 of them had spontaneous teratomas. This incidence was markedly higher than from other matings we had observed and it proved heritable. The descendants of that mating were bred by brother times sister mating to produce a new inbred subline of strain 129, designated 129/Sv-*ter* (27). One-third of the males of this new subline have spontaneous testicular teratomas. Apparently a mutation had occurred, and the increased incidence is assumed to be due to a single gene designated *ter*. It was shown by reciprocally transplanting ovaries between 129/Sv and 129/Sv-*ter* that the effect of *ter* was on the genotype of the primordial germ cell rather than the maternal environment.

Early in the course of investigating testicular teratomas it became apparent that there was a strong laterality influence (28). There were about twice as many teratomas in the left testis as in the right. There is still no explanation for this laterality influence. However, in an attempt to resolve this problem, the gene situs inversus viscerum (*iv*) which causes left to right transposition of the thoracic and abdominal viscera and associated blood vessels including the origin of the spermatic artery (14) was introduced onto the strain 129 genetic background in order to observe its affect on the laterality of teratomas. The penetrance of *iv* was incomplete. About half of the animals resulting from *iv/iv* × *iv/iv* matings had normally oriented viscera. The other half had reversed viscera. In the normal appearing *iv/iv* males there were about twice as many teratomas on the left as on the right side. In the reversed animals the right side was affected about twice as frequently as the left.[1] It is possible that the difference in the origin of the spermatic artery is causatively related to the reversal of laterality of teratomas.

The undifferentiated stem cells (embryonal carcinoma) of some malignant transplantable teratocarcinomas are totipotent (15, 19). Embryonal carcinoma cells from a transplantable teratocarcinoma designated OTT6050 were injected into the inner cell mass of blastocysts and the resulting mosaic embryos were transferred into the uteri of pseudopregnant females. The embryonal carcinoma cells participated in normal development. The mosaic embryos developed normally in the uterus, were born, and matured. The embryonal carcinoma cells contributed to the formation of all tissues and organs including melanoblasts, hair follicle dermis, erythrocytes, leukocytes of diverse kinds, liver, thymus, kidneys, and most striking of all—functional sperm. One male sired hundreds of normal offspring, and they were all derived from sperm which originated from embryonal carci-

noma cells injected into a blastocyst. At the time the cells were injected into the blastocyst, OTT6050 had been a transplantable highly malignant tumor for 8 years and about 200 transplant generations. The orderly expression of many genes occurred *in vivo* after they had been "silent" or undetected in the tumors for 8 years.

The capacity of embryonal carcinoma cells to form normally functional adult tissues demonstrates that conversion to neoplasia did not involve structural changes in the genome, but rather a change in gene expression. Perhaps this nonmutational basis for neoplastic transformation, involving changes in gene expression due to tissue disorganization, may apply to some other malignancies of partially specialized stem cells of particular tissues.

Illmensee[2] transferred embryonal carcinoma cells from a transplantable LT/Sv ovarian teratocarcinoma (see below) into the inner cell mass of blastocysts and obtained mosaic individuals composed of cells derived from the tumor and others from normal cells. One female had offspring derived from ova that originated from the injected tumor cells and other offspring that originated from the normal cells of the inner cell mass. The production of sperm and eggs in mosaics composed of normal and embryonal carcinoma cells demonstrates that embryonal carcinoma cells may be totipotent. Apparently teratocarcinogenesis entails changes in gene function rather than gene structure.

About half of strain LT females have ovarian teratomas at 3 months of age (30). These tumors originate from parthenogenetically activated ovarian ova after the first meiotic division (9). All stages from cleavage to primitive streak formation have been observed. Until the egg cylinder stage, the ovarian embryos appear normal (Fig. 31.10). At about 6 days of gestation, the embryos become disorganized and the cells lose their normal relationships with each other. They are similar in composition to the testicular teratomas described above. They are also similar to the testicular tumors in that most are benign. Occasionally they are malignant and can be maintained as transplantable teratocarcinomas.[1]

When large numbers of virgin strain LT females are examined, about 10% of them are found to be in early stages of pregnancy. The eggs are parthenogenetically activated after ovulation. They undergo cleavage and implant in the uterus. As in the ovary, they appear to de-

---

[1] L. C. Stevens and D. S. Varnum, unpublished data.

[2] K. Illmensee, personal communication.

velop normally to the egg cylinder stage, but then they become disorganized and are expelled from the uterus.

We attempted to "rescue" parthenogenetic embryos by removing them from the uterus and grafting them to the testes of adults. The grafted parthenogenetic cells proliferated and survived indefinitely as teratomatous growths. This means that parthenogenetic cells are viable at the cellular but not the organismic level.

In another attempt to "rescue" parthenogenetic cells, 8-cell pigmented parthenogenetic embryos were fused with normal albino 8-cell embryos and transferred to the uteri of pseudopregnant females (2, 31). Chimeric mice with pigmented and white hairs were produced. They were also chimeric with respect to alleles at the glucose-phosphate-isomerase-1 locus.

Chimeric females were mated to normal albino males. One produced five litters of albino offspring indicating that they were derived from ova from the normal member of the chimera. In the sixth litter there were 3 albino and 2 pigmented offspring. The pigmented offspring must have been derived from ova that developed from the parthenogenetic cells.[1] Parthenogenetic cells survived and participated in normal development. It is still a mystery why parthenogenetic embryos will not survive *in utero*.

In an effort to identify genetic factors involved in parthenogenesis and ovarian teratocarcinogenesis, strain LT mice were crossed with mice of several other inbred strains. When crossed to C57BL/6 about 6% of the offspring had ovarian teratomas. Teratomas were not observed when LT mice were crossed with other strains. Apparently C57BL/6 is genetically different from other strains with respect to susceptibility to ovarian teratocarcinogenesis.

We attempted to combine genes that were responsible for susceptibility to ovarian teratocarcinogenesis by creating recombinant inbred strains derived from strains LT/Sv and C57BL/6. Twenty-six pairs of F_1 hybrids were mated brother times sister. All subsequent generations were also mated brother times sister. One strain designated LTXBJ had a higher incidence of teratomas than any of the other strains involved including the original strain LT/Sv. Apparently a gene or genes had been fixed from C57BL/6 that was lacking in LT/Sv that increased the susceptibility to ovarian teratocarcinogenesis.

Spontaneous and induced gonadal tumors in general are strain specific indicating that there is a genetic basis for susceptibility. In most cases susceptibility has shown to be influenced by multiple genes. In a few cases, however, single genes have been identified which affect their development.

Acknowledgment. The Jackson Laboratory is fully accredited by the American Association of Laboratory Animal Care. The work was supported by research grant CA02662 from the National Cancer Institute.

References

1. Andervont, H. B., Shimkin, M. B., and Canter, Y. (1960): Susceptibility of seven inbred strains and the F_1 hybrids to estrogen-induced testicular tumors and occurrence of spontaneous testicular tumors in strain BALB/c mice. *J.N.C.I.*, 25:1069–1082.
2. Azim, H. S., Barton, S. C., and Kaufman, M. H. (1977): Development to term of chimaeras between diploid parthenogenetic and fertilized embryos. *Nature*, 270:601–602.
3. Bielschowsky, M., and D'Ath, E. F. (1973): Spontaneous granulosa cell tumors in mice of strains NZC/BI, NZO/BI, NZY/BI and NZB/BI. *Pathology*, 5:303–310.
4. Bollengier, W. E., Eisenfeld, S. J., and Gardner, W. U. (1972): Accumulation of ^{3}H-estradiol in testes and pituitary glands of mice of strains differing in susceptibility to testicular interstitial cell and pituitary tumors after prolonged estrogen treatment. *J.N.C.I.*, 49:847–852.
5. Deringer, M. K. (1959): Occurrence of tumors, particularly mammary tumors in agent-free mice. *J.N.C.I.*, 22:995–1002.
6. Deringer, M. K. (1970): Influence of the lethal-yellow (A^Y) gene on development of reticular neoplasms. *J.N.C.I.*, 45:1205–1210.
7. Dickie, M. M. (1954): The use of F_1 hybrid and backcross generations to reveal new and/or uncommon tumor types. *J.N.C.I.*, 15:791–799.
8. Dixon, F. J., Jr., and Moore, R. A. (1953): Testicular tumors; a clinicopathological study. *Cancer*, 6:427–454.
9. Eppig, J. J., Kozak, L. P., Eicher, E. M., and Stevens, L. C. (1977): Ovarian teratomas in mice are derived from oocytes that have completed the first meiotic division. *Nature*, 269:517–518.
10. Franks, L. M. (1968): Spontaneous interstitial cell tumors of a testis in a C3H mouse. *Cancer Res.*, 28:125–127.
11. Heston, W. E. (1963): Genetics of neoplasia, in *Methodology in Mammalian Genetics*, pp. 247–268, edited by W. J. Burdette. Holden-Day, San Francisco.
12. Hooker, C. W., Strong, L. C., and Pfeiffer, C. A. (1946): A spontaneous transplantable testicular tumor in a mouse. *Cancer Res.*, 6:503.
13. Hummel, K. P. (1954): A spontaneous transplantable testis tumor in a mouse. *Cancer Res.*, 1:21.
14. Hummel, K. P., and Chapman, D. B. (1959): Visceral inversion and associated anomalies in the mouse. *J. Hered.*, 50:9–13.
15. Illmensee, K., and Mintz, B. (1976): Totipotency and normal differentiation of single teratocarcinoma cells cloned by injection into blastocysts. *Proc. Natl. Acad. Sci. U.S.A.*, 73:549–589.
16. Jull, J. W. (1973): Ovarian tumorigenesis. *Methods Cancer Res.*, 7:131–186.
17. Krarup, T. (1970): Effect of 9,10-dimethyl-1,2-benzanthracene on the mouse ovary. Ovarian tumorigenesis. *Br. J. Cancer*, 24:168–186.
18. Meier, H., Myers, D. D., Fox, R. R., and Laird, C. W. (1970): Occurrence, pathologic features, and propagation of gonadal teratomas in inbred mice and rabbits. *Cancer Res.*, 30:30–34.
19. Mintz, B., and Illmensee, K. (1975): Normal genetically mosaic mice produced from malignant teratocarcinoma cells. *Proc. Natl. Acad. Sci. U.S.A.*, 72:3585–3589.
20. Murphy, E. D. (1966): Characteristic tumors, in *Biology of the Laboratory Mouse*, pp. 521–562, edited by E. L. Green. McGraw-Hill, New York.
21. Murphy, E. D. (1972): Ovarian tumors in W^v/W^v mice. *J.N.C.I.*, 48:1288.
22. Pierce, G. B. (1967): Teratocarcinoma; model for a developmental concept of cancer, in *Current Topics in Developmental Biology*, Vol. 2, pp. 223–246, edited by A. A. Moscona. Academic Press, New York.
23. Russell, E. S., and Fekete, E. (1958): Analysis of W-series pleiotropism in the mouse; effect of W^v/W^v substitution on definitive germ cells and on ovarian tumorigenesis. *J.N.C.I.*, 21:365–381.
24. Slye, M., Holmes, H. F., and Wells, H. G. (1919): Primary spontaneous tumors of the testicle and seminal vesicles in mice and other animals; XII. Studies on the incidence and heritability of spontaneous tumors in mice. *J. Cancer Res.*, 4:207–228.
25. Stevens, L. C. (1967): Origin of testicular teratomas from primordial germ cells in mice. *J.N.C.I.*, 549–552.
26. Stevens, L. C. (1970): Experimental production of testicular teratomas in mice of strains 129, A/He, and their F_1 hybrids. *J.N.C.I.*, 44:923–929.
27. Stevens, L. C. (1973): A new inbred subline of mice (129/terSv) with a

high incidence of spontaneous congenital testicular teratomas. *J.N.C.I.,* 50:235–242.

28. Stevens, L. C., and Little, C. C. (1954): Spontaneous testicular teratomas in an inbred strain of mice. *Proc. Natl. Acad. Sci. U.S.A.,* 40:1080–1087.

29. Stevens, L. C., and Mackensen, J. A. (1961): Genetic and environmental influences on teratocarcinogenesis in mice. *J.N.C.I.,* 27:443–453.

30. Stevens, L. C., and Varnum, D. S. (1974): The development of teratomas from parthenogenetically activated ovarian mouse eggs. *Dev. Biol., 37:* 369–380.

31. Stevens, L. C., Varnum, D. S., and Eicher, E. M. (1977): Viable chimaeras produced from normal and parthenogenetic mouse embryos. *Nature,* 269:515–517.

32. Vlahakis, G., and Heston, W. E. (1971): Spontaneous cholangiomas in strain C3H-A^{vy} mice and their hybrids. *J.N.C.I., 46:*677–683.

32

Influence of the Major Histocompatibility Complex (H-2) on Oncornavirus-induced Neoplasia in Mice

Bruce Chesebro

INTRODUCTION

The influence of the mouse major histocompatibility gene complex (H-2) on virus-induced leukemia was first confirmed in studies of Gross virus leukemogenesis (22). H-2 has since been shown to influence a number of other oncornavirus-induced tumor systems (23). The following specific questions are now of particular concern: Do the same genetic subregions of H-2 influence virus-induced leukemia in different systems? Do genetic effects which map at similar locations have similar mechanisms of action? What are the mechanisms of H-2-associated influence on leukemia and other tumors?

Since the initial observations of the influence of H-2 on leukemia, knowledge of the genetic complexity of H-2 has expanded considerably (18, 35). The identification of recombinations within the H-2 complex has made genetic mapping possible. So far H-2 has been divided into 10 subregions, each identifiable by marker loci. Correlation of different H-2 subregions with biological phenomena has helped considerably in dissection of many aspects of cellular interactions involved in the immune response. As knowledge about the functions of H-2 subregions increases, it is likely that precise genetic localization of H-2-associated genes involved in leukemogenesis will lead to additional ideas concerning the mechanisms of action of these genes.

GENETIC MAPPING OF H-2-ASSOCIATED GENES

H-2-associated resistance to Gross leukemia virus was first demonstrated in a C3H × C57BL F_2 cross (1). $H-2^{b/b}$ and $H-2^{b/k}$ mice had a much lower incidence of leukemia than $H-2^{k/k}$ mice. It was subsequently shown that $H-2^{a/a}$, $H-2^{k/k}$, and $H-2^{d/d}$ mice were highly susceptible to Gross virus leukemogenesis, and $H-2^{b/b}$ mice were highly resistant (20, 22) (Table 32.1). The H-2-associated gene responsible for these effects was called Rgv-1 (resistance to Gross virus-1). The location of the Rgv-1 gene within the H-2 complex was studied by testing two mouse strains, HTH and HTI, with genetic recombinations within H-2 (20). These strains differed markedly in incidence of leukemia after Gross virus inoculation (96% and 8%, respectively). In both strains the recombination position was between the H-2S and H-2D regions, and thus the Rgv-1 gene appeared to be located to the left of the H-2D region as shown in Figure 32.1. More precise mapping studies will be necessary to determine the exact location of this gene within the H-2 complex.

More recently Sato et al. (34) demonstrated H-2-associated resistance to leukemia-associated transplantation antigens (X.1 system). In this model H-2 recombinant strains HTI and HTG were crossed with BALB/c mice, and the F_1

475

Table 32.1
Influence of Different H-2 Haplotypes on Oncornavirus-induced Primary Tumor Incidence

Virus	Primary Tumor Incidence of H-2 Haplotypes		Gene Position within H-2	References
	High	Low		
Friend leukemia	a,d	b,q,s	H-2D	11, 13, 19
Mammary tumor	f,a,d,k,r	b,q	H-2D	29
Kaplan-radiation leukemia	q,s,k	d,a,b	H-2D	28
Balb/Tennant-leukemia	d,a,k	b	?	38, 39
A-radiation leukemia	b,d,k,r	s	H-2I (A,B,J)	25
Gross leukemia	a,k,d	b	H-2K, H-2I, H-2S	20, 22
Rous sarcoma	a,b	s,d	?	15, 41

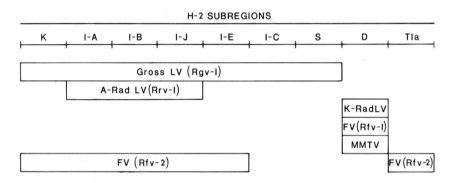

Figure 32.1. Possible map positions of H-2-associated genes influencing oncornavirus-induced neoplasia. *Bars* denote possible map positions of H-2-associated genes influencing oncornavirus-induced neoplasia in mice. *Smaller bars* indicate more precise gene localization. Data from references as follows: Gross LV (Rgv-1 gene), Ref. 20; A strain-Radiation LV, Ref. 25; Kaplan strain-Radiation LV, Ref. 28; Friend virus (Rfv-1 and Rfv-2 genes), Refs. 11 and 13; mouse mammary tumor virus, Ref. 29. *Note added in proof:* The H-2G region was previously defined by a marker only expressed in certain mouse strains, and could not be typed in H-2^d or H-2^a haplotypes. Recent data indicated that this marker was actually located in the H-2S region (15a, 42). Thus there is now no evidence for the existence of the H-2G region.

offspring were found to differ in resistance to transplantation of a BALB/c radiation-induced leukemia cell line (RL♂1). These results indicated that the H-2 region responsible for resistance was located to the left of the H-2D region, i.e., somewhere between H-2K and H-2S. Since this location was the same as that of the Rgv-1 gene (Fig. 32.1), the authors suggested that Rgv-1 was probably responsible for the effect observed in the X.1 system. Further analysis of both the Gross virus and X.1 systems would be highly desirable in order to locate more accurately the positions of the gene(s) involved, as well as to provide evidence concerning their possible identity.

Recovery from Friend virus (FV)-induced erythroleukemia was strongly influenced by H-2-associated genes (19). H-2$^{a/b}$ and H-2$^{d/b}$ genotypes were associated with a low incidence of recovery, and the H-2$^{b/b}$ genotype predisposed to high recovery incidence (Table 32.1). Genetic mapping studies (13) indicated that the predom-

inant effect in this system was due to a gene (Rfv-1) located in the H-2D region (22) (Fig. 32.1). Precise localization of this gene was possible since a number of different H-2 recombinants were tested. The results showed that the main H-2 effects in the Gross virus and Friend virus systems were mediated by genes located in different positions. A second H-2-associated gene which influenced recovery from FV leukemia also has been identified (11). This gene, Rfv-2, was located either in the H-2K, H-2I or Tla region (Fig. 32.1). The Rfv-2 effect was seen in H-2D$^{d/b}$ mice (low recovery) but was not noted in H-2D$^{b/b}$ mice (high recovery). Therefore, it seemed likely that Rfv-2 had a much weaker effect on recovery than Rfv-1. Complementation between these two genes did not appear to be important in the strains studied.

Resistance to transplantation of an FV-induced erythroleukemia cell line from BALB.G mice also appeared to be influenced by a gene in the H-2D region (3). BALB.G mice (H-2$^{g/g}$) could reject this tumor, however congenic (BALB.G × BALB/c)F$_1$ mice (H-2$^{g/d}$) could not. BALB.G and the F$_1$ hybrid mice are identical (d/d genotype) at all H-2 subregions except H-2D. BALB.G are H-2D$^{b/b}$, and (BALB.G × BALB/c)F$_1$ are H-2D$^{b/d}$ (22). Since these same H-2D genotypes also gave rise to the different Rfv-1 recovery phenotypes, it seemed likely that Rfv-1 was the main H-2-associated gene involved in influencing rejection of the FV-induced BALB.G leukemia cells.

Mouse mammary tumor virus (MMTV) oncogenesis was also influenced by a gene located in the H-2D region (Fig. 32.1) (29). Susceptibility and resistance associated with different H-2 alleles appeared to be similar to that seen in the FV system (Table 32.1). It is unclear at the present time whether the same gene is involved in both the FV and MMTV systems.

Susceptibility to leukemia induced by the Kaplan strain of radiation leukemia virus (K-RadLV) has been known for some time to be influenced by H-2 (16). Genetic mapping studies by Meruelo et al. (28) indicate that a single gene located in the H-2D region was involved (Fig. 32.1). H-2$^{q/q}$, H-2$^{k/k}$, and H-2$^{s/s}$ mice were susceptible to leukemogenesis, and H-2$^{d/d}$, H-2$^{a/a}$, and H-2$^{b/b}$ mice were resistant (Table 32.1). These observations were most interesting for two reasons. First, this gene was located in the same region as the Rfv-1 gene and the gene influencing MMTV. This suggested that a common gene might influence the RadLV, FV, and MMTV systems. Second, the H-2 genotypes most resistant to RadLV (H-2$^{d/d}$ and H-2$^{a/a}$) were the most susceptible genotypes to FV and MMTV (Table 32.1). Thus, either the different H-2 genotypes show a great deal of selectivity in terms of their effects on different viruses, or within the H-2D region there are several different but closely associated genes which influence oncornavirus-induced neoplasia (Fig. 32.1).

Using the A strain of radiation leukemia virus (A-RadLV), Lonai and Haran-Ghera (25) found H-2-associated resistance to leukemia which was quite different from that reported for the Kaplan RadLV (28). H-2$^{b/b}$, H-2$^{d/d}$, H-2$^{k/k}$, and H-2$^{r/r}$ mice were susceptible to A-RadLV leukemogenesis, and H-2$^{s/s}$ mice were resistant (Table 32.1). Mapping studies suggested that the gene involved (Rrv-1) was located in the H-2I-A, H-2I-B, or H-21-J regions (Fig. 32.1). Since the Kaplan-RadLV and A-RadLV strains were derived independently by different procedures, the apparent contradiction in the results of these two groups is likely due to the differences in the viruses used.

As shown in Figure 32.1, the combined genetic mapping data on H-2-associated genes which influence oncornavirus-induced neoplasia in mice suggests the presence of at least two separate genes or clusters of genes within the H-2 complex. One is in the H-2D region, and another in the H-2K and H-2I regions. The presence of these clusters may indicate that either the same gene can operate in several different virus systems or that groups of separate genes with similar functions exist in each cluster. One possible implication from either of these situations is that the genes within each group may operate through similar mechanisms.

H-2-associated effects on tumor incidence have been noted in four other oncornavirus-induced tumor systems. In the B/T-L virus (Balb/Tennant-leukemia) model, H-2$^{b/b}$ was resistant, and H-2$^{d/d}$, H-2$^{a/a}$, and H-2$^{k/k}$ were susceptible (Table 32.1) (38, 39). Studies of spontaneous leukemia (?endogenous MuLV-induced) in (BALB/c × AKR)F$_1$ × AKR backcross mice indicated that H-2$^{k/k}$ mice had a higher incidence of leukemia than H-2$^{k/d}$ mice (24). In the Rous sarcoma virus (RSV) system in mice H-2$^{s/s}$ and H-2$^{d/d}$ were resistant, and H-2$^{a/a}$ and H-2$^{b/b}$ were susceptible (Table 32.1) (15, 41). Resistance to transplantation of a Moloney leukemia virus-induced H-2$^{a/a}$ lymphoma was found to be greater in H-2$^{a/b}$ than in H-2$^{a/a}$ mice (17, 33). No mapping data were available from any of these systems.

Indirect evidence for an H-2 influence on virus-induced leukemia has also been obtained by several groups. Aoki et al. (1, 2) found that H-2$^{k/k}$ mice had a high incidence of Gross virus soluble antigen (GSA) in their plasma and a low incidence of antibody to Gross virus-induced cell surface antigens compared to H-2$^{b/b}$ mice. Similarly, Nowinski and Doyle (32) found a higher incidence of antibody to endogenous MuLV in H-2$^{u/b}$ mice than in H-2$^{u/u}$ mice. Tucker et al. (40) observed higher titers of endogenous B-tropic MuLV after infection in H-2$^{a/a}$, H-2$^{d/d}$, and H-2$^{k/k}$ mice than in H-2$^{b/b}$ or H-2$^{q/q}$ mice. Except in the Gross virus system these observations have not yet been related to incidence of primary virus induction of tumors.

GENETIC DOMINANCE OF H-2-ASSOCIATED RESISTANCE OR SUSCEPTIBILITY

The genetic dominance of the H-2-associated effects on susceptibility or resistance to leukemia has been studied in heterozygous crosses

Table 32.2
Genetic Dominance of Different H-2 Genotypes in Terms of Relative Tumor Incidence in Oncornavirus-Induced Tumor Models

Virus or Tumor	Relative Tumor Incidence of H-2 Genotypes	Mice Tested	References
Gross LV	k/k > k/b = b/b	C3H × C57BL F$_2$	22
	k/k > k/b	(B10.BR × C57BL)F$_1$ × B10.BR	20
	k/k > > b/b	B10.BR vs. C57BL	20
	d/d > d/b	(BALB/c × C57BL)F$_1$ × BALB/c	20
	d/d > > b/b	B10.D2 vs. C57BL	20
AKR spontaneous leukemia	k/k > k/d	(BALB/c × AKR)F$_1$ × AKR	24
RL♂1 tumor (X.1 antigen)	d/d > d/b	(B10.D2 × BALB/c)F$_1$ vs. (C57BL/10 × BALB/c)F$_1$	34
BALB/Tennant-LV	k/k = k/b > > b/b	C57BL/10 congenic mice	39
	d/d > d/b > > b/b	ʼ ʼ	
	a/a > a/b > b/b	ʼ ʼ	
	d/d > d/k = k/k	ʼ ʼ	
	d/d = a/d > a/a	ʼ ʼ	
Kaplan-Radiation LV	q/q > q/d = d/d	C57BL/10 congenic mice	28
Friend LV	a/a > a/b > > b/b	(C57BL/10 × A)F$_1$ congenic mice	11, 13, 19
Rous sarcoma virus	a/a > a/s > > s/s	A congenic mice	15, 41
	b/b = b/d > > d/d	C57BL/10 congenic mice	
Mammary tumor virus	i/i = i/b > > b/b	C57BL/10 congenic mice	29
YAC tumor (Moloney LV)	a/a > a/b	(A × C57BL)F$_1$ × A	17, 33
HFL/b tumor (Friend LV)	b/d > b/b	BALB congenic mice	3
HFL/g tumor (Friend LV)	g/d > g/g	BALB congenic mice	3

between high and low susceptibility H-2 genotypes in several systems. No clear pattern of results has emerged. Heterozygous mice have shown all three possibilities (susceptibility dominant, resistance dominant, and heterozygotes intermediate) in crosses between different H-2 alleles in different systems, and even within the same system (B/T-L virus) (Table 32.2). One possible unifying concept is illustrated by the situation with FV leukemia (11, 19). The initial FV dose inoculated appears to have a profound effect on the ultimate incidence of recovery from leukemia observed (Table 32.3). By using a wide range of FV doses, H-2$^{b/b}$, H-2$^{a/b}$, and H-2$^{a/a}$ mice can each be distinguished. At a high FV dose (1500 focus-forming units, FFU) H-2$^{b/b}$ mice have a high recovery incidence (76%), and H-2$^{a/b}$ and H-2$^{a/a}$ mice have low recovery incidences (21% and 16%). Thus at this FV dose *low* recovery (susceptibility) appears dominant. However, at a low FV dose (15 FFU) both H-2$^{b/b}$ and H-2$^{a/b}$ mice have high recovery incidences (91% and 81%), and H-2$^{a/a}$ mice have a low recovery incidence (21%). In this case *high* recovery (resistance) appears dominant. At an intermediate FV dose (150 FFU) the recovery incidence of all three H-2 genotypes are distinguishable (H-2$^{b/b}$>H-2$^{a/b}$>H-2$^{a/a}$).

Table 32.3
Effect of H-2 Genotype on Incidence of Recovery from FV-induced Splenomegaly in Congenic F$_1$ Mice

Mouse Strain	H-2 Genotype	FFU Inoculated[a]		
		1500	150	15
(C57BL/10 × A.BY)F$_1$	b/b	34/45(76%)[b]	25/31(81%)	29/32(91%)
(B10.A × A.BY)F$_1$	a/b	7/33(21)%	15/38(40%)	32/39(81%)
(B10.A × A/WySn)F$_1$	a/a	5/31(16%)	8/61(13%)	12/58(21%)

[a] Focus-forming units (FFU) of Friend virus inoculated intravenously.
[b] Number of mice recovered from splenomegaly 60–90 days after FV inoculation/total number of mice inoculated. Value in parentheses = percent recovery.

The above findings with FV suggest that in other systems in which only one virus dose was tested, heterozygotes might appear resistant or susceptible depending on the actual potency of the virus used. The results of studies on Gross virus leukemogenesis in a (B10.BR × C57BL)F$_1$ × B10.BR backcross are in agreement with this possibility (20). In these experiments using virus preparations with a short latent period, H-2$^{k/k}$

and H-2$^{k/b}$ mice both had a high incidence of leukemia. However, with virus preparations having longer latent periods, H-2$^{k/k}$ mice had much higher leukemia incidence than H-2$^{k/b}$ mice. It is likely that in the above experiments the virus inoculum with the shorter latent period contained a higher virus dose than the preparation with the longer latent period. If so, the different responses of the H-2$^{k/b}$ heterozygotes to the two virus preparations might be a result of the different virus doses used. Thus H-2$^{k/b}$ mice would be intermediate between H-2$^{b/b}$ and H-2$^{k/k}$ mice in susceptibility to Gross virus leukemogenesis, since H-2$^{k/b}$ mice had a high leukemia incidence after a high virus dose and a low leukemia incidence after a low virus dose. A similar effect of virus dose on incidence of leukemia has also been seen with B/T-L virus (38). It is possible that H-2 heterozygotes have an intermediate susceptibility in all oncornavirus systems, but that different virus doses must be studied in order to observe this intermediate status. This would explain the apparently contradictory results regarding genetic dominance of H-2-associated effects on resistance to leukemia which have been observed in different model systems (Table 32.2). This hypothesis leaves open the possibility that many of the genes involved in these models may be similar or identical.

NON-H-2 GENES NECESSARY FOR H-2-ASSOCIATED RESISTANCE EFFECTS

H-2-associated resistance to leukemia can be strongly influenced by non-H-2 genes. For both FV and the Kaplan-RadLV, H-2-associated effects have been demonstrated to be completely dependent on single non-H-2 genes (10, 13, 27). Similarly H-2 influence on B/T-L virus-induced leukemia is influenced by non-H-2 gene(s), although the number of genes involved is unknown (39).

In the course of studying resistance to Kaplan RadLV-induced leukemia, Meruelo et al. (27, 28) found that a partially congenic mouse strain B10.AQR(n4) was highly susceptible to leukemia in spite of the fact that this strain had the H-2D$^{d/d}$ genotype usually associated with resistance. Breeding of B10.AQR(n4) mice with B10.A mice (H-2D$^{d/d}$ genotype, resistant to RadLV leukemia) gave rise to F$_1$ progeny which were sus-

ceptible to leukemia. Therefore, the non-H-2 effect seen in B10.AQR(n4) mice appeared to be dominant. Segregation analysis of the F$_2$ generation indicated that the B10.AQR(n4) mice had a single non-H-2 gene (Srlv-1) responsible for increased susceptibility to Kaplan-RadLV and which could override the H-2D$^{d/d}$-associated resistance to Kaplan RadLV. The Srlv-1 gene was not linked to other genes known to influence MuLV leukemogenesis.

Studies of recovery from Friend virus leukemia have also revealed the importance of non-H-2 genes in facilitating the H-2-associated resistance effect. In (C57BL × BALB/c) × C57BL backcross mice the H-2$^{b/b}$ genotype was associated with a high incidence of recovery from FV leukemia (19), but two H-2$^{b/b}$ mouse strains, BALB.B and A.BY, failed to show this resistance (13). When either of these two strains were crossed with C57BL/10 mice, the H-2$^{b/b}$ F$_1$ progeny displayed a high degree of resistance. Subsequent studies of the H-2$^{b/b}$ backcross, (C57BL/10 × A.BY)F$_1$ × A.BY, showed that the dominant C57BL allele of a single autosomal non-H-2 gene (Rfv-3) was necessary for the H-2$^{b/b}$-associated recovery effect (10). In an H-2$^{a/a}$ backcross (low recovery from leukemia), (B10.A × A)F$_1$ × A, the B10.A allele of the Rfv-3 gene, was associated with cure of FV viremia in the presence of ongoing progressive leukemia (12). Thus in H-2$^{a/a}$ mice the presence of the Rfv-3 resistant allele appeared to be sufficient for elimination of viremia, but not sufficient for recovery from leukemia. However, in H-2$^{b/b}$ mice (i.e., in combination with the high recovery H-2-associated Rfv-1$^{b/b}$ genotype) the Rfv-3 resistant allele was found necessary for recovery from both viremia and leukemia. Rfv-3 is not associated with the Fv-1 or Fv-2 genes (12, 23), and its location in the genome is unknown.

Rfv-3 and Srlv-1 appear to be similar since both can override the H-2-associated resistance effects of FV and Kaplan-RadLV respectively. However, they differ in that resistance is dominant for Rfv-3 and susceptibility is dominant for Srlv-1. Possible genetic association between these genes has not yet been examined, and the mechanisms of action of both genes are not known.

MECHANISMS OF H-2-ASSOCIATED INFLUENCE ON LEUKEMIA

The ways in which genes of the H-2 complex influence virus-induced leukemia are not understood. Results from several systems suggest that H-2 influences late events in leukemia, possibly rejection of transformed cells, rather than the early events of oncogenesis. This has been most clearly shown in the FV system where the very short latent period allows a separation of leukemia induction from the process of recovery from leukemia (13, 19). This finding has been supported by the results obtained in studies of resistance to leukemia cell transplantation (3, 17, 33, 34). In view of the role of the host immune response in rejection of many types of tumors (particularly those of viral origin) the influence of H-2 on leukemia has often been ascribed to an influence on the host anti-viral and anti-leukemia cell immune response (1, 15, 19, 25, 31). After the initial documentation of the influence of the H-2I region on the specific immune response to several protein antigens (26), it was hypothesized that the Rgv-1 gene, which may be located in this region, could act as an immune response gene controlling the response to Gross virus antigens (21). This idea was supported by the observation that mice which rejected RL♂1 tumor had high cytotoxic antitumor antibody titers after rejection and that these antibodies passively protected other mice from tumor challenge (34). Unfortunately, these studies were unable to prove that antitumor antibodies were a *cause* rather than an *effect* of the original tumor rejection observed.

In the FV leukemia system the roles of anti-leukemia cell antibody and cell-mediated immunity have been studied. Neutralizing antiviral antibodies and cytotoxic antileukemia cell antibodies appear to be necessary but not sufficient for recovery from leukemia in this system (8, 12). Mice which recover from leukemia have splenic T-lymphocytes which can specifically lyse FV leukemia cells *in vitro* (9). Again the cause-effect relationship between this cell-mediated immunity and recovery from leukemia has not been determined. Nevertheless, all individual mice who recover from leukemia have virus-specific immune T-lymphocytes in their spleens following recovery, regardless of their H-2 genotype (9). There is no H-2-associated inability to make virus-specific cytotoxic T-lymphocytes, only a difference in the incidence with which recovery and immune lymphocytes appear.

Using FV-induced tumors of congenic BALB mice with various H-2 types, Blank et al. (5) have found a strong correlation between primary tumor rejection and appearance of T-lymphocytes as well as non-T lymphocytes which specifically kill FV leukemia cells *in vitro*. Furthermore, this group has found that the T-lymphocytes involved must recognize both viral and H-2-associated antigenic determinants for successful *in vitro* killing to occur, and that viral and H-2-D^b antigens are physically associated both on the cell surface and in the virus particles (4, 6, 7). Possibly leukemia cells with FV antigens in association with H-2-D^b antigens are highly immunogenic and easily eliminated. This might explain the effect of the H-2D (Rfv-1) gene. However, this interpretation would not explain the lower recovery incidences noted in H-2$^{a/b}$ and H-2$^{d/b}$ heterozygotes who have ample H-2-D^b antigen on their leukemia cells, nor would it explain the occurrence of potent cytotoxic T-lymphocytes in recovering H-2$^{a/a}$ mice (9). In addition, these hypotheses probably have no bearing on the role of non-T immune lymphocytes present in the BALB mice after primary tumor rejection. These non-T cells also appear to be important in the tumor rejection phenomenon, and they do not require simultaneous recognition of viral and H-2 antigens on the leukemia cells they kill. In summary, the possibility exists that H-2 influences FV leukemia by its involvement in immune recognition of virus-induced leukemia cells by T-lymphocytes; however this interpretation will undoubtedly require future refinement as additional findings become available.

Another possible mechanism of H-2-associated resistance to leukemia is through the action of "natural killer" cells. These cells which are different from B-lymphocytes, T-lymphocytes and macrophages have been found in the spleens of various mouse strains and can lyse various tissue culture lines of mouse leukemia cells *in vitro* (17). A good correlation has been found between H-2 genotype, the presence of natural killer cells and *in vivo* resistance to leukemia cell transplantation (33).

Since immunosuppression is known to influence susceptibility to virus-induced leukemia (37) and since MuLV is known to have an immunosuppressive action of its own (36), it is tempting to speculate that H-2-associated genes might also act by influencing virus-induced immunosuppression. So far the immunosuppression effects demonstrated have been nonspecific, *i.e.*, reduced immune responsiveness to heterologous antigens such as sheep erythrocytes (14). In some mouse strains this effect appears to be minimal, or at least does not influence the immune response to viral antigens (8). To date there is no data available on the role of antigen-specific suppressor cells in modulating the host susceptibility to leukemia. However, in view of the influence of H-2I subregions on the biology of suppressor lymphocytes (30), it seems likely that this will be an important area for future investigations.

Another possible point of H-2-associated genetic influence on leukemogenesis is on virus growth (and/or viral antigen expression). H-2 was shown to influence expression of plasma Gross soluble antigen (GSA) by Aoki *et al.* (2). Mice with the H-2$^{k/k}$ genotype (susceptible to leukemogenesis) expressed more GSA than mice with the H-2$^{k/b}$ genotype (resistant to leukemogenesis). Tucker *et al.* (40) have shown a striking H-2 influence on titers of B-tropic endogenous MuLV found in the spleens of congenic mice 10 weeks after virus inoculation. In the FV system using congenic F$_1$ mice H-2$^{b/b}$ (high recovery) mice were able to clear FV viremia several days faster than H-2$^{a/b}$ (low recovery) mice (8). All these examples suggest the possibility that H-2-associated genes could influence the rate of spread of MuLV infection *in vivo*, which in turn could influence the ultimate incidence of leukemia observed. However, it is still unclear whether the H-2 influence on virus growth is mediated by immunological mechanisms such as anti-viral antibody or by some non-immunological mechanism such as virus receptors or rate of growth of infected cells.

In conclusion, although much new information is available concerning location of H-2-associated genes which influence virus-induced leukemia in mice, the mechanism(s) of these genetic effects are very poorly understood. Most evidence suggests that H-2 genes influence expression or control of transformed and infected cells rather than the transformation event itself. It seems likely that the host immune response against the virus and viral-induced cellular antigens is an important mediator of H-2 influence. However, nonimmunological mechanisms of influence may also be important.

Acknowledgment. The author thanks Mrs. Helen Blahnik for preparation of the manuscript.

References

1. Aoki, T., Boyse, E. A., and Old, L. J. (1966): Occurrence of natural antibody to the G (Gross) leukemia antigen in mice. *Cancer Res.*, 26: 1415–1419.
2. Aoki, T., Boyse, E. A., and Old, L. J. (1968): Wild-type Gross leukemia virus; II. Influence of immunogenetic factors on natural transmission and on the consequences of infection. *J.N.C.I.*, 41:97–101.
3. Blank, K., and Lilly, F. (1977): Personal communication.
4. Blank, K., and Lilly, F. (1977): Evidence for an H-2/viral protein complex

on the cell surface as the basis for the H-2 restriction of cytotoxicity. *Nature*, 269:808–809.
5. Blank, K., Freedman, H. A., and Lilly, F. (1976): T lymphocyte response to Friend virus-induced tumor cell lines in strains of mice congenic at H-2. *Nature*, 260:250–252.
6. Bubbers, J. E., and Lilly, F. (1977): Selective incorporation of H-2 antigenic determinants into Friend virus particles. *Nature*, 266:458–459.
7. Bubbers, J. E., Blank, K. J., Freedman, H. A., and Lilly, F. (1977): Mechanisms of the H-2 effect on viral leukemogenesis. *Scand. J. Immunol.*, 6: 533–539.
8. Chesebro, B., and Wehrly, K. (1976): Studies on the role of the host immune response in recovery from Friend virus leukemia; I. Anti-viral and anti-leukemia cell antibodies. *J. Exp. Med.*, 143:73–84.
9. Chesebro, B., and Wehrly, K. (1976): Studies on the role of the host immune response in recovery from Friend virus leukemia; II. Cell-mediated immunity. *J. Exp. Med.*, 143:85–99.
10. Chesebro, B., and Wehrly, K. (1977): A single non-H-2 gene is required for H-2$^{b/b}$-associated recovery from Friend virus leukemia in mice. *Adv. Comp. Leuk. Research, Bibl. Haematol.*, p. 69–73, eds. Bentvelzen *et al.*, Elsevier/North Holland Biomedical Press.
11. Chesebro, B., and Wehrly, K. (1978): Rfv-1 and Rfv-2, two H-2-associated genes which influence recovery from Friend leukemia virus-induced splenomegaly. *J. Immunol.*, 120:1081–1085.
12. Chesebro, B., and Wehrly, K. (1979): Identification of a non-H-2 gene (Rfv-3) influencing recovery from viremia and leukemia induced by Friend virus complex *Proc. Natl. Acad. Sci. U.S.A.*, 76:425–429.
13. Chesebro, B., Wehrly, K., and Stimpfling, J. (1974): Host genetic control of recovery from Friend leukemia virus-induced splenomegaly. Mapping of a gene within the major histocompatibility complex. *J. Exp. Med.*, 140: 1457–1467.
14. Friedman, H., and Ceglowski, W. (1971): Immunosuppression by tumor viruses; effects of leukemia virus infection on the immune response, in *Progress in Immunology*, pp. 815–830, edited by B. Amos. Academic Press, New York.
15. Haughton, G., and Whitmore, A. C. (1976): Genetics, the immune response and oncogenesis. *Transplant. Rev.*, 28:75–97.
15a. Huang, C. M., and Klein, J. (1979): Murine H-2.7; its genetics, tissue expression, and strain distribution. *Immunogenetics*, 9:233–243.
16. Kaplan, H. S. (1967): On the natural history of the murine leukemias: presidential address. *Cancer Res.*, 27:1325–1340.
17. Kiessling, R., Petranyi, G., Klein, G., and Wigzell, H. (1975): Genetic variation of *in vitro* cytolytic activity and *in vivo* rejection potential of non-immunized semi-syngeneic mice against a mouse lymphoma line. *Int. J. Cancer*, 15:933–940.
18. Klein, J. (1975): *Biology of the Mouse Histocompatibility-2 Complex.* Springer-Verlag, New York.
19. Lilly, F. (1968): The effect of histocompatibility-2 type on response to the Friend leukemia virus in mice. *J. Exp. Med.*, 127:465–473.
20. Lilly, F. (1969): The role of genetics in Gross virus leukemogenesis. *Bibl. Haematol.*, 36:213–220.
21. Lilly, F. (1971): H-2, membranes and viral leukemogenesis, in *Second International Convocation on Immunology*, Buffalo, N. Y., pp. 103–108, edited by Cohen, S., Cudkowicz, G., and McCluskey, R., Karger, Basel.
22. Lilly, F., Boyse, E. A., and Old, L. J. (1964): Genetic basis of susceptibility to viral leukaemogenesis. *Lancet*, 2:1207–1209.
23. Lilly, F., and Pincus, T. (1973): Genetic control of murine viral leukemogenesis. *Adv. Cancer Res.*, 17:231–277.
24. Lilly, F., Duran-Reynals, M. L., and Rowe, W. P. (1975): Correlation of early murine leukemia virus titer and H-2 type with spontaneous leukemia in mice of the BALB/c × AKR cross; a genetic analysis. *J. Exp. Med.*, 141:882–889.
25. Lonai, P., and Haran-Ghera, N. (1977): Resistance genes to murine leukemia in the I immune response gene region of the H-2 complex. *J. Exp. Med.*, 146:1164–1168.
26. McDevitt, H. O., Deak, B. D., Shreffler, D. C., Klein, J., Stimpfling, J. H., and Snell, G. D. (1972): Genetic control of the immune response. Mapping of the Ir-1 locus. *J. Exp. Med.*, 135:1259–1278.
27. Meruelo, D., Lieberman, M., Deak, B., and McDevitt, H. O. (1977): Genetic control of radiation leukemia virus tumorigenesis; II. Influence of Srlv-1, a locus not linked to H-2. *J. Exp. Med.*, 146:1088–1095.
28. Meruelo, D., Lieberman, M., Ginzton, N., Deak, B., and McDevitt, H. (1977): Genetic control of radiation leukemia virus-induced tumorigenesis; I. Role of the major murine histocompatibility complex, H-2. *J. Exp. Med.*, 146:1079–1087.
29. Mühlbock, O., and Dux, A. (1974): Histocompatibility genes (the H-2 complex) and susceptibility to mammary tumor virus in mice. *J.N.C.I.*, 53:993–996.
30. Murphy, D. B., Herzenberg, L. A., Okomura, K., Herzenberg, L. A., and McDevitt, H. O. (1976): A new I subregion (I-J) marked by a locus (Ia-4) controlling surface determinants on suppressor T lymphocytes. *J. Exp. Med.*, 144:699–712.
31. Nowinski, R. C. (1976): Genetic control of natural immunity to ecotropic

mouse leukemia viruses; immune response genes. *Infect. Immun.*, 13:1098–1102.

32. Nowinski, R. C., and Doyle, T. (1976): Antibody to murine leukemia virus; genetic control linked to the H-2 locus in PL mice. *J. Immunol.*, 117:350–351.

33. Petranyi, G., Kiessling, R., Povey, S., Klein, G., Herzenberg, L., and Wigzell, H. (1976): The genetic control of natural killer cell activity and its association with *in vivo* resistance against a Moloney lymphoma isograft. *Immunogenetics*, 3:15–28.

34. Sato, H., Boyse, E. A., Aoki, T., Tritani, C., and Old, L. J. (1973): Leukemia-associated transplantation antigens related to murine leukemia virus. *J. Exp. Med.*, 138:593–606.

35. Shreffler, D. C., and David, C. S. (1975): The H-2 major histocompatibility complex and the I immune response region; genetic variation, function and organization. *Adv. Immunol.*, 20:125–195.

36. Stutman, O. (1975): Immunodepression and malignancy. *Adv. Cancer Res.*, 22:261–422.

37. Stutman, O., and Dupuy, J. (1972): Resistance to Friend leukemia virus in mice; effect of immunosuppression. *J.N.C.I.*, 49:1283–1293.

38. Tennant, J., and Snell, G. (1966): Some experimental evidence for the influence of genetic factors on viral leukemogenesis. *Natl. Cancer Inst. Monogr.*, 22:61–72.

39. Tennant, J. R., and Snell, G. D. (1968): The H-2 locus and viral leukemogenesis as studied in congenic strains of mice. *J.N.C.I.*, 41:597–604.

40. Tucker, H., Weens, J., Tsichlis, P., Schwarz, R., Hiroya, R., and Donnally, J. (1977): Influence of H-2 complex on susceptibility to infection by murine leukemia virus. *J. Immunol.*, 118:1239–1243.

41. Whitmore, A. C., and Haughton, G. (1975): Genetic control of susceptibility of mice to Rous sarcoma virus tumorigenesis; I. Tumor incidence in inbred strains and F_1 hybrids. *Immunogenetics*, 2:379.

42. Yokota, S., Beisel, K. W., and David, C. S. (1980): The S region controls expression of H-2-7. *Transplantation*, in press.

33

Genetic Tumors in Plants with Special Emphasis on *Nicotiana* Hybrids

Ira H. Ames

INTRODUCTION

Neoplastic growths in plants vary from somewhat exaggerated but self-limiting overgrowths at one extreme to rapidly proliferating non-self-limiting tumors at the other. The latter develop in numerous plant species just as they do in many animals. In such situations the tumor is composed of altered, randomly growing cells that reproduce true to type. The tumor cells become autonomous and thereby gain the ability to direct their own metabolic activities independent of the control mechanisms that regulate the growth of normal cells. There are three major non-self-limiting diseases of plants, each of which has a different and quite distinct etiology. These are: crown gall disease, tumors of viral origin, and genetic tumors. Crown gall is initiated by a specific bacterium, *Agrobacterium tumefaciens*. In addition to the presence of the bacterium, a second requirement for the initiation of the disease is that the plant must suffer a wound. A number of viruses produce tumors in plants, but the wound tumor virus has been studied most extensively (20). This is an RNA-containing virus that is transmitted in nature by insects. As was the case with crown gall, wounding plays an important role in the initiation of this disease.

Crosses between related species of plants, as well as animals, often result in genetic imbalances that, in some instances, lead to the formation of neoplastic growths. Such tumors, which presumably occur because of an upset in the balance between growth and the regulation of growth, have become known as genetic tumors. They arise spontaneously and are not thought to be incited by environmental agents. In animals the best known examples of genetic tumors are the melanomas that form in the F_1 hybrids of certain species of the subgenera *Platypoecilus* and *Xiphophorus* (28) and the melanotic tumors in *Drosophila* (25). An interesting example of this type of tumor in mammals occurs in the cross between *Mus bactrianus* (wild mouse) and *Mus musculus*, an inbred strain of domestic mouse (38). In this case the incidence of tumors in the hybrid is 10-fold higher than is the sum of the parental incidence.

The first report of genetically determined plant tumors was that of Lund and Kjaerskov (40) in 1885. They noted that certain reciprocal hybrids between *Brassica* species were characterized by the presence of root tumors. As indicated in the review by Smith (54), genetic tumors have been subsequently described in a number of plant genera. However, the genus that has been most extensively studied in this respect is *Nicotiana*. Kostoff (34) first reported in 1930 the occurrence of spontaneous tumors in interspecific hybrids of *Nicotiana*. Subsequently, it has been shown that over 30 species hybrids produce spontaneous tumors in entire progeny populations, and that about 25 additional species combinations give variable tumor expression in the F_1 (33, 59). This chapter will be limited to a consideration of tumor formation in *Nicotiana* species hybrids, since little work has been done on spontaneous tumors in other plant genera. It will be further limited to those aspects of tumorigenesis in the *Nicotiana* system that are considered germane for a book of this type.

TUMOR MORPHOLOGY

The gross morphology of genetic tumors in *Nicotiana* hybrids was thoroughly covered by Smith (54); and, therefore, I shall merely summarize his description. Such tumors appear most frequently on mature plants during and after the flowering period. However, they can also be observed on seedlings and young plants. Tumors may appear on stems, leaves, roots, and floral parts, but they usually develop first at leaf scars, leaf axils, the bases of branches, or at the ground line on the main stem. More often than not, nodal tumors make their appearance before there are any signs of internodal tumors. The first morphological indication of tumorigenesis is the appearance of small, light green excrescences, which eventually attain various forms and sizes. Genetic tumors in *Nicotiana* have a tendency to differentiate and organize (see Fig. 33.4), and often shoots bearing fertile flowers originate from the tumor mass. In the largest tumors necrotic areas sometimes develop.

Whitaker (61) reported that tumors formed on the hybrid *Nicotiana glauca* × *Nicotiana langsdorffii* were composed largely of parenchymatous cells associated with scattered vascular elements. At the surface of the tumor mass there were numerous active meristematic areas. Levine (37) essentially confirmed these findings. He noted that tumors of *Nicotiana* hybrids arose from a callus-like mass of parenchymatous tissue with cells frequently filled with starch and other bodies. The fibrovascular elements were poorly developed. Brieger and Forster (24) reported that the first sign of tumor formation in *N. glauca* × *N. langsdorffii* was the activation of cells in tissues between the epidermis and collenchyma. Some cells, adjacent to dead or dying cells, started to divide and later the whole region became activated and the cortical layers degenerated. At this stage the tumors could be quite large, but they lacked connection to the xylem. Subsequently, the cambium and secondary medullary rays developed irregularly but finally connected the tumors with vascular bundles.

Tissue from genetic tumors at an early stage

of development on seedlings of *Nicotiana suaveolens* × *N. langsdorffii* has been examined with the electron microscope (6). Such tumors are composed essentially of three cell types. They are covered by a single layer of epidermal cells including guard cells and trichomes. The majority of cells in the tumors are large, irregularly shaped, highly vacuolated, parenchymal cells (Fig. 33.1). These cells have relatively thin walls with numerous plasmodesmata. The cellular organelles are confined to a layer of cytoplasm which surrounds a large central vacuole. The most conspicuous organelles are the chloroplasts, which are larger and have more extensive lamellar systems than those in the other tumor cell types. These chloroplasts contain few, if any, osmiophilic globules. Mitochondria are not numerous, the endoplasmic reticulum is not extensively developed, and dictyosomes are rare in parenchymal cells. Meristematic cells, which are found in clusters close to the surface of the tumor, are the third cell type (Fig. 33.2). They have large, centrally placed nuclei and a considerably greater nuclear-cytoplasmic ratio than other tumor cells. Mitochondria, which do not differ structurally from those observed in the

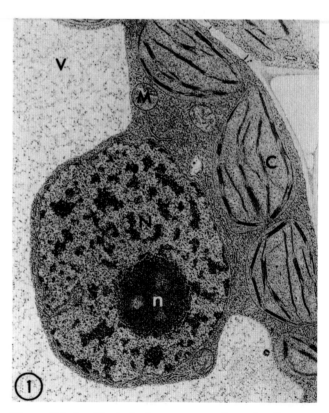

Figure 33.1. Part of a tumor parenchymal cell, showing several chloroplasts (*C*), a few mitochondria (*M*), a portion of the vacuole (*V*), and the nucleus (*N*) with a prominent nucleolus (*n*) (×9,800).

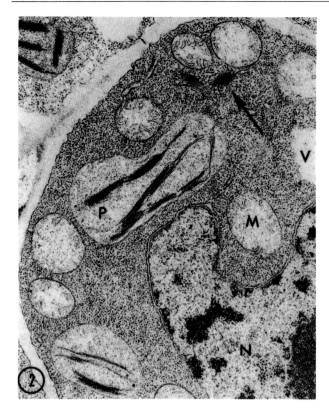

Figure 33.2. Part of a tumor meristematic cell showing numerous mitochondria (*M*), several dictyosomes (*arrow*), two proplastids (*P*), and a portion of the nucleus (*N*) and of the vacuolar system (*V*) (×17,050).

other tumor cell types, are the most prominent of the cytoplasmic organelles. Plastids within meristematic cells are smaller and their lamellar systems are less well developed than in parenchymal cells. They could properly be called proplastids. The cytoplasm is more richly endowed with elements of the rough endoplasmic reticulum, and dictyosomes are more numerous in meristematic cells than in parenchymal cells.

The most significant finding of this study by Ames (6) is that there are no major differences at the ultrastructural level between parenchymal cells of genetic tumors and their normal counterparts from stems without any signs of tumor formation. This is in contrast to the situation reported for crown gall cells (41), in which differences in fine structure between normal mesophyll cells and tumor cells have been reported. Tumor cells induced by *A. tumefaciens* show an extensive development of the endoplasmic reticulum, stimulated activity of dictyosomes, and a more frequent occurrence of multivesicular bodies (41). In other words, bacterial induction transforms mesophyll cells into actively dividing meristematic cells. On the other hand, in the

case of *Nicotiana* hybrid tumors, only some cortical parenchymal cells are transformed into cells that are capable of mitotic activity. These transformed meristematic cells presumably give rise to the parenchymatous cell, which is the major cell type of the tumor mass. Since the epidermal cells of the tumor can divide, one would assume that as the tumor enlarges, cells are added to the surface by division of preexisting epidermal cells.

A membrane-bound inclusion similar to that observed in other plants by numerous investigators (see Ames and Pivorun (12)) was found within plastids of some tumor cells (6). This structure consists of electron-dense granular material which is enclosed by a single membrane. The inclusion is often associated with the thylakoid membrane system (Fig. 33.3) and has become known as the thylakoidal body. The results of a cytochemical investigation indicate that protein is the major chemical constituent of this membrane-bound plastid inclusion (12). This, together with the work of Hurkman and Kennedy (29), supports the view that the thylakoidal body represents stored material utilized in the formation of plastid lamellae.

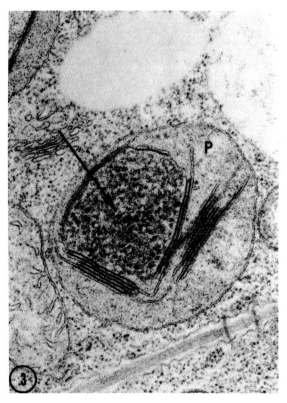

Figure 33.3. A membrane-bound inclusion (*arrow*) within a plastid (*P*) of a tumor meristematic cell (×33,150).

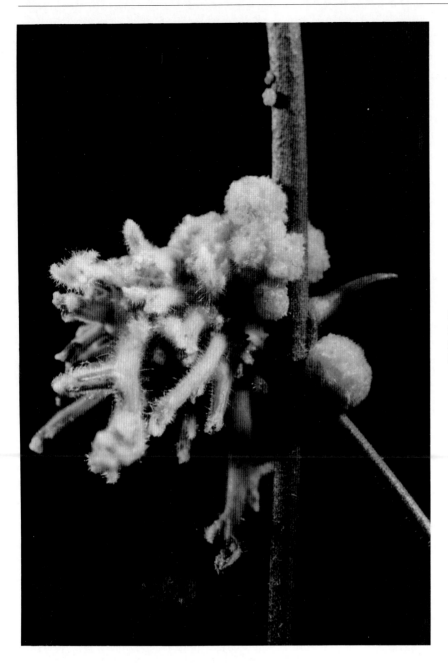

Figure 33.4. Spontaneous tumors formed on the stem of the amphiploid *Nicotiana suaveolens* × *Nicotiana langsdorffii.*

GENETIC CONTROL OF TUMOR FORMATION

Evidence supporting the conclusion that tumor formation in certain *Nicotiana* hybrids is under genetic control is quite good and was most recently reviewed by Smith (54). The following is a synopsis of the major arguments for nuclear gene control of tumorigenesis in this system.

1. More than 300 interspecific hybrids have been reported in the genus *Nicotiana*, but in only about 30 of these are spontaneous tumors produced in all of the progeny. The fact that tumors appear on only certain hybrids is general evidence of genetic control.

2. In spite of the efforts of numerous investigators to do so, it has not been possible to isolate a pathogen from *Nicotiana* hybrid tumors (32). In addition, grafting experiments have failed to reveal the presence of a transmissible agent (1, 33, 35, 56, 57).

3. Tumor formation is the same in reciprocal hybrids (32, 35). This indicates that tumorigenesis is controlled by nuclear elements contributed equally by both parents.

4. Interspecific hybrids are usually characterized by the presence of a complete set of chro-

mosomes from each parental species. It has been shown, however, with one tumor-prone *Nicotiana* hybrid that genetic manipulation of the ratio of genomes does not alter qualitatively the potential to form tumors as long as an appropriate contribution of chromosomes from each parent is present the hybrid (33).

5. Attempts have been made to detect association between tumorigenesis and specific chromosomes. Work with the hybrid *N. glauca* × *N. langsdorffii* (33) demonstrated that tumors do not form on plants with only one or a few *N. glauca* chromosomes on a diploid *N. langsdorffii* background. It has not as yet been shown which of the *N. glauca* chromosomes are required for tumor formation. However, recent unpublished work from Smith's laboratory indicates that the genetic information from *N. glauca* that causes tumors in combination with diploid *N. langsdorffii* resides in any one of two or three chromosomal sites. A similar cytogenetic analysis has been carried out in crosses between *Nicotiana longiflora* and the amphiploid *Nicotiana debneyi-tabacum* (1). In this case it was possible to show that only a single chromosome or a fragment of that chromosome from one parent is sufficient to cause tumor formation when combined with the complete genome of the other parent.

6. The closely related species *N. langsdorffii* and *Nicotiana sanderae* have different effects on tumor formation. On the one hand, *N. langsdorffii* contains genes that enhance tumorigenesis, while the complement of *N. sanderae* seems to inhibit tumor formation (24, 53, 56). By hybridizing *N. langsdorffii* × *N. sanderae* with a variety of other species, Smith and Stevenson (56) were able to demonstrate segregation for the tumor controlling genes.

7. A nontumorous fertile mutant of the tumor-prone amphiploid *N. glauca* × *N. langsdorffii* has been induced with x-rays (30). Smith and Stevenson (56) were able to show that this mutant has the same chromosome number as the parent, is dominant to the tumorous condition, and segregates in the F_2 and first backcross generation.

Initiation of Tumor Formation

Several hypotheses have been put forward to explain the cause of genetically controlled tumors. In 1930 Kostoff proposed that the phenomenon could be explained in terms of an immunological reaction. However, he discarded this postulate in 1943 when he suggested that tumorigenesis in the cross *N. glauca* × *N. langsdorffii* was due to heterogeneity of tissues and abnormal mitoses. Kehr (32) cited considerable evidence which indicated that this hypothesis was inadequate to account for tumor formation in *Nicotiana* hybrids. Whitaker (61) advanced the concept that tumor formation in this system was the result of a cytoplasmic disturbance caused by the introduction of the genome of *N. langsdorffii* as a male into the cytoplasm of *N. glauca*. This explanation can also be ruled out, since it has been demonstrated conclusively that the progeny of the reciprocal cross between these two species do form tumors (32).

Tumors appear most frequently on mature plants during and after the flowering period when growth of the shoot apex is reduced. This observation led Kehr and Smith (33) to point out that active meristematic elongation is inversely related to the development of tumors and to suggest that an alteration in normal metabolic processes, particularly auxin metabolism, is associated with spontaneous tumor formation. It also prompted Whitaker (61) to conclude that when terminal growth ceased, meristematic activity was transferred to other growth centers resulting in tumor formation, and Ahuja (2) to suggest that a shift in hormonal relationships may provide the trigger for abnormal growth.

It has been proposed that the trigger for tumor induction in tumor-prone *Nicotiana* hybrids is a reduction in the endogenous level of auxin (13). There is considerable evidence in support of this hypothesis, and it appears that the mechanism of tumor induction in this system is similar to that by which axillary buds are released from the dominance of the apical meristem. The following is a summary of this evidence.

1. It has been demonstrated that correlative inhibition of axillary buds diminishes as a plant gets older (39). As mentioned above, tumors appear most frequently on mature hybrids during and after the flowering period when growth of the shoot apex is reduced (33).

2. Growth of inhibited axillary buds can be stimulated by decapitation of the apical bud, and this loss of apical dominance can be prevented by applying indoleacetic acid (IAA) to the cut surface of decapitated plants (60). Decapitation of primary and secondary shoots accelerates tumor formation in the *Nicotiana* system, and the appearance of internodal tumors can be suppressed with exogenous IAA (13).

3. Triiodobenzoic acid has been shown to break apical dominance in a variety of plants and to increase tillering in grasses (see Ames (9)). This auxin antagonist also markedly accelerates the rate of tumorigenesis in two tumor-prone *Nicotiana* amphiploids (4).

4. Cytokinins are also capable of releasing axillary buds from apical dominance (49, 51) as well as enhancing tumor formation in genetically tumor-conditioned *Nicotiana* hybrids (7).

5. Gibberellic acid, which is known to increase the amount of extractable or diffusible auxin in a variety of plants (44) and to enhance apical dominance (21, 23, 48), significantly reduces the rate of tumor formation in the amphiploid *N. suaveolens* × *N. langsdorffii* (5).

6. Correlative inhibition of axillary buds is enhanced when plants are grown under low light intensity (45), and the rate of tumorigenesis is reduced when plants are grown under reduced illumination (8).

7. The rate of tumor formation in flask-grown *Nicotiana* seedlings has been decreased significantly by raising them on medium supplemented with IAA (11).

8. There is a close correlation in time between the decline in endogenous level of IAA and onset of tumor formation in seedlings of a tumor prone *Nicotiana* amphiploid grown on nutrient medium in a growth chamber (9) as well as in greenhouse-grown plants (11).

9. Ames and Mistretta (11) have shown that plants grown under conditions that favor tumorigenesis (high light intensity) have a lower endogenous level of IAA than those grown under conditions that suppress the rate of tumor formation (low light intensity).

The hypothesis that the trigger for tumor induction in *Nicotiana* hybrids is a reduction in the endogenous level of auxin must be viewed in the context of other reports of the auxin levels in *Nicotiana* species and their tumor-prone hybrids. Bayer (15, 16) and Bayer and Ahuja (19) have shown that tumorous genotypes have a higher level of auxin than their non-tumor-forming species and that tumor-prone hybrid tissues show an increased auxin uptake and a lower transport capacity for IAA than do the parent non-tumor tissues (18). It has been suggested that these elevated levels of auxin are responsible for the abnormal type of growth that one sees in the tumors. Bayer (17) has also demonstrated a qualitative difference in auxins in extracts prepared from tumorous and nontumorous plants. However, such quantitative and qualitative differences in extractable auxin exist

at all stages of the plant life cycle, and do not explain why the tumors only appear at a rather specific time. It seems logical to conclude that there must be some signal to which cells in potential centers of growth respond by becoming meristematic. Once this initial response is made, the abnormal quantities or different types of auxin found in tumor-prone genotypes may result in the formation of non-self-limiting tumors rather than in a more normal manifestation of growth. As suggested by Ames (4), the association of two different genotypes in specific *Nicotiana* hybrids may confer upon cells in potential growth centers the ability to respond to decreased endogenous levels of auxin by becoming meristematic. Once they have been triggered to active meristematic growth, the cells in the adventitious growth centers produce abnormal quantities of growth regulating substances, especially auxin, resulting in the formation of tumors.

It is interesting to note that a hormonal trigger has been suggested in the case of one of the animal genetic tumors. The work of Sang (50) suggests that the trigger for tumor formation in the case of hereditary tumors in *Drosophila* is the balance between juvenile hormone and the pupation hormone, ecdysone. It seems from the available data that anything that lowers either ecdysone synthesis or release will increase the frequency of tumors in a population. Since apical dominance in plants may depend, at least in a general way, on an antagonism between the inhibiting influence of auxin and the effect of cytokinins (49), it may be that tumorigenesis in the tumor-prone *Nicotiana* amphiploids depends not so much on the level of a single hormone, but rather on the ratio of the endogenous levels of auxin and cytokinin.

Cyclic 3′,5′-adenosine monophosphate (cyclic AMP) is recognized as an important regulatory agent in animals and many microorganisms. Its best known function in animals is that of a second messenger, serving as an amplifying system in endocrine responses (47). Recent studies of the role of cyclic AMP in animal cancer have revealed that this compound may play an important role in the control of tumor development (see Ames (10)). Attempts to demonstrate the presence of cyclic AMP in tissues of higher plants have frequently been made. Much of the early evidence for the presence of this cyclic nucleotide is purely of a presumptive nature, its presence being deduced from an observed physiological effect after the addition of the compound. Recently, however, considerable direct evidence for the presence of cyclic AMP in plants has been presented (see Ames (10)). It has been shown that this compound is present at the level of 12–25 pmol/g fresh weight in stem tissue of *N. suaveolens* × *N. langsdorffii*. Furthermore, treatment of young seedlings of this tumor-prone amphiploid with cyclic AMP caused a significant reduction in the rate of tumor formation (10). It is interesting to note in this connection that Babula and Galsky (14) have reported that cyclic AMP inhibited the formation of crown gall tumors induced by infectious strains of *A. tumefaciens* on the primary leaves of Pinto beans.

TISSUE CULTURE AND SOMATIC CELL HYBRIDIZATION

In 1939 White (62) succeeded in culturing tissue from *N. glauca* × *N. langsdorffii* on a chemically defined medium. Since that time numerous investigators have utilized tissue culture in order to study differences in the growth requirements of normal and tumorous plant cells. In most cases, normal plant cells require the addition of one or both of the growth promoters auxin and cytokinin for *in vitro* growth. This has been shown to be true for tissues from *N. suaveolens* and *N. langsdorffii* (52). However, tissue from the tumor-conditioned hybrid made by crossing these species gave little growth response to either auxin or kinetin. A similar situation was also demonstrated for tissues from the tumor-forming hybrid *N. glauca* × *N. langsdorffii* and its nontumorous mutant (52) as well as for tissues of the tumor-prone F$_1$ of *N. debneyi-tabacum* × *N. longiflora* (3). Braun (22) had previously shown that tissue from bacterially induced crown gall tumors was able to grow on a minimal nutrient medium, while untransformed cells required exogenous auxin and kinetin. Therefore, it seems that in both crown gall and genetic tumors similar metabolic alterations have occurred at the cellular level so that they can synthesize the factors that are required for growth *in vitro*. This is the type of evidence that led to the conclusion mentioned above that, once cells have been triggered to active meristematic growth, they produce greater than regulatory amounts of growth regulating substances leading to the formation of tumors. The work of Cheng (27) is interesting in this connecton. She showed that IAA synthetases could be induced

by IAA in pith explants from the hybrid *N. glauca* × *N. langsdorffii* but not in similar explants from *N. glauca*. This observation indicates that IAA may cause continued production of itself in a tumor-prone hybrid but not in one of the parental species.

The use of protoplasts isolated from higher plant cells has opened up numerous areas of investigation. One of these is the production of hybrid plants without involving a normal sexual cycle. This was made possible because isolated protoplasts can be caused to fuse (46) and the fusion products can be induced to regenerate into entire plants (43, 58). The first interspecific plant hybrid to be produced by parasexual means was between *N. glauca* and *N. langsdorffii* (26). One of the major difficulties in this type of work is the availability of a technique for the selection and recovery of fused hybrid cells. The regeneration medium used in this case contained no hormones. Since tissue from both *N. glauca* and *N. langsdorffii* require an exogenous supply of auxin and cytokinin in order to grow *in vitro*, the regeneration medium selected for cells that contained the genetic information of both parental species. This work has been confirmed and extended further by Smith *et al.* (55). They noted that the parasexual hybrids they obtained differed morphologically from the amphiploid produced by sexual means. Cytogenetic analysis of the somatic cell hybrids revealed that they contained from 56 to 64 chromosomes rather than the expected 42. This could have been the result of triple fusions followed by the subsequent loss of chromosomes. Smith's group have taken somatic cell hybridization one step further (31). They have succeeded in fusing human HeLa cells with protoplasts of the amphiploid *N. glauca* × *N. langsdorffii*, and by so doing have opened many new avenues of research.

POSSIBLE ROLE OF A VIRUS IN GENETIC TUMOR FORMATION

I would like to conclude this limited review of plant genetic tumors by returning and commenting upon a point made earlier. No investigator has succeeded in isolating an environmental causative agent from *Nicotiana* tumors. In addition, all attempts to transmit an entity from tumor-forming plants to normal plants by grafting experiments have failed (32). Therefore, the consensus is that a viral etiology is not a likely possibility in the case of *Nicotiana* tumors. However, in view of the complexity of viral reproduction and genetics, one cannot entirely rule out the involvement of a viral entity in tumorigenesis in this system. Kovács (36), in a remarkably short but thought-provoking paper, suggested that genetic tumors may be caused by a virus or an episome-like factor. He noted that tumor-prone *Nicotiana* hybrids display many of the features of virus-infected plants. He went on to speculate that some species of *Nicotiana* may be characterized by the presence of a viral genome which is integrated into one of the host cell chromosomes. The release of this provirus, which presumably contains the genes responsible for causing the tumors, and the expression of its genetic content have at least two requirements. The first is the establishment of a specific genetic milieu. It was mentioned above that tumors appear on only certain hybrids. Näf (42) had earlier proposed that *Nicotiana* species involved in tumorous combinations could be divided into two groups, which he referred to as plus and minus. He further predicted that only hybrids between a plus species and a minus species would be tumorous. This prediction has, with a few exceptions, stood the test of time. Ahuja (2) extended this line of thinking one step by postulating that species in the plus group of Näf carry genes for tumor initition (I), while those in the minus group carry genes (ee) modifying the expression of the (I) genes. Tumors will only form when both the (I) and (ee) factors are present. In other words, the tumor initiation genes require the appropriate genetic background for their expression. Biochemical characterization of (I) and (ee) has not been reported, but Kovács (36) feels that one or the other may exist in the form of a provirus. This would be similar to the situation with oncogenic viruses in animals.

The second requirement for tumorigenesis in *Nicotiana* hybrids is tumor induction. As mentioned above tumors usually appear at a specific time during the life cycle of the plant. This argues for the existence of a trigger mechanism for tumor induction in this system. It has been suggested that this signal is a reduction in the endogenous level of auxin (13), and this hypothesis has been rigorously tested and found to be correct (11). Therefore, the development of tumors in the *Nicotiana* system may depend upon the expression of the genetic information of a provirus. This can only occur in the proper genetic milieu that is established by hybridization and is triggered by a shift in the hormonal balance within the plant. It is interesting, in this connection, that the genes responsible for causing crown gall tumors seem to reside on a plasmid present in the causal microorganism (63).

NOTE ADDED IN PROOF

During the time in which the materials for this chapter were being assembled and processed for publication, several papers appeared which cast new light upon some of the points that have been discussed. First, the oncogenic virulence of *A. tumefaciens* in crown gall disease has been shown to be associated with a large plasmid. Part of this plasmid is stably incorporated and transcribed in the plant tumor cells. This work was most recently reviewed by Drummond (2). Second, Ames *et al.* (1) have demonstrated a close correlation between onset of tumorigenesis and elevation in endogenous cytokinin activity in *Nicotiana suaveolens* × *N. langsdorffii*. They also reported that abscisic acid does not appear to be involved in regulation of tumorigenesis in the *Nicotiana* system. Therefore, it is now felt that the balance between the endogenous levels of auxin and cytokinin is the major factor which determines when tumors will be formed in tumor-prone *Nicotiana* amphiploids. Third, Liu *et al.* (3) found that tumorous *Nicotiana* hybrids synthesize bound IAA more rapidly and efficiently than nontumorous parental species. They suggested, therefore, that IAA conjugates may play a role in tumorigenesis in *Nicotiana* genetic tumors.

Additional References

1. Ames, I. H., Hill, C. A., Walton, D. C., and Dashek, W. V. (1979): Hormonal regulation of genetic tumor induction; cytokinin and abscisic acid. *Plant Cell Physiol.*, 20:1055–1061.
2. Drummond, M. (1979): Crown gall disease. *Nature*, 281: 343–347.
3. Liu, S.-T., Gruenert, D., and Knight, C. A. (1978): Bound form indole-3-acetic acid synthesis in tumorous and nontumorous species of *Nicotiana*. *Plant Physiol.*, 61:50–53.

Acknowledgments. I am grateful to Dr. Harold H. Smith and Dr. Herbert B. Tepper for their many helpful suggestions and to Dr. Smith for providing one of the photographs. Sincere thanks are also due to Mrs. Karen Sammartino and Mrs. Margarete Denis for their assistance with the manuscript.

References

1. Ahuja, M. R. (1962): A cytogenetic study of heritable tumors in *Nicotiana* species hybrids. *Genetics*, 47:865–880.
2. Ahuja, M. R. (1968): An hypothesis and evidence concerning the genetic components controlling tumor formation in *Nicotiana*. *Mol. Gen. Genet.*, 103:176–184.

3. Ahuja, M. R., and Hagen, G. L. (1966): Morphogenesis in *Nicotiana debneyi-tabacum, N. longiflora* and their tumor-forming hybrid derivatives *in vitro. Dev. Biol., 13:*408–423.

4. Ames, I. H. (1970): Induction of tumor formation in *Nicotiana* amphiploids with triiodobenzoic acid. *Can. J. Bot., 48:*2209–2212.

5. Ames, I. H. (1971): Gibberellic acid; effect on genetic tumor induction. *Can. J. Bot., 49:*1699–1701.

6. Ames, I. H. (1972): The fine structure of genetic tumor cells. *Am. J. Bot., 59:*341–345.

7. Ames, I. H. (1972): The influence of cytokinins on genetic tumor formation. *Can. J. Bot., 50:*2235–2238.

8. Ames, I. H. (1973): The effect of light intensity on tumorigenesis in a *Nicotiana* amphiploid. *Can. J. Bot., 51:*639–641.

9. Ames, I. H. (1974): Endogenous levels of auxin and tumorigenesis in a *Nicotiana* amphiploid. *Plant Physiol., 54:*953–955.

10. Ames, I. H. (1976): The possible role of cyclic AMP in the control of genetic tumor induction. *Plant Cell Physiol., 17:*1059–1066.

11. Ames, I. H., and Mistretta, P. W. (1975): Auxin; its role in genetic tumor induction. *Plant Physiol., 56:*744–746.

12. Ames, I. H., and Pivorun, J. P. (1974): A cytochemical investigation of a chloroplast inclusion. *Am. J. Bot., 61:*794–797

13. Ames, I. H., Rice, T. B., and Smith, H. H. (1969): Inhibition of tumor induction by auxin in totally debudded *Nicotiana glauca* × *N. langsdorffii. Plant Physiol., 44:*305–307.

14. Babula, M. J., and Galsky, A. G. (1975): Effects of cyclic-AMP on the formation of crown-gall tumors on the primary leaves of *Phaseolus vulgaris* var. Pinto. *Plant Cell Physiol., 16:*357–360.

15. Bayer, M. H. (1965): Paper chromatography of auxins and inhibitors in two *Nicotiana* species and their hybrid. *Am. J. Bot., 52:*883–890.

16. Bayer, M. H. (1967): Thin-layer chromatography of auxin and inhibitors in *Nicotiana glauca, N. langsdorffii* and three of their tumor-forming hybrids. *Planta, 72:*329–337.

17. Bayer, M. H. (1969): Gas chromatographic analysis of acidic indole auxins in *Nicotiana. Plant Physiol., 44:*267–271.

18. Bayer, M. H. (1972): Transport and accumulation of IAA-^{14}C in tumor-forming *Nicotiana* hybrids. *J. Exp. Bot., 23:*801–812.

19. Bayer, M. H., and Ahuja, M. R. (1968): Tumor formation in *Nicotiana*; auxin levels and auxin inhibitors in normal and tumor-prone genotypes. *Planta, 79:*292–298.

20. Black, L. M. (1972): Plant tumors of viral origin. *Prog. Exp. Tumor Res., 15:*110–137.

21. Bradley, M. V., and Crane, J. C. (1960): Gibberellin-induced inhibition of bud develpment in some species of *Prunus. Science, 131:*825–826.

22. Braun, A. C. (1958): A physiological basis for autonomous growth of the crown-gall tumor cell. *Proc. Natl. Acad. Sci. U.S.A., 44:*344–349.

23. Brian, P. W., Hemming, H. G., and Lowe, D. (1959): The effect of gibberellic acid on shoot growth of cupid sweet peas. *Physiol. Plant., 12:*15–29.

24. Brieger, F. G., and Forster, R. (1942): Tumores em certos hibridos do gênero *Nicotiana. Bragantia, 2:*259–274.

25. Burdette, W. J. (1952): Tumor incidence and lethal mutation rate in *Drosophila* treated with 20-methylcholanthrene. *Cancer Res., 12:*201–205.

26. Carlson, P. S., Smith, H. H., and Dearing, R. D. (1972): Parasexual interspecific plant hybridization. *Proc. Natl. Acad. Sci U.S.A., 69:*2292–2294.

27. Cheng, T.-Y. (1972): Induction of indoleacetic acid synthetases in tobacco pith explants. *Plant Physiol., 50:*723–727.

28. Gordon, M. (1927): The genetics of a vivaparous top-minnow *Platypoecilus;* the inheritance of two kinds of melanophores. *Genetics, 12:*253–283.

29. Hurkman, W. J., and Kennedy, G. S. (1977): Development and cytochemistry of the thylakoidal body in tobacco chloroplasts. *Am. J. Bot., 64:*86–95.

30. Izard, C. (1957): Obtention et fixation de lignées tumorales et non tumorales a partir de mutations experimentales de l'hybride *N. glauca* × *N. langsdorffii. C. R. Acad. Agric., 43:*325–327.

31. Jones, C. W., Mastrangelo, I. A., Smith, H. H., Liu, H. Z., and Meck, R. A. (1976): Interkingdom fusion between human (HeLa) and tobacco hybrid (GGLL) protoplasts. *Science, 193:*401–403.

32. Kehr, A.E. (1951): Genetic tumors in *Nicotiana. Am. Nat., 85:*51–64.

33. Kehr, A. E., and Smith, H. H. (1954): Genetic tumors in *Nicotiana* hybrids. *Brookhaven Symp. Biol., 6:*55–78.

34. Kostoff, D. (1930): Tumors and other malformations on certain *Nicotiana* hybrids. *Zentralbl. Bakteriol. Parasitenk., 81:*244–260.

35. Kostoff, D. (1943): Cytogenetics of the genus *Nicotiana,* pp. 1071. State Printing House, Sofia, Bulgaria.

36. Kovács, E. I. (1972): A new theory of genetic tumor formation in plants. A viroid explanation. *Bot. Közlem., 59:*251–257.

37. Levine, M. (1937): Tumors of tobacco hybrids. *Am. J. Bot., 24:*250–256.

38. Little, C. C. (1939): Hybridization and tumor formation in mice. *Proc. Natl. Acad. Sci. U.S.A., 25:*452–455.

39. Lockhart, J. A., and Gottschall, V. (1961): Fruit-induced and apical senescence in *Pisum sativum* L. *Plant Physiol., 36:*389–398.

40. Lund, S., and Kjaerskov, H. (1885): Morphological and anatomical description of *Brassica oleracea* L., *B. campestris* (L.) and *B. napus* (L.) (garden cabbage, rutabaga and rape) with accounts of pollination and cultivation experiments with these species. *Bot. Tidsskr., 15:*1–150.

41. Manocha, M. S. (1970): Fine structure of sunflower crown gall tissue. *Can. J. Bot., 48:*1455–1458.

42. Näf, U. (1958): Studies on tumor formation in *Nicotiana* hybrids; I. The classification of the parents into two etiologically significant groups. *Growth, 22:*167–180.

43. Nagata, T., and Takebe, I. (1971): Plating of isolated tobacco mesophyll protoplasts on agar medium. *Planta, 99:*12–20.

44. Paleg, L. G. (1965): Physiological effects of gibberellins. *Annu. Rev. Plant Physiol., 16:*291–322.

45. Phillips, I.D.J. (1969): Apical dominance, in *The Physiology of Plant Growth and Development,* edited by M. B. Wilkins. McGraw-Hill, New York.

46. Power, J. B., Cummins, S. E., and Cocking, E. C. (1970): Fusion of isolated plant protoplasts. *Nature, 225:*1016–1018.

47. Robison, G. A., Butcher, R.W., and Sutherland, E. W. (1971): *Cyclic AMP.* Academic Press, New York.

48. Ruddat, M., and Pharis, R. P. (1966): Participation of gibberellin in the control of apical dominance in soybean and redwood. *Planta, 71:*222–228.

49. Sachs, T., and Thimann, K. V. (1967): The role of auxins and cytokinins in the release of buds from dominance. *Am. J. Bot., 54:*136–144.

50. Sang, J. H. (1969): Biochemical basis of hereditary melanotic tumors in *Drosophila. Natl. Cancer Inst. Monogr., 31:*291–301.

51. Schaeffer, G. W., and Sharpe, F. T., Jr. (1969): Release of axillary bud inhibition with benzyladenine in tobacco. *Bot. Gaz., 130:*107–110.

52. Schaeffer, G. W., and Smith, H. H. (1963): Auxin-kinetin interaction in tissue cultures of *Nicotiana* species and tumor conditioned hybrids. *Plant Physiol., 38:*291–297.

53. Smith, H. H. (1958): Genetic plant tumors in *Nicotiana. Ann. N.Y. Acad. Sci., 71:*1163–1177.

54. Smith, H. H. (1972): Plant genetic tumors. *Prog. Exp. Tumor Res., 15:*138–164.

55. Smith, H. H., Kao, K. N., and Combatti, N. C. (1976): Interspecific hybridization by protoplast fusion in *Nicotiana. J. Hered., 67:*123–128.

56. Smith, H. H., and Stevenson, H. Q. (1961): Genetic control and radiation effects in *Nicotiana* tumors. *Z. Vererbungsl., 92:*100–118.

57. Steitz, E. (1963): Untersuchungen über die Tumorbildung bei Bastarden von *Nicotiana glauca* und *N. langsdorffii.* Dok. Diss., Univ. Saarlands, Saarbrücken.

58. Takebe, I., Labib, G., and Melchers, G. (1971): Regeneration of whole plants from isolated mesophyll protoplasts of tobacco. *Naturwissenschaften, 58:*318–320.

59. Takenaka, Y., and Yoneda, Y. (1962): Tumorous hybrids in *Nicotiana. Annu. Rep. Natl. Inst. Genet. Japan, 13:*63–64.

60. Thimann, K. V., and Skoog, F. (1934): On the inhibition of bud development and other functions of growth substance in *Vicia faba. Proc. R. Soc. Ser. B., 114:*317–339.

61. Whitaker, T. W. (1934): The occurrence of tumors on certain *Nicotiana* hybrids. *J. Arnold Arbor., 15:*144–153.

62. White, P. R. (1939): Potentially unlimited growth of excised plant callus in an artificial nutrient. *Am. J. Bot., 26:*59–64.

63. Zaenen, I, van Larebeke, N., Teuchy, H., van Montagu, M., and Schell, J. (1974): Supercoiled circular DNA in crown gall inducing *Agrobacterium* strains. *J. Mol. Biol., 86:*109–127.

34

Species-Specific Aspects of Immunity in Cancer

Ronald B. Herberman

INTRODUCTION

Most of the available information on immunity in relation to cancer has been obtained in studies of various mammalian species, especially rodents and man. Lesser amounts of data exist on immunity against tumors in birds. In this chapter, because of these restrictions on our knowledge and also because of space limitations, I will concentrate mainly on selected studies in mice, rats, and man. However, when possible, I will also comment on related findings in other species, especially nonmammalian species. Each tumor system, even within the same species or inbred strain, has its own peculiarities, and predominant factors in one system may be minor in others. However, by performing studies on immunity in a variety of tumor models in different species, it would seem possible to identify common features in the immunologic reactivity of the host. Such information on comparative aspects of tumor immunology might help to provide more insight into some of the general principles involved in host resistance against tumor growth. These general principles would be more likely to be directly relevant to the problem of immunity in cancer patients than would any particular animal model, no matter how well studied.

This chapter will deal mainly with the following issues: the possible relationship between the evolution of the immune system and neoplasia, particularly with regard to concepts of immunologic surveillance, the development of immune depression in tumor-bearing individuals, and the various lines of evidence for immune reactions, systemically and locally, of the host against the tumor.

POSSIBLE RELATIONSHIP BETWEEN EVOLUTION OF IMMUNE SYSTEM AND NEOPLASIA

The general role of the immune system in preventing or limiting tumor growth has been emphasized by many investigators, perhaps beginning with Ehrlich in 1908 (14). Burnet (6) formulated the theory of immune surveillance, stating that "it is by no means inconceivable that small accumulations of tumor cells may develop and because of the possession of new antigenic potentialities provoke an effective immunological reaction with regression of the tumor and no clinical hint of its existence." In other words, it has been proposed that neoplastic transformations occur with considerable frequency but that the immune response is able to eliminate most of these, with only the rare escapes from surveillance leading to detectable tumors. Although this theory has aroused considerable controversy in the last few years (36, 39, 41, 43), there is no doubt that this concept has had a fundamental impact on thinking and experimentation in tumor immunology. One aspect of the theory which has generated much discussion is the relationship between malignant growth and the evolution of the immune system. It has been suggested that the appearance of tumors in vertebrates led to the evolution of the immune system. Although this causal link between tumors and development of the immune system is often considered to be the central issue in the theory of immune surveillance, Burnet (7) himself has granted that this is the least amenable to experimental proof. Good and Finstad (21) have pointed to the correlation between the first appearance of malignant tumors in lower vertebrates and the development of the cellular immune system. They placed a particular emphasis on the phylogenetic development of thymus-like functions. However, there is substantial evidence for the occurrence of tumors in invertebrates (13) and also for more primitive immune systems in invertebrates which might mediate resistance against tumors (11). Thomas (45) postulated that the mechanisms for the homograft rejection were evolved primarily as a natural defense against neoplasia. If so, this would place the beginnings of this defense mechanism at the level of more primitive invertebrates, since rejection of foreign tissue grafts has been demonstrated even in earthworms (10). There has probably been a considerable overemphasis placed on the importance of thymic-dependent immunity in surveillance against tumors. The modification of the immune surveillance theory, to cast T cells in a central role, has been made only recently (7), and it is actually this modification of the concept that has aroused most of the criticism and which even led to a counter theory of immune stimulation of tumor growth (40). In several well-studied rodent tumor systems, T cells do appear to be a major defense mechanism against tumors. However, in the absence of mature T cells, either in immune deficiency states in vertebrates or in species lacking thymic development, alternative immune mechanisms may play an effective role in resistance against tumor growth. There may be some merit to the concept advanced by Good and Finstad (21) that tumors in higher vertebrates tend to be more aggressive and malignant, with a higher predilection toward metastases, and, to deal with such tumors, a more highly developed and diversified immune system had to be developed.

Most of the above arguments are based on the presumption that some form of immune surveillance has the capacity to prevent tumor development. However, this is also very difficult to conclusively verify. One of the predictions of the immune surveillance theory is that in the absence of immunologic reactivity, more tumors would be detectable and they might behave more aggressively. Therefore a main approach has been to examine the incidence of tumors in immunosuppressed individuals. With certain types of tumors, this has been demonstrated, but with other tumor types, little or no effects have been seen (44). However, as will be discussed later, this may be related to the fact that most forms of immunosuppression are not complete and some effector mechanisms may remain intact.

Klein and Klein (33) have recently discussed the issue of the effectiveness of surveillance and its relationship to evolution from a different viewpoint. They propose that there have been evolutionary pressures to develop immune mechanisms to deal with only certain types of tumors, primarily those induced by oncogenic viruses. They point out that certain species have become highly resistant to the effects of known oncogenic viruses, and that in those systems, immunosuppression does lead to a much higher tumor incidence. In contrast, tumors induced by other carcinogens or occurring spontaneously usually develop late in life, after the reproductive period, and therefore these might not be expected to select for effective surveillance. The host might have considerably more difficulty in responding immunologically to such tumors, and it might be harder to show an effect of immune suppression on the growth of these tumors.

DEVELOPMENT OF IMMUNE DEPRESSION IN TUMOR-BEARING INDIVIDUALS

The issue of most practical importance in regard to immune surveillance is what occurs under "normal conditions," rather than in experimental situations or in deliberately immunosuppressed individuals. Do many or most spontaneous tumors arise because of preceding genetic defects or environmental suppression of the immune response, or because of the immunosuppressive effects of the carcinogenic agent? Or alternatively, as suggested by Klein and Klein (33) do the tumors which become detectable represent those which in some way have evaded the constraints of an intact immune system? There is not much experimental evidence directly relating to this. However, regardless of whether immune depression is a primary event or secondary to the presence of tumor, it is clear that immune depression occurs frequently in tumor-bearing individuals, both in experimental animals (44) and in cancer patients (24).

The immune depression in tumor-bearing

hosts may be manifested by a decrease in either the number of lymphoid cells of a given type or in the functional activity of the immune system. There have been several indications that many cancer patients, including some with localized, early disease, have decreased proportions of T cells forming rosettes with sheep erythrocytes (reviewed by West (48)). Some studies have indicated that many of these patients have a decrease in a subpopulation of T cells with high affinity receptors for sheep erythrocytes, rather than a depression in total numbers of T cells.

Until recently, it has been generally assumed that depressions in measurable amounts of a particular cell type or of functional activity were due to quantitative depletion of cells or to intrinsic defects in the cells. However, in an increasing number of instances, immune depression in tumor-bearing rodents and patients has been attributable to the presence of inhibitory factors or cells. Depressed levels of rosette-forming T cells in patients with Hodgkin's disease were reported to be due to suppressive serum factors (16). Other serum factors from animals and humans with tumors have been found to inhibit lymphocyte functions (5). Similarly, suppressor cells, mainly cells with properties of macrophages or monocytes (2, 4, 32) but also T cells (8, 15), have been shown to inhibit proliferative responses and some other functions of lymphocytes of tumor-bearing individuals.

MORPHOLOGICAL AND FUNCTIONAL EVIDENCE OF IMMUNE REACTIONS AT THE SITES OF TUMOR GROWTH

A frequent histopathological feature of tumors is their infiltration by host lymphocytes and macrophages (reviewed by Haskill et al. (23)). This phenomenon has been recognized with some human tumors for about 70 years, and has often been taken as evidence for an immune reaction against the tumors. Some characteristic patterns of lymphoid cell infiltration within the primary tumors or in regional lymph nodes have been associated with prolonged survival (3). It has become apparent that many tumors in mice and rats are infiltrated by large numbers of lymphoid cells and that the presence of infiltrating cells, particularly macrophages, is associated with regression or lack of metastases (23). Although there are relatively few reports of such infiltration in tumors of other species, it is prob-

ably a very widespread phenomenon. Ghelelovitch (17) noted an intense inflammatory element in melanotic tumors of Drosophila and suggested that this was a more primitive form of immune reaction against the tumor.

In the past few years, techniques have been developed to isolate the host cells from tumors in viable and functional conditions. These procedures have permitted more detailed characterization of the infiltrating cells and examination of their antitumor activity (23). These studies should lead to important advances in the understanding of the relevant immune reactions against tumors, since some effector cells which are found in the central lymphoid system may not accumulate at the tumor site. In some rodent and human tumors, cytotoxic T cells (e.g., Holden et al. (29) and Jondal et al. (30)); macrophages (e.g., Holden et al. (29) and Haskill et al. (23)); and natural killer cells (Becker and Klein (1)) have been detected.

CELL-MEDIATED IMMUNITY AGAINST TUMORS

Although the recent studies on effector cells within tumors are quite promising, the data are quite scarce compared to the very extensive information which has been accumulated on systemic cell-mediated immunity against tumors. As noted above, thymic-dependent T lymphocytes have usually been focused on the important cells mediating immunological surveillance and resistance against tumor growth. The major role of T cells in protection against tumor growth in mice and rats has been supported by the observations of increased growth of some tumors in thymectomized hosts (reviewed by Stutman (44)) and by the protective effects of systemic adoptive transfer of T cells (9, 19). In chickens, it has been possible to assess the relative roles of T cells and B cells, since removal of the bursa of Fabricius causes impairment of B cell functions. Lam and Linna (34), in studies of two different tumor systems, found that thymectomy had a strong effect on tumor growth, but that bursectomy also led to some increase in oncogenicity. This illustrates one of the important features of the immune response to tumors, that a variety of effector mechanisms are often involved.

In the past few years, a large variety of assays have been developed to study in detail the antitumor effector mechanisms. For example, it has been possible to detect T cell-mediated reactivity against tumors *in vitro* by cytotoxicity assays and by assays of proliferative responses by lymphocytes or their production of lymphokines, especially migration inhibitory factor. A central issue is which assays best reflect *in vivo* resistance against tumor growth. One of the principal assays for study of T cell immunity has been the ^{51}Cr-release cytotoxicity assay and it was expected that such an assay would indicate important antitumor reactivity. However, there was an apparent lack of correlation between the kinetics of *in vitro* reactivity and *in vivo* resistance against tumor growth, with cytotoxic reactivity being considerably more transient after immunization. Recent studies have provided a simple answer to this. In *in vivo* experiments to demonstrate resistance against tumors, the challenge with tumor cells actually represents the second exposure of the immune host to tumor antigens. A key factor in resistance to challenge may be the ability of the host to mount a rapid secondary immune response, particularly in the region of challenge. In three different rodent tumor systems, rapid development of T cell-dependent cytotoxic reactivity after secondary tumor challenge has been demonstrated (18, 28, 47).

Macrophages represent another effector cell mechanism for reactivity against tumor cells. As pointed out by Cooper (11), phagocytic cells may represent the oldest form of defense mechanism, being present even in protozoans. Macrophages may have significant *in vivo* antitumor effects, and even tumors which are usually considered nonimmunogenic may be able to stimulate this mechanism or be susceptible to the effects of macrophages.

Yet another effector cell mechanism, which is of considerable interest and potential significance for *in vivo* resistance against tumor growth, is natural cell-mediated cytotoxicity (reviewed by Herberman and Holden (26)). Mice and rats spontaneously develop this reactivity for a transient period, and humans have apparent long term persistence of this reactivity. High levels of natural cytotoxicity were found in nude mice, which congenitally lack a thymus, and although the effector cells were initially found to have no detectable cell surface markers, recent studies have indicated that both mouse and human natural killer cells may be in the T cell lineage, although not thymus dependent. There are several preliminary indications that natural killer cells may play a significant *in vivo* role.

Kiessling *et al.* (31) found a correlation between levels of natural reactivity in different strains of mice and the relative resistance to growth of transplantable leukemia cells. Our laboratory has recently found that some tumor cells which are very sensitive to NK reactivity grew less well in nude mice than in conventional mice with intact thymuses. As discussed in detail elsewhere (26), these findings may have important implications for concepts of immune surveillance.

HUMORAL RESPONSES AGAINST TUMORS

In mammals and in birds, B cells have been shown to react against tumor antigens by formation of specific antibodies. The extensive literature on antibodies to tumors has been reviewed (27, 46) and for the purposes of the present discussion, only a few selected points will be emphasized. It is important to note that in addition to the induction of antibodies by immunization with tumor cells, natural or spontaneously appearing antibodies may be seen, with reactivity against a variety of tumor-associated or virus-associated antigens (reviewed by Herberman (25)). Such natural antibodies might be viewed as a type of first line defense against tumors. It seems possible that even more primitive humoral defense mechanisms may exist.

Although antibody synthesis is purely an attribute of vertebrates (11), Dawe (12) has pointed out some invertebrates have humoral antitumor factors (e.g., Schmeer (42)) and it is conceivable that such factors may play a role maintaining a very low incidence of neoplasia in such species.

In addition to the direct effects of antibodies on tumor cells, antibodies to tumor antigens may act in cooperation with certain lymphocytes or macrophages bearing receptors for immunoglobulins, to produce antibody-dependent cell-mediated cytotoxicity. Such antibodies have been found to play a role in the immune response against tumors in mice (38), rats (37), and in man (22).

References

1. Becker, S., and Klein, E. (1977): Decreased "natural killer"-NK-effect in tumor bearing mice and its relation to the immunity against oncornavirus determined cell surface antigens. *Eur. J. Immunol*, 6:892–898.
2. Berlinger, N. T., Lopez, C., and Good, R. A. (1976): Facilitation or attenuation of mixed leukocyte culture responsiveness by adherent cells. *Nature*, 260:145–146.
3. Black, M. M., Barclay, T. H. C., and Hankey, B. F. (1975): Prognosis in breast cancer utilizing histologic characteristics of the primary tumor.

Cancer, 36:2048–2055.

4. Broder, S., Humphrey, R., Durm, M., Blackman, M., Meade, B., Goldman, C., Strober, W., and Waldmann, T. (1975): Impaired synthesis of polyclonal (non-paraprotein) immunoglobulins by circulating lymphocytes from patients with multiple myeloma. *N. Engl. J. Med.*, 293:887–892.

5. Brooks, W. H., Netsky, H. G., Normansell, D. E., and Horwitz, D. A. (1972): Depressed cell-mediated immunity in patients with primary intracranial tumors. *J. Exp. Med.*, 136:1631–1647.

6. Burnet, F. M. (1957): Cancer—a biological approach. *Br. Med. J.*, 1:779–786, 841–847.

7. Burnet, F. M. (1970): The concept of immunological surveillance. *Prog. Exp. Tumor Res.*, 13:1–27.

8. Carnaud, C., Ilfeld, D., Levo, Y., and Trainin, N. (1974): Enhancement of 3LL tumor growth by autosensitized lymphocytes independent of the host lymphatic system. *Int. J. Cancer*, 14:168–175.

9. Collavo, D., Colombatti, A., Chieco-Bianchi, L., and Davies, A. J. S. (1974): T lymphocyte requirement for MSV tumour prevention or regression. *Nature*, 249:169–170.

10. Cooper, E.L. (1969): Neoplasia and transplantation immunity in annelids. *Natl. Cancer Inst. Monogr.*, 31:655–669.

11. Cooper, E. L. (1976): *Comparative Immunology*, p. 338. Prentice-Hall, Englewood Cliffs, N.J.

12. Dawe, C. J. (1969): Phylogeny and oncogeny. *Natl. Cancer Inst. Monogr.*, 31:1–40.

13. Dawe, C. J., and Harshbarger, J. C. (1969): Neoplasms and related disorders of invertebrates and lower vertebrate animals. *Natl. Cancer Inst. Monogr.*, 31:1–772.

14. Ehrlich, P. (1957): Über den jetzigen Stand der Karzinomforschung, in *The Collected Papers of Paul Ehrlich, Vol. II*, pp. 550–562, edited by F. Himmelweit. Permagon Press, London.

15. Fujimoto, S., Greene, M. I., and Sehon, A. H. (1976): Regulation of the immune response to tumor antigens; II. The nature of immunosuppressor cells in tumor-bearing hosts. *J. Immunol.*, 116:800–806.

16. Fuks, Z., Strober, S., and Kaplan, H. S. (1976): Interaction between serum factors and T lymphocytes in Hodgkins's disease. *N. Engl. J. Med.*, 295:1273–1278.

17. Ghelelovitch, S. (1969): Melanotic tumors in *Drosophila melanogaster*. *Natl. Cancer Inst. Monogr.*, 31:263–275.

18. Glaser, M., and Herberman, R. B. (1976): Secondary cell-mediated cytotoxic response to challenge of rats with syngeneic Gross virus-induced lymphoma. *J.N.C.I.*, 56:1211–1215.

19. Glaser, M., Lavrin, D. H., and Herberman, R. B. (1976): In vivo protection against syngeneic Gross virus-induced lymphoma in rats; comparison with in vitro studies of cell-mediated immunity. *J. Immunol.*, 116:1507–1511.

20. Glasgow, A. H., Nimberg, R. B., Menzoian, J. O., Saporoschetz, I., Cooperband, S. R., Schmid, K., and Mannick, J. A. (1974): Association of anergy with an immunosuppressive peptide fraction in the serum of patients with cancer. *N. Engl. J. Med.*, 1291:1263–1267.

21. Good, R. A., and Finstad, J. (1969): Essential relationship between the lymphoid system, immunity, and malignancy. *Natl. Cancer Inst. Monogr.*, 31:41–58.

22. Hakala, T. R., Lange, P. H., Castro, A. E., Elliott, A. Y., and Fraley, E. E. (1974): Antibody induction of lymphocyte-mediated cytotoxicity against human transitional-cell carcinomas of the urinary tract. *N. Engl. J. Med.*, 291:637–641.

23. Haskill, J. S., Häyry, P., and Radov, L. A. (1978): Systemic and local immunity in allograft and cancer rejection. *Contemp. Top. Immunobiol.* 8:107–170.

24. Herberman, R. B. (1974): Cell-mediated immunity to tumor cells. *Adv. Cancer Res.*, 19:207–263.

25. Herberman, R. B. (1980): Immunology of oncornaviruses, in *Immunology of Human Infections, Vol. II*, edited by A. J. Nahmias and R. J. O'Reilly. Plenum, New York (in press).

26. Herberman, R. B., and Holden, H. T. (1978): Natural cell-mediated immunity. *Adv. Cancer Res.*, 27:305–377.

27. Hirshaut, Y. (1979): Immune responses of patients to tumor associated antigens; humoral immunity, in *Handbook of Clinical Immunology, Vol. 1*, Section F, Part 2, pp. 237–268, edited by A. Baumgarten and F. Richards. CRC Press, Cleveland.

28. Holden, H. T., Kirchner, H., and Herberman, R. B. (1975): Secondary cell-mediated cytotoxic response to syngeneic mouse tumor challenge. *J. Immunol.*, 115:327–331.

29. Holden, H. T., Haskill, J. S., Kirchner, H., and Herberman, R. B. (1976): Two functionally distinct anti-tumor effector cells isolated from primary murine sarcoma virus-induced tumors. *J. Immunol.*, 117:440–446.

30. Jondal, M., Svedmyr, E., Klein, E., and Singh, S. (1975): Killer T cells in a Burkitt's lymphoma biopsy. *Nature*, 225:405–407.

31. Kiessling, R., Petranyi, G., Klein, G., and Wigzell, H. (1975): Genetic variation of in vitro cytolytic activity and in vivo rejection potential of nonimmunized semisyngeneic mice against a mouse lymphoma line. *Int. J. Cancer*, 15:933–940.

32. Kirchner, H., Glaser, M., Holden, H. T., Fernbach, B. R., and Herberman, R. B. (1976): Suppressor cells in tumor bearing mice and rats. *Biomedicine*, 24:371–373.

33. Klein, G., and Klein, E. (1977): Rejectability of virus induced tumors and non-rejectability of spontaneous tumors—a lesson in contrasts. *Transplant. Proc.*, 9:1095–1104.

34. Lam, K. M., and Linna, T. J. (1976): Impaired host defense against XC cell-induced tumors in thymectomized and in bursectomized chickens. *Cancer Res.*, 36:1710–1713.

35. McMaster, R., Buhler, K., Whitney, R., and Levy, J. G. (1977): Immunosuppression of T lymphocyte function by fractionated serum from tumor-bearing mice. *J. Immunol.*, 118:218–222.

36. Möller, G., and Möller, E. (1975): Guest editorial: Considerations of some current concepts in cancer research. *J.N.C.I.*, 55:755–759.

37. Ortiz de Landazuri, M., Kedar, E., and Fahey, J. L. (1974): Antibody-dependent cellular cytotoxicity to a syngeneic Gross virus-induced lymphoma. *J.N.C.I.*, 52:147–152.

38. Pollack, S., Heppner, G., Brawn, R. J., and Nelson, K. (1972): Specific killing of tumor cells in vitro in the presence of normal lymphoid cells and seen from hosts immune to the tumor antigens. *Int. J. Cancer*, 9:316–324.

39. Prehn, R. T. (1971): Immunosurveillance, regeneration and oncogenesis. *Prog. Exp. Tumor Res.*, 14:1–24.

40. Prehn, R. T., and Lappe, M. A. (1971): An immunostimulation theory of tumor development. *Transplant. Rev.*, 7:26–54.

41. Rygaard, J., and Povlsen, C. O. (1976): The nude mouse vs. the hypothesis of immunological surveillance. *Transplant. Rev.*, 28:43–61.

42. Schmeer, A. C. (1969): Mercenene; an antineoplastic agent extracted from the marine clam, *Mercenaria mercenaria*. *Nat. Cancer Inst. Monogr.*, 31:581–591.

43. Schwartz, R. S. (1975): Another look at immunologic surveillance. *N. Engl. J. Med.*, 293:181–184.

44. Stutman, O. (1975): Immunodepression and malignancy. *Adv. Cancer Res.*, 22:261–422.

45. Thomas, L. (1959): Discussion, in *Cellular and Humoral Aspects of the Hypersensitive State*, pp. 529–530, edited by H. S. Lawrence. Harper, New York.

46. Ting, C. C., and Herberman, R. B. (1976): Humoral host defense mechanisms against tumors. *Int. Rev. Exp. Pathol.*, 15:93–152.

47. Ting, C. C., Kirchner, H., Rodrigues, D., Park, J. Y., and Herberman, R. B. (1976): Cell-mediated immunity to Friend virus-induced leukemia; III. Characteristics of secondary cell-mediated cytotoxic response. *J. Immunol.*, 116:244–252.

48. West, W. H. (1979): Rosette formation in immunodiagnosis, in *Immunodiagnosis of Cancer* pp. 704–721, edited by R. B. Herberman and K. R. McIntire. Marcel Dekker, New York.

35

Epidemiology of Selected Aspects of Dog and Cat Neoplasms and Comparison with Man

Howard M. Hayes, Jr.

INTRODUCTION

There are a myriad of factors implicated in the etiology of cancer. Singly or in combination, determinants such as viruses, genetic susceptibility, alterations of endocrine metabolism, and exposures to solar radiation, x-radiation, certain chemicals, radioactive elements, inorganic substances, foods and drugs have been identified (41). Yet, there is considerably more research to be done. Who is at risk for cancer, when and why? Some of the answers may lie in gaining new knowledge about disease processes in domesticated animals.

Proof of the kinship of animal and human cancer is easily demonstrated by the work of Holsti an Ermala (62). These investigators attempted to induce lung cancer by painting the oral mucosa of mice with tobacco tar. Rather than producing tumors of the lung, they induced carcinomas of the bladder. The association of tobacco usage and subsequent bladder cancer in humans has now been established and quantified (75, 76).

Etiologic mechanisms for naturally occurring tumors have been identified in many diverse laboratory and domestic animal species. Viruses have been implicated in the etiology of papillomas in wild cottontail rabbits (118), renal adenocarcinomas in leopard frogs (80, 95), and sarcomas in chickens (110). Parasites, such as *Spirocerca lupi* which causes esophageal tumors in the dog (107), have also been incriminated in tumorigenesis.

Exposure to sunlight is known to cause squamous cell carcinomas of the skin and oral mucosa in white cats (30), the unpigmented skin on the end of the nose of collies and Shetland sheepdogs (92), and is involved with the etiology of ocular carcinoma in Hereford cattle (5). Interesting to note, the frequency of occurrence of these ocular tumors is correlated with the level of protein nutrition in Hereford cattle—the higher the amount of protein in the diet, the greater the frequency (4).

GENERAL CONSIDERATIONS

Investigators have become increasingly aware of the usefulness of animal models to depict and understand the human counterpart of disease. Early veterinary reports about naturally occurring neoplasms were generally descriptions of single cases. Subsequently, investigators assembled groups of cases together for presentation, such as the studies by Goodpasture (48), Crocker (25), Feldman (36), Mulligan (93), and Cotchin (22). While offering a greater array of descriptive data, these studies could not present the epidemiologic features of the disease. Domestic animals, especially pet dogs and cats, have not been the subject of census counts, birth and death records, or other enumerations that are applicable to humans. Thus, descriptive data about the general population from which diseased animals evolved was unavailable.

In the early 1960s several data registries were formed which collected information about diseased and nondiseased animals seen by veterinarians. The largest was the Veterinary Medical Data Program (VMDP) sponsored by the National Cancer Institute (124). Similar programs are operated by the World Health Organization and various veterinary universities in Europe, Africa, and Australia (9).

The VMDP is a computerized registry composed of a standarized case abstract about each patient's visit to hospitals and clinics operated by 14 veterinary schools of medicine in the United States and Canada (as of July, 1976). Diagnoses and operative procedures are coded from the outline in the *Standard Nomenclature of Veterinary Diseases and Operations* (96). Besides unique patient number, descriptive characteristics of the patient are abstracted (*i.e.*, age, breed, sex). Thus, definitive information is available about the zoographical characteristics of the complete hospital/clinic population.

The measure of association for disease with a particular patient characteristic in epidemiologic studies from the VMDP and alike registries has been an estimate of relative risk (44, 84, 123). This statistic, as used in the VMDP studies, refers to a hospital-based prevalence value.

The term "incidence" has often been used in veterinary studies with little regard to its actual meaning. If the general population was undefined, the incidence rate of the disease cannot have been determined. Associations between the disease and particular patient characteristics, such as sex or breed, can not be ascertained without data about the companion population at-risk from which the cases were drawn. The reference population used in some veterinary studies has been based upon samples taken of the general population. This approach requires that calculated incidence rates be presented as estimates, with appropriate standard errors, so as not to be misleading.

Retrospective studies about veterinary hospital data may be subject to several biases. Some of these include: 1) Did the medical history contain data about all of the patient's diseases and abnormalities? 2) Is there a differing owner impetus to bring the animal to medical attention, depending upon age, breed, sex, and economic value? 3) Do diagnostic criteria differ substantially between clinicians within one medical facility or between different medical facilities?

The problem of missing data results in an underreporting of the disease prevalence. However, it may be reasonable to assume that missing data, like owner impetus to bring purebred animals to the veterinarian for medical attention, is a random phenomenon.

Random samples of the VMDP data registry have failed to show appreciable differences between veterinary teaching facilities for the frequency of tumor diagnoses, relative to the zoographical characteristics of their patients. It is true that some veterinary teaching institutions pursue the study of oncology with more vigor than others (106); yet, this interest seems to have been focused across all types of neoplasms and breeds of pets.

An investigator should be cautious in the interpretation of veterinary data about the occurrence of spontaneous neoplasms, and when possible, attempt to minimize the effects of known bias. For instance, in calculating an estimate of relative risk for a particular disease in one canine breed compared to that in all hospitalized dogs, the results could possibly be subject to gross error if adjustment is not made for variations in age and sex between the test and comparison groups.

The study of spontaneous occurring neoplasms in pets has recently gained new impetus. With the identification of excessive mortality rates of particular human cancers in specific U.S. counties (85, 86), it has now become very important to pursue the epidemiology of the lesion in similarly exposed pets. Pets could be an ideal sentinel for monitoring the effects of low level environmental determinants. They share their owner's environment except for work related exposures and tobacco usage. These two confounding variables presently bias many human surveys.

Specific tumor sites discussed in this chapter are the skin, testis, ovary, mammary gland, bladder, kidney, thyroid gland, chemoreceptor system, brain, and blood-lymphatic system. These sites were chosen for review because the descriptive features of the lesion have evolved from recent studies and were based upon credible statistical analyses. Comparisons are drawn between the human and veterinary epidemiology when possible.

ALL SITES

The dog and cat develop neoplasms in almost every anatomical site found in man (106). The more common canine sites are shown in Table

35.1, and the feline sites in Table 35.2. A recent estimate of the annual incidence of malignant neoplasms for all body sites, from one tumor registry, was 381/100,000 dogs and 156/100,000 cats (31). The estimated annual prevalence of cancer recently seen in 12 veterinary teaching hospitals was 687 cases per 100,000 dogs and 311 per 100,000 cats (106). Both sets of data, independent of each other, indicate that the dog has about twice as much cancer as the cat.

BREED RISK

Familial predispositions for specific tumors and tumor syndromes have played an increasing role in understanding the etiology of human cancer. One can look upon the canine and feline species as being composed of numerous separate families (breeds) whose genetic pools have been maintained relatively homogeneous through time. As such, it is important to identify breeds with an excessive risk for neoplasms and like-wise those breeds which are markedly spared.

It is also important to note that among canines, the boxer breed appears unique because of its diathesis for neoplasia (106). The excessive risk in this dog family (breed) involves many different tumors and suggests that this breed has some basic genetic defect, e.g., immunologic or enzymatic, which favors tumorigenesis (104). Comparison of the biochemical or cytogenic profiles during the various stages of neoplastic development in the boxer with that of other breeds experiencing significantly less neoplasia may shed light on factors responsible for the familial risk seen in related humans for multiple types of neoplasms.

Other breeds have been identified with excessive risk for tumors (Table 35.3). Notable is the Great Dane, whose high risk for generalized cancer can be largely attributed to its propensity for osteosarcoma. Several breeds appear to be spared from neoplasia, as are mongrel dogs, if considered as one family unit (106).

The risk for generalized tumors in cats and specifically malignant tumors appears to be evenly distributed among the common pure-breeds (Table 35.4). However, because of the smaller number of cases, considerably less work has been done in the field of epidemiology of feline neoplasia than canine neoplasia.

Table 35.1
Distribution of Canine Neoplasms Reported to the Veterinary Medical Data Program, March 1964 through December 1969[a]

Anatomical Site	No. of Neoplasms	Percentage of All Neoplasms	Percentage of Malignant Neoplasms within Site
Skin	1691	28	20
Mammary gland	732	12	46
Digestive	574	10	33
Hemic and lymphic system	445	7	95
Genitourinary system	429	7	37
Oral cavity (soft tissue)	362	6	49
Bone	295	5	81

[a] Modified from Priester and Mantel (106).

Table 35.2
Distribution of Feline Neoplasms Reported to the Veterinary Medical Data Program, March 1964 through December 1969[a]

Anatomical Site	No. of Neoplasms	Percentage of All Neoplasms	Percentage of Malignant Neoplasms within Site
Hemic and lymphic system	170	35	98
Skin	86	18	41
Oral cavity (soft tissue)	37	8	65
Digestive	35	7	71
Mammary gland	23	5	78
Respiratory	23	5	78
Bone	19	4	47

[a] Modified from Priester and Mantel (106).

SEX RISK

The overall relative risk (R) for tumors is higher ($R = 1.2$; $P < 0.001$) in female dogs. This has been attributed to the high frequency of mammary tumors. If sex-specific tumors are excluded, there is no marked sex differential. In cats, there is no evidence of a sex risk for all tumors combined. For malignant tumors only, a sex ratio of about 1:1 is seen in both species (106).

In contrast, the U.S. incidence (27) and mortality (85, 86) from cancer is much higher in men than in women, with the exception among American Indians (86). Excluding carcinoma *in situ* and nonmelanoma skin cancers, the average annual age-adjusted incidence for all sites in males (all races combined) in 347/100,000 population; for females of all races combined, the rate is 270/100,000 (27). Exclusion of sex-specific cancers widens this differential.

The greater risk in men has been, in part, attributed to the much higher frequency of lung

Table 35.3
Estimated Relative Risk (R) of Primary Tumors in Dogs for Those Breeds with 30 or More Tumors Observed or Expected, or with Risk Values Significantly (0.1%) Different than 1[a]

Breed	All Tumors		R[b]	Malignant Tumors		R[b]
	Observed	Expected		Observed	Expected	
Boxer	469	223.4	**4.0**	222	92.4	**3.3**
Kerry blue terrier	35	18.4	**3.0**	13	7.1	2.2
Great Dane	57	23.7	**2.8**	31	9.7	**3.6**
Airdale terrier	41	23.2	**2.6**	22	9.2	**3.2**
Bulldog, English	66	33.0	**2.5**	30	13.1	**2.6**
Weimaraner	124	73.4	**2.3**	55	30.6	**2.1**
Saint Bernard	70	36.6	**2.2**	38	15.0	**2.9**
Golden retriever	101	64.9	**2.1**	59	26.2	**2.9**
Scottish terrier	80	50.5	**2.0**	36	18.8	**2.2**
Irish setter	94	61.5	**1.9**	46	24.4	**2.1**
English setter	134	88.5	**1.8**	62	34.9	**2.0**
Pointer	137	88.7	**1.8**	61	33.6	**2.0**
Basset hound	71	47.1	**1.7**	31	19.6	1.7
Poodle, standard	118	82.8	**1.7**	41	33.0	1.3
German short-hair pointer	91	69.0	1.5	43	28.9	1.6
Norwegian elkhound	33	24.7	1.5	15	9.7	1.7
Doberman pinscher	58	46.0	1.4	22	18.6	1.2
English springer	78	61.3	1.4	35	24.5	1.5
Boston terrier	130	157.1	1.2	56	63.2	0.9
Labrador retriever	174	156.6	1.2	81	64.6	1.3
Cocker spaniel	383	371.2	1.1	135	152.2	0.9
Dalmatian	48	46.1	1.1	13	18.6	0.7
Other purebred	224	231.9	1.0	111	96.4	1.2
Miniature schnauzer	53	52.1	1.0	13	20.9	0.6
All canine species	6,009	6,009	1	2,431	2,431	1
Beagle hound	229	239.8	0.9	83	96.9	0.8
Brittany spaniel	65	72.3	0.9	24	28.3	0.8
German shepherd	338	353.2	0.9	183	146.6	**1.3**
Manchester terrier	41	48.6	0.8	14	19.7	0.7
Shetland sheepdog	47	53.5	0.8	23	21.8	1.1
Crossbreed	1,034	1,230.9	**0.8**	399	481.7	**0.8**
Colie	159	200.4	**0.7**	75	83.2	0.9
Pug	27	34.4	0.7	9	13.4	0.6
Poodle, miniature or toy	346	477.8	**0.6**	102	193.2	**0.5**
Dachshund	312	463.7	**0.6**	76	185.2	**0.4**
Pekingese	50	90.2	**0.5**	18	34.6	0.5
Fox terrier	79	132.4	**0.5**	24	52.2	**0.4**
Chihuahua	76	158.3	**0.4**	18	58.6	**0.3**
Pomeranian	27	60.3	**0.4**	4	24.0	**0.1**

[a] R of tumors for all breeds = 1. Adjustment was made for teaching facility, age, and sex. Cases reported to the Veterinary Medical Data Program, March 1964 through December 1969 (modified from Priester and Mantel (106)).
[b] R values which differed significantly ($P \leq 0.001$) from $R = 1$ are in **boldface** type.

Table 35.4
Estimated Relative Risk (R) of Primary Tumors in Cats for Those Breeds with 30 or More Tumors Observed or Expected, or with Risk Values Significantly (0.1%) Different than 1[a]

Breed	All Tumors		R[b]	Malignant Tumors		R[b]
	Observed	Expected		Observed	Expected	
Domestic short hair	294	288	1.0	211	205	1.1
Other feline species	64	64	1.0	41	40	1.0
All feline species	488	488	1	339	339	1
Siamese	92	98	0.9	60	67	0.9
Persian	34	36	0.9	24	27	0.9

[a] R of tumors for all breeds = 1. Adjustment was made for teaching facility, age, and sex. Cases reported to the Veterinary Medical Data Program, March 1964 through December 1969 (modified from Priester and Mantel (106)).
[b] R values did not differ significantly ($P \leq 0.001$) from $R = 1$.

cancer (much of which is the result of longer tobacco usage). The incidence of lung cancer in men is 81/100,000; women experience only one-fifth this rate (27). Less important, but still a risk factor have been occupational exposures experienced by men and generally not by women. Some of the male risk for lung cancer can be attributed to worker exposure to coal soot, tar, products of coal burning, petroleum products, mustard gas, arsenic, nickel, and uranium. Some other sites where cancer developes from worker exposure are 1) the nasal cavity and sinuses—chromium, wood, and leather; 2) bone marrow (leukemia)—benzene, radioactive elements, and x-rays; and 3) urinary bladder—aromatic hydrocarbons, tobacco, and leather (41). At this time, it is not known whether men would have greater risk for nonsex-specific tumors than women if the factors of tobacco usage and occupational exposures could be excluded.

SKIN

The early studies of human skin cancer have been considered "landmarks" of cancer epidemiology. Chronic exposure to sunlight was demonstrated in 1907 as one of the etiologic factors of these lesions (32). Today we known that there is a gradient effect between the amount of skin cancer and the host factor of skin pigmentation (81). The annual incidence rate can double for each 10 degrees decrease in latitude of an individual's environment (26). As expected, the lesion is very rare in black Americans (86). Although in the United States, skin cancer is inversely related to both social class and urbanization (41). Besides exposure to ultraviolet rays, chemicals such as arsenic, nitrates, and petroleum products are documented as etiologic agents.

Skin tumors are the most frequently diagnosed neoplasm in dogs and second most frequent in cats. Skin tumors (excluding those of the eyelids and perianal glands) accounted for 28% of all canine tumors in one study (106), 20–27% in other studies (31, 97).

Skin cancer (excluding melanoma) is the most frequently diagnosed malignancy of all cancers among humans (27). The magnitude of incidence can be extremely high. For instance, in Dallas-Fort Worth, Texas, the annual incidence of skin cancer has been greater than all other forms of cancer combined (26).

Familial (breed) predispositions to generalized skin tumors and skin cancer have been detected in several canine breeds (Table 35.5), but not in feline breeds. The diversity of anatomic characteristics of the canine breeds (e.g., different body conformation, hair coat density, and hair coat) deems it improbable that these characteristics have any strong association with risk for the lesion (103).

The boxer breed has consistently elevated risks for different skin tumors of mesodermal origin, particularly those cell-types derived from primitive hemangioblastic tissue—mastocytoma, hemangioma, hemangiopericytoma, and histocytoma (103). Aggregations of skin tumors have been reported in certain human families. An autosomal dominant form of inheritance is suggested for associations of multiple nevoid basal cell lesions with basal cell carcinoma, benign cystic epithelioma with basosquamous cell carcinoma, and other aggregations of skin tumors (49).

Bitch dogs have greater risk for skin tumors overall than males ($P < 0.01$). The excess is attributed to benign lesions. Apparently there is no increased risk among bitches for benign tumors under 4 and over 14 years of age, suggesting a possible etiologic role for ovarian hormones (or a protective role for testicular hormones). Both sexes have about equal risk for skin cancer (103). The risk for skin cancer in humans is twice as great in white men than white women (27). This finding has been attributed to the greater work-related exposure to ultraviolet rays in outdoor occupations generally dominated by males.

The most frequent tumor cell-types of human skin cancer are basal and squamous cell carcinomas (27). In dogs, the most common skin cancers are mastocytomas, followed by squamous cell carcinomas (103). The proportionally lower frequency of basal and squamous cell carcinomas in dogs, compared with humans, may be indicative of the natural protection offered by the dog's hair coat to the effects of ultraviolet rays. However, basal and squamous cell carcinomas do commonly occur on the unpigmented nose of collies and Shetland sheepdogs (92).

TESTIS

The mortality rate from testicular neoplasms has doubled in men in the last 20 years (91). This

Table 35.5
Estimated Relative Risk (R) of Primary Tumors of Skin by Breed among Dogs, for All Breeds with 10 or More Tumors Observed or Expected, or with Risk Values Significantly ($P < 0.01$) Different from 1[a]

Breed	All Tumors		Malignant Tumors	
	Observed	R[b]	Observed	R[b]
Kerry blue terrier	15	**4.4**	2	2.2
Norwegian elkhound	19	**2.7**	5	3.5
Basset hound	32	**2.6**	5	1.9
Boxer	124	**2.4**	43	**3.7**
Weimaraner	40	**2.2**	9	2.1
Scottish terrier	27	**2.1**	10	**3.8**
Bulldog	15	1.7	5	3.2
Pug	14	1.6	3	1.9
Poodle, standard	33	1.5	6	1.2
German shorthair pointer	28	1.5	5	1.2
Pointer	28	1.4	5	1.5
Golden retriever	25	1.3	6	1.6
Miniature schnauzer	20	1.3	4	1.3
Dalmatian	15	1.3	0	—[c]
Doberman pinscher	16	1.2	2	0.8
Shetland sheep dog	18	1.2	4	1.3
Boston terrier	50	1.2	14	1.6
Irish setter	20	1.2	6	1.8
English setter	25	1.1	4	1.0
Cocker spaniel	116	1.1	23	1.0
Saint Bernard	12	1.1	4	2.0
English springer	19	1.0	5	1.2
All canine breeds	16	1	337	1
Brittany spaniel	19	0.9	3	0.7
Labrador retriever	44	0.9	10	1.1
Crossbred	317	**0.9**	66	0.9
Dachshund	117	0.9	13	**0.5**
Beagle hound	57	0.9	8	0.6
Manchester terrier	12	0.8	2	0.6
Poodle, miniature or toy	121	0.8	16	0.6
Collie	42	0.8	13	1.2
Other purebred	46	0.7	10	0.8
German shepherd	66	**0.6**	9	0.5
Fox terrier	21	**0.6**	0	—[c]
Pekingese	13	0.5	4	0.9
Chihuahua	22	**0.5**	1	**0.1**
Pomeranian	5	**0.3**	0	—[c]

[a] R of tumors for all breeds combined equals 1. Adjusted for institution, age, and sex. Cases reported to the Veterinary Medical Data Program, March 1964 through December 1969 (modified from Priester (103)).
[b] R values significantly different from $R = 1$ ($P < 0.01$) are in **boldface** type.
[c] R was not calculated because there were no cases.

lesion is now the leading cause of cancer death among white Americans between the ages of 25 and 29 (85). These neoplasms are second in hospital prevalence to skin neoplasms in the male dog (60), but are very rare in the cat (106).

Men and dogs share many of the epidemiologic features of testicular tumors; the primary exception is the different frequency of occurrence of certain cell types. Embryonal carcinomas and teratomas predominate in children and

seminomas in adults, but Sertoli cell and interstitial cell tumors in humans are quite rare (91). In the dog, seminomas, Sertoli cell tumors, and interstitial cell tumors occur with about equal frequency; teratomas have been unreported (60).

Several canine breeds have been identified with an excessive risk for one or more cell types of testis tumors (Table 35.6). However, it is difficult to determine the magnitude of the effect from inheritance on the etiology of these tumors. In one report, of the 3 predominant cell types, 17.5%, 22%, and 16.7% of the cases of Sertoli cell tumors, seminomas, and interstitial cell tumors

Table 35.6
Estimated Relative Risk (R) for Dogs with Testicular Neoplasms by Breed[a]

Tumor Type/Breed	Cases Observed	R[b]	95% Confidence Interval
Sertoli cell tumor only (137)			
Shetland sheepdog	8	5.4	2.40–12.65
Weimaraner	6	4.8	1.98–11.92
Boxer	10	2.7	1.38–5.57
Poodle, standard	5	1.8	0.67–4.71
Boston terrier	5	1.7	0.61–4.38
German shepherd	14	1.5	0.89–2.88
Fox terrier	4	1.5	0.48–4.31
Labrador retriever	3	0.8	0.21–2.71
Poodle, miniature or toy	11	0.8	0.41–1.52
Mixed breed	15	0.5	0.26–0.80
Dachshund	3	0.3	0.07–0.87
Beagle	1	0.2	0.01–1.34
Seminoma only (127)			
German shepherd	20	2.6	1.75–4.85
Weimaraner	3	2.5	0.63–8.22
Boxer	8	2.1	1.01–4.73
Beagle	8	1.8	0.83–3.89
Fox terrier	5	1.8	0.68–4.83
Shetland sheepdog	2	1.7	0.29–7.04
Poodle, miniature or toy	15	1.2	0.71–2.25
Dachshund	8	0.8	0.36–1.70
Poodle, standard	2	0.7	0.13–3.04
Mixed breed	18	0.7	0.34–0.99
Labrador retriever	1	0.3	0.02–2.06
Boston terrier	1	0.3	0.02–2.16
Interstitial cell tumor only (96)			
Boxer	16	5.7	3.71–11.83
Boston terrier	5	2.2	0.81–5.87
Labrador retriever	5	1.8	0.55–5.07
Shetland sheepdog	1	1.1	0.06–7.50
Weimaraner	1	1.1	0.06–7.39
Fox terrier	2	1.0	0.17–3.93
Poodle, miniature or toy	8	0.8	0.33–1.77
Mixed breed	18	0.8	0.48–1.40
German shepherd	4	0.8	0.23–2.09
Beagle	3	0.6	0.10–2.43
Dachshund	4	0.5	0.17–1.50
Poodle, standard	1	0.5	0.03–3.25

[a] Modified from H. M. Hayes, Jr., and T. W. Pendergrass (60).
[b] R values were calculated for breeds with ≥ 5 cases of either Sertoli cell tumors, seminomas, or interstitial cell tumors; R was adjusted for age.

occurred, respectively, in high risk breeds. But, the boxer breed alone accounted for 7.3%, 6.2%, and 16.7% of these tumor cases (60). Familial occurrences of testicular tumors have been observed very infrequently in man (119).

What is intriguing is that the factor(s) responsible for the familial risk in boxers expressed itself in three different tumor cell types, whereas in the weimaraner, just two cell types were present excessively, and in the Shetland sheepdog and German shepherd dog only one cell type. In about half of the familial aggregates of testicular neoplasia in man, more than one tumor cell type was exhibited (119). This may be another opportunity for studies of the cytogenetic and immunogenetic constitution of high risk dog families that could offer clues applicable to similar conditions in man.

It does seem apparent, though, that other factors besides inheritance play a large role in testicular tumorigenesis. There is some evidence to suggest that enviornmental exposures associated with rural or urban living contribute to the origin of seminomas in man (18, 50, 78, 117). Unfortunately, comparative data for dogs are not currently available.

Cryptorchism has long been recognized as a contributing factor to testicular neoplasia. Whether the etiology of the tumor(s) is founded only upon the dysgenetic gonad or is also the result of the inguinal and intra-abdominal environment is debatable (119). Cryptorchid dogs have a risk for testis tumors 13.6 times that of normal dogs (60). In cryptorchid men, the relative risk has been estimated to be 14 by Mostofi (91) and 8.8 by Morrison (90). However, tumor cell types associated with the defect are different in each species. Among cryptorchid men, seminomas are the major cell type (90, 91), while seminomas and Sertoli cell tumors share about equal risk in cryptorchid dogs (60). Interstitial cell tumors have not been observed with cryptorchism in humans and only very rarely in dogs. The Shetland sheepdog has been proposed as an appropriate model for further research into testicular maldescent and tumorigenesis (60); they have excessive risk for each independent factor (60, 99).

OVARY

Ovarian malignancies represent 5% of the cancers diagnosed in U.S. women (27). Black Amer-

ican women experience about ¾ the mortality of white women. Similarly, American Indians, Chinese and Japanese American women have less mortality from ovarian cancer than white Americans (86). Most studies of human ovarian cancer have been based upon death certificates. Criticisms have been levied that these sources of data lacked information about "borderline" malignancies. Tumors that appear as benign lesions but later have tendencies to become malignant are not recorded (77). Thus, ovarian cancer could be a greater problem than may be currently realized. Ovarian tumors are uncommon in the dog and very rare in the cat.

There is a strong histologic similarity between ovarian neoplasms in dogs and those in women with the exception of granulosa-theca cell tumors. These tumors show considerably more morphological variation in bitch dogs than in women. This finding led Willis (129) to suggest that granulosa-theca cell tumors and epithelial ovarian tumors in the dog may share a common etiology. However, this hypothesis is not consistent with the presently known epidemiologic features of these tumors in dogs (61).

The epidemiologic features of human ovarian cancer vary widely in different countries (77). Epithelial neoplasms account for about 75% of the U.S. incidence of ovarian cancer in white females (27). Second most frequent are granulosa-theca cell tumors. In the dog, epithelial neoplasms account for 60% and granulosa-theca cell tumors 27% of the classifiable tumors (Table 35.7).

Epithelial ovarian cancers, as a group, show consistently increasing rates of incidence with age through 75 years in women. In contrast, the incidence rates for malignant granulosa-theca cell tumors present two relatively static levels of occurrence with 45 years being the age when risk increases (27) (Fig. 35.1). Similarly in dogs, risk increases strikingly with age for bitches with epithelial ovarian tumors. Whereas, those with granulosa-theca cell tumors have a generally constant risk between 4 and 15 years of age, followed by an increase (Fig. 35.2).

There is little evidence of a familial association of ovarian neoplasms in women (77). However, the incidence of ovarian cancer is much higher in white than black women. The difference here is attributed to the much higher incidence of epithelial ovarian cancer in whites over 45 years of age than experienced by blacks (127). Inheritance plays only a small role, at most, in the etiology of the canine lesion (Table 35.8) (61).

The pathogenesis for spontaneous ovarian tu-

Table 35.7
Distribution of 92 Canine Ovarian Neoplasms Reported to the Veterinary Medical Data Program, March, 1964 to June, 1976[a]

Histogenetic Origin	No. of Cases
Tumors of germinal epithelium (53)	
Adenocarcinoma	15
Cystadenocarcinoma	11
Cystadenoma	10
Adenoma	7
Serous papillary cystadenoma	4
Serous papillary cystadenocarcinoma	2
Carcinoma, type unspecified	2
Cystadenoma (malignancy not determined)	1
Brenner tumor (malignant)	1
Tumors of sex cord stroma (23)	
Granulosa cell tumor	3
Benign	8
Malignant	11
Malignancy not determined	1
Theca cell tumor (malignancy not determined)	
Tumors of germ-cell origin (7)	
Teratoma	1
Benign	1
Malignant	3
Malignancy not determined	2
Dysgerminoma (malignancy not determined)	
Tumors of soft tissue not specific to ovary (5)	
Fibroma	2
Fibrosarcoma	1
Leiomyoma	1
Sarcoma, type unspecified	1
Unclassified tumors	4

[a] Modified from H. M. Hayes, Jr., and J. L. Young, Jr. (61).

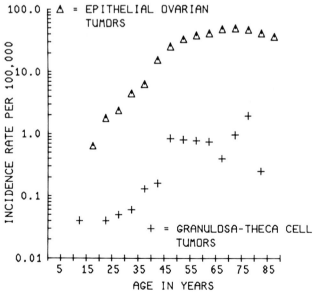

Figure 35.1. Annual incidence rate per 100,000 women by age for epithelial ovarian tumors and granulosa-theca cell tumors in the United States in 1969–1971 (127). Rates plotted at the midpoint for 5 year intervals from 10 through 84 years; ≥85 years was plotted at 87.5 years.

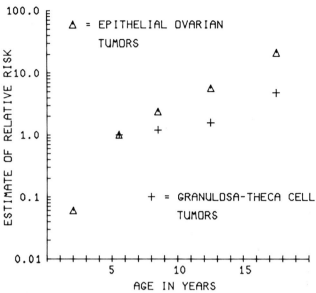

Figure 35.2. Estimated relative risk (R) by age for dogs with epithelial ovarian tumors and granulosa-theca cell tumors. The age interval 4–6 years was used as the standard reference ($R = 1$). R values for the age intervals 0–3, 4–6, 7–9, and 10–14 years were plotted at the midpoint of each interval; ≥15 years was plotted at 17.5 years. (Reproduced with permission from H. M. Hayes, Jr., and J. L. Young, Jr.: *Gynecologic Oncology*, 6:348–353, 1978 (61).)

Table 35.8
Estimated Relative Risk (R) of Ovarian Tumors by Breed Among Dogs Seen by Veterinary Medical Data Program Participants, March 1964—June 1976[a]

Ovarian Neoplasm	Breed	No. of Cases	R	99% Confidence Intervals
Tumors of germinal epithelial origin (N = 55)[b]	Pointer	3	4.0	1.04–13.84
	Cocker spaniel	5	2.3	0.84–6.34
	Dachshund	4	2.0	0.64–5.99
	Poodles[c]	10	1.6	0.80–3.50
	German shepherd	4	1.2	0.37–3.48
	Mixed breed	5	0.4	0.11–0.86
Granulosa-theca cell tumors (N = 23)[d]	English bulldog	3	20.8	4.47–82.28
	Poodles[c]	4	1.7	0.52–5.61
	Mixed breed	3	0.3	0.14–2.03

[a] Modified from H. M. Hayes, Jr., and J. L. Young, Jr. (61).
[b] R calculated for breeds represented by 3 or more cases.
[c] Includes miniature and toy poodles.
[d] R calculated for breeds represented by 2 or more cases.

mors in humans and animals is obscure. Suspected causes among women include hormonal imbalances and environmental carcinogens. Lingeman (77), in her treatise on human ovarian cancer, suggests the latter as the most prominent cause of the lesion, although few definitive clues exist. Unfortunately, the presently known epidemiologic features of canine ovarian cancer shed no new light on etiology (61). Yet, the bitch dog does appear to be a suitable model for testing suspected ovarian carcinogens in women because of the similarities of the disease in both subjects.

MAMMARY GLAND

In the United States, white women have about 10% greater mortality from breast cancer than do blacks; American Indians, Chinese and Japanese Americans have less than half the mortality rate of whites (86). Tumors of the mammary gland are the most common neoplasm in the female dog and are not infrequent in the cat (106), although less is known about the epidemiology of the feline lesion. The ratio of female cats to male dogs with the lesion is about 50:1 (unpublished data from the VMDP, 1980), which is about the same ratio in humans (86). The distribution of mammary cancer by age in bitch dogs seems similar to that in women, using Lebeau's (72) dog-years to human-years formula (115).

Feline mammary carcinomas are more readily recognized histologically as malignant than canine mammary carcinomas. Occasionally in the cat, and often in the dog, mammary carcinomas are not uniform in histologic apperance. As in humans, it appears that a correlation exists in the cat between histologic grading and prognosis (52).

Intact and spayed female cats have similar patterns of age risk for mammary carcinoma. This may be notable since spayed females show only 60% of the cancer risk of intact females. While oophorectomy is protective, the optimum age for surgery is unclear (unpublished data from the VMDP, 1980).

The relationship between tumor risk and parity in the bitch dog has been disputed (13, 37, 115, 126). Schneider *et al.* (115) have reported that a significant sparing effect for mammary cancer occurs in the bitch who has had an oophorectomy prior to 2.5 years of age. Studies of human breast cancer show that 1) risk increases with age at giving first birth, 2) women under 30 years of age who complete a full term pregnancy have less cancer risk than nulliparous women, although cancer protection is generally not enhanced by additional births (83), and 3) oophorectomy in women under 40 years of age has a protective effect (35).

Familial factors play some role in the etiology of breast cancer. Female relatives of women with breast cancer have 2–3 times risk for the lesion than the general population (83). The increased risk is especially evident in the patient's children of either sex (33, 82).

Siamese cats have twice the risk ($P=0.01$) of other breeds for mammary carcinoma. They also tend to be younger than other breeds of cats at the time of cancer diagnosis (unpublished data from the VMDP, 1980).

In dogs, an excessive risk for mammary cancer has been identified in four canine breeds—miniature poodle, English setter, German shorthair pointer, and pointer (unpublished data from the VMDP, 1977). It is important to note that the Pointer breed is also at high risk for ovarian cancer (Table 35.8). The occurrence of both cancers appears to be linked in some human families (42).

More investigation is needed to delineate factors possibly affecting canine and feline mammary cancer (*i.e.*, obesity, presence of benign mammary neoplasms). Yet, there appears to be ample reason to use the dog and cat as research models to better understand human breast cancer.

BLADDER

In man, bladder cancer accounts for 4.3% of the incidence of all malignancies (27). In dogs, it represents 1% of the hospital prevalence of malignant tumors (54) and is very rare in cats (106). Racial differences in mortality exist in the United States; American Indians have about half

Table 35.9
Canine Bladder Cancer by Sex Reported to the Veterinary Medical Data Program March 1964 to July 1975[a]

Tumor Group	No. of Cases	Sex	
		Male	Female
Epithelial tissue			
Transitional cell carcinoma	87	33	54
Squamous cell carcinoma	7	4	3
Adenocarcinoma	6	4	2
Unclassified carcinoma	1	1	0
Muscular tissue			
Leiomyosarcoma	5	3	2
Connective tissue			
Fibrosarcoma	3[b]	0	2
Unclassified sarcoma	2	0	2
Vascular tissue			
Hemangiosarcoma	3	2	1
Total	114[b]	47	66

[a] Modified from H. M. Hayes, Jr. (54).
[b] Sex not reported in one case.

Table 35.10
Estimated Relative Risk (R) of Transitional Cell Carcinoma in Dogs by Breed[a]

Breed Category	Cases Observed		R[b]	95% C.I.[c]	P
	Male	Female			
Scottish terrier	1	7	12.9	6.3–30.5	< 0.001
Shetland sheepdog	3	3	7.6	3.2–19.5	< 0.001
Beagle	2	7	3.0	1.5–6.6	< 0.001
Collie	5	2	2.7	1.2–6.5	< 0.01
Cocker spaniel	1	3	0.9	0.3–2.7	> 0.1
Mix breed (mongrel)	9	7	0.8	0.4–1.3	> 0.1
Poodle, toy and miniature	2	5	0.7	0.3–1.5	> 0.1

[a] Modified from H. M. Hayes, Jr. (54).
[b] Adjustment made for age and sex.
[c] Confidence interval; when C.I. does not include 1, breed R is significantly different from that in all breeds combined $P < 0.05$.

the death rate from bladder cancer than whites or blacks (86). Transitional cell carcinoma is the most common malignant tumor of the human (20) and canine (54) bladder (Table 35.9).

Four canine breeds show a marked propensity for the malignancy (Table 35.10). There is little evidence for an inheritance role in humans although two families have been identified with an unusual aggregation of bladder tumors (43, 87). One characteristic investigated in the living members of these families was their level of urinary tryphophan metabolites, a suspected cause of bladder cancer (20). The similarities in the tryphophan metabolism between humans and dogs (14,101) suggest that further studies using high risk breeds of dogs could be helpful.

Female dogs have been detected with 1.5 times the risk of male dogs ($P < 0.05$) for transitional cell carcinoma (54). This sex differential probably has its etiology in the patterns of infrequent urination on a daily basis by the female dog as compared to the male (122). Urine-borne carcinogenic agents would thus have longer exposure to the bladder epithelium of the female than the male dog. McDonald and Lund (88) have demonstrated that urine containing the carcinogenic agent must come into contact with the bladder epithelium to initiate tumorigenesis.

The sex risk is reversed in humans (27). About half of the incidence of bladder cancer in men is reportedly associated with cigarette smoking (40, 76) and occupational exposures to chemicals, e.g., aromatic amines (20).

Recent canine trials indicate a dose-time relationship exists for the lesion. The total dose of carcinogen required to produce tumors is considerably less if given in small amounts over an extended period of time (21). The latent period has been as long as 10 years in some trials. Yet, once carcinogenesis has been initiated, removal of the exposure does not inhibit the growth of the tumor (88). The overall low frequency of bladder cancer in dogs is consistent with a low dose response to general environmental exposures over an extended period of time (54).

It has been proposed that transitional cell carcinoma in the dog should be made a reportable disease in the United States (54). Increasing case counts over time, a method used by the Center for Disease Control, U.S. Public Health Service, to monitor and control rabies in animal wildlife (69), would possibly identify geographic areas where emerging environmental hazards to humans are now present.

KIDNEY

Very little is known about the etiology of renal carcinoma. Wynder (132) has proposed nutritional factors, e.g., animal fats and cholesterol, as a possible cause.

The epidemiology of feline renal carcinoma is unknown. The epidemiologic features of canine renal carcinoma are very similar to those in humans. Renal carcinoma accounts for 2% of human malignancies (27). They represent slightly less than 1% of malignancies in the dog. In neither species are genetic determinants conspicuous, although men and male dogs are at high risk for the lesion (27, 57).

Interestingly, the male predominance of canine renal carcinoma by age also resembles that in man (57). The canine male risk peaks at 7–9 years of age. Using LeBeau's conversion of dog-years to human-years (72), the mean of this age group approximates 49 years of age in humans. Similarly, the sex differential (male:female incidence rates) in humans is the highest in the age bracket of 45–49 years (27) (Fig. 35.3).

The reason for the male predominance of human renal carcinoma is obscure. Environmental factors are suggested by the rising incidence among American men, but not among women (68) and call for further studies to evaluate the role of tobacco, nutrition, and occupational determinants. However, these factors cannot account for the male excess in dogs (and similar trends in sex ratio with age) and suggest the influence of host susceptibility, including the endogenous production or metabolism of sex hormones. There is evidence of remission in some human patients treated with progestrone (70, 112).

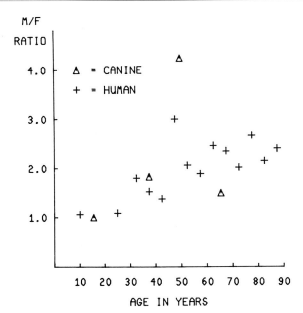

Figure 35.3. Distribution of the male/female ratio of renal carcinoma in humans (27) and dogs by midpoint age intervals using the dog-years to human-years conversion formula (72). (Reproduced with permission from H. M. Hayes, Jr., and J. F. Fraumeni, Jr.: *Cancer Research,* 37:2253–2256, 1977 (57).)

THYROID GLAND

Endocrine malignancies compose 1.4% of all cancers in humans (27), 3.7% and 0.9% of the cancer in hospitalized dogs and cats (106). Carcinoma of the thyroid is the predominant lesion. An environmental influence, linked with endemic goiter, has been disputed as an etiologic factor in human beings (34) and dogs (55). X-radiation, a well known etiologic agent for the human lesion (98), has not been implicated in the spontaneous neoplasia of the thyroid gland of domestic animals (55).

The morbidity and mortality from thyroid cancers is about 2 times greater in women than in men (34, 85); an exception is the 1:1 sex ratio among Japanese Americans (86). The diagnostic frequency in dogs shows no sex differential (55); the epidemiology in cats is unknown.

Medullary thyroid carcinoma, singularly or in combination with other endocrine abnormalities, has been reported in familial agregates in man (38). Familial predispositions to thyroid carcinoma have been detected in several canine breeds (Table 35.11), however medullary carcinoma is relatively rare in dogs (16).

The excess risk among boxers is thought to be partly due to the anomalous follicular patterns commonly seen in their thyroid glands. More

Table 35.11
Estimated Relative Risk (*R*) of Canine Thyroid Carcinoma for Breeds in Which ≥5 Cases Were Reported to the VMDP March 1964 through June 1975[a]

Breed	Cases	*R*[b]	95% Confidence Interval
Boxer	19	8.1	5.59–15.80
Golden retriever	5	4.1	1.51–10.68
Beagle	10	2.3	1.21–4.83
Labrador retriever	6	1.9	0.79–4.70
Dachshund	10	1.1	0.52–2.22
All dogs	119	1.0	
Mixed breed	20	0.7	0.41–1.14
Poodle (miniature and toy)	5	0.4	0.14–0.98

[a] Modified from H. M. Hayes, Jr., and J. F. Fraumeni, Jr. (55).
[b] R adjusted for age and sex.

interesting is the finding of excessively high risk among the beagle breed (55). Investigators have reported an unexplained high prevalence of thyroiditis in several beagle colonies used in laboratory research (8,125). This type of thyroiditis is indistinguishable from Hashimoto's thyroiditis in man (94).

Hashimoto's disease is an autoimmune disorder with familial aggregation, at times suggesting an autosomal dominant form of inheritance in humans (109). A question yet to be resolved is whether or not Hashimoto's disease increases the risk for thyroid carcinoma in humans (23, 24, 45, 131). Follow-up studies of beagles with thyroiditis may clarifiy this relationship.

Certain other primary neoplasms have been identified in man as occurring in association with thyroid carcinoma. Multiple endocrine adenomatosis, type 1 (MEA$_1$) syndrome is a dominantly inherited constellation consisting of hyperplasia, adenomas, and occasionally carcinomas of several endocrine glands, including the thyroid, adrenal cortex, and pituitary (7). Multiple lipomas have also been implicated as part of MEA$_1$ (10, 120). Dogs have also been reported with these same aggregates of lesions (55). However, the etiology of the syndrome in dogs is unclear. Another tumor complex that occurs in humans (2) and dogs (56) involves tumors of chemoreceptor tissue and the thyroid.

CHEMORECEPTOR SYSTEM

The chemoreceptor system consists of numerous morphologically similar glomera located throughout the body. The larger clusters of cells have been named the glomus jugulare, glomus pulmonale, aortic body, and carotid body. Although the function and mode of action is not completely understood, the aortic and carotid bodies have been shown to be responsive to changes in the oxygen and carbon dioxide tensions, pH, and temperature of the circulating blood (15).

These bodies can initiate an increase in the depth, minute volume, and rate of respiration via parasympathetic innervation. Also, via the sympathetic nervous system, they can increase the heart rate and elevate the arterial blood pressure. The human and canine chemoreceptor systems are quite similar.

Tumors of these structures (chemodectomas) are uncommon in humans and dogs, and very rarely occur in cats. In people, they occur twice as often in the carotid body as in other sites (111). Conversely, about 80% of the chemodectomas in dogs are located at the aortic body (56). Chemodectomas, regardless of location however, are histologically indistinguishable. There is usually no correlation between histologic appearance of this tumor and its malignancy potential (17).

The number of human chemodectomas observed in each sex has been about the same; one exception are Peruvians living in the Andes. They experience a 6-fold excess among their women (100, 101). In dogs, males have about 2 times the risk of females (53). In neither humans nor dogs are the reasons for this sex differential known. However, an association of seminomas and interstitial cell tumors in conjunction with chemodectomas has been reported in dogs (56, 67).

Genetic factors have been implicated, by familial aggregations, in about 8% of humans with carotid body tumors (100, 130). Further, chronic hypoxia was implicated in the etiology among Peruvians living at high altitudes in the Andes (111).

In dogs, only breeds of English bulldog ancestry (i.e., boxer, Boston terrier) have been detected with significantly high risk (53). Brachycephalic breeds frequently have soft tissue anomalies of the oral and nasal cavities which restrict and impede respiration (39, 73). However, other brachycephalic breeds, e.g., Pekingese and pug, show no particular affinity for chemodectomas. Thus, for bulldog breeds, a genetic predisposition plus the aggravation of respiratory distress may be the basic factors responsible for the tumorigenesis of their chemoreceptor systems (53).

BRAIN

Intracranial neoplasms have held a special interest for researchers over many centuries.

Irrespective of the tumor's behavior (benign or malignant), these neoplasms have an insidious effect caused by the increase in intracranial pressure due to displacement by the tumor's growth.

The annual age-adjusted incidence of brain tumors in humans is about 5 per 100,000 in the United States (27). These tumors are rare in domestic animals with the exception of the dog (59). Gliomas, astrocytomas, and glioblastomas are the predominant tumor types of the brain in adult humans and dogs. Medulloblastomas predominate in children. Little is known about the types of brain tumors that occur in puppies.

The age distribution in humans is biphasic. The childhood peak is under 10 years of age and the adult peak is 65–69 years (27). The highest risk plateau in dogs is between 10 and 14 years of age (59), the median of which approximates the second peak in humans (72). Men have higher mortality from brain tumors than women and the rate is uniform in different races in the United States (86). No sex risk has been noted in dogs (59).

The etiology of naturally occurring brain tumors is obscure. An association of reticulum cell sarcoma in the human brain following renal transplant and immunosuppression has been observed (114). In dogs, gliomas have been induced with Rous sarcoma virus (51).

Familial excesses for astrocytomas have been reported in humans (89, 128). In dogs, only breeds of English bulldog ancestry show high risk (59). As mentioned in the discussion of chemodectomas, this composite dog family commonly have soft tissue anomalies of the nose and mouth which may result in chronic hypoxia.

Chronic hypoxia in humans can be a stimulus for fibrillary gliosis in the neonatal and infantile brain (11), the severity of which appears to be correlated with the length of time of prolonged hypoxia (12). Gliosis may be a precursor of gliomas and other related tumors. Or, the conditions may share a common etiology, since the entire spectrum of nodular and diffuse gliosis, gliomatosis, astrocytomas, and glioblastoma has been concurrently observed in people with neurofibromatosis (1, 6, 79), a known genetically determined disease (3).

BLOOD-LYMPHATIC SYSTEM

Tumors of the hematopoietic system are the most common neoplasms diagnosed in cats and rank fourth in occurrence in dogs. The leukemia-lymphoma complex ranks first in cats and dogs for the percentage of malignancies (106). Leukemia accounts for about half of the incidence of cancer in children under 5 years of age. Lymphomas account for about 3% of the cancers in the same age group. Each lesion represents 3.25% of the annual age-adjusted incidence of cancer in the United States (27). Among racial groups in the United States, whites have the highest mortality from leukemia; black, Chinese, and Japanese Americans have about two-thirds of the white rate (86). The age distribution of feline lymphosarcoma is biphasic (28) and similar in age pattern to human leukemia (27).

Lymphoid tumors constitute most of the hematopoietic neoplasms in dogs and cats, and lymphosarcoma is the most common form of malignancy of the system. It should be noted that the term "leukemia" in the veterinary literature has often been used as a general term to represent, in fact, lymphosarcoma. Lymphosarcoma is a solid tumor while leukemia denotes free neoplastic cells in the vascular system. Histologically, lymphosarcomas in the dog and cat are similar and resemble the disease in man.

The boxer (19, 29, 102) and English pointer (102) have been identified with significantly high risk for canine lymphosarcoma. No sex-specific features are evident in the dog (102). Transmission of the canine disease has not been successful with cell-free distillates of the tumor (63).

Lymphosarcoma is the most prevalent malignant tumor in cats. No breed predisposition has been established. Males appear to have a 2-fold risk compared with females (28).

The etiology of the feline lesion is a C-type RNA virus (66), commonly referred to as feline leukemia virus (FeLV). FeLV has been transmitted by cat-to-cat contact in the laboratory (65). This is also the likely mode of transmission in the general population (116). The errant and often hostile instincts of the male (noncastrated) cat to other male cats may subject them to sufficient cat-to-cat contact that could explain their 2-fold risk for FeLV infection. Feline lymphosarcoma has been associated with at least one other infectious disease, feline infectious anemia (FIA). FIA is caused by *Hemobartonella felis*, a protozoan, and can result in severe anemia.

Cats with acute clinical expression of FIA have 12 times the risk of development of feline lymphosarcoma as matched controls (105). The exact association between FIA and feline lymphosarcoma (105) or between severe anemia and subsequent lymphosarcoma is unclear (71). As in experiments with rats and mice (46, 47), severe anemia may trigger clinical lymphosarcoma in the cat. However, the causal organisms of FIA and FeLV could, in some way, be linked. Similar

to lymphosarcoma, FIA appears to be naturally transmitted by cat-to-cat contact; male cats have a 2.5 fold risk for acute clinical disease (58).

Evidence has been presented to show FeLV can cross species barriers. Newborn and young puppies inoculated with FeLV will develop lymphosarcoma (108, 121). Of great importance is the fact that FeLV will replicate in human cells (64, 113). Many studies have evaluated the possibility of cat-to-human transmission of FeLV; none have shown the FeLV is a hazard to man (74).

CONCLUSIONS

Recent data about the epidemiologic features of all neoplasms and those specifically occurring at 10 different sites in dogs and cats have been reviewed. Far more information is currently known about oncology in dogs than cats. The epidemiologic features for canine tumors at most of the body sites showed marked similarity to those in humans. Although, the frequency of particular cell-types at some organs often differs. Considerable research is underway to determine which cancers in the dog are correlated with environmental factors that affect human beings. Identification and monitoring the frequency of these canine cancers may provide a prognostic resource about subsequent environmentally influenced cancer in human beings.

References

1. Aita, J. A. (1968): Genetic aspects of tumors of the nervous system. *Nebr. Med. J.*, 53:121–124.
2. Albores-Saavedra, J. and Duran, M. E. (1973): Association of thyroid carcinoma and chemodectoma. *Am. J. Surg.*, 116:887–890.
3. Anderson, D. E. (1970): Genetic varieties of neoplasia, in *Genetic Concepts and Neoplasia*, pp. 85–104. Williams & Wilkins, Baltimore.
4. Anderson, D. E., Pope, L. S., and Stephens, D. (1970): Nutrition and eye cancer in cattle. *J.N.C.I.*, 45:697–707.
5. Anderson, D. E., and Skinner, P. E. (1961): Studies on bovine ocular squamous cell carcinoma ("cancer eye"); XI. Effects on sunlight. *J. Anim. Sci.*, 20:474–477.
6. Barnard, R. O., and Lang, E. R. (1964): Cerebral and cerebellar gliomas in a case of von Recklinghausen's disease with adrenal phaeochromocytomas. *J. Neurosurg.*, 21:506–511.
7. Bartuska, D. (1973): Evolving concepts of the genetics of thyroid disease—a review. *Am. J. Med. Sci.*, 266:249–252.
8. Beierwaltes, W. H., and Nishiyama, R. H. (1968): Dog thyroiditis; occurrence and similarity to Hashimoto's struma. *Endocrinology*, 83:501–508.
9. Beveridge, W. I. B. (1972): Data storage and retrieval systems for disease information, in *Proceedings of the International Summer School on Computers and Research in Animal Nutrition and Veterinary Medicine*, pp. 329–337, edited by A. Madsen and P. Willeberg. Frederiksberg Bogtrykkeri, Copenhagen.
10. Bolande, R. P. (1974): The neurocristopathies. A unifying concept of disease arising in neural crest maldevelopment. *Hum. Pathol.*, 5:409–429.
11. Brand, M. M., and Bignami, A. (1969): The effects of chronic hypoxia on the neonatal and infantile brain. *Brain*, 92:233–254.
12. Brand, M. M., Durbridge, T. C., Rosan, R. C., and Northway, W. H., Jr. (1972): Neuropathological lesions in respiratory disease syndrome; acute and chronic changes during hypoxia and oxygen therapy. *J. Reprod. Med.*, 8:267–279.

13. Brodey, R. S., Fidler, I.J., and Howson, A. E. (1966): The relationship of estrous irregularity, pseudopregnancy, and pregnancy to the development of canine mammary neoplasms. *J. Am. Vet. Med. Assoc.*, 149: 1047–1049.

14. Brown, R. R., and Price, J. M. (1956): Quantitative studies on metabolites of tryptophan in the urine of the dog, cat, rat, and man. *J. Biol. Chem.*, 219:985–997.

15. Burman, S. O. (1956): The chemoreceptor system and its tumor—the chemodectoma. *Surg. Gynecol. Obstet*, 102:330–341.

16. Casey, H. W. (1975): Unpublished data from the Armed Forces Institute of Pathology.

17. Cheville, N. F. (1972): Ultrastructure of canine carotid body and aortic body tumors. *Pathol. Vet.*, 9:166–189.

18. Clemmesen, J. (1968): A doubling of morbidity from testis carcinoma Copenhagen, 1943–1962. *Acta Pathol. Microbiol. Scand.*, 72:348–349.

19. Cohen, D., Booth, S., and Sussman, O. (1959): An epidemiological study of canine lymphoma and its public health significance. *Am. J. Vet. Res.*, 20:1026–1031.

20. Cole, P. (1975): Lower urinary tract, in *Cancer Epidemiology and Prevention*, pp. 233–262, edited by D. Schottenfeld. Charles C Thomas, Springfield, Ill.

21. Conzelman, G. M., Jr., and Moulton, J. E. (1972): Dose-response relationships of the bladder tumorigen 2-naphthylamine; a study in beagle dogs. *J.N.C.I.*, 49:193–200.

22. Cotchin, E. (1951): Neoplasms in small animals. *Vet. Rec.*, 63:67–72.

23. Crile, G., and Fisher, E. W. (1953): Simultaneous occurrence of thyroiditis and papillary carcinoma. *Cancer*, 6:57–62.

24. Crile, G., and Hazard, J. B. (1962): Incidence of cancer in struma lymphomatosa. *Surg. Gynecol. Obstet.*, 115:101–103.

25. Crocker, W. J. (1919): Three thousand autopsies. *Cornell Vet.*, 9:142–161.

26. Cutler, S. J., Scotto, J., Devesa, S. S., et al. (1974): Third national cancer survey—an overview of available information. *J.N.C.I.*, 53:1565–1575.

27. Cutler, S. J., and Young, J. L., Jr. (eds.) (1975): National Cancer Institute Monograph 41: Third National Cancer Survey Incidence Data. DHEW Pub. No. (NIH) 75–787, Washington, D.C.

28. Dorn, C. R., Taylor, D. O. N., and Hibbard, H. H. (1967): Epizootiologic characteristics of canine and feline leukemia and lymphoma. *Am. J. Vet. Res.*, 28:993–1001.

29. Dorn, C. R., Taylor, D. O. N., and Schneider, R. (1970): The epidemiology of canine leukemia and lymphoma. *Bibl. Haematol.*, 36:403–415.

30. Dorn, C. R., Taylor, D. O. N., and Schneider, R. (1971): Sunlight exposure and risk of developing cutaneous and oral squamous cell carcinomas in white cats. *J.N.C.I.*, 46:1073–1078.

31. Dorn, C. R., Taylor, D. O. N., Schneider, R., et al. (1968): Survey of animal neoplasms in Alameda and Contra Costa Counties, California; II. Cancer morbidity in dogs and cats from Alameda County. *J.N.C.I.*, 40:307–318.

32. Dubreuilh, W. (1907): Epitheliomatose d'origine solaire. *Ann. Dermato-Syphiligr. (Paris)*, 8:387–416.

33. Everson, R. B., Fraumeni, J. F., Jr., Wilson, R. E., et al. (1976): Familial male breast cancer. *Lancet*, 1:9–12.

34. Farooki, M. A. (1968): Epidemiology and pathology of cancer of the thyroid; Part 2. Discussion. *Int. Surg.*, 51:317–333.

35. Feinleib, M. (1968): Breast cancer and artificial menopause; a cohort study. *J.N.C.I.*, 41:315–329.

36. Feldman, W. H. (1927): The primary situation of 133 spontaneous tumors in the lower animals. *J. Cancer Res.*, 11:436–462.

37. Fidler, I. J., Abt, D. A., and Brodey, R. S. (1967): The biological behavior of canine mammary neoplasms. *J. Am. Vet. Med. Assoc.*, 151:1311–1318.

38. Fletcher, J. R. (1970): Medullary (solid) carcinoma of the thyroid gland. *Arch. Surg.*, 100:257–262.

39. Fox, M. W. (1963): Developmental abnormalities of the canine skull. *Can. J. Comp. Vet. Sci.*, 27:219–222.

40. Fraumeni, J. F., Jr. (1968): Cigarette smoking and cancers of the urinary tract; geographic variation in the United States. *J.N.C.I.*, 41:1205–1211.

41. Fraumeni, J. F., Jr. (ed.) (1975): *Persons at High Risk of Cancer. An Approach to Cancer Etiology and Control*. Academic Press, New York.

42. Fraumeni, J. F., Jr., Grundy, G. W., Creagan, E. T., et al. (1975): Six families prone to ovarian cancer. *Cancer*, 36:364–369.

43. Fraumeni, J. F., Jr., and Thomas, L. B. (1967): Malignant bladder tumors in a man and his three sons. *J.A.M.A.*, 201:507–509.

44. Gart, J. J. (1970): Point and interval estimation of the common odds ratio in the combination of 2×2 tables with fixed marginals. *Biometrika*, 57:471–475.

45. Glass, H. G., Waldron, G. W., and Brown, W. G. (1956): Coexistent sarcoma, adenocarcinoma and Hashimoto disease in a thyroid gland. *Cancer*, 9:310–316.

46. Gong, J. K. (1971): Anemic stress as a trigger of myelogenous leukemia in rats rendered leukemia-prone by x-ray. *Science*, 174:833–835.

47. Gong, J. K., Braunschweiger, P. G., and Glomski, C. A. (1971): Anemic stress as a trigger of myelogenous leukemia in the unirradiated RF mouse. *Science*, 177:274–276.

48. Goodpasture, E. W. (1918): An anatomical study of senescence in dogs with especial reference to relation of cellular changes of age to tumors. *J. Med. Res.*, 38:127–190.

49. Gorlin, R. J., and Sedano, H. O. (1972): The multiple nevoid basal cell carcinoma syndrome revisited, in *Skin, Heredity, and Malignant Neoplasms*, pp. 149–164, edited by H. T. Lynch. Medical Examination Pub., Flushing, N.Y.

50. Graham, S., and Gibson, R. W. (1972): Social epidemiology of cancer of the testis. *Cancer*, 29:1242–1249.

51. Haguenau, F., Rabotti, G. F., Lyon, G., et al. (1971): Gliomas induced by Rous sarcoma virus in the dog—an ultrastructural study. *J.N.C.I.*, 46: 539–545.

52. Hampe, J. F., and Misdorp, W. (1974): Tumours and dysplasias of the mammary gland. *Bull W.H.O.*, 50:111–113.

53. Hayes, H. M., Jr. (1975): An hypothesis for the aetiology of canine chemoreceptor system neoplasms, based upon an epidemiological study of 73 cases among hospital patients. *J. Small Anim. Pract.*, 16: 337–343.

54. Hayes, H. M., Jr. (1976): Canine bladder cancer: epidemiologic features. *Am. J. Epidemiol.*, 104:673–677.

55. Hayes, H. M., Jr., and Fraumeni, J. F., Jr. (1975): Canine thyroid neoplasms; epidemiologic features. *J.N.C.I.*, 55:931–934.

56. Hayes, H. M., Jr., and Fraumeni, J. F., Jr. (1974): Chemodectomas in dogs; epidemiologic comparisons with man. *J.N.C.I.*, 52:1455–1458.

57. Hayes, H. M., Jr., and Fraumeni, J. F., Jr. (1977): Epidemiologic features of canine renal neoplasms. *Cancer Res.*, 37:2253–2256.

58. Hayes, H. M., Jr., and Priester, W. A. (1973): Feline infectious anaemia. Risk by age, sex and breed; prior disease; seasonal occurrence; mortality. *J. Small Anim. Pract.*, 14:797–804.

59. Hayes, H. M., Jr., Priester, W. A., and Pendergrass, T. W. (1975): Occurrence of nervous-tissue tumors in cattle, horses, cats and dogs. *Int. J. Cancer*, 15:39–47.

60. Hayes, H. M., Jr., and Pendergrass, T. W. (1976): Canine testicular tumors; epidemiologic features of 410 dogs. *Int. J. Cancer*, 18:482–487.

61. Hayes, H. M., Jr., Young, J. L., Jr. (1978): Epidemiologic features of canine ovarian neoplasms. *Gynecol. Oncol.* 6:348–353.

62. Holsti, L. R., and Ermala, P. (1955): Papillary carcinoma of the bladder in mice, obtained after peroral administration of tobacco tar. *Cancer*, 8:679–682.

63. Jarrett, O. (1970): Evidence for the viral etiology of leukemia in the domestic mammals. *Adv. Cancer Res.*, 13:39–62.

64. Jarrett, O., Laird, H. M., and Hay, D. (1969): Growth of feline leukemia virus in human cells. *Nature*, 224:208–1209.

65. Jarrett, W., Jarrett, O., Mackey, L., et al. (1973): Horizontal transmission of leukemia virus and leukemia in the cat. *J.N.C.I.*, 51:833–841.

66. Jarrett, W. F. H., Martin, W. B., Crighton, G. W., et al. (1964): A virus-like particle associated with leukaemia (lymphosarcoma). *Nature*, 202: 556–567.

67. Johnson, K. H. (1968): Aortic body tumors in the dog. *J. Am. Vet. Med. Assoc.*, 152:154–160.

68. Kantor, A. L. F., Meigs, J. W., Heston, J. F., et al. (1976): Epidemiology of renal cell carcinoma in Connecticut, 1935–1973. *J.N.C.I.*, 57:495–500.

69. Kappus, K. D. (1976): Canine rabies in the United States, 1971–1973: study of reported cases with reference to vaccination history. *Am. J. Epidemiol.*, 103:242–249.

70. Kelley, R. M. (1973): Progestins, in *Cancer Medicine*, pp. 923–929, edited by J. F. Holland and E. Frei, III. Lea & Febiger, Philadelphia.

71. Kowall, N., Stansbury, R., Charman, H., et al. (1971): A current look at feline lymphoma. *Vet. Clin. North Am.*, 1:355–365.

72. Lebeau, A. (1953): L'age duchien et celui de l'homme, essa' de statistique sur la mortalité canine. *Bull. Acad. Vet. Fr.*, 26:229–232.

73. Leonard, H. C. (1960): Collapse of the larynx and adjacent structures in the dog. *J. Am. Vet. Med. Assoc.*, 137:360–363.

74. Levy, S. B. (1974): Cat leukemia; a threat to man? *N. Engl. J. Med.*, 290: 513–514.

75. Lilienfeld, A. M. (1964): The relationship of bladder cancer to smoking. *Am. J. Public Health*, 54:1864–1875.

76. Lilienfeld, A. M., Levin, M. L., and Moore, G. E. (1956): The association of smoking with cancer of the urinary bladder in humans. *Arch. Intern. Med.*, 98: 129–135.

77. Lingeman, C. H. (1974): Etiology of cancer of the ovary; a review. *J.N.C.I.*, 53:1603–1618.

78. Lipworth, L., and Dayan, A. D. (1969): Rural preponderance of seminoma of the testis. *Cancer*, 23:1119–1121.

79. Lu, A. T., and Eisenstein, B. E. (1963): Papillary subependymal gliosis (gliomatyosis) associated with von Recklinghausen's disease and subependymal glioma. *Bull. Los Angeles Neurol. Soc.*, 28:151–156.

80. Lucké, B. (1938): Carcinoma in the leopard frog. Its probable causation by a virus. *J. Exp. Med.*, 68:457–468.

81. MacDonald, E. J. (1976): Epidemiology of skin cancer, 1975, in *Neoplasms of the Skin and Malignant Melanoma*, pp. 27–42. Year Book Medical Pub., Chicago.

82. Macklin, M. T. (1959): Comparison of the number of breast-cancer

deaths observed in relatives of breast-cancer patients, and the number expected on the basis of mortality rates. *J.N.C.I.*, 22:927–951.

83. MacMahon, B., Cole, P., and Brown, J. (1973): Etiology of human breast cancer. *J.N.C.I.*, 50:21–42.

84. Mantel, N., and Haenszel, W. (1959): Statistical aspects of the analysis of data from retrospective studies of disease. *J.N.C.I.*, 22:719–748.

85. Mason, T. J., McKay, F. W., Hoover, R., et al. (1975): Atlas of Cancer Mortality for U.S. Counties: 1950–1969. DHEW Pub. No. (NIH) 75–780, Washington, D.C.

86. Mason, T. J., McKay, F. W., Hoover, R., et al. (1976): Atlas of Cancer Mortality Among U.S. Nonwhites: 1950–1969. DHEW Pub. No. (NIH) 76-1204, Washington, D.C.

87. McCullough, D. L., Lamm, D.L., McLaughlin, A. P., et al. (1975): Familial transitional cell carcinoma of the bladder. *J. Urol.*, 113:629–635.

88. McDonald, D. F., and Lund, R. R. (1954): The role of the urine in vesical neoplasm; 1. Experimental confirmation of the urogenous theory of pathogenesis. *J. Urol.*, 71:560–570.

89. Miller, R. W. (1971): Deaths from childhood leukemia and solid tumors among twins and other sibs in the United States, 1960–67. *J.N.C.I.*, 46:203–209.

90. Morrison, A. S. (1976): Cryptorchidism, hernia, and cancer of the testis. *J.N.C.I.*, 56:731–733.

91. Mostofi, F. K. (1973): Testicular tumors. Epidemiologic, etiologic, and pathologic features. *Cancer*, 32:1186–1201.

92. Muller, G. H. (1967): Basal cell epithelioma and squamous cell carcinoma in animals. *Arch. Dermatol.*, 96:386–389.

93. Mulligan, R. M. (1948): Statistical and histologic study of one hundred and twenty canine neoplasms. *Arch. Pathol.*, 45:216–228.

94. Musser, E., and Graham, W. R. (1968): Familial occurrence of thyroiditis in purebred beagles. *Lab. Anim. Care*, 18:58–68.

95. Naegele, R. F., Granoff, A., Darlington, R. W. (1974): The presence of the Lucké herpesvirus genome in induced tadpole tumors and its oncogenicity; Koch-Henle postulates fulfilled. *Proc. Natl. Acad. Sci. U.S.A.*, 71:830.

96. National Cancer Institute, U.S. Department of Health, Education, and Welfare. (1966): *Standard Nomenclature of Veterinary Diseases and Operations*, Rev. Ed., PHS No. 1466, Washington, D.C.

97. Orlova, L. V., and Terekhov, P. E. (1969): Statistical data on neoplastic diseases in dogs in Moscow (1962–1966). *Vop. Onkol.*, 15:91–95 (cited in *Carcinogenesis Abst.*, 8:395, 1970).

98. Parker, L. N., Belsky, J. L., Yamamoto, T., et al. (1974): Thyroid carcinoma after exposure to atomic radiation. *Ann. Int. Med.*, 80:600–604.

99. Pendergrass, T. W., and Hayes, H. M., Jr. (1975): Cryptorchism and related defects in dogs. *Teratology*, 12:51–55.

100. Pratt, L. W. (1973): Familial carotid body tumors. *Arch. Otolaryngol.*, 97:334–336.

101. Price, J. M., Wear, J. B., Brown, R. R., et al. (1960): Studies on etiology of carcinoma of urinary bladder. *J. Urol.*, 83:376–382.

102. Priester, W. A. (1967): Canine lymphoma; relative risk in the boxer breed. *J.N.C.I.*, 39:833–845.

103. Priester, W. A. (1973): Skin tumors in domestic animals. Data from 12 United States and Canadian colleges of veterinary medicine. *J.N.C.I.*, 50:457–466.

104. Priester, W. A., Goodman, G. D., and Theilen, G. H. (1977): Nine simultaneous primary tumors in a boxer dog. *J. Am. Vet. Med. Assoc.*, 170:823–826.

105. Priester, W. A., and Hayes, H. M., Jr. (1973): Feline leukemia after feline infectious anemia. *J.N.C.I.*, 51:289–291.

106. Priester, W. A., and Mantel, N. (1971): Occurrence of tumors in domestic animals. Data from 12 United States and Canadian colleges of veteri-

nary medicine. *J.N.C.I.*, 47:1333–1344.

107. Ribelin, W. E., and Bailey, W. S. (1958): Esophageal sarcoma associated with *Spirocerca lupi* infection in the dog. *Cancer*, 11:1242–1246.

108. Rickard, C. G., Post, J. E., Noronha, F., et al. (1969): A transmissible virus-induced lymphocytic leukemia of the cat. *J.N.C.I.*, 42:987–1014.

109. Rimoin, D. L., and Schimke, R. N. (1971): *Genetic Disorders of the Endocrine Glands*, pp. 126–128. C. V. Mosby, St. Louis.

110. Rous, P. (1911): A sarcoma of the fowl transmissible by an agent separable from the tumor cells. *J. Exp. Med.*, 13:397–411.

111. Saldana, M. J., Salem, L. E., and Travezen, R. (1973): High altitude hypoxia and chemodectomas. *Hum. Pathol.*, 4:251–263.

112. Samuels, M. L., Sullivan, P., and Howe, C. D. (1968): Medroxyprogesterone acetate in the treatment of renal cell carcinoma (hypernephroma). *Cancer*, 22:525–532.

113. Sarma, P. S., Huebner, R. J., Basker, J. F., et al. (1970): Feline leukemia and sarcoma viruses; susceptibility of human cells to infection. *Science*, 168:1098–1100.

114. Schneck, S. A., and Penn, I. (1971): De-novo brain tumours in renal transplant recipients. *Lancet*, 1:983–986.

115. Schneider, R., Dorn, C. R., and Taylor, D. O. N. (1969): Factors influencing canine mammary cancer development and postsurgical survival. *J.N.C.I.*, 43:1249–1261.

116. Schneider, R., Frye, F. L., Taylor, D. O. N., et al. (1967): A household cluster of feline malignant lymphoma. *Cancer Res.*, 27:1316–1322.

117. Sharma, K. C., Gaeta, J. F., Bross, I. D., et al. (1972): Testicular tumors. *N.Y. State J. Med.*, 72:2421–2425.

118. Shope, R. E. (1933): Infectious papillomatosis of rabbits. *J. Exp. Med.*, 58:607–624.

119. Simpson, J. L., and Photopulos, G. (1976): Hereditary aspects of ovarian and testicular neoplasia. *Birth Defects*, 12:15–50.

120. Snyder, N., Scurry, M. T., and Deiss, W. P. (1972): Five families with multiple endocrine adenomatosis. *Ann. Int. Med.*, 76:53–58.

121. Snyder, S. P., and Theilen, G. H. (1969): Transmissible feline fibrosarcoma. *Nature*, 221:1074–1075.

122. Sprague, R. H., and Anisko, J. J. (1973): Elimination patterns in the laboratory beagle. *Behaviour*, 67:257–267.

123. Thomas, D. C. (1975): Exact and asymptotic methods for the combination of 2×2 tables. *Comput. Biomed. Res.*, 8:423–446.

124. Tjalma, R. A., Priester, W. A., Adelstein, E. H., et al. (1964): Clinical records systems and data retrieval function in veterinary medicine; a proposal for systematic data programming. *J. Am. Vet. Med. Assoc.*, 145:1189–1197.

125. Tucker, W. E. (1962): Thyroiditis in a group of laboratory dogs. A study of 167 beagles. *Am. J. Clin. Pathol.*, 38:70–74.

126. Überreiter, O. (1966): Effect of pregnancy and false pregnancy on the occurrence of mammary tumors in the bitch. *Berl. Münch. Tieraerztl. Wochenschr.*, 79:451–456.

127. Weiss, N. S., Homonchuck, T., Young, J. L., Jr. (1977): Incidence of the histologic types of ovarian cancer; the U.S. third national cancer survey, 1969–71. *Gynecol. Oncol.* 5:161–167.

128. Wiel, H. J., van der (1960): *Inheritance of Glioma*. Elsevier, Amsterdam.

129. Willis, R. A. (1960): *Pathology of Tumours*, Ed. 3, pp. 512, 515. Butterworth, Washington, D.C.

130. Wilson, H. (1970): Carotid body tumors-familial and bilateral. *Ann. Surg.*, 171:843–848.

131. Woolner, L. B., McConahey, W. M., and Beahrs, O. H. (1959): Struma lymphomatosa (Hashimoto's thyroiditis) and related thyroidal disorders. *J. Clin. Endocrinol.*, 19:53–83.

132. Wynder, E., Mabuchi, K., Whitmore, W. F., Jr. (1974): Epidemiology of adenocarcinoma of the kidney. *J.N.C.I.*, 53:1619–1634.

Addendum. Since this chapter was prepared new information is available which should be brought to the reader's attention.

The Veterinary Medical Data Program (VMDP) is presently managed by a consortium of its 16 participants; data are maintained at Cornell University. The abstracted data items have been expanded to include the postal zip code associated with the home address of the animal's owner (133). This information will permit correlation of animal disease occurrence with general environmental considerations. Further studies in this direction may yield additional clues into environmental health hazards.

Testis

Two distinct patterns of hormone activity are often associated with canine testicular tumors. In many instances, particularly among cryptorchid dogs, Sertoli cell tumors are accompanied by clinical signs of feminization, such as gynecomastia, alopecia, pendulous penile sheath, and atrophy of the unaffected testicle (134).

Canine interstitial cell tumors, however, are rarely seen with signs of feminization. Instead, they often give the clinical impression that they are responsible for a systemic androgen increase. An association ($P < 0.05$) between interstitial cell tumor and perianal gland adenoma has been described (135). This is a tumor, located most often about the anal ring, of the circumanal glands which possesses androgen binding receptors and responds favorably to castration (136). Because the perianal gland adenoma is rarely lethal and is readily recognizable, further study of its association with hormone imbalances could offer leads applicable to human aggregations of hormone-related tumors.

Bladder

Cancer at sites of the lower urinary tract, other than the bladder, occur infrequently in the dog. A study of 40 urethral cancer cases identified most to be transitional cell carcinomas (137). Although the number of cases was small, a significant ($P < 0.05$) excess was seen in beagles even after the exclusion of 13 cases with concomitant bladder cancer. Female dogs showed 1.5 times the risk of males, but the value was not statistically significant.

The association between bladder and urethral cancer has been recognized in people, especially men (138). The causal mechanisms of urethral cancer are unclear. The disease in humans appears positively associated with chronic irritation of the urethral mucosa, possibly due to venereal infection, stricture, coitus, or parturition (139). It also seems reasonable that the etiology may be the same as that for bladder cancer—urine-borne carcinogenic agents.

Tarvin and others (140) suggest that female dogs have more urethral cancer than males because the female urethra is more susceptible to the effects of carcinogens. This observation is probably true, but it is suggested that the resting prostatic secretion is responsible for many male dogs being spared the lesion (137). Huggins (141) observed that mature noncastrated dogs discharge resting prostatic secretion into their urethra, without aid of parasympathetic stimulation, at a rate approaching 2 ml/hr. It seems likely that this quantity of fluid would dilute the residual urine in the urethra and alter the mucosal exposure to urine-borne carcinogens. In man, it is estimated 2 ml/day of resting prostatic secretion is discharged. Whether this imparts a sparing effect in man has not been determined.

Thyroid

A study of canine hypothyroidism (142) (including myxedema and thyroiditis) shows that certain breeds are at high risk. These high risk breeds clinically display a sig-

nificant ($P < 0.01$) proportion of their disease under 4 years of age. Conversely, low risk breeds experience a linearly increasing hospital prevalence through age 9. This strongly suggests the activity of genetic factors in the high risk breeds. The beagle was not one of the high risk breeds although they have been observed before with a propensity for clinically silent Hashimoto-like thyroiditis (8, 125). Several endocrine related conditions were diagnosed subsequent to the diagnosis of hypothyroidism in this case series. One of these, thyroid carcinoma, was particularly evident.

Blood-Lymphatic System

Recent analysis of mortality, 1966–1977, among practicing U.S. veterinarians (143) indicates they have experienced significantly ($P < 0.05$) more leukemia and Hodgkin's disease than expected based on the mortality distribution of the general U.S. population. This increased mortality may be related to occupational exposures such as ionizing radiation. The potential of zoonotic animal viruses (e.g., FeLV) should also be a consideration.

Additional References

133. Hayes, H. M., Jr., Wilson, G. P., and Moraff, H. (1979): The veterinary medical data program (VMDP): past, present, and future, in *Proceedings of International Symposium on Animal Health and Disease Data Banks, December 4–6, 1978*, pp. 127–132, APHIS, USDA Misc. Pub. No. 1381, Washington, D.C.
134. Lipowitz, A. J., Schwartz, A., Wilson, G. P., et al. (1973): Testicular neoplasms and concomitant clinical changes in the dog. *J. Am. Vet. Med. Assoc.*, 163:1364–1368.
135. Hayes, H. M., Jr., and Wilson, G. P. (1977): Hormone-dependent neoplasms of the canine perianal gland. *Cancer Res.*, 37:2068–2071.
136. Wilson, G. P., and Hayes, H. M., Jr. (1979): Castration for treatment of perianal gland neoplasms in the dog. *J. Am. Vet. Med. Assoc.*, 174:1301–1303.
137. Wilson, G. P., Hayes, H. M., Jr., and Casey, H. W. (1979): Canine urethral cancer. *J. Am. Anim. Hosp. Assoc.*, 15:741–744.
138. Grabstald, H. (1973): Tumors of the urethra in men and women. *Cancer*, 32:1236–1255.
139. Sullivan, J., and Grabstald, H. (1978): Management of carcinoma of the urethra. In: *Genitourinary Cancer*, pp. 419–429, edited by D. G. Skinner and J. B. de Kernion. W. B. Saunders, Philadelphia.
140. Tarvin, G., Patnaik, A., and Greene, R. (1978): Primary urethral tumors in dogs. *J. Am. Vet. Med. Assoc.*, 172:931–933.
141. Huggins, C. (1945): The physiology of the prostate gland. *Physiol. Rev.*, 25:281–295.
142. Milne, K. L., and Hayes, H. M., Jr. (1981): Epidemiologic features of canine hypothyroidism. *Cornell Vet.* (in press).
143. Blair, A., and Hayes, H. M., Jr. (1980): Cancer and other causes of death among U.S. veterinarians, 1966–1977. *Int. J. Cancer*, 25:181–185.

36

Selected Aspects of Racial and Geographic Occurrence of Neoplasms in Man

S. Boonyanit and Hans E. Kaiser

INTRODUCTION

The rate of occurrence of many diseases varies extensively (36, 37, 57, 62, 118, 155, 180, 232, 257, 264) from one race of people to another, due to considerable differences in habits, socioeconomic (56, 63) status, customs (49), religion (242), nutrition (71), and also physical environment. Geographic distribution of diseases is also important and has led scientists to seek underlying factors that may influence the occurrence of neoplasms in humans (Tables 36.1 and 36.2) (115, 189).

Race (8, 82, 86, 122, 158, 236, 261) is an important influential factor. In countries such as the United States, to which people have migrated from many other parts of the world, although the environment is common to all, the incidence of diseases among the immigrant races may vary. Examples of migrant races are the Chinese (124) who have resettled in many parts of the world; the Parsi, who migrated a thousand years ago from Persia to India; the Japanese, to Hawaii (157) and Brazil; the Negroes to the United States, etc. In each of these races the incidence of diseases differs between the people who remained in their original homeland and the immigrants, and differs yet again among the people born of migrant parents in the new countries, and within new environments. An obvious example is the nasopharyngeal carcinoma which occurs frequently both among the Chinese in Asia and among the Chinese who migrated to the United States, but has a very low incidence among the Chinese born in the United States.

From 1950 to 1969 5713 American Chinese died from cancer in the United States (79). The death rate for cancer was remarkably higher than in white males but comparable to black males. The rate of death in Chinese females was remarkably lower when compared to white and black females (Fig. 36.1).

Especially high was the mortality from nasopharyngeal cancer with an elevation of 26 times in Chinese males and 22 times in Chinese females, but declined during the study. Lung and primary liver cancer, especially in Chinese females was also high. A low mortality was seen for prostate and bladder cancer in Chinese males. The Chinese males had a higher mortality of cancer of the large intestine than the Chinese females. (See also Ref. 221.)

In many countries there are good examples for the study of different races occupying the same environment: in the United States the Negroes, Mongols, Puerto Ricans (150), Mexicans, Filipinos and Caucasians (for example, cancer of the Spanish surnamed population in Texas differs from cancer among other ethnic groups by topographic location, cell type and geographic location (142); in Hawaii the Japanese, the Chinese, the old natives and Caucasians; in Singapore and Malaysia the Chinese, Indians and Caucasians.

Striking differences occur in some of specific cancer sites when the conditions in Japan were compared to those in the San Francisco bay

Table 36.1
Comparison of Incidence of Cancer between Selected Countries in Asia, Europe, and America[a]

Cancer Site		Singapore (All Races) (1968–70)	Japan (Miyagi) (1962–64)	India (Bombay) (1964–66)	England (Birmingham) (1963–66)	Norway 1964–66	U.S.A. (Connecticut) (1963–65)	U.S.A. Hawaii (Chicago) (1960–64)
Mouth	M	3.3	1.1	6.5	1.4	0.9	4.0	0.6
(143–145)	F	0.6	0.6	5.9	0.6	0.5	1.4	0.0
Nasopharynx	M	16.3	0.1	0.6	0.5	0.4	0.5	10.4
(147)	F	6.8	0.1	0.5	0.2	0.1	0.1	4.6
Oesophagus	M	16.3	14.5	13.0	4.7	2.8	4.1	7.6
(150)	F	6.8	4.9	11.3	2.6	0.9	1.4	0.0
Stomach	M	38.1	95.3	10.0	25.2	28.8	15.3	9.5
(151)	F	16.4	44.7	6.5	13.2	15.4	6.8	14.2
Colon	M	9.6	4.1	4.1	15.3	12.0	24.0	35.9
(153)	F	7.4	4.0	3.4	14.9	11.6	26.7	23.5
Rectum	M	8.4	4.8	4.3	15.8	6.8	15.5	15.8
(154)	F	6.6	0.8	0.1	9.3	4.7	10.7	9.4
Liver	M	27.1	1.3	0.5	0.8	1.0	?	7.3
(155.0)	F	6.9	0.8	0.1	0.3	0.4	?	0.0
Nasal cavity	M	1.2	3.4	1.4	0.7	0.8	2.1	2.4
(160)	F	0.2	1.9	1.0	0.6	0.3	1.3	2.4
Larynx	M	6.6	2.4	13.8	3.8	2.0	7.5	0.6
(161)	F	0.7	0.3	2.8	0.5	0.2	0.8	0.0
Lung	M	44.3	15.6	13.3	73.3	16.5	44.0	27.2
(162)	F	14.9	6.0	3.7	8.4	3.1	7.8	16.7
Melanoma skin	M	0.6	0.3	0.2	1.1	3.6	3.5	3.0
(172)	F	0.2	0.2	0.5	1.8	4.0	3.2	0.0
Skin (other)	M	5.0	1.5	1.3	27.9	?	?	0.6
(173)	F	4.6	1.4	1.6	17.6	?	?	0.0
Breast	M	18.3	11.0	20.4	51.1	41.0	62.3	44.3
(174)	F							
Cervix uteri	F	16.2	?	24.7	13.6	16.2	10.3	13.4
(180)								
Corpus uteri	F	4.8	1.3	1.5	9.0	8.2	15.3	19.5
(182)								
Prostate	M	3.6	3.2	6.5	18.4	29.8	33.0	9.8
(185)								
All sites	M	217.5	196.0	139.5	254.5	174.8	257.8	207.0
(140–205)	F	143.6	142.8	131.1	196.3	164.9	220.0	228.3

[a] The rate shown is per 100,000 persons per year and age is standardized to world population.

area. Most obvious were the differences of the gastrointestinal tract and the sex organs. The high gastric rates of Japanese immigrants and American born Japanese adapted to comparable conditions of the United States population. In contrast, the higher rates of colon cancer, of the breast, of uterine corpus, ovary and prostate of Japanese living or born in the United States approached the higher but common rates in the United States (70).

Autopsy specimen of Japanese who lived in Hawaii showed in comparison to those living in Japan an increase of adenomatous and hyperplastic polyps and diverticula associated with atherosclerosis. The rate of gastric cancer is similar in both geographic location according to

this study (217). A total of 16,492 cancer cases in the Philippines from July 1968 to June 1973 indicated as the leading neoplasm for males lung cancer and for females breast cancer; also a higher frequency was observed in the cancers of the oral cavity, nasopharynx, liver, lung, breast, cervix, ovary, thyroid and malignant lymphoma (13).

In Thailand, variations between the old natives and the Mongol immigrants, and in India, variations between the natives and the Parsis, are worthy of study. In Singapore and Hong Kong also the variations among the Chinese of different dialects are of interest, as is the variation among local tribes in African countries. The inhabitants in developing countries, when compared with those in industrialized countries such as Europe and the United States can also be useful.

One study has revealed that sickle cell anemia is more common among Negroes than among Caucasians in the United States. Another, in Thailand, shows that the native people have a higher frequency of abnormal hemoglobin (E-trait) than do the Mongols, who migrated to that country from the north. Burkitt lymphoma is more common among the Negroes in Africa than those in the United States: the distribution of this tumor, which is related to temperature and rainfall, is now known to reflect also the distribution of hyperendemic malaria (25). Meanwhile, cancers of the stomach and liver are more common among Negroes in the United States than among their African counterparts.

In India the incidence of cancer among Parsis was found to be lower than that for the total Indian population, dramatically so in Bombay. Furthermore, their specific site risk differs radically from the greater Bombay pattern. Cancers of the buccal cavity, pharynx, larynx, esopha-

gus, and uterine cervix, which have a high frequency in the Bombay population as a whole, were less commonly observed in the Parsi community. On the other hand, the rate of cancers of the female breasts, body of the uterus, ovary, prostate and skin, and for all types of leukemias, were higher among the Parsis in the same environment. However, the incidence of carcinoma of the esophagus among these formerly Persian people (who emigrated long ago from Iran to India and who still keep their own traditions and customs and seldom intermarry) is much lower than among the people of Iran along the Caspian littoral (Table 36.3).

The Japanese living in Japan have the highest rates of severe cancer of the stomach in the world, closely followed by the Chinese in Singapore; but among the Chinese and Japanese in Hawaii this disease is not prevalent. The incidence of nasopharyngeal carcinoma and trophoblastic disease among the Chinese and Japanese in Southeast Asia is exceptionally high, but very low among the Chinese in Hawaii and California. The accumulated evidence suggests that both race and geographic location have an influence upon the occurrence of malignant neoplasms in humans (Fig. 36.2).

A renewal of interest in a geographical approach to medicine is urged for the following reasons: (a) It will enable us to make an estimate of the frequency with which most diseases can be expected to occur, even in areas with relatively poorly developed medical services. (b) It proves to us that under certain conditions a disease will not occur, or occurs rarely, or occurs only under particular conditions. (c) As living conditions are rapidly becoming similar throughout the world the opportunity for studying the frequency with which any given disease will occur under different conditions will soon be lost forever.

The concept that cancer is a rare condition in

Table 36.2
Relationship between Man and Carcinogenic Stimulus Showing Various Levels at Which Carcinogenic Stimuli Can Be Investigated in the Environment[a]

Carcinogenic Stimulus		Nature	Type of Study
Environment	Distant	Geography Agriculture Level of sociological development	Historic and geographic
	Intermediate	Specific foods Cultural habits Occupations	Cultural
	Immediate	Carcinogen	Analytic (chemical or biological)

[a] Source: Hippinson (99).

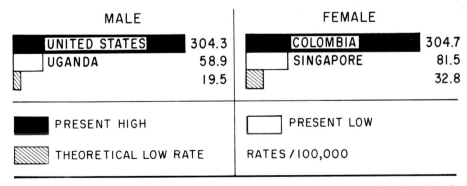

MALE

UNITED STATES	304.3
UGANDA	58.9
	19.5

FEMALE

COLOMBIA	304.7
SINGAPORE	81.5
	32.8

■ PRESENT HIGH

□ PRESENT LOW

▨ THEORETICAL LOW RATE

RATES / 100,000

Figure 36.1. Age-adjusted cancer morbidity rate with theoretical low rate, indicating the theoretical low rate which could pertain if the lowest incidence rate were summated from all countries. (Source: Higginson (99).)

Table 36.3
Summary of Highest Rate (First to Third Rank) of Cancer Incidence by Site, Area, and Population, Age Standardized Rates per 100,000 Population Based on World Population

Tumour Site	Male		Female	
	Country	Rate	Country	Rate
Lip	Canada, Newfoundland	27.1	Brazil, São Paulo	1.7
	Canada, Saskatchewan	16.4	Brazil, Recife	1.4
	Malta	13.0	Israel, all Jews	1.4
Tongue	India, Bombay	12.6	Singapore, Indian	3.8
	Puerto Rico	7.5	India, Bombay	3.1
	Brazil, São Paulo	5.7	Hawaii, Hawaiian	2.4
Mouth	Singapore, Indian	8.6	Singapore, Indian	16.9
	Puerto Rico	7.8	India, Bombay	5.4
	Brazil, São Paulo	7.0	Brazil, Recife	3.3
Oropharynx	India, Bombay	5.6	Singapore, Indian	2.3
	El Paso, other White	4.8	El Paso, Spanish	1.9
	Swiss, Geneva	4.7	Colombia, Cali	1.2
Larynx	Brazil, São Paulo	14.1	India, Bombay	2.6
	India, Bombay	13.6	Alameda, Black	1.7
	Alameda, Black	12.9	Colombia, Cali	1.6
Trachea, bronchus, and lung	UK, Liverpool	89.5	New Zealand, Maori	35.4
	UK, SMCR	78.5	Bay Area, Chinese	22.2
	Detroit, Black	77.1	Hawaii, Hawaiian	20.6
Bone	Spain, Zaragoza	3.0	Israel Born AFK.Asia	2.2
	El Paso, Spanish	2.3	Germany, Saarland	2.0
	Germany Hamburg	2.2	Spain, Zaragoza	2.0
Connective tissue	Hawaii, Hawaiian	8.1	Hawaii, Hawaiian	4.1
Other soft tissue	Hawaii, Caucasian	4.2	Israel, born in Israel	3.2
	El Paso, Spanish	3.8	New Mexico, American Indian	2.9
Melanoma of skin	New Zealand, Non-Maori	7.4	New Zealand, Non-Maori	11.7
	Hawaii, Caucasian	6.8	Israel, born in Israel	7.0
	Norway, Urban	6.7	USA, Bay area, white	6.6
Nasopharynx	USA, Bay area, Chinese	19.1	Singapore, Chinese	7.1
	Singapore, Chinese	18.7	USA, Bay area, Chinese	6.4
	Hawaii, Chinese	10.3	Hawaii, Hawaiian	5.1
Hypopharynx	India, Bombay	7.7	Singapore, Indian	2.5
	Puerto Rico	4.4	India, Bombay	1.8
	Singapore, Indian	4.1	UK, Liverpool	0.9
Oesophagus	Bulawayo, African	63.8	India, Bombay	10.8
	Singapore, Chinese	20.1	Singapore, Chinese	6.4
	USA, Bay area, black	15.2	Singapore, Indian	5.9
Stomach	Japan, Osaka	91.4	Japan, Okayama	48.3
	Japan, Okayama	90.3	Japan, Osaka	45.1
	Japan Miyagi	84.6	Japan, Miyagi	40.1
Large Intestine	USA, Connecticut	30.1	Connecticut	26.1
	Hawaii, Chinese	28.7	Iowa	25.0
	USA, Bay area	28.3	Canada, Newfoundland	24.2
Rectum	Hawaii, Chinese	20.4	Hawaii, Caucasian	12.0
	USA, Bay area, Chinese	19.5	Israel, born in Europe, America	11.2
	Connecticut	18.2	Connecticut	11.1
Liver and intrahepatic bile ducts	Bulawayo, African	64.6	Bulawayo, African	25.4
	Singapore, Chinese	34.2	Brazil, Recife	10.3
Sp. as primary	USA, Bay area, Chinese	21.1	Singapore, Chinese	8.0
Gallbladder and bile ducts	Israel, born in Africa, Asia	8.8	Israel, born in Europe, America	15.9
	Israel, all Jews	7.5	Poland, Warsaw city	13.8
	Israel, born in Europe, America	7.0	New Mexico, American Indian	13.5
Pancreas	Hawaii, Hawaiian	15.8	Alameda, Black	9.9
	USA, Bay area, black	15.2	El Paso, Spanish	9.2
	Detroit, black	14.9	Bay area, black	9.0
Other skin	El Paso, other white	144.9	El Paso, other white	73.3
	Canada, British Columbia	101.3	Canada, British Columbia	67.6
	New Mexico, other white	96.7	Canada, Saskatchewan	59.5
Breast			Hawaii, Caucasian	80.3
			Canada, British Columbia	80.0
			USA, Bay area, white	79.9

Table 36.3—*continued*

Tumour Site	Male		Female	
	Country	Rate	Country	Rate
Cervix uteri			El Paso, Spanish	80.9
			Colombia, Cali	62.8
			Brazil, Recife	58.1
Corpus uteri			Alameda, white	33.3
			Hawaii, Hawaiian	31.8
			USA, Bay area, white	29.9
Ovary, fallopian tube, and broad ligament			Denmark	15.1
			Sweden	15.1
			Norway	15.0
Other unspecified female genital organs			Japan, Okayama	5.6
			Germany, Saarland	4.1
			Brazil, Recife	3.5
Prostate	USA, Bay area, black	77.0		
	Alameda, black	75.0		
	Detroit, black	67.1		
Testis	Denmark	4.9		
	Germany, Hamburg	4.7		
	Norway, urban	4.6		
Brain and nervous system	Israel, born in Israel	11.4	Israel, born in Israel	11.3
	Israel, all Jews	10.5	Israel, all Jews	10.4
	Israel, born in Europe, America	10.5	Israel, born in Europe, America	9.2
Thyroid gland	Iceland	5.0	Hawaii, Filipino	18.7
	Israel, born in Israel	4.8	Hawaii, Hawaiian	16.0
	Hawaii, Chinese	4.7	Iceland	15.0
Lymphosarcoma	Nigeria, Ibadan	9.1	Nigeria, Ibadan	7.7
Reticulum cell sarcoma	Israel, all Jews	8.8	Israel, all Jews	7.2
	USA, Bay area, white	8.2	Hawaii, Caucasian	7.1
Other lymphoid tissue	USA, Bay area, Chinese	2.5	Canada, Manitoba	2.4
	New Mexico, other white	2.3	Canada, British Columbia	2.1
	Norway, urban	2.3	Norway, urban	1.8
Multiple myeloma	USA, Bay area, black	8.2	USA, Bay area, black	6.5
	Alameda, black	6.1	New Mexico, American Indian	6.3
	Detroit, black	5.4	Alameda, Black	5.3
Lymphatic leukemia	Utah	9.1	Utah	6.3
	Bulawayo, African	7.5	Finland	5.3
	Finland	7.2	New Mexico, other white	4.1
Myeloid leukemia	Alameda, white	4.6	N'Mexico, Amer. Indian	3.5
	Connecticut	4.6	Bay Area Chinese	3.4
	Alameda, black	4.5	G.D.R.	3.4
Other and unspecified sites	Canada, British Columbia	3.2	Canada, Brit-Col.	2.6
	Norway, urban	2.7	El Paso, other white	2.1
Leukemia	Norway	2.6	Canada, New Foundland	2.0
Other and unspecified sites	Malta	24.9	Japan, Osaka	22.7
	Israel, born in Israel	24.1	Spain, Zaragoza	22.6
	Japan, Osaka	22.3	Brazil, Sao Paulo	19.4

Source: IARC, Cancer Incidence in Five Continents, Vol. III, 1976.

the underdeveloped areas of the world has already been proven to be erroneous. The evidence suggests, despite lack of medical data for many parts of the world, that basic patterns and incidences of cancer have existed for hundreds of years. The cancer pattern in sub-Saharan Africa shows the greatest differences from what is seen in Europe or America, and similar patterns can be seen in areas such as New Guinea. While it is possible to make certain generalizations about the sub-Saharan pattern, it is important to stress that the distribution of certain cancers, such as those of esophagus, nasopharynx, stomach, etc., shows foci of either high or low incidence; generally, in Africa, cancers of the lungs, the colon, the rectum, the body of the uterus, and the breast have a low frequency, while cancers of the liver and cervix and choriocarcinoma have a higher frequency than in Europe and America.

These contrasts in cancer frequency may again be explained by differences in geographical location, racial and socioeconomic status, and cultural influences.

The common types of malignant disease in

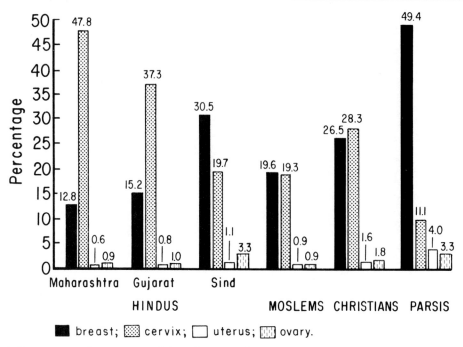

Figure 36.2. Relative cancer frequency of female reproductive organs according to ethnic groups of India. (Source: Jussawalla (117).)

many developing countries differ radically from those observed in the West. In the industrial world these diseases occur in greatest numbers in that portion of the digestive tract which lies below the level of the cardio-esophageal junction and in the bronchus and the female breast.

In developing countries, such as India, on the other hand, it is the upper digestive tract, oral cavity, pharynx and esophagus, as well as the uterine cervix which are the most frequently affected. In some parts of India, the tongue is the common organ affected in the male, followed by the larynx, esophagus, stomach and hypopharynx. Age-adjusted incidence in women is seen to be the highest in the uterine cervix, followed by the breast, esophagus, stomach, and ovary (76, 118).

In Malaysia and Singapore the ethnic or racial differences in cancer incidence are obvious between the native Malays, the Chinese, the Indians and the Caucasians. The incidence rate for cancer of most sites is lower for Malays than for the Chinese and Indians. At the same time there are also some diseases which are more prevalent among the Malays than among the Chinese or Indian populations. Malay women have a significantly higher risk of cancer of the mouth than Chinese women, this finding being related to their habit of chewing betel nut. The Malays also have higher incidence rates for cancer of the nasopharynx, liver, and lungs than the Indians. Chinese also have higher rates for most

cancer than Indians: the incidence rates for cancers of the esophagus, stomach, liver, lung, and nasopharynx in particular are significantly higher among the Chinese than among the Indians. By contrast, the rates for cancers of the tongue, mouth, and hypopharynx are significantly higher among Indians than Chinese.

Of the major ethnic groups in Singapore, the Chinese have the highest incidence of cancer. Thus, the generally high incidence of cancer in Singapore may be due to the predominantly Chinese composition of the population. In comparison with immigrant Chinese in Hawaii, the Chinese in Singapore have a lower incidence of cancer of the colon, rectum, and breast and a higher incidence of cancer of the liver and stomach (Table 36.4).

China-born immigrants in Singapore were found to have a significantly higher risk of liver cancer than local-born Chinese, but no such difference was found for cancer of the nasopharynx. From an epidemiological standpoint the high risk of nasopharyngeal cancer among the Chinese may be due to a genetic predisposition arising out of geographical or environmental factors.

The differences in cancer incidence among Chinese of different dialects is of further interest. Epidemiological studies of the Chinese revealed that cancer of the nasopharynx occurs with highest frequency in the southern provinces, especially in Kwangtun and Kwangsi,

Table 36.4
Basis of Diagnosis of Selected Cancer among Singapore Chinese, by Both Dialect and Sex

Dialect and Site	Basis of Diagnosis									
	Necropsy		Biopsy		Cytology		Exploration x-ray		Clinical	
	M	F	M	F	M	F	M	F	M	F
Hokkien										
Nasopharynx	—	—	83	24	—	—	—	—	6	4
Oesophagus	2	—	67	32	—	—	27	8	21	14
Stomach	10	1	142	55	2	1	63	19	60	38
Rectum	—	2	35	39	—	—	1	—	5	7
Lung	29	3	131	29	10	4	122	21	30	11
Breast[a]	—	—	—	80	—	—	—	2	—	12
Other sites	29	13	386	345	36[b]	23[b]	45	30	136	79
Teochew										
Nasopharynx	1	1	56	22	—	—	—	—	5	2
Oesophagus	5	—	50	17	1	—	25	7	9	11
Stomach	3	2	67	28	5	—	31	11	41	19
Rectum	—	—	22	24	—	—	2	—	2	1
Lung	15	2	72	18	3	2	67	11	16	2
Breast	—	—	—	39	—	—	—	1	—	11
Other sites	16	10	164	161	19[b]	13[b]	18	8	67	33
Cantonese										
Nasopharynx	1	—	83	45	—	—	—	—	7	4
Oesophagus	—	—	6	9	—	—	3	3	3	4
Stomach	2	3	26	27	1	—	8	11	11	16
Rectum	—	—	20	16	—	—	1	1	1	3
Lung	12	9	48	53	9	8	65	45	5	9
Breast	—	2	—	100	—	—	—	—	—	8
Other sites	20	20	131	263	13[b]	16[b]	28	18	44	37

[a] Excludes 2 male patients.
[b] Includes hematology.
Source: Shanmugaratnam (204).

while carcinoma of the esophagus is more prevalent in the north, particularly in the Lin County in Honan province. Differences in cancer incidences among the specific Chinese communities or dialect groups has been reported mostly in connection with nasopharynx cancer. Studies in China, Hong Kong, and Singapore have shown that this neoplasm has higher frequency among the Cantonese than among other dialect groups.

In the United States, the incidence of all malignancies among Negroes is lower than among Caucasians. Differences in the frequency of cancer incidence still exist among Negroes in Africa, the West Indies and the United States. These differences appear to be the result of environmental changes consequent upon migration. Negroes have lived in the United States for more generations than any of the other groups except the Caucasians and some of Mexican origin. The Japanese in the United States have lived there for a relatively short time, and peculiarities of site involvement for the migrants remain similar to those of native Japanese.

Cancer frequency is also found to be low among the Chinese in the United States: the striking peculiarities of site distribution reported by some authors from China are not seen.

A low frequency of cancer among Filipinos in the United States is also observed, but it is impossible to determine at present whether there has been any change produced by the new environment.

In the United States malignant tumors are also less common among Mexicans and Negroes than among the Caucasians.

Among the Chinese the age-connected cancer frequency is half that among Caucasians, and in Filipinos it is 40% of the Caucasian rate. The differences between the Mongoloid group cancer frequency is extremely low.

CANCER OF DIGESTIVE ORGANS

Variation in the incidence of carcinoma of the gastrointestinal tract between countries of relatively similar ethnological background is wide (33, 87, 201), and the change in frequency observed within immigrant populations indicates that environmental factors are significantly involved. However, there has so far been a failure to demonstrate any condition in terms of geographical distribution between carcinoma of the esophagus, stomach, and large intestine.

Comparatively the impact of Westernization of nutrition of Japanese with the change of their physique, cancer, longevity and centenarians as described by Kagawa in 1978 (121) showed the following. Between 1950 and 1975 a drastic change of Japanese diet took place, with an increase of intake of milk (10 times); meat, poultry, and eggs (7.5 times); and fat (6 times). There was a decrease of barlay (1.40), potatoes (1.2) and rice (0.7). Especially the younger generation is affected from these changes. At the same time the Japanese became taller and heavier. Breast, colon, and lung cancer increased 2–3 times. Those of stomach and uterus decreased (0.6 to 0.3), respectively. Life expectancy increased for males and females (12 and 14 years, respectively). In 1977, 888 centenarians were known. The Japanese in Okinawa had the lowest total energy, sugar and salt, the smallest physique, healthy longevity and the most centenarians (Table 36.5).

Esophagus (145)

Carcinoma of the esophagus is rare in Caucasians under 40 years of age. In a series of 207 cases in the United States the youngest patient was 35 years old (2).

Table 36.5
Factors Reported to Be Associated with High Incidence of Stomach Cancer[a]

Soil
  Acidic soil
  Meadow soil
  Peat Soil
  Low lying clay areas
  Igneous rocks near the surface
  Deep ground water
  Mineral balance high zinc/copper ratio
  Inorganic dust with free silica
Occupation
  Farmers
  Workers in quarries
  Low social class
Diseases
  Stomach ulcer
  Chronic gastritis
  Adenomatoid polyps
  Intestinal metaplasia
  Hyposecretion
  Pernicious anemia
  Plummer Vinson
  Dental caries
Heredity
  Blood group A
  Race (Mongolian, Japanese, Finnish, etc.)

Climate
  Northern countries
  Heavy rainfall
  Low temperature
Environment
  Rural areas
  Grain dust
  Iron dust
Dietary Factors
  Irregular meal times
  Excessive zinc, copper
  Deficiency in iron
  Molybdenum
  Deficiency in vitamins A, B, B_{12}, C
  Tobacco
  Alcohol
  Liquid paraffin (purgative)
Diet
  High intake of starchy foods: rice, cereals, potatoes
  Highly brined food, home-cured bacon, salami, sausage
  Smoked food, salted food, fried food
  Hot food
  Low protein diet
  Low consumption of fruit and fresh vegetables

[a] Source: Saxen and Hakama (191).

Mortality of esophageal cancer of Caucasian males and females from 1935 to 1974 remained stable in contrast to the non-Caucasian population of the United States; especially blacks showed an 8-fold increase in males and a 5-fold increase in females (141).

The diet has not only an effect on racial differences of intestinal cancer but also on pituitary and adrenal activity as shown with regard to North American black and white and South African Bantu men (102).

In some black areas of South Africa an unprecedented rise of the disease occurred. Umtata Hospital (Transkei) reported three cases between 1925 and 1933, but 378 between 1965 and 1969. Transval black women are less affected than those in the Transkei. Mortality figures show an increase for colored men and Indian women between 1949 and 1969 (187).

A 5-fold increase in each decade has been shown at the University of Natal, South Africa, since 1955 and have now reached 500 admissions per year (12). This tumour ranked as the eighth commonest site of cancer among Koreans and Thais, and rates as number three among the Chinese in Hong Kong and Singapore, number one in Mainland China, and number four in Formosa and Malaysia. India is also a country with high incidence. Occurrences in other countries are rather low.

The pathology department of the Tripoli Central Hospital in its studies from 1968 to 1972 investigated 7,585 biopsies of which 996 showed malignant lesions. This was 13.13% of all malignancies, of which 56.22% were male and 43.7% female. Sixty-eight cases were 6.83% of all malignancies and 0.90% of all biopsies. The sequence of incidence was 33.82% rectum, 22.06% large intestine, 19.12% esophagus, 16.18% stomach, and 8.82% small intestine. Of all malignant neoplasms 73.53% were in male patients and 26.47% in female patients (237). A total of 21,128 cases of gastrointestinal cancer during the period of 1941–1975 was observed in Tata Memorial Hospital, Bombay. Of these 71% were esophageal cancer, 12% stomach cancer, 9% rectal cancer, 4% cancer of the colon, and 4% cancer of the anal canal (83). If compared to the years 1973–1977, the studies showed that changes occurred in cancer incidence some types increasing, other decreasing (237). The incidence differs markedly to comparable reports from the Tata Memorial Hospital, Bombay, India. Esophageal cancer was more common in Western India, stomach cancer in the southern part of the country, particularly the coastal states in the southwest. It is interesting that gastric cancer was infrequent in Gujaret, a coastal state north of Bombay. Squamous cell cancer of the anal canal was especially high in patients from northern states of India. This may be due to some implications of socioreligious habits (83).

The highest incidence of the disease occurs in the Caspian littoral of Iran (8). The causes are unknown (nutritional and vitamin deficiency, sheep's milk and hot tea are suspected stimulants) (145). The suspected reasons of the causes of the disease vary from chemical carcinogens with organotropism to the esophagus in experimental animals, trauma, hot or spicy foods, nass (special chewing substance) also used in Soviet Central Asia, to ethnic factors, stress, psychic depression and food toxins of which the implications vary in different areas (141, 145).

A study of malignant tumors in North China revealed esophageal carcinoma to have the highest incidence there. The rate was found to be 24.5% in Tsinan and 16% in Sian. In Tsinan it ranked first while in Tiensin and Peking it was second in frequency among carcinomas in men (110). Carcinoma of the esophagus is also common in southern China but not prominent as in the North. In Hong Kong it was found to be the most frequently biopsied cancer among men over 55 years old.

In Singapore a study revealed a high risk of esophagus and stomach cancer among Hokkiens and Teochews. The composition and high temperature of food consumed and the use of strong alcohol are among some of the factors that have been postulated in the etiology of cancer of the upper gastrointestinal tract.

Hokkiens and Teochews are descendants of groups that had migrated to Fukien between A.D. 713 from the province of Honan, more specifically from the Kwangchow and Ku Shinh districts. Surveys of the incidence of esophagus cancer in North China (137) have shown that the highest incidence of this neoplasm is found in the Lin County of Honan province. The researchers speculated that the high incidence of esophagus cancer observed among Hokkiens and Teochews in Singapore may be linked to their originating from this part of China.

Mahboubi et al (146) and Aramesh (9) have shown a 20- to 30-fold variation in the incidence of esophageal cancer along the Caspian littoral. Preliminary case history studies have excluded any possible role of alcohol or tobacco, but nutritional factors involving the consumption of nitrosamine-rich food may have an influence. Such evidence of high incidences of esophageal carcinoma is also found in the northern part of France, where the people drink apple cider which is known to be rich in nitrosamines.

Among Caucasians in the United States, cancer of the esophagus is not prevalent. However, the incidence is high among Negro males in Washington, D.C., and intermediate in Alameda county in California (6). White males also showed low rates of incidence in Alameda county. Rates for both Negro and White females are low throughout the United States. Carcinoma of the esophagus exhibits an extremely variable geographic distribution of incidence. Isolated areas of high incidence are also found in eastern and southern Africa. Otherwise, in Africa, this malignancy is practically unknown.

The age-standardized incidence rate for males is 75.6/100,000 in Rhodesia, 40.9/100,000 in Nabal, South Africa, but only 0.8/100,000 in Ibedan, Nigeria. Esophageal cancer has increased significantly among the Bantus in large urban areas in South Africa within the last decade. The disease pattern of Southern Africa reflects the heterogeneous cultures and varying climatic geographical areas (187).

Analysis of mortality rates in the United States between 1960 and 1967 showed rapidly increasing rates in the non-white population, while those for the white population remained relatively unchanged.

The increasing rate was associated with cigarette smoking and alcohol consumption. A considerably higher percentage of urban non-white cases than white were found to be heavy smokers. Also heavy drinking in urban areas was found to be twice as common in Negroes as in whites of a similar socioeconomic class. The geographic distribution of esophageal cancer in Africa reflects the use of maize as a major ingredient of alcoholic beverages—the same as in North China and some countries in Europe, e.g., Germany.

Stomach

The incidence of gastric cancer varies from one country to another. A comparison of autopsy material from stomach cancer from Japan, the United States, Korea, New Zealand, Chile and Poland was done to autopsy material from patients with stomach metaplasia from Japan, the United States, New Zealand and Chile (Tables 36.6 and 36.7). The age-standardized calculations of stomach metaplasia for males were: 36,785/100,000 in Japan, 28,177 in Chile, 12,394 in New Zealand, and 9,000 in the United States (Caucasians). The death rates for gastric cancer per 100,000 were 66 for Japanese males, 56 for Chileans, 15 for New Zealanders and 17 for Caucasians in the United States. The positive correlation of metaplasia and gastric cancer was $r = 0.990$. The ratio of persons with cancer to those with metaplasia was 0.00179 in Japan, 0.00198 in Chile, 0.00121 in New Zealand, and 0.00172 in the United States (Caucasians). The calculated figure for Poland was 0.00166. It could be concluded that 0.17% of persons with metaplasia develop stomach cancer (Figs. 36.3–36.5) (129); see also Ref. 90. The effect of genetics in the development of stomach cancer was in general greater in young persons (except the under 30-year-old female group), whereas the environmental factor was more pronounced in older persons (except the over 59-year-old male groups) (130). The highest incidences are found in Japan (about the application of mass surveys, see Ref. 151, for gastric cancer of Japanese in Hawaii, see Ref. 218, for long standing food habits, Ref. 163).

Gastric cancer in Venezuela, as in one of the countries with the highest rate of this disease in South America, occurs in an especially high rate in the Andean mountain region (states of Táchira and Mérida) and in the neighboring region (as in the Falcón state) (156); for Colombia see Refs. 42, 48, and 91.

In the USSR stomach cancer is one of the most widespread cancers. A decrease of morbidity was noted in recent years. The rate in old people was increased in contrast to young people. The highest rate of stomach cancer occurs in Russia, followed by the Pre-Baltic republics, and is lowest in Georgia and Armenia. The standard of living is almost similar in all regions but particularities in nutrition occur (19). However, the incidence rate is now decreasing in most countries (87).

The case of gastric cancer also varies by country and also by regions within countries. Thus, a substantial change in the regional peculiarities coincident with high rates of stomach cancer should result in a change in the incidence of the cancer. Clemmesen (33) pointed in 1965 to many such factors: soil, climate, environment, occupation, dietary factors, and heredity. However, the most natural explanation for differences in incidence of stomach cancer is that they reflect differences in habits.

In a joint study undertaken concurrently in New York, Iceland, Japan and Yugoslavia, by Wynder, Kmet *et al.*, Dungal and Segi, respectively, in order to compare dietary factors among populations in different races, high consumption of cereal, low intake of vegetables and fruits and a high consumption of rice, cereals and potatoes (that is of starchy foods with low protein diet) was correlated with a high incidence of stomach cancer (259) (Fig. 36.6).

According to these findings we would expect that the consumption of cereals in populations with high stomach cancer incidence would be higher than in populations with low stomach cancer incidence. The high consumption of cereals correlates with many other factors connected often with a low standard of living. Increasing consumption of milk in the new standard of diet in Japan with more western style of food tends to decrease the incidence of stomach cancer. A role for host factors in this disease has been suggested by two types of observation: (a) an excess risk for persons of blood group A (5, 18, 23, 211, 244) and (b) clustering of stomach cancer within families, the collective evidence from several studies suggesting that stomach cancer risk among relatives of probands are 2–3 times those for relatives of control groups (143, 251).

Table 36.6
Age-adjusted Death Rates for Ulcer of the Stomach in 25 Countries (1962–1963)

Male		Female	
Country	Death rate	Country	Death rate
1. Japan	16.00	1. Japan	5.85
2. Portugal	9.65	2. Portugal	2.52
3. South Africa	6.98	3. Ireland	2.39
4. Chile	6.89	4. Chile	2.39
5. Finland	6.27	5. South Africa	2.15
6. Germany, F.R.	5.43	6. Austria	2.06
7. Austria	5.17	7. Denmark	2.00
8. Ireland	4.90	8. England and Wales	1.99
9. Italy	4.74	9. Sweden	1.99
10. USA, nonwhite	4.49	10. Scotland	1.97
11. England and Wales	4.41	11. Finland	1.70
12. Sweden	4.40	12. Australia	1.67
13. Scotland	4.40	13. Switzerland	1.64
14. Denmark	4.28	14. Northern Ireland	1.59
15. Belgium	4.22	15. New Zealand	1.55
16. Northern Ireland	4.16	16. USA, nonwhite	1.49
17. USA, white	3.91	17. USA, white	1.42
18. Australia	3.57	18. Canada	1.31
19. Canada	3.57	19. Germany, F.R.	1.26
20. New Zealand	3.53	20. Norway	1.20
21. Switzerland	3.46	21. Netherlands	1.16
22. France	3.20	22. Israel	1.13
23. Netherlands	3.11	23. Belgium	1.11
24. Israel	2.38	24. Italy	0.97
25. Norway	2.29	25. France	0.74

[a] Source: Saxen and Hakama (191).

Table 36.7
Age-adjusted Death Rates for Cancer of the Stomach among Various Countries

Male		Female	
Country	Rate	Country	Rate
1. Chile	71.00	1. Chile	45.79
2. Japan	69.50	2. Japan	36.80
3. Hungary	46.50	3. Austria	26.11
4. Austria	45.55	4. Hungary	26.11
5. Finland	45.17	5. Finland	26.07
6. Czechoslovakia	43.59	6. Czechoslovakia	23.97
7. Germany, F.R.	39.95	7. Germany, F.R.	23.22
8. Poland	39.79	8. Venezuela	21.96
9. Italy	34.56	9. Poland	19.39
10. Venezuela	33.00	10. Italy	18.49
11. West Berlin	32.72	11. Colombia	18.35
12. Belgium	31.44	12. Belgium	18.14
13. Portugal	31.30	13. Spain	18.09
14. Netherlands	31.10	14. Switzerland	17.60
15. Switzerland	30.41	15. West Berlin	17.54
16. Spain	30.37	16. Norway	17.45
17. Norway	29.11	17. Portugal	17.37
18. South Africa	28.62	18. Ireland	16.74
19. Northern Ireland	27.88	19. Netherlands	16.45
20. Scotland	26.83	20. Northern Ireland	16.35
21. Sweden	26.12	21. Denmark	16.26
22. Denmark	25.96	22. Scotland	16.09
23. England and Wales	25.44	23. South Africa	15.84
24. France	25.44	24. Israel	14.97
25. Ireland	23.79	25. Sweden	14.30
26. Israel	22.29	26. England and Wales	13.26
27. Taiwan	21.86	27. France	12.74
28. Yugoslavia	21.72	28. Yugoslavia	12.70
29. Colombia	21.20	29. Taiwan	11.93
30. USA, nonwhite	20.14	30. Australia	9.65
31. Canada	19.45	31. Canada	9.61
32. New Zealand	19.01	32. Greece	9.47
33. Australia	18.38	33. New Zealand	9.22
34. Greece	15.17	34. USA, nonwhite	8.89
35. USA, white	11.46	35. Mexico	8.58
36. Mexico	8.72	36. Ceylon	8.16
37. Ceylon	5.21	37. USA, white	5.81
38. Egypt	2.43	38. Egypt	1.40

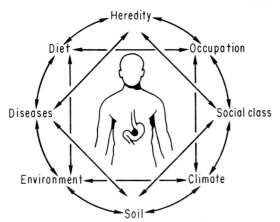

Figure 36.3. Schematized presentation of the interrelationships of etiological factors as they affect incidence of stomach cancer. Source: Saxen and Hakama (191).

Among various ethnic groups in Japan, the age-standardized death rate for stomach cancer was noted to be much higher among Japanese and Koreans than among Caucasians and Chinese (Fig. 36.7).

Socioeconomic Variation

Both mortality and morbidity rates were found to become higher with the decrease in socioeconomic status, resembling the tendency in the United States, England, Wales, Denmark, and Japan (32, 67, 103, 105, 183).

Just as among the Japanese in the United States, the age-specific death rates of stomach cancer in Japan have also shown a decrease since 1955, except in the age group over 70.

For sarcomas of the stomach, see Ref. 8.

Regional Variation

The observation of age-standardized death rate of stomach cancer by villages, towns, and cities clearly indicates a significant geographical aggregation showing a high endemicity in the northern district facing the Japan Sea (103). Recently a decrease in stomach cancer appeared in Japan.

All of these epidemiologic phenomena suggest a significant effect of environmental factors which appear to operate more strongly in males, also among the Japanese, especially from the northern part of Japan, and among people of lower socioeconomic status. The decreasing

trend in recent years also indicate the strong effect of post-war environmental changes.

Biliary Passage and Liver

Primary cancer of the biliary passage and liver are more common in Asia than in Europe and the United States. The incidence is high in Thailand, Singapore, Hong Kong and Malaysia, but low among the Chinese in these countries, and in Japan and Europe. In Thailand it is also associated with hepatic cirrhosis (41%, 8%), a further 18.9% being associated with infestation of liver fluke (*Opisthorchis viverrini*). Races with a high incidence of liver cancer also display a high incidence of cirrhosis. The association with *Clonorchis sinensis* (249) and *Opisthorchis viverrini* infestation of the liver is also well established. These parasites are common in Korea

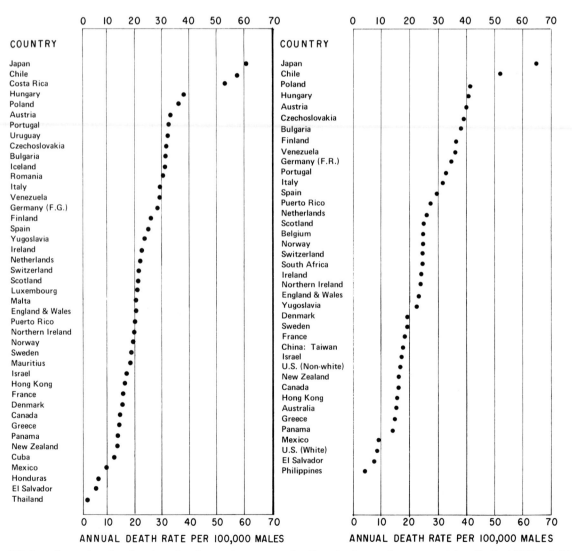

Figure 36.4. Age standardized male stomach cancer death rate for various countries (left, 1972; right, 1967) (Source: Segi and Kurihara (201); WHO Statistics Annual 1968 (246), Segi 1972, WHO Statistics Annual 1972/73).

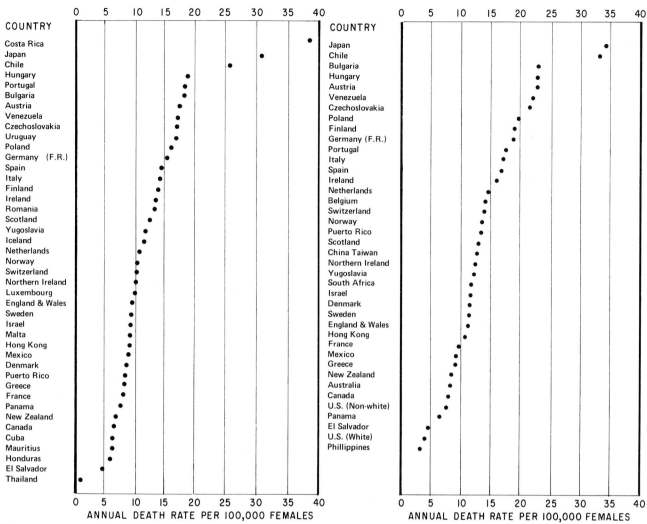

Figure 36.5. Age standardized female stomach cancer death rate for various countries (left, 1972; right, 1967). (Source: Segi (200); Segi and Kurihara (201); WHO Statistics Annual 1968 (246).)

and Thailand. Primary cancer of the liver shows a particularly high incidence in other parts of the Orient as well as in regions of Africa and South America, the tumor usually being superimposed upon a background of nutritional cirrhosis or parasitic infestation of the liver (185). Significant differences have also been observed among the major Chinese groups in Singapore, with Cantonese males having lower relative incidence rates than the pool Hokkien and Teochew groups. By contrast, the rates of female Cantonese are higher than for these latter two groups. Most primary hepatic carcinomas occur at average age of 50–60 years in the United States, but in Africa the peak incidence is the third and fourth decade of lives (184) (Tables 36.8 and 36.9). Primary carcinoma of the liver represents only about 2.5% of all malignancies in the United States, but in certain regions of Africa it is said to constitute over 50% of all malignancies in women. Some of this difference may not be due to racial factors, but rather to

the fact that the life span in Africa is much shorter, so that the individual may not live long enough to develop the other types of malignancy encountered in the Northern hemisphere (184). The frequency of liver cirrhosis is also high in Mexico, but the incidence of primary liver carcinoma is low in this and other Latin American countries.

The epidemiology of cancer found in 177 vinyl chloride workers was investigated because this substance causes angiosarcoma of the liver. Biochemical and immunological tests have been developed in this high risk population (Table 36.10) (171). See also Refs. 176 and 177.

Colon (235) and Rectum

Reddy *et al.* (182) compared the fecal constituents of a high risk North American and a low risk Finnish population for the chance to develop large bowel cancer. Adenomatosis coli is a condition increasing the risk of colon cancer in Japan, as before reported for other countries. It is considered the best example of development of genetic cancer in the human (233). For reports on colon cancer in India compare Ref. 119.

All countries report a prevalence of males in rectal cancer cases (245). However, many data suggest that this cancer is relatively uncommon in the developing areas of the world (255). Cancer of the colon and rectum ranks second among malignant tumors in the United States (39) and equals that of the stomach in frequency among Hawaiians of Japanese ancestry. An older study

has shown that rectal cancer is as common in Japan as it is in the United States (256). Cancer of the colon is, however, significantly less common in Japan, and is associated with a higher socioeconomic status and a more western type of diet.

There is, on the whole, a positive correlation between colonic and rectal cancers, countries with a high rate of cancer of the colon usually also having a high rate of cancer of the rectum. Exceptions to this rule are Canadian and U.S. Caucasians, who have high rates of colonic cancer but relatively low rates of rectal cancer. In Japan the rates are reversed (255), as they are in Korea.

Among the Chinese in Hong Kong cancer of the colon ranks fifth among males. In Malaysia the incidence is high among the Chinese and Indians, but low among the Malays. This is correlated with the Chinese in Hawaii, who had almost as high an incidence of colorectal cancer as Caucasians. The incidence of colorectal cancer remains low among the Chinese in Thailand, Formosa, and Indonesia who still eat old Chinese style food, and moderate among the Chinese in Singapore and Hong Kong only some of whom still eat old style Chinese food. These findings suggest an oncogenic effect of more western style food among the Chinese. See also Ref. 46.

RESPIRATORY ORGANS

Nasal and Paranasal Regions (161)

These locations represent the most commonly encountered primary site (Fig. 36.9) among the Chinese in Singapore, Formosa, Hong Kong, Thailand, and Korea. The increased risk in

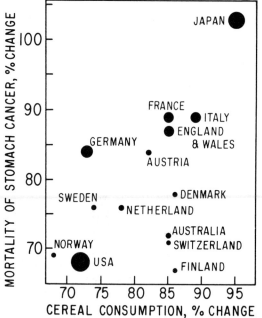

Figure 36.6. Mortality rate in incidence of stomach cancer, correlated to the cereal consumption of various countries. Source: Saxen and Hakama (191).

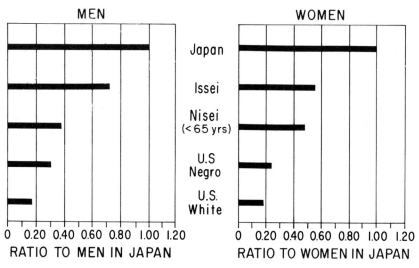

Figure 36.7. Incidence of stomach cancer among the Japanese in Japan, Hawaii, and the United States, compared with non-Japanese people of the United States. Source: Saxen and Hakama (191).

Chinese toward developing nasopharyngeal carcinoma is suspected to be associated with a Chinese-related HL-A profile (A2, Singapore 2) (210).

Nasopharyngeal cancer, very common among Chinese, especially in Southern China and also frequent in other mongoloid groups in Southeast Asia, exhibits also a remarkable high incidence among eskimos of the western Canadian arctic and Alaska. An eskimo population with some mixture of Caucasians presented during 1955–

Table 36.8
Geographic Distribution of Primary Cancer of the Liver in Men[a]

Age-standardized Incidence (rates per 100,000 males)			
Group I		*Group II*	
Mozambique	106.9	New Zealand	4.3
South Africa (Bantu)	22.0	Puerto Rico	3.8
Nigeria	10.5	Sweden	3.8
Singapore (Chinese)	9.6		
Colombia	8.3	*Group III*	
USA, 10 cities, white	7.2	Finland	2.7
Kyadondo, Uganda	7.2	Norway	1.1
USA, 10 cities, nonwhite	6.3		
Jamaica	6.0		

[a] Source: L. Dunham and J. C. Bailar (69).

1976, 35 cases of nasopharyngeal cancer, of which 34 cases or 94% were squamous cell carcinomas, including lymphoepitiomas. Research to clarify a possible racial susceptibility to Epstein-Barr (EB) virus infection is recommended (166).

The mortality caused by cancers of the respiratory system in white males in Louisiana is one of the highest in the United States but seems to depend heavily on wet lands and certain industries (240). Various investigators have found the nasopharynx is the primary site of 1% to 2% of cancers in the United States, but malignant conditions of the nasopharynx account for 18% of cancer sites in Hong Kong. The reason for the high prevalence among the Chinese (excluding Mainland China) is still unknown, but existence of EB virus in the nasopharynx of these peoples may be a cause.

The epidemiology of nasopharyngeal carcinoma in four provinces in South China covering a period from 1970 to 1975 and a population of 170 million showed a significantly limited localization of risk, a higher susceptibility of certain groups of people, a lower occurrence of the disease among children in the high risk area

Table 36.9
Relative Frequencies of Liver Cancer among Histologically Confirmed Cases in Selected Asian Countries

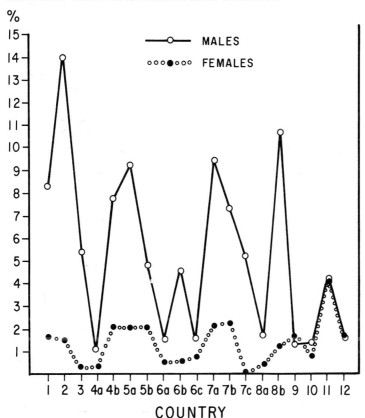

Source: Proceedings, 2nd Asian Cancer Congress, Manila.

Table 36.10
Frequency of Hepatocellular Carcinoma and Cholangiocarcinoma among Autopsy Cases in the World

| Author(s) | Country | No. of Autopsies | Hepatocellular Carcinoma | | No. of Cholangiocarcinomas |
			No.	%	
Edmondson and Steiner (1954)	USA	48,900	75	0.15	18
Kohn, K. (1955)	Germany	35,745	80	0.22	
MacDonald, R. A. (1956)	USA	23,114	80	0.34	24
Roulet, F. C. (1957)	Switzerland	23,470	93	0.40	16
Berman, C. (1958)	South Africa	15,280	248	1.62	
Gall, E. A. (1960)	USA	12,200(over 21 years)	76	0.62	20
Becker and Chatgidakis (1961)	South Africa	4,949(white)	9	0.18	0
		4,893(native)	84	1.72	6
Wainwright, J. (1961)	South Africa	2,560	102	3.98	14
Shanmugaratnam, K. (1961)	Singapore	9,893	103	1.04	9
Glennert, J. (1961)	Denmark	14,881	50	0.34	36
Tiktinskii, O. L. (1961)	USSR	6,163	17	0.28	
Ying et al. (1963)	China	3,497	87	2.49	10
Elkington et al. (1963)	England	7,366	39	0.53	
Sagebiel et al. (1963)	USA	23,275	100	0.43	
Sundarsanam et al. (1963)	India	3,400	22	0.65	2
Miyai and Reubner (1963)	USA	25,000	64	0.26	8
Ervasti, J. (1964)	Finland	15,545	45	0.29	29
Patton and Horn (1964)	USA	12,980	47	0.36	13
Epstein, S. (1964)	USA	3,079	50	1.62	
Saragoca et al. (1964)	Portugal	168	6	3.57	
		4,338	14	0.32	
Ohlsson and Norden (1965)	Sweden	8,837	120	1.36	1
San Jose et al. (1965)	USA	12,687	73	0.58	6
Manderson et al. (1965)	England	6,586	41	0.62	
Ottolenghi, A. (1966)	Italy	6,241	94	1.51	
		4,000	124	3.10	
Pequignot et al. (1967)	France	2,540	42	1.65	
Voigt and Helbig (1968)	Germany	26,235	75	0.29	42
Scrinivasa and Sharma (1968)	India	1,293	29	2.24	2
Wockel and Altrock (1968)	Germany	15,568	40	0.26	
Stitnimankarn (1970)	Thailand	12,265	287	2.421	42
Sievers, B.-U. (1973)	Germany	4,411	36	0.82	11
Purtilo and Gottlieb (1973)	USA	14,000	84	0.60	12
Elsner and Jauregui (1974)	Argentina	22,170	54	0.24	10

From T. Miyaji: In *Gann Monograph 18, Cancer in Asia,* University of Tokyo Press, Tokyo, 1976.

than the low risk area, and a general stability of the incidence of this type of cancer (56). In the United States the incidence of nasopharynx carcinoma is also higher among the immigrant Chinese than in those born of immigrant parents. While this does not exclude a racial factor, it does, in the opinion of Sturtor *et al.* (220), suggest a strong possibility of factors due to environment or habits (e.g. sputum spitting among these peoples). Chemical and spectroscopic reports on condensate from joss sticks were also mentioned: the incense smoke may be a factor in the etiology of this malignant disease. The burning of Buddhist incense is also practiced in Korea, Thailand, Formosa, Malaysia, and Singapore, but prohibited in Mainland China. This may be the reason for the higher incidence of this disease in these countries.

Cancer arising in the lymphoepithelium of the nasopharynx is particularly common in the Mongoloid races, and occurs on average in younger individuals than carcinoma developing in the Schneiderian mucosa of the nose and paranasal sinus. Nasal and paranasal carcinoma are otherwise unusual in young people and most prevalent in the sixth and seventh decade. Most series of cases show more males affected than females.

A study of early cases may reveal information on whether nasopharyngeal carcinoma is the product of the environment. Clifford (38) claims that the disease has afflicted man since antiquity. It was certainly mentioned in ancient Chinese medical writing, but whereas most of the old Chinese medical writings were written by physicians in Northern and Central China, nasopharyngeal carcinoma is prevalent only in the Southern part today.

High risk of nasopharyngeal carcinoma is not associated with the Mongoloid race as a whole, but only with Chinese originating from the southern provinces. This ethnic risk has not been found to be influenced by geographical factors where migrants are concerned.

Among the Mongoloid people, the Malays throughout Southeast Asia have a risk somewhere between those of the Southern Chinese and low risk Caucasoids and Indians living in Singapore. The Malays in Southeast Asia have had a long period of cultural and some racial

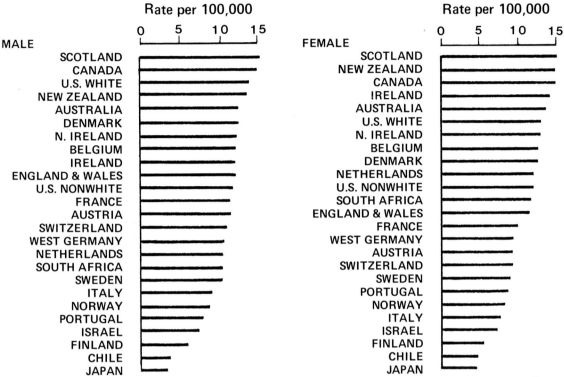

Figure 36.8. Age-adjusted mortality rate from cancer of the colon in various parts of the world. (Source: Segi and Kurihara (201).)

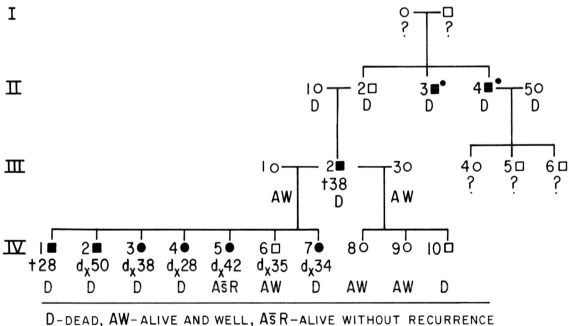

Figure 36.9. Pedigree study of a family with multiple case of nasopharyngeal carcinoma extending over three successive generations. (Source: Ho (108).)

intermingling with Chinese, mainly those from the South in more recent times, but earlier predominantly with Chinese from the North. There has been practically no racial intermingling between Chinese and the indigenous Mongoloid people living in Sarawak and Sabah, but some cultural intermingling can not be ruled out: a comparatively high incidence of nasopharyngeal carcinoma has been found in both. Among the people in the Highlands of Papua New Guinea, largely of Melanesian stock with practically no racial or social intermingling with Chinese, the disease is rare. It would seem that a high risk is not necessary associated with racial intermingling with Chinese, but this could not be said for the sharing of certain cultural traits, especially dietary, as a result of social intermingling. In the case of the Indians in Singapore, there is definite social but practically no racial intermingling. It may be that the social intermingling did not result in the sharing of those cultural traits which are of importance in the etiology of nasopharyngeal carcinoma. If there are such traits, religion is unlikely to be involved. This is indicated by the finding of Ho that in Hong Kong, Macaonese descendants of Portuguese settlers in Macao who intermarried with Chinese from Kwangtung had a much higher frequency of nasopharyngeal carcinoma than the rest of the non-Chinese population, and the finding by Garnjana-Goonchorn and Chanterakul that in Thailand, Thais with part Chinese ancestry have a relative frequency of nasopharyngeal carcinoma intermediate between Thais and Chinese. Macaonese are traditionally Catholics and Thais and Sino-Thais are traditionally Buddhists. Portuguese are of Caucasoid stock and Thais are Mongoloid. In both, the progeny resulting from their intermarriage with Chinese share one thing in common: a part of the high risk of nasopharyngeal carcinoma of their Chinese ancestors.

Ho (108) found a significantly higher frequency of nasopharyngeal carcinoma in close blood relatives of nasopharyngeal carcinoma patients suffering from other cancers, and that the familial clustering of nasopharyngeal carcinoma was quite random and appeared to be as likely to occur in the vertical as in the horizontal direction, and was not sex-linked. This impression is further reinforced by an up-to-date study of the pedigree of a southern Chinese family with nasopharyngeal carcinoma affecting three successive generations.

Occurrences of nasopharyngeal cancer in twins, with the onset of the disease at the same age, are rare but have been observed occasionally as the following case. An instance of nasopharyngeal carcinoma with simultaneous clinical onset at the age of 21 in a pair of dizygotic twins, the youngest of 10 siblings was reported. (The family migrated to Israel from Morocco.)

Of some 7000 cases of nasopharyngeal carcinoma diagnosed at the Medical and Health Department, Institute of Radiology, Hong Kong, there were only two verified instances of nasopharyngeal carcinoma occurring in twins. One dizygotic pair were born of a wealthy family in Kwangtung, where they had schooling together. They also studied medicine together, qualified at the same time, and migrated to Hong Kong at about the age of 29. One migrated to Canada at 30 and had clinical onset of nasopharyngeal carcinoma at 49, whereas his twin brother who remained in Hong Kong had clinical onset at 40. They had two other brothers and three sisters. The homozygotic pair were born in a village at Nam Hoi of poor peasant parents with eight sons. The twins were always together, even sharing the same bed until they left school at age 10. One migrated to Hong Kong at 17 and has been working as a Chinese teahouse waiter since. He had clinical onset at 45. His twin brother migrated to Hong Kong first at 23 and worked as a laborer. He returned home 2 years later to work for the parents until he was 38 when he returned to Hong Kong and has also been working as a teahouse waiter since. He had clinical onset at 48. In none of the three instances was there a family history of nasopharyngeal carcinoma. The Chinese twins consumed Cantonese salted fish, which is known to contain nitrosamines, frequently in their childhood.

In Hong Kong people who spend most of their lives in their boats and cook their food in the open air are prone to nasopharyngeal carcinoma. Besides, salted marine fish prepared ungutted contains appreciable quantities of dimethylnitrosamine and is commonly consumed by southern Chinese, especially those from Kwangtung, wherever they may subsequently reside. In Northern China, where salted fish is seldom used, nasopharyngeal carcinoma is rare.

In Asia, Japan is the one country with the low incidence of nasopharyngeal carcinoma comparable to that of the United States and other western countries.

The tribal distribution of cases of nasopharyngeal carcinoma in the Sudan points to a possible genetic susceptibility for this tumor (147).

Oral and oropharyngeal carcinomas provide a notable example of widely differing prevalence in different parts of the world. In many cases, areas of high incidence have been shown to be associated with the existence of particular habits which might be considered to exert a carcinogenic effect. Such habits particularly associated with high incidence are tobacco clearing and chutta smoking in India. Such habits also appear to influence the predilection to a particular site as well as histologic types of cancer.

Oral and Oropharyngeal Cavities (80)

In Malaysia, oral cancer appears to be the second commonest histologically confirmed malignant tumor. The peak incidence for the Indian male, Indian female, and Malay female was between 50 and 59 years, and for the Malay male and Chinese male it was between 60 and 65 years.

Racial variations in the pattern of carcinoma are evident. Except among Malaysians and Indians the average age of the females was generally higher than the corresponding males. The buccal mucosa in the females was generally more abundant than in the corresponding males. The buccal mucosa are the commonest site for oral carcinoma in the Indian and Malay females, but are the least common site in Caucasian and Chinese males. Carcinoma of the lips and the floor of the mouth is very common among Caucasians but relatively uncommon in Malaysians. In the Indian male, Chinese male, and Chinese female the upper half of the mouth was more commonly involved than the lower half, whereas in the Malay male and female and the Indian female, the upper and lower half of the mouth were equally affected.

In Sri Lanka cancer of the oropharynx forms 47% of all cancer cases admitted to the Cancer Institute. The breakdown of these cancers shows that 10% occur in the lower alveolus. This is caused by the chewing of betel with tobacco and slake like. The reason for the incidence is the abnormal flow of saliva in the mouth.

Larynx

Carcinoma of the larynx, like that of the mouth and pharynx, has a decided class gradient among males, being highest in the unskilled classes (249). The tumors are common among the Indian, Korean, and Thai peoples. The victims belong to lower socioeconomic strata and are often among the older age groups. For mor-

tality statistics relative to Oklahoma from 1950–1970, see Ref. 41.

Of all cancers observed in the Fundacao Antonio Prudente, Sao Paulo, Brazil, 4.8% were laryngeal cancers. The average age for man was 57.3 and 57.5 years for women (53).

It was again concluded in a study in Buenos Aires that there exists a very strong connection between cancer of the larynx and smoking, with statistical evidence reaching up to $p\ 5 \times 10^{-13}$ (231).

A study of Libya during 1968–1972 showed the detection of malignancy in 13.3% of 7585 biopsies (996); 56.22% of the malignancy occurred in males and 43.77% in females. The malignancies of the larynx occurred in 39.85%, followed by those of the nasopharynx with 12.03%, and those of maxilla and nose each with 10.53%. The incidence of all malignancies was much higher in males with 75.19% than in females with 24.81% concerning the upper respiratory tract. The neoplasms of the larynx and nasopharynx showed a continued increase. Most occurred in the age group from 40 to 49 years. A sex variation is indicated by the fact that the most frequent malignant neoplasms in males were those of the nasopharynx followed by maxilla, nose, pharynx, epiglottis, and tonsil, whereas in females the most frequent malignant neoplasms occurred in the nose followed by larynx, maxilla, and hypopharynx (238).

Trachea, Bronchus and Lung (101)

There are high rates of lung cancer in industralized countries such as England, the United States, Singapore, and Israel, but the incidence is low in Japan and Hong Kong. In Africa and South America the incidence is generally higher among males than among females, and cigarette smoking, polluted air, exhaust gas from engines, and industries are believed to be the causes (Table 36.11).

A high incidence rate of lung cancer occurs in Chinese women in Singapore (124).

Israeli studies indicated that tuberculosis patients have a higher risk of developing lung, esophageal, and primary liver cancer (214).

For conditions of the bronchiogenic carcinoma in Greece, see Ref. 66.

The incidence of lung cancer among Negroes in Washington, D.C., and Alameda County, California, is very high in males and intermediate in females, while throughout Africa the rates are

Table 36.11
Incidence of Lung Cancer in Selected Countries, Population Morbidity Rates per 100,000 Persons per Year, Age-adjusted to World Population[a]

Males		Females	
Countries/population	Rates	Countries/population	Rates
UK, Liverpool	86.6	New Zealand, Maori	37.7
UK, Birmingham region	73.3	Singapore, Chinese (Cantonese)	25.6
USA, Hawaii: Hawaiian	70.3	USA, Hawaii, Hawaiian	22.3
New Zealand, Maori	70.1	USA, Hawaii, Filipino	17.4
Finland	70.0	USA, Hawaii, Chinese	16.7
Singapore, Chinese (Hokkien)	69.2	Singapore, Chinese (all groups)	15.9
UK, Scotland	67.0	Singapore, Chinese (Hokkien)	12.8
Federal Republic of Germany, Hamburg	66.0	UK, Liverpool	11.8
Singapore, Chinese (Cantonese)	53.6	Singapore, Chinese (Teochew)	10.2
Singapore, Chinese (all groups)	53.5	South Africa, Natal, African	10.2
Singapore, Chinese (Teochew)	52.9	Federal Republic of Germany, Hamburg	10.2
German Democratic Republic (GDR)	48.8	USA, Hawaii, Caucasian	10.2
USA, California, white	47.8	UK, Scotland	9.9
Rhodesia, Bulawayo, African	47.1	Singapore, Indian	9.7
Poland, Warsaw City	46.9	USA, California, Negro	9.0
New Zealand, European	45.1	Israel, Jews	8.7
South Africa, Cape Prov., white	44.7	Poland, Warsaw City	8.4
USA, Connecticut	44.0	UK, Birmingham Region	8.4
USA, California, Negro	43.8	USA, Connecticut	7.8
USA, Hawaii, Caucasian	43.8	USA, Hawaii, Japanese	7.6
South Africa, Cape Prov., colored	42.8	Singapore, Malay	7.6
Canada, Manitoba	42.2	Jamaica, Kingston and St. Andrew	7.5
South Africa, Natal, African	41.2	USA, California, white	7.4
Yugoslavia, Slovenia	38.5	Canada, Manitoba	7.3
Denmark	31.4	New Zealand, European	6.1
Hungary, Miskolc	28.4	Japan, Miyagi Prefecture	6.0
USA, Hawaii, Chinese	27.2	Hungary, Miskolc	5.6
South Africa, Cape Prov., Bantu	26.9	South Africa, Cape Prov., white	5.3
Israel, Jews	26.4	Japan, Okayama Prefecture	5.2
USA, Hawaii, Japanese	26.3	Denmark	5.2
Poland, four rural areas	26.2	Puerto Rico	5.0
Canada, Alberta	25.8	South Africa, Cape Prov., Bantu	4.9
Romania, Banat region	24.9	Rhodesia, Bulawayo, African	4.7
Jamaica, Kingston and St. Andrew	24.6	Finland	4.4
Israel, non-Jews	24.6	Sweden	4.4
South Africa, Natal, Indian	20.0	Yugoslavia, Slovenia	4.4
Sweden	19.2	German Democratic Republic (GDR)	4.3
Colombia, Cali	17.5	South Africa, Cape Prov., Colored	4.2
USA, Hawaii, Filipino	17.1	Canada, Alberta	4.1
Norway	16.5	Poland, four rural areas	3.8
Japan, Miyagi Prefecture	15.6	Colombia, Cali	3.8
Japan, Okayama Prefecture	15.3	India, Bombay	3.7
Singapore, Malay	14.6	Romania, Banat region	3.5
Puerto Rico	13.6	South Africa, Natal, Indian	3.3
India, Bombay	13.3	Norway	3.1
Singapore, Indian	4.8	Israel, non-Jews	3.1
Nigeria, Ibadan	1.2	Nigeria, Ibadan	1.0

[a] Source: K. Shanmugaratnam (204).

quite low (except in South Africa where the incidence of lung cancer has increased 6-fold in urban Bantu-speaking African males in the last decade).

Variations in the incidence of lung cancer between different races in the same environment have been recorded in Hawaii, Singapore, Hong Kong, and mainland China. In Hawaii the incidence among the native Hawaiians is more prevalent than among the Caucasians, Japanese, and Chinese. In the southern United States, e.g., New Orleans, lung cancer is twice as common in whites as in Negroes, but in the North the incidence is the same in both groups. The Negro migrant elsewhere has a lung tumor frequency which resembles that of the Negro in the United States rather than the low rate which appears to prevail in Africa.

The Japanese in the United States have the same frequency of lung cancer as the Caucasians, but among the Filipinos this disease is less common than among the Caucasoids. In Malaysia the incidence among the Chinese there is much higher than among the Malays and Indians.

The incidence of lung cancer in Singapore is higher than in other Asian countries and is roughly at the same levels as in Europe and North America. The highest rates are found in England (Birmingham) and among females in Singapore. There are significant differences in lung cancer incidence among the major ethnic groups in the latter country: Chinese males have appreciably higher relative incidence rates than Malay males and Indian males, and Chinese females also have significantly higher relative incidence rates than their Malay and Indian counterparts.

The incidence among the Chinese in Singapore is higher than among the Chinese in Malaysia, Hong Kong, Formosa, and Peking (where the indicence is very low), and in Singapore the incidence among Chinese of the Hokkien dialect is almost double the incidence among the Teochew and the Cantonese.

In Korea pulmonary carcinoma affects younger people more often than other types of carcinoma, and is found preponderantly in males (249). This type of tumor has a high rate of occurrence in the United States, Hong Kong and Malaysia, but a low incidence in Japan, Scandinavia, and Africa. For the epidemiology of lung cancer in Tokyo, see Ref. 107 and regarding Argentina, Ref. 17.

FEMALE GENITAL ORGANS

Breast (258)

The evidence for genetic influence and the role of viruses is minimal or largely inferential compared with hormonal and environmental factors. Emphasis, however, has been placed on environmental factors since such influences must be identified to explain the ethnic and geographic difference in the incidence of breast cancer (Fig. 36.10).

Many countries in Asia have a very low incidence of breast cancer, especially Japan, Singapore, and India, the exceptions, however, are Thailand and Korea, where the rate of incidence is high. In Thailand it represents 6.8% of all cancers and ranks third, and in Korea it is 8%

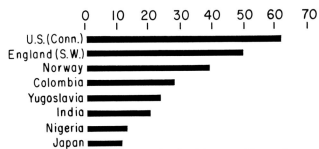

Figure 36.10. Comparative incidence of breast cancer rate per 100,000 persons. Source: O'Connor (169).

and said to be the commonest site, comparable to the United States and Western Europe. Factors influencing breast cancer are more hormonal than genetic, viral or environmental. Hormonal and racial influences may operate as the positive risk factors related to ovarian function in early menarche, multiparous states, anovulatory cycles, increasing age of first parity, and increasing age of menopause. These factors which increase risk, studied by Lemon, revealed that ovarian estragens are a major factor in breast cancer. This may help explain the high incidence of breast cancer among the Semites in Israel, who have early menarche and have also a high incidence of breast cancer. The geographic and ethnic variation in total incidence and particularly in the age-specific incidence rates of breast cancer are striking (117, 213, 230); for Denmark, see Ref. 35.

These differences, the extremes of which are represented by the United States and Japan, are most indicative of environmental influences as are the data for migrant studies. The latter shows a rising incidence and a changing age distribution pattern for breast cancer in the Japanese living in Hawaii and California, but the rate nevertheless suggests persisting cultural factors (Fig. 36.11).

There have been thus far only two environmental factors of importance identified, and these are related in part to geographic and ethnic differences. They are socioeconomic status and diet. There are striking geographical differences in the incidence of this disease (184). Thus, while cancer of the breast is the most common cancer among women in the United States (207) the death rate recorded for mammary cancer in Japan is remarkably low (249) being only 3.8 per 100,000 (184).

In India ethnic comparison has enabled frequency ratios to be prepared for cancer of the breast and female genital organs in different religious communities. Among the Parsis of Bombay and the Hindu migrants from Sind, the

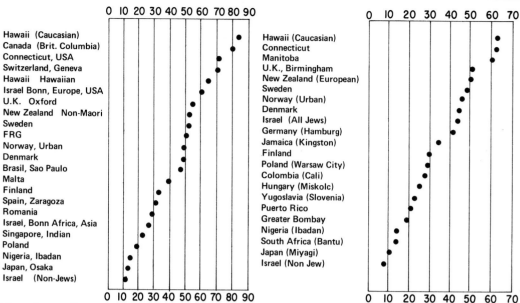

Figure 36.11. Age-adjusted world incidence rates for cancer of the female breast for various registries (left, 1976; right, 1966). (Source: UICC, Cancer Incidence in Five Continents, 1966 and 1976, IARC.)

frequency ratios of breast cancer were found to be higher than that of the cervix, whereas among the rest of the population cervical cancer was by far the most frequent. The incidence among Parsis was greater than among the Sindhis, which was in turn greater than the rate in the general population. This difference in frequency ratios arises from the different origins of the peoples affected. The Parsis are the sole survivors of the ancient Persians, followers of Zarathustra, who fled their homeland to escape religious persecution during successive waves of invasion by Moslems. The community is highly inbred and the rate of incidence of breast cancer is 1.7 times higher than in other Greater Bombay women, although lower than among the Norwegian and English. The Sindhis migrated to India after partition of their country and settled down in different parts, the majority of them choosing to stay in areas around Greater Bombay.

It is concluded that a large percentage of all breast cancers grow very fast and metastasis is more likely than in the slow growing and not as common breast cancers as indicated by mammography (212).

The main risk factors of breast cancer are: (a) sex with 99% in the female, (b) age with 85% over the age of 40, (c) family history of breast cancer, (d) previous benign breast disease, (e) precancerous mastopathy, (f) previous cancer in one breast, and (g) adverse hormonal milieu as related to parity. Additional factors playing a role are given by the hormonal milieu reduction of immunologic competence, the exposure to

carcinogens, adverse personal factors, risk patterns of the parenchyma on breast x-rays, and abnormal thermograms (Fig. 36.12) (136).

Breast cancer in Czechoslovakia is the second most frequent tumor in women, exhibiting a continued increase from 2,348 new registered cases in 1965 to 3,477 new cases in 1975 (222).

Breast cancer in women is more common in overweight individuals. The blood level of estradiol in the postmenopausal women would be below 25 pg/ml of the plasma (78).

The average weight in body surface area is larger in women with breast cancer than in controls as investigated in Tokyo. The risk factors have been similar as in the United States (136). The risk is, for example, high in women who were never married, who had no children, or who had a first child very late with late menopause. They were tall and heavy, too overweight, with a large body surface and with relatives afflicted by the same disease. Hypersensitive women have a low risk (223).

Hormonal and other factors delaying marriage and the birth of children seem to have an influence on the development of breast cancer as indicated by studies of cancer patients and their sisters (265); see Chapter 37.

Similar findings were observed in São Paulo, Brazil, regarding gynecological and breast cancers (190).

Obese patients with too high body weight have a higher risk for the recurrence of mammary cancer after mastectomy (65).

Indian women undergoing mastectomy after preoperative counseling accepted the situation

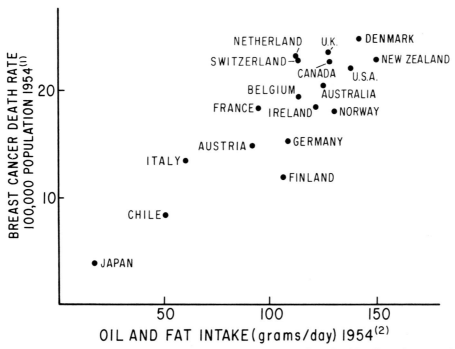

Figure 36.12.   Rate of death from breast cancer, correlated with oil and fat intake.

psychologically with more ease (55). See also Ref. 15. The relationship of breast cancer and religion in greater Bombay area was investigated by Jussawalla and Jain (120).

Breast cancer in British Columbia exhibited a continued increase from 55 to 120/100,000 and more during the past 20 years. The increase concerns women from the fourth to sixth decades. The incidence was highest in British Columbia and lowest in New Foundland. The mortality rate remains stable in British Columbia, Canada, Japan, Chile, Australia and the United States (Caucasians), but increased in England, Denmark, Scotland, Belgium, Netherlands, Sweden, West Germany and the United States (non-Caucasians). Epidemiologically the disease is related to age, sex, geographic distribution, and diet (estrogen), especially milk (Figs. 36.13 and 36.17) (54).

Uterine cervix

In all countries with mortality statistics, carcinoma of the uterus appears as one of the three commonest causes of death from cancer in women, the other two being in most countries carcinomas of the stomach and breast (249). Cervical carcinoma is twice as common in American Negroes as in whites, but is rare among Jews (184).

In India the estimated crude average annual

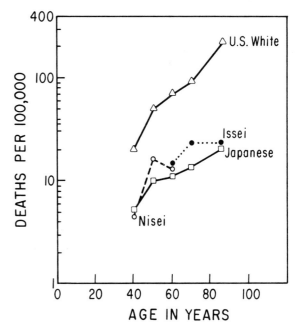

Figure 36.13.   Age-specific death rates for breast cancer in women in Issei, Nisei, and the United States white population. (Source: Haenszel and Kurihara (88).)

prevalence rate for the Agra put them among the populations of highest risk for uterine cancer in the world. Early marriage and multiple pregnancies are significant factors, together with a higher prevalence of cervical cancer than among Hindu females.

In Thailand and Vietnam the disease ranks

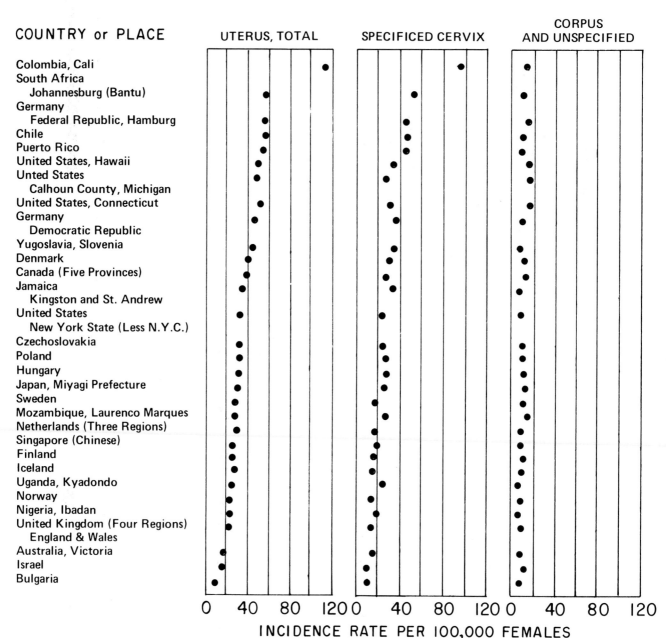

Figure 36.14. Age-standardized incidence rate of uterus cancer from registries in various countries. (Source: Doll *et al.* (64), Seidman *et al.*, and WHO Epidemiological Statistic Reports (248).)

first, whereas in Singapore, Japan, Norway, and the United States it occurs at lower rates.

In Malaysia the incidence of carcinoma of the cervix is twice as high among the Chinese as the Malays and Indians.

Cervical carcinoma is the most common cancer in Chinese women. The highest relative frequencies were reported from Tientsin in North China, accounting for 72.6% of carcinomas in women. It is also frequent in other northern regions: Sian 69.9%, and Tsinen 56% (110). In Hong Kong it accounts for 34.9% of carcinomas affecting women. The figure is similar to the

incidence in Southern China: Canton 35.3%, Fukien 37.2%, and Kwangsi 31.4%.

A report from Taiwan also revealed 58.2% (260), but in Singapore a rate of only 11.2% is encountered among Chinese females. In Malaysia it accounted for only 24.4% of carcinomas in Chinese women (149). The peak relative frequency in China is in the 40–44-year age group, while in Hong Kong it is in the 55–59-year group (Table 36.12 and Fig. 36.16).

The ratio of cervical to endometrial carcinoma in Chinese is high. This is due to the high proportion of young women and the high parity among the Chinese. In Nanking there were as many as 47 cervical carcinomas for each endometrial carcinoma (138). Reports from the Chinese Academy of Medical Science in Peking and from Taiwan put the ratio at 22.3 to 1 and 18.9 to 1, respectively. In overseas Chinese Marsden found 6.4 to 1 in Malaysia, in Thailand 18.3 to 1 and in Hong Kong 10.2 to 1.

Cancer of the uterine cervix was also high both in American and African Negro women, but intermediate in white women. The high risk of cancer among African women is in contrast to the general cancer pattern; among Negro females the age standardized rates were highest in Bantu-speaking South Africans. Concerning a screening program of cervical cancer in Manitoba, see Ref. 30.

Uterine Corpus

There is a strong suggestion that endometrial carcinoma (Fig. 36.14) has a life history resembling that of cervical carcinoma. Retrospective studies on the development of carcinomas following endometrial hyperplasia indicate a progressive series of glandular atypicalities that precede by many years the development of overt malignancy (50, 184).

Carcinoma of the corpus has a high rate of occurrence among the Jews. The ratio between carcinoma of the cervix and corpus is 4:1 in Singapore, 15:1 in India, 1:5 in England, 2:1 in Norway, and 1:1.5 in the United States. Among the Chinese in Malaysia it is 1:1.2, and in India

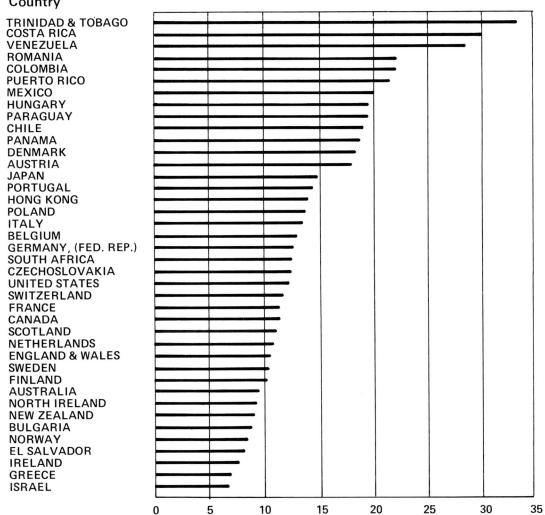

Figure 36.15. Age-standardized death rate from cancer of the uterus for various countries. (Source: Segi and Kurihara (201) and WHO Statistics Annual (246).)

POPULATION GROUP

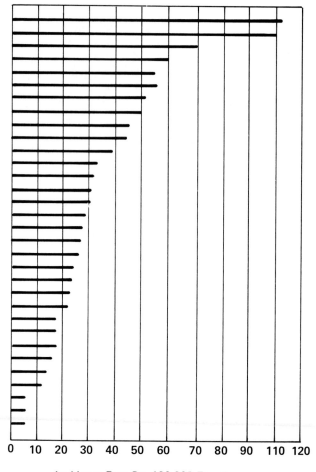

Figure 36.16. Age-standardized incidence rate of cancer of cervix for various groups. (Source: Dunham and Bailar (69).)

3:1. In Thailand the rate is markedly different from the other countries at 16.1 (Fig. 36.15).

Generally cervical cancer in Kazakhstan is second to gastric cancer but also the most common cancer in some areas. There is no difference concerning urban and rural areas and women in the age from 50 to 59 exhibit the highest risk. From 1960 to 1964 the incidence increased in rural areas, whereas in urban areas a decrease occurred. After 1965, incidence and mortality decreased especially in women under 60 (168).

Ovary

The rate and magnitude of increase of malignant ovarian tumors is stated to be almost identical in Caucasians and non-Caucasians until about the age of menopause, when the non-Caucasian rate levels off and begins to decline at around age 60-65. The rate in Caucasians, how-

ever, continues to rise sharply for another decade (243).

A study of ovarian carcinomas from New South Wales, Australia, in the years 1960–1970 and 1970–1977 revealed in age incidence of 55.2 years from 1960–1970 and 54.55 years from 1970–1977. It is the eighth and most lethal of the cancers in women; bilateral occurrence is 10%. The most frequent tumors are the serous ones followed by endometrioid, mucinous, undifferentiated, mesonephroid, germ cell, granulosa, unclassified, mixed mesodermal, unclassified epithelial, and mixed epithelial (153).

The incidence of ovarian cancer is low in Japan, though recently increasing, but it is high in the Scandinavian countries, notably in Denmark. This malignancy accounted for 6.7% of the Caucasian and 5% of the non-Caucasian reported cancer deaths among American women in 1965. Age-adjusted death rates from all parts of the world ranged from 1.69 in Japan to 11.02 in Denmark (254). Malignancies of the ovaries are less common in Japan than in the United States, this racial difference also applying to the Japanese population in the United States, including Hawaii (243).

Cancer of the ovary seems to be considerably more prevalent in South Korea, Thailand, and Malaysia, while the incidence among the Chinese in those countries is higher than among the natives and the Indians. In Korea ovarian tumors rank fifth in the series (Table 36.13).

Trophoblastic Disease

This disease is relatively frequent in the Chinese (249) and the frequency is generally stated to be high in all parts of Asia (21, 111, 228); for Ibadan, see Ref. 114.

The incidence of trophoblastic disease in Asia, Africa, and South America is higher than in the United States and Europe. The average number of pregnancies was consistently higher in Asian than in U.S. and European women, as indicated

by the population samples investigated (97) and there were considerably more pregnancies in the older Asian age groups. The average age of the Asian patients was found to be higher, and in the current series the estimated highest liability choriocarcinoma was found in individuals within the 40–49 age bracket.

Of 750 cases of trophoblastic diseases documented in Singapore in 16 years the majority was benign, but 106 cases were malignant. The latter ones were histologically diagnosed as villous or avillous, a third category (persistence of HCG activity after evacuating or secondaries with no histology) were classified as clinical choriocarcinoma. The histologic classification was related to prognosis (28).

Geographic and ethnic factors are not thought to be related to the cause of trophoblastic tumors. The reason for the high incidence of trophoblastic disease in Asia, Africa, and South America has not been clearly elucidated, but interest is concentrated on the low socioeco-

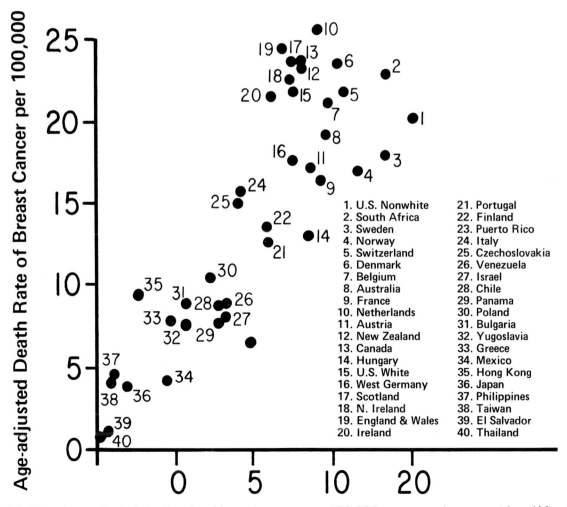

Figure 36.17. Age-adjusted death rate of breast cancer per 100,000 among various countries. (After Wynder et al.: *Cancer Detection and Prevention*, Vol. II, © Excerpta Medica, 1974.)

Table 36.12
Age-standardized Cervical Cancer Death Rate and also Supplementary Ratios of Cervical Cancer, Shown as Percentage of Total Cancer Deaths for Various Population Groups

Death Rates per 100,000 Females		Percentage Cervix of Total Cancer Deaths	
Population group	Rate	Population group	%
Cali, Colombia	64.2	Taiwan	62.3
Lima, Peru	59.8	Recife, Northeast Brazil	49.8
Mexico City, Mexico	42.3	Surinam	47.6
Guatemala City, Guatemala	37.8	South Vietnam	47.2
Santiago, Chile	31.3	Shanghai, China	46.2
Caracas, Venezuela	29.9	Morocco	45.0
Bogota, Colombia	29.4	Korea	44.2
		South Africa, Bantu	42.2
USA, North Central, nonwhite	22.1	Paraiba, Northeast Brazil	40.6
USA, South, nonwhite	20.5	Ceylon	37.7
São Paulo, Brazil	20.0	Madagascar	35.5
Ribeirao Preto, Brazil	18.0	Fiji, E. Indian	31.6
USA, Northeast, nonwhite	17.2	Assam, India	31.3
USA, West, nonwhite	15.8	Jamaica	30.9
Denmark	15.2	Tunisia	28.7
Portugal	12.1	Ghana	28.6
La Plata, Argentina	11.7	North Vietnam	28.5
Puerto Rico	11.0	Cuba	27.3
		Kyadondo, Uganda	27.1
Austria	10.5	Bulawayo, Rhodesia	26.9
Switzerland	9.8	Iran	26.3
Scotland	9.1	Paraguay	26.0
USA, South, white	9.0	Kenya	23.4
Canada	8.9	Mozambique	23.4
Romania	8.8	Thailand	22.2
Belgium	8.4	Yugoslavia	22.2
Italy	8.4	Fiji, Fijian	21.3
England and Wales	7.9	Bombay, India	21.1
Sweden	7.9		
USA, North Central, white	7.9	Hungary	19.9
New Zealand	7.7	Philippines	19.9
USA, West, white	7.7	Lebanon	19.8
Germany (West)	7.4	Congo (Kinshasa)	19.7
Netherlands	7.3	Katana area, Congo (Kinshasa)	19.5
Finland	7.1	Nigeria	18.5
Norway	6.8	Costa Rica	18.0
USA, Northeast, white	6.7	Czechoslovakia	16.5
France	6.6	Ex-French Equatorial Africa states	15.9
Northern Ireland	6.6	UAR (Egypt)	14.3
Australia	5.3	Papua and New Guinea	14.1
Ireland	4.0	Turkey	13.5
Poland	3.6	Ex-French West Africa states	13.2
Israel	3.3		
		Hawaii, Hawaiian	10.7
		Antigua	9.1
		Hawaii, Japanese	8.3
		Hawaii, Caucasian	5.7

[a] Source: L. Dunham and J. C. Bailar (69).

nomic status and the high number of multiparous women, especially among the old (218). The peak of incidence coinciding with winter and the dry season in Thailand suggests the possibility of viral infection as a cause of the disease (21).

The joint project for study of choriocarcinoma and hydatidiform mole in Asia revealed by clinical observations showed that tumors in Asian women and those from the United States be-

haved similarly, but incidence of trophoblastic tumors in Asian women is higher than among women in the United States. The average age of the Asian patients was found to be older than the age of women from the United States in each diagnostic group.

Geographic and ethnic factors are not usually thought to be related to the cause of trophoblastic tumors, socioeconomic status usually being selected as the one cultural factor. Frequency of pregnancy in older age groups has been the important associated finding in preliminary studies. However, the total number of pregnancies may not account for all of the cases of trophoblastic tumors appearing in Asian women.

The geographic location therefore may in fact have an influence on trophoblastic disease. Differences in race, culture and climate are as great as the more obvious differences between populations of Asian countries and the United States. The socioeconomic status of the people in the United States and in Europe is much higher than in Asia and Africa. Within Asia, hydatidiform mole occurs very rarely among the people in affluent districts (21). Evidence of trophoblastic disease among the Irish, Italian, Negro, and Puerto Rican groups in the United States did not occur in as remarkable a frequency as the Far East, even in the lowest socioeconomic groups.

Evidence of a greater frequency of hydatidiform mole in the broad geographic area is consistent with the possibility that one significant factor in the production of a mole may be a gene of nonselective value. An outstanding example of such a nonselective gene would be the familiar gene for blood group B. This gene for B is of worldwide distribution, being especially common in East Central Asia. A gene of similar nonselective character and analogous world distribution might be a significant factor in the

Table 36.13

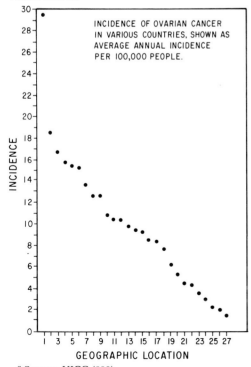

INCIDENCE OF OVARIAN CANCER IN VARIOUS COUNTRIES, SHOWN AS AVERAGE ANNUAL INCIDENCE PER 100,000 PEOPLE.

a Source: UICC (230).

production of moles, and this could be one way to explain the interesting fact of the geographic pathology of trophoblastic disease. For vulva cancer see Refs. 20 and 84.

MALE GENITAL ORGANS

Penis

In China, 18.3% of all cancers in men arise in the penis while the figure is less than 2% in the United States. The disease is also common in Korea. Squamous cell carcinoma of the penis is the only common tumor in the male genital organ but has shown a decreasing trend in recent years. The figure, however, is 3–4 times more frequent in Negroes than in Whites (178).

In Malaysia the disease is 5½ times more common among the Chinese and Indians than among the native circumcised Malays, and the ethnic factor concerning different customs is clearly an influence of pathogenesis of the disease.

Prostate

A viral etiology of prostate cancer has not been proven up to date (174).

Willis (249) found that prostatic carcinoma has only occasionally been recorded in the Chinese and is of little significance, as the peak of the age distribution curve for this disease is toward the end of the seventh decade. The observed number of cases is also low in China, Korea, Hong Kong, Singapore, India, and among the Chinese in Hawaii. It seems difficult to exclude at least some racial and ethnic differences. In 1960–1961, 13.6% of all deaths from malignant neoplasms in the United States among nonwhites and in Norwegian males were caused by prostatic carcinoma (201). The corresponding sex-specific level in the United States white population was 9.17%, in England and Wales 6.9%, but in Japan only 0.9%.

Prostate cancer in the United States shows the highest morbidity among black males and is similar to lung cancer in white males. There is a greater risk in patients who experienced a late development of secondary sexual characteristics as well as other factors such as exposure to fertilizers and auto exhaust fumes (188). See also Ref. 112.

Table 36.14
Distribution of Gestational Trophoblastic Disease in Various Parts of the World

Geographic Region	Reference	Incidence of Hydatidiform Mole (Rate per Pregnancy
America, South	Fernandes and Marques (76)	
Brazil		1:1071
Argentina		1:829
Australia	Coppelson (41)	1:320
Benelux	De Snoc (54)	1:1200
Hong Kong	Chun et al. (31)	1:242
India	Rao	1:361
Japan	Hasegawa (94)	1:232
Malaysia	Llewellyn-Jones (139)	1:600
Mexico	Marquez-Monter (148)	1:200
Philippines	Acosta Sison (3)	1:126
Scandinavia	Kolstad and Hognestadt (126)	1:300
Singapore	Lean	1:703
Taiwan	Wei and Ouyang (241)	1:125
Thailand	Boonyanit (20, 21)	1:383
UK	Jeffcoate (113)	1:1500
USA	Chesley (27)	1:1321
	Novak and Seah (167)	1:2000

The low incidence of prostatic carcinoma among the Japanese was studied by Strahan (219). Examination at autopsy of 12,227 prostatic glands from Japanese men uncovered carcinoma of the prostate gland in only 15 cases, or in 0.125% of those examined (165, 184). In Korea from 1,714 cases of malignant neoplasm only 3 cases of carcinoma of the prostate were diagnosed, i.e., on overall incidence of 0.175% of all gene-specific malignancies. The corresponding incidence was 0.508% in this large Korea autopsy.

Testis

The highest rates of testicular malignancies have been reported from Denmark, Norway, New Zealand, Canada, Sweden, and Connecticut in the United States; cancer of the testis is thus particularly prevalent in Scandinavian countries, with the exception of Finland (34). During the years 1943–1962 morbidity from carcinoma of the testis for the age groups between 20 and 55 years increased in Danish urban areas to the extent of a doubling of rates for the capital, resulting in higher rates than elsewhere. There is also an excess in Norway for urban areas over rural districts. There was no evidence or any association of the increase in morbidity with the smoking of tobacco or the use roentgen rays (34). Incidence of carcinoma of the testis is very low among the Chinese, Koreans, and Japanese.

OTHER COMMON PRIMARY SITES

Urinary Organs

Cancers of these primary sites are common among the people in Northern Africa, Egypt, and Sudan, but are uncommon among the Japanese, Chinese or Norwegian.

In Korea malignant neoplasms of the kidney were approximately as common in men as in women. Those of the bladder and other urinary organs revealed a decidedly higher frequency in males (corrected male to female ratio 5.7%) the highest being Mozambique, the United States (Connecticut), Canada, and among the Caucasians in Hawaii.

Thyroid Gland

There is no proof that thyroid carcinoma is more common in one geographic region than in another (7), but Willis (249) states that the frequency of cancer of the thyroid differs according to the prevalence of goiter. There seem to be exceptions to this general statement, at least within some Scandinavian regions. A comparatively large amount of autopsy and biopsy material seen by Willis and obtained from inland districts of South-east Sweden showed a high frequency of goiter, but a surprisingly low incidence of thyroid carcinoma. On the other hand, it is also through the review of 62,000 biopsies obtained mainly from coastal districts of western Norway that these regions reveal an overall low prevalence of goiter, but comparatively many cases of thyroid malignancy.

Investigations in Taj Cancer Institute at Teheran University showed a sex difference of thyroid cancer insofar as 39% of men with thyroid disease had cancer but only 18.7% of the females. The overall incidence was 23.4%. This is considered to be the highest percentage of thyroid cancer published in the literature up to date (96).

In the United States there is no difference in incidence between the white and colored races, the incidence of thyroid cancer being the same as in Japan i.e., 0.5%. In England and Wales, and in Australia (excluding full-blood aboriginals) the rate is 0.6%, while the figure reaches 1% among Norwegian females.

Cancer of the thyroid gland in females was the only malignancy showing an estimated bimodal incidence curve in adult age groups, with a transient decrease approximately corresponding to the age at the onset of menopause. Malignant tumors of the thyroid gland predominate in patients 40–70 years of age, but are also found in young people, usually 10 years of age or older (1). The median age observed among the females was 35.0 years, with 63.3% below the age of 40 years. Hawaiian ethnic and Caucasians had among the highest incidences, the same as occurred among people of Colombia, South America.

Skin

Malignant neoplasms of the skin, excluding malignant melanoma were quite common among Koreans.

In a study covering the years 1968–1972 7,585 biopsies in Lybia resulted in 186 malignancies of the skin, this is 2.45% of the total biopsies. Of all malignant neoplasms of the skin 54.30% were basal cell cancer, 24.19% squamous cell cancer followed by undifferentiated cancer, malignant melanoma, and sweat gland cancer. There were more malignant melanomas in males; sweat gland carcinoma and lymphoma were more common in females. Kaposis' sarcoma was diagnosed only in women. There was a continued increase of basal cell and squamous cell carcinomas in each sex. The highest incidence occurred in individuals between 60 and 64 years of age. A topographic difference existed concerning the location of the mentioned tumor types in relation to their frequency. Most basal cell car-

cinomas were found at the head and neck, squamous cell cancers at the head, neck and limbs, and malignant melanomas were most frequent at lower limbs (239). Malignant melanoma, although found in all races was rare among Negroes (184).

Malignant melanoma most often occurring in white Caucasians has a lower frequency in blacks where it mainly appears on the sole of the feet. Pigmentation seems to be important for prevention and repeated injury on the surface of the feet seems to explain the increased frequency in this region. The most common location in Argentina are face, lower limb, and back; in Brazil trunk and lower limb; in Mexico the feet followed by face and lower limb and back; this topographical preference is similar in Venezuela. The most often affected region in Peru are the toes. In Paraguay and South Africa the sole of the feet is the most frequent site affecting the South African blacks and the Paraguayan Brunettes (186). It is an uncommon tumor in Japan and also appears to be uncommon in South Korea. The current series included remarkably few cases of malignant melanoma: only 10 were diagnosed in males and 3 in females. Malignant melanoma in Germany is of higher incidence than other malignant neoplasms of the skin in England.

Spanish speaking Americans of the southwestern United States have particular food habits which may result in differences if compared to other groups. Spanish men have a higher risk for malignancies of esophagus, stomach, rectum, liver, gallbladder, prostate, kidney, and thyroid if compared to other Caucasians. Black males have a higher risk for cancer of esophagus, lung, and prostate. The risk for lung cancer and skin melanomas was lower than in other Caucasians. Spanish females exhibited a high risk for cancers of stomach, rectum, gallbladder, pancreas, lung, cervix, ovary, kidney, thyroid, and for leukemias. They had a low risk for cancers of the buccal cavity esophagus and melanomas of the skin (75, 197) and for the epidemiology of melanomas in Mexico (229).

Malignant Lymphomas

Lymphosarcoma and reticulosarcoma constituted together the second most commonly observed type of malignant disease within the current series in Korean males, and ranked as number six in encountered frequency among females. The study of 190 autopsy and biopsy cases of malignant lymphomas in Koreans during the period from 1955 to 1964 revealed that the incidence of these types of malignant tumors ranked as the second in frequency in males and as the sixth in females. The highest incidences of the disease are found in Canada, New Zealand, and among the Caucasians in Hawaii, respectively.

Less than 1 per 100,000 people in India suffer from Hodgkin's disease. This is one-fourth of the number seen in the United States. The disease increases in children; it is the second common type of lymphoma in India. The most frequent variation is this one of mixed cellularity with 54% followed by lymphocytic predominance (20%), lymphocytic depletion 15% and nodular sclerosis 11%.

The correlation of beef and milk consumption with the incidence of leukemias and lymphomas in Norway, Sweden, Finland, Denmark, German Democratic Republic, Malta, Israel, Singapore, Cuba, and New Zealand in the period from 1968 to 1972 showed a high correlation with milk consumption and lymphatic leukemia and multiple myeloma.

Nervous System

The ethnic distribution of primary central nervous system tumors in the United States from 1958 to 1970 was reviewed (73). Primary neoplasms of the nervous system in 61 population groups worldwide showed a higher mortality rate in males than females. A small peak appeared in childhood and a taller one between 60 and 80 years of age (195). The same authors had indicated some discrepancies concerning the reported incidence of primary neoplasms of the nervous system in 1976 (195) and concerning brain tumors in 1978 (194). Heshmat et al. (98) reported about the incidence and population selectivity in the Washington, D.C., metropolitan area of the neoplasms of the central nervous system in 1976 stating that: 990 primary neoplasms of the central nervous system in Washington, D.C., metropolitan area exhibited obviously important racial differences. The incidence rates for Caucasians were 5.5 in males and 3.6 in females and for blacks 4.8 in males and 3.6 in females per 100,000 annual population. Caucasians had a higher proportion of gliomas, the blacks in Washington and of a comparative group of West African blacks. Blacks had a

higher occurrence of meningiomas and pituitary adenomas (98).

A comparison intracranial neoplasms in children of North America, Europe, Africa and Asia (59) in 1976 showed that astrocytomas were the most frequently observed neoplasms in all series with the exception of the Japanese. Pinealomas were 3 times as frequent in Japan and Africa as elsewhere. Craniopharyngiomas were twice as high in Japan and Africa than in other areas; whereas medulloblastomas in contrast were relatively rare. Ependymomas were twice as frequent in India than in the other series.

Glioblastoma multiforme in a series of 488 children with CNS neoplasms described at Yale University in 1976 (60) showed 43 (8.8%) with glioblastomas (22 in the cerebral hemispheres, 16 in the brainstem, 2 in the cerebellum, and 3 in the spinal cord). The sexual ratio male to female was 3:2. The most frequent site in the cerebral hemispheres was the frontal lobe, the main age 12.7 years. Glioblastomas of the brain stem had as most frequent site the pons, and as the most common age 6.7 years.

CHILDHOOD NEOPLASMS

For the incidence and mortality of childhood cancer in Sweden from 1958 to 1974, see Ericsson et al. (72), and concerning malignant neoplasms in African infants, Owor (170).

BCG vaccination and cancer mortality rate for leukemia and other neoplastic diseases from 1957 to 1969 in 85,356 vaccinated newborns, and 534,870 nonvaccinated blacks had the following results: 13 deaths under 20 years of age occurred in the vaccinated group and 306 among the nonvaccinated. The statistics showed a reduction of 74% in the vaccinated group. The types of neoplasms for this age group were leukemia, central nervous system neoplasms, lymphoma and bone and connective tissue neoplasms (45).

Another series from 1975 from India (173), dealing with malignant neoplasms in children showed the highest frequency of embryonal tumors, confirmed that the malignant epithelial tumors are uncommon in infancy and childhood, and that the majority is formed by the neoplasms occurring in head and neck. (See also Chapter 13.)

See for comparison Ref. 263 regarding autoantibodies.

CANCER EPIDEMIOLOGY OF ATOMIC BOMB SURVIVORS (123)

The late effects of atomic bomb (A bomb) radiation on 109,000 persons exhibited a decrease of the risk of leukemia after the peak years from 1950 to 1954, but is still higher than in control groups. There were age differences. From 1960 to 1965, persons exposed to 100 rads or more after a latent period of 15–20 years showed an increased risk. A definite relation period of 15–20 years. A definite relation occurred to cancers of thyroid, lung and breast, and a possible to salivary glands and stomach cancers.

CONCLUSIONS

Survival rate of 5 years of all cancers increased only by 2%. For the past 100 years man has searched in an enforced and continued endeavor to find just what are the exact causes of cancer in humans and animals. Even today many factors and causes both direct and indirect are being investigated in humans and animals alike. Experiments *in vivo* and *in vitro*, including the study of oncogenic mechanism, heredity, racial and environmental influences are being carried out throughout the world.

We cannot pinpoint the exact causes of oncogenesis, but we do believe the influence of race and environment to be salient among the many factors undoubtedly involved. This belief is based on the observation of numerous cancer cases which have been seen to differ between races with habits and environments varying according to geographic location, custom, traditions, nutrition, socioeconomic status, and physical environment.

We live in a world made constantly smaller by advances in communications, a world in which there is a continuous movement of people from one country to another, sometimes in huge numbers. These people are resettling in new environments where they are subjected to new influence of foods, climate, and custom. We hope that in the future these immigrants will provide a good source of information for comparative study with the sedentes.

The influence of race and environment on oncogenesis is likely to remain of unique importance for a long time to come.

In general, the numerous race-linked differences in the incidence of cancer tend, on critical analysis, to indicate environmental rather than hereditary factors in their etiology. Geographical differences also tend to prove to be environmental rather than racial in origin. Hereditary differences tend to be explicable by cultural rather than genetic factors. Genetic factors require to be considered in a completely separate analysis and interpretation, except in the case of a few well-known neoplasms. These genetic factors, however, should not be ignored because they may be important in determining whether environmental factors are at sub- or superthreshold oncogenic levels.

It appears that the frequency of some tumors changes in the migrating generation, but for other types of tumor there may be persistent etiological factors in migrants.

In conclusion, it is considered that the value of study into the etiology of cancers within widely differing environments, such as has been witnessed and recorded in populations both before and after migration, lies in its enabling us to discriminate between hereditary cancer, environmental cancer, and cancers of other possible sources.

References

1. Ackerman, L. V., and Del Regato, J. A. (1954): *Cancer Diagnosis, Treatment and Prognosis,* Ed. 2. C. V. Mosby, St. Louis.
2. Ackerman, L., and Del Regato, J. A. (1962): *Cancer, Diagnosis, Treatment and Prognosis,* Ed. 3. C. V. Mosby, St. Louis.
3. Acosta Sisson, H. (1963): Studies in choriocarcinoma from 88 patients admitted to the Philippine General Hospital from 1950–51. *Philippine J. Cancer,* 4:197–203, or *Cancer,* 20:144, 1967.
4. Adelusi, B., Smith, J. A., and Junaid, T. A. (1978): Histopathological studies of carcinoma of cervix uteri in Ibadan. *Afr. J. Med. Sci.,* 7:9–16.
5. Aird, I., and Bentall, H. H. (1953): A relationship between cancer of stomach and the ABO blood groups. *Br. Med. J.,* 1:799–801.
6. Alameda County Cancer Registry (1967): Incidence of cancer in Alameda County, California, 1960–64. State of California Department of Public Health, Berkeley.
7. Anderson, W. A. D. (1966): Thyroid gland, in *Pathology,* Ed. 5, Vol. 2, pp. 1094–1101. C. V. Mosby, St. Louis.
8. Appelman, H. D., and Helwig, E. B. (1977): Sarcomas of the stomach. *Am. J. Clin. Pathol.,* 67:2–10.
9. Aramesh, B. (1978): Prevalent cancer cases during 9 years registration (1968–1977) in Caspian littoral of Iran, p. 78. XIIth International Cancer Congress, Buenos Aires, Workshop 6:18.
10. Armstrong, B., Garrod, A., and Doll, R. (1976): A retrospective study of renal cancer with special reference to coffee and animal protein consumption. *Br. J. Cancer,* 33:127–36.
11. Aromaa, A., Hakama, M., Hakulinen, T., Saxen, E., Teppo, L., Ida, A., and Lan-Heikkil, A. J. (1976): Breast cancer and use of rauwolfia and other antihypertensive agents in hypertensive patients; a nationwide case-control study in Finland. *Int. J. Cancer,* 18:727–38.
12. Baker, L. W. (1978): Carcinoma of the oesophagus; experience in a high-incidence area, pp. 216–217. XIIth International Cancer Congress, Buenos Aires, Workshop 39:2
13. Basa, G. F., Hirayama, T., and Cruz-Basa, A. G. (1977): Cancer epidemiology in the Philippines. *Natl. Cancer Inst. Monogr.,* 47:45–56.
14. Belamarie, J. (1969): Malignant tumours in Chinese. *Int. J. Cancer,* 4:560–573.
15. Bender, H. C., and Faber, P. (1978): Organization and efficiency of follow-up-care for gynaecological cancer-patients, p. 84. XIIth International Cancer Congress, Buenos Aires, Workshop 7:6.
16. Ben-Hur, M., Costin, C., and Steinitz, R. (1978): Clusters of cancer in families, a pilot study from a population-based cancer registry; prob-

lems of methodology, p. 159. XIIth International Cancer Congress, Buenos Aires, Workshop 34:10.

17. Biagini, R., Rivero, M., Salvador, M., and Cordoba, S. (1978): Hidroarsenicismo cronico y cancer de pulmon, p. 82. XIIth International Cancer Congress, Buenos Aires, Workshop 7:2.

18. Billington, B. P. (1956): Gastric cancer relationships between ABO bloodgroups, site and epidemiology. *Lancet,* 2:859–862.

19. Blokhin, N. N. (1978): Epidemiology of stomach cancer in USSR, p. 132. XIIth International Cancer Congress, Buenos Aires, Abstract, panel 12.

20. Boonyanit, S., and Kaiser, H. E. (1977): Malignant neoplasms of the vulva. *Anat. Rec.,* 187:538–539.

21. Boonyanit, S., and Kaiser, H. E. (1977): Geographic variation in the occurrence of cancer in Thailand compared with other countries. *Cancer Res.,* AACR Abstract, 726.

22. Bradshaw, F., and Harington, J. S. (1975): The changing pattern of cancer mortality in South Africa, 1949–1969, *S. Afr. Med. J.,* 49:919–925.

23. Buckwalter, J. A., et al. (1957): The association of the ABO blood groups to gastric carcinoma. *Surg. Gynecol. Obstet.,* 104:176–179.

24. Burkitt, D. P. (1969): A study of cancer patterns in Africa. *Sci. Basis Med.,* 82–94.

25. Burkitt, D. P., and Kafuko, G. W. (1970): Burkitt's lymphoma and malaria. *Int. J. Cancer,* 6:1–9.

26. Chabalko, J. J., Creagan, E. T., and Fraumeni, J. F., Jr. (1974): Epidemiology of selected sarcomas in children, *J.N.C.I.,* 53:675–679.

27. Chesley, L. S., et al. (1946): Hydatidiform mole, with special reference to recurrence and associated eclampsia. *Am. J. Obstet. Gynecol.,* 52:311–320.

28. Chew, S. C., and Ratnam, S. S. (1976): Treatment of choriocarcinoma in Singapore. *Int. J. Gynaec. Obstet. (Sweden),* 14:173–176.

29. Chiazze, L. Jr., Silverman, D. T., and Levin, D. L. (1976): The cancer mortality scare. Problems of estimation using monthly data, *J.A.M.A.,* 236:2310–2312.

30. Choi, N. W., and Nelson, N. A. (1978): Some epidemiologic aspects of cervical cancer and cytology screening program in Manitoba, Canada, pp. 83–84. XIIth International Cancer Congress, Buenos Aires, Workshop 7:4.

31. Chun, D., et al. (1967): Choriocarcinoma in Hong Kong, in *Proceedings of the 5th World Congress of Gynaecology & Obstetrics,* pp. 398–465, edited by C. Wood and W. A. W. Walters. Butterworth, London.

32. Clemmesen, J., and Nielsen, A. (1951): The racial distribution of cancer in Copenhagen 1943–47. *Br. J. Cancer,* 5:159–71.

33. Clemmesen, J. (1965): *Statistical Studies in the Aetiology of Malignant Neoplasms.* Munksgaard, Kobenhavn.

34. Clemmesen, J. (1969): Statistical studies in the aetiology of malignant neoplasms; III. Testis cancer, Denmark 1958–62. *Acta Pathol. Scand. Supp. 209.*

35. Clemmesen, J. (1976): [Letter: Survival in breast neoplasm patients in Denmark, 1960–1966.] *UGESKR Laeger,* 138:1527–1528.

36. Clemmesen, J. (1976): Danish cancer occurrence 1968–72. *UGESKR Laeger,* 138:2991–2996.

37. Clemmesen, J. (1977): Statistical studies in the aetiology of malignant neoplasms; V. Trends and risks, Denmark 1943–72. *Acta Pathol. Microbiol. Scand. [Suppl.]* 261:1–286.

38. Clifford, P. C. (1970): The epidemiology of NPC. *Int. J. Cancer,* 5:287–309.

39. Cole, J. W., and McKalen, (1963): Studies on the morphogenesis of adenomatous polyps in the human colon. *Cancer,* 16:998–1002.

40. Cook, P. (1971): Cancer of the oesophagus in Africa; a summary and evaluation of the evidence for the frequency of occurrency and a preliminary indication of the possible association with the consumpton of alcoholic drinks made from maize. *Br. J. Cancer,* 25:853–880.

41. Coppleson, M. (1958): Hydatidiform mole and its complications. *J. Obstet. Gynaecol. Br. Emp.,* 65:238–252.

42. Correa, P., Cuello, C., Duque, E., Burbano, L. C., Garcia, F. T., Bolanos, O., Brown, C., and Haenszel, W. (1976): Gastric cancer in Colombia; III. Natural history of precursor lesions. *J.N.C.I.,* 57:1027–1035.

43. Corwitz, K., and Dennis, R. (1976): On the decrease in the life expectancy of black males in Michigan. *Public Health Rep.,* 91:141–145.

44. Cox, P. J., Farmer, P. B., Foster, A. B., Gilby, E. D., and Jarman, M. (1976): The use of deuterated analogs in qualitative and quantitative investigations of the metabolism of cyclophosphamide (NSC-26271). *Cancer Treat. Rep.,* 60:483–491.

45. Crispen, R. G., and Rosethal, S. R. (1976): BCG vaccination and cancer mortality (Ger.). *Cancer Immunol. Immunother.,* 1:139–142.

46. Crowther, J. S., Drasar, B. S., Hill, M. J., Maclennan, R., Magning, D., Peach, S., and Teoh-Chan, C. H. (1976): Faecal steroids and bacteria and large bowel cancer in Hong Kong by socio-economic groups. *Br. J. Cancer,* 34:191–198.

47. Cuchiara, A. J., and Asal, N. R. (1976): Laryngeal neoplasm mortality in Oklahoma: 1950–1970. *South Med. J.,* 69:908–910.

48. Cuello, C., Correa, P., Haenszel, W., Gordillo, G., Brown, C., Archer, M., and Tannenbaum, S. (1976): Gastric cancer in Colombia; I. Cancer risk and suspect environmental agents. *J.N.C.I.,* 57:1015–1020.

49. Curnen, M. G., McCrea, M. B., Skovron, M., Turgeon, L., and Shrout, P. (1978): Cancer risk in physicians and lawyers, p. 87. XIIth International Cancer Congress, Buenos Aires, Workshop 7:11.

50. Currie, G. A. (1970): The conceptus as an allograft: immunological reactivity of the mother. *Proc. R. Soc. Med.,* 63:61–64.

51. Cutler, S. J., Scotto, J., Devesa, S. S., and Connelly, R. R. (1974): Third national cancer survey—an overview of available information. *J.N.C.I.,* 53:1565–1575.

52. De Lustig, E. S., Puricelli, L., De Kier Joffe, E. Bal, and Lanzetti, J. C. (1978): Chagas disease associated with tumoral processes, p. 86. XIIth International Cancer Congress, Buenos Aires, Workshop 7:9.

53. de Padua Bertelli, A., Roxo Nobre, M. O., Alecrim, D., Castro, S., Kestel, K. G., and Sanvit, L. C. (1978): Laryngeal cancer—epidemiological study and analysis of the evolution and treatment in 741 cases, p. 203. XIIth International Cancer Congress, Buenos Aires, Workshop 38:3.

54. De Snoc, K. (1946): Appearance and disappearance of endometriosis. *Nederl. Tijdschr. Geneesk.,* 90:480–483.

55. De Souza, C., and De Souza, L. J. (1978): The psychological impact of mastectomy in Indian women, pp. 126–127. XIIth International Cancer Congress, Buenos Aires, Workshop 32:11.

56. Devesa, S. S. (1978): The association of cancer incidence and socioeconomic status, p. 85. XIIth International Cancer Congress, Buenos Aires, Workshop 7:8.

57. De Waard, F. (1978) Epidemiology and geographic pathology, p. 100. XIIth International Cancer Congress, Buenos Aires, Abstract, panel 5.

58. Dietert, S. E. (1975): Papillary cystadenoma lymphomatocum (Warthin's tumor) in patients in a general hospital over a 24-year period. *Am. J. Clin. Pathol.,* 63:866–875.

59. Dohrmann, G. J., and Farwell, J. R. (1976): Intracranial neoplasms in children; a comparison of North America, Europe, Africa and Asia. *Dis. Nerv. Syst.,* 37:696–697.

60. Dohrmann, G. J., Farwell, J. R., and Flannery, J. T. (1976): Glioblastoma multiforme in children. *J. Neurosurg.,* 44:442–448.

61. Doll, R. (1973): Tumours in a tropical country—foreword recent results. *Cancer Res.,* 41:V.

62. Doll, R. (1978): An epidemiological perspective of the biology of cancer. *Cancer Res.,* 38:3573–3583.

63. Doll, R., and Peto, R. (1977): Mortality among doctors in different occupations. *Br. Med. J.,* 1:1433–1436.

64. Doll, R., Payne, P., and Waterhouse, J. (1966): *Cancer Incidence in Five Continents.* Springer-Verlag, New York.

65. Donegan, W. L., Jayich, S., Koehler, M., and Donegan, J. H. (1978): The association of body weight and obesity with recurrence of mammary cancer after mastectomy, pp. 90–91. XIIth International Cancer Congress, Buenos Aires, Workshop 7:18.

66. Dontas, N., and Papachristopoulos, G. (1978): Epidemiological studies of bronchogenic carcinoma in Greece, p. 91. XIIth International Cancer Congress, Buenos Aires, Workshop 7:19.

67. Dorn, H. F., and Cutler, S. J. (1959): Morbidity from Cancer in the U.S. *Public Health Monogr.,* 56:1–207.

68. Drasar, B. S., and Hill, M. J. (1972): Intestinal bacteria and cancer. *Am. J. Clin. Nutr.,* 25:1399–1404.

69. Dunham, L., and Bailar, J. C. (1968): World maps of cancer mortality rates and frequency ratios. *J.N.C.I.,* 41:155–203.

70. Dunn, J. E., Jr. (1977): Breast cancer among American Japanese in the San Francisco Bay area. *Natl. Cancer Inst. Monogr.,* 47:157–160.

71. Enstrom, J. E. (1978): Cancer mortality among Mormons, p. 158. XIIth International Cancer Congress, Buenos Aires, Workshop 34:8.

72. Ericsson, J. L. E., Karnstrom, L., and Mattsson, B. (1978): 1958–1974. I. Incidence and mortality. *Acta Paediatr. Scand. (SE),* 67:425–432.

73. Fan, K. J., Kowi, J., and Earl, K. M. (1977): The ethnic distribution of primary central nervous system tumors: AFIP, 1958–1970. *J. Neuropathol. Exp. Neurol.,* 36:41–49.

74. Fears, T. R., Scotto, J., and Schneiderman, M. A. (1976): Skin cancer, melanoma, and sunlight. *Am. J. Public Health,* 66:461–464.

75. Fears, T. R., Scotto, J., and Schneiderman, A. M. (1977): Mathematical models of age and ultraviolet effects on the incidence of skin cancer among whites in the United States. *Am. J. Epidemiol.,* 105:420–427.

76. Fernandes, M., and Marques, C. (1957): *Rev. Gynecol. Obstetr.,* 100:15.

77. Fratkin, L. B. (1978): The epidemiology of breast cancer in British Columbia and Canada with comparison to world data. p. 74. XIIth International Cancer Congress, Buenos Aires, Workshop 6:11.

78. Fratkin, L. B. (1978): The influence of diet on breast cancer and the relationship to blood estradiol levels, p. 82. XIIth International Cancer Congress, Buenos Aires, Workshop 7:1.

79. Fraumeni, Jr., J. F., and Mason, T. J. (1974): Cancer mortality among Chinese Americans, 1950–69. *J.N.C.I.,* 52:659–665.

80. Fu, K. K., Lichter, A., and Galante, M. (1976): Carcinoma of the floor of mouth; an analysis of treatment results and the sites and causes of failures. *Int. J. Radiat. Oncol. Biol. Phys.,* 1:829–837.

81. Fu, K. K., Newman, H., and Phillips, T. L. (1975): Treatment of locally recurrency carcinoma of nasopharynx. *Radiology,* 117:425–431.

82. Fujimoto, I., and Hanai, A. (1978): Cancer incidence and survival rates in Japan, pp. 72–73. XIIth International Cancer Congress, Buenos Aires, Workshop 6:8.

83. Gangadharan, P., Nagaraj, R. D., and Jussawalla, D. J. (1978): Some epidemiological observations on the gastrointestinal cancer in India. XIIth International Cancer Congress, Buenos Aires, Abstracts 1/W 6 #14:76.

84. Garau, J. M., Orsini, W., Franzani, W., Elizalde, R., and Soulages, G. (1978): Epidemiologia del cancer vulvar. XIIth International Cancer Congress, Workshop 65:271, Abstract 12.

85. Grigore, M. (1978): Some correlations between cattle products consumption and human leukemia-lymphoma, p. 89. XIIth International Cancer Congress, Buenos Aires, Workshop 7:15.

86. Habibi, A. (1978): Some epidemiological aspect of cancer in Iran, p. 75. XIIth International Cancer Congress, Buenos Aires, Workshop 6:12.

87. Haenszel, W. (1958): Variation in incidence and mortality from stomach cancer, with particular reference to the United States, *J.N.C.I., 21*:213–262.

88. Haenszel, W. M., and Kurihara, M. (1968): Studies of Japanese migrants; I. Mortality from cancer among Japanese in the U.S. *J.N.C.I., 40*:43–68.

89. Haenszel, W., Kurihara, M., Segi, M., and Lee, R. K. C. (1972): Stomach cancer among Japanese in Hawaii. *J.N.C.I., 49*:969.

90. Haenszel, W., Kurihara, M., Locke, F. B., Shimuzu, K., and Segi, M. (1976): Stomach cancer in Japan. *J.N.C.I., 56*:265–274.

91. Haenszel, W., Correa, P., Cuello, C., Guzman, N., Burbano, L. C., Lores, H., and Munoz, J. (1976): Gastric cancer in Colombia; II. Case-control epidemiologic study of precursor lesions. *J.N.C.I., 57*:1021–1026.

92. Hakama, M., and Saxen, E. A. (1967): Cereal consumption and gastric cancer. *Int. J. Cancer, 2*:265–268.

93. Hakama, M., and Pukkala, E. (1977): Selective screening for cervical cancer. Experience of the Finnish mass screening system. *Br. J. Prev. Soc. Med., 31*:238–244.

94. Hasegawa, T. (1971): TROPHOBLASTIC NEOPLASIA; *Its Basic and Clinical Aspects.* Williams & Wilkins, Baltimore.

95. Hasegawa, Y. (1974): The association of aplastic anemia and PNH, in *Aplastic Anemia, Vol. 2,* pp. 227–31, edited by S. Hibino. Aplastic Anemia Research Commission of Japan, Nagoya, Japan.

96. Hashemian, H. (1978): Carcinoma of the thyroid gland in Iran, p. 78. XIIth International Cancer Congress, Buenos Aires, Workshop 6:17.

97. Hertig, A. T., and Mansell, H. (1956): Tumors of the female sex organs. Part I. Hydatidiform mole and choriocarcinoma, Sect. 9, Fasc. 33, *Atlas of Tumor Pathology.* Armed Forces Institute of Pathology, Washington, D.C.

98. Heshmat, M. Y., Kovi, J., Simpson, C., Kennedy, J., and Fan, K. J. (1976): Neoplasms of the central nervous system. Incidence and population selectivity in the Washington, D.C. metropolitan area. *Cancer, 38*:2135–2142.

99. Higginson, J. (1972): *Proceedings of Second DEPECA Conference, 1972.* North-Holland, Amsterdam.

100. Higginson, J., and Svoboda, D. J. (1970): Primary carcinoma of the liver as a pathologist's problem. *Pathol. Anna, 5*:61–89.

101. Higginson, J., and Jensen, O. M. (1977): Epidemiological review of lung cancer in man. *IARC. Sci. Publ., 16*:169–189.

102. Hill, P., Wynder, E., Whitmore, J. F., Garnes, H., and Walker, A. R. P. (1978): Effect of diet, LRF/TRH and HCG administration on plasma hormone levels in North American black and white and South African Bantu men, p. 214. XIIth International Cancer Congress, Workshop 16:1.

103. Hirayama, T. (1963): A study of epidemiology of stomach cancer with special reference to the effect of the diet factor. *Bull. Inst. Pub. Health (Tokyo), 12*:85–96.

104. Hirayama, T. (1966): An epidemiological study of oral and pharyngeal cancer in Central and South-East Asia. *Bull. W.H.O., 34*:41–69.

105. Hirayama, T. (1963): The occupational-social class risks of cancer in Japan. *Jpn. J. Cancer Clin., 9*:66–74.

106. Hirayama, T. (1977): Changing patterns of Japan with special reference to the decrease in stomach cancer mortality, in *Incidence of Cancer in Humans, Proceedings of the Cold Spring Harbor Conferences on Cell Proliferation, Vol. 4,* pp. 55–75, edited by H. H. Hiatt, J. D. Watson, and J. A. Winsten. Cold Spring Harbor Laboratory, Cold Spring Harbor.

107. Hitosugi, M., Yamaguchi, K., Nagasaki, M., and Hirayama, T. (1978): Epidemiology of lung cancer in Tokyo, pp. 84–85. XIIth International Cancer Congress, Buenos Aires, Workshop 7:7.

108. Ho, H. C. (1976): Epidemiology of nasopharyngeal carcinoma. *Gann Monogr. Cancer Res., 18.*

109. Ho, H. C. (1976): Epidemiology of nasopharyngeal carcinoma, in *Cancer in Asia,* pp. 49–61, edited by T. Hirayama. University Park Press, Baltimore.

110. Hu, C. H., and Yang, C. (1959): A decade of progress in morphologic pathology. *Clin. Med. J., 79*:409–422.

111. Iversen, O. H. (1967): Kinetics of cellular proliferation and cell loss in human carcinomas. *Eur. J. Cancer, 3*:389–394.

112. Jackson, M. A., Ahluwalia, B. S., Herson, J., Heshmat, M. Y., Jackson, A. G., Jones, G. W., Kapoor, S. K., Kennedy, J., Kovi, J., Lucas, A. O., Nkposong, E. O., Olisa, E., and Williams, A. O. (1977): Characterization of prostatic carcinoma among blacks; a continuation report. *Cancer Treat. Rep., 61*:167–172.

113. Jeffcoate, T. N. A. (1967): Trophoblastic tumours, in *Principles of Gynecology,* Ed. 3, pp. 282–295. Appleton-Century-Crofts, New York.

114. Junaid, T. A., De Hendrickse, J. P., Williams, A. O., and Osunkoya, B. O. (1976): Choriocarcinoma in Ibadan; clinicopathologic studies. *Hum. Pathol., 7*:215–222.

115. Junaid, T. A., De Hendrickse, J. P., Oladiran, B., Edington, G. M., and Williams, A. O. (1974): Choriocarcinoma in Ibadan, Nigeria; Epidemiologic aspects, *J.N.C.I., 53*:1597–1602.

116. Jung, P. F., and Yu, C. (1963): Nasopharyngeal carcinoma in China. *Postgrad. Med. J., 33*:77–82.

117. Jussawalla, D. J. (1976): Breast cancer in India. *Gann Monogr. Cancer Res., 18*:187–193.

118. Jussawalla, D. J. (1976): The problem of cancer in India; an epidemiological assessment, in *Cancer in Asia,* pp. 265–73, edited by T. Hirayama. University Park Press, Baltimore.

119. Jussawalla, D. J., and Gangadharan, P. (1977): Cancer of the colon; 32 years of experience in Bombay, India. *J. Surg. Oncol., 9*:607–622.

120. Jussawalla, D. J., and Jain, D. K. (1977): Breast cancer and religion in greater Bombay women; an epidemiological study of 2,130 women over a 9-year period. *Br. J. Cancer, 36*:634–638.

121. Kagawa, Y. (1978): Impact of westernization on the nutrition of japanese; changes in physique, cancer, longevity and centenarians. *Dept. Biochem. Jichi Med. Sch. Prev. Med., 7*:205–217.

122. Kaplan, H. S., and Jones Tsuchitani, P. (eds.) (1978): *Cancer in China.* Alan R. Liss, Inc., New York.

123. Kato, H. (1977): Cancer study on a cohort of atomic bomb survivors. *Natl. Cancer Inst. Monogr., 47*:31–32.

124. King, H., and Locke, F. B. (1978): Cancer mortality among foreign- and native-born Chinese in the United States; a follow-up study, p. 79. XIIth International Cancer Congress, Buenos Aires, Workshop 6:20.

125. Kmet, J., and Mahboubi, E. (1972): Esophageal cancer in Caspian Littoral of Iran—initial studies. *Science, 175*:846.

126. Kolstad, P., and Hognestadt, J. (1965): Trophoblastic tumours in Norway. *Acta Obstetr. Gynecol. Scand., 44*:80–88.

127. Kori, J., et al. (1973): Incidence of cancer in Negroes in Washington, D.C., and selected African cities. *Am. J. Epidemiol., 96*:401–413.

128. Kratochvil, O. (1976): [Medical geography in the problem of cancer] (Rus.). *Zdrav. Prac., 26.*

129. Kubo, T. (1978): The risk of developing cancer from "intestinal metaplasia" of the stomach, a geographical-pathological approach, pp. 75–76. XIIth International Cancer Congress, Buenos Aires, Workshop 6:13.

130. Kurita, H. (1978): The interrelationship between genetic and environmental factors in stomach cancer, pp. 91–92. XIIth International Cancer Congress, Buenos Aires, Workshop 7:20.

131. Larsson, L.-G., and Sandström, A. (1978): Studies on cancer incidences in Northern Sweden, p. 72. XIIth International Cancer Congress, Buenos Aires, Workshop 6:7.

132. Law, C. H., Day, N. E., and Shanmugaratnam, K. (1976): Incidence rates of specific histological types of lung cancer in Singapore Chinese dialect groups, and their aetiological significance. *Int. J. Cancer, 17*:1304–1309.

133. Lee, A. T. C., and Siegel, I. (1965): Hydatidiform mole with rupture of the uterus. Report of a case. *Obstetr. Gynecol., 26*:133–134.

134. Lee, K. T., Kim, D. N., and Thomas, W. A. (1965): Ultrastructural changes in liver of rats fed high fat diets. *Fed. Proc., 27*:576.

135. Leeder, J. R. (1964): Metastasing hydatidiform mole. *Am. J. Obstet. Gynecol., 88*:833–835.

136. Leis, H. P., Jr. (1978): Patients at risk for breast cancer, p. 93. XIIth International Cancer Congress, Buenos Aires, Workshop 7:23.

137. Li, K.-H., Kao, J. C., and Wu, Y. K. (1962): A survey of the prevalence of carcinoma of the oesophagus in North China. *Chinese Med. J., 81*:489–494.

138. Liu, R. L., and Tien, C. Y. (1964): Gynecologic malignancy registration in Nanking area. A 5-½ year statistical survey. *Chin. Med. J., 83*:171–173.

139. Llewellyn-Jones, D. (1965): Trophoblastic tumours; geographical variations in incidence and possible aetiological factors. *J. Obstetr. Gynaecol. Br. Cwlth., 72*:242–248.

140. Lowenfels, A. B. (1973): Etiological aspects of cancer of the gastrointestinal tract, *Surg. Gynecol. Obstet., 137*:291–292.

141. Lyon, J. L. (1978): Esophageal cancer mortality, pp. 146–147. XIIth International Cancer Congress, Buenos Aires, Abstract, panel 15.

142. Macdonald, E. J. (1978): Regional differences in cancer among the Spanish surnamed population in Texas, pp. 73–74. XIIth International Cancer Congress, Buenos Aires, Workshop 6:9.

143. Macklin, M. T. (1955): The role of heredity in gastric and intestinal cancer. *Gastroenterology, 29*:509–514.

144. Maclennan, R., Da Costa, J., Day, N. E., Law, C. H., Ng, Y. K., and Shanmugaratnam, K. (1977): Risk factors for lung cancer in Singapore Chinese, a population with high female incidence rates. *Int. J. Cancer, 20*:854–860.

145. Mahboubi, E. (1978): Etiological factors and esophageal cancer, p. 146. XIIth International Cancer Congress, Buenos Aires, Abstract, panel 15.

146. Mahboubi, E., Kmet, J., Cook, P. J., Day, N. E., Ghadirian, P., and Salmasizadeh, S. (1973): Oesophageal cancer studies in the Caspian littoral of Iran; the Caspian cancer registry. *Br. J. Cancer, 28*:197–214.

147. Malik, M. O. A. (1978): Nasopharyngeal carcinoma (NPC) in the Sudan, p. 207. XIIth International Cancer Congress, Buenos Aires, Workshop 38:11.

148. Marquez-Monter, H. (1963): Epidemiology and pathology of hydatidi-

form mole in the General Hospital of Mexico. *Am. J. Obstet. Gynecol.,* 85:856.

149. Marsden, A. T. (1958): The geographical pathology of cancer in Malaya. *Br. J. Cancer, 12:*161–176.

150. Martinez, I. (1978): Factores asociados con adenocarcinomas del intestino grueso en Puerto Rico, p. 92. XIIth International Cancer Congress, Buenos Aires, Workshop 7:21.

151. Masuda, Y., Hisamichi, S., Mochizuki, F., Oshiba, S., and Sugawara, N. (1978): 10-year relative survival rate of stomach cancer detected by gastric mass survey, p. 227. XIIth International Cancer Congress, Buenos Aires, Workshop 40:6.

152. Maurer, G. (1975): [Possibilities and limitations of the surgical treatment of cancer] (Ger.). *Langenbecks Arch. Chir., 339:*65–74.

153. McGarrity, K. A. (1978): Carcinoma of the ovary, p. 143. XIIth International Cancer Congress, Buenos Aires, Abstract, panel 14.

154. McMichael, A. J., Spirtas, R., Gamble, J. F., and Tousey, P. M. (1976): Mortality among rubber workers; relationship to specific jobs. *J. Occup. Med., 18:*178–185.

155. Merabishvili, V. M., Napalkov, N. P., and Tserkovnyi, G. F. (1978): Status and developmental prospects of oncological statistics in the USSR. *Vopr. Onkol., 24:*38–44.

156. Merino, F. (1978): Immunological and epidemiological studies of gastric cancer in Venezuela, pp. 228–229. XIIth International Cancer Congress, Workshop 40:9.

157. Mi, M. P., Onizuka, S., and Kagawa, J. (1978): A statistical analysis of cancer incidence and mortality rates in Hawaii, pp. 71–72. XIIth International Cancer Congress, Buenos Aires, Workshop 6:6.

158. Miyaji, T. (1978): Statistical analysis of malignancies among 298,907 autopsies in Japan, pp. 78–79. XIIth International Cancer Congress, Buenos Aires, Workshop 6:19.

159. Müller, N. R., Remizov, A. L., Belogorodski, I., V. V., and Filov, V. A. (1975): [Some characteristics of the biological action of D,L-1,4-dibromo-1,4-dideoxy-2,3-butanediol], *Farmakol. Toksikol., 38:*590–591.

160. Muir, C. S. (1978): On-going research and needs in cancer epidemiology—a worldwide survey, p. 146. XIIth International Cancer Congress, Buenos Aires, Abstract, panel 15.

161. Muir, C. S. (1975): The epidemiology of cancer of the nasopharynx *Bull. Cancer (Paris), 62:*251–264.

162. Myers, M. H., White, P. L., and Bundy, B. N. (1978): Trends in survival rates for all cancer sites combined, p. 75. XIIth International Cancer Congress, Buenos Aires, Workshop 6:10.

163. Nakano, G., and Nakamura, T. (1978): High incidence of multiple gastric cancer in the aged patients admitted to Tokyo geriatric hospital, p. 77. XIIth International Cancer Congress, Buenos Aires, Workshop 6:16.

164. Napalkov, N. P., Tserkovnyi, G. F., Merabishvili, V. M., and Preobrazhenskaia, M. N. (1978): Malignant neoplasms in the USSR in 1975. *Vopr. Onkol., 24:*8–37.

165. Napalkov, N. P., Tserkovny, G. R., Preobrazhenskaia, M. N., Berezkin, D. P., and Shabashova, N. I. (1975): [The incidence of malignant neoplasms among the population of the USSR], *Vopr. Onkol., 21:*3–28.

166. Nielsen, N. H., Mikkelsen, F., and Hansen, J. P. H. (1977): Nasopharyngeal cancer in Greenland. The incidence in an arctic eskimo population. Dept. Pathol., Rigshosp, Copenhagen. *Acta Pathol. Microbiol. Scand. Denmark, 85:*850–858.

167. Novak, E., and Seah, C. S. (1954): Choriocarcinoma of the uterus. Study of 74 cases from the Mathieu Memorial Chorionepithelioma Reigistry. *Am. J. Obstet. Gynecol., 67:*933–957.

168. Nugmanov, S. N. (1978): Epidemiology of cancer of the uterine cervix in Kazakhstan, p. 71. XIIth International Cancer Congress, Buenos Aires, Workshop 6:5.

169. O'Conor, G. T. (1976): A perspective for collaborative studies of breast cancer in human population groups. *Gann Monogr. Cancer Reg., 18:*179–186.

170. Owor, R.: Malignant neoplasms in African infants. (1977), East African Med. J., 54, (1), 9–13.

171. Page, M., Theriault, L., and Delorme, F. (1978): Biomedical surveillance of vinyl chloride workers, p. 84. XIIth International Cancer Congress, Buenos Aires, Workshop 7:5.

172. Pai, K. N. (1967): A study of choriocarcinoma; its incidence in India and its aetiopathogenesis, in *Choriocarcinoma: Transactions of a Conference of the International Union against Cancer,* pp. 54–57, edited by J. F. Holland and M. M. Hreshchyshyn. Springer-Verlag, Berlin.

173. Pathak, I. C., Datta, B. N., Aikat, B. K., et al. (1975): Pattern of neoplastic disease in children with special reference to malignant tumors. *Indian J. Cancer, 12*(1 Suppl.):46–55.

174. Paulson, D. (1978): Etiology and epidemiology of prostate cancer, p. 136. XIIth International Cancer Congress, Buenos Aires, Abstract, panel 13.

175. Pekkarinen, M., Seppanen, R., and Roine, P. (1964): Naringsforskning Nr. 4, 139–149.

176. Perez-Arias, E., and Feller, J. (1978): Epidemiologia del cancer en la Provincia de Buenos Aires—estructura y tendencia de la mortalidad, pp. 79–80. XIIth International Cancer Congress, Buenos Aires, Workshop 6:21.

177. Perez-Arias, E., and Feller, J. J. (1978): Epidemiologia del cancer en la Provincia de Buenos Aires—estructura y tendencia de los egresos hospitalarios, p. 80. XIIth International Cancer Congress, Buenos Aires, Workshop 6:22.

178. Pessin, S. B. (1961): Lower urinary tract and male genitalia, in *Pathology,* Ed. 4, pp. 636–640, edited by W. A. D. Anderson. C. V. Mosby, St. Louis.

179. Pitt, H. A., and Zuidema, G. D. (1975): Factors influencing mortality in the treatment of pyogenic hepatic abscess. *Surg. Gynecol. Obstet., 140:*228–234.

180. Qassab, Kh. (1978): A study of cancer epidemiology, p. 70. XIIth International Cancer Congress, Buenos Aires, Workshop 6:3.

181. Reddy, C. R. R. M., Reddy, V. C., and Rao, M. S. (1967): Distribution of malignant tumors in Kurnool. *Indian J. Cancer, 4:*64–71.

182. Reddy, B. S., Hedges, A., Laakso, K., and Wynder, E. L.: Fecal constituents of a high-risk North American and a low-risk Finnish population for the development of large bowel cancer. *Cancer Lett.,4:*217–222.

183. Registrar General's Decennial Supplement, England and Wales (1958): *1951 Occupational Mortality, Part II, Vol. 2.* Her Majesty's Stationery Office, London.

184. Robbins, S. L. (1967): *Pathology,* Ed. 3, pp. 922–925. W. B. Saunders, Philadelphia.

185. Rockwell, G., et al. (1966): Cholangiocarcinoma of the liver. *Cancer, 19:*1177–1184.

186. Rolon, P. A. (1978): The geographical distribution of melanoma in Latin America, p. 94. XIIth International Cancer Congress, Buenos Aires, Abstract, panel 4.

187. Rose, E. F. (1978): Epidemiology of oesophageal cancer in Southern Africa, p. 147. XIIth International Cancer Congress, Buenos Aires, Abstract, panel 15.

188. Rotkin, I. D., Cooper, J. F., Grayhack, J. T., and Clark, S. S. (1978): Effect of selected epidemiologic variables upon risk of prostatic cancer, pp. 86–87. XIIth International Cancer Congress, Buenos Aires, Workshop 7:10.

189. Saleh, J. S., Pourmand, K., and Mojaradi, N. (1966): A study of the trophoblastic disease among the Iranian population. *Br. J. Clin. Pract., 20:*119–127.

190. Salvatore, C. A. (1978): Epidemiological factors for gynecological and breast cancer, p. 90. XIIth International Cancer Congress, Buenos Aires, Workshop 7:17.

191. Saxen, E. A., and Hakama, M. (1976): The different incidence of gastric cancer all over the world and possible reasons for this difference. *Gann Monogr. Cancer Res., 18.*

192. Schoenberg, B. S. (1978): Epidemiology of primary nervous system neoplasms. *Adv. Neurol., 19:*475–495.

193. Schoenberg, B. S., Bailar, J. C., 3rd, and Fraumeni, J. F., Jr. (1971): Certain mortality patterns of esophageal cancer in the United States, 1930–67, *J.N.C.I., 46:*63–73.

194. Schoenberg, S., Christine, B. W., and Whisnant, J. P. (1978): The resolution of discrepancies in the reported incidence of primary brain tumors. *Neurology, 28:*817–823.

195. Schoenberg, B. S., Christine, B. W., and Whisnant, J. P. (1976): Discrepancies in the reported incidence of primary neoplasms of the nervous system; international comparisons. *Am. J. Epidemiol., 104:*332.

196. Schulze, R., and Kasten, F. (1975): [Effect of the atmospheric ozone layer on the biologically active ultraviolet radiation on the earth's surface] (Ger.). *Strahlentherapie, 150:*219–226.

197. Scotto, J., and Fraumeni, J. (1978): Patterns of cancer incidence among Spanish Americans in the Southwestern United States, pp. 80–81. XIIth International Cancer Congress, Buenos Aires, Workshop 6:23.

198. Scotto, J., Kopf, A. W., and Urbach, F. (1974): Non-melanoma skin cancer among caucasians in Kour areas of the United States. *Cancer, 34:*1333–1338.

199. Sedlacek, H. H., Meesmann, H., and Seiler, F. R. (1975): Regression of spontaneous mammary tumors in dogs after injection of neuraminidase-treated tumor cells. *Int. J. Cancer 15:*408–416.

200. Segi, M. (1976): A statistic study of mortality from cancer of the stomach in selected countries. *Gann Monogr. Cancer Res., 18.*

201. Segi, M., and Kurihara, M. (1964): Cancer mortality for selected sites in 24 countries, No. 3, 1960/61. Dept. Public Health, Tohoku Univ., School of Med., Sendai, Japan.

202. Seidl, S., and Junge, W. D. (1970): Zum Krankheitsbild der klinischen Choriomatose. *Wien. Klin. Wochenschr., 82:*235–237.

203. Shanmugaratnam, K. (1973): Cancer in Singapore ethnic and dialect group variations in cancer incidence. *Singapore Med. J., 14.*

204. Shanmugaratnam, K. (1976): Epidemiological studies of lung cancer in Singapore. in *Cancer in Asia,* pp. 153–158, edited by T. Hirayama. University Park Press, Baltimore.

205. Shanmugaratnam, K., and Muir, C. S. (1967): Cancer incidence in Singapore, in *Racial and Geographic Factors in Tumour Incidence,* pp. 133–146, edited by A. A. Shivas. Edinburg University Press.

206. Shanmugaratnam, K., and Tye, C. Y. (1970): A study of nasopharyngeal cancer among Singapore Chinese with special reference to migrant status and specific community (dialect group). *J. Chron. Dis., 23:*433–441.

207. Shimkin, M. B. (1963): Cancer of the breast; some old facts and new prospectives. *Cancer, 13*:109–112.

208. Shore, R. E., Albert, R. E., and Pasternack, B. S. (1976): Follow-up study of patients treated by x-ray epilation for *Tinea capitis*; resurvey of post-treatment illness and mortality experience. *Arch. Environ. Health, 31*:21–28.

209. Sierra, L. M., Gland, M., and de Levin, R. W. (1978): Cancer incidence in the "Great Buenos Aires," p. 69. XIIth International Cancer Congress, Buenos Aires, Workshop 6:1.

210. Simons, M. J., Wee, G. B., Goh, E. H., Chan, S. H., Shanmugaratnam, K., Day, N. E., and De-The, G. (1976): Immunogenetic aspects of nasopharyngeal carcinoma; IV. Increased risk in Chinese of nasopharyngeal carcinoma associated with a Chinese-related HLA Profile (A2, Singapore 2). *J.N.C.I., 57*:977–980.

211. Speiser, P. (1956): Bestehen mathematisch gesicherte Beziehungen der ABO-Blutgruppen, des Rhesusfaktors Rh$_o$(D) und des Geschlechtes zu Carcinoma ventriculi, Ulcus ventriculi und Ulcus duodeni? *Krebsarzt, 11*:344.

212. Spratt, J. S., Jr., Heuser, L., and Polk, H., Jr. (1978): The spectrum of growth rates of mammary cancers in a population of 10,000 women, p. 83. XIIth International Cancer Congress, Buenos Aires, Workshop 7:3.

213. Steiner, P. E. (1954): *Cancer: Race and Geography*. Williams & Wilkins, Baltimore.

214. Steinitz, R. C. C., and Ogen, Y. (1978): Malignant neoplasms in tuberculosis patients, pp. 159–160. XIIth International Cancer Congress, Buenos Aires, Workshop 34:11.

215. Stell, P. M. (1973): Cancer of the hypopharynx. *J. R. Coll. Surg. Edinb., 18*:20–30.

216. Stemmerman, G. N. (1966): Cancer of the colon and rectum discovered at autopsy in Hawaiian Japanese. *Cancer, 19*:1567–1572.

217. Stemmermann, G. N., Nomura, A., Mower, H. F., and Mandel, M. (1977): Gastrointestinal carcinoma in the Japanese of Hawaii; a status report. *Natl. Cancer Inst. Monogr., 47*:169–174.

218. Stemmermann, G., Haenszel, W., and Locke, F. (1977): Epidemiologic pathology of gastric ulcer and gastric carcinoma among Japanese in Hawaii. *J.N.C.I., 58*:13–20.

219. Strahan, R. W. (1963): Carcinoma of the prostate; incidence, origin, pathology. *J. Urol., 89*:875–880.

220. Sturton, G. D., Wen, H. L., and Sturton, O. G. (1966): Etiology of cancer of the nasopharynx. *Cancer, 19*:1666–1669.

221. Sung, J. L., Wang, T. H., Chen C. S., *et al.* (1976): [Epidemiological study on peptic ulcer and gastric cancer in the Chinese] (Chin.). *J. Formosan Med. Assoc., 75*:116–119.

222. Svejda, J. (1978): Breast cancer in Czechoslovakia, pp. 30–31. XIIth International Cancer Congress, Buenos Aires, Workshop 46:4.

223. Takatani, O., Wakabayashi, Y., and Hirayama, T. (1978): Clinical epidemiology of breast cancer with special reference to the relationship with height, weight and body surface area, pp. 87–88. XIIth International Cancer Congress, Buenos Aires, Workshop 7:3.

224. Talvalkar, G. V., Sampat, M. B., and Gangadharan, P. (1978): Hodgkin's disease in Western India; a clinico-pathologic review of 576 cases seen in Tata Memorial Hospital, Bombay, India, pp. 89–90. XIIth International Cancer Congress, Buenos Aires, Workshop 7:16.

225. Templeton, A. C. (1976): Superficial vascular tumours in Ugandan Africans. *East Afr. Med. J., 53*:130–135.

226. Templeton, A. C., and Hutt, M. S. (1973): Distribution of tumours in Uganda; recent results. *Cancer Res., 41*:1–22.

227. The People's Republic of China (Kwangchow, China) (1978): A preliminary investigation on the epidemiology of nasopharyngeal carcinoma (NPC) in four provinces and an autonomous region in South China, p. 215. XIIth International Cancer Congress, Buenos Aires, Workshop 38: 28.

228. Thorborg, J. V., and Kim, Y. K. (1964): On hydatitiform mole and choriocarcinoma in Korea. Proceedings of the 14th Scandinavian Congress on Pathology and Microscopy, Oslo.

229. Tiscareno, A. M., Ortega, A. B., and Angeles, A. A. (1978): Epidemiology of melanoma in Mexico. XIIth International Cancer Congress, Workshop 65:270, Abstract 11.

230. UICC (Union internationale contre le cancer) (1970): *Cancer Incidence in Five Continents, Vol. 11*, edited by R. Doll, C. S. Muir and J. Waterhouse. Springer-Verlag, Berlin.

231. Urquijo, C., Guardo, A., Eleta, G., Saco, P., and Pradier, R. (1978): A study of some environmental factors related to the incidence of larynx cancer, p. 92. XIIth International Cancer Congress, Buenos Aires, Workshop 7:22.

232. Uslenghi, C., Centenaro, G., Sigurta, D., and Volterrani, F. (1978): A computerized cancer patient information system, pp. 158–159. XIIth International Cancer Congress, Buenos Aires, Workshop 34:9.

233. Utsunomiya, J., Murata, M., Iwama, T., Miyanaga, T., Tanimura, M., and Murakami, T. (1978): Colonic cancer arising in adenomatosis coli in Japanese, p. 256. XIIth International Cancer Congress, Buenos Aires, Workshop 42:9.

234. Venzmer, G. (1975): [The geography of cancer] (Ger.). *Krankenpflege, 29*:320–321.

235. Walker, A. R., and Burkitt, D. P. (1976): Colon cancer; epidemiology. *Semin. Oncol., 3*:341–350.

236. Wassef, S. A. (1978): Cancer epidemiology in the Libyan Arab popular and socialist Gamahiryah, p. 161. XIIth International Cancer Congress, Buenos Aires, Workshop 34:13.

237. Wassef, S. A., and El Fergani, M. (1978): Malignant neoplasms of the gastro-intestinal tract in Libyan patients. A clinicopathological study, pp. 161–162. XIIth International Cancer Congress, Workshop 34:14.

238. Wassef, S. A., and El Retiemi, S. (1978): Malignant neoplasms of the upper respiratory tract in Libyan patients, pp. 69–70. XIIth International Cancer Congress, Buenos Aires, Workshop 6:2.

239. Wassef, S. A., and Sassi, I. (1978): Malignant neoplasms of the skin in Libyan patients, p. 160. XIIth International Cancer Congress, Buenos Aires, Workshop 34:12.

240. Weed, S. G., Johnson, W. D., Vial, L. J., Du Sapin, K., and Rothschild, H. (1978): Trends in mortality due to respiratory system cancers in Louisiana, pp. 70–71. XIIth International Cancer Congress, Buenos Aires, Workshop 6:4.

241. Wei, P. Y., and Ouyang, P. C. (1963): Trophoblastic diseases in Taiwan, a review of 157 cases in a 10-year period. *Am. J. Obstet. Gynecol., 58*: 844–849.

242. Wellington, D. G., MacDonald, E. J., and Wolf, P. F. (1978): Ethnic effects in U.S. cancer mortality models, p. 88. XIIth International Cancer Congress, Buenos Aires, Workshop 7:13.

243. West, R. O. (1966): Epidemiologic study of malignancies of the ovaries. *Cancer, 19*:1001–1007.

244. White, C., and Eisenberg, H. (1959): ABO blood groups and cancers of the stomach. *Yale J. Biol. Med., 32*:58–61.

245. WHO (1960): Research Committee on Gastroenterology.

246. WHO Statistics Annual (1968): World Health Organization, Geneva, 1971.

247. WHO Statistics Annual (1970): World Health Organization, Geneva, 1973.

248. WHO Epidemiological and Vital Statistics Report. World Health Organization, Geneva.

249. Willis, R. A. (1967): *Pathology of Tumours*, Ed 4. Butterworth, London.

250. Wiskemann, A. (1975): [Light-induced cancer] (Ger.). *Strahlentherapie, 150*:195–198.

251. Woolf, B. (1955): On estimating the relation between blood group and disease. *Ann Hum. Genet., 19*:251–253.

252. Woolf, C. M. (1956): A further study on the familial aspects of carcinoma of the stomach. *Am. J. Hum. Genet., 8*:102–109.

253. Wright, D. H. (1973): Lymphoreticular neoplasms; recent results. *Cancer Res., 41*:270–291.

254. Wynder, E. L., Dodo, H., and Barber, H. R. K. (1969): Epidemiology of neoplastic cancer of the ovary human. *Cancer, 23*:352–370.

255. Wynder, E. L., and Shigematsu, T. (1967): Environmental factors of the colon and rectum cancer. *Cancer, 20*:1520–1561.

256. Wynder, E. L., Kagitami, T., Ishikawa, S., Dodo, H., and Takano, A. (1969): Environmental factors of cancer of the colon and rectum; II. Japanese epidemiological data. *Cancer, 23*:1210–1220.

257. Wynder, E. L., and Hirayama, T. (1977): Comparative epidemiology of cancers of the United States and Japan. *Prev. Med., 6*:567–594.

258. Wynder, E. L., Maccornack, F. A., and Stellman, S. D. (1978): The epidemiology of breast cancer in 785 United States Caucasian women. *Cancer, 41*:2341–2354.

259. Wynder, E. L., Kmet, I., Dungal, N., and Segi, M. (1963): An epidemiological investigation of gastric cancer. *Cancer, 16*:1461–1496.

260. Yeh, S. (1966): Some geographic pathology aspects of common disease in Taiwan; II. Infection and cancer. *Int. Pathol., 7*:24–28.

261. Yeh, S. D. J. (1973): Experimental and clinical oncology in People's Republic of China. *Am. J. Chin. Med., 1*:193–224.

262. Yo, K., Nakamura, K., Kitagawa, T., Sugano, H. (1978): Change in the histological types of gastric carcinoma in Japan during 1955 to 1974, pp. 238–239. XIIth Congreso Internacional del Cancer, Buenos Aires, Workshops 2, No. 23/43.

263. Yoshida, T. O. (1974): Autoantibodies in the sera of various cancer patients. *Nagoya Gann Mongr. Cancer Res. (Jpn.), 16*:63–70.

264. Young, J. L., Jr. (1978): International trends in cancer mortality, 1950–1974. XIIth International Cancer Congress, Buenos Aires, Workshop 6: 15, pp. 76–77.

265. Zippin, C., and Petrakis, N. L. (1978): Marital and reproductive history of breast cancer patients and their sisters, pp. 88–89. XIIth International Cancer Congress, Buenos Aires, Workshop 7:14.

References for Table 36.10

1. Becker, B. J., and Chatgidakis, C. B. (1961): Cirrhosis of the liver in Johannesburg. *Acta Unio Int. Contra Cancrum, 17*:639–649.

2. Becker, B. J., and Chatgidakis, C. B. (1961): Primary carcinoma of the liver in Johannesburg. *Acta Unio Int. Contra Cancrum, 17*:650–653.

3. Berman, C. (1958): Primary carcinoma of the liver. *Adv. Cancer Res., 5*: 55–96.

4. Edmonson, H. A., and Steiner, P. E.: Primary carcinoma of liver; study

of 100 cases among 48,900 necropsies. *Cancer, 7:*462–503.

5. Elkington, S. G., McBrien, D. J., and Spencer, H. (1963): Hepatoma in cirrhosis. *Br. Med. J., 4:*1501–1503.

6. Elsner, B., and Jauregui, E. M. (1974): Autopsy study of primary liver carcinoma in Buenos Aires, Argentina. *Acta Hepatogastroenterol., 21:* 26–34.

7. Ervasti, J. (1964): Primary carcinoma of the liver. A pathologic and clinical study of 100 cases. *Acta Chir. Scand. Supp. 334:*1–65.

8. Frumin, A., and Kohn, A. (1955): Autoimmune hemolytic disease in acute leukemia. *Arch. Intern. Med., 95:*326–327.

9. Gall, E. A. (1960): Primary and metastiatic carcinoma of the liver. Relationship to hepatic cirrhosis. *Arch. Pathol., 70:*226–232.

10. Glennert, J. (1961): Primary carcinoma of the liver. A postmortem study of 104 cases. *Acta Pathol. Microbiol. Scand., 53:*50–60.

11. MacDonald, E. J. (1955): Epidemiology of cancer. *Tex. Rep. Biol. Med., 13:*826–839.

12. Manderson, W. G., Patrick, R. B., and Peters, E. E. (1965): Primary carcinoma of liver; a survey of cases admitted to Glasgow Royal Infirmary during 1949–63. *Scot. Med. J., 10:*60–64.

13. Miyai, K., and Reubner, B. H. (1963): Acute yellow atrophy, cirrhosis and hepatoma. Their incidence at the Johns Hopkins Hospital 1917–1960. *Arch. Pathol., 75:*609–617.

14. Ohlsson, E. G., and Norden, J. G. (1965): Primary carcinoma of the liver. A study of 121 cases. *Acta Pathol. Microbiol. Scand., 64:*430–440.

15. Ottolenghi, A. (1966): Brain biopsy and histopathology of extrapyramidal disease. *J. Neurosurg., 24:* Suppl. 256.

16. Patton, R. B., and Horn, R. C., Jr. (1964): Primary liver carcinoma. Autopsy study of 60 cases. *Cancer, 17:*757–768.

17. Pequignot, H., Etienne, J. P., Delavierre, P., et al. (1967): Cancers primitifs du foie sur cirrhose augmentation de frequence et observation chez des cirrhotiques connus et suivis. *Presse Med., 75:*2595–2600.

18. Purtilo, D. T., and Gottlieb, L. S. (1973): Cirrhosis and hepatoma occurring at Boston City Hospital (1917–1968). *Cancer, 32:*458–462.

19. Roulet, F. C. (1957): Anatomico-pathological considerations on primitive cancer of the liver. *Act Unio Int. Contra Cancrum, 13:*623–627.

20. Sagebiel, R. W., McFarland, R. B., and Taft, E. B. (1963): Primary carcinoma of the liver in relation to cirrhosis. *Am. J. Clin. Pathol., 40:* 516–520.

21. San Jose, D., Cady, A., West, M., et al. (1965): Primary carcinoma of the liver; analysis of clinical and biochemical features of 80 cases. *Am. J. Dig. Dis., 10:* 657–674.

22. Saragoca, A., Barros, B., and Soares, C. S. (1964): Primary neoplasms of the liver; the possibility of biochemical diagnosis. *Am. J. Dig. Dis., 9:* 337–344.

23. Shanmugaratnam, K. (1961): Liver cancer and cirrhosis in Singapore. *Acta Unio Int. Contra Cancrum, 17:*898–902.

24. Sievers, B. U. (1973): Liver cirrhosis and liver carcinoma—findings from a department of pathology extending over 1 year. *Acta Hepatogastroenterol., 20:*483–490.

25. Stitnimankaran, T., and Thakerngpol, K. (1969): Enzyme histochemical study of primary hepatic carcinoma in Thailand. *Cancer, 24:*1064–1067.

26. Tiktinskii, O. L. (1961): On the problem of primary liver cancer. *Sov. Med., 25:*107–109.

27. Voigt, K. G., and Helbig, W. (1968): Zur Pathologie des primären Leberkarzinoms Obduktionsbefunde von 124 Fällen. *Arch. Geschwulstforsch., 31:*39–71.

28. Voigt, K. G., and Helbig, W. (1968): Zur Klinik des primären Leberkarzinoms Katamnestische Untersuchungen von 124 Patienten. *Arch. Geschwulstforsch., 31:*158–183.

29. Wainwright, J. (1961): Malignant hepatoma in the African in Natal. *Acta Unio Int. Contra Cancrum, 17:*677–679.

30. Wainwright, J. (1961): Cirrhosis in the African in Natal. *Acta Unio Int. Contra Cancrum, 17:*667–676.

31. Wöckel, W., and Altrock, H. (1968): Zur Häufigkeit der Leberzirrhose und des Leberkrebses im Obduktionsgut. *Dtsch. Gesundheitswes., 23:* 165–169.

32. Ying, Y. Y., Ma, C. C., Hsu, Y. T., Lei, H. H., Liang, S. F., Lin, C. H., and Ku, C. Y. (1963): Primary carcinoma of the liver with special reference to histogenesis and its relationship to liver cirrhosis. *Chin. Med. J., 82:* 279–294.

Addendum. Very recently there appeared a number of epidemiologic studies which deserve brief attention. One of the largest epidemiologic studies dealing with 600,000 workers among the population of 840 million Chinese during a 3-year period was undertaken. This study showed that esophageal cancer was prevalent in northern China. Cancer was the cause of 620,000 deaths/year in the studied population of 840 million (ref: P. E. Frederick and Elaine L. Shiang: Cancer Mortality in China, *J.N.C.I., 65(2):*217–221, see also Research on Esophageal Cancer in China: A Review, *Cancer Res., 40:*2633–2644, 1980, in which the human cancer was compared to gullet cancer in chickens especially in the Taihang Mountain range of northern China believed due to carcinogens in moldy food and pickled vegetables). Another study dealt with hepatocellular carcinoma in Chinese patients (S. H. Chan, M. J. Simons, and C. J. Oon: HLA Antigen in Chinese Patients with Hepatocellular Carcinomas, *J.N.C.I., 65(1):*21–23, 1980). An international study dealt with leukemia in women following radiotherapy (Leukemia in Women following Radiotherapy for Cervical Cancer: Ten-Year Follow-up of an International Study, *J.N.C.I., 65(1):*115–127, 1980). Other studies of importance are R. Saracci and F. Repetto: Time Trends of Primary Liver Cancer: Indication of Increased Incidence in Selected Cancer Registry Populations, *J.N.C.I., 65(2):*241–247, 1980; S. Preston-Martin *et al.:* Case Control Study of Intracranial Meningiomas in Women in Los Angeles County, California, *J.N.C.I., 65(1):*67–73, 1980; E. Matsunaga: Hereditary Retinoblastoma: Host Resistance and Second Primary Tumors, *J.N.C.I., 65(1):*47–51, 1980; D. Trichopoulos *et al.:* Estrogen Profiles of Primiparous and Nulliparous Women in Athens, Greece, *J.N.C.I., 65(1):*43–51, 1980; J. M. Guileyardo *et al.:* Prevalence of Latent Prostate Carcinoma in Two U.S. Populations, *J.N.C.I., 65(2):*311–319, 1980; Z. E. Land *et al.:* Breast Cancer Risk from Low-Dose Exposures to Ionizing Radiation: Results of Parallel Analysis of Three Exposed Populations of Women, *J.N.C.I., 65(2):*353–376, 1980. In the last study, breast cancer incidence was analyzed in women who were survivors of the Hiroshima and Nagasaki atomic bombs, patients in Massachusetts tuberculosis sanitoria (multiple chest fluoroscopies) and patients treated by x-rays for postpartum mastitis in Rochester, New York. Finally the distribution of non-Hodgkin's lymphoma in the United States between 1950 and 1975 was reviewed by Cantor and Fraumeni (*Cancer Res., 40:*2645–2652, 1980). In November 1980, the NCI monograph *Populations at Low Risk of Cancer J.N.C.I., 65(5):*1055–1195 appeared, dealing with cancer and mortality among religious groups; cancer patterns among ethnic groups and cancer mortality among non-smokers in the United States.

37

International Geographic Studies of Oncological Interest on Chronobiological Variables[*]

Franz Halberg, Germaine Cornélissen, Robert B. Sothern, Lee Anne Wallach,
Erna Halberg, Andrew Ahlgren, Marilyn Kuzel, Alan Radke, Jose Barbosa,
Frederick Goetz, Joseph Buckley, Jack Mandel, Leonard Schuman
(Minneapolis, Minnesota, USA);
Erhard Haus, David Lakatua, Linda Sackett, Harriet Berg, Hans W. Wendt (St.
Paul, Minnesota, USA);
Terukazu Kawasaki, Michio Ueno, Keiko Uezono, Midori Matsuoka, Teruo
Omae (Fukuoka, Japan);
Brunetto Tarquini, Mario Cagnoni (Florence, Italy);
Mauricio Garcia Sainz, Edmee Perez Vega (Mexico City, Mexico);
Douglas Wilson, Keith Griffiths, (Cardiff, Wales, Great Britain);
Luciano Donati, Patrizio Tatti, Mario Vasta, Jacopo Locatelli, A. Camagna
(Urbino, Italy);
Renato Lauro (Rome, Italy);
George Tritsch (Buffalo, New York, USA);
Lennard Wetterberg (Stockholm, Sweden)

INTRODUCTION

For a given variable of oncologic interest displaying rhythmicity the more prominent and predictable is its variability with time, the greater is the urgency of procuring reference intervals ("normal values") that are time-qualified. Many oncologic variables show predictable changes recurring at similar intervals in similar sequences—in brief, rhythms. Actually, more often than not, statistically validated rhythms of several frequencies are found to characterize a series of data. Some of these rhythms are more prominent than others (18). Circadian rhythms in plasma cortisol, among the more prominent ones, have already been analyzed by special rhythmometric procedures on healthy human beings living on different continents. Good agreement of the circadian acrophase characterized the results from such studies (15), whether it was determined for an individual or for a group.

It seems important to extend studies on the individual assessability (i.e. inferential statistical quantification) of a given rhythm in conjunction with studies of the corresponding rhythm in peer groups. What is yet more important in dealing with rhythmic functions is to provide an optimal specification for serial sampling times and also for single samples (14). The latter qualification for single samples (that are currently almost exclusively used for oncologic interpretation) is the most valuable, when cost-effective and appropriate, but may not substitute in all cases for an eventual requirement of cost-effective repetitive sampling. The clinical interpretation of single samples or time series from rhythmic variables is best done, whenever possible, on an individualized basis, in addition to comparisons with corresponding distributions from a peer group. Whether one's interest is in the epidemiology of cancer, in its early diagnosis, or in its treatment, time-qualified reference intervals may avoid many pitfalls (55, 56). Stud-

[*] Senior investigators italicized.

ies along these several lines[1] are under way with cooperation among investigators in Italy (8, 55), India (16, 19), United Kingdom (35), Sweden (62), Mexico (13), Japan, and the United States. The design of cooperative work in the latter two locations and in Italy concerning the epidemiology of breast cancer, and some early results, may be of methodologic interest more broadly to oncologists. In this cooperative endeavor, blood samples for hormonal evaluation along with other physiologic variables were taken around the clock several times a year in different geographic locations from subjects with different ethnic backgrounds. This strategically placed sampling assessed a set of bioperiodicities in variables of potential interest to research on cancer in the context of diseases with so-called competing risks. In so doing, a data base was secured so that eventually sampling requirements may be specified for a cost-effective time-qualified evaluation, clinical as well as epidemiologic, of individuals as well as of groups.

Methodology for sampling and analysis thus becomes available to implement research on a rational prevention and/or treatment of disease relying on an individualized, rather than a group, definition of health by the establishment of time-qualified reference intervals and characteristics. In several variables, large differences were detectable among groups being compared by rhythmometric procedures. By contrast, correlation matrices limited, for instance, to data from a single season led to confusing and, therefore, contradictory results

Sampling of blood around the clock four times a year and the application of rhythmometric procedures revealed why previous results on but a single hormone, prolactin, could be so controversial (20, 25). Differences in characteristics of circadian and circannual rhythms in prolactin and other hormones were observed between Japanese and North American women, as well as between women with fibrocystic mastopathy and healthy controls in Italy.

Correlations were found in this study between the breast cancer risk represented (according to conventional criteria) by individuals and some of the hormonal end points gathered (with proper regard for rhythms or as rhythm characteristics at one or the other frequency). Some correlations will be presented without any causal implications primarily for the purpose of illustrating possible relationships that have to be investigated with much larger numbers of individuals, yet with fewer strategically placed samples. Eventually, this task, in view of the results presented, will be feasible on one or the other of the hormones investigated with far fewer time-specified single or multiple samples.

A risk scale was needed which, as opposed to the usual approach conventionally aimed at assessing the risk of a population, attempts to use population experience in an individualized fashion. The results from the use of such a scale will await much additional study with more rigorous data applicable to a given population. It cannot be overemphasized that it is premature at this time to extrapolate beyond the scope of these data, which are still awaiting intensive scrutiny, or to account for any geographic-ethnic, climatic, dietary, or other underlying factors. It is within our scope to emphasize, first, that differences demonstrated by the chronoepidemiologic approach are not only statistically significant but also are partly replicated and, second, that these differences, e.g. in certain circannual rhythm amplitudes, are not detectable by sampling at certain hours or seasons fixed by convenience rather than pertinence.

SUBJECTS AND METHODS

Three age groups totalling about 12 women volunteers were selected in Kyushu, Japan, and nearly twice that number in Minnesota. The group of Japanese women was considered to have a low risk of breast cancer, whereas in Minnesota two groups were formed according to then conventional epidemiologic criteria to distinguish low and high risk of breast cancer (using breast cancer in the immediate family, e.g. mother or sister = high risk; lack of any cancer in the immediate family = low risk). Each group consisted of three age groups: early postpubertal, young adult, and postmenopausal women.

The comparison of hormonal function in Japanese and North American women brought together samples from two populations (a) differing greatly with respect to death rates from breast cancer and (b) documented as such by a reasonable number of autopsies. However, one has to be aware of regional differences in breast cancer risk that may characterize a given country, notably when limitations on the number of subjects sampled restrict the use of subjects to a single region. Takeshi Hirayama (27) points out that adjusted and crude death rates for breast cancer in Fukuoka (where the Japanese subjects were sampled) were 4.9 and 6.3/100,000, respectively, as compared to 4.6 and 5.8 for all

[1] Eventually, international studies of much larger scope seem to be indicated and have begun (8, 13, 49, 55, 56, 62, 63).

Japan. Similarly, the age-adjusted death rate from breast cancer per 100,000 in 1956-1967 in Minnesota for white women was 26.360 as compared to 25.287 for the U.S.A.

Risk also depends upon age. In this study, it was our goal to cover different ages and to attempt to include as early an age as practicable. This choice was made in view of the assumption that, notably with respect to endocrine factors, there may be two possible sets of hormonal influences. One set could consist of inherited hormonal influences and the other of acquired ones.

Another important risk factor concerns marital status, since single women in Japan carry a higher risk of breast cancer than do U.S.A. white women—as revealed by Figure 37.1. This finding certainly points to the need for studying women in the two countries at different times after marriage.

Limitations in sample size prompted compromise in the design of sampling schedules for variables characterized by rhythms with different frequencies. Cost and considerations of practicality prevented the proper assessment of all components in this spectrum, yet attempts were made to take their contribution into consideration. Most subjects were sampled throughout a 24-hr span four times a year, once in each season, and in a different menstrual stage (early follicular, late follicular, early luteal, and late luteal) in each season, according to a Latin square design (47). Figures 37.2 and 37.3 display the design. During each 24-hour span 1 ml of blood was withdrawn through an i.v. catheter every 20 min and an additional 12.5 ml (for a total of 13.5 ml) of blood was taken every 100 min. Pituitary, adrenal, ovarian, thyroidal, and pancreatic functions were assessed by chemical analyses of these blood samples. Plasma prolactin and cortisol were determined every 20 min, while values for other hormones (thyroid-stimulating hormone (TSH), thyroxine (T4), triiodothyronine (T3), insulin, luteinizing hormone (LH), dehydroepiandrosterone sulfate (DHEA-S), estrone (E1), estradiol (E2), estriol (E3), aldosterone, and 17-OH-progesterone) were determined every 100 min, each by radioimmunoassay. Reagents for the determinations of human prolactin were obtained from Calbiochem, Calif., with human pituitary prolactin used as standard, 1 ng being equivalent to 0.6 ng WHO 75/504 human prolactin reference standard. Reagents for plasma cortisol were obtained from Clinical Assays, Cambridge, Mass. E1, E2, E3, and 17-OH-progesterone were determined following LH-20 column chromatography with antiserum obtained from Steranti, Ltd., England, and ^{3}H-labeled purified steroid standards from Steraloids. This method has been modified after Jaffe and Berson (29). Plasma insulin was determined with reagents obtained from Becton, Dickinson. Total DHEA-S was determined directly in plasma with reagents obtained from Radioassay Systems Laboratories using 7-^{3}H-DHEA as standard. Plasma aldosterone determinations were modified by reducing sample and reagent volumes and by using a double antibody instead of a charcoal separation technique. Reagents were obtained from Diagnostics Products and ^{125}T-labeled aldosterone standard. Reagents for the determination of human luteinizing hormone (hLH) in plasma were obtained from BIORIA, Montreal, Canada. The method is adapted from Midgley (41).

Plasma T4 and T3 were determined by radioimmunoassay with reagents obtained from Bio-Rad Laboratories, Richmond, Calif. and Pantex Laboratories, Santa Monica, Calif., respectively. Human TSH in plasma was determined by solid-phase radioimmunoassay, reagents obtained from Beckman Instruments, Fullerton, Calif. Quality control lyophilized serum speci-

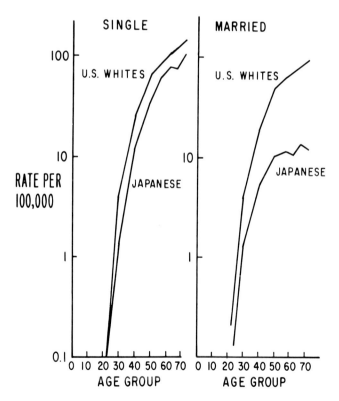

From Dr. T. Hirayama

Figure 37.1. Geographic ethnic difference in age-specific death rate for breast cancer with respect to marital status for U.S. white (1959–1961) and Japanese (1970) women. Data from Dr. T. Hirayama.

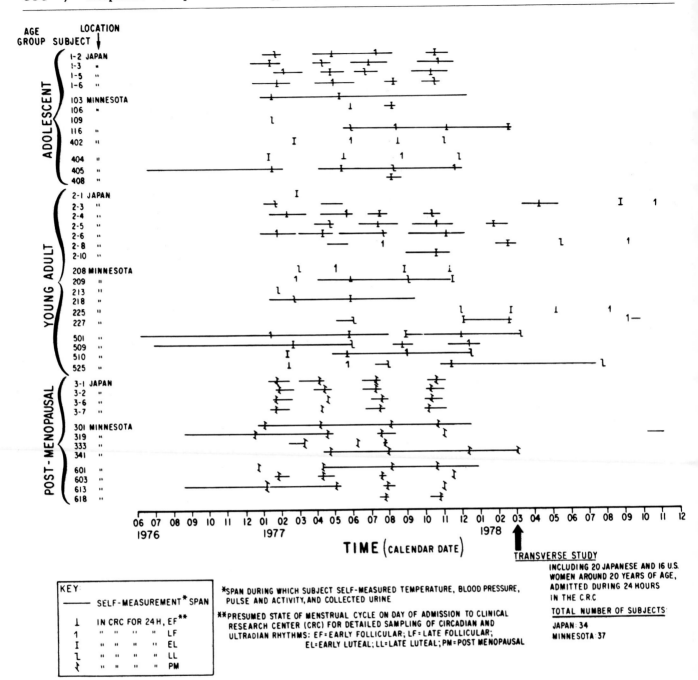

Figure 37.2. Individual sampling schemes (spans) for assessment of hemic, urinary, and other rhythms. Experimental design of Minnesota-Japan chronoepidemiologic study: schedule of hospital admission and at-home self-measurements of subjects classified according to age and geographic location, with specification of menstrual cycle stage on day of admission. (See Figure 37.3 for sampling intervals during sampling spans shown.)

mens were obtained from the following manufacturers:

Ortho Diagnostics: Ortho-V and Ortho-VI for aldosterone, Ortho-I, II, III, and IV for cortisol, E1, E2, E3, and 17-OH-progesterone, insulin, TSH, T3, and LH.

Nuclear Medical Systems: NMS-IIa for human prolactin, E1, E2, and E3, 17-OH-progesterone.

Beckman: Beckman control for serum TSH, Monitrol-I and Monitrol-II for the determination

of serum T4. References to the methods and coefficients of variation are summarized in Table 37.1.

In addition to blood hormones, adenosine deaminase activity in red blood cells was determined for some of the subjects (59). Blood was centrifuged at 500 × g for 10 min and plasma removed. The red cells were gently washed with saline, recentrifuged at 500 × g for 10 minutes; the supernatant saline was removed and the

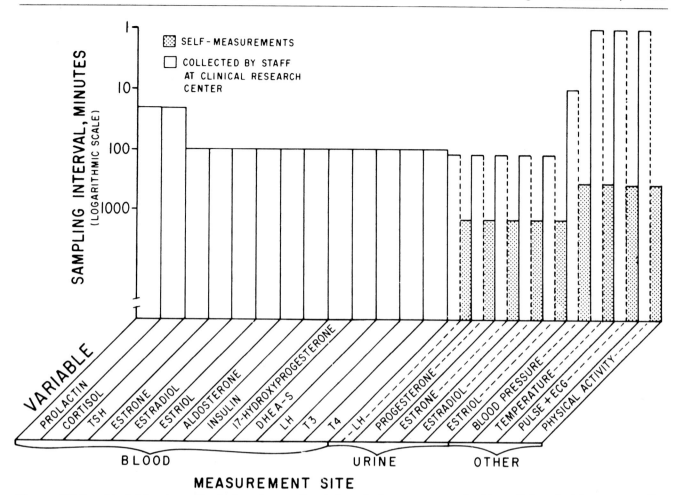

Figure 37.3. Variables investigated and sampling intervals for assessment of hospital and at-home sampling rates of hemic, urinary, and other rhythms investigated in the Minnesota-Japan chronoepidemiologic study. (See Fig. 37.2 for spans documented at intervals shown above.) *TSH*, thyroid-stimulating hormone; *DHEA-S*, dehydro-epiandrosterone sulfate; *LH*, luteinizing hormone; *T3*, triiodothyronine; *T4*, thyroxine; and *ECG*, electrocardiogram.

packed red cells were frozen at −20°C until analysis for adenosine deaminase by an automated procedure developed by Tritsch and Mittelman (60). Ammonia produced during the conversion of adenosine into inosine by the enzyme was quantified by Nesslerization. Erythrocyte adenosine deaminase activity at 37°C was expressed as µmol of NH_3/h per milliliter of packed erythrocytes and also per gram of hemoglobin.

Several physiologic variables also were monitored in the hope of elaborating relations among factors directly relevant to cancer, on the one hand, and of providing information on potential marker rhythms, on the other. The marker rhythm information is needed not only because it is more easily accessible but, what is critical, because it can be obtained with a density and over spans that may not be practicable for hormones—for economic or other reasons, such as an excessive requirement for blood or an undue interference with the daily routine of the individual investigated.

Blood pressure, breast surface temperature, activity, and EKG were automatically monitored and urine was collected every 2 hr throughout the 24-hr stay in a research center, in Minneapolis, Minn., and Fukuoka, Kyushu, Japan. Breast surface temperature was measured automatically with a so-called Medilog (Ambulatory Monitoring Inc., Ardsley, New York), and/or was self-measured with a telethermometer manufactured by the Yellow Springs Instrument Company (Yellow Springs, Ohio,), and blood pressure was measured with an Arteriosonde (Roche Medical Electronics Division, Hoffmann-La Roche, Inc., Cranbury, New Jersey). Breast surface temperature data automatically recorded on tape in an analog form were digitized and edited. Data thus were available for a given subject for one or several spans of about 24 hr, with a sampling interval of 1 min. In order to improve the signal-to-noise ratio, these data were averaged over 15-min spans.

Wrist activity was measured for 24 hr at each

Table 37.1
Coefficients of Variation (CV) for Hormonal
Determinations and References to Methods Used

Variable	CV	Reference
	%	
Aldosterone	21.2	Drewes, P. A., et al. (1973): Clin.
	14.6	Biochem., 6:88.
Cortisol	11.8	Foster, L. B., and Dunn, R. T.
	9.2	(1974): Clin. Chem., 20:365.
DHEA-S[a]	20.8	Buster, J. E., and Abraham, G. E.
	19.6	(1972): Anal. Lett., 5:543.
E1	31.1	Orczyk, G. P., et al. (1974): Meth-
	17.3	ods of Hormone Radioimmu-
	21.3	noassay, Chapt. 19, edited by
		B. Jaffe and H. Berson, Aca-
		demic Press (1974).
E2	36.0	Orczyk, G. P., et al. (1974): Meth-
	14.2	ods of Hormone Radioimmu-
	17.6	noassay, Chapt. 19, edited by
		B. Jaffe and H. Berson. Aca-
		demic Press, New York.
E3	26.7	Orczyk, G. P., et al., (1974): In
	20.3	Methods of Hormone Radioim-
	13.7	munoassay, Chapt. 19, edited
		by B. Jaffe and H. Berson, Aca-
		demic Press (1974).
Insulin	12.1	Herbert, F., Lau, K. S., Gottlieb,
	14.3	C. W., and Bleicher, S. J., (1965):
		J. Clin. Endocrinol., 25:1375–
		1384.
LH	27.0	Midgley, A. R. (1966): Endocri-
	12.3	nology, 79:10–18.
	16.0	
17-OH-Proges-	21.6	Powell, J. E., and Stevens, V. C.
terone	19.8	(1973): Clin. Chem. 19:210–215.
	19.4	
Prolactin	9.9	Sinha, Y., Selby, F. W., Lewis, U.
	10.0	J., and Vanderlaan, W. P.
		(1973): J. Clin. Endocrinol. Me-
		tab. 36:509.
TSH	10.7	Hall, R. J., Amos, J., and Ormston,
	10.9	B. (1972): Br. Med. J., 1:582.
	14.9	
T3	8.1	Chopra, I. J., and Lam, R. (1972):
	7.4	Clin. Res. 20:216.
	8.6	
T4	7.7	Chopra, I. (1972): J. Clin. Endocri-
	7.8	nol. Metab., 34:938.

[a] DHEA-S, dehydroepiandrosterone sulfate; E1, estrone; E2, estradiol; E3 estriol; LH, luteinizing hormone; TSH, thyroid-stimulating hormone; T4, thyroxine; and T3, triiodothyronine.

admission to hospital, using a piezo-electric transducer and Medilog recorder. Activity recordings were replayed in a computer system in order to digitize at 16 times a second the recorded voltages and to compute successive 5-min cumulations (33). The waking and rest and/or sleep portions of the recordings were analyzed separately by variance spectra (30).

In addition, each subject self-measured her blood pressure, pulse, and oral temperature and collected morning (and in a few cases, around-the-clock) urines for at least one menstrual cycle

(or 1 month) bracketing the hospital admission.

To complement this main investigation, a study was also carried out during a second winter season on 20 Japanese and 16 Minnesotan young women, mostly low risk, between 18 and 24 years of age. In this study, blood was sampled every 4 hr during a 24-hr span and analyzed for plasma prolactin. In addition, urine was collected every 2 hr during wakefulness and whenever a subject awoke from sleep, for assay of melatonin.

Four-hourly blood sampling throughout a 24-hr span was also applied to 22 women with fibrocystic mastopathy and to 18 clinically healthy controls in a study in Florence, Italy (55).

With the same design as that of the Kyushu-Minnesota chronoepidemiologic study, blood also was sampled through an i.v. catheter every 20 min for 24 hr at the Center for Social Medicine of the Ospedale di Urbino, in Urbino, Italy, for plasma prolactin determination by radioimmunoassay, but this assay was carried out in the Department of Medicine at the University of Rome, Italy. Hence the data of this parallel study are not strictly comparable in terms of radioimmunoassay for prolactin determination.

The single cosinor procedure (21) was used to assess any rhythmic (e.g. circadian or circannual) variation. In this procedure, a cosine curve with a period selected on the basis of a priori knowledge is fitted to the data, using the method of least squares. An F-statistic is then used to test the zero-amplitude hypothesis for a circadian, circannual, and other rhythm. For statistically validated rhythms ($P \leq 0.05$), the following parameters are estimated: the mesor (rhythm-adjusted mean), the amplitude (half the total extent of predictable change) and the acrophase (crest time of the best-fitting cosine function, in relation to a given reference time—such as local midnight or preferably midrest (midsleep) at the outset for circadian rhythms and midnight on December 22 of the year preceding data collection for circannual rhythms).

It is often desirable, with a small sample size available, to consider all rhythm characteristics from the time series on hand, whether or not the zero-amplitude assumption is rejected. As discussed earlier by Halberg et al. (24), the rhythm characteristics are then regarded as imputations, i.e. as intermediate calculations. In this case, additional methods along more classical lines are desired whenever possible. A mesor, for instance, could be replaced by the series mean; in the actual cases discussed (since the vast majority of samples, except for a few missed time points, was obtained at equidistant intervals over integral multiples of at least the circadian period being analyzed) means and mesors will differ rarely and if so only slightly. In any event, in dealing with "imputed" amplitudes, one can gain insight into the statistical significance of a relationship between dynamic indices that would go unassessed in a conventional analysis of variance. It is pertinent, further, that the use of imputation in an operation bootstrap may lead to statistically significant conclusions for the group in cases when sampling is insufficient to establish the corresponding relation for the individual.

Wave-form may also be portrayed by plotting a plexogram (5) whenever data covering several cycles are available. In this procedure, the different cycles are folded onto one, thus providing confidence intervals for the mean at each time-point within that (folded) cycle. When only short but equidistant time series can be obtained, a harmonic interpolation serves to compute a paraphase, *i.e.* the lag from a reference time of the peak in the harmonically interpolated function (6). This method reconstructs a continuous function from the samples on the basis of a spectral decomposition, using all harmonics. Whenever information is available concerning the variance of the noise affecting the data, it is also possible to derive confidence limits around the reconstructed curve or wave-form.

Several authors have previously defined breast cancer risk factors and have suggested their use. Robert L. Egan (10) estimated risk for asymptomatic and minimally symptomatic breast cancer patients, demonstrating the feasibility of using simultaneously large numbers of risk factors in a systematic way to pinpoint patients with mammary cancer. Breast cancer patients have been found to marry later, have shorter lactational histories, and have fewer children when compared to controls (37). A study by Sartwell *et al.* (53) showed breast cancer to be associated with nulliparity, first pregnancy over 20 years of age, premenopausal status, and frequency of artificial menopause.

Hormonal status has also been repeatedly considered as a risk factor. Farewell *et al.* (11) included etiocholanolone excretion with three historical risk factors—age of menarche, family history, and age at first pregnancy. In studying menstrual patterns, Wallace *et al.* (61) suggested that late menopause may be a breast cancer risk factor resulting from relative estrogen excess and progesterone lack. Cole and Cramer (4) suggested the saturated fatty acid component of the diet as another risk factor. Miller (42) furthers

this idea by suggesting that dietary factors mediated through a hormonal mechanism play a major role in breast cancer etiology.

The risk scale for this chronoepidemiologic breast cancer study was developed using risk factors as identified by MacMahon *et al.* (36) and Choi *et al.* (3). The risk factor scale is based upon the following items:

1. Geographic area of residence		
	North America and Northern Europe	+5
	South America and Southern Europe	+2.5
2. Benign breast disease		+4
3. Other primary cancers		
	Cancer of major salivary glands	+4
	Cancer of colon and/or uterus	+2
4. Familial aggregation		+3
5. Obesity		
	≥ 68 kg in postmenopausal women ≥ 70 years	+3
6. Age		
	After 30 years of age (for every decade)	+2
7. Late first pregnancy		
	After 30 years of age	+2
8. Early menarche		
	Before 16 years of age	+2
9. Late menopause		
	After 55 years of age	+2
a. Early pregnancy		
	Before 25 years of age	−0.5
b. Surgical menopause		−0.4

The total risk for an individual was calculated by simply adding all the risk numbers relevant to that individual from the foregoing risk scale.

We illustrate below the procedure used to assign a risk number to an individual: if none of the above listed factors apply, the individual's total breast cancer risk is equated to unity. The risk number of 5 is assigned to a woman in North America, without any other pertinent characteristic listed above. If this woman has benign breast disease, her risk (+4) becomes 9, as long as she lives most of the time in North America.

A statistical correlation was computed between the individual's total risks and certain first order statistics, such as circannual prolactin or TSH amplitudes. Using a linear regression procedure, the total risk can thus be correlated with the circannual amplitude expressed in nanograms per milliliter and also as percentage of mesor.

To explore the potential clinical usefulness of thermorhythmometry, breast surface temperatures also were monitored with a 10-channel Yellow Springs telethermometer from the nipple and four quadrants of each breast during wakefulness, at 2-hr intervals, for 4 days from three groups each composed of eight women; 1, presumably healthy; 2, with nonmalignant conditions; and 3, with breast cancer, at the Hospital de Oncologia, Mexico City, Mexico. A so-called chronobiologic window (22)—with 0.2-hr intervals between consecutive trial periods ranging from 20 to 28 hr—was fitted to the ten series from each woman.

RESULTS

Individualized Circadian Rhythm Assessment for Cortisol and Prolactin

For each hormone, in each season, the 24-hr series from each subject was analyzed by the single cosinor. Figure 37.4 portrays the observed hierarchy of statistical significance for individualized circadian variation in 13 of the hormones studied. For prolactin and cortisol, the characteristics of a 24-hr synchronized rhythm were confidently measured with their probable errors on an individual basis for almost all subjects, in Kyushu and Minnesota as well as in Italy.

A Spectrum of Rhythms

Circadian Hormonal Rhythms

The estimates of circadian rhythm parameters were similar for most subjects sampled from each population. This was statistically verified by applying the population-mean cosinor procedure (24) to each group as a whole. Table 37.2 indicates that for each group of subjects a statistically significant circadian rhythm could be demonstrated for most of the hormones investigated, including those for which circadian rhythms were difficult to assess on an individual basis.

Table 37.2 also reveals that a population circadian rhythm could be demonstrated in all four seasons in both Japanese and Minnesotan subjects, for prolactin, cortisol, and DHEA-S and, with very few exceptions, for insulin, TSH, T3, T4, 17-OH progesterone, and aldosterone. In the case of E1, E2, E3, and LH, a statistically significant cosine-fitting to describe a group rhythm was not achieved. This finding suggests, if not a

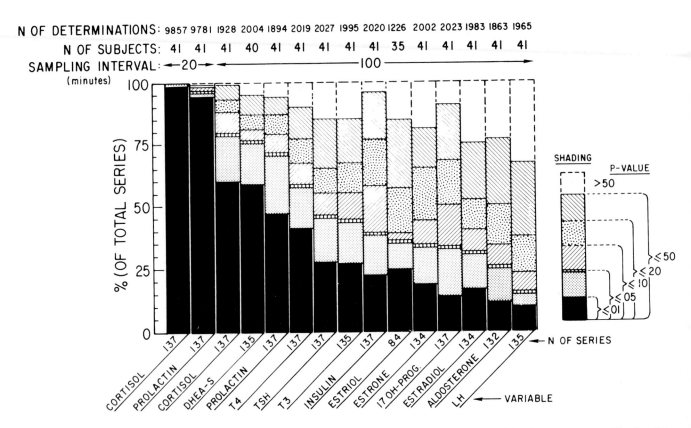

Figure 37.4. Comparison of statistical significance of circadian rhythm, assessed by least-squares fit of a 24-hour cosine curve for 13 hormones in plasma of healthy women sampled for *individualized* rhythm assessment. *P* from F-test of zero-amplitude hypothesis. Since the hierarchical statistical significance represented by *P*-values is sampling-dependent, prolactin and cortisol, measured every 20 min, were also analyzed at 100-min intervals as for the other hormones. Total number (*N*) of determinations = 40765.

Table 37.2
Circadian Mean Cosinors of Several Hormones in Human Plasma from Two Populations (Japan and Minnesota) at Four Different Seasons

Hormone (units)	Japan (N ≅ 12)[a]				Minnesota (N ≅ 24)			
	P	M (±SE)	A	φ	P	M (±SE)	A	φ
			Winter	Deg				Deg
Prolactin (ng/ml)	<0.001	24.8 (±2.4)	16.6	−47	<0.001	18.4 (±1.8)	8.0	−46
Cortisol (µg/dl)	<0.001	6.9 (±0.4)	4.2	−134	<0.001	9.0 (±0.4)	4.9	−138
Insulin (µU/ml)	0.06	23.7 (±3.6)	7.8	−243	<0.001	18.3 (±1.5)	9.2	−235
TSH (µIU/ml)	0.02	4.3 (±3.6)	0.3	−21	0.27	6.4 (±1.3)	1.1	−47
DHEA-S (ng/ml)	<0.001	1390.0 (±200.0)	250.0	−221	<0.001	1980.0 (±260.0)	290.0	−230
T3 (ng/dl)	0.76	104.0 (±7.1)	3.4	−229	0.002	96.8 (±4.2)	6.6	−211
17-OH-Progesterone (pg/ml)	0.09	552.0 (±182.0)	42.0	−80	0.23	518.0 (±91.0)	46.0	−185
T4 (µg/dl)	<0.001	7.1 (±0.3)	0.4	−212	<0.001	6.4 (±0.3)	0.5	−235
Aldosterone (ng/dl)	0.002	5.2 (±0.4)	1.5	−113	0.07	8.9 (±1.1)	1.3	−135
E1 (pg/ml)	0.16	81.0 (±15.5)	6.5	−235	0.93	86.1 (±9.6)	0.9	−93
E2 (pg/ml)	0.64	94.8 (±33.2)	7.3	−94	0.31	76.3 (±14.0)	4.4	−211
E3 (pg/ml)	0.86	18.9 (±3.8)	1.1	−257	0.38	13.5 (±3.1)	2.2	−285
LH (mIU/ml)	0.83	34.4 (±7.3)	1.1	−105	0.66	34.9 (±6.4)	1.4	−243
			Spring					
Prolactin (ng/ml)	<0.001	19.3 (±2.4)	14.2	−42	<0.001	17.2 (±1.5)	7.8	−45
Cortisol (µg/dl)	<0.001	10.0 (±0.6)	5.3	−120	<0.001	9.3 (±0.4)	5.3	−134
Insulin (µU/ml)	0.007	23.3 (±2.7)	8.9	−195	<0.001	21.7 (±1.6)	10.6	−225
TSH (µIU/ml)	0.006	4.1 (±0.3)	0.5	−1	0.07	5.2 (±0.8)	0.5	−21
DHEA-S (ng/ml)	0.05	1860.0 (±350.0)	280.0	−182	<.001	2250.0 (±420.0)	270.0	−236
T3 (ng/dl)	0.02	105.0 (±5.3)	12.0	−270	.005	94.0 (±7.1)	5.8	−255
17-OH-Progesterone (pg/ml)	0.85	423.0 (±85.0)	38.0	−309	.002	368.0 (±45.0)	75.0	−130
T4 (µg/dl)	0.04	7.2 (±0.3)	0.3	−187	<0.001	7.2 (±0.4)	0.3	−232
Aldosterone (ng/dl)	0.02	4.9 (±0.6)	1.7	−85	0.05	5.5 (±0.9)	1.3	−117
E1 (pg/ml)	0.83	91.4 (±12.6)	2.6	−84	0.006	67.2 (±11.6)	9.9	−122
E2 (pg/ml)	0.48	62.1 (±17.5)	4.2	−350	0.03	57.8 (±13.4)	5.2	−47
E3 (pg/ml)	0.19	26.7 (±6.5)	11.1	−354	0.11	34.4 (±4.8)	4.3	−237
LH (mIU/ml)	0.17	30.5 (±6.9)	2.8	−316	0.49	39.9 (±9.1)	1.5	−157
			Summer					
Prolactin (ng/ml)	0.003	15.1 (±1.2)	9.5	−39	<0.001	15.9 (±1.2)	7.7	−61
Cortisol (µg/dl)	<0.001	8.3 (±0.5)	5.7	−128	<0.001	9.8 (±0.4)	5.8	−143
Insulin (µU/ml)	<0.001	26.4 (±4.0)	11.2	−243	<0.001	24.4 (±2.4)	15.5	−234
TSH (µIU/ml)	<0.001	4.2 (±0.4)	0.7	−31	0.13	5.4 (±0.09)	0.8	−40
DHEA-S (ng/ml)	0.002	1070.0 (±220.0)	140.0	−206	<0.001	1370.0 (±190.0)	270.0	−223
T3 (ng/dl)	0.03	92.0 (±6.7)	4.8	−249	<0.001	95.0 (±3.6)	6.8	−248
17-OH-Progesterone (pg/ml)	0.006	600.0 (±219.0)	71.0	−107	0.004	543.0 (±115.0)	72.0	−132
T4 (µg/dl)	0.06	7.5 (±4.2)	0.2	−208	<0.001	7.0 (±0.3)	0.4	−238
Aldosterone (ng/dl)	0.003	4.2 (±0.7)	1.1	−115	0.54	6.3 (±1.0)	0.5	−242
E1 (pg/ml)	0.35	45.4 (±8.8)	1.3	−202	0.96	61.5 (±8.2)	0.3	−47
E2 (pg/ml)	0.10	50.7 (±14.1)	11.1	−67	0.15	65.8 (±15.2)	5.2	−350
E3 (pg/ml)	0.71	9.4 (±3.2)	1.2	−40	0.03	18.4 (±2.6)	5.3	−217
LH (mIU/ml)	0.13	39.5 (±11.0)	3.6	−278	0.67	46.6 (±10.5)	0.9	−138
			Fall					
Prolactin (ng/ml)	0.003	20.4 (±4.4)	9.8	−47	<0.001	15.0 (±1.0)	7.8	−45
Cortisol (µg/dl)	<0.001	8.8 (±0.5)	5.1	−122	<0.001	8.7 (±0.3)	5.2	−135
Insulin (µU/ml)	0.002	23.5 (±3.0)	13.5	−234	<0.001	29.1 (±2.3)	19.1	−238
TSH (µIU/ml)	0.008	3.1 (±0.2)	0.5	−24	<0.001	4.9 (±0.7)	0.8	−33
DHEA-S (ng/ml)	<0.001	1410.0 (±200.0)	200.0	−231	<0.001	1370.0 (±230.0)	230.0	−234
T3 (ng/dl)	0.01	104.0 (±4.9)	5.4	−249	<0.001	105.0 (±3.1)	5.6	−233
17-OH-Progesterone (pg/ml)	<0.001	414.0 (±117.0)	78.0	−107	0.47	570.0 (±139.0)	41.0	−114
T4 (µg/dl)	0.004	7.6 (±2.8)	0.4	−235	<0.001	7.1 (±0.2)	0.4	−221
Aldosterone (ng/dl)	<0.001	5.3 (±0.6)	1.9	−108	0.45	7.3 (±0.9)	0.5	−206
E1 (pg/ml)	0.64	72.6 (±12.7)	1.6	−157	0.58	61.0 (±9.0)	2.7	−92
E2 (pg/ml)	0.32	69.9 (±18.8)	4.2	−113	0.07	81.0 (±17.7)	7.6	−5
E3 (pg/ml)	0.99	13.4 (±3.0)	0.3	−50	0.15	13.9 (±1.8)	2.3	−212
LH (mIU/ml)	0.74	29.5 (±7.8)	2.8	−346	0.46	43.5 (±8.5)	1.0	−246

[a] N, number of subjects; P, P-value derived from the zero amplitude test; M, mesor; SE, standard error: A, amplitude; φ, acrophase (360° ≡ 24 hr; 0° = 00.00); TSH, thyroid-stimulating hormone; DHEA-S, dehydroepiandrosterone sulfate; T3, triiodothyronine; T4, thyroxine; E1, estrone; E2, estradiol; E3, estriol; LH, luteinizing hormone; mIU, milli-international unit.

different behavior of the estrogens and the luteinizing hormone as compared to the other hormones, at least an unfavorable signal-to-noise ratio, wherein the uncertainties associated with the technique of hormone determination may play a sizable role and more refined techniques will have to scrutinize the noise term.

Circannual Hormonal Rhythms

For each hormone, circannual mean-cosinors (24) were obtained from the least squares fit of a 365.25-day cosine curve to the circadian mesors of those clinically healthy women who contributed data during four seasons. Table 37.3 shows that in Minnesota a circannual rhythm could be demonstrated at or near the 5% level for plasma insulin, TSH, E1, aldosterone and DHEA-S. In Japan, a statistically significant circannual rhythm was found for plasma prolactin and estriol while any circannual variation in plasma TSH and DHEA-S was associated with a P of only ~0.10.

Circatrigintan Hormonal Variation

Apart from circadian and circannual rhythms in human plasma hormones, other components may also contribute to the variability of the data. A circatrigintan (about 30-day) prolactin rhythm, difficult to assess in this investigation, was demonstrated by our analysis of longitudi-

nal, if sparse, data published by Gala et al. (12). Gala et al. sampled blood from a 27-year-old woman once weekly between 09:00 and 10:00 hr starting June 1975 and continuing for 13 months. Serum prolactin was analyzed in chronobiologic windows (17) with trial periods between 40 and 20 days, with a decrement of 6 hr between consecutive trial periods, and then by a nonlinear least squares procedure (52) following Marquardt's program (39).

The results from spectral analysis of these data suggested that a circatrigintan component was present in the time series, with a period fluctuating from about 30 days (the average length of the menstrual cycle of this woman) at the beginning of the observation span up to about 38 days, which is the prevailing component in the overall observation span. The validity of the circatrigintan component in more appropriately sampled time series and the possibility of internal circatrigintan desynchronization of the prolactin rhythm from the menstrual cycle certainly deserve follow-up.

In our investigation, circatrigintan variation has thus far been examined only for prolactin and cortisol, by fitting individual circadian mesors estimated at different stages of the menstrual cycle with an arbitrary 28-day cosine curve, using the least squares method. For the case of prolactin in North American subjects, a circatrigintan variation of borderline statistical significance could be demonstrated in this way. In this approach, interindividual variability, some uncertainty about the actual menstrual stage at the time of sampling and other factors

Table 37.3
Circannual Variation Investigated by Population-Mean Cosinor Procedure on 13 Hormones in Clinically Healthy Women[a]

Variable (units)	JAPAN (N = 11)[b]				MINNESOTA (N ≅ 17)			
	PR	M (±SE)	A/M	ϕ	PR	M (±SE)	A/M	ϕ
			%				%	
Prolactin (ng/ml)	74	26.8 (±8.3)	19.9	−331	65	16.7 (±1.4)		
Cortisol (μg/dl)	41	8.6 (±0.5)			70	9.3 (±0.3)		
Insulin (μU/ml)	64	24.0 (±2.8)			64	21.8 (±1.4)	18.5	−214
T4 (μg/dl)	70	7.4 (±0.3)			74	6.9 (±0.3)		
TSH (μIU/ml)	72	4.1 (±0.2)			80	5.8 (±1.0)	14.4	−325
17-OH Progesterone (pg/ml)	70	474.0 (±111.0)			81	512.0 (±74.0)		
E1 (pg/ml)	62	69.9 (±11.1)			75	71.7 (±7.6)	29.0	−72
E2 (pg/ml)	73	70.4 (±17.2)			66	71.1 (±11.4)		
E3 (pg/ml)	74	14.1 (±2.5)	72.0	−70	77	13.0 (±1.9)		
Aldosterone (ng/dl)	81	4.9 (±0.4)			78	7.1 (±0.8)	25.5	−11
DHEA-S (ng/ml)	57	1519.0 (±253.0)			69	1697.0 (±227.0)	22.2	−74
T3 (ng/dl)	63	103.3 (±4.6)			77	98.8 (±3.1)		
LH (mIU/ml)	63	35.6 (±8.8)			71	38.8 (±6.9)		

[a] Each contributing 72 plasma samples during four or more seasons.
[b] N, number of subjects; PR, percentage rhythm; M, mesor (or mean); SE, standard error; A, amplitude; ϕ, acrophase (reference: December 22; 360° ≡ 365.25 days); A/M and ϕ given only when P-value (from zero amplitude test) ≤ 0.05.

contribute a very large error term. Moreover, circatrigintan rhythms may differ in frequency among different individuals or at least may exhibit less frequency and/or acrophase synchronization than circadian rhythms. From the viewpoint of intra- as well as interindividual synchronization, they may compare unfavorably with circannual and circadian rhythms.

Ultradian Hormonal Variation

On prolactin and cortisol, sampled every 20 min, ultradian frequencies were investigated also. Using the same zero-amplitude test as that used in the cosinor procedure, each harmonic of the 24-hr period was tested for statistical "significance" over the possible spectral range. All statistically significant "candidate" harmonics were then ranked by increasing amplitude: the most prominent frequency was thus assigned rank 1, the second most prominent was assigned rank 2, and so on. These ultradian ranks were highly variable.

It is interesting to search for differences in the spectral representations of cortisol and prolactin. For both hormones, the circadian component accounted for the largest share of variability in the data (~46% for prolactin and ~53% for cortisol). The circadian rhythm was the most prominent in 86% of all individual profiles on prolactin, and in 97% of the cortisol profiles. Whatever its origin, nonsinusoidality or other, a statistically "significant" 12-hr harmonic was present in 78% of the series for prolactin, accounting for ~18% of the total variance, and in only 44% of the series for cortisol, accounting for only ~10% of the total variance. A statistically "significant" component with a period less than 6 hr could be demonstrated in 22% of the prolactin profiles and in 33% of the cortisol profiles. The mean period of all ultradians with a period less than 6 hr was between 3 and 4 hr for both prolactin and cortisol.

Circadian Hormonal Wave-Form

In order to obtain a better idea of the waveform for prolactin and cortisol rhythms, data from all volunteers sampled during the winter in Japan and in Minnesota were averaged over consecutive 3-hr spans to yield circadian "plexograms." Figures 37.5 and 37.6 portray the plexograms for prolactin and cortisol, respectively, in each of the two geographic locations, while

Figures 37.7 and 37.8 give the corresponding curves reconstructed (from the 3-hr averages) by harmonic interpolation. Figures 37.5 and 37.6 reveal that, at night, prolactin concentrations are higher in Japanese than in Minnesotan women. With harmonic interpolation, a second peak in late afternoon (prolactin) or early afternoon (cortisol) also could be found for the Japanese subjects. This result is interesting in regard to a publication by Kwa et al. (34) reporting an evening elevation of plasma prolactin in postmenopausal women and to another publication by Tarquini et al. (54) on abnormalities in evening plasma prolactin concentrations in nulliparous women with benign or malignant breast disease. Table 37.4 compares acrophases (from the fit of a 24-hr cosine curve) and paraphases (from harmonic interpolation) for prolactin and cortisol in both geographic locations. Very good agreement of these two indices is achieved in the case of prolactin, while a difference of about 2 hr is observed in the case of cortisol. This may be explained by the fact that the cortisol peak is much sharper than the prolactin peak. Of inter-

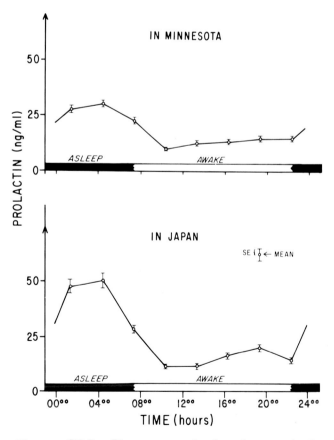

Figure 37.5. Plexogram of circadian prolactin rhythms obtained by pooling, over 3-hr spans, winter data for women from all Minnesotans (*above*) and all Japanese (*below*).

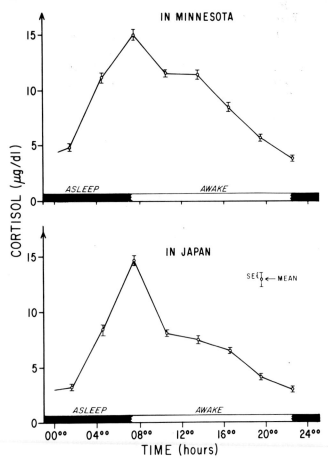

Figure 37.6. Plexogram of circadian cortisol rhythms obtained by pooling, over 3-hr spans, winter data for women from all Minnesotans (*above*) and all Japanese (*below*).

est is the good agreement of acrophases and paraphases between the two populations.

Potential Marker Rhythms: Blood Pressure, Breast Temperature, and Wrist Activity

In the case of a physiologic variable, it is interesting to note that with blood pressure data taken every 10 min, the circadian rhythm could be assessed in most subjects. The acrophases, however, were quite different from one individual to another. This was not observed for the circadian rhythm in prolactin or cortisol (see Figures 37.9–37.11) and may indicate the action of a completely different mechanism in the physiology of the individual.

A population-mean cosinor analysis was performed on blood pressure data in each season (considering all subjects sampled) to yield the results shown in Table 37.5. From the systolic and diastolic blood pressures, the pulse pressure and mean arterial pressure were computed and analyzed. The acrophases for all four variables

occurred in the early afternoon. It can also be seen from Table 37.5 that the mesor and the amplitude of the circadian rhythm in systolic blood pressure underwent circannual changes.

Figures 37.12 and 37.13 summarize the blood pressure results for all Minnesotan subjects pooled over all seasons.

Table 37.6 gives an account of the number of individual series for which a statistically significant circadian rhythm could be demonstrated by rejecting the zero-amplitude hypothesis (single cosinor procedure).

A circadian rhythm of breast surface temperature was demonstrated. Frequency analysis, similar to a discrete Fourier transform, applied to the standard deviations of the 15-min averages yielded ultradians with a period of about 2 hr, at least in some of the series analyzed thus far. Further analyses will have to be carried out to investigate any possible rhythmicity in the noise term.

Daytime wrist activity was analyzed by computing an averaged spectrum. The percentage variance at 12–16 cycles/day was found to be more than double the random expectation. This

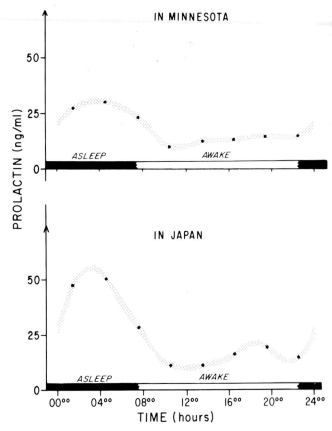

Figure 37.7. Wave-form of circadian prolactin rhythms reconstructed by harmonic interpolation, from data for women from Minnesota (*above*) and Japan (*below*), summarized as plexograms in Figure 37.5.

result was also confirmed by a *t*-test and Wilcoxon signed rank test comparing the variance at this frequency for the group of subjects investigated with the random expectation, which was exceeded significantly ($P < 0.005$). Plots of the wrist activity data analyzed thus far, however, revealed no regular or stable ultradian rhythms, and the spectral analyses demonstrated no variance peaks in the predicted 12–16 cycles/day frequency band. Thus, there was no well-defined ultradian rhythm, although most of the variance was concentrated below four cycles/day, in the circadian range and its harmonics.

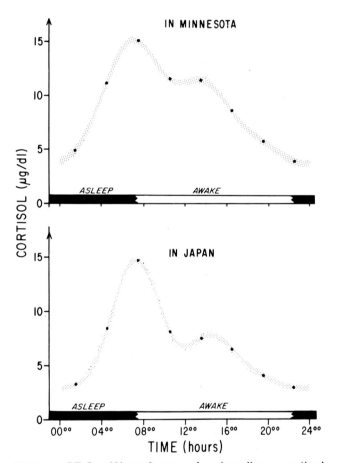

Figure 37.8. Wave-form of circadian cortisol rhythms reconstructed by harmonic interpolation, from data for women from Minnesota (*above*) and Japan (*below*), summarized as plexograms in Figure 37.6.

Time-Specified Reference Intervals

Against the background of such a spectrum of rhythms, one can determine proper reference intervals. Time-unqualified tolerance intervals will not be appropriate since a large share of variability can be accounted for by circadian, circannual, or other variations. On a short-term basis, circadian time-specified tolerance intervals—so-called chronodesms (17, 23)—can be determined to provide reference intervals against which time-qualified single samples can be interpreted cost-effectively. Chronodesms present the advantage of being usually narrower than time-unqualified "normal ranges," since part of the variance on the latter is due to the rhythmic behavior of the physiologic variable. This means that a given value can be too high at one time, too low at another, or "normal" at yet another time (Fig. 37.14).

The fact that 7 out of 13 hormones could be shown to exhibit marked circannual variation (Table 37.3), even with relatively few subjects, suggests the need for supplementary circannual chronodesms, in addition to circadian ones, as reference standards in cancer epidemiology and probably in the clinic quite broadly.

Observed Differences

Prolactin in Kyushu and Minnesota—First Study

Age-specific mortality and morbidity rates attributed to breast cancer (27, 28) are 6 times larger in the U.S.A. than they are in Japan. Among the hormones suspected of playing a role in the development of human breast cancer, prolactin has aroused much interest. Prolactin was indeed shown (1, 40, 48) to be essential for the promotion of both spontaneous and carcinogen-induced mammary tumors in rodents. The role of prolactin in the pathogenesis of human breast cancer, however, is uncertain (2) and controversial,

Table 37.4
Comparison of Acrophases and Paraphases[a] for Circadian Rhythms in Prolactin and Cortisol

Hormone	Acrophase		Paraphase			
	Japan	Minnesota	Japan			Minnesota
			Main Peak	Second Peak		
	($\pm$SE)[b]		deg	deg		deg
Prolactin	-48 ± 17	-51 ± 15	$-36 < -45 < -57$	$-225 < -279 < -297$		$-30 < -51 < -95$
Cortisol	-135 ± 17	-144 ± 10	$-105 < -110 < -114$	$-195 < -217 < -232$		$-97 < -107 < -119$

[a] Acrophases and paraphases expressed in degrees; $360° \equiv 24$ hr; reference time, local midnight (*P*-values all ≤0.05).
[b] SE, standard error

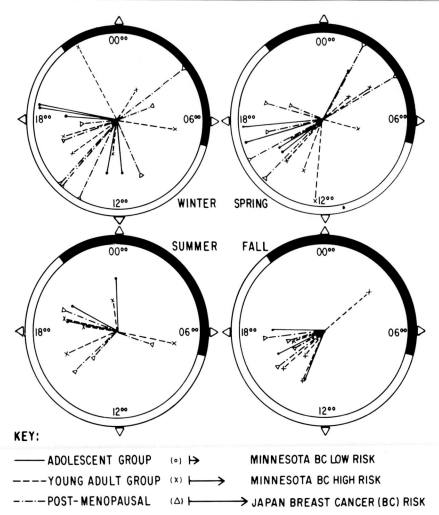

KEY:

——— ADOLESCENT GROUP　(∘) ⊢▷　　MINNESOTA BC LOW RISK

– – – – YOUNG ADULT GROUP　(x) ⊢——→　MINNESOTA BC HIGH RISK

– · – · – POST-MENOPAUSAL　(△) ⊢———→ JAPAN BREAST CANCER (BC) RISK

Figure 37.9. Circadian acrophases of systolic blood pressure in adolescent, young adult, and postmenopausal women from Japan and the two breast cancer risk groups from Minnesota in each of the four seasons show high variability despite individual statistical significance of circadian rhythm.

This chronoepidemiologic study has demonstrated differences between women from different ethnic-geographic backgrounds in plasma prolactin, with the magnitude and even the sign of some of these differences dependent upon circadian and circannual rhythm stage. The mesor and amplitude of the circadian rhythm in prolactin and the circannual variations in circadian prolactin mesor and amplitude are much more prominent in Japanese women than in Minnesotan women (Fig. 37.15 and 37.16). Moreover, the circannual prolactin mesors in Japanese are higher than the corresponding values in Minnesotan women.

These differences can also be seen from Figure 37.17, displaying mean prolactin circadian profiles for subjects in Minnesota and in Japan for all four seasons. Here again, one can see that Minnesotan women tend to have lower prolactin values than Japanese women when prolactin concentrations are high, i.e. during the night. This difference is more accentuated in winter

and can hardly be discerned in summer.

A large but time-restricted difference in plasma prolactin concentration between Japanese and Minnesotan subjects could be observed during the winter season. The difference was less prominent during the other seasons and was statistically not significant during summer. This finding indicates the importance of sampling time in investigations of the role of certain hormones in oncogenesis. It also may explain previous discrepancies and controversies reported in the literature and provides a clue to possible differences in circadian physiological time structure of groups of women with different risks of developing breast cancer.

Kyushu-Minnesota Replication of Prolactin Study

This large but strictly time-dependent difference between Japanese and Minnesotan women

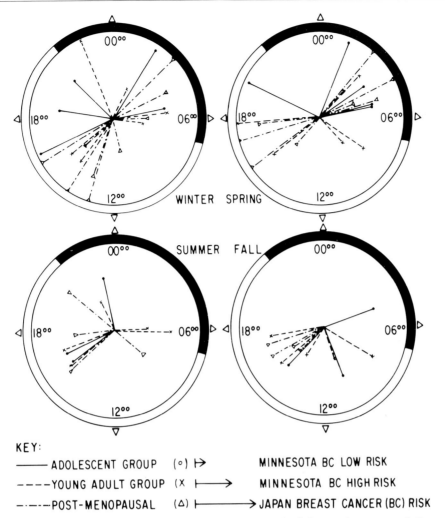

KEY:
——— ADOLESCENT GROUP (○) ⊢→   MINNESOTA BC LOW RISK
---- YOUNG ADULT GROUP (× ⊢——→   MINNESOTA BC HIGH RISK
–·–· POST-MENOPAUSAL (△) ⊢———→ JAPAN BREAST CANCER (BC) RISK

Figure 37.10. Circadian acrophases of diastolic blood pressure of adolescent, young adult, and postmenopausal women from Japan and the two breast cancer risk groups from Minnesota in each of the four seasons show high variability despite individual statistical significance of circadian rhythm.

was confirmed in groups of 20 young and 15 adult subjects examined at one circannual stage (first part of March) in Fukuoka City, Kyushu, Japan and Minneapolis, Minnesota, respectively, the Japanese showing higher average circadian prolactin mesors and a higher circadian amplitude than did the Minnesotans, Figure 37.18. This observation emphasizes the critical importance of appropriate timing of sampling of endocrine functions of potential interest for oncogenesis by single or by a limited number of samples chosen on the basis of chronobiologic individual or group reference values.

Prolactin Study in Urbino, Italy

The circadian prolactin amplitude and mesor of a postmenopausal woman, 55 years of age, were lower than the mesors and amplitudes of three series from a 23-year-old woman, Table 37.8 and Figure 37.19. This result is in keeping

with a statistically significant decrease in prolactin mesor found in groups of women studied in Minnesota before and after menopause.

Prolactin Study in Florence, Italy

A statistically significant mean circadian rhythm in serum prolactin was observed in groups of 22 women with fibrocystic mastopathy and of 18 clinically healthy women, sampled in Italy with circadian but not circannual idiocyclicity (see below) (55). The circadian amplitude and acrophase were similar in the two groups but the mesor was statistically significantly higher in patients with fibrocystic mastopathy as compared to the controls. This result suggests that circadian mesor-hyperprolactinemia is a feature associated with fibrocystic mastopathy (Fig. 37.20).

A circannual rhythm in circadian mesors of

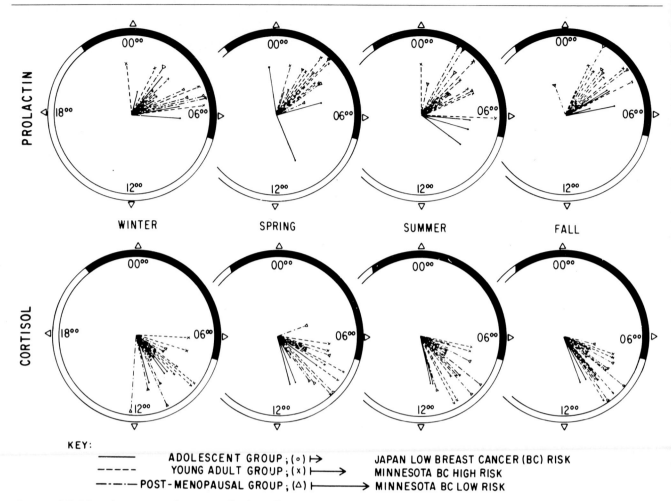

KEY:

————	ADOLESCENT GROUP; (○) ↦	JAPAN LOW BREAST CANCER (BC) RISK
– – – –	YOUNG ADULT GROUP; (×) ⟼	MINNESOTA BC HIGH RISK
–·—·–	POST-MENOPAUSAL GROUP; (△) ⟼	MINNESOTA BC LOW RISK

Figure 37.11. As opposed to systolic (see Fig. 37.9) and diastolic (see Fig. 37.10) blood pressure, circadian acrophases of plasma prolactin, and cortisol of adolescent, young adult, and postmenopausal women from Japan and the breast cancer risk groups from Minnesota in each of the four seasons show a higher degree of synchronization.

Table 37.5
Comparison of Circadian Rhythm Characteristics With Respect to Seasons in Minnesotan Women

Season	P-value	Number of series	Mesor	Amplitude	Acrophase[a]
				torr	deg
		Systolic Blood Pressure			
Winter	0.02	19	105.2	3.2	−225
Spring	0.07	20	101.3	2.4	−227
Summer	0.07	20	100.5	2.6	−252
Fall	<0.01	18	105.3	7.8	−235
		Diastolic Blood Pressure			
Winter	0.03	19	66.7	1.5	−197
Spring	0.11	20	66.8	1.5	−199
Summer	0.33	20	66.6	1.5	−250
Fall	<0.01	18	66.2	4.2	−229

[a] 360° ≡ 24 hr; 0° = local midnight.

serum prolactin also was detected in healthy Italian women (55). With the same sampling schedule, a circannual rhythm in serum prolactin was not detected in women with fibrocystic mastopathy, although circadian rhythms could be found also in this group of subjects, which on the basis of a different risk factor show a higher likelihood of developing breast cancer. As in the comparison of women in Kyushu and Minnesota, the extent of predictable circannual prolactin variation in these Italian subjects decreased as the risk of breast cancer increased.

Circannual Prolactin Amplitude and Breast Cancer Risk

In correlating the total breast cancer risk in any one subject in the Minnesota-Kyushu study with her circannual amplitude of prolactin, expressed as nanograms per milliliter, a negative correlation (-0.42; $P = 0.025$) was clearly apparent and is visualized in Figure 37.21A. When the circannual amplitude of prolactin is expressed as percentage of mesor (rather than nanograms per milliliter), its correlation coefficient with the

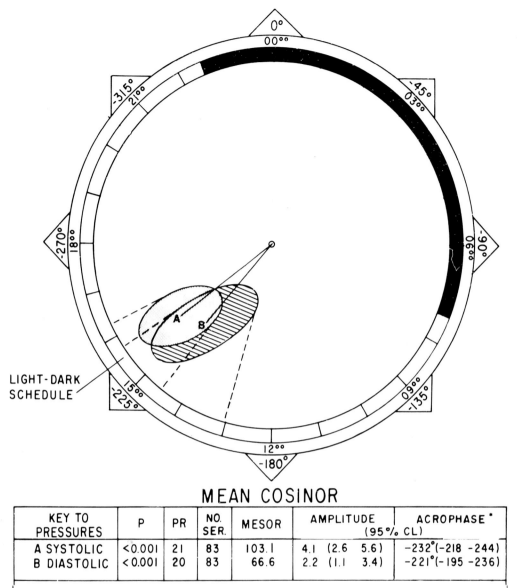

MEAN COSINOR

KEY TO PRESSURES	P	PR	NO. SER.	MESOR	AMPLITUDE (95% CL)		ACROPHASE* (95% CL)
A SYSTOLIC	<0.001	21	83	103.1	4.1	(2.6 5.6)	−232°(−218 −244)
B DIASTOLIC	<0.001	20	83	66.6	2.2	(1.1 3.4)	−221°(−195 −236)

P=PROBABILITY OF HYPOTHESIS AMPLITUDE =0 ; PR=PERCENT RHYTHM
NO. SER. = NUMBER OF SERIES USED FOR MEAN COSINOR;
95% CL=CONSERVATIVE 95% CONFIDENCE LIMITS

*360°=24H ; 0°=LOCAL MIDNIGHT

Figure 37.12. When pooling over all subjects and all seasons, a circadian population-mean cosinor yields a statistically significant ($P < 0.05$) circadian rhythm of systolic and diastolic blood pressure.

risk of breast cancer is of borderline statistical significance ($P \sim 0.06$). It also can be seen from Figure 37.21A that, from the viewpoint of the total risk, some of the women who were grouped originally as high risk in Minnesota, on the basis of a relative with breast cancer, were actually at no higher risk than some of the women rated as low risk for breast cancer, when all factors are considered. When, however, a t-test was applied to compare total breast cancer risks between the two groups of Minnesotan subjects a statistically significant difference was found ($P < 0.05$). Re-

ferring to Figure 37.21A, a possible relationship between the circannual amplitude of prolactin and total breast cancer risk deserves scrutiny in larger samples of women. This can now be done with more cost-effective sampling aimed at assessing over a longer time-span serum prolactin rhythms with a better optimization schedule than was maintained in this investigation.

Although Figure 37.21A suggests a negative correlation for prolactin and a positive one for TSH as a function of total breast cancer risk load, one should be aware of statistical difficul-

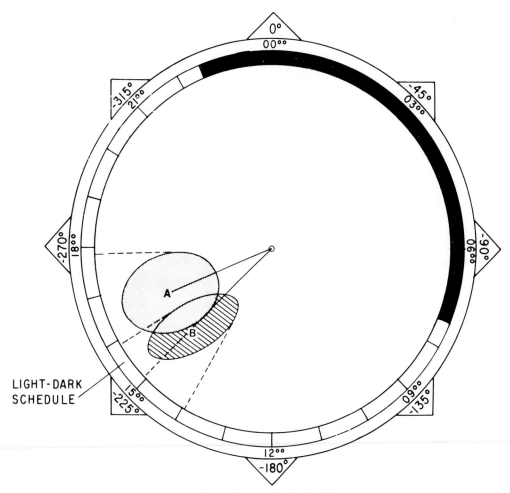

MEAN COSINOR

KEY TO PRESSURES	P	PR	NO. SER.	MESOR	AMPLITUDE (95% CL)	ACROPHASE* (95% CL)
A PULSE	<0.001	10	83	36.4	2.0 (1.1 2.8)	−247°(−226 −268)
B MEAN ARTERIAL	<0.001	22	83	78.7	2.8 (1.6 4.1)	−227°(−209 −239)

P=PROBABILITY OF HYPOTHESIS AMPLITUDE = 0 ; PR=PERCENT RHYTHM
NO. SER. = NUMBER OF SERIES USED FOR MEAN COSINOR;
95% CL=CONSERVATIVE 95% CONFIDENCE LIMITS

*360°=24H ; 0°=LOCAL MIDNIGHT

Figure 37.13. When pooling over all subjects and all seasons, a circadian population-mean cosinor yields a statistically significant ($P < 0.05$) circadian rhythm of pulse pressure and mean arterial pressure.

ties associated with the assignment of a P-value for these correlations. A test of lack of fit indicates the inappropriateness of a linear model of TSH ($F (11,15) = 2.67$, $P = 0.05$). Moreover, in addition to the hypothesis of "no error" in the independent variable (total breast cancer risk load), the usual assumptions are those of normality and homogeneity of variance of the error term. These assumptions have been tested by χ^2 for goodness of fit and Bartlett's test for homogeneity of variance. The normality hypothesis was rejected for the case of TSH ($\chi^2(3) =$

13.6, $P < 0.05$) but not for prolactin ($\chi^2(3) = 5.9$, $P > 0.05$). Homogeneity of variance along the independent variable was not satisfied for either prolactin ($F(3,1037) = 5.33$, $P < 0.05$) or TSH ($F(3,1037) = 5.39$, $P < 0.05$).

Broader Circannual Hormonal Rhythmometry

Quite apart from any negative correlation between the circadian amplitude of plasma prolactin on the one hand, and breast cancer risk on

Table 37.6
Rhythometric Summary of Blood Pressure in Women of Various Ages in Different Seasons and Different Geographic Locations

Group	% Rhythm (±SE)	Mesor (Torr ±SE)	Double Amplitude (Torr ±SE)	% of series with P-values > 0.10	0.10 ≥ P > 0.05	0.05 ≥ P > 0.01	< 0.01	% of series with P-values <0.05
			U.S. Systolic					
Ad	14.0 (±2.8)	98.4 (±1.8)	9.7 (±1.2)	4 (18)	2 (9)	0 (0)	16 (73)	16 (73)
YA	23.5 (±2.8)	102.1 (±1.4)	13.1 (±1.3)	0 (0)	0 (0)	2 (6)	30 (94)	32 (100)
PM	22.1 (±3.3)	109.2 (±1.8)	15.2 (±1.7)	1 (4)	1 (4)	0 (6)	25 (92)	25 (92)
W	21.8 (±3.1)	106.2 (±2.0)	13.4 (±1.5)	0 (0)	1 (4)	1 (4)	22 (92)	23 (96)
Sp	15.2 (±3.1)	101.3 (±2.4)	9.4 (±1.4)	4 (20)	0 (0)	0 (0)	16 (80)	16 (80)
S	16.4 (±2.7)	100.5 (±1.7)	11.5 (±1.2)	1 (5)	2 (10)	0 (0)	17 (85)	17 (85)
F	29.3 (±4.9)	105.5 (±2.1)	18.1 (±2.4)	0 (0)	0 (0)	1 (6)	16 (94)	17 (100)
			U.S. Diastolic					
Ad	10.0 (±2.5)	62.4 (±0.9)	5.8 (±0.9)	7 (32)	2 (9)	2 (9)	11 (50)	13 (59)
YA	21.7 (±3.0)	65.5 (±0.8)	9.4 (±1.0)	3 (9)	0 (0)	5 (16)	24 (75)	29 (91)
PM	24.1 (±3.8)	71.7 (±1.1)	10.6 (±1.4)	4 (15)	2 (7)	0 (0)	21 (78)	21 (78)
W	20.0 (±3.5)	67.1 (±1.2)	9.0 (±1.2)	4 (17)	1 (4)	2 (8)	17 (71)	19 (79)
Sp	16.6 (±3.5)	66.8 (±1.5)	7.8 (±1.3)	4 (20)	1 (5)	2 (10)	13 (65)	15 (75)
S	19.1 (±3.8)	66.6 (±1.3)	8.8 (±1.3)	3 (15)	1 (5)	2 (10)	14 (70)	16 (80)
F	21.9 (±5.1)	66.3 (±1.6)	9.9 (±1.8)	3 (18)	1 (6)	1 (6)	12 (70)	13 (76)
			Japan Systolic					
Ad	20.3 (±4.1)	105.2 (±3.2)	9.1 (±1.5)	1 (13)	0 (0)	1 (13)	6 (75)	7 (88)
YA	4.3 (±2.6)	102.0 (±2.2)	4.3 (±1.6)	3 (50)	2 (33)	0 (0)	1 (17)	1 (17)
PM	22.6 (±4.5)	110.2 (±4.4)	14.9 (±1.7)	1 (13)	0 (0)	0 (0)	7 (88)	7 (88)
W	21.8 (±3.9)	105.7 (±3.3)	11.8 (±1.8)	1 (9)	1 (9)	0 (0)	9 (82)	9 (82)
Sp	11.7 (±3.5)	106.5 (±2.7)	7.9 (±1.7)	4 (36)	1 (9)	1 (9)	5 (45)	6 (55)
			Japan Diastolic					
Ad	10.1 (±2.7)	63.8 (±2.7)	6.9 (±1.0)	2 (25)	0 (0)	0 (0)	6 (75)	6 (75)
YA	13.8 (±5.4)	66.1 (±0.8)	8.6 (±2.0)	1 (17)	0 (0)	2 (33)	3 (50)	5 (83)
PM	15.4 (±4.0)	75.3 (±2.8)	8.6 (±1.6)	1 (25)	0 (0)	1 (13)	6 (75)	7 (88)
W	10.4 (±1.7)	69.1 (±2.4)	7.7 (±0.9)	1 (9)	0 (0)	2 (18)	8 (73)	10 (91)
Sp	15.7 (±4.0)	68.1 (±2.7)	8.3 (±1.5)	3 (27)	0 (0)	1 (9)	7 (64)	8 (73)

Ad, adolescent; YA, young adult; PM, postmenopausal woman; W, winter; Sp, spring; S, summer, F, fall.

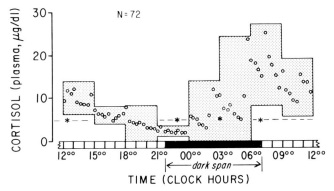

*Note that a value of 5 µg/dl is suspiciously high for a blood sample taken at 23⁰⁰, but suspiciously low for one taken during the morning or at noon (between 06⁰⁰ and 13⁰⁰). The same value is "usual" (or "normal") at certain other times.

Figure 37.14. Individual circadian merodesm. Tolerance intervals determined separately for 3-hr spans indicate limits within which 90% of measurements would be expected to fall with 90% confidence. A cortisol value such as 5 µg/dl may be too low at one time (e.g. 06:00), too high at another time (e.g. 23:00), or normal at yet another time (e.g. 03:00).

the other hand, it seemed of interest to explore more broadly the imputations (17) of circannual mesor and amplitude in relation to breast cancer risk for the thirteen hormones examined systematically in the Kyushu-Minnesota study. Table 37.9 summarizes the statistically significant aspects of a correlation matrix computed between breast cancer risk and imputations of circannual rhythm characteristics from data on those volunteers who provided blood for four different seasons. This matrix revealed, in addition to the negative correlation with breast cancer risk of the prolactin amplitude, a negative correlation with the prolactin mesor and a positive correlation with the LH mesor and the TSH amplitude. Thyroidal function has been discussed in relation to breast cancer risk by Mittra (43) and Mittra and Hayward (44, 45). Hence, the circumstance that it is the circannual amplitude of TSH which seems to discriminate between the groups with high and low risk is of particular interest, notably since a relation of the TSH mesor to

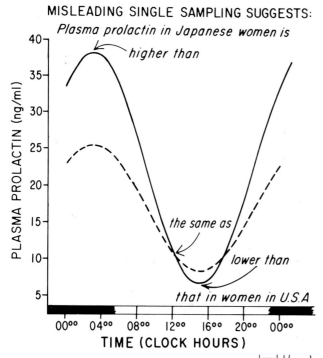

MISLEADING SINGLE SAMPLING SUGGESTS:

Plasma prolactin in Japanese women is

higher than

the same as

lower than

that in women in U.S.A

	JAPAN (—)	U.S. (- -)
NUMBER OF SUBJECTS	11	19
NUMBER OF SERIES (SOME SUBJECTS PROVIDED 2 SERIES)	15	26
TOTAL NUMBER OF DETERMINATIONS (IN DUPLICATE)	1070	1824

Figure 37.15. Circadian rhythms of plasma prolactin in Japanese and North American women in winter. Dense sampling on plasma prolactin suggests both a larger circadian amplitude and a larger rhythm-adjusted mean or mesor in Japanese as compared to North American women ($P < 0.002$ from Hotelling T^2 test).

breast cancer risk is only of borderline statistical significance, whereas relation to the circannual amplitude, indeed, seems to be established and should be checked in further work.

Urinary Melatonin

We here summarize results discussed elsewhere (62). Urine specimens, analyzed for melatonin, revealed statistically significant differences between groups ($P < 0.01$) as well as a statistically significant time-group interaction, thereby attesting to the fact that the intergroup difference depends upon time. It can be seen from Figure 37.22 that Japanese have consistently lower values of melatonin excretion than do North Americans. Analyses of values from the night span confirmed the fact, already observed in earlier studies (for review, see Refs. 19 and 51), that melatonin excretion is higher during the time of darkness (habitual rest). Figure 37.22 also summarizes the results from a

population mean-cosinor analysis after pooling data from Minnesota and Japan, thus documenting a statistically significant circadian rhythm in urinary melatonin.

Other Hormones

Differences in other hormones were less obvious. In contrast to prolactin, plasma cortisol during the winter has a larger circadian mesor and amplitude in Minnesota than in Japan (Table 37.10). In the early morning hours (~09:00), a difference in cortisol of about 4 µg/dl may be observed between the two populations. During the other seasons, a statistically significant difference in all characteristics of the cortisol rhythm was also observed between Japanese and Minnesotan low-risk subjects, as shown by a Hotelling T^2 test.

North American women had a higher circadian aldosterone mesor in the winter than did Japanese subjects. In the summer, Minnesotans also had a higher circadian DHEA-S amplitude than did Japanese subjects. Differences between Japanese and Minnesotans (both risk categories) also were observed in the amplitude/mesor ratio for plasma insulin during the summer.

Age-Related Differences

Langlands *et al.* (35) report that deaths occurring in patients with breast cancer show a circannual pattern differing in relation to menopause. When analyses are carried out separately for women diagnosed before and after menopause, circannual rhythms were found to be in antiphase.

The investigation that is the subject of this report was planned to include four subjects from each of the three age categories and each of the three risk categories for a total of 36 subjects, so that sampling at different seasons and menstrual stages could proceed according to a balanced Latin-square design. For a variety of reasons, some subjects had to be replaced part-way through the study, and for some 24-hr sampling sessions, not all the planned blood samples could be obtained or analyzed. To avoid possible bias from unbalanced sampling of the various rhythms, the analyses for an age effect included only those subjects sampled in all four seasons (and menstrual stages) from whom most, if not all, of the planned blood samples were obtained

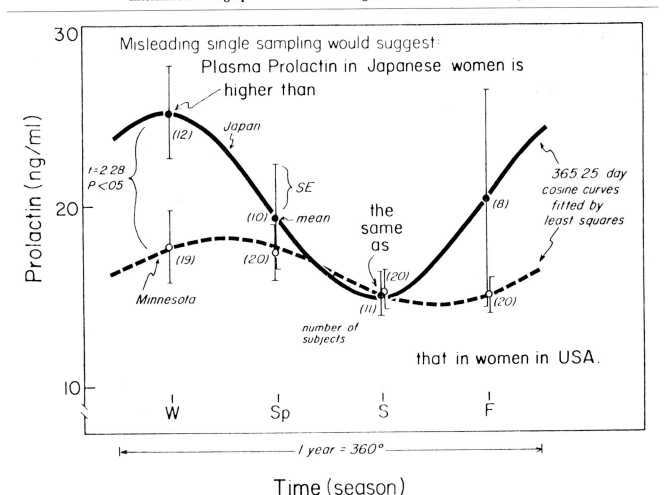

Figure 37.16. Geographic difference in circannual rhythm of human plasma prolactin. Contradictory comparisons of circadian mesor could be obtained by sampling in different seasons. Moreover, controlling time of year (or time of day, Fig. 37.15) may not avoid misleading results due to circannual (or circadian, as the case may be) variations, whereas assessment of circannual (or circadian) rhythm characteristics may reveal important chronoepidemiologic or chronoprotopathologic results. Conclusions from single samples obtained in different seasons (or times of day) can be resolved as differences of circannual (circadian) prolactin rhythm between Japanese and American women. Each subject provided 72 blood samples (8640 determinations, each in duplicate). *W*, Winter; *Sp*, Spring; *S*, Summer; *F*, Fall.

during each 24 hr span. An added consideration in the latter case was whether missing samples were more or less evenly distributed through the 24 hr so that their absence would not be expected to bias results.

Rather than simply analyzing the overall mean value for a given hormone on each subject, we chose to use estimates based on the fit of a 24-hr cosine (see above) so that the hormone's circadian amplitude as well as its mesor could be examined. It should be noted that the mesor estimate in this procedure is identical with the 24-hr arithmetic mean if the data are equally spaced throughout an entire cycle.

For each subject, the mean value of a circadian parameter (e.g. mesor) for a given hormone across all four seasons (menstrual stages) rep-

resented that subject in a two-way analysis of variance (ANOVA) for age and risk factors. In dealing with uneven numbers of values in different age versus risk cells, the conventional experimental approach (46) was used to partition the total sum of squares in testing the statistical significance of main effects and interaction.

Results concerning the effects of age on circadian mesors and circadian amplitudes of 12 hormones (including prolactin) are summarized in Tables 37.11A and 37.11B, respectively. Estriol (E3) was not included because of inadequate data satisfying the criteria indicated above. Inferences as to the statistical significance of main effects (age and risk) are not valid if there is interaction or if inhomogeneity of variance is

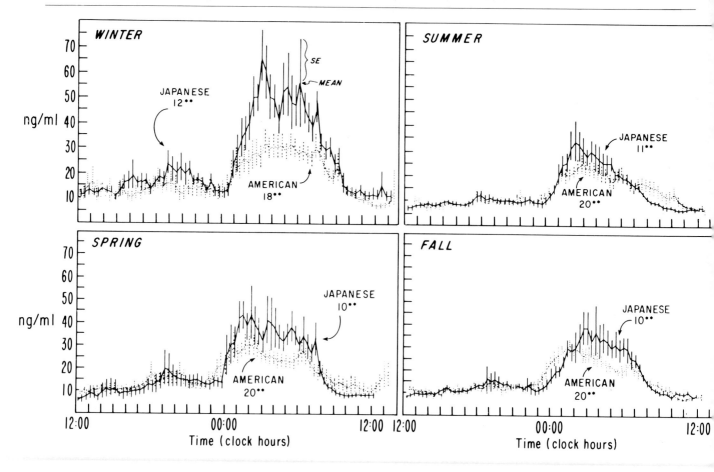

**NO. OF SUBJECTS.

Figure 37.17. Comparison of plasma prolactin in clinically healthy Japanese and Minnesotan women in four seasons. Samples taken at 20-min intervals over a 24-hr span in Fukuoka City, Japan and Minneapolis, Minn.

indicated. In such cases, resort was made to a contrast test using separate variance estimates from each cell involved in the contrast to estimate the standard error. Such a test of an age effect for these hormones exhibiting inhomogeneity of variance or an interaction effect involved a contrast (46) between the mature-adult (age 29–36) and the postmenopausal (age 44–59) groups. A contrast involving the young-adult group as a whole could not be made because the U.S.A. low-risk, young-adult cell had only one value for all hormones.

Even allowing for an effect of multiple inference, an effect of age is clearly apparent for the circadian mesors of LH, prolactin, estrone (E1), estradiol (E2), and 17-OH-progesterone. In the case of DHEA-S, an interaction between age and risk effects plus inhomogeneity of variance among the nine age-versus-risk cells invalidate the indication of an apparently highly significant age effect in the ANOVA. A P-value of 0.09 in the contrast between the mature adult and postmenopausal age groups does not lend much sup-

port to the conclusion of an age effect on DHEA-S, especially if one considers multiple inferences. For these five hormones exhibiting a clear age effect, LH undergoes a marked *increase* while prolactin, the estrogens, and 17-OH-progesterone *decrease* between the age classes of 29–36 and 44–59 years.

LH, E2, and 17-OH-progesterone also exhibit a clear effect of age on the circadian *amplitude*, with an increase for LH and a decrease for the other two hormones. In addition, the results indicate a statistically significant decrease in amplitude of DHEA-S while an age effect on the amplitudes of circadian rhythms in prolactin, E1, and aldosterone may be considered of borderline statistical significance. It should be borne in mind that amplitude estimates were obtained by fitting a 24-hr cosine curve to the data from each 24-hr sampling span. For these hormones with 15 or fewer samples/24-hr span (*i.e.* all hormones except prolactin and cortisol), the cosine fit often was not statistically significant, as indicated by a zero-amplitude test; nevertheless,

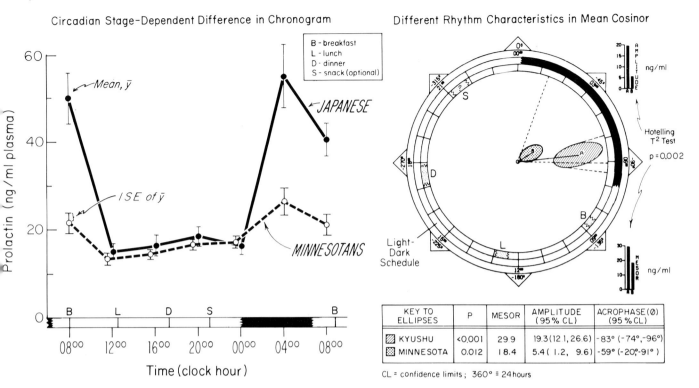

Circadian Stage-Dependent Difference in Chronogram

Different Rhythm Characteristics in Mean Cosinor

Figure 37.18. Difference of plasma prolactin between clinically healthy Japanese and American women in March, 1978 when circadian rhythm is near its maximum, confirmed by complementary study. Fifteen whites of mixed ethnic background (18–24 years old) in Minnesota and 20 Japanese (~20 years old) in Kyushu, Japan.

the estimates were considered indicative of the extent of variation on the circadian time scale, for the purposes of investigating the age effect.

Results from testing of a possible breast cancer risk effect on circadian mesors and amplitudes are not tabulated, since there are only two cases (the aldosterone mesor and the prolactin amplitude) in which interpretation of a low P-value was not compromised by the presence of an interaction effect. The P-value for an effect of risk status on the aldosterone mesor was 0.01 while that for an effect of risk on the prolactin amplitude was 0.03.

A comparison of circannual amplitudes of the adolescent (15–21 year old) and the young adult (29–36 year old) groups consisting of 8 and 10 subjects, respectively, with those of the postmenopausal (44–59 year old) group (10 subjects) reveals a decrease in mean circannual amplitude as a function of age for aldosterone, 17-OH-progesterone, estrone, estradiol and prolactin and an increase for LH. These changes were statistically significant below the 5% level (Table 37.7). These finding are qualified by possible effects of unbalanced representation of menstrual stages, limited numbers of circadian mesors provided for the fit of a 1-year cosine curve and by any novelty effect biasing the data.

Table 37.7

Circannual Amplitude of Plasma Aldosterone, 17-OH-Progesterone, Estradiol, Estrone, Prolactin, and LH in Women after Menopause

Hormone (units)	Age Group[a]		
	I	II	III
Aldosterone (ng/dl)	2.84	4.85	1.68
17-OH-Progesterone (ng/ml)	491	615	73
Estradiol (pg/ml)	66.97	71.73	12.08
Estrone (pg/ml)	47.19	45.41	21.19
Prolactin (ng/ml)	7.11	8.82	2.38
LH (mIU/ml)	11.48	7.14	16.74

[a] I, II and III indicate mean values for amplitude of subjects in age groups 15–21, 29–36, and 44–59 years.

Population-mean-cosinor analyses were also applied to blood pressure data from subjects of different ages (pooling over all seasons). Results are summarized in Table 37.12. The circadian blood pressure mesor increases with age. This statement is rhythm-qualified and hence seemingly secure since it is based on measurements made about every 10 min for 24 hr. This circumstance, however, does not solve the obvious problem associated with transverse observations involving sampling on different groups of individuals (defined as anidiocyclic below).

Table 37.8
Circadian Prolactin Rhythm in a Premenopausal and A Post-menopausal Woman (Urbino, Italy)

Series			Fit of 24-hr period				Acrophase[b]	
No.	Age (yr)	Date (mo/day)	P	PR[a] %	M (ng/ml) (±SE)	A (ng/ml) (±SE)	deg (±SE)	hr/min
1	55	07/26	0.021	14	4.24 (±0.12)	0.51 (±0.18)	−64 (±17)	04:19
2	23	10/17	0.125	6	16.09 (±1.60)	4.70 (±2.26)	−69 (±26)	04:39
3	23	01/23	0.001	28	12.16 (±0.72)	5.40 (±1.03)	−81 (±10)	05:28
4	23	04/08	0.001	36	6.74 (±0.41)	3.68 (±0.58)	−105 (±9)	07:00

[a] P-value in testing zero-amplitude hypothesis, PR, percentage rhythm; M, mesor; SE, standard error; A, amplitude
[b] From local 00:00; 360° ≡ 24 hr

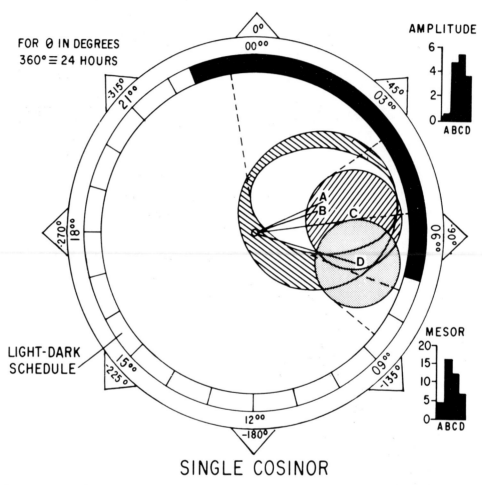

SINGLE COSINOR

KEY TO ELLIPSES		P	NO. OBS.	PR	MESOR SE	AMPLITUDE (95% CL)	ACROPHASE (Ø) (95% CL)
A	F 1,55Y 07/26	0.021	54	14.1	4.2 0.1	0.5 (0.1 1.0)	−65°(−351 −110)
B	FS,23Y 10/17	0.125	69	6.1	16.2 1.6	4.7 ( )	−70°( )
C	" 01/23	<0.001	73	28.1	12.2 0.7	5.4 (2.8 8.0)	−82°(−54 −110)
D	". 04/08	<0.001	73	36.2	6.7 0.4	3.7 (2.2 5.1)	−105°(−82 −129)

Figure 37.19. Lower circadian mesors and amplitudes in serum prolactin of a postmenopausal woman as compared to a 23-year old woman, both sampled in Urbino, Italy.

Sampling on the same individual (idiocyclicity) is required to explore the possibility that the mesor of some individuals may not change with age and that the age-associated increase seen in transverse studies may result from the circumstance that, with advancing age, some individuals develop mesor-hypertension.

Table 37.12 shows further that a circadian

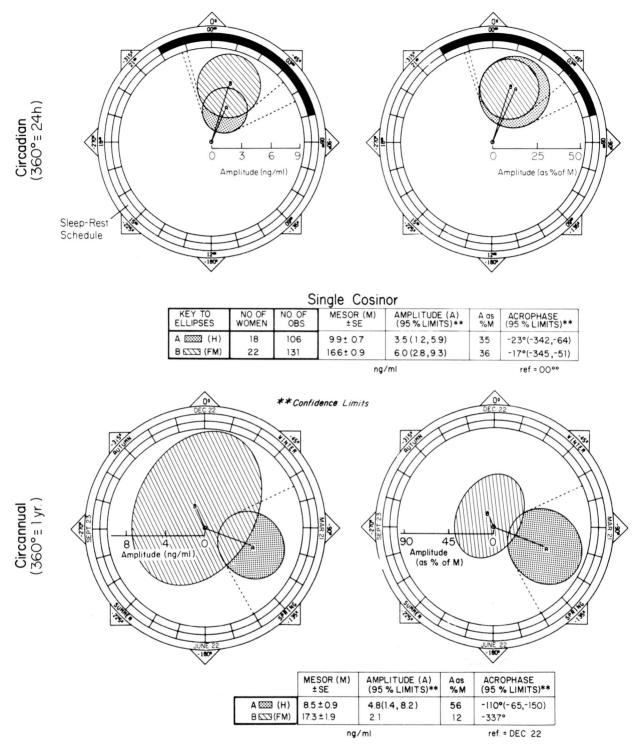

Single Cosinor

KEY TO ELLIPSES	NO. OF WOMEN	NO. OF OBS.	MESOR (M) ±SE	AMPLITUDE (A) (95 % LIMITS)**	A as %M	ACROPHASE (95 % LIMITS)**
A ▨ (H)	18	106	9.9± 0.7	3.5 (1.2, 5.9)	35	-23°(-342,-64)
B ▧ (FM)	22	131	16.6± 0.9	6.0 (2.8, 9.3)	36	-17°(-345,-51)

ng/ml   ref = 00°°

**Confidence Limits

	MESOR (M) ±SE	AMPLITUDE (A) (95 % LIMITS)**	A as %M	ACROPHASE (95 % LIMITS)**
A ▨ (H)	8.5±0.9	4.8(1.4, 8.2)	56	-110°(-65,-150)
B ▧(FM)	17.3±1.9	2.1	12	-337°

ng/ml   ref. = DEC 22

Figure 37.20. Circannual chronopathology. Obliteration of circannual but not of circadian rhythm in serum prolactin in fibrocystic mastopathy (*FM*) as compared to clinical health (*H*) for women sampled in Florence, Italy. While the circadian amplitude (expressed in ng/ml or as percentage of mesor) is not affected in presence of benign disease of the breast, the circannual amplitude is drastically reduced. The alteration of a circannual prolactin rhythm might thus be a harbinger of increased breast cancer risk.

amplitude increases with age in these clinically healthy subjects, in keeping with an early observation made on mesor-hypertensive patients by Menzel (personal communication). The circadian acrophase seems to remain unchanged.

Hormonal Models

From the Latin-square design of this study, it was possible to assess circannual or circatrigin-tan (menstrual) rhythms. Most subjects were

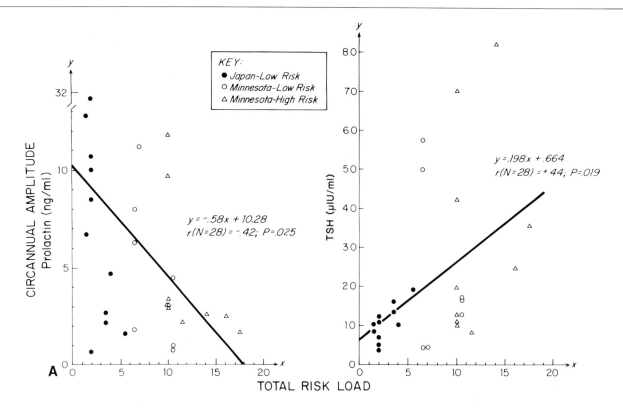

Figure 37.21A A *negative* correlation between the total relative breast cancer risk evaluated from epidemiologic criteria and the circannual prolactin amplitude corroborates the finding that an elevation of breast cancer risk is associated with a decrease in circannual amplitude (based on least squares fit of 365.25-day cosine curve to circadian mesors assessed in each of the four seasons.) (see Fig. 37.16 and 37.20). Note further the *positive* correlation between epidemiologically assessed breast cancer risk and the circannual amplitude of thyroid-stimulating hormone (TSH). Clinical hypothyroidism has empirically been associated with breast cancer risk. If, then, this topic is still controversial, this may, perhaps, be accounted for by the circannual-stage-dependence of the correlation.

It is also noteworthy that in prostatic cancer (38) (a condition characterized by geographic differences in morbidity and mortality similar to those of breast cancer), the extent of circannual variation also changes as a function of risk and/or cancer. In blood sampled with serial independence in the morning at different times of the year, a prominent circannual rhythm in TSH of healthy subjects is lost in prostatic cancer (and perhaps even in men at high risk of prostatic cancer). For prolactin, a circannual rhythm becomes demonstrable in the case of prostatic cancer, while it is not demonstrable with serially independent sampling in healthy men of low or high prostatic cancer risk.

Thus, TSH and prolactin show opposite behavior along the 1-yr scale in cancers of both breast and prostate (rather than responding in the same fashion, as is the case along the scale of minutes to hours—following the application of stimuli such as Thyrotropin Releasing Hormone (26)). It is yet more interesting that the circannual relations of plasma TSH and prolactin to the risk of breast cancer are opposite to those with respect to prostatic cancer (and, as noted, opposite to each other in each cancer).

The two correlations shown in the figure are but part of a large correlation matrix. The circumstance is noted that correlations emerged as statistically significant for the very hormones which clinicians have long considered had some relation to breast cancer, yet thus far could not rigorously establish such a relation as biologically significant, perhaps because of all-too-limited sampling.

While these conclusions rest on large samples, they describe only a small number of subjects. Moreover, all conditions required to apply a linear regression between two variables are not satisfied. A test for lack of fit indicates that the model is not adequate for TSH: the error term is not normally distributed. In addition, the assumption of homogeneity of variance is not verified for prolactin as well as for TSH. Finally, in the case of prolactin, there seems to be an age effect on both this circannual amplitude (decreases with age) and the breast cancer risk (increases with age). This may account for the negative correlation illustrated in the figure. Hence the correlations in the figure are of ordering rather than documenting value. They are intended to emphasize that circannual rhythmicity deserves further study in relation to carcinogenesis. If such correlations can be confirmed and if the circannual rhythms involved should prove to be determinants of carcinogenesis in the human breast, these same correlations will point to the possibility of a chemoprevention of breast cancer.

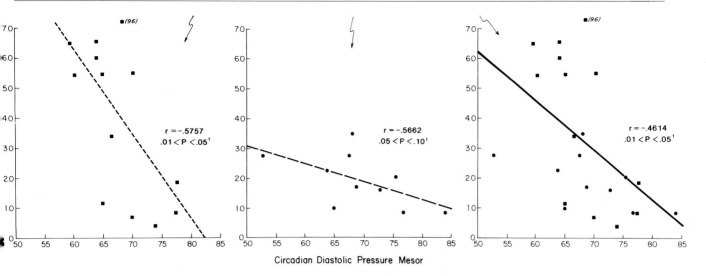

Figure 37.21B Negative correlation between the circannual aldosterone amplitude (based on least squares fit of 365.25-day cosine curve to circadian mesors assessed in each of the four seasons on each of the women investigated in Minnesota and Japan) and the circadian diastolic blood pressure mesor (in winter, the season when blood pressure profiles at about 10-min intervals were obtained in both locations) observed in women in Minnesota (N = 13, - - -, *left*), in Kyushu, Japan (N = 10, — — —, *center*), and both (N = 23, ——, *right*). † Results from heterogeneous sample, ostensibly not meeting conditions for significance testing.

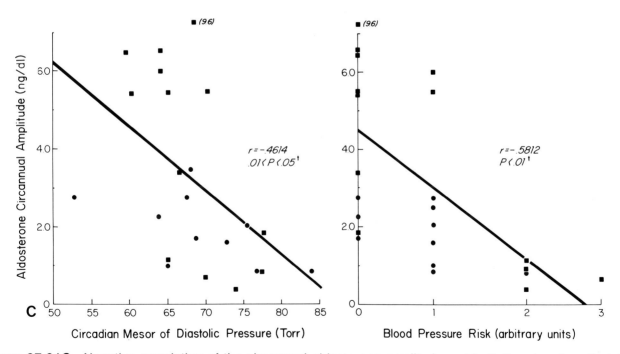

Figure 37.21C Negative correlation of the circannual aldosterone amplitude and both the circadian diastolic blood pressure mesor and the individual risk of diseases associated with high blood pressure. Results from 23 presumably healthy women, 13 in the USA (■) and 10 in Japan (●); estimate of circadian diastolic pressure mesor based on appropriate data obtained only in winter; circannual aldosterone amplitude determined by fit of 365.25-day cosine curve to circadian mesors assessed in each of the four seasons; factors determining risk value included familial morbidity or mortality, obesity, "high" heart rate and a history of blood pressure "spiking." The same restrictions as outlined for Figure 21A apply to Figures 21B and C. † Results from heterogeneous sample, ostensibly not meeting conditions for significance testing.

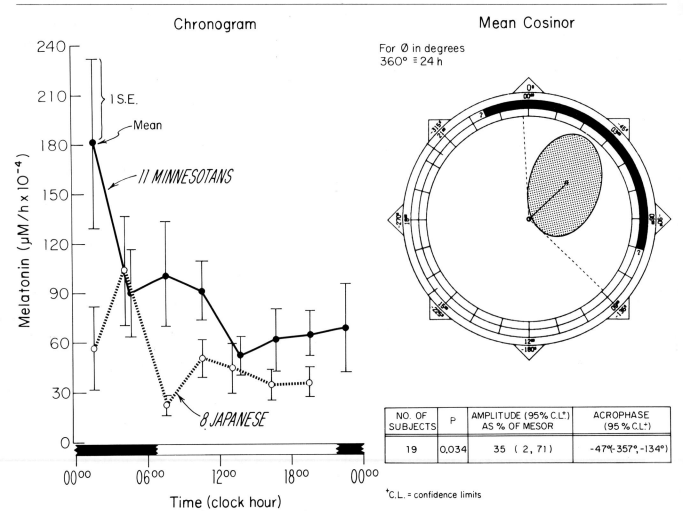

Figure 37.22. Circadian variation in urinary excretion of melatonin in 11 white women of mixed ethnic background in Minnesota and 8 Japanese women in Kyushu, Japan. Chronogram (*left*) shows urinary melatonin excretion by Japanese and Minnesotan women at several timepoints during 1-day span. Each woman contributed six to eight samples collected over a single 24-hr span; data for each population averaged across all subjects for 3-hr intervals (no Japanese samples between 21:00 and 24:00 hr). Amplitude and acrophase estimates from all subjects were combined in population-mean cosinor (*right*).

Table 37.9
Correlations Between Relative Breast Cancer Risk and (Imputations of) Circannual Rhythm Characteristics

Characteristic	Variable	r^a	P
Amplitude	TSH	+0.44	0.019
	Prolactin	−0.42	0.025
Mesor	TSH	+0.34	0.076
	Prolactin	−0.34	0.080
	LH	+0.39	0.045

[a] r, correlation coefficient; P, probability; TSH, thyroid-stimulating hormone; LH, luteinizing hormone.

Table 37.10
Circadian Mesor and Amplitude of Cortisol in Winter

	Japan	Minnesota	Comparison (*P*-value from *t*-test)
		(μg/dl)	
Mesor	7.0 ± 0.4	9.0 ± 0.4	0.003
Amplitude	4.4 ± 0.3	5.4 ± 0.4	0.07

indeed sampled four times a year, once in each season and in each of four different menstrual stages. Although we observed an effect of age and risk status on some hormones (see above), a consideration of such effects would leave only one individual per season and menstrual stage. For obvious reasons, even the most powerful statistical tools would not enable us to take this approach. Instead, for a given site and risk status we pooled over all ages to examine the effect of one factor at a time. Although such an approach is far from being rigorous and would lead to only a very rough approximation, it was our goal to investigate any possible effects in order to determine sampling requirements for further studies.

The data on hand (four spans of 24 hr—about 3 months apart—during which the sampling rate was three times an hour) were not sufficient to allow us to fit concomitantly the different frequencies of interest. The alternative was to analyze the circadian rhythm characteristics over the year and over the menstrual cycle separately. In the case of the circannual rhythm, individual circadian parameter estimates could be assigned to the actual date of sampling. In attempting to characterize a circatrigintan rhythm, however, it was necessary to pool individuals according to menstrual stage (early follicular, late follicular, early luteal or late luteal) at the time of sampling, without regard for differences in length of menstrual cycle.

Based on the results and considerations of the analyses mentioned above, the following composite model was constructed, mainly for didactic purposes:

$$y(t) = M_1 + A_1 \left[1 + \frac{A_2}{A_1} \cos \frac{2\pi}{\tau_2} \left(t - \varphi_2 \right) \right.$$
$$\left. + \frac{A_3}{A_1} \cos \frac{2\pi}{\tau_3} \left(t - \varphi_3 \right) \right] \cdot \cos \frac{2\pi}{\gamma_1} \left(t - \varphi_1 \right) \qquad (1)$$
$$+ A_4 \cos \frac{2\pi}{\tau_4} \left(t - \varphi_4 \right) + A_5 \cos \frac{2\pi}{\tau_5} \left(t - \varphi_5 \right)$$

The subscript 1 refers to the circadian component; subscripts 2 and 3, respectively refer to the

Table 37.11A
Results from Two-Way ANOVA[a] for Effects of Age on Circadian Mesor (~24-Hr Mean) of 12 Plasma Hormones in Women Sampled in Each of Four Menstrual Stages and Four Seasons

Hormone (units)	N[b]	Age[c]			ANOVA[d]		Contrast (II vs. III)	
		I	II	III	F	P	t	P
LH (mIU/ml)	27	14.9	18.6	80.1	74.80	<0.001		
Prolactin (ng/ml)	29	22.9	19.5	12.7	10.37	<0.001		
E1 (pg/ml)	27	75.0	94.9	38.3	14.66	<0.001		
E2 (pg/ml)	26	81.3	113.2	17.0	14.52	<0.001[e]	6.46	0.001
17-OH Progesterone (pg/ml)	29	602.0	716.0	158.0	22.50	<0.001[e]	7.90	<0.001
Cortisol (μg/dl)	30	8.7	9.0	9.4	0.12			
Aldosterone (ng/dl)	25	6.1	6.6	4.9	2.16			
DHEA-S (ng/ml)	28	3090.0	1400.0	960.0	20.65	0.001[g]	1.93	
TSH (μIU/ml)	29	3.3	6.4	5.0	1.51			
T3 (ng/dl)	28	94.7	98.7	101.7	0.35			
T4 (μg/dl)	29	6.8	7.0	7.2	0.15			
Insulin (μU/ml)	29	26.9	19.3	22.5	3.08			

[a] ANOVA, analysis of variance, F = value taken by F-test in ANOVA, P = corresponding P-value, LH, luteinizing hormone; E1, estrone; E2, estradiol; DHEA-S, dehydroepiandrosterone sulfate; TSH, thyrotropic hormone; T3, triiodothyronine; T4, thyroxine.

[b] N, number of subjects satisfying the criteria of having adequate data (see text) throughout a 24-hr span in each of four seasons and four menstrual stages; each subject contributed one value, her average circadian mesor, to the analysis.

[c] I, II, and III indicate mean values for ages 15–21, 29–36, and 44–59 yr, respectively; each value is the mean of means from the three risk categories.

[d] Only P-values < 0.05 are indicated.

[e] Inhomogeneity of variance (P < 0.05).

[f] Interaction between age and risk (P < 0.05).

[g] Both inhomogeneity of variance (P < 0.05) and interaction between age and risk (P < 0.05).

Table 37.11b
Results from Two-way ANOVA[a] for Effects of Age on Circadian Amplitude of 12 Plasma Hormones in Women Sampled in Each of Four Menstrual Stages and Four Seasons

Hormone (units)	N[b]	Age[c]			ANOVA[d]		Contrast (II vs. III)	
		I	II	III	F	P	t	P
LH (mIU/ml)	27	4.0	4.8	13.4	38.99	<0.001[e]	7.13	<0.001
Prolactin (ng/ml)	29	12.4	16.5	11.0	4.34	0.027		
E1 (pg/ml)	27	17.6	15.9	11.4	4.30	0.03[e]		
E2 (pg/ml)	26	28.0	28.4	8.1	10.00	<0.001[g]	5.30	0.001
17-OH Progesterone (pg/ml)	29	181.0	196.0	128.0	10.00	<0.001		
Cortisol (μg/dl)	30	7.1	7.5	7.0	1.23			
Aldosterone (ng/dl)	25	4.1	2.5	1.8	11.49	<0.001[e]	2.36	0.056
DHEA-S (ng/ml)	28	580.0	370.0	230.0	19.62	<0.001[f]	3.42	0.006
TSH (μIU/ml)	29	0.73	1.95	1.04	2.48			
T3 (ng/dl)	28	12.9	12.5	13.2	0.17			
T4 (μg/dl)	29	0.58	0.59	0.67	2.01			
Insulin (μU/ml)	29	20.5	15.6	18.0	2.85			

[a] See footnotes for Table 37.11A; substitute "circadian amplitude" for "circadian mesor." Adapted from W. Nelson et al., J. Gerontology, 35: 512–519, 1980.

Table 37.12
Comparison of Circadian Rhythm Characteristics with Respect to Age in Minnesotan Women

Age	P-value	Number of series	Mesor	Amplitude	Acrophase[a]	P-value	Number of series	Mesor	Amplitude	Acrophase[a]
				torr	deg				torr	deg
			Systolic blood pressure (S)					Diastolic blood pressure (D)		
Adolescent	<0.01	22	98.4	3.0	−254	>0.05	22	62.4	0.1	−105
Young adult	<0.01	32	102.1	3.1	−215	<0.01	32	65.5	1.8	−205
Postmenopausal	<0.01	28	108.9	6.2	−234	<0.01	28	71.5	4.3	−230
			Pulse pressure[b] (PP)					Mean arterial pressure[c] (MAP)		
Adolescent	<0.01	22	36.0	3.1	−256	>0.05	22	74.3	0.9	−250
Young adult	0.08	32	36.6	1.3	−231	<0.01	32	77.6	2.3	−209
Postmenopausal	0.02	28	37.3	1.9	−247	<0.01	28	83.9	4.9	−232

[a] $360° \equiv 24$ hr; $0° =$ local midnight.

[b] PP = S − D.

[c] $MAP = D + \dfrac{PP}{3}$.

circatrigintan and circannual rhythms modulating the circadian amplitude; subscripts 4 and 5 refer to the superimposed circatrigintan and circannual rhythms (modulating the circadian mesor). In other words, waves 2 and 3 were obtained by considering the circadian amplitudes (A) while waves 4 and 5 were obtained by considering the circadian mesors (M). The phases φ_i in equation (1) are related to the respective acrophases ϕ_i by the equation

$$\phi_i = \frac{2\pi}{\tau_i} \varphi_i \text{ (where } \varphi_i \text{ and } \phi_i \text{ are expressed in radians)} \quad (2)$$

For two hormones—prolactin and cortisol—six groups were considered: the three risk groups (pooled over age), *i.e.* Japan, Minnesota low-risk, and Minnesota high-risk; and the three age groups (pooled over risk and geographic location), *i.e.* adolescents, young adults, and postmenopausal women. The sequence considered in Figure 37.23 consists of: (a) the circadian rhythm over a 60-day span; (b) the circatrigintan rhythm (wave 4) superimposed on the circadian rhythm (modulating the circadian mesor) during a 60-day span; (c) the circatrigintan rhythms modulating both the circadian mesor and amplitude (waves 2 and 4) over a 60-day span; (d) the latter model extended over a 365-day span; (e) the same model as in (d) but with the circannual rhythm superimposed (wave 5: mesor modulation); and (f) the final model consisting of all 5 waves over a full year span.

It has to be noted that in order to visualize the full range of variation and to give a better idea of the envelope, the circadian phase (φ_i) was fixed to −0.5. Because of the finite number of points used to construct the model, the amplitude may be clipped if φ_i is not fixed to this value. Tables 37.13 and 37.14 show the parameter values used for waves 1–5 in the theoretical models. Since the postmenopausal women were

admitted irrespective of any circatrigintan rhythm, this component was not evaluated.

In the case of prolactin, the circadian mesor and amplitude tended to be higher in Japanese than in Minnesotan subjects. The amplitudes of circannual rhythms in the circadian mesor and amplitude were also larger in the Japanese.

Prolactin concentrations were higher in adolescents and young adults than in postmenopausal women. The circatrigintan rhythms modulating both the circadian mesor and amplitude were more pronounced in young adults than in adolescents, Figure 37.24.

In the case of cortisol, the mesors and relative amplitudes were about the same for the Japanese and the two Minnesota risk categories. As a result of phase relationships among the different components, however, the lower limit of variation of cortisol was almost constant in Minnesotans, whereas in the Japanese it was influenced by the circannual rhythm. Only slight differences were observed among age categories. For young adults, the lower limit of cortisol variation throughout the year remained almost constant, whereas the circannual variation was clearly visible at the two other age categories.

Change in Circadian Period of Human Breast Surface Temperature

Breast surface temperatures, measured with a 10-channel Yellow Springs telethermometer in Mexico City (from the nipple and four quadrants of each breast during wakefulness, at 2-hr intervals, for 4 days from three groups each composed of eight women)—in health (H), benign breast disease (B), and breast cancer (C)—indicate a shortening of the circadian period in the presence of benign disease and further in the presence of cancer—Figures 37.25 and 37.26. One

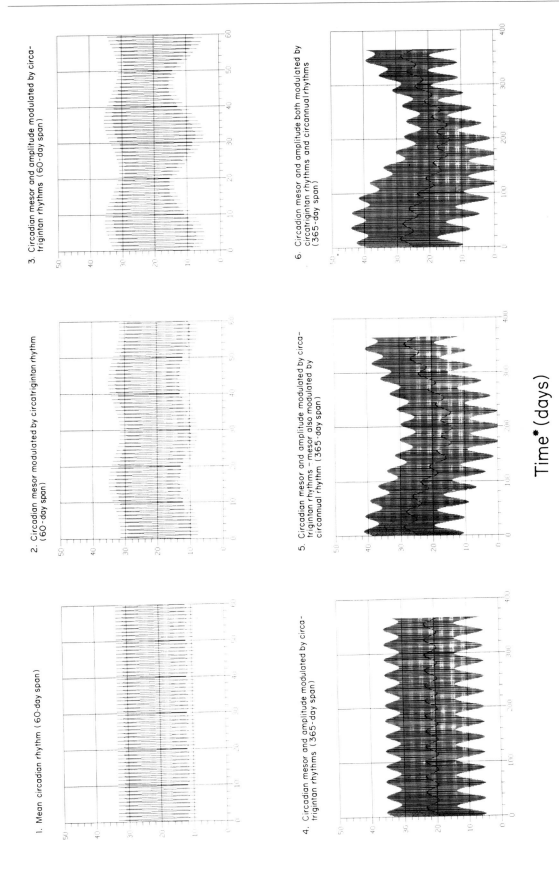

Figure 37.23. Stepwise theoretical reconstruction of partial spectral structure of human plasma prolactin for group of Japanese women (based on parameter estimates obtained from separate least-squares fittings of cosine curves with periods of 24 hours (circadian), 28 days (circatrigintan) and 365 days (circannual) to data on plasma prolactin obtained every 20 min for 24 hours, ~4 times a year on a few women). Didactic example modeling the interaction of human plasma prolactin rhythms with different frequencies, including modulation of circadian mesor and amplitude by circatrigintan and circannual rhythms.

Table 37.13
Parameter Values Used in Theoretical Reconstruction of Cortisol Variability Due to Circadian, Circatrigintan, and Circannual Rhythms

M^a	A	τ	φ		M	A	τ	φ
Japan					Adolescent			
1. 8.37	5.03	1	−0.35 (−0.5)		1. 8.69	5.43	1	−0.40 (−0.5)
2. 0.5	0.17	28	−5.29		2. 0.5	0.11	28	−10.11
3. 0.5	0.15	365	−223.06		3. 0.5	0.11	365	−251.44
4. 0.0	0.54	28	−1.40		4. 0.0	0.41	28	−14.31
5. 0.0	1.27	365	−172.36		5. 0.0	0.93	365	−171.35
Minnesota low risk					Young adult			
1. 9.44	5.46	1	−0.39 (−0.5)		1. 8.83	5.38	1	−0.35 (−0.5)
2. 0.5	0.06	28	−18.12		2. 0.5	0.02	28	−25.82
3. 0.5	0.15	365	−215.96		3. 0.5	0.14	365	−221.03
4. 0.0	0.18	28	−23.96		4. 0.0	0.24	28	−24.03
5. 0.0	0.95	365	−208.86		5. 0.0	0.75	365	−223.06
Minnesota high risk					Postmenopausal			
1. 8.91	5.20	1	−0.37 (−0.5)		1. 9.18	5.01	1	−0.37 (−0.5)
2. 0.5	0.04	28	−17.42		2. 0.0	0.0	28	0.0
3. 0.5	0.07	365	−256.51		3. 1.0	0.08	365	−15.48
4. 0.0	0.84	28	−15.63		4. 0.0	0.0	28	0.0
5. 0.0	0.62	365	−200.75		5. 0.0	1.06	365	−161.21

^{a} M, mesor; A, amplitude; τ, period; φ, phase, related to acrophase ϕ by equation $\phi = (2\pi/\tau)\varphi$, expressed in radians. Circadian φ adjusted to −0.5 for comparison of groups.

Table 37.14
Parameter Values Used in Theoretical Reconstruction of Prolactin Variability Due to Circadian, Circatrigintan and Circannual Rhythms

M^a	A	τ	φ		M	A	τ	φ
Japan					Adolescent			
1. 21.35	11.93	1	−0.12 (−0.5)		1. 20.31	7.99	1	−0.16 (−0.5)
2. 0.5	0.26	28	−5.52		2. 0.5	0.12	28	−22.17
3. 0.5	0.41	365	−86.18		3. 0.5	0.23	365	−70.97
4. 0.0	1.82	28	−15.79		4. 0.0	3.50	28	−25.20
5. 0.0	5.8	365	−13.18		5. 0.0	2.94	365	−75.03
Minnesota Low Risk					Young Adult			
1. 15.47	6.92	1	−0.15 (−0.5)		1. 20.58	11.10	1	−0.12 (−0.5)
2. 0.5	0.27	28	−10.97		2. 0.5	0.33	28	−9.80
3. 0.5	0.11	365	−131.81		3. 0.5	0.23	365	−114.57
4. 0.0	1.69	28	−7.00		4. 0.0	5.07	28	−13.46
5. 0.0	2.59	365	−140.93		5. 0.0	3.55	365	−22.31
Minnesota High Risk					Postmenopausal			
1. 17.13	8.89	1	−0.13 (−0.5)		1. 12.95	8.58	1	−0.13 (−0.5)
2. 0.5	0.11	28	−13.38		2. 0	0.0	28	0.0
3. 0.5	0.13	365	−29.40		3. 1	0.23	365	−57.79
4. 0.0	1.57	28	−17.42		4. 0	0.0	28	0.0
5. 0.0	2.58	365	−44.61		5. 0	1.51	365	−53.74

^{a} M, mesor; A, amplitude; τ, period; φ, phase, related to acrophase ϕ by equation $\phi = (2\pi/\tau)\varphi$, expressed in radians. Circadian φ adjusted to −0.5 for comparison of groups.

might question the validity of these results, since they were based on "imputations" rather than on statistically validated rhythm characteristics. Nevertheless, the same finding is observed when the mean "best-fitting" circadian period is computed after (a) disregarding period imputations that yielded best-fitting periods at one of the limits of the chronobiologic window investigated (20 or 28 hr) and (b) considering only the best-

fitting periods that showed a rhythm significant at the 5% level.

The circadian acrophases were found to be similar for groups H, B, and C when a 24-hr cosine was fitted to the data. In this connection, it is important to note that when the population-mean cosinor was first proposed (24), it was emphasized that a given precise period such as the 24-hr period was fitted with the expectation

1-Adolescent Women

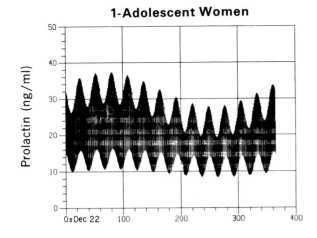

2-Young Adult Women

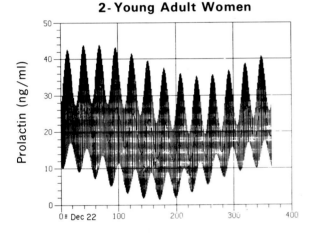

3- Post-menopausal Women

(possible residual circatrigintan component not investigated)

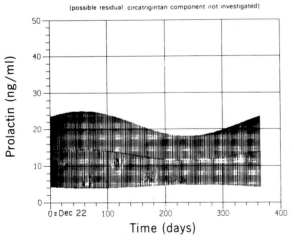

Time (days)

Figure 37.24. Theoretical reconstruction of partial spectral structure of human plasma prolactin in three age groups (based on parameter estimates obtained from separate least-squares fittings of cosine curves with periods of 24 hr (circadian), 28 days (circatrigintan) and 365 days (circannual) to data on plasma prolactin obtained very 20 min for 24 hr, four times a year on a few women). Didactic example modeled on the basis of data collected in the Japan-Minnesota investigation, suggests age-related differences in the

that the period best characterizing the data set on any one day would almost certainly differ from precisely 24 hr. It was further emphasized that no implication was made as to any precise period length by the fit of, say, a 24-hr period; it was thereby solely assumed that an *a priori* 24-hr period would be close enough to the actual period to demonstrate substantially the same parameters and significance; the 24-hr period would thus serve only as a simple representative of the circadian region of the spectrum.

The fact that acrophases for different groups of subjects—H, B, and C—are close to each other when a 24-hr period is being fitted to the data on human breast temperatures is likely due to the fact that all subjects lived on a regular 24-hr routine. The conclusions to be promptly derived from the results of these fits are: (a) that there is a high likelihood that a circadian period characterized the data; (b) that this period was in the neighborhood of 24 hr in all three groups; (c) that, nonetheless, the circadian period differed among the several groups investigated, H, B, and C; and (d) that the technical limitations of analyses based upon only a few days' data are not likely to account for this intergroup difference. (These limitations will be amplified later in this paper.) Study of more individuals for longer spans, including recordings under conditions of isolation from any 24-hr routine, will be desirable to clarify the question whether multiple periods may underlie the results.

DISCUSSION

In this first report of a large international cooperation, many problems arise that are not solved. They are here presented as an indication of the need to control seemingly trivial factors such as the inequalities of the samples of blood withdrawn at different consecutive times and the need to establish for each of the variables being examined that any differences in amount do not play a role. Such illustrative problems serve to indicate the tasks on hand in devising pertinent sampling procedures and thus may serve others who may build upon the results of this study.

interaction of human plasma prolactin rhythms with different frequencies, including circadian mesor and amplitude both modulated by circatrigintan rhythms (except for postmenopausal group) and by circannual rhythms.

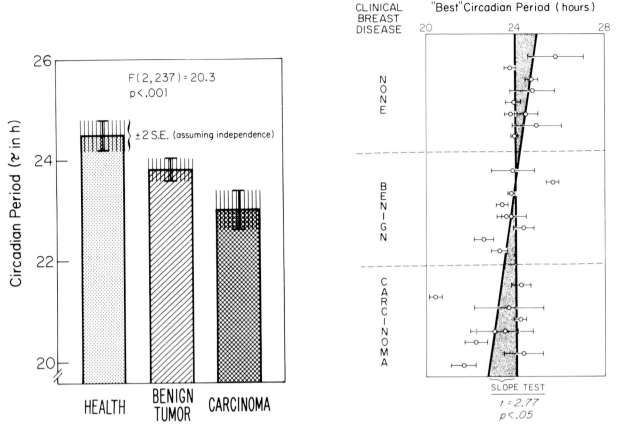

Figures 37.25. (*left*) and **37.26.** (*right*): Average period of circadian temperature rhythm on human breast surface in health, benign disease, and cancer. Shortening of circadian period length of breast surface temperature rhythm in women with carcinoma as compared to healthy controls, with intermediate result obtained from women with benign disease of the breast. Ordinates on Figure 37.26 were scaled in an admittedly arbitrary fashion by assigning one for the healthy controls, two to women with benign disease, and three to women with carcinoma. Thereby, it was assumed, for the purpose of this computation, that there was an even change from health to benign disease to cancer. All period values in a given ordinate category were equally weighted for the computation of a *slope-test*. The linear trend thus formed constitutes a rough approximation. It suggests a shortening of circadian period with increasing severity of the disease. Based on least squares fitting of cosine curves with periods ranging from 20-28 hr. Best circadian period: that of cosine with smallest residual error. Recordings at five sites (four quadrants and nipple) from each breast. Ten series/subject, each series covering 96 hr, at 2-hr intervals daily from 08:00 to 22:00 hr. *F*, F-test; *p*, P-value (associated to F-test), S.E., standard error; *t*, t-[*t*-test] and *p*, P-value (associated to t-test).

Sampling

In turning to the effect of blood sample size, several differences relative to the amount of blood withdrawn were observed. According to the original protocol, small amounts of blood (1 ml) were withdrawn every 20 min in order to evaluate prolactin and cortisol concentration, whereas every 100 min a larger amount of blood (13.5 ml) was withdrawn so that eleven additional hormones could also be evaluated. Thus it was possible to investigate the effect of sampling by comparing results obtained from the large and small blood samples for prolactin and cortisol.

Circadian rhythm characteristics were derived from all samples ($\Delta t = 20$ min) and from the 100-min samples only, in each of the four seasons. The differences between the rhythm characteristics from the two series ($\Delta t = 100$ min; $\Delta t = 20$ min) were computed for each season. A highly statistically significant linear correlation between the rhythm characteristics determined from the 20-min and 100-min samples was demonstrated. Figure 37.27 illustrates the goodness of the linear regression in the case of prolactin mesors, determined in the four seasons, in the classical regression problem, and when the straight line is constrained to pass through the origin. Although very good correla-

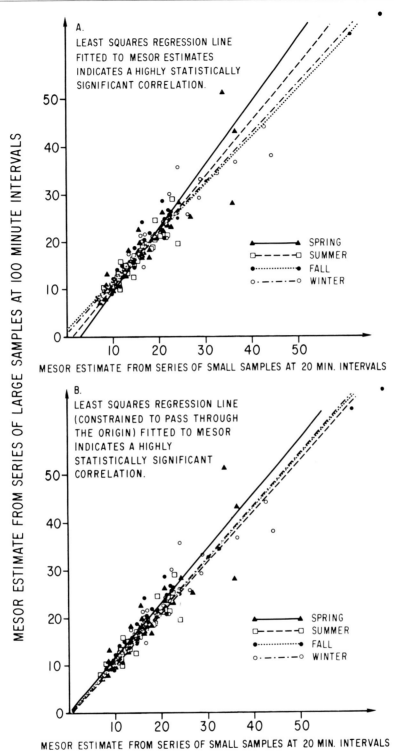

Figure 37.27. Statistically highly significant correlation of prolactin circadian mesors evalutated from all blood samples, collected at 20-min intervals, and from larger amounts of blood withdrawn every 100 min throughout a 24-hr span in each of four seasons; least-squares regression line fitted to data without (A) and with (B) the constraint that the straight line must pass through the origin.

tion coefficients were obtained, a *t*-test for paired "observations" demonstrates a consistent, statistically significant difference in mesor for all seasons except for cortisol in summer,

Tables 37.15A and 37.16A. This finding is corroborated by two nonparametric inferential statistical tests, *i.e.* the sign test (Tables 37.15B and 37.16B) and Wilcoxon's signed ranked test (Ta-

Table 37.15
Detection of Differences Between Circadian Parameter Estimates for Prolactin Determined with Large Blood Samples (every 100 min) and Small Blood Samples (every 20 min)

Parameter	Winter		Spring		Summer		Fall	
A. Test (t, P) on differences in rhythm characteristics obtained with large and small samples (paired "observations")[a]								
Mesor	(3.68,	<0.05)	(2.68,	<0.05)	(2.76,	<0.05)	(5.93,	<0.05)
Amplitude	(0.68,	>0.05)	(1.71,	>0.05)	(2.09,	~0.05)	(3.84,	<0.05)
Acrophase	(0.67,	>.05)	(1.69,	>0.05)	(−1.11,	>0.05)	(−.26,	>0.05)
Percentage Rhythm	(3.27,	<0.05)	(2.23,	<0.05)	(1.07,	>0.05)	(2.02,	>0.05)
B. P-values resulting from sign test (nonparametric test)								
Mesor		<0.01		<0.01		0.01		<0.01
Amplitude		>0.05		0.10		0.10		<0.01
Acrophase		>0.05		>0.05		>0.05		>0.05
Percentage Rhythm		0.10		0.10		>0.05		>0.05
C. Wilcoxon's signed ranked test (T, P)[b]								
Mesor	(435.0,	<0.05)	(402.0,	<0.05)	(403.0,	<0.05)	(507.0,	<0.05)
Amplitude	(302.5,	>0.05)	(346.5,	<0.05)	(354.5,	<0.05)	(453.5,	<0.05)
Acrophase	(163.0,	>0.05)	(144.5,	>0.05)	(180.5,	>0.05)	(163.5,	>0.05)
Percentage Rhythm	(400.5,	<0.05)	(280.0,	<0.05)	(291.5,	>0.05)	(329.5,	~0.05)

[a] $t = \bar{D}/S_{\bar{D}}$ where $\bar{D}$ is the mean difference observed between the two series of data and $S_{\bar{D}}$ is the standard error of $\bar{D}$. P is the P-value associated with t.
[b] T = value taken by the test statistic in the Wilcoxon's signed ranked test; P = associated P-value.

Table 37.16
Detection of Differences Between Circadian Parameter Estimates for Cortisol Determined with Large Blood Samples (every 100 min) and Small Blood Samples (every 20 min)

Parameter	Winter		Spring		Summer		Fall	
A. Test (t, P) on differences in rhythm characteristics obtained with large and small samples (paired "observations")[a]								
Mesor	(5.17,	<0.05)	(3.01,	<0.05)	(0.90,	>0.05)	(5.95,	<0.05)
Amplitude	(2.75,	<0.05)	(2.37,	<0.05)	(0.27,	>0.05)	(3.39,	<0.05)
Acrophase	(−2.79,	<0.05)	(−.66,	>0.05)	(0.66,	>0.05)	(0.33,	>0.05)
Percentage Rhythm	(1.14,	>0.05)	(0.35,	>0.05)	(0.16,	>0.05)	(2.65,	<0.05)
B. P-value resulting from sign test (nonparametric test)								
Mesor		<0.01		<0.01		>0.05		<0.01
Amplitude		0.05		>0.05		>0.05		0.10
Acrophase		0.10		0.05		0.10		>0.05
Percentage Rhythm		>0.05		>0.05		>0.05		>0.05
C. Wilcoxon's signed ranked test (T, P)[b]								
Mesor	(486.0,	<0.05)	(421.0,	<0.05)	(388.0,	<0.05)	(491.5,	<0.05)
Amplitude	(394.0,	<0.05)	(364.0,	<0.05)	(308.5,	>0.05)	(424.0,	<0.05)
Acrophase	(110.0,	<0.05)	(134.5,	<0.05)	(213.0,	>0.05)	(262.5,	>0.05)
Percentage Rhythm	(269.5,	>0.05)	(205.5,	>0.05)	(233.5,	>0.05)	(361.0,	<0.05)

[a] $t = \bar{D}/S_{\bar{D}}$ where $\bar{D}$ is the mean difference observed between the two series of data and S_D is the standard error of $\bar{D}$. P is the P-value associated with t.
[b] T, value taken by the test statistic in the Wilcoxon's signed ranked test; P, associated P-value.

bles 37.15C and 37.16C). It can thus be concluded that a slightly and statistically significantly larger mesor estimate is obtained with prolactin and cortisol data from larger volumes of blood withdrawn every 100 min, as compared to smaller volumes taken every 20 min.[2]

A similar finding was obtained for adenosine deaminase activity (ADA), an enzyme evaluated in samples of packed erythrocytes from some of the subjects. A t-test for comparison of effect due to the amount of blood withdrawn was carried out. In the series investigated, there was a highly statistically significant difference ($P <$

[2]The chemical analyses of the 20-min and 100-min samples were done at the same time in the same series of samples and with equal sample size in each assay. A relatively larger degree of evaporation from the tubes containing the smaller (0.5 ml) amount of plasma as compared with the three 2-ml samples of the 100-min specimen cannot be responsible for the differences, for the values obtained in the 100-min samples are slightly larger than those in the 20-min

samples. Hormone absorption to the glass tube, however, may be relatively more important in the smaller samples, which were kept in the same type of tubes. Further investigation is being conducted to pinpoint the cause of this difference. An ultradian rhythm with a frequency near 100 min also can be considered, although so far only speculatively, as possibly contributing to the results.

0.001) between mean values determined on samples representing different amounts of withdrawn blood: when a larger amount of blood was withdrawn, the values tended to be higher. This effect was observed only for ADA expressed in terms of μmole of NH_3 produced per milliliter of packed red cells and not for ADA expressed in terms of μmole of NH_3 produced per hr per gram of hemoglobin. Differences in values observed when expressed as enzyme activity per milliliter of packed cells as compared to enzyme activity per gram of hemoglobin are likely to be due to differences in the packing of red cells during centrifugation.

In discussing the apparently inverse relationship between circannual prolactin amplitude and the total risk of developing breast cancer, the shortcomings of the risk scale must be emphasized. First, the value for risk used may be a poor measure of risk. It is an estimate of increased risk linearly combined from weighted dichotomization of the characteristics investigated in separate epidemiological studies. Information has been lost in the dichotomizations, and the total risk ignores any interactions among the various risk factors. Furthermore, no consideration is given to relationships between breast cancer factors on the one hand, and possibly competing and interacting risks of other diseases on the other hand. Since epidemiological data for a risk interaction equation are not known to us, no attempt was made to correlate the risk factors with each other.

The advantage of the risk scale is that it uses the available data on risk factors as completely as possible, not only by ascertaining the presence or absence of a given risk factor but also by scaling it according to the information on increased risk determined by prior epidemiological studies. The risk scale is amenable to adjustment as epidemiological data on new risk factors are ascertained and corroborated. This method of individualized risk assessment and correlation deserves further testing and development with special endeavors to account for interactions (50).

With regard to an individual assessment of risk, it is interesting to note recent results obtained by Toti et al. (58). In an analysis of a screening program for the detection of breast cancer in Italy, 15 biological variables extracted from the subjects' histories were used to construct discriminant functions between women with breast cancer and control women without breast cancer. Four variables (age at first examination, number of pregnancies, number of sucklings, symptoms in breast at any time) were found to provide adequate separation of the two groups of women. Although there were problems with false positives and false negatives, Toti et al. state that "...individual values of a discriminant function may be associated with the risk of developing breast cancer in normal women." They suggest that it may be possible in screening programs to consider those women having a discriminant value below a given threshold as being at a higher risk than those above the threshold and therefore requiring follow-up.

Methodologic Considerations

Rhythms with many frequencies in each of several body functions create a dynamic hormonal environment. The complexity of this situation determines from a methodologic viewpoint a given study's minimum duration and sampling frequency in certain cases, such as in work on prolactin. In order to shed light on reproductive and other hormonal processes, as well as on causes of breast cancer and other major diseases, research projects must eventually account for the spectrum of rhythms, from ultradian over circadian to circannual.

Important effects are likely to be missed if sampling is inappropriate. Differences between Japanese and Minnesotans in overall prolactin circadian mesor or amplitude would not have been detected if sampling had been restricted to the summer. Even on the scale of a single day, differences between Japanese and Minnesotans might not have been detected if sampling were limited to a single clock-hour chosen by convenience rather than pertinence.

When dealing with a spectrum of rhythms with different frequencies, several intricate methodologic problems arise, mainly related to sampling rate and size. Straightforward testing of the zero-amplitude assumption with the cosinor procedure on autoregressive data will employ an overestimated number of degrees of freedom and thus lead to a too-optimistic P-value. Methods for arriving at the correct number of degrees of freedom are therefore needed. Moreover, if the time series on hand is not sinusoidal and short, the estimation of a best-fitting period may be the more misleading, the smaller the number of cycles covered by the data. In order to obtain a reasonable estimation of the period length, four to five complete cycles of data are needed (Fig 37.28).

Whenever the period length is known, methods other than the cosinor procedure are avail-

Waveform

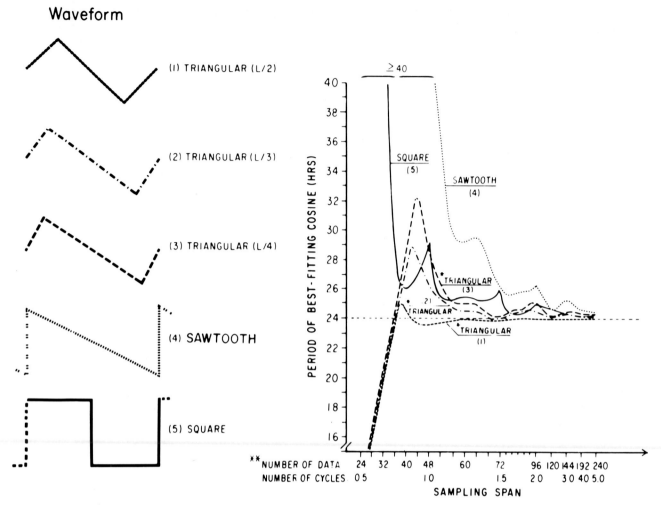

*PERIOD OF TRIANGULAR FUNCTION = 2L (≡ 24 hours) IN EACH CASE ; L/2, L/3 AND L/4 INDICATE DIFFERENT TIMES NEEDED FOR THIS FUNCTION TO REACH ITS PEAK, ON THE UPSLOPE, STARTING FROM THE MEAN

**DATA AT 30-MINUTE INTERVALS.

Figure 37.28. Effect of sampling span and wave-form upon period of best fitting cosine in chronobiological window. Cosine curve fitted by least-squares: at least five consecutive cycles should be considered in order to obtain a reasonable evaluation (within ~5%) of the true period length.

able to account for any asymmetry in the waveform. Such methods include harmonic interpolation (6), where the data on hand are used to reconstruct a continuous time function, thus allowing visualization of the shape of the bioperiodicity. Other methods are also available, where, for instance, more complex models (*e.g.* models including higher harmonics) are fitted by least squares to the data on hand (57).

When designing demanding and expensive experiments in biology or medicine, it is important to examine all possible benefits from different sampling schemes, whether from repeated measurements on the same individual in a longitudinal survey or from sampling transversely in groups of similar individuals. A practical solution may be achieved when a compromise between the two sampling schedules is followed;

in such a hybrid approach, several individuals are followed-up longitudinally while new groups of subjects are added, thus providing simultaneously for longitudinal and transverse samples. Sampling is further complicated if the experiments are carried out in several locations, leading to an additional source of variation. In some cases, for instance in animal experiments synchronized with several different lighting regimens, it is possible to achieve serially independent "around-the-clock" data by experiments done only during working hours; this is achieved by using different rooms, each being set to a different lighting regimen, in which the animals have been stabilized with validated different timing.

Since specifications concerning the experimental set-up are usually lengthy, some terms are here proposed to facilitate precise and concise experimental descriptions. Clear, succinct composite terms seem efficient for this purpose. They can be built according to part or all of the following pattern. All the proposed new compounds would end with "-cyclic" to denote repetitive sampling:

Prefixes (if needed)		Required Stems	Uniform Suffix
met- (if staggered)	an- (negation)	-idio- (individual)	-cyclic
		-eco- (related to location)	
(1)	(2)	(3)	(4)

(1) The prefix "met-" allows the choice among several staggered schedules instead of a regular (not staggered) regimen.

(2) The prefix "an-" indicates the absence of the next part of the word.

(3) The main specification in relation to an individual is the "-idio-" and in relation to a location the "-eco-".

(4) The final "-cyclic" implies specified equidistant or unequidistant placement of repeated observations.

One could consider for future work subjects (e.g. permanent night workers) with a consistently changed temporal placement along the 24-hr scale of certain of their circadian rhythms. Thus, one could institute certain "metanidioanecocyclic" schemes to compare different circadian stages of a given rhythm, measured simultaneously in different individuals in different locations—in an approach to an idealized circadian cycle. The "met-," in this case, would indicate the use of staggered work environments.[3]

Correlation matrices were computed first without eliminating outliers because of the small total numbers of subjects in the groups being compared. Further investigations will have to clarify whether and if so to what extent outliers bias the results obtained thus far.

For some analyses beyond our scope, tests for

---

[3] I (for idio) also can stand for an individual and thus for idiocyclicity. By the same token E (for eco) stands also for the environment. Once sampling is serially independent, it is usually staggered and the staggering can be indicated by an M (for meta). Thus abbreviations are logical and etymologically correct: MI stands for serially independent sampling of individuals at different (staggered) times and ME indicates different environments studied in a staggered fashion. Combinations may also be used, such as MEMI, indicating serial independence with respect to both the environment and the individual. It is possible that sampling is MI in relation to circannual rhythms but not to circadian ones. In the latter case, the convention is that it does not have to be indicated. Sampling that may be serially dependent as to individuals for a circadian profile, but serially independent for a circannual profile, would be circannual MI; this would imply the entire sentence of circadian serial dependence of individuals.

outliers were performed. Thus, in a summary of results obtained by applying the population-mean cosinor to the risk or age categories, the Hotelling's T^2 statistic was utilized to test for any statistically significant differences between two populations with respect to parameters of circadian rhythms (mesors, amplitudes, and acrophases), jointly considered. A preliminary examination of circadian parameters, however, revealed that some subjects had an unusually high mesor compared to others in their respective categories. Assuming multivariate normality of parameters, a simple test for detecting outliers (7) was applied to the mesors in each category compared. To apply the test, the mesors in a given category were ordered from the smallest to the largest and denoted as $M_{(1)}$, $M_{(2)}$, and $M_{(n)}$, where n was the total number of mesors. The test statistic, r, was then computed for the largest or smallest value, as follows:

$$r_{(n)} = \frac{M_{(n)} - M_{(n-1)}}{M_{(n)} - M_{(1)}} \quad \text{for} \quad M_{(n)}$$

$$r_{(1)} = \frac{M_{(2)} - M_{(1)}}{M_{(n)} - M_{(1)}} \quad \text{for} \quad M_{(1)}$$

The calculated $r_{(n)}$ or $r_{(1)}$ was then compared with tabulated critical values of r (9). If an outlier was detected it was deleted and the procedure was repeated on remaining values.

Indeed, the inclusion of outliers in a first analysis does not lessen the need to eliminate those outliers which, in retrospect, indicate that some

Table 37.17
Schedule for Stepwise Seasonal Sampling for Estimation of Circannual and Circadian Parameters[a]; Endocrine Rhythm Parameters Correlated with the Risks of Developing Breast Cancer (BC) and/or Diseases Associated with an Elevated Blood Pressure (BP)

	Hormone	Fall	Winter	Spring	Summer	
BP	Aldosterone	←------- Circannual Amplitude --------→				
	DHEA-S[b]		M*			
	E2			A*		
	E3		M, A**		M, A**	
	Prolactin	M**	<u>M</u>, A**	<u>M</u>, A*		
	Prolactin	←------- Circannual Amplitude --------→				
	LH	<u>M</u>		M**	M*	
	LH	←------ Circannual Mesor -------→				BC
	E1	M**			M**	
	T4	M**				
	TSH	M**				
	TSH	------- Circannual Amplitude -------→				

[a] If not specified, frequency is circadian.

[b] DHEA-S, dehydroepiandrosterone sulfate; M, mesor; E2, estradiol; A, amplitude; E3, estriol; LH, luteinizing hormone; E1, estrone; T4, thyroxine; TSH, thyroid-stimulating hormone; *, correlation with blood-pressure-associated disease risk; **, correlation with breast cancer risk; =, correlation with both risks; ←----, circannual urinary sampling; ←——, circannual blood sampling.

subjects may lie remote from the mean in one or several respects.

Much has been written about biochemical individuality without taking rhythms into account. These authors do not wish to commit the reverse mistake in not considering biochemical individuality while considering rhythms. Rhythms have long been recognized as a feature of biochemical and other individuality. Individuality, as it may appear from consecutive comparisons of subjects, is more readily pursued when, for example, a circadian rhythm in cortisol can be documented by sampling on a single day for 132 out of 133 series. Many more individuals on many more days will have to be assessed to segregate at each pertinent frequency the biochemical individuality of a single subject, qualified as to the rhythms' mesor, acrophase, amplitude, and wave-form. Finally, it may be noted that the comparison of healthy populations with no known disease also constitutes an attempt to define health positively and in an individualized fashion. Thus, this approach complements the continued definition of an index of health tied to causes of death (sic), an approach that continues to be used at this time.

This study was based on relatively few individuals. It had to be carried out (for economic reasons) without the originally planned inclusion of a high-risk group in Japan. Nonetheless, it has sufficed to yield suggestions for further work that can be supported by a set of statistically significant results (Table 37.17). The many samples from each of a very few individuals lead to conclusions that can now be properly tested on many more individuals with relatively few samples and even with single samples for one or the other variable, as the case may be. Various breast cancer risk factors that could not be separated because of the lack of a Japanese high-risk group and because dietary and other conditions, including climate, were not controlled, confound the results. For this reason the circumstance is noteworthy that all of these factors are controlled to some extent in the Italian study involving groups of subjects exposed to the same climate of Tuscany, presumably a comparable diet, and but a single risk factor. The agreement of certain results that are comparable in the Italian and Kyushuan-Minnesotan studies is the more noteworthy.

CONCLUSION

Apart from the slight differences observed in the amounts of blood withdrawn that still need further investigation, reliable determination of a spectrum of rhythms could be made for most of the hormones evaluated in these international studies. It can thus be concluded that rhythms with many frequencies in several body functions together create a dynamic hormonal environment. The complexity of this environment determines from a methodologic viewpoint the desirable minimum duration and sampling frequency of a certain study in certain circumstances, such as in work on cortisol and prolactin, in order to shed light on reproductive and other hormonal processes, as well as on causes of breast cancer and other major diseases.

An increasingly rational individualized prevention and/or treatment of disease requires an individualized and time-qualified definition of health by the establishment of reference intervals and rhythm characteristics of hormonal and other physiologic variability. With these reference intervals and rhythm characteristics available, one can better interpret with single samples or time series an increased risk of a certain disease or the inception of the disease. The practitioner needs rhythm-qualified peer-group and individualized reference intervals for the study of single samples, and estimates of rhythm characteristics for reference in the study of time series. Diagnostic nihilism and over-prescription of tests are equally probable consequences of sampling without proper qualifications as to individualized timing—whenever it is unambiguously demonstrated that without a rhythm-qualified interpretation, a single sample may be interpreted as too high at one time, too low at another, and "normal" at a third time.

From the viewpoint of benefit versus cost, time-specified single samples and time series interpreted against appropriately time-qualified tolerance intervals constitute for several variables a highly rational approach in medical research and practice (Table 37.18). This approach is desirable, in any event, in order to avoid misinterpretation. By contrast, without (individualized or at least peer-group) reference intervals that are qualified by a spectrum of rhythms, the interpretation of single samples is likely to be an undiscriminating endeavor, often wasteful because useless, and occasionally harmful. Figures 37.29 and 37.30 describe tolerance intervals along the scales of a day and Figures 37.30 and 37.31 with seasons. While circadian mesors of aldosterone estimated for the Minnesotan subjects should not get higher than ~12.5 ng/dl, in spring, values as high as ~22 ng/dl are still included in the (0.90, 0.90) winter tolerance interval. With rhythmometric precautions "sins of omission" such as relying on time-unspecified single samples can be avoided and, as this chronoepidemiologic study has revealed, large differences may be found in rhythms among certain populations, also characterized by large differences in morbidity and mortality from breast cancer among other conditions.

SUMMARY

Several hormones as well as other physiologic variables of potential interest for breast cancer research have been shown to undergo rhythmic variation. The bioperiodicities involved concern

Table 37.18
Circadian Chronodesm for Plasma Prolactin Concentration Established on the Basis of Data from 4 Adolescent Japanese Women in Winter (Group I) and Validated ~1 Year Later on a Larger Group of 20 Women of Same Age and Ethnicity (Group II)[a]

Time Interval	Circadian Prolactin Concentration Chronodesm (Group I) (ng/ml)		Percent of Data from Group II Outside Chronodesm
	Lower limit	Higher limit	
$00^{00}-02^{00}$	10.7	158.5	15%
$02^{00}-04^{00}$	15.8	112.2	0%
$04^{00}-06^{00}$	10.7	134.9	
$06^{00}-08^{00}$	10.7	102.3	17.5%
$08^{00}-10^{00}$	2.6	63.1	
$10^{00}-12^{00}$	2.6	40.7	10%
$12^{00}-14^{00}$	5.6	28.8	
$14^{00}-16^{00}$	5.3	31.4	10%
$16^{00}-18^{00}$	5.0	33.9	
$18^{00}-20^{00}$	4.3	89.1	5%
$20^{00}-22^{00}$	5.5	50.1	
$22^{00}-24^{00}$	3.4	50.1	10.7% overall

[a] It seems pertinent that in a recent issue of the *New England Journal of Medicine*, Zervas and Martin (64) state that excessive prolactin secretion (by pituitary adenomas) can be readily detected by measuring basal (morning) plasma concentration. For these authors prolactin concentrations larger than 100 ng/ml are considered abnormal and indicative of a tumor, whereas normal values are considered to be less than 15 ng/ml. Time-specified tolerance intervals such as those reported in this table indicated that prolactin concentration in the morning is still decreasing from overnight high values. Prolactin assessment will be more discriminating, in the diagnosis of tumors and other disorders, if careful consideration is given to rhythms, *i.e.*, if samples are obtained at appropriate times. The problem on hand should also be taken into account. One must consider with the expected change (*e.g.*, elevation of prolactin in patients with certain pituitary tumors) also the physiologic timing of the sleep-wakefulness or activity-rest pattern. By taking rhythmic variations into account, chronodesms will usually yield narrower intervals than conventional "normal ranges". The set of time-specified tolerance intervals shown in this table is expected to contain at least about 90% of the distribution of data with 90% confidence. As expected, on the average, in a replication about 90% of the data fall within the chronodesm.

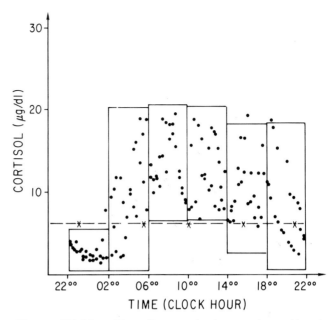

Figure 37.29. Circadian cortisol merodesm (*bars*) established from data (•) on young women (15–21 yr) in winter. As for an individual (Fig. 37.14), a value may be found for a pair of young women that is well within the reference interval at several times, yet below or above the tolerance interval at other times.[4]

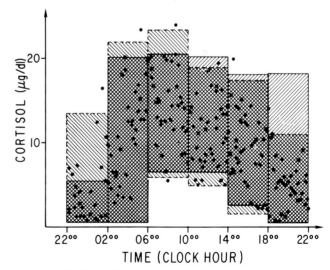

Figure 37.30. Extent of agreement of chronodesms constructed for two seasons.[4]

[4] When applied directly to the data collected, chronodesms may sometimes yield a zero lower limit when no zeros recur in the original data and may yield even negative lower limits. In these cases, it is recommended to compute the chronodesm after log-transformation of the data. Limits thus obtained are then retransformed into original units. These limits usually are different from those obtained without log-transformation.

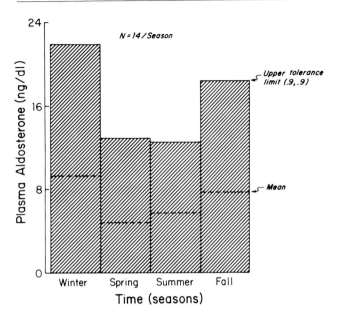

Figure 37.31. Circannual merodesm for aldosterone in blood plasma. Circannual and circadian chronodesms may have to be derived, as suggested by large differences in upper tolerance limits established for plasma aldosterone of healthy Minnesotan women. (In each season circadian mesor of each subject estimated by fitting 24-hr cosine curve to data obtained throughout 24 hr. Tolerance interval (with 90% chance of including 90% of distribution) for circadian mesors was then computed. Only upper tolerance limits are pertinent (lower limits are computational artifacts: zero).) Statistically-significant effect of season on circadian mesor indicated by ANOVA (analysis of variance) (with repeated measures). *F*, 4.16; *P*, 0.02.[4]

several frequencies, indicating the need to investigate, when pertinent, not only single samples and not even solely a circadian rhythm, but multiple frequencies. Exploration of a spectrum of rhythms with several frequencies suggested differences between Japanese (mostly Kyushuan) and North American (mostly Minnesotan) women in plasma prolactin, aldosterone, insulin, estrone and estriol, and urinary melatonin. Rhythmometry on strategically placed and sequenced time series allowed the individualized quantification of circadian rhythms in plasma prolactin and cortisol for most (>90%) Japanese and Minnesotan subjects. Statistically significant differences in circadian parameters between the two populations were thus demonstrated. In addition, rhythm-qualified tolerance intervals could be derived for a cost-effective interpretation of subsequent time-qualified single samples. Circannual rhythms had to be taken into consideration as well, since circannual (about-yearly) variation in several plasma hormones could be described in one geographic

location but not in another—insulin, estrone, aldosterone, and DHEA-S in Minnesota, prolactin and estriol in Japan. A reduction in extent of predictable circannual variation in plasma prolactin of Minnesotan, as compared to Kyushuan, women—differing in breast cancer risk—was paralleled by lesser circannual variation in patients with fibrocystic mastopathy, as compared to clinically healthy women, found in a separate study of serum prolactin in Italy. The geographic-ethnic and/or otherwise determined differences between Kyushuans and Minnesotans were shown to be statistically significant and were partly replicated, yet they would not have been detectable by sampling at certain hours or seasons fixed only by convenience rather than pertinence.

The paper emphasizes, in fact, the importance of sampling at a time chosen according to clinical pertinence rather than to convenience. Important hormonal differences between populations differing in risk of breast cancer are detectable only if bioperiodicities are properly assessed. Sampling requirements concerning density, duration of observation span, cost-effectiveness of spot-checks or adequate time-qualified single samples and other sampling problems related to clinical protocols are thoroughly examined in a few cases. In so doing, a feasibility check of the chronobiologic approach is provided. Added service by chronobiologists to oncologists must be extended 1) in depth and scope, 2) to additional frequencies, 3) to more hormonal and other variables, and 4) with (a) strategically placed but fewer samples and (b) for more individuals. The rhythmometric highways yet to be laid are ambitious and demanding endeavors. Once completed, they promise to facilitate rapid traffic to the goals, among others, of cancer prevention and treatment.

Addendum. Further work on the samples from the Japanese-American chronoepidemiologic study has revealed differences in plasma renin activity associated in part with differences in diet. Further evidence from the same samples also was obtained on geographic differences in plasma aldosterone and was complemented by findings of differences in urinary aldosterone and electrolytes (31, 32). These findings are of interest for students of diseases associated with high blood pressure as well as of breast cancer and allow considerations of competing risks—to be considered in any chronoepidemiologic endeavor. Such risks come to the fore in circannual rhythm parameters at a time when evidence from casual single samples or even from circadian rhythm parameters is noncontributory.

A recent clinical symposia issue published by CIBA (Volume 32, 2, 1980, 32 pp.) in discussing "breast lumps" reflects caution toward thermography. The latter procedure is not even mentioned—a decision apparently justified in view of the experience thus far with diagnostic uses of thermography for dealing with breast lumps. As yet that publication does not refer to thermorhythmometry, a decision again justified since the promise of this procedure discussed in the foregoing chapter and elsewhere notwithstanding, large-scale tests are essential before it may be advocated for practical application.

Acknowledgment. Supported by United States Public Health Service (GM-13981), National Cancer Institute (CA-14445 and CP-55702), National Institute of Occupational Safety and Health (OH-00631), National Institute of Aging (AG-00158), Environmental Protection Agency (R804512), and the St. Paul-Ramsey Medical Education and Research Foundation. The authors are most indebted for invaluable help to the subjects of this study who gave amply of their time in an unusually motivated and consistent fashion; to the staff of the Clinical Research Center at the University of Minnesota, notably Ms. Jane Gergan, Ms. Grace Anderson, and Ms. Dawn Cressey; to many volunteers who helped in the recruitment and screening of subjects; to Elliot Weitzman (Professor and Chairman, Department of Neurology, Albert Einstein College of Medicine, New York) who kindly demonstrated the three stopcock technique used for sampling blood without awareness of the subject; to Kurt Amplatz (Professor of Radiology, University of Minnesota) who reviewed the same technique and provided training for a fellow; and to Charles Ehret (Argonne National Laboratory, Lamont, Illinois) who read the manuscript and provided helpful comments.

References

1. Boot, L. M. (1970): Prolactin and mammary gland carcinogenesis—problem of human prolactin. *Int. J. Cancer,* 5:167.
2. Cappelaere, P. (1975): Prolactine et cancers mammaires. *Pathol. Biol.,* 23: 161.
3. Choi, N. W., Howe, E. R., Miller, A. B., Matthews, V., Morgan, R. W., Munan, L., Bursh, J. D., Feather, J., Jain, M., and Kuley, A. (1978): An epidemiologic study of breast cancer. *Am. J. Epidemiol.,* 107:510–521.
4. Cole, P., and Cramer, D. (1977): Diet and cancer of endocrine target organs. *Cancer,* 40:434–437.
5. Cornélissen, G., Carandente, F., and Halberg, F. (1980): Data collection and analysis, in *Biological Rhythms, Documenta Geigy,* pp. 6–8. Ciba-Geigy Ltd., Basel, Switzerland.
6. De Prins, J., Cornélissen, G., Hillman, D., Halberg, F., and Van Dyck, C. (in press): Harmonic interpolation yields paraphases and orthophases for biologic rhythms, in *Proc. XIII Int. Conf. Int. Soc. Chronobiol.,* D. K. Hayes, F. Halberg, L. E. Scheving (eds) Il Ponte, Milan, Italy.
7. Dixon, W. J. (1953): Processing data for outliers. *Biometrics,* 9:74–89.
8. Donati, L., Lauro, R., Vasta, M., Locatelli, I., Camagna, A., Tatti, P., and Halberg, F. (1979): Circadian plasma prolactin hemopsy—variation assessed individually in a menstrually-cycling and a post-menopausal Italian woman. *Chronobiologia,* 6:93.
9. Dunn, O. J., and Clark, V. A. (1974): *Applied Statistics: Analysis of Variance and Regression.* John Wiley & Sons, New York.
10. Egan, R. L. (1979): Estimated risk and occurrence of breast cancer in assymptomatic and minimally symptomatic patients. *Cancer,* 43:871–877.
11. Farewell, V. T., Math, B., and Math, M. (1977): The combined effect of breast cancer risk factors. *Cancer,* 40:931–936.
12. Gala, R. R., Van de Walle, C., Hoffman, W. H., Lawson, D. M., Pieper, D. R., Smith, S. W., and Subramanian, M. G. (1977): Lack of a circannual cycle of daytime serum prolactin in man and monkey. *Acta Endocrinol.,* 86:257–262.
13. Garcia Sainz, M., Tarquini, B., Cagnoni, M., Castellanos, J. M., Garcia Pena, J., and Halberg, F. (1979): Thermorrhythmometry in health (H), benign breast disease (B) and breast cancer (C) and obliteration of circannual, but not of circadian rhythm in serum prolactin in fibrocystic mastopathy. *Proc. AACR/ASCO,* 20:110.
14. Halberg, F. (1965): Some aspects of biologic data analysis; longitudinal and transverse profiles of rhythms, in *Circadian Clocks,* pp. 13–22, edited by J. Aschoff. North-Holland Publishing Company, Amsterdam.
15. Halberg, F. (1969): Chronobiology. *Annu. Rev. Physiol.,* 31:675–725.
16. Halberg, F. (1977): Biological as well as physical parameters relate to radiology. Guest Lecture, *Proc. 30th Ann. Cong. Rad.,* January, 1977, Post Graduate Institute of Medical Education and Research, Chandigarth, India.
17. Halberg, F., Carandente, F., Cornélissen, G., and Katinas, G. S. (1977): Glossary of chronobiology. *Chronobiologia,* 4: Suppl. 1.
18. Halberg, F., Engeli, M., Hamburger, C., and Hillman, D. (1965): Spectral resolution of low-frequency, small-amplitude rhythms in excreted 17-ketosteroid; probable androgen-induced circaseptan desynchronization. *Acta Endocrinol.,* 50: Suppl. 103, 5–54.
19. Halberg, F., Gupta, B. D., Haus, E., Halberg, E., Deka, A. C., Nelson, W., Sothern, R. B., Cornélissen, G., Lee, J. K., Lakatua, D. J., Scheving, L. E., and Burns, E. R. (1977): Steps toward a cancer chronopolytherapy, in *Proc. XIVth Int. Cong. Therapeutics,* pp. 151–196, Montpellier, France, L'Expansion Scientifique Française, Paris.
20. Halberg, F., Haus, E., Tarquini, B., Cagnoni, M., Cornélissen, G., Lakatua, D., Kawasaki, T., Wallach, L. A., Halberg, E., and Omae, T. (1979): Circannual and circadian variations in some blood hormones, notably prolactin. In: Internal Medicine, Proc. XIVth Int. Cong. Internal Medicine, ISM Rome, Italy, held in October, 1978, L Condorelli, U. Teodori, M. Sangiorgie and R. Neri Semeri, Eds., Excerpta Medica, Amsterdam/Oxford, pp. 5–11.
21. Halberg, F., Johnson, E. A., Nelson, W., Runge, W., and Sothern, R. (1972): Autorhythmometry—procedures for physiologic self-measurements and their analysis. *Physiol. Teacher,* 1:1–11.
22. Halberg, F., Katinas, G. S., Chiba, Y., Garcia Sainz, M., Kovats, T. G., Künkel, H., Montalbetti, N., Reinberg, A., Scharf, R., and Simpson, H. (1973): Chronobiologic glossary of the International Society for the Study of Biologic Rhythms. *Int. J. Chronobiol.,* 1:31–63.
23. Halberg, F., Lee, J. K., and Nelson, W. (1978): Time-qualified reference intervals—chronodesms. *Experientia,* 34:713–716.
24. Halberg, F., Tong, Y. L., and Johnson, E. A. (1967): Circadian system phase—an aspect of temporal morphology; procedures and illustrative examples, in *The Cellular Aspects of Biorhythms,* pp. 20–48, edited by H. von Mayersbach. Springer-Verlag, Berlin.
25. Haus, E., Lakatua, D. J., Halberg, F., Halberg, E., Cornélissen, G., Sackett, L. L., Berg, H. G., Kawasaki, T., Ueno, M., Uezono, K., Matsuoka, M., and Omae, T. (1980): Chronobiologic studies of plasma prolactin in women in Kyushu, Japan and Minnesota, USA *J. Clin. Endocrinal Metab.* 51:632–640, 1980.
26. Hershman, J. M. (1974): Clinical application of thyrotropin-releasing hormone. *N. Engl. J. Med.,* 290:886–890.
27. Hirayama, T. (ed.) (1977): *Comparative Epidemiology of Cancer in the U.S. and Japan—Mortality.* The U.S.-Japan Cooperative Cancer Research Program, Japan Society for the Promotion of Science.
28. Hirayama, T. (ed) (1978): *Comparative Epidemiology of Cancer in the U.S. and Japan—Morbidity.* The U.S.-Japan Cooperative Cancer Research Program, Japan Society for the Promotion of Science.
29. Jaffe, B. M., and Berson, H. R. (1974): *Methods of Hormone Radioimmunoassay.* Academic Press, New York.
30. Jenkins, G. M., and Watts, D. G. (1968): *Spectral Analysis and Its Applications.* Holden Day, New York.
31. Kawasaki, T., Ueno, M., Uezono, K., Matsuoka, M., Omae, T., Halberg, F., Wendt, H., Taggett-Anderson, M. A., and Haus, E. (1980): Different circadian mesors for plasma renin activity in healthy young women in Japan and U.S.A. *Am. J. Med.,* 68:91–96.
32. Kawasaki, T., Ueno, M., Uezono, K., Omae, T., Haus, E., and Halberg, F. (1979): Plasma and urinary aldosterone and urinary electrolytes in healthy young women in Japan and U.S.A. *Chronobiologia,* 6:116.
33. Kripke, D. F., Mullaney, D. J., Messin, S., and Wyborney, V. G. (1978): Wrist actigraphic measures of sleep and rhythms. *Electroencephalogr. Clin. Neurophysiol.,* 44:674–676.
34. Kwa, H. G., Bulbrook, R. D., Cleton, F., Verstraeten, A. A., Hayward, J. L., and Wang, D. Y. (1978): An abnormal early evening peak of plasma prolactin in nulliparous and obese post-menopausal women. *Int. J. Cancer,* 22:691–693.
35. Langlands, A. O., Simpson, H., Sothern, R., and Halberg, F. (1977): Different timing of circannual rhythm in mortality of women with breast cancer diagnosed before and after menopause, in *Proc. 8th Int. Scientific Mtg. Int. Epidemiological Assoc.,* San Juan, Puerto Rico, September 17–23.
36. MacMahon, B., Cole, P., and Brown, J. (1973): Etiology of human breast cancer: a review. *J. Natl. Cancer Inst.,* 50:21–42.
37. Malhotra, S. L. (1977): A study of cancer of the breast with special reference to its causation and prevention. *Medical Hypotheses,* 3:21–24.
38. Mandel, J., Halberg, F., Radke, A., Seal, U., and Schuman, L. (1979): Circannual variation in serum TSH and prolactin of prostatic cancer patients. Proc. 3rd Conf. Indian Soc. Chronobiolo., Varanasi, India, December 27–29, 1979.
39. Marquardt, D. W. (1963): An algorithm for least squares estimation of non-linear parameters. *J. Soc. Industrial Appl. Math.,* 11:431–441.
40. Meites, J. (1972): Relation of prolactin to mammary tumorigenesis and growth in rats, in *Prolactin and Carcinogenesis,* 4th Tenovus Workshop, edited by A. R. Boyns and K. Griffiths. Alpha Omega Alpha Publications, Cardiff, Wales.
41. Midgley, A. R. (1966): Radioimmunoassay: a method for human chorionic gonadotropin and human luteinizing hormone. *Endocrinology,* 79:10–18.
42. Miller, A. B. (1978): An overview of hormone-associated cancers. *Cancer Res.,* 38:3985–3990.
43. Mittra, I. (1974): Mammotropic effect of prolactin enhanced by thyroidectomy. *Nature,* 248:525–526.

44. Mittra, I., and Hayward, J. L. (1974): Hypothalamic-pituitary-thyroid axis in breast cancer. *Lancet*, 1:885–889.

45. Mittra, I., and Hayward, J. L. (1974): Hypothalamic-pituitary-prolactin axis in breast cancer. *Lancet*, 1:889–891.

46. Nie, N., Hull, C., Jenkins, J., Steinbrenner, K., and Bent, D. (1975): *Statistical Package for the Social Sciences*, 2nd Ed. McGraw Hill Co., New York.

47. Ostle, B. (1963): *Statistics in Research*. Iowa State University Press.

48. Pearson, O. H., Llurna, O., Llurna, L., Molina, A., and Butler, J. (1969): Prolactin dependent rat mammary cancer: a model for man. *Assoc. Am. Physicians*, 82:225.

49. Perez-Vega, E., Halberg, E., Halberg, F., and Garcia-Sainz, M. (1979): Circannual population rhythm of serum prolactin in serially independent samples from women in Mexico City, Mexico—further steps toward chronopsies. *Proc. Minn. Acad. Sci.*, p. 20.

50. Radke, A. Q., Hillman, D. C., Cornelissen, G., Mandel, J. S., Schuman, L., and Halberg, F. (1979): Correlation between individualized total breast cancer risk and imputed circannual amplitude of plasma prolactin. *Proc. Minn. Acad. Sci.* 19–20.

51. Reiter, R. J. (1974): Circannual reproductive rhythms in mammals related to photoperiod and pineal function: a review. *Chronobiologia*, 4:365–395.

52. Rummel, J. A., Lee, J. K., and Halberg, F. (1974): Combined linear-nonlinear chronobiologic windows by least squares resolve neighboring components in a physiologic rhythm spectrum, in *Biorhythms and Human Reproduction*, pp. 53–82, edited by M. Ferin, F. Halberg, R. M. Richart, and R. Vande Wiele. John Wiley & Sons, New York.

53. Sartwell, P. E., Arthes, F. G., and Tonascia, J. A. (1977): Exogenous hormones, reproductive history and breast cancer. *J. Natl. Cancer Inst.*, 59:1589–1592.

54. Tarquini, A., di Martino, L., Malloci, A., Kwa, H. G., Van der Gugten, A. A., Bulbrook, R. D., and Wang, D. Y. (1978): Abnormalities in evening plasma prolactin levels in nulliparous women with benign or malignant breast disease. *Int. J. Cancer*, 22:687–690.

55. Tarquini, B., Gheri, R., Romano, S., Costa, A., Cagnoni, M., Lee, J. K., and Halberg, F. (1979): Circadian mesor-hyperprolactinemia in fibrocystic mastopathy. *Am. J. Med.* 66:229–237.

56. Tarquini, B., Gheri, R., Romano, S., Costa, A., Cagnoni, M., Lee, J. K., and Halberg, F. (1980): Circadian variation of serum prolactin and TSH of women in health or with mammary carcinoma, fibroadenoma or fibrocystic mastopathy. *Int. J. Chronobiol* (in press).

57. Tong, Y. L., Nelson, W. L., Sothern, R. B., and Halberg, F. (1977): Estimation of the orthophase—timing of the high values on a non-sinusoidal rhythm—illustrated by the best timing for experimental cancer chronotherapy, in *Proc. XII Int. Conf. Int. Soc. Chronobiol.*, Wash., D.C., pp. 765–769. Il Ponte, Milan, Italy.

58. Toti, A., Piffanelli, A., Pavanelli, T., Buriani, C., Nenci, I., Arslan-Pagnini, C., Zanardi, P., Pecorari, S., Rossi, R., and Barrai, I. (in press): Possible indication of breast cancer risk through discriminant functions. *Cancer*.

59. Tritsch, G. L., and Halberg, F. (1979): Individualized circadian rhythmometry of adenosine deaminase activity in red blood cells of healthy women. *Chronobiologia*, 6:164–165.

60. Tritsch. G. L., and Mittelman, A. (1975): Automated determination of adenosine aminohydrolase in human plasma and erythrocytes by continuous flow analysis. *Biochem. Med.*, 12:66–71.

61. Wallace, R. B., Sherman, B. M., Bean, J. A., Leeper, J. P., and Treolar, A. E. (1978): Menstrual cycle patterns and breast cancer risk factors. *Cancer Res.*, 38:4021–4024.

62. Wetterberg, L., Halberg, F., Tarquini, B., Cagnoni, M., Haus, E., Griffiths, K., Kawasaki, T., Wallach, L. A., Ueno, M., Uezono, K., Matsuoka, M., Kuzel, M., Halberg, E., and Omae, T. (1979): Circadian variation in urinary melatonin in clinically healthy women in Japan and U.S.A. *Experientia*, 35:416–419.

63. Wilson, D. W., Groom, G. V., Pierrepoint, C. G., Phillips, F., Fahmy, D. R., Simpson, H., Halberg, F., and Griffiths, K. (1979): Breast skin temperature rhythms throughout the menstrual cycle. *J. Endocrinol.*, 81:118P–119P.

64. Zervas, N. T., and Martin, J. B. (1980): Current concepts in cancer; management of hormone-secreting pituitary adrenomas. *N. Engl. J. Med.*, 302:210.

38

Selected Aspects of the Comparative Pathology of Neoplastic Growth: The Melanomas

Alfonso Giordano, Piergiovanni Grigolato, and Umberto Binda

The melanotic tumors constitute a singular example of neoplastic pathology (13, 15). Several points have to be discussed (1), beginning with their natural, primitive sites.

COMPARATIVE ASPECTS

The melanotic tumors are named after the endogenous pigments known as melanins (7) which have a very wide distribution in invertebrates, vertebrates, and plants. They constitute a group of chemically not well enough known black, dark brown, tan, also yellowish, and reddish pigments. They can be located intercellularly as in chromatophores, or extracellularly. As pointed out by Pierre Masson (14) and others, they occur in different types of tissues, epithelial or nonepithelial, in animals and plants alike. Also, they produce important racial differences in man because they are more abundant in the black race, less common in the yellow races, and least prevalent in the Caucasian race. The pigments are responsible for the dark skin areas, such as the nipple of the breast, the anus, and variations in hair and skin colors. In the Caucasian race, the nipples of dark-haired women or, in general, of dark-haired persons, in the same ontogenetic stage, are more strongly pigmented and therefore darker than the pink nipples in the natural blond. This lead to the observation that melanins are most common in superficial body regions and, therefore, superficial tissues

because they may serve as a protection against intense sunlight—they can also play a role in the heat exchange between organisms and the environment. The many relations and the additional fact that melanomas are generally highly malignant neoplasms, are summarized in Table 38.1. The melanin-containing cells and the neoplasms developing from them are an excellent example for particular aspects of comparative pathology and of great importance for future research.

NEOPLASTIC CHARACTERISTICS OF MELANOMAS

In all neoplasms, relevant enzymatic cellular variations are widely described, which end in metabolic alterations which are sometimes deep. It is rare to find functional deviations which, although serious, allow such a differentiation as to permit the elaboration, even if incomplete, of a proteinaceous substratum as relevant as the melanin.

Unlike almost all other malignant tumors (e.g., pulmonary Ca, gastric Ca) which are grown from a particular organ and follow their own evolution, the melanomas can originate in numerous areas of the body out of the cutis of mucous linings depending on the many terminal sites of the primitive neuroectodermic nodes (8). The melanocytes (2) actually constitute a widely distributed system which contains numerous and unforeseeable potential sites for the appearance of malignant neoplasms which, therefore, within certain limits, could be regarded as a systemic disease, at least potentially. Nevertheless, while the pluricentrism of the melanomas is still to be explained, some aspects referable to an illness of a complicated system remain. To this extent, let us consider the imposing metabolic modifications that the melanomas undergo in the neoplasm and its metastases, up to the extreme reduction of the melanic pigment. This can be documented histologically and chemically.

MELANIN SYNTHESIS

Among the numerous substances involved in this synthesis, two are of greatest importance:

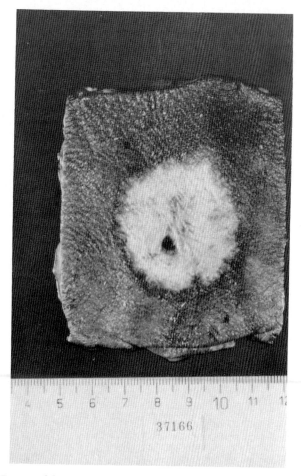

Figure 38.1. Irradiated melanoma of the back (man, age 62 years) (autopsy n. 37166 Ist. An. Pat. Univ. Milan).

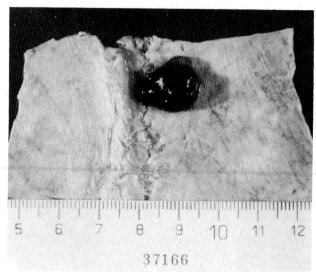

Figure 38.3. Same case as above: subdural metastasis.

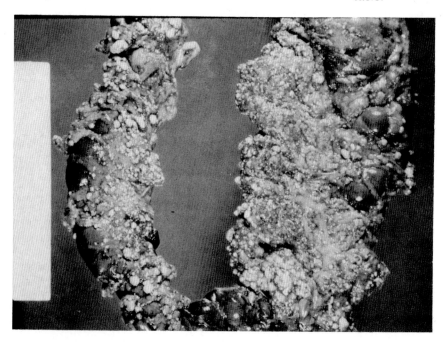

Figure 38.2. Same case as above: peritoneal and intestinal metastases, almost achromatical.

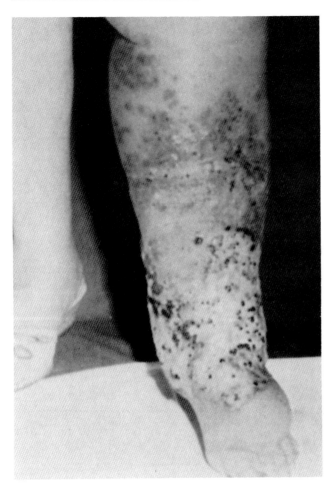

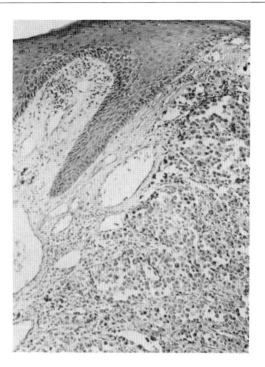

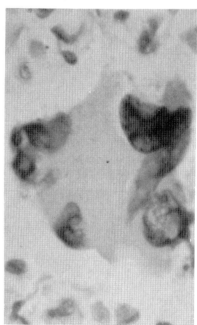

Figure 38.4. Voluminous melanotic lesion of the lower limb without appreciable loco-regional metastatic diffusions.

Figures 38.5 and 38.6. Histological aspects of a melanoma almost achromatic with apparent nuclear movements.

tyrosinase and dopa. The former is an enzyme of the phenolases group which can act on the tyrosine so that after going through other stages, it will form melanin. The latter is a substance which not only constitutes the substrate for the transformation of tyrosine into melanin, but also activates the tyrosinases by subtracting hydrogen atoms, and by oxidizing the enzyme, activates it in the same way as ultraviolet rays would.

As we look at the data objectively, we must consider the following: in albinism, a condition characterized by hereditary lack of pigment, the tyrosinase enzyme is lacking, while in the melanomas we find an increase in the tyrosinases in proportion to the degree of their differentiation.

Nevertheless, the metabolic consequences also can produce, in addition to the specific pathology of the melaninic replacement, other illnesses.

One example is *phenylpyruvic imbecillity*, which includes a brief period of melanin for-

mation; some investigators believe that this is due to a competitive condition where the high concentration of phenylpyruvic acid present in the blood and in the tissues prevents the tyrosine from contacting the tyrosinases and melanin from being synthesized from tyrosine.

Much of our knowledge of the metabolic activity of the tyrosinases has been obtained, in recent years, through the use of tyrosine-containing ^{14}C. In any case, it is possible that many

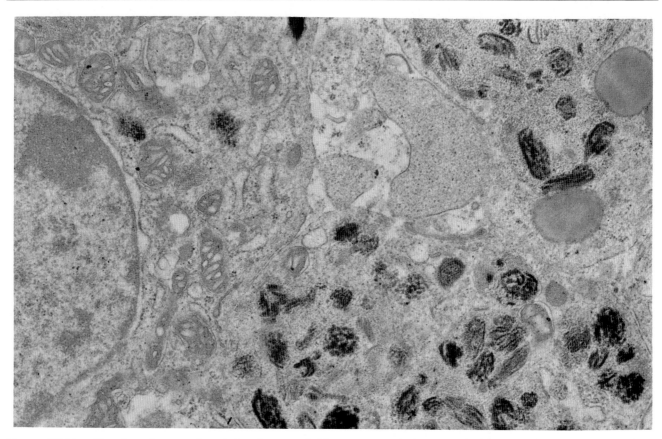

Figure 38.7. Cloudman's experimental melanoma S 91: component pigmented with premelanosomas in various stages of evolution.

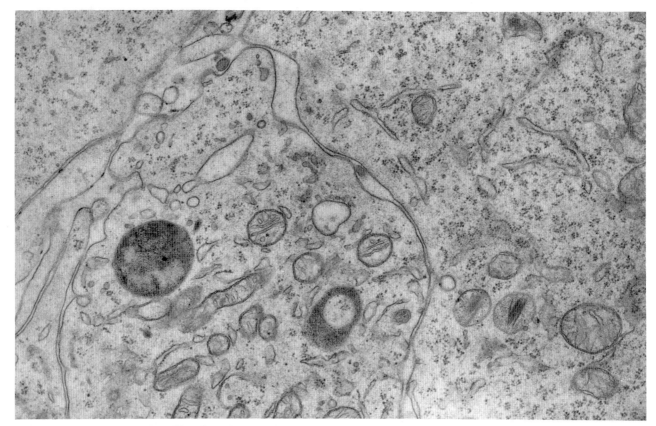

Figure 38.8. Cloudman's experimental melanoma S 91: achromatic component.

Table 38.1
Selected Aspects of the Normal and Pathological Species-Specific Relationship of the Melanogenic System[a]

Melanin Pigments	Class of Compounds	Cells	Normal Appearance in Human Body	Neoplasms in Human Body where Melanin is Involved		Racial Differences	Appearance in Other Structures (Cellular Distribution)	Phyla	Remarks
				Benign	Malignant				
Melanins are built by the stepwise oxidation of tyrosine through the enzyme tyrosinase. The process seems to be similar in insects and, for example, in mammals	Nitrogenous compounds in solution or granular form	Chromatophores Melanophores Melanocytes Stroma cells of iris and choroid Retina Nerve cells of particular nuclei in the brain (Nucleus niger, Nucleus ruber)	Epidermis of skin stratum germinativum; in black races stratum granulosum also Melanocytes transform the pigment to basal cells Melanocytes in stroma of iris and choroid Retina Nervous system	Junctional nevus (dermo-epidermal nevus) Intradermal nevus (common mole or neuronevus) Compound nevus Juvenile melanoma Blue nevus (Jadassohn-Tieche nevus) Melanoameloblastoma (see p.15/histogenesis)	Malignant melanoma (melanocarcinoma): 1. from lentigo 2. maligna 3. superficial 4. spreading 5. nodular Melanoma of rectum: Anorectal junction or anus (highly malignant) Melanoma of vulva (rare) Melanoma of vagina	More common in Caucasian or white race than in black or yellow races (see section of Boonyanit)	General: Integument and other tissues of invertebrates Melanin containing cells: Chromatophores Melanophores Coelomocytes Melanin from coelomocytes may transfer to epidermal chromatophores Extracellular distribution: Molluscan shells and arthropod cuticles, mainly between endocuticle and exocuticle Distribution in plants	Fossil: Ichthyosaurs Cephalopoda ink sac Echinodermata: Cl.: Echinoidea Diadema antillarum Phillippi Mollusca Arthropoda Other kingdoms beside animals such as Fungi and Plants.	Intermedin produced by the anterior lobe of the pituitary stimulates melanocytes in mammals Albinos result partly from a lack of the enzyme tyrosinase.

[a] Courtesy of H. E. Kaiser.

other factors are involved in melanogenesis; the actions performed by numerous hormones in the pigmentation of the cutis have been established and documented. We must only consider the increase of pigmentation in particular zones such as the mammary aureola, linea alba, etc., during pregnancy. It is also known that ACTH interferes with the pigmentation process. As an example, Addison's disease comes to mind.

The premelanosoma, the site of pigment synthesis, is always present, even in the "white" melanocytes of the achromic melanomas although modified by the above mentioned factors; and it is the sole morphological substrate that is really "diagnostic."

The presence of this singular proteinous crystalline intracellular structure singularly marks a cell which, even in the most malignant evolutions evident, retains a morphological equivalent of sure value as ultrastructural marker. It is a known fact that the most common malignant neoplasms are nearly always lacking cytoplasmatic components which would be useful for the purpose of establishing a sure trend (pulmonary cancer, mammary cancer, gastric cancer, uterine cancer) and, except for some rare examples of neoplasms of endocrine nature, are supplied with nonspecific components anyway. It is often difficult, even through an electron microscope, to positively distinguish an epithelial from a mesenchymatic tumor. In the histopathological diagnosis of the melanotic tumors, a new method has been proposed recently which uses a type of immunological technique.

It seems that the chimpanzee may furnish an antihuman melanoma serum specific enough to indicate the pigmented malignant neoplasms without reacting to interferences by other tumors (11). The reactivity between immune serum and melanoma can be evaluated in two ways: the first relies on the determination of the different degrees of cytotoxicity which are naturally high for the "target" pigmented cells; the second, which is perhaps more elegant, is based on the known principle of immunological deviation.

During the neoplastic differentiation process, the melanocytes undergo significant changes, morphological as well as functional, with relevant variations of the complicated series of enzymatic reactions which make the melanomic pigment mature.

Thus, the melanin, although immature, and a singular example for a typically structured cellular "secretion," is always perfectly recognizable, at least as a site of maturity (the premelanosama).

A morphological ultrastructural equivalent does not exist for most of the cellular secretions except for certain incretions produced by cells with endocrine activity. But, even in this case, a structural standard specific to each hormone is not available. This unique characteristic of the melanocytes can be appreciated in all its singularity when we consider the reproduction at a distance, i.e., the formation of metastases, which often are achromatic.

THE MELANOCYTE AND THE MELANOGENIC SYSTEM

The complex terminology once used to define the single types of cells containing melanomic pigment has been simplified by Fitzpatrick (6) who has proposed four types of elements: *the melanocyte*, a specialized cell which produces melanomic pigment and contains melanosomas; *the melanoforum*, a particular type of melanocyte which intervenes in the variations of the color of the skin with intracytoplasmatic movements of melanosomas; *the melanoblast*, forerunner of melanocyte and melanofora; *the Langerhans cell*, epidermic and, in the mammals, dermic cells whose functions are still unclear, but they are a component of the melanocytory system.

HUMAN MELANOMAS AND THE METASTATIC SPREAD

The human melanomas act like neoplasms—they invade rapidly with imposing metastatic diffusions and frequently resemble the phenomenon known as *satellitosis*. This seems to be due to the great facility with which the neoplastic cells pass through, repeatedly and in opposite directions, the walls of lymphatic vessels: thus, neoplastic nests can be recognized which colonize short distances from each other and are the morphological expression of the so-called "metastasis in transit" phenomenon. The location of a melanoma at the lymph node is, in the early stage, represented by neoplastic infiltrations into the central zone. They do not adhere to the criteria of invasion generally followed by other neoplasms. But, with regards to hematogenous diffusion, the melanoma is not different from other tumors. Within the range of the biological aggressiveness of the melanomas, one common characteristic is the disproportion between the mass, which is sometimes very exiguous of the primitive neoplasms and the extent of the metastases: we have observed cases of metastasis formation after diffusion to all the organs, the heart, lungs, meninges, etc., for melanomas that, with difficulty, can be shown as evidence (little melanoma of the uvea).

Nevertheless, exceptions and aspects do exist which contrast more with this behavior. For example, very large pigmented tumors can be observed (in one case the tumor encompassed the entire lower limb) which are apparently devoid of metastasic locations. Within the range of the biological complexity of the melanomas we can find cases of spontaneous regression through which numerous elements traceable to a valid result of immunitory type have become evident. The melanoma is a tumor which attacks not only the human being but, though with different methods and degrees of expression, many animal species.

GENETIC BACKGROUND AS A COMPARATIVE PROBLEM

Usually the melanoma originates from the melanocytes contained in the derma, but cases where the tumor arose from the epidermic stratum have been described. It may represent only an occasional event and may be due to genetic factors or may be transmitted by an infecting agent.

Melanomas with strong genetic conditioning can be produced, as is shown by the classical experiments of Gordon who, crossing two similar species of fish (*Xiphophorus maculatus* and *Xiphophorus hellerii*) (see Chapter 29), developed hybrids which showed a very high incidence rate for melanomas (10).

Gordon was the first to show genetically that it was the macromelanocytes rather than the micromelanocytes which produce tumors; thereafter, he succeeded in pointing out that the melanocytes were controlled by two genes, one responsible for the pigmented spots, the other for the black stripes. The development of the melanoma in the hybrids depended upon the reception of a macromelanocytory gene derived from the first kind, and a gene modifying the growth of the macromelanocyte derived from the second. Further, five alleles of the macromelano-

cytory gene were discovered which determine the location of the tumor.

From the primitive hybrids two separate strains were obtained, one with a double recessive gene for albinism, producing amelanotic tumors, and another with a dominant gene for pigmentation, producing pigmented tumors.

But a genetic origin cannot be found to explain all animal melanomas, particularly since it was discovered that in a colony of *Drosophila melanogaster* (see Chapter 30) more than 80% of the members had a melanoma. The factor that seemed to perpetuate the diffusion of the tumors showed many characteristics similar to those of a virus and it was transmitted from generation to generation through gonad tissue.

MELANOMAS IN SELECTED DOMESTICATED ANIMALS

The relative rarity with which the melanomas can be observed in animals is probably due to the fact that many of those are slaughtered before reaching an age in which the tumor could develop more easily. For this reason, particular attention has been given to horses and dogs because they normally have a longer life span.

As far as the horse (4) is concerned, Virchow already had noted that gray or albino animals developed melanoma more frequently in the region of perineum and at the tail base than others.

The melanomas of the dog (5) show some characteristics similar to the human melanoma; for example, in both, the tumor originates more easily from the junctional nevos. Further, we must not forget that if many histological sections are affected many nevi may never be connected. As far as the formation of metastases is concerned, either lymphatic or hematogenous, there is no difference between human and canine lesions.

In some aspects, on the other hand, the melanoma of the dog is different from that of humans; while in man both sexes are attacked equally, in dogs, for reasons not yet clear, the male is attacked more frequently. The zones where the melanoma attacks also are different: in man it is the lower limbs and feet that are attacked more frequently, while in dogs it is the oral mucous membrane.

Finally, in the human race, fair men with clear cutis and eyes incur the melanoma more easily, while in dogs this disease seems to prefer subjects with accented pigmentation. In dogs, particularly, the blue nevi are lacking; their absence depends perhaps on a more superficial location of the nevi or on the higher degree of pigmentation in the cutis of the animal as compared to that of man. In dogs the dermic nevus seems to be the equivalent of the blue nevus in man.

The cellular differentiation and the metabolic disorder which always follows it, lead to a significant quantitative reduction of the content to ripe pigment, but the premelanosomas, in their characteristic proteinaceous structure, remain visibly well. The results are that the metastases of the melanoma are sometimes achromatic and, therefore, often unrecognizable in their true nature from a histological and histochemical standpoint. Nevertheless, it is still possible to identify them with an electron microscope through the verification of the typical premelanosoma. In this respect, we must refer to recent studies which take into account some particular evolutionary aspects which can recall characteristic structures of other cells of the so-called melanocytory system. Actually, the body-racket, considered as the ultrastructural equivalent of the Langerhans' cell, has a morphology and a very complicated maturative evolution with intermediate aspects which recall, in the opinion of some authors, immature stages of the premelanosoma.

If one considers the actual histogenetic theories concerning the melanoma which, as Masson says, derive from the neural crest, and those for the Langerhorns' cell which are istiocyte of mesodermic origin, then the importance of these ultrastructural analogies, although the subject of dispute and contrary to the most valid and qualified histogenetic hypothesis, become evident. But they are interesting and seem to stimulate new research towards yet unexpected results.

References

1. Birbeck, M. S. C., Breathnach, A. S., and Everall, J. D. (1961): An electron microscope study of basal melanocytes and high-level clear cells (Langerhans cells) in vitiligo. *J. Invest. Derm.*, 37:51.
2. Breathnach, A. S., and Wyllie, L. M. (1965): Electron microscopy of melanocytes and Langerhans cells in human fetal epidermis at 14 weeks. *J. Invest. Derm.*, 44:51.
3. Cantaboni, A., Grigolato, P., Ceresa-Castellani, L., and Bestetti-Bo, M. (1969): Ultrastruttura ed enzimologia del melanoma di Cloudman. (Ultrastructure and enzyomology of Cloudman melanoma). *Atti Soc. Ital. Patol.*, 11(Parte I):65–103.
4. Conroy, J. D. (1967): Melanocytic tumors of domestic animals. *Arch. Derm.*, 96:372.
5. Cotchin, E. (1955): Melanotic tumours of dogs. *J. Comp. Pathol.*, 65:115–129.
6. Fitzpatrick, T. B., *et al.* (1966): Terminology of Vertebrate Melanin-containing Cells, their Precursor, and Related Cells. A report of the Nomenclature Committee of the Sixth International Pigment Cell Conference. (Structure and control of the melanocyte.) Springer-Verlag, Berlin, p. 1.
7. Giordano, A. (1966): Natural history of tumor pigmenta. *Ras. Clin. Sci.* 42:201–206.
8. Giordano, A. (1966): Pathology of the melanoma. Short Course, VI International Congress, International Academy of Pathology, Kyoto.
9. Giordano, A. (1968): Ultrastructure of melanocytes. *Morgagni*, 1:23–36.
10. Gordon, M. (1948): Effects of five primary genes of the site of melanomas in fishes and the influence of two color genes on their pigmentation. *N. Y. Acad. Sci.* (Special Publ.), 4:216.
11. Gori, M., Stuhlmiller, P. D., Boylston, J. A., Seigler, H. F., and Fetter, B. F. (1977): Immunodiagnosis of melanoma using chimpanzee antihuman melanoma antiserum. *Am. J. Clin. Pathol.*, 67:573–79.
12. Langerhans, P. (1868): The nerves of the human skin. *Arch. Pathol. Anat. Phys.*, 44:325.
13. Levene, A. L. (1965): The comparative pathology of melanomas, The Comparative Physiology and Pathology of the Skin, p. 759. Blackwell, Oxford.
14. Masson, P. (1970): *Human Tumors*, translated by S. D. Kobernick. Wayne State University Press.
15. Sutton, J. B. (1885): Tumours in animals. *J. Anat. Phys. (Lond.)*, 19:415–475.
16. Zelickson, A. S., and Hartman, J. E. (1961): The fine structure of the melanocyte and melanin granule. *J. Invest. Derm.*, 36:23.

39

Regression of Neoplasms From a Species-Specific Point of view

Hans E. Kaiser

INTRODUCTION

A neoplasm, especially a malignant one, is defined as a type of abnormal growth in which a stimulus can disappear after initiation, but where growth itself will not cease. This phenomenon is known as autonomous growth; each neoplastic autonomous growth can be seen as a pathological variation of one or the other type of normal growth. It was reviewed briefly in preceding sections of this book as it relates to the different organismic groups.

Neoplastic growth is only possible through an easing of normal growth control which, in its main aspects, is still unknown today.

In recent years, a regaining of the control over neoplastic growth in one way or another has been reported in cases of observed spontaneous and experimentally produced regression of cancer. It is of importance to investigate the species-specific pattern of this phenomenon. It will be reviewed briefly. (For general reports, see (381), for case reports (303) and for reports on long survival of cancer patients (126, 304).) Also genetic susceptibility will at least play a part in regression (324) (see also Chapters 29 by Schwab and Anders and Chapter 33 by Ames).

Psychological factors may also be involved which are not pure illusions but are based on the fact that the psychological impact on the patient may make him independent through his mind. This, in turn, may weaken the whole body by exerting a wide influence on the whole system, including metabolism. In this way it acts on neoplasms or their development (also preliminary stages). Our knowledge of this is extrapolated from the fact that a choleric condition may raise the blood pressure or that anger may have an effect on appetite and stomach secretion or fear on hormonal secretions. These facts have to be investigated and evaluated in detail.

Weinstock (380) has summarized recent progress in cancer psychobiology and psychiatry. Janssen and Weiszbach (173) have reported on the psychosomatics of treated testicular tumor patients; Meares on ataveistic regression as a factor in the remission of cancer (235), and on regression of cancer after intensive meditation (234). A better and earlier recognition of paraneoplastic syndromes should also be anticipated if dealing with neoplastic therapy (326); concerning chemotherapy, see (9).

DEFENSE BY IMMUNITY IN THE HEALTHY ORGANISM

Neoplastic transformation usually occurs in organisms with advanced age. For the human population, the evidence is founded on a broad statistical basis. Table 39.1 shows age dependence for some common cancers.

It is currently thought that at the beginning of neoplastic growth, that is for primary tumor formation, approximately 1,000 neoplastically transformed cells are required. This finding suggests that quite often single neoplastic cells occur in everyone's life through mutations but that these cells are destroyed by the defense mechanism of the healthy body. It is perhaps realistic to state that in a healthy condition the human body is able to bring about the destruction of singly occurring neoplastically transformed

Table 39.1
Age Dependence of Selected Neoplasms with Some Remarks on Sex and Racial Differences[a]

Neoplasms	Most Common Age	Benign	Malignant	Remarks
Squamous cell cancer	After 5 decades		+	Beside the skin, this neoplasm occurs in other regions where stratified squamous cell epithelium or transitional epithelium is present
Melanoma	Between 30 and 60 yr	+	+	This tumor group is less common in the black and yellow races; it occurs predominantly in the less pigmented regions
Wilms' tumor	Commonly 3 yr of age		+	This neoplasm is a mixed tumor
Hepatoblastoma	Infancy and childhood		+	Among most frequent neoplasms of this age group
Mammary cancer	Peak 50–59 yr; again increase in older age		+	Remarkable variations with regard to racial differences
Cancer of thyroid			+	Papillary carcinoma, the most common, occurs at a younger age group than follicular or medullary carcinoma as well as anaplastic carcinoma; the latter occurs generally in older persons
Brenner tumor	After 50 yr of age	+		Generally unilateral
Dysgerminoma of ovary	Before 35 yr of age		+	
Seminoma of testis	Older age group		+	
Embryonal cancer of testis	Adult type; infantile type			
Granulosa cell tumor of ovary	Any age		+	
Renal tubular cancer	5th to 6th decade		+	
Osteochondroma	2nd decade	+		Predominance in male
Osteoma	6th decade	+		
Nonossifying bone fibroma	2nd decade	+		
Osteoclastoma	2nd decade	+		
Chondrosarcoma	Between 30 and 50 yr		+	
Osteogenic sarcoma	Between 10 and 30 yr		+	
Rhabdomyosarcoma	Embryonic variation occurs in children		+	
	Pleomorphic variation in adults		+	
Astrocytoma	Children and young adults		+	These tumors comprise one half of all gliomas
Oligodendroglioma	Adults		+	
Medulloblastoma	Children		+	
Retinoblastoma	Children		+	

[a] *Sources:* R. W. Evans: *Histological Appearance of Tumours.* Williams & Wilkins, Baltimore, 1966; H. J. Fischbier and H. U. Lohbeck (eds.): Früdiagnostik des Mammakarzinoms. Klinische, Röntgenologische, thermographische und zytologische Untersuchungsmethoden und ihre Wertigkeit. Georg Thieme Verlag, Stuttgart, 1977; W. Frommhold and P. Gerhardt: Klinisch-radiologisches Seminar, Band 10: Knochentumoren. George Thieme Verlag, Stuttgart, 1980; P. Masson: *Human Tumors, Histology, Diagnosis, Technique* (translated by S. D. Kobernick). Wayne State University Press, Detroit, 1970; G. Meuret: *Mammakarzinom, Grundlagen, Diagnostik, Therapie, Komplikationen, Rehabilitation.* Georg Thieme Verlag, Stuttgart, 1980; A. Von Albertini: Histologische Geschwülstdiagnostik. Systematische Morphologie der menschlichen Geschwülste als Grundlage für die klinische Beurteilung, Ed. 2. Georg Thieme Verlag, Stuttgart, 1974.

cells. The question remains, however, whether this capability can persist in its effectiveness, once it has been broken down, or whether a complete recovery of the defense mechanism of the body is possible after the development of a malignant tumor. A recovery resulting in the regression is generally not sufficiently understood. It is suggested that these processes must be conceived as a reactivation of the defense system of the body following damage it has suffered or temporary failure of its defense activity. It is further submitted that a fresh understanding of these processes may result from a new approach to the problem—the comparison of the different defense mechanisms of the var-

ious species against neoplastic cell transformation.

DEFENSE OF THE BODY IN DIFFERENT SPECIES

Theoretical Aspects

The defense mechanisms in the bodies of different species vary considerably, as does reaction to injury. The currently known facts as they apply to the most important phyla are briefly reviewed in Table 39.2.

Table 39.2
Defense Mechanisms in Major Animal Phyla[a]

Phyla	Reaction to Injury		Immunology	
	Structures	Remarks	Structures	Remarks
Cnidaria	Interstitial cell	Phagocytosis, response to injury differs from sponges	Autografts survive, allografts and xenografts are rejected	Quasi-immuno recognition[b]
Platyhelminthes	General	High regenerative capacity	Transplantation immunity	Circulating antigens
Nemertinea	? Interstitial cells, mesenchymatic and phagocytic cells	High regenerative capacity	Unknown	Unknown
Rotifera[c]	General cell invariability	Incapable of healing an injury	Nearly unknown	Nearly unknown
Mollusca	Phagocytic cells	Wide variety of characteristics	Phagocytic cells	Wide variation
Annelida	Coelomocytes	Importance of peritoneal endothelia and segmental confinement of the wound	—	Accelerated or curtailed rejection
Arthropoda	Phagocytes	Wide variety of characteristics due to species number	Haemolymph	Immune reactions
Brachiopoda	Unknown	Unknown	Unknown	Unknown
Echinodermata	Intestinal tract	Highest regenerative capacity in holothurians	Hemocytes	—
Vertebrata	Connective tissues (macrophages)	Easily comparable to mollusca	Reticuloendothelial system	Understanding of the comparability of vertebrate and invertebrate immunology has increased over the last decade

[a] For review see: H. E. Kaiser: *Species-Specific Potential of Invertebrates for Toxicological Research*. University Park Press, Baltimore, 1980; and A. K. Sparks: *Invertebrate Pathology. Noncommunicable Diseases.* Academic Press, New York, London, 1972.
[b] Invertebrates have not shown to produce immunoglobulin antibodies as vertebrates do.
[c] Rotifera have been included due to their cell invariability.

Practical Cases Reported From Different Species, a Selection

A few cases of neoplastic regression in different species have been reported. These will be discussed and evaluated.

DEFENSE MECHANISMS IN AN ADVANCED STATE OF NEOPLASTIC TRANSFORMATION

General Considerations

It is currently widely accepted that after surgical removal of the primary cancer or of other malignant neoplasms, the host body and its metabolism, including the mechanisms of defense, return more or less to normal, until such time as newly developing neoplastic (metastatic) cells regain their overwhelming power. As pointed out in the previous chapter by Krokowski, there are situated different centers of gravity where a return to normal could be achieved.

The knowledge of neoplastic immunology is important for surgery (150). In the extreme statistical rarity of neoplastic regression it is not necessary to give a pessimistic outlook as pointed out by Hewitt (152). Also, the fact that the failure to demonstrate that a tumor-specific antigen in humans exists is no reason for such an assumption, because in the author's opinion we know little about species-specific and neoplasm-specific variations of immunology of neoplasms.

The Impact of Comparative Aspects and New Approaches for Research

To put the cases of neoplastic regression in the wider comparative picture will enable us to understand certain aspects, unexplainable by themselves or seen from a single point of view. This will result in a combined knowledge of normal as well as pathologic aspects of growth in various species. Events occurring normally in one species may be present under abnormal conditions in another species (e.g., normal and abnormal autolysis as described in Chapter 6 or normal and abnormal regression/regeneration treated in this and other chapters). It will be possible to learn this approach especially concerning cancer therapy enhancing the understanding of spontaneous regression.

IMPACT OF THE COMPARATIVE APPROACH UPON RESEARCH IN DEFENSE MECHANISMS

A review of the literature on spontaneous regression of cancer in man seems in order. On May 9 and 10 of 1974 a conference on the spontaneous regression of cancer was already held at the Medical Institutions of Johns Hopkins University in Baltimore. By October 14, 1977, a literature of approximately 260–270 (267) recent citations had accumulated, a number which increased to 353 useful citations at the time of first draft completion of this chapter in 1978. The most significant facts emerging from these sources and other materials is summarized below.

Instances of general cancer regression have been reported by Cole (69, 72), Nossal (265), Thomas (359), Hellström and Hellström (149) and of specific types of cancer by Atuk et al. (11) involving pheochromocytoma, and Briuzgin (47) on peripheral lung cancer.

The perspectives of tumor immunology in relation to host-neoplasms (parasites) have been brought into focus by Weiss (383); aspects of an immune surveillance by Klein (179, 180); and immunology-related reactions on large tumor masses by Alexander (5).

The migration of splenic T and B lymphocytes into syngeneic tumors undergoing immunologic rejection was investigated by Elboim et al. (101) using T and B lymphocytes from either normal or MSV tumor-bearing BALC/c mice. They concluded that T and B lymphocytes in normal or tumor-bearing mice migrate to a syngeneic tumor which undergoes immunologic rejection where assymigration of these cells was decreasing to the peripheral lymph nodes when the tumor grew most intensively.

Horstmann et al. (159), in the case of pulmonary leiomyomas, reported that the pulmonary nodules regressed spontaneously during pregnancy and the postpartum period. Trnka (365, 366) described spontaneous healing of histologically completely removed basaliomas and Stutman (349) the effect of age on the regression of

M-MSV tumors in CBA/H mice. In 1976 Cole (72) pointed out that although we know more about cellular immunity at present than about humoral immunity, greater possibilities can be expected from the latter. He pointed especially to the role played by immunoglobulins.

The immune response to Rauscher virus-induced leukemia in DBA mice and especially the connection of disease regression to the role of tumor-specific antibodies was discussed by Toth et al. (362) whereas Meigs et al. (240) evaluated the regression of carcinoma in situ and a second form of invasive cervical cancer in cases reported from 1953 to 1973 in Connecticut.

Factors such as old age, genetic defects, and postradiologic and postchemotherapeutic metabolism, will influence the ability of the neoplasm to bypass the consequences of immunogenecity, Schneeweiss (316). The role of the estrogen-binding capacity following endocrine ablation therapy was compared by using breast cancer in the rat and man (263). For details on a spontaneous reversion of neoplastic cells see Krueger and Raferty (188) and for metabolic aspect of the problem in general, Cole (69).

A special problem of cancer therapy in the future will be the use of therapeutic methods against metastases; this was pointed out in the contribution of Krokowski (Chapter 40). A spontaneous regression of metastatic growth has been reported in several cases and shall be reviewed briefly. In hepatic metastases, regression of the secondary lesion followed the removal of the primary renal cell cancer (87). The first and second remission after first and second relapse radiotherapy in Hodgkin's disease, and based on the study of 175 patients, showed that the prognostic significance depends on a partial or full previous remission, the site of recidivism, the histology, and the age of the patient, to name only some factors in addition to activity B (255). Boasberg et al. (37) reported on the regression of metastatic renal cell carcinoma in relation to immunocompetence, whereas Komatsu et al. reported on the regression of tumor metastasis of the lymph nodes of a transplanted rat lymphosarcoma (185). Maiskii and Lomakin published reports on factors of bodily resistance and metastasis (217).

EXPERIMENTAL REGRESSION

Gross and Dreyfuss (134) investigated the early and late effects of immunization of guinea pigs against L2C leukemia with live leukemic cells by intradermal inoculation. Thiobendazole was found to be a new immunopotentiator if used in the therapy of murine fibrosarcoma (209). In a study involving 15 generations of C3 H/ST mice, Strong and Matsunaga (346) found that after 15 generations a transmissible entity was found producing a second sudden reversal of effect on cancer growth. This change increased from a very low effect to a maximum one and finally to a complete regression in a high percentage. The effects of spontaneous tumors of the mammary gland were obtained in a single lineal descent of this strain. Aylsworth et al. (13) concluded due to their experiments (bilateral adrenalectomy or estradiol benzoate treatment affecting the growth of 7,12-dimethylbenz[a]anthracene-induced mammary tumors during postpartum lactation) that adrenocortical activity in rats is primary responsible for reduced growth of mammary neoplasms during postpartum lactation.

Age as a modifying factor of 7,12-dimethylbenz[a]anthracene-induced mammary carcinogenesis in the rat was investigated by Haslam (145).

Furmanski et al. (121) observed the effects of radiation and athymia on the spontaneous regression on Friends murine leukemia virus-induced erythroleukemia. Irradiation prior to Friend murine leukemia virus complex inoculation inhibited the spontaneous regression of the erythroleukemia as well as the treatment of the mice with the bone seeking isotope ^{89}Sr implicating the same effector mechanisms in the resistance to Friend murine leukemia virus or Friend murine leukemia virus-induced immunosuppression. This data suggested the involvement of the immune system in erythroleukemia regression and the specific participation of thymus cells and an ^{89}Sr-susceptible function, perhaps marrow-dependent cells, in the process of regression.

Dietz et al. (90) found that thymectomy of newborn but not adult outbred Swiss mice inhibited regression. The rejection of murine sarcoma virus (Moloney strain) leaves the animals immune to tumor induction. Growth and regression of experimental tumor S180 was investigated by volume measurements and cytophotometric studies in mice by Techer et al. (355) and the reversibility and irreversibility of liver tumors in mice initiated by the alpha isomer of 1,2,3,4,5,6-hexochlorocyclohexane by Ito et al. (169). The latter study indicated that mesenchymal cells may play an important role in reversing the growth of liver tumors produced by this compound. Nonimmunological regression of dimethylbenz[a]anthracene-induced 17 experimentally keratoacanthomas in 9 rabbits were observed by Ramselaar and van der Meer (294). No significant staining patterns nor delayed cutaneous hypersensitivity reactions could be detected.

THEORETICAL ASPECTS OF DIFFERENT WAYS FOR THE EVALUATION OF CANCER REGRESSION

It is worthwhile to ask if the recent accumulation of knowledge on regression of malignancies in particular and neoplasms in general indicate any specific pattern.

Such a specific regression pattern could be seen either as tissue-specific, cell-specific, tumor-specific, and species-specific. Looking at tumor regression in this way we may come closer to the specific elements involved in tumor regression. Such handling may also be applicable to new experiments and even more important to new trends in therapy. This will be the case because we evaluate these cases in which the growth control of the body declined, enabling the growth of malignancy, even metastasis, to develop and was regained at a later stage (multistage processes in cancer development, neoplastic growth). It underlines our general thesis that abnormal growth may start from each phase of normal organismic development, but at least theoretically may be regained at each phase of pathologic growth, because the whole metabolism and the defense of the body is connected with this possible process. The comparability of the role of autolysis as part of normal ontogenetic growth process and cancer regression as self-defending autolysis is summarized in Table 39.3.

Spontaneous, nonpigmented benign epitheliomas (histologically noninvasive, hyperblastic epidermal and characterized by loss of basal, subdermal melanocytes lesions) were found in 44 of 1586 (2.8% adult newts, Cynops pyrrhogaster, of central Japan). The sexes were equally affected with single tumors which regressed or disappeared under laboratory conditions (283).

In the canine, venereal neoplasm spontaneous regression is combined with the production of a

Table 39.3

Comparison of Hormonally and Immunological Regulated Normal and Nonregulated Abnormal Growth Processes on a Species Specific Platform in Regard to the Neoplastic Regression

Types of Neoplasms	Continued Embryonal Potential	Partially Continued Embryonal Potential	Normal Catastrophic Development	Normal Continued Development	Neoplastic Regression
Epithelial animal neoplasms	100% meristems	Larval tissues of invertebrates, up to 95%	Regulated by hormone and immune systems		
Mixed animal neoplasms			**Role of autolysis as part of normal ontogenetic growth process.** Selected examples: The peak of autolytic processes (destruction processes) among crustaceans, where a combination of synthetic processes and destruction (dissimilation) processes occur is reached in cirriped crustaceans	Species-specific switch from indirect continued to direct continued development as in crustaceans where up to 24 nauplii (larvae) occur, sometimes direct development in related species as in *Astacus* (throughout superorders Peracarida and Phyllocarida) is interesting: These varying ontogenetic processes occur side by side in related species if viewed taxonomically. This fact makes the comparison between normal ontogenetic growth and individual abnormal ontogenetic growth even more valuable	Regulated by: immune system, hormone system, nervous system, circulatory system
Mesenchymal or nonepithelial animal neoplasms					
True neoplasms of vascular plants					**Cancer regression as self-defending autolysis** as regaining hormonal and immunologic control of the diseased organism (therapy: treatment of certain prostatic cancers)
Certain hypertrophic plant neoplasms					Theoretically neoplastic regression is possible at each phase of neoplastic development; and seems to occur permanently in the early stages of neoplastic development before formation of a primary tumor

serum factor inhibiting *in vitro* neoplasm colony-forming units in agar (33).

EVALUATION OF THE NEOPLASTIC REGRESSION ACCORDING TO THE PARENT TISSUES OF TUMORS

The reports on regression are now presented in a tissue specific arrangement.

Regression of Epithelial Neoplasms

Neoplasms Arising From Lining Membranes

The arrangement, according to specific epithelial tissues, is not always completely accurate

because the exact tracing of tumors is not always possible, sometimes different tissues regress together; thus, it may be possible to assume that the reaction of the "malignant regressive cell" is responding, not the tissue in the center of the reaction. Among the cases reported are one by Odintsova and Bukthoiarova (266) where skin papillomas and a gastric polyp disappeared after the removal of a corticosteroma, or at border areas involving stratified squamous epithelium and simple columnar epithelium at the cervix where malignancies develop frequently (16).

Simple Squamous Epithelium (Pseudoepithelia of Blood Vessels). The author lists the hemangiomas here only with great reservation because of the composition of these tumors or tumorlike structures made up of different components and the cell types involved (see Masson (222)). Hemangiomas (19, 20, 22, 153, 175, 361, 364) may be benign, benign metastasizing (semimalignant) and malignant and have been observed in at least the following organs of man: mamma, ovary, urinary bladder, urethra, skin, cardiac muscle, bone system, liver, stomach, spleen, adrenal cortex, kidney, parotis, pharynx, pleura, ureter, and uterine wall (larynx, intestine, lung, nose and sinuses as far as angiomas (255, 177) are concerned). A large, slightly elevated choroidal hemangioma along the superior temporal arcade was seen in a 30-year-old white woman with two month history of decreased vision and in the fifth month of pregnancy. The neoplasm regressed after the delivery of the child (286).

For hemangioma of the transverse colon see (249).

Stratified Squamous Epithelium. *Skin.* The report on the disappearance of skin papillomas by Odintsova and Bukhtoiarova (266) has already been mentioned. Other reports are those by Stenbäck (341) on the spontaneous regression of skin tumors, Trnka (366) on spontaneous regression of basalioma portions treated by partial excision in stages, Carapeto (59) on multiple trichoepithelioma with variable evolution of its lesions (but two lesions in the same person exhibited the development of malignancy (basal cell epithelioma)); and Leicher (198) on organ resistance and organ disposition involving the upper airways, digestive tract and the ear.

Esophagus. Regression of multiple squamous papillomatosis involving the hypopharynx and the entire length of the oesophagus was described by Frootko and Rogers (116).

Simple Cuboidal/Columnar Epithelium. Tsukamoto and coworkers (368) have reported spontaneous disappearance of gastric polyps; Witek *et al.* (387) on gallbladder carcinoma regression; De Cosse *et al.* (84) on familial polyposis; and Hrushesky and Murphy (161) on the therapy of advanced renal carcinoma.

Regression of kidney cancer is reviewed in several papers: Luderer *et al.* (207) and Ludwig *et al.* (208); and of kidney cancer with metastases, Dubrow (94) has reported on a case of regression of metastatic hypernephroma; Freed and coworkers (115) on idiopathic regression from renal cell carcinoma; Artibani and collaborators (10) also on renal carcinoma, as well as Deweerd *et al.* (87); the current status of advanced renal carcinoma therapy was discussed by Hrushesky and Murphy (161). Another study involving human renal cell carcinoma in the "nude" mouse was reported by Groscurth and Kistler (132).

Pseudostratified Columnar Epithelium. A case involving local spontaneous regression of bronchial cancer was described by Dahl *et al.*

(81), one on peripheral lung cancer by Briuzgin (47) which is included here for simplicity.

Spontaneous regression of pulmonary metastases of a renal cell carcinoma after preoperative arterial embolization and infarction of the neoplasm followed by radical nephrectomy 7 days later was seen by Mohr and Whitesel. A cerebral metastasis requiring craniotomy appeared 14 months after surgery. Twenty-one months after original surgery the patient was alive and without sign of disease (247). The status of adjuvant therapy for renal cell cancer is given in (310); uterine cervix (46).

Neoplasms Arising From Glandular Epithelium

Exocrine Glandular Epithelia (Salivary Glands, Mammary Glands and Liver). For details related to a study on spontaneous regression of induced parotid gland tumors in rats, see El-Mofty (103). Cho-Chung *et al.* (65) have investigated the inverse relationship of estrogen-receptors with cyclic AMP-binding proteins in hormone-dependent mammary tumor regression. Regression of breast cancer was reported by Lewison (203). Benign breast lumps may regress with change in diet (62).

Studies involving beagles were performed by Giles and coworkers (124); rats, Lagova (192); and mice, Strong and Matsunaga (346). Baum and Coyle (23) evaluated the behavior of untreated axillary nodes in relation to simple mastectomy for early breast cancer. A case of resolution after discontinuation of oral contraceptive use was reported by Ramseur and Cooper (295), another on the treatment of primary liver carcinoma by Lee (197).

Endocrine Glandular Epithelia (Adrenal Glands, Testes, Ovaries) Avascular necrosis of a large pheochromocytoma led to a spontaneous remission (11). Cases of spontaneous regressions of metastases from testicular tumors are described by Franklin (114), Bär and Hedinger (15) and Hassenstein (146). Luteoma of the ovary which occur only during pregnancy, but which regress spontaneously after birth, were described by Böhm (39). Regarding the surveillance of hydatidiform moles and choriocarcinomas see Roger *et al.* (300).

Regression of Tumors of the Melanogenic System

Several reports about regression of neoplasms of the melanogenic system exist (45). These are valuable for various reasons: (1) the multi-tissue sphere of action (membership) of the tumor-forming cells present in epithelia, connective tissues, and neural tissues (systems) in mammals and by a wide species distribution in other animal phyla and plants; also occurring in the cells of plectenchymata of fungi. (2) Different reaction of the cells during transformation to and during malignancy itself. Malignant melanoma or melanosarcomas are one of the most unpredictable types of tumor. (This characteristic applies also to metastatic growth, e.g., as described by Rampen (293) about spontaneous regression of metastatic malignant melanoma.) The reason for this unpredictability may offer new research challenges to immunologists, chronobiologists, biochemists, biophysicists and others. They may offer new insight as a model for species-specific variations of regression by their wide taxonomic distribution. (3) Furthermore, important racial differences with regard to epidemiology exist. The black races are less exposed to a majority of skin diseases than members of the Caucasian race, for example. In the dark races the areas with less pigmentation as, for example, in the sole of the foot, are the primary sites of these tumors (67, 127, 187, 216, 218, 227, 228, 320).

Regression of Neoplasms of Connective Tissues (including Hematogenic and Supporting Tissues)

Connective Tissues Per SE

Investigations on the resolution of fibromatoses were performed by Allen (6), Sturzaker et al. (347), Benjamin and co-workers (25) and Kennedy et al. (176).

Hematogenic (Hematopoietic) Tissues

Remy et al. described a case of spontaneous remission of congenital histiocytosis X, with solely skin involvement (297). Congenital self-healing reticulohistiocytosis composed of congenital skin neoplasms and disseminated papules on the trunk, without other organ involvement regressed during the first two months of life. The disease similar to the congenital self-healing reticulohistiocytosis of Hashimoto and Pritzker exhibits histiocytic cells characterized

by large irregularly nuclei and partially opaque foamy cytoplasm (305). For hepatitis and leukemia see (73) and the pattern of lymphoid infiltrate in the canine cutaneous histiocytoma (68); Saman et al. regarding histiocytoma of the corneal limbus (312).

Certain cells of hematopoietic tissues belong to the reticuloendothelial system, which can be considered as being the cellular police force of the body. Selected studies show that particular circumstances are working in at least certain regression of malignancies. For details consult the reports of Cron (80) on phagocytic activities of leucocytes and of Gross and Dreyfuss (135).

The infection of macrophages with Friend virus exhibits a relationship to the spontaneous regression of viral erythroleukemia (220), on which Marcelletti & Furmanski reported on the immunization of guinea pigs against L2C leukemia with live cells.

Neoplastic cells are often considered to be parasites or other foreign agents, because they behave anarchistically when compared with the normal body cells. The reticuloendothelial system of the organism, for example, attacks foreign bodies like dust particles, bacteria, protozoa and other intruders into the internal environment of the organism. These special cells, such as the lymphocytes or macrophages, have the ability to move not only within the body fluids but also in the tissue spaces and between the other tissue cells. It is important to note that there exist large variations in these cells with regard to the body fluids of different animals. A regression similar to that in animals cannot exist in plants because the body fluids of plants do not have movable cells. (An exception may be seen in cells which have been freed from tissue connections by injury, but these cells float in body fluids for only a very short time and are without any functional significance.)

If we look at the important capability of cells such as the lymphocytes (sometimes also called killer lymphocytes) and macrophages with regard to their action during the regression of neoplasms, then three aspects or capabilities of these cells become weighty: (1) the distribution of these cells and their migration: T and B lymphocytes migrate either to a syngeneic tumor undergoing rejection or especially during excessive tumor growth they concentrate at the lymph nodes where the drainage for this tumor occurs (101); (2) the second point of importance is the toxicity of those reticuloendothelial cells with respect to the tumor cells under attack (306); (3) cytologic characteristics of attacking reticuloendothelial cells are visible through a polar accumulation of organelles at the point of contact between the lymphocytes and the neoplastic target cell (279).

A number of recent studies, taken at random from the literature, indicate the spectrum of research which is currently being performed on this subject: Elboim et al. (101) have investigated T and B lymphocyte migration into syngeneic tumors. Russell et al. (306) have reported on the cytotoxicity mediated in vitro by macrophages recovered from disaggregated regressing Moloney sarcomas. This is part of a larger study on inflammatory cells in solid murine neoplasms. Tumors induced in mice by MSV and the distribution of MSV-immune cytolytic T lymphocytes in vivo were studied by Plata and Sordat (287). As part of a long-term project on the spontaneous regression of Friend virus-induced erythroleukemia, Marcelletti and Furmanski (219) have investigated the role of macrophages. McGrail and co-workers (229) have reported on the lymphocytic toxicity of chickens bearing Rous' sarcoma; they found that lymphocytes from chickens whose tumors were regressing were significantly more cytotoxic than those from hosts with progressing tumors. Perry et al. (279) found that regressing tumors contained moderate to marked lymphocyte infiltration while lymphocytes from progressing tumors lacked the polar organization of organelles. A very rare case of lymph node anticarcinoma reaction was discussed by Popa et al. (289) and lymphomatoid papulosis by MacAuley (212). Further immune responses of chickens with Rous' sarcoma were reported in two papers by Gyles and co-workers (138, 139). Early immune response excreted by genes for regression is considered the key to spontaneous regression of Rous' sarcomas. Adzhigitov (2) used the Rous' virus on primates for the modelling of sarcomas. See also Seto et al. (323) for development and regression of experimentally produced Shope papillomas of newborn domestic rabbits.

Supporting Tissues—Adipose Tissue (27), Cartilage and Bone

The spontaneous regression of an unusual metastasis of a chondrosarcoma was seen by McLaughlin et al. (233).

A report by Dissing and coworkers (91) mentions an inoperable primary bone tumor in the pelvis which underwent spontaneous regression.

Regression of Neoplasms of Muscular Tissues

Smooth Musculature

A case of spontaneous regression of pulmonary leiomyomas during pregnancy has been observed by Horstmann et al. (159). It was found that all tumors were metastases of a primary uterine neoplasm. The regression of the pulmonary nodules indicated an apparent hormonal dependence.

Congenital angioleiomyomatosis also exhibited spontaneous regression (142).

Regression of Neoplasms of the Nervous System

Neuron Series

Neuroblastoma. Several studies have been described in the recent literature dealing with the regression of these neoplasms: McLaughlin and Urich (232) have reported on four cases of maturing neuroblastoma and ganglioneuroblastoma with long survival periods of the patients. Other cases of regression were seen by Schwartz (317), Takeda and Sotooka (352), Maurus (224), and Groncy and Finklestein (131).

Retinoblastoma. For details of recent studies see Benson and co-workers (28), Gallie et al. (123) who showed that histocompatibility typing in Caucasian patients failed to show any differences in antigen frequency as compared to a control population; other reports on regression of this neoplasm include Constantinides et al. (74), Axelsen (12) and Dhir et al. (88). Among 52 cases of retinoblastoma which were diagnosed at the Ophthalmology Department of Lausanne, Switzerland, was one case of spontaneous cure of bilateral retinoblastoma (18). The establishment of retinoblastoma protocols was suggested, due to the importance of this rare neoplasm for an understanding of general biology of neoplasms (34) and immunologic mechanisms in spontaneous regression of retinoblastoma were reviewed by Gallie et al. (122).

In General

Studies of note on the regression of tumors also include the following: El-Domeiri (102) has reported on delayed hypersensitivity reactions and its relation to tumor spread and diagnoses; Edmondson *et al.* (98) on regression of liver cell adenomas, Kobori and co-workers (181) and Rosen (301) on dystrophic xanthomatosis in mycosis fungoides; Davies and Marks (82) on multiple xanthogranulomata in an adult. A study on tumor regression after administration of alkoxyglycerols was described by Brohult *et al.* (48). An agent for immunotherapy was used by Meier and Lobuglio (239) and a regression of bronchial epidermoid carcinoma by Dahl *et al.* (81). Woodruff and Warner (392) have discussed the effect of *Corynebacterium parvum* on tumor growth in normal and athymic mice, and Burby (51) vanishing lesions, mycosis fungoides.

CONCLUSIONS

Surely, regression of cancer and other malignancies occurred also in earlier decades of this century and in the preceding centuries. But only continuously increased diagnostic efficiency and experimentation has brought the problem of neoplastic regression into focus. It is the author's belief that the facts already known have a threefold impact: (1) they give the theoretical basic platform for the assumption that cancer and allied diseases will be curable in the future; (2) a continued increase in our knowledge of the immunologic background and the specific cellular interactions between attacking cells, for example macrophages (from biochemical, biophysical, chronooncological and additional aspects) and neoplastic cells seen before the background of species specific function and evaluated for specific tumors will dramatically increase our arsenal for the therapy of cancer and allied diseases; (3) the fact that a small number of malignancies regresses spontaneously widens our chance for a comparison between the animal and plant neoplasms in the sense of the two kingdom approach because some yet rather unknown influences in the host of the malignancy must disappear before it can return from autonomous to controlled growth (endogenous regression), just as abnormal growth regresses when the stimulus for nonautonomous growth, known as a gall, regresses in a plant (exogenous regression). This leads to the conclusion that a fluent connection exists between stimulus-dependent, benign, semimalignant (intermediate, Gateff, see Chapters 43 and 48) and malignant growth when seen from a comparative platform.

After having briefly reviewed the regression of neoplasm on hand with selected examples, it can be stated that further studies on the basis of tumor specificity and species specificity may reveal new insights into species-specific immunology and other defense mechanisms of the organisms. The problem is closely linked to a gaining of understanding about destruction of neoplastically transformed cells before the development of a primary tumor, multiple tumor development, metastatic growth and cachexia in the frame of species-specific growth control and body defense. Comparative problems in nonautonomous and autonomous plant growth tumors have not been considered here because they are basically different.

References

1. Adenis, L., Cappelaere, P., Dulaquais, M. C., Coulombel, G., and Triplat, I. (1976): Are spontaneous cures, regressions and remissions of cancers possible? Clinical study. *Lille Med., 21*:29–36.
2. Adzhigitov, F. I. (1977): Modelling of sarcomas using the Rous virus on primates. *Vestn. Akad. Med. Nauk. SSSR, 8*:88–91.
3. Ahuja, M. R., and Anders, F. (1976): A genetic concept of the origin of cancer, based in part upon studies of neoplasms in fishes. *Prog. Exp. Tumor Res., 20*:380–97.
4. Aldrich, C. D., and Pedersen, N. C. (1974): Persistent viremia after regression of primary virus-induced feline fibrosarcomas. *Am. J. Vet. Res., 35*:1383–7.
5. Alexander, P. (1976): Some immunologically based reactions that can cause the regression of large tumor masses. *Natl. Cancer Inst. Monogr., 44*:105–8.
6. Allen, P. W. (1977): The fibromatoses: A clinicopathologic classification based on 140 cases. *Am. J. Surg. Pathol., 1*:255–70.
7. Andreev, V. C., Petkov, I., Berova, N., and Mustakov, G. (1975): Isolated lymphogranulomatosis of the skin. *Dermatol. Monatsschr. 161*:209–14.
8. Arenson, E. B., Jr., Hutter, J. J., Jr., Restuccia, R. D., and Holton, C. P. (1976): Neuroblastoma in father and son. *J. A. M. A., 235*:727–9.
9. Armitage, J. O., and Sidner, R. D. (1979): Antitumour effect of cimetidince (letter). *Lancet, 1*:882–3.
10. Artibani, W., Breda, G., Zattoni, F., Graziotti, P., Vancini, P., and Mazza, G. (1978): Treatment of renal carcinoma with metastases. *Chir. Ital., 30*: 81–105.
11. Atuk, N. O., Teja, K., Mondzelewski, P., Turner, S. M., and Selden, R. F. (1977): Avascular necrosis of pheochromocytoma followed by spontaneous remission. *Arch. Intern. Med., 137*:1073–5.
12. Axelsen, I. (1978): Retinoblastoma in a microphthalmic eye. *Ophthalmologica, 176*:27–33.
13. Aylsworth, C. F., Hodson, C. A., Berg, G., Kledzik, G., and Meites, J. (1979): *Cancer Res., 39*:(Pt. 1):2436–9.
14. Bachi, C., Coda, R., and Jona, B. (1976): Observations on a case of immunopathy in the course of acute leukemia. *Minerva Med., 66*:2697–9.
15. Bär, W., and Hedinger, C. (1977): Burned-out: Testicular tumors. Testicular lesions in germ cell tumors of clinically presumed extratesticular origin. *Virchows Arch. (Pathol. Anat.), 377*:67–78.
16. Bajardi, F. (1977): Etiology and distribution of intraepithelia cervical neoplasms. *Gynaekol. Rundsch.*: The treatment of capillary hemangiomas. *Dermatol. Monatsschr., 164*:375–7.
17. Baker, R. R. (1976): Spontaneous regression of bronchogenic carcinoma. *Natl. Cancer Inst. Monogr., 44*:31–3.
18. Balmer, A., and Gailloud, C. (1979): Treatment of retinoblastoma (author's transl.). *Klin. Monatsbl. Augenheilkd., 174*:922–6.
19. Bamberg, M., and Scherer, E. (1978): Low-dose x-ray treatment of 44 haemangiomas of the lid. *Dtsch. Med. Wochenschr., 103*:1293–7.
20. Bamberg, M., and Scherer, E. (1978): Radiotherapy of blastomatous hemangiomas—under special consideration of 44 eyelid hemangiomas. *Strahlentherapie 154*:233–9.
21. Bandhauer, K., and Obermayer, W. (1974): Nephrectomy in metastatic renal cancer. *Urol. Int., 29*:421–30.
22. Basta, L. L., Anderson, K. S., and Acers, T. E. (1977): Regression of orbital hemangioma detected by echography. *Arch. Ophthalmol., 95*: 1383–6.
23. Baum, M., and Coyle, P. J. (1977): Simple mastectomy for early breast cancer and the behaviour of the untreated axillary nodes. *Bull. Cancer (Paris), 64*:603–10.

24. Becker, J. M. (1978): Case of the summer season. *Semin. Roentgenol.,* 13:189–90.

25. Benjamin, S. P., Mercer, R. D., and Hawk, W. A. (1977): Myofibroblastic contraction in spontaneous regression of multiple congenital mesenchyma hamartomas. *Cancer,* 40:2343–52.

26. Bennett, B. T., Debelak-Fehir, K. M., and Epstein, R. B. (1975): Tumor-blocking and -inhibitory serum factors in the clinical course of canine venereal tumor. *Cancer Res.,* 35:(Pt. 1):2942–7.

27. Benny, P. S., and MacVicar, J. (1979): Multiple lipomas in pregnancy. *Br. Med. J.,* 1:1679–80.

28. Benson, W. E., Cameron, J. D., Furgiuele, F. P., Felberg, N. T., and Yanoff, M. (1978): Presumed spontaneously regressed retinoblastoma. *Ann. Ophthalmol.,* 10:897–9.

29. Berger, B. W., and Hori, Y. (1978): Multicentric Bowen's disease of the genitalia: spontaneous regression of lesions. *Arch. Dermatol.,* 114:1698–9.

30. Berlinger, N. T., and Good, R. A. (1974): Contemporary immunologic considerations in head and neck tumors. *Otolaryngol. Clin. North Am.,* 7:859–83.

31. Bernard, J. (1974): Generalities concerning therapy of acute leukemias. *Cah. Sociol. Demogr. Med.,* 15:613–5.

32. Bernstein, I. D. (1973): Immunologic defenses against cancer. *J. Pediatr.,* 83:906–18.

33. Beschorner, W. E., Hess, A. D., Nerenberg, S. T., and Epstein, R. B. (1979): Isolation and characterization of canine venereal tumor-associated inhibitory and blocking factors. *Cancer Res.,* 39:3920–7.

34. Bishop, J. O. (1979): Retinoblastoma. *Pediatr. Ann.,* 8:12–33.

35. Bloem, J. J., Vuzevski, V. D., and Huffstadt, A. J. (1974): Recurring digital fibroma of infancy. *J. Bone Joint Surg.,* 56(B):746–51.

36. Bluming, A. Z. (1976): Spontaneous regression of sarcoma. *Natl. Cancer Inst. Monogr.,* 44:55–7.

37. Boasberg, P. D., Eilber, F. R., and Morton, D. L. (1976): Immunocompetence and spontaneous regression of metastatic renal cell carcinoma. *J. Surg. Oncol.,* 8:207–10.

38. Bodurtha, A. J., Berkelhammer, J., Kim, T. H., Laucius, J. F., and Mastrangelo, M. J. (1976): A clinical histologic and immunologic study of a case of metastatic malignant melanoma undergoing spontaneous remission. *Cancer,* 37:735–42.

39. Böhm, J. (1977): Luteoma of the ovary during pregnancy. *Zentralbl. Allg. Pathol.,* 121:404–8.

40. Bolande, R. P. (1971): Benignity of neonatal tumors and concept of cancer regression in early life. *Am. J. Dis. Child.,* 122:12–4.

41. Bolt, H. M. (1975): The importance of estrogen receptors in the pharmaco-therapy of mammary carcinoma. *Münch. Med. Wochenschr.,* 117:33–6.

42. Booth, G. (1977): A "spontaneous" recovery from cancer. *J. Am. Acad. Psychoanal.,* 5:207–14.

43. Bove, K. E., and McAdams, A. J. (1975): Letter: Management of neuroblastomas. *N. Engl. J. Med.,* 292:593–4.

44. Brennan, M. J. (1975): Endocrinology in cancer of the breast. Status and prospects. *Am. J. Clin. Pathol.,* 64:797–809.

45. Briele, H. A., and Das Gupta, T. K. (1979): Natural history of cutaneous malignant melanoma. *World J. Surg.,* 3:255–70.

46. Briggs, R. M. (1979): Dysplasia and early neoplasia of the uterine cervix. A review. *Obstet. Gynecol. Surv.,* 34:70–99.

47. Briuzgin, V. V. (1977): Clinical features of the course of peripheral lung cancer with degeneration. *Ter. Arkh.,* 49:99–102.

48. Brohult, A., Brohult, J., and Brohult, S. (1978): Regression of tumor growth after administration of alkoxyglycerols. *Acta Obstet. Gynecol. Scand.,* 57:79–83.

49. Brown, T. (1977): Cytostatic treatment of gastro-intestinal cancer. *Tidsskr. Nor. Laegeforen,* 97:1737–39.

50. Bulkley, G. B., Cohen, M. H., Banks, P. M., Char, D. H., and Ketcham, A. S. (1975): Long-term spontaneous regression of malignant melanoma with visceral metastases. Report of a case with immunologic profile. *Cancer,* 36:485–94.

51. Burby, V. P. (1977): The case of the vanishing lesions: *Myosis fungoides. Arch. Dermatol.,* 113:513.

52. Burnet, F. M. (1970): The concept of immunological surveillance. *Prog. Exp. Tumor Res.,* 13:1–27.

53. Burnet, F. M. (1973): Implications of cancer immunity. *Aust. N. Z. J. Med.,* 3:71–7.

54. Burns, F. J., VanderLaan, M., Sivak, A., and Albert, R. E. (1976): Regression kinetics of mouse skin papillomas. *Cancer Res.,* 36:1422–7.

55. Caldwell, E. H. (1976): Desmoid tumor: Musculoaponeurotic fibrosis of the abdominal wall. *Surgery,* 79:104–6.

56. Callan, J. E., Wood, V. E., and Linda, L. (1975): Spontaneous resolution of an osteochondroma. *J. Bone Joint Surg.,* 57:723.

57. Calnek, B. W., Higgins, D. A., and Fabricant, J. (1975): Rous sarcoma regression in chickens resistant or susceptible to Marek's disease. *Avian Dis.,* 19:473–82.

58. Cappelaere, P., Demaille, A., and Adenis, L. (1973): Immunological exploration of cancer patients. II. Tumoral immunity. *Lille Med.,* 18:179–201.

59. Carapeto, F. J. (1977): Multiple trichoepithelioma with variable evolution of its lesions (malignancy and spontaneous remission). *Med. Cutan. Iber. Lat. Am.,* 5:65–9.

60. Cerni, C. M. (1974): Tumor immunology. *Wien Med. Wochenschr.,* 124: (Suppl. 2): 21–5.

61. Cerny, J., Essex, M., Rich, M. A., and Hardy, W. D., Jr. (1975): Expression of virus-associated antigens and immune cell functions during spontaneous regression of the Friend viral murine leukemia. *Int. J. Cancer,* 15:351–65.

62. Check, W. (1979): Benign breast lumps may regress with change in diet (news). *J. A. M. A.* 241:1221.

63. Chesebro, B., Wehrly, K., and Stimpfling, J. (1974): Host genetic control of recovery from Friend leukemia virus-induced splenomegaly: Mapping of a gene within the major histocompatability complex. *J. Exp. Med.,* 140:1457–67.

64. Chieco-bianchi, L., Colombatti, A., Collavo, D., Sendo, F., Aoki, T., and Fischinger, P. J. (1974): Tumor induction by murine sarcoma virus in AKR and C58 mice. Reduction of tumor regression associated with appearance of Gross leukemia virus pseudotypes. *J. Exp. Med.,* 140: 1162–79.

65. Cho-Chung, Y. S., Bodwin, J. S., and Clair, T. (1978): Cyclic amp-binding proteins: Inverse relationship with estrogen-receptors in hormone-dependent mammary tumor regression. *Eur. J. Biochem.,* 86:51–60.

66. Cho-Chung, Y. S., Clair, T., and Zubialde, J. P. (1978): Increase of cyclic AMP-dependent protein kinase type II as an early event in hormone-dependent mammary tumor regression. *Biochem. Biophys. Res. Commun.,* 85:1150–5.

67. Clark, W. H., Jr., Mastrangelo, M. J., Ainsworth, A. M., Berd, D., Bellet, R. E., and Bernardino, E. A. (1977): Current concepts of the biology of human cutaneous malignant melanoma. *Adv. Cancer Res.,* 24:267–338.

68. Cockerell, G. L., and Slauson, D. O. (1979): Patterns of lymphoid infiltrate in the canine cutaneous histiocytoma. *J. Comp. Pathol.,* 89: 193–203.

69. Cole, W. H. (1974): Spontaneous regression of cancer: the metabolic triumph of the host? *Ann. N.Y. Acad. Sci.,* 230:111–41.

70. Cole, W. H. (1974): Spontaneous regression of cancer. *Cancer,* 24:274–9.

71. Cole, W. H. (1976): Spontaneous regression of cancer and the importance of finding its cause. *Natl. Cancer Inst. Monogr.,* 44:5–9.

72. Cole, W. H. (1976): Relationship of causative factors in spontaneous regression of cancer to immunologic factors possibly effective in cancer. *J. Surg. Oncol.,* 8:391–411.

73. Conrad, M. E., and Barton, J. C. (1979): Hepatitis and leukemia (letter). *Ann. Intern. Med.,* 90:988.

74. Constantinides, G., Guilbert, Bolvin, M. J. (1977): Retinoblastoma with spontaneous regression (apropos of 2 cases). *Bull. Soc. Ophthalmol. Fr.,* 77:547–9.

75. Corbett, A. C., Collins, W. M., and Dunlop, W. R. (1975): Effect of regression of Rous sarcoma tumors upon egg production in an inbred line of White Leghorns. *Poult. Sci.,* 54:136–9.

76. Cotter, P. F., Collins, W. M., Dunlop, W. R., and Corbett, A. C. (1976): The influence of thymectomy on Rous sarcoma regression. *Avian Dis.,* 20:75–9.

77. Cotter, P. F., Collins, W. M., Dunlop, W. R., and Corbett, A. C. (1976): Detection of cellular immunity to Rous tumors of chickens by the leukocyte migration inhibition reaction. *Poult. Sci.,* 55:1008–11.

78. Crittenden, (1975): Two levels of genetic resistance to lymphoid leukosis. *Avian Dis.,* 19:281–92.

79. Cron, J. (1970): Antineoplastic defense of the organism. *Vnitr. Lek.,* 16: 659–63.

80. Cron, J. (1977): Phagocytic activity of leucocytes in cancer remission. *Cas. Lek. Cesk.,* 116:1343–5.

81. Dahl, R., Lindgren, A., Lindholm, C. E., Nou, E., and Ollman, B. (1978): Local spontaneous regression of bronchial cancer. *Lakartidningen,* 75: 325–6.

82. Davies, M. G., and Marks, R. (1977): Multiple xanthogranulomata in an adult. *Br. J. Dermatol.,* 97(Suppl. 15):70–2.

83. de Brux, J., Trevoux, R., and Willemin, A. (1978): Breast cancer diagnosed in the pre-clinical stage with the phenomena of histological regression. *J. Gynecol. Obst. Biol. Reprod. (Paris),* 7:945–51.

84. DeCosse, J. J., Adams, M. B., and Condon, R. E. (1977): Familial polyposis. *Cancer,* 39:267–73.

85. DeLanney, L. E. (1970): Lymphosarcoma in the Mexican axolotl, *Ambystoma mexicanum. Bibl. Haematol.,* 36:642.

86. DeVita, V. T., Jr., and Fisher, R. I. (1976): Natural history of malignant melanoma as related to therapy. *Cancer Treat. Rep.,* 60:153–7.

87. Deweerd, J. H., Hawthorne, N. J., and Adson, M. A. (1977): Regression of renal cell hepatic metastasis following removal of primary lesions. *J. Urol.,* 117:790–2.

88. Dhir, S. P., Jain, I. S., and Das, S. K. (1977): Regressed retinoblastoma. *Indian J. Ophthalmol.,* 24:35–6.

89. Dhoine, G., Woillez, M., and Beal, F. (1973): Orbital thyroid metastasis (cure after 10 years). *Bull. Soc. Ophthalmol.,* 73:1229–31.

90. Dietz, M., Furmanski, P., Clymer, R., and Rich, M. A. (1976): Effects of thymectomy and antithymocyte serum on spontaneous regression of Friend virus-induced erythroleukemia. *J. Natl. Cancer Inst.,* 57:91–5.

91. Dissing, I., Heerfordt, J., and Schidt, T. (1978): Spontaneous regression

of a malignant primary bone tumour. *Acta Orthop. Scand.*, 49:49–53.

92. Dotsenko, A. P. (1966): On the spontaneous regression of malignant neoplasms. *Vopr. Onkol.*, 12:103–11.

93. Downing, V., and Levine, S. (1975): Erythrocytosis and renal cell carcinoma with pulmonary metastases: Case report with 18-year follow-up and brief discussion of literature. *Cancer*, 35:1701–5.

94. Dubrow, E. L. (1977): Regression of metastatic hypernephroma. *J. Am. Geriatr. Soc.*, 25:454–7.

95. Dunham, W. B., and Waymouth, C. (1976): Intradermal transplantation in mice of small numbers of sarcoma cells followed by tumor growth and regression. *Cancer Res.*, 36:189–93.

96. Durand, M., Hoerni, B., and Chauvergne, J. (1974): Conditions of appreciation of efficiency in treatments of cancers. *Bull. Cancer (Paris)*, 61:229–34.

97. Editorial (1975): Spontaneous regression of primary cutaneous melanoma. *Med. J. Aust.*, 2:761.

98. Edmondson, H. A., Reynolds, T. B., Henderson, B., and Benton, B. (1977): Regression of liver cell adenomas assoc contraceptives. *Ann. Intern. Med.*, 86:180–2.

99. Edwards, H. (1975): Alternative medicine: The science of spiritual healing. *Nurs. Times*, 71:2008–10.

100. Ehrensperger, J., and Genton, N. (1970): Cancer in the new-born. *Acuel. Probl. Chir.*, 14:329–44.

101. Elboim, C. M., Reinisch, C. L., and Schlossman, S. F. (1977): T and B lymphocyte migration into syngeneic tumors. *J. Immunol.*, 118:1042–8.

102. El-Domeiri, A. A. (1977): Delayed hypersensitivity reaction: Its relation to tumor spread and diagnosis. *Surg. Annu.*, 9:343–350.

103. El-Mofty, S. (1978): Spontaneous regression of induced parotid gland tumors in rats. *Oral Surg.*, 45:431–40.

104. Erb, H. (1976): Diagnostic and therapeutic procedures for small ovarian tumors. *Praxis*, 65:167–71.

105. Essex, M., Snyder, S. P., and Klein, G. (1973): Relationship between humoral antibodies and the failure to develop progressive tumors in cats injected with feline sarcoma virus (FSV). *Bibl. Haematol.*, 39:771–7.

106. Evans, A. E., Gerson, J., and Schnaufer, L. (1976): Spontaneous regression of neuroblastoma. *Natl. Cancer Inst. Monogr.*, 44:49–54.

107. Everson, T. C. (1967): Spontaneous regression of cancer. *Prog. Clin. Cancer*, 3:79–95.

108. Fabricant, J., Calnek, B. W., Schat, K. A., and Murthy, K. K. (1978): Marek's disease virus-induced tumor transplants: development and rejection in various genetic strains of chickens. *Avian Dis.*, 22:646–58.

109. Fairley, G. H. (1971): Immunity to malignant disease in man. *Sci. Basis Med.*, 17–38.

110. Firminger, H. I. (1976): A pathologist looks at spontaneous regression of cancer. *Natl. Cancer Inst. Monogr.*, 44:15–8.

111. Fisher, B. (1971): The present status of tumor immunology. *Adv. Surg.*, 5:189–254.

112. Fortner, J. G., and Shiu, M. H. (1974): Organ transplantation and cancer. *Surg. Clin. North Am.*, 54:871–6.

113. Fox, P. S., Hofmann, J. W., Decosse, J. J., and Wilson, S. D. (1974): The influence of total gastrectomy on survival in malignant Zollinger-Ellison tumors. *Ann. Surg.*, 180:558–66.

114. Franklin, C. I. (1977): Spontaneous regression of metastases from testicular tumours. A report of six cases from one centre. *Clin. Radiol.*, 28:499–502.

115. Freed, S. Z., Halperin, J. P., and Gordon, M. (1977): Idiopathic regression of metastases from renal cell carcinoma. *J. Urol.*, 118:538–42.

116. Frootko, N. J., and Rogers, J. H. (1978): Oesophageal papillomata in the child. *J. Laryngol. Otol.*, 92:823–7.

117. Fryns, J. P., Eggermont, E., and Eeckels, R. (1974): Multiple diffuse hemangiomatosis. Case report and review of the literature. *Z. Kinderheilkd.*, 117:115–9.

118. Fudge, T. L., and McKinnon, W. M. (1976): Fibroadenoma of the breast during pregnancy and lactation—disappearance postpartum: Report of a case. *J. La. State Med. Soc.*, 128:157–8.

119. Furmanski, P., Baldwin, J., Clymer, R., and Rich, M. A. (1975): Spontaneous regression of Friend virus induced leukemia: Coinfection with regressing and conventional strains of virus. *Science*, 187:72–3.

120. Furmanski, P., Juni, S., Hall, L., and Rich, M. A. (1975): The role of interferon in the spontaneous regression of Friend virus induced leukemia. *Proc. Soc. Exp. Biol. Med.*, 150:11–13.

121. Furmanski, P., Dietz, M., Fouchey, S., Hall, L., Clymer, R., and Rich, M. A. (1979): Spontaneous regression of Friend murine leukemia virus-induced erythroleukemia. IV. Effects of radiation and athymia on leukemia regression in mice. *J. Natl. Cancer Inst.*, 63:449–54.

122. Gallie, B. L., Wong, J. J., Ellsworth, R. M., Dupont, B., and Good, R. A. (1978): Immunological mechanisms in spontaneous regression of retinoblastoma. In *Immunology and Immunopathology of the Eye*, pp. 190–6, edited by A. M. Silverstein and G. R. O'Connor, New York, Masson.

123. Gaillie, B. L., Dupont, B., Whitsett, C., Kitchen, F. D., Ellsworth, R. M., and Good, R. A. (1977): Histocompatibility typing in spontaneous regression of retinoblastoma. *Prog. Clin. Biol. Res.*, 16:229–37.

124. Giles, R. C., Kwapien, R. P., Geil, R. G., and Casey, H. W. (1978):

Mammary nodules in beagle dogs administered investigational oral contraceptive steroids. *J. Natl. Cancer Inst.*, 60:1351–64.

125. Gille, J. (1975): Choriocarcinoma. *Med. Klin.*, 70:532–43.

126. Glasser, M., Rosenberg, M. A., and Gaito, R. (1979): Widespread adenocarcinoma of the colon with survival of 28 years. *J.A.M.A.*, 241:2542–3.

127. Golbert, Z. V., Romanova, O. A., and Chervonnaia, L. V. (1977): Spontaneous regression of malignant melanoma. *Arkh. Patol.*, 39:36–42.

128. Goldwyn, R. M., and Kasdon, E. J. (1978): The "disappearance" of residual basal cell carcinoma of the skin. *Ann. Plast. Surg.*, 1:286–9.

129. Gregor, R. T. (1976): Vitiligo and malignant melanoma: A significant association? *S. Afr. Med. J.*, 50:1447–9.

130. Gromet, M. A., Epstein, W. L., and Blois, M. S. (1978): The regressing thin malignant melanoma: a distinctive lesion with metastatic potential. *Cancer*, 42:2282–92.

131. Groncy, P., and Finklestein, J. Z. (1978): Neuroblastoma. *Pediatr. Ann.*, 7:548–59.

132. Groscurth, P., and Kistler, G. (1977): Human renal cell carcinoma in the "nude" mouse: Long-term observations. *Beitr. Pathol.*, 160:337–60.

133. Gross, L. (1971): Transmission of cancer in man. Tentative guidelines referring to the possible effects of inoculation of homologous cancer extracts in man. *Cancer*, 28:785–8.

134. Gross, L., and Dreyfuss, Y. (1974): The role of the skin in active specific immunization against leukemia in guinea pigs. *Proc. Natl. Acad. Sci.*, 71:3550–4.

135. Gross, L., and Dreyfuss, Y. (1977): Immunization of guinea pigs against L2C leukemia with live leukemic cells by intradermal inoculation: Early and late effects. *Fed. Proc.*, 36:2272–6.

136. Guinan, P., Sadoughi, N., Bush, I. M., John, T., Eghrari, F., and Ablin, R. J. (1972): Immunology of genitourinary tumors. *Urology*, 2:493–9.

137. Gunale, S., and Tucker, W. G. (1975): Regression of metastatic melanoma. *Mich. Med.*, 74:697–8.

138. Gyles, N. R., Marini, P. J., and Smith, J. L. (1977): The infectivity of fluid from regressing Rous sarcomas. *Poult. Sci.*, 56:1315–7.

139. Gyles, N. R., Blythe, M., Test, P., Bowanko, A., and Brown, C. J. (1977): Immune response in progressor and regressor strains of chickens at specific intervals after a primary challenge with Rous sarcoma virus. *Poult. Sci.*, 56:758–66.

140. Happle, R., Schotola, I., and Macher, E. (1975): Spontaneous regression and leukoderma in malignant melanoma. *Hautarzt*, 26:120–3.

141. Harada, M., Pearson, G., Redmon, L., Winters, E., and Kasuga, S. (1975): Antibody production and interaction with lymphoid cells in relation to tumor immunity in the Moloney sarcoma virus system. *J. Immunol.*, 114:1318–22.

142. Harms, D., and Hornstein, O. P. (1979): Spontaneous regression of congenital angioleiomyomatosis. *Monatsschr. Kinderheilkd.*, 127:313–4.

143. Harrington, W. J. (1969): Curable forms of disseminated cancer. *Adv. Intern. Med.*, 15:317–37.

144. Harwood, R. A., and Abreu, F. B. (1975): Benign lymphoma and diffuse lymphoid hyperplasia. A case report. *Am. J. Protocol.*, 26:63–6.

145. Haslam, S. Z. (1979): Age as a modifying factor of 7,12-dimethylbenz[a]anthrazene-induced mammary carcinogenesis in the Lewis rat. *Int. J. Cancer*, 23:374–9.

146. Hassenstein, E. O. (1977): An unusual regression of pulmonary metastases from embryonal carcinoma of the testis. *Br. J. Radiol.*, 50:668–70.

147. Hattori, T. (1974): A review of clinical tumor immunology. An approach to immunochemotherapy. *J. Jpn. Soc. Cancer Ther.*, 9:381–90.

148. Hellström, K. E., and Hellström, I. (1972): Immunity to neuroblastomas and melanomas. *Annu. Rev. Med.*, 23:19–38.

149. Hellström, K. E., and Hellström, I. (1976): Spontaneous tumor regression: Possible relationship to in vitro parameters of tumor immunity. *Natl. Cancer Inst. Monogr.*, 44:131–4.

150. Herfarth, C. (1979): Knowledge of tumor immunology—consequences for surgery. *Chirurgie*, 50:1–4.

151. Hertz, R. (1976): Spontaneous regression in choriocarcinoma and related gestational trophoblastic neoplasms. *Natl. Cancer Inst. Monogr.*, 44:59–60.

152. Hewitt, H. B. (1979): A critical examination of the foundations of immunotherapy for cancer. *Clin. Radiol.*, 30:361–9.

153. Himmelberger, E. S., Miller, S. H., Davis, T. S., and Graham, W. P. (1978): Involuting hemangiomas. *Am. Fam. Physician*, 17:99–102.

154. Höffken, K., and Schmidt, C. G. (1978): Tumor antigens. *Dtsch. Med. Wochenschr.*, 103:1187–90.

155. Holland, J. M. (1973): Proceedings: Cancer of the kidney—natural history and staging. *Cancer*, 32:1030–42.

156. Holland, J. M. (1973): Natural history and staging of renal cell carcinoma. *Cancer*, 25:121–33.

157. Holtermann, O. A., Papermaster, B., Rosner, D., Milgrom, H., and Klein, E. (1975): Regression of cutaneous neoplasms following delayed-type hypersensitivity challenge reactions to microbial antigens or lymphokines. *J. Med.*, 6:157–68.

158. Honore, L. H., and Moloney, P. J. (1976): Malignant germ cell tumor of the testis: Spontaneous regression of pulmonary metastases with 7-year survival. *J. Urol.*, 116:382–4.

159. Horstmann, J. P., Pietra, G. G., Harman, J. A., Coie, N. G., and Grinspan, S. (1977): Spontaneous regression of pulmonary leiomyomas during pregnancy. *Cancer*, 39:314–21.

160. Hozumi, M. (1971): Instability of phenotypes of tumor cells—on decarcinogenesis. *Tanpakushitsu Kakusan Koso*, 16:599–612.

161. Hrushesky, W. J., and Murphy, G. P. (1977): Current status of the therapy of advanced renal carcinoma. *J. Surg. Oncol.*, 9:277–88.

162. Hudym-Levkovych, K. A., Surkina, I. I., Sherban, S. D., and Kovbasiuk, S. A. (1976): Cytological characteristics of mouse lymphatic nodes in viral cancerogenesis. *Mikrobiol. Zh.*, 38:722–6.

163. Hula, M. (1975): Spontaneous regression of primary melanoblastoma. *Cesk. Dermatol.*, 50:156–68.

164. Humphrey, L. J. (1970): Tumor immunity. *J. Surg. Res.*, 10:493–512.

165. Hutter, J. J., Jr., Hays, T., and Holton, C. P. (1975): Letter: Spontaneous regression in neuroblastoma. *J. Pediatr.* 86:820.

166. Iakimov, M. (1975): Complement-dependent immune cytolysis of cells from transplantable myeloid tumor. *Acta Microbiol. Virol. Immunol.*, 2:52–6.

167. Ikawa, Y., Yoshikura, H., and Sugano, H. (1970): Transformation of a cloned renal epithelial cell line by Moloney murine sarcoma virus (M-MSV). *Bibl. Haematol.*, 36:312–22.

168. Inglot, A. D., and Oleszak, E. (1978): Effect of non-steroidal anti-inflammatory drugs of Moloney sarcoma virus inoculated mice. *Experientia*, 34:1615–7.

169. Ito, N., Hananouchi, M., Sugihara, S., Shirai, T., and Tsuda, H. (1976): Reversibility and irreversibility of liver tumors in mice induced by the alpha isomer of 1,2,3,4,5,6-hexachlorocyclohexane. *Cancer Res.*, 36(Pt. 1):2227–34.

170. Iwasaki, H., Tsuneyoshi, M., and Enjoji, M. (1974): Infantile digital fibromatosis. Histopathological and electron microscopic study with a review of the literature. *Acta Pathol. Jpn.*, 24:717–32.

171. Jacobs, J. B., Edelstein, L. M., Snyder, L. M., and Fortier, N. (1975): Ultrastructural evidence for destruction in the halo nevus. *Cancer Res.*, 35:352–7.

172. Jakowski, R. M., Fredrickson, T. N., Schierman, L. W., and McBride, R. A. (1974): A transplantable lymphoma induced with Marek's disease virus. *J. Natl. Cancer Inst. Monogr.*, 53:783–9.

173. Janssen, P. L., and Weiszbach, L. (1978): To psychosomatics of treated testicular tumor patients. *Z. Psychosom. Med. Psychoanal.*, 24:1–86.

174. Julian, C. G. (1976): Spontaneous regression in gynecologic neoplasia. *Natl. Cancer Inst. Monogr.*, 44:27–30.

175. Jung, E. G., and Köhler, U. (1977): Regression of haemangiomata in infants after x-ray treatment and mock-radiation. *Arch. Dermatol. Res.*, 259:21–8.

176. Kennedy, J. R., Yang, T. J., and Allen, P. L. (1977): Canine transmissible venereal sarcoma: Electron microscopic changes with time after transplantation. *Br. J. Cancer*, 36:375–85.

177. Kik, A., and Lyko, M. M. (1977): Spontaneous regression of true angiomas. *Przegl. Dermatol.*, 64:741–6.

178. Klein, E., and Cochran, A. J. (1971): Immunology and malignant disease. *Haematologia*, 5:179–203.

179. Klein, G. (1976): Immune surveillance—a powerful mechanism with a limited range. *Natl. Cancer Inst. Monogr.*, 44:109–113.

180. Klein, G. (1976): Mechanisms of escape from immune surveillance. *Natl. Cancer Inst. Monogr.*, 44:135–6.

181. Kobori, O., Adachi, S., Kusama, S., and Shimazu, H. (1977): Statistical analysis of 1186 cases of gastric carcinoma: With special reference to advanced lesion. *Langenbeck's Arch. Chir.*, 344:83–92.

182. Koch, K., Bloom, G. E., and Wolfson, S. L. (1971): Chemotherapy in childhood malignancies. *J. Fla. Med. Assoc.*, 58:24–35.

183. Kodama, T., Goto, T., and Kobayashi, H. (1974): Proceedings: Immunological study of regression of metastatic neoplasm in lymph nodes. *Hokkaido J. Med. Sci.*, 49:153–4.

184. Kodama, T., Gotohda, E., Takeichi, N., Kuzumaki, N., and Kobayashi, H. (1975): Histopathology of regression of tumor metastasis in the lymph nodes. *Cancer Res.*, 35:1628–36.

185. Komatsu, Y., Sakata, Y., Ishizawa, M., Aizawa, T., and Yanagiya, S. (1975): A case of metastatic tumor in the liver with spontaneous regression. Metastatic tumor, spontaneous regression. *J. Jpn. Soc. Intern. Med.*, 64:1160–6.

186. Koop, C. E. (1972): The neuroblastoma. *Prog. Pediatr. Surg.*, 4:1–28.

187. Kopf, A. W., Bart, R. S., and Rodriguez-Sains, R. S. (1977): Malignant melanoma: a review. *J. Dermatol. Surg. Oncol.*, 3:41–125.

188. Krueger, G., and Raferty, B. (1975): Proceedings: Spontaneous reversion of neoplastic cells. *Verh. Dtsch. Ges. Pathol.*, 59:485.

189. Krutchik, A. N., Buzdar, A. U., Blumenschein, G. R., and Lukeman, J. M. (1978): Spontaneous regression of breast carcinoma. *Arch. Intern. Med.*, 138:1734–5.

190. Kurrle-Knapp, U., and Kurrle, G. (1975): Growth and spontaneous remission of a tumor—a nine-year observation. Clinical diagnosis: *Epulis gigantocellularis*. *Quintessence Int.*, 6:9–12.

191. Kvakina, E. B., Shibkova, S. A., and Isadzhanova, S. Kh. (1974): Morphological changes in the hypothalamus during tumor resorption under the influence of an alternating magnetic field. *Vopr. Onkol.*, 20:89–92.

192. Lagova, N. D. (1978): Mechanism of mammary cancer regression in lactating rats. *Biull. Eksp. Biol. Med.*, 85:582–5.

193. Laird, W. P., Friedman, S., Koop, C. E., and Schwartz, G. J. (1976): Hepatic hemangiomatosis. Successful management by hepatic artery ligation. *Am. J. Dis. Child.*, 130:657–9.

194. Lamon, E. W., Skurzak, H. M., Andersson, B., Whitten, H. D., and Klein, E. (1975): Antibody-dependent lymphocyte cytotoxicity in the murine sarcoma virus system: Activity of IgM and IgG with specificity for MLV determined antigen(s). *J. Immunol.*, 114:1171–6.

195. Largiader, F., Uhlschmid, G., and Gattiker, H. H. (1975): Cryosurgery of lung metastases. *Thoraxchirurgie*, 23:515–22.

196. Lee, Y. T. (1972): Prognostic factors in surgical treatment of bronchogenic carcinoma. *Surg. Gynecol. Obstet.*, 135:961–75.

197. Lee, Y. T. (1977): Systemic and regional treatment of primary carcinoma of the liver. *Cancer Treat. Rev.*, 4:195–212.

198. Leicher, H. (1978): The origin of malignant tumors of the upper-airways, the digestion tract and the ear. Organ-resistance and organ-disposition (organotrophy) by the origin of malignant primary tumors. *Laryngol. Rhinol. Otol.*, 57:162–76.

199. Lenstrup, C. (1975): Spontaneous regression of lung cancer. *Ugeskr. Laeger*, 137:1470–1.

200. Levy, J. P., and Kourilsky, F. M. (1973): Tumor-associated membrane antigens and the antitumor immune reactions. *Transplant. Proc.*, 5:1435–40.

201. Levy, R. B., St. Pierre, R. L., and Waksal, S. D. (1976): Macrophage participation in a spontaneously regressing syngeneic tumor. *Adv. Exp. Med. Biol.*, 73(B):415–21.

202. Lewi, M. G. (1972): Circulating humoral antibodies in cancer. *Med. Clin. North Am.*, 56:481–99.

203. Lewison, E. F. (1977): Spontaneous regression of breast cancer. *Prog. Clin. Biol. Res.*, 12:47–53.

204. Likhite, V. V. (1975): Rejection of mammary adenocarcinoma cell tumors in DBA/2 mice immunocompromised by thymectomy and treatment with antithymocyte serum. *J. Immunol.*, 114:1736–42.

205. Lindley, J., and Smith, S. (1974): Histology and spontaneous regression of retinoblastoma. *Trans. Ophthalmol. Soc.*, 94:953–67.

206. Louw, J. H. (1974): Flank tumours in infants and children. *S. Afr. J. Surg.*, 12:5–18.

207. Luderer, R. C., Opipari, M. I., and Perrotta, A. L. (1978): Treatment of metastatic renal cell carcinoma: Review of experience and world literature. *J.A.O.A.*, 77:590–603.

208. Ludwig, G., Jentzsch, R., and Nuri, M. (1977): Spontaneous regression of pulmonary metastases from hypernephroma: Report of a case and review of literature. *Med. Klin.*, 72:2118–21.

209. Lundy, J., and Lovette, E. J. (1976): Thiabendazole: A new immunopotentiator effective in therapy of murine fibrosarcoma. *Surg. Forum*, 27:132–4.

210. Luosto, R., Koikkalainen, K., and Sipponen, P. (1974): Spontaneous regression of a bronchial carcinoid tumour following pregnancy. *Ann. Chir. Gynaecol. Fenn.*, 63:342–5.

211. Lynch, H. T., Frichot, B. C., 3rd, Fisher, J., Smith, J. L., Jr., and Lynch, J. F. (1978): *J. Med. Genet.*, 15:357–62.

212. MacAuley, W. L. (1978): Lymphomatoid papulosis. *Int. J. Dermatol.*, 17:204–12.

213. MacDougal, B. A., Weeks, P. M., and Wray, R. C., Jr. (1976): Spontaneous regression of the primary lesion of a metastatic malignant melanoma. *Plast. Reconstr. Surg.*, 57:355–8.

214. Macher, E., Sorg, C., and Seibert, E. R. (1976): Immunology of malignant melanoma. *Langenbecks Arch. Chir.*, 342:533–8.

215. Mackie, B. S. (1976): Hutchinson's melanotic freckle: Partial regression of lesion and surrounding actinic keratoses. *Australas. J. Dermatol.*, 17:49–51.

216. Mahrle, C., Bolling, R., and Gartman, H. (1977): Verrucous malignant melanoma, spontaneous regression and simultaneous development of a secondary tumor. *Z. Hautkr.*, 52:897–905.

217. Maiskii, I. N., and Lomakin, M. S. (1976): Factors of bodily resistance and metastasis. *Usp. Sovrem. Biol.*, 82:63–76.

218. Manelis, G., Shasha, S. M., Manelis, J., Suprun, H., and Robinson, E. (1978): Spontaneous regression of malignant melanoma. *Oncology*, 35:83–6.

219. Marcelletti, J., and Furmanski, P. (1978): Spontaneous regression of friend virus-induced erythroleukemia. III. The role of macrophages in regression. *J. Immunol.*, 120:1–8.

220. Marcelletti, J., and Furmanski, P. (1979): Infection of macrophages with Friend virus: relationship to the spontaneous regression of viral erythroleukemia. *Cell*, 16:649–59.

221. Markarian, D. S., Adzhigitov, F. I., and Gubeladze, D. A. (1974): Sarcoma induction in Dzungarian hamster using Rous sarcoma virus (Carr-Zilber strain). *Vopr. Virusol.*, 2:137–9.

222. Masson, P. (1970): *Human Tumors* (Translated by D. Kobernick), 2nd Ed., Wayne State University Press, Detroit.

223. Matsuzawa, A., and Yamamoto, T. (1974): A transplantable pregnancy-dependent mammary tumor line (TPDMT-4) in strain DDD mice. *GANN*, 65:307–15.

224. Maurus, R. (1977): Present strategy of treatment of neuroblastoma: Recent results. *Cancer Res.*, 62:210–2.
225. Mauss, J. (1978): Follow-up of a disfiguring hemangiolymphangioma of the face. *Hautarzt*, 29:94–5.
226. McCarthy, W. H., Shaw, H. M., and Milton, G. W. (1978): Spontaneous regression of metastatic malignant melanoma. *Clin. Oncol.*, 4:203–7.
227. McGovern, V. J. (1975): Spontaneous regression of melanoma. *Pathology*, 7:91–9.
228. McGovern, V. J. (1977): Epidemiological aspects of melanoma: A review. *Pathology*, 9:233–41.
229. McGrail, T. P., Collins, W. M., Dunlop, W. R., and Zsigray, R. M. (1978): Lymphocytotoxicity of chickens bearing Rous sarcomas. *Poult. Sci.*, 57: 90–4.
230. McKhann, C. F., and Yarlott, M. A., Jr. (1975): Tumor immunology. *CA*, 25:187–97.
231. McLaughlin, A. P., 3d, and Gittes, R. F. (1974): Spontaneous tumor regression. Experimental aspects. *Urology*, 3:544–51.
232. McLaughlin, J. E., and Urich, H. (1977): Maturing neuroblastoma and ganglioneuroblastoma: A study of four cases with long survival. *J. Pathol.*, 121:19–26.
233. McLaughlin, R. E., Wang, G. J., Ritchie, W. P., Jr., and Sweet, D. E. (1979): Protracted survival in chondrosarcoma despite an unusual metastasis that regressed spontaneously. *J. Bone Joint Surg.*, 61:137–9.
234. Meares, A. (1977): Regression of cancer after intensive meditation followed by death (letter). *Med. J. Aust.*, 2:374–5.
235. Meares, A. (1977): Atavistic regression as a factor in the remission of cancer. *Med. J. Aust.*, 2:132–3.
236. Meares, A. (1978): Regression of osteogenic sarcoma metastases associated with intensive meditation. *Med. J. Aust.*, 2:433.
237. Mehra, K. S., and Gupta, I. M. (1974): Unilaterally regression retinoblastoma with massive optic nerve involvement in a bilateral lesion. *Ann. Ophthalmol.*, 6:919–22.
238. Mehta, F. S., and Pindborg, J. J. (1974): Spontaneous regression of oral leukoplakias among Indian villagers in a 5-year follow-up study. *Community Dent. Oral Epidemiol.*, 2:80–4.
239. Meier, C. R., and Lobuglio, A. F. (1977): Transfer factor: A potential agent for immunotherapy of cancer. *World J. Surg.*, 1:617–23.
240. Meigs, J. W., Laskey, P. W., and Flannerei, J. T. (1976): Evidence for regression of carcinoma-in-situ and for a second form of invasive cervical cancer, Connecticut 1935–73. *Geburtshilfe Frauenheilkd.*, 36: 554–69.
241. Merkin, L. (1978): The aetiology of cancer: Clues from spontaneous recovery. *Med. Hypotheses*, 4:136–40.
242. Micksche, M., Cerni, C., Gebhart, W., and Kokoschka, E. M. (1975): Halo Nevus (Morbus Sutton): Model of an immunological tumor regression. *Oesterr. Z. Onkol.*, 2:73–81.
243. Milas, L., Hunter, N., Basic, I., and Withers, H. R. (1974): Complete regressions of an established murine fibrosarcoma induced by systemic application of *Corynebacterium granulosum*. *Cancer Res.*, 34:2470–5.
244. Milton, G. W. (1975): The surgeon's dilemma. *Med. J. Aust.*, 2:229–30.
245. Mobley, W. C., Server, A. C., Ishii, D. N., Riopelle, R. J., and Shooter, E. M. (1977): Nerve growth factor (third of three parts). *N. Engl. J. Med.*, 297:1211–8.
246. Moggian, G., Barboni, F., and Sabetta, C. (1974): Immunologic study of a case of spontaneous regression of metastatic carcinoma of the portio. *Cancro*, 27:165–8.
247. Mohr, S. J., and Whitesel, J. A. (1979): Spontaneous regression of renal cell carcinoma metastases after preoperative embolization of primary tumor and subsequent nephrectomy. *Urology*, 14:5–8.
248. Monks, F. T. (1975): Central angioma of the mandible: A possible treatment. *Br. J. Oral Surg.*, 12:296–7.
249. Morita, Y., Shinohara, M., Ishikawa, K., and Kato, Y. (1979): Hemangioma of the transverse colon; diagnosis by angiography (author's transl.). *Rhinsho Hoshasen*, 24:311–4.
250. Morris, W. E., and LaPiana, F. G. (1974): Spontaneous regression of bilateral multifocal retinoblastoma with preservation of normal visual acuity. *Ann. Ophthalmol.*, 6:1192–4.
251. Morton, D. L., Eilber, F. R., and Malmgren, R. A. (1971): Immune factors in human cancer: Malignant melanomas, skeletal and soft tissue sarcomas. *Prog. Exp. Tumor Res.*, 14:25–42.
252. Morton, D. L., Eilber, F. R., Holmes, E. C., Hunt, J. S., Ketcham, A. S., Silverstein, M. J., and Sparks, F. C. (1974): BCG immunotherapy of malignant melanoma: Summary of a seven-year experience. *Ann. Surg.*, 180:635–43.
253. Moscovici, C. (1975): Leukemic transformation with avian myeloblastosis virus: Present status. *Curr. Top. Microbiol. Immunol.*, 71:79–101.
254. Muldoon, C. J. (1975): Squamous cell carcinoma with bony reaction. *J. Surg. Oncol.*, 7:17–9.
255. Musshoff, K., Hartmann, C., Niklaus, B., and Rossner, R. (1976): The prognostic significance of first and second remission after first and second relapse radiotherapy in Hodgkin's disease. *Z. Krebsforsch.*, 85: 243–70.
256. Nakahara, C., and Tanaka, M. (1978): Acute lymphocytic leukemia with jaw tumor formation after a short period of spontaneous remission. *Rhinsho Ketsueki*, 19:1086–94.

257. Nasiell, K., Nasiell, M., Vaclavinkova, V., Roger, V., and Hjerpe, A. (1976): Follow-up studies of cytologically detected precancerous lesions (dysplasia) of the uterine cervix. In *Health Control in Detection of Cancer*, pp. 244–56, edited by H. Boström *et al.* Almqvist and Wiksell, Stockholm.
258. Nathanson (1976): Spontaneous regression of malignant melanoma: A review of the literature on incidence, clinical features, and possible mechanisms. *Natl. Cancer Inst. Monogr.*, 44:67–76.
259. Nehen, J. H. (1975): Spontaneous regression of retinoblastoma. *Acta Ophthalmol.*, 53:647–51.
260. Niethe, U. (1975): Spontaneous healing of a malignoma? (author's transl.) *Klin. Monatsbl. Augenheilkd.*, 166:137–8.
261. Nilsson, T., and Jönsson, G. (1975): Clinical results with estramustine phosphate (NSC-89199): A comparison of the intravenous and oral preparations. *Cancer Chemother. Rep.*, 59:229–32.
262. Nitta, K., and Umezawa, H. (1975): Presence of immunosuppressive agents with various activities in Ehrlich ascites fluid. *GANN*, 66:459–60.
263. Nomura, Y., Abe, Y., Yamagata, J., and Takenaka, K. (1976): Possible retention of the estrogen-binding capacity after endocrine ablation therapy in the rat and human breast cancer. *GANN*, 67:101–4.
264. Nose, K., and Sakakibara, K. (1975): Carcinogenesis in tissue culture 25: reduced tumorigenicity of alkaline phosphatase-constitutive variants from Chinese hamster ovary cells. *Jpn. J. Exp. Med.*, 45:326–34.
265. Nossal, G. J. (1976): Spontaneous regression of cancer: summary and profile for the future. *Natl. Cancer Inst. Monogr.*, 44:145–8.
266. Odintsova, T. A., and Bukhtoiarova, S. S. (1978): Case of disappearance of skin papillomas and gastric polyp after removal of corticosteroma. *Ter. Arkh.*, 50:131–2.
267. Old, L. J. (1976): Tumor necrosis factor. *Clin. Bull.*, 6:118–20.
268. Olenov, Iu. M. (1970): Comparison of carcinogenesis and differentiation processes in normal cells. *Vopr. Onkol.*, 16:94–101.
269. Oliver, R. T. (1975): The immunological aspects of malignant disease. *Practitioner*, 214:511–21.
270. Papermaster, B. W., Holtermann, O. A., Klein, E., Djerassi, I., Rosner, D., Dao, T., and Costanzi, J. J. (1976): Preliminary observations on tumor regressions induced by local administration of a lymphoid cell culture supernatant fraction in patients with cutaneous metastatic lesions. *Clin. Immunol. Immunopathol.*, 5:31–47.
271. Papermaster, B. W., Holtermann, O. A., Klein, E., Parmett, S., Dobkin, D., Laudico, R., and Djerassi, I. (1976): Lymphokine properties of a lymphoid cultured cell supernatant fraction active in promoting tumor regression. *Clin. Immunol. Immunopathol.*, 5:48–59.
272. Papp, S. (1975): Multiple (five-fold) synchronous and asynchronous primary malignant tumors with spontaneous regression. *Orv. Hetil.*, 116:27–9.
273. Parish, C. (1971): Complications of mediastinal neural tumours. *Thorax*, 26:392–5.
274. Parks, L. C., Baer, A. N., Pollack, M., and Williams, G. M. (1974): Alpha fetoprotein: An index of progression or regression of hepatoma, and a target for immunotherapy. *Ann. Surg.*, 180:599–605.
275. Pattillo, R. A. (1976): Tumor immunology. *Obstet. Gynecol.*, 48:374–80.
276. Pawlikowski, M., and Podkul, D. (1975): Unusual remission of an intracellar tumor in a 10-year-old boy. *Endokrynol. Pol.*, 26:645–60.
277. Pennelli, N., Chieco-Bianchi, L., Collavo, D., and Cecchetto, A. (1975): Histopathologic and ultrastructural study of tumors induced by murine sarcoma virus (msv) (author's transl.). *Tumori*, 61:–29–50. (Ita.)
278. Perk, K., Sims, H. (1975): Some pathogenic aspects of murine sarcoma virus (Moloney) in rats. *Lab. Anim.*, 9:9–17.
279. Perry, L. L., Wight, T. N., Collins, W. M., and Dunlop, W. R. (1978): Differentiation of progressive versus regressive Rous virus-induced avian sarcomas according to tumor and infiltrating lymphocyte fine structure. *Poult. Sci.*, 57:80–4.
280. Peters, T. G., Lewis, J. D. (1976): Treatment of breast cancer with danazol. *Surg. Forum*, 27:97–8.
281. Petersen, K. R., Pless, J., and Christensen, H. E. (1976): Cystic hygroma of the neck. *Ugeskr. Laeger*, 138:1818–1821.
282. Pettengill, O. S., and Sorenson, G. D. (1974): Effect of 5-bromodeoxyuridine on mouse neuroblastoma cells. *In Vitro*, 10:274–80.
283. Pfeiffer, C. J., Nagai, T., Fujimura, M., and Toba, T. (1979): Spontaneous regressive epithelioma in the Japanese newt, *Cynops pyrrhogaster*. *Cancer Res.*, 39 (Pt. 1):1904–10.
284. Pierce, G. B., and Fennell, R. H., Jr. (1976): Latent carcinoma and carcinoma *in situ*. *Natl. Cancer Inst. Monogr.*, 44:99–102.
285. Pinsard, N., De Micco, C., Garcin, M., and Bernard, R. (1975): Regressive neonatal neurofibromatosis and late nerve tumor. *Pediatrie*, 30:831–6.
286. Pitta, C., Bergen, R., and Littwin, S. (1979): Spontaneous regression of a choroidal hemangioma following pregnancy. *Ann. Ophthalmol.*, 11: 772–4.
287. Plata, F., and Sordat, B. (1977): Murine sarcoma virus (MSV)-induced tumors in mice. I. Distribution of MSV-immune cytolytic T lymphocytes *in vivo*. *Int. J. Cancer*, 19:205–11.
288. Polak, E. (1967): A few thoughts on the present state of treatment of malignant tumors. *Bratisl. Lek. Listy*, 47:666–72.
289. Popa, G., Dobrescu, G., and Hanganu, E. (1977): A peculiar lymph node

anticarcinoma reaction. *Folia Haematol.* 104:216–21.

290. Post, J. E., Noronha, F., and Richard, C. G. (1970): Canine mast cell leukemia. *Bibl. Haematol.,* 36:425–9.

291. Pratt, L. W. (1978): Unusually long survival of patients with cancer. *J. Main Med. Assoc.,* 69:33–4.

292. Puri, S., and Spencer, R. P. (1978): Hepatic scans in spontaneous regression of neuroblastoma. *Int. J. Nucl. Med. Biol.,* 5:129.

293. Rampen, F. (1979): Spontaneous regression of metastatic malignant melanoma. *Clin. Oncol.,* 5:91–2.

294. Ramselaar, C. G., and Van der Meer, J. B. (1979): Non-immunological regression of dimethylbenz[a]anthracene-induced experimental keratoacanthomas in the rabbit. *Dermatologica,* 158:142–51.

295. Ramseur, W. L., and Cooper, M. R. (1978): Asymptomatic liver cell adenomas. Another case of resolution after discontinuation of oral contraceptive use. *J.A.M.A.,* 239:1647–8.

296. Ratzkovski, E., and Walach, N. (1977): Spontaneous regression of tumors (editorial). *Harefuah,* 92:327–9.

297. Remy, R., Göbel, U., Goerz, G., and Müntefering, H. (1979): A case of spontaneous remission of congenital histiocytosis X. *Klin. Paediatr.,* 191:225–7.

298. Ridley, C. M. (1974): Giant halo naevus with spontaneous resolution. *Trans. St. Johns Hosp. Dermatol. Soc.,* 60:54–8.

299. Rieche, K. (1975): The present state of chemotherapy of gastric cancer (author's transl.). *Arch. Geschwulstforsch,* 45:566–71.

300. Roger, M., Feinstein-Soldat, M. C., Emmanuel, J., and Scholler, R. (1977): Biological criteria for the surveillance of hydatidiform moles and choriocarcinomas. *J. Gynecol. Obstet. Biol. Reprod.,* 6:207–25.

301. Rosen, T. (1978): Dystrophic xanthomatosis in mycosis fungoides. *Arch. Dermatol.,* 114:102–3.

302. Ruben, L. N. (1970): Lymphoreticular disorders and responses in Xenopus laevis the South African clawed toad. *Bibl. Haematol.,* 36:638–9.

303. Rudowski, W. (1978): Spontaneous neoplasm regression. *Nowotwory,* 28:161–71.

304. Rudowski, W. (1978): 2 cases of spontaneous neoplasm regression extending over many years. *Nowotwory,* 28:173–7.

305. Rufli, T., and Fricker, H. S. (1979): Congenital, self-heeling reticulohistiocytosis. *Z. Hautkr.,* 54:554–8.

306. Russell, S. W., Gillespie, G. Y., and McIntosh, A. T. (1977): Inflammatory cells in solid murine neoplasms. III. Cytotoxicity mediated in vitro by macrophages recovered from disaggregated regressing Moloney sarcomas. *J. Immunol.,* 118:1574–9.

307. Rygard, J., and Hansen, H. S. (1975): Use of chemotherapy—bleomycin. *Can. J. Otolaryngol.,* 4:21–5.

308. Saby, R., Chate, M., Hypousteguy, D., and Baste, J. C. (1978): Malignant melanoma of the small intestine arising from a regressive skin lesion. Survival after 4 years. *Chirurgie,* 104:913–20.

309. Saegesser, F., Besson, A., Kafai, F. (1970): Pulmonary coin lesions nd metastases. *Aktuel. Probl. Chir.,* 14:539–610.

310. Sagalowsky, A., and Donohue, J. (1979): Status of adjuvant therapy or renal cell cancer. *J. Ind. State Med. Assoc.,* 72:521–4.

311. Sakakibara, K., and Ooto, K. (1975): Metastasis formation of Yoshida sarcoma heterotransplanted in adult golden hamsters treated with anti-hamster thymocyte serum. *Cancer Res.,* 35:548–53.

312. Saman, K., and Tesinsky, H. V. (1979): Histiocytoma of the corneal limbus. *Cesk. Oftalmol.,* 35:89–92.

313. Sardemann, H., and Tygstrup, I. (1974): Prolonged obstructive jaundice and haemangiomatosis. Report of 2 cases. *Arch. Dis. Child,* 49:665–7.

314. Sato, S., and Sugimura, T. (1970): Decarcinogenesis and carcinostasis. *Saishin Igaku,* 25:996–1002.

315. Schirmer, H. K. (1976): Spontaneous regression of genitourinary cancers. *Natl. Cancer Inst. Monogr.,* 44:19.

316. Schneeweiss, U. (1975): Immunological aspects of chemotherapy or bronchial carcinomas. (author's transl.). *Z. Erkr. Atmungsorgane,* 142:116–26.

317. Schwartz, A. D. (1977): Neuroblastoma and Wilms' tumor. *Med. Clin. North. Am.,* 61:1053–71.

318. Schwartz, A. D., Dadash-Zadeh, M., Lee, H., and Swaney, J. J. (1974): Spontaneous regression of disseminated neuroblastoma. *J. Pediatr.,* 85:760–3.

319. Sedlacek, H. H., Meesmann, H., and Seiler, F. R. (1975): Regression of spontaneous mammary tumors in dogs after injection of neuraminidase-treated tumor cells. *Int. J. Cancer,* 15:409–16.

320. Seigler, H. F., and Fetter, B. F. (1977): Current management of melanoma. *Ann. Surg.,* 186:1–12.

321. Selenkow, H. A., and Karp, P. J. (1971): An approach to diagnosis and therapy of thyroid tumors, *Semin. Nucl. Med.,* 1:461–73.

322. Serpick, A. A. (1976): Spontaneous regression of colon carcinoma. *Natl. Cancer Inst. Monogr.,* 44:21.

323. Seto, A., Notake, K., Kawanishi, M., and Ito, Y. (1977): Development and regression of Shope papillomas induced in newborn domestic rabbits (39876). *Proc. Soc. Exp. Biol. Med.,* 156:64–7.

324. Shaport, V. S., and Likhtenshtein, A. V. (1978): Genetic nature of neoplastic transformation. *Tsitol. Genet.,* 12:73–84.

325. Shimoyama, M. (1971): Problems of tumor immunity and the possibility of immunotherapy in tumor. *Jap. J. Clin. Med.,* 29:1515–29.

326. Shnider, B. I., and Manalo, A. (1979): Paraneoplastic syndromes: unusual manifestations of malignant disease. *DM,* 25:1–6U.

327. Silber, S. J., Chen, C. Y., and Gould, F. (1975): Regression of metastases after nephrectomy for renal cell carcinoma. *Br. J. Urol.,* 47:259–61.

328. Simmons, R. L.; Rios, A. (1973): Neuraminidase treated cells and their role in cancer immunotherapy. *Birth Defects,* 9:223–8.

329. Sindelar, W. F. (1976): Regression of cancer following surgery. *Natl. Cancer Inst. Monogr.,* 44:81–4.

330. Sinha, D., and Dao, T. L. (1974): A direct mechanism of mammary carcinogenesis induced by 7, 12-dimethyl-benz[alpha]anthracene. *J. Natl. Cancer Inst.,* 53:841–6.

331. Slauson, D. O., Osburn, B. I., Shifrine, M., and Dungworth, D. L. (1975): Regression of feline sarcoma virus-induced sarcomas in dogs. I. Morphologic investigations. *J. Natl. Cancer Inst.,* 54:361–70.

332. Slauson, D. O., Osburn, B. I., Shifrine, M., and Dungworth, D. L. (1975): Regression of feline sarcoma virus-induced sarcomas in dogs. II. Immunologic investigations. *J. Natl. Cancer. Inst.,* 54:371–7.

333. Smith, R. T. (1968): Tumor-specific immune mechanisms. *N. Engl. J. Med.,* 278:1326–31.

334. Smith, R. T., and Bausher, J. C. (1972): Epstein-Barr virus infection in relation to infectious mononucleosis and Burkitt's lymphoma. *Annu. Rev. Med.,* 23:39–56.

335. Smoes-Charles, J. (1972): Papulous reticulosis with spontaneous resolution. *Arch. Belg. Dermatol.,* 29:213–5.

336. Sophocles, A. M., Jr., and Nadler, S. H. (1971): Immunologic aspects of cancer. *Surg. Gynecol. Obstet.,* 133:321–31.

337. Stansly, P. G. (1975): Is there another approach to cancer therapy? Workshop on suppression of the malignant phenotype. *Cancer Res.,* 35:1599–600.

338. Stecher, G., Bloemertz, H., and Pfitzer, P. (1976): Sarcoma 180: growth and regression. Comparative investigations using flow-through and scanning cytophotometers as well as histological, cytological and autoradiographic techniques (author's transl.). *Beitr. Pathol.,* 158:255–86.

339. Steffin, J. (1975): Immunological factors in the origin and development of neoplasms. I. *Nowotwory,* 25:123–33.

340. Steg, A., and Boccon-Gibod, L. (1973): From the image to the metastasis. Doubts and errors. *J. Urol. Nephrol.,* 79(Pt. 2):392–7.

341. Stenbäck, F. (1978): Tumor persistence and regression in skin carcinogenesis. An experimental study. *Z. Krebsforsch,* 91:249–59.

342. Stephens, F. O. (1974): Tumour immunology: A review of the present situation with particular reference to solid tumours and surgical implications. *Aust. N.Z. J. Surg.,* 44:321–9.

343. Stephenson, H. E., Jr. (1976): Spontaneous regression of cancer evaluated by computerized data. *Natl. Cancer Inst. Monogr.,* 44:43–7.

344. Storck, H., and Schwarz, K. (1967): Should evolutive hemangiomas be treated? *Schweiz. Med. Wochenshr.,* 97:469–77.

345. Stromberg, B. V., Weeks, P. M., and Wray, R. C., Jr. (1976): Treatment of cystic hygroma. *South Med. J.,* 69:1333–5.

346. Strong, L. C., and Matsunaga, H. (1977): Increased effect of a transmissible entity on the control of cancer in C3 H/St mice. *J. Surg. Oncol.,* 9:99–103.

347. Sturzaker, H. G., Berry, C. L., and McColl, I. (1977): Spontaneous resolution of a mesenteric fibromatosis. *J. R. Coll. Surg. Edinb.,* 22:395–9.

348. Stutman, O. (1975): Delayed tumour appearance and absence of regression in nude mice infected with murine sarcoma virus. *Nature,* 253:142–4.

349. Stutman, O. (1976): Age-dependent regression of M-MSV tumors in CBA/H mice: Requirement for a macrophage-adherent cell population. *Adv. Exp. Med. Biol.,* 73(B):371–8.

350. Svirnovskii, A. I. (1974): Interrelationship between regeneration and carcinogenesis. *Usp. Sovrem. Biol.,* 77:133–52.

351. Svirsky, S., Milbauer, B., Weisman, I., and Langer, L. (1957): Vascular tumor of the liver in a newborn. *Harefuah,* 88:272–4.

352. Takeda, T., and Sotooka, T. (1977): Spontaneous regression of neuroblastoma. *Hokkaido J. Med. Sci.,* 52:12–5.

353. Tarquini, A., Di Martino, L., and Caporelli, S. (1975): Treatment of penile neoplasms by means of loco-regional intra-arterial therapy. *Minerva Chir.,* 30:817–24.

354. Tchertkoff, V., and Hauser, A. D. (1979): Carcinoma of head of pancreas with spontaneous regression. *N.Y. State J. Med.,* 74:1814–7.

355. Techer (1975):

356. Terry, W. D. (1975): BCG in the treatment of human cancer. *CA,* 25:198–203.

357. Test, P., Gyles, N. R., and Patterson, L. T. (1976): The interaction between *Microbacterium bovis* (BCG) and genotype of chicken in increasing the percentage of regression of Rous sarcomas. *Poult. Sci.,* 55:779–85.

358. The T. H. (1972): Some recent developments in human tumour immunology. *Folia Med. Neerl.,* 15:279–90.

359. Thomas, L. (1976): Possible mechanisms in regression. *Natl. Cancer Inst. Monogr.,* 44:137–9.

360. Thomas, W. R., Aw, E. J., Papadimitriou, J. M., and Simons, P. J. (1974): Effect of tissue injury on tumorigenesis induced by murine sarcoma virus (Harvey). *J. Natl. Cancer Inst.,* 53:763–6.

361. Thormann, T. (1978): The treatment of capillary hemangiomas (authors transl). *Dermatol. Monatsschr., 164*:375–7.

362. Toth, F. D., Gomba, S., Vaczi, L., Kasa, M., and Jako, J. (1976): Immune response to Rauscher virus-induced leukemia in DBA mice. I. Role of cellular and humoral immunity in spontaneous regression. *Neoplasm, 23*:471–81.

363. Trepel, F. (1971): Tumor antigens and immune reactions against tumors. *Med. Klin., 66*:215–22.

364. Tresserra, L., Martinez-Mora, J., and Boix-Ochoa, J. (1977): Haemangiomas of the parotid gland in children. *J. Maxillofac. Surg., 5*:238–41.

365. Trnka, J. (1976): Spontaneous healing of histologically incompletely excised basaliomas (author's transl.). *Cesk. Dermatol., 51*:327–8.

366. Trnka, J. (1977): Spontaneous regression of basalioma portions treated by partial excision in stages. *Cesk. Dermatol., 52*:193–6.

367. Tsubura, E., Hirao, F., Fujisawa, T., Ogura, T., and Masaki, S. (1967): Tumor and infection. *Saishin Igaku, 22*:2281–90.

368. Tsukamoto, Y., Nishitani, H., Oshiumi, Y., and Okawa, T. (1977): Spontaneous disappearance of gastric polyps: Report of four cases. *AJR, 129*: 893–7.

369. Tulzer, H., and Ulm, R. (1976): A very large lutecoma gravidarum. *Zentralbl. Gynaekol., 98*:1659–63.

370. Tumours of the sympathetic nervous system (1975): Round-table conference (author's transl.) *Probl. Med. Wieku Rozwoj, 4*:175–202.

371. Vasilev, Iu. M. (1973): Nature and mechanisms of changes in cells during neoplastic evolution. *Arkh. Patol., 35*:3–13.

372. Verger, P., Guillard, J. M., Fontan, D., and Laigle, J. L. (1974): Multimodular hemangliomastosis of the liver. Favorable course in infancy. *Med. Chir. Dig., 3*:347–52.

373. Vinokurov, V. L. (1976): Dissemination of ovarian cancer. *Vogr. Onkol., 22*:106–16.

374. Vintergalter, S. F., and Levitskaia, N. A. (1975): Value of repeated lymphography in the diagnosis of lymphogranulomatosis and its recurrences. *Med. Radiol., 20*:57–9.

375. Wahren, B., and Edsmyr, F. (1974): Fetal proteins occurring in testicular teratomas. *Int. J. Cancer, 14*:207–14.

376. Wasko, R. (1976): Regression of pulmonary metastases from renal carcinoma. *Urology, 7*:299–301.

377. Watanabe, M. (1970): Experiences with complement ascitic tumor derived from a mouse with moloney sarcoma: Tumorigenic, antigenic and virologic properties (author's transl.). *Z. Immunitaetsforsch, 148*:151–61.

379. Weinert, C. R., Jr., McMaster, J. H., Ferguson, R. J. (1974): Immune response to sarcomas. A review. *Clin. Orthop., 102*:207–16.

380. Weinstock, C. (1977): Recent progress in cancer psychobiology and psychiatry. *J. Am. Soc. Psychosom. Dent. Med., 24*:4–14.

381. Weinstock, C. (1977): Notes on "spontaneous" regression of cancer. *J. Am. Soc. Psychosom. Dent. Med., 24*:106–10.

382. Weinstock, C. (1977): Spontaneous cancer regression (letter). *J. Am. Acad. Psychoanal., 5*:285–6.

383. Weiss, D. W. (1976): Neoplastic disease and tumor immunology from the perspective of host-parasite relationships. *Natl. Cancer Inst. Monogr., 44*:115–22.

384. Weissel, V. W., Garbsch, H., and Schmetz, E. (1974): Tumor regression in hypokalemia, *Acta Med. Austriaca, 2*:69–71.

385. Whitmore, W. F., Jr. (1973): Proceedings: The natural history of prostatic cancer. *Cancer, 32*:1104–12.

386. Wiernik, P. H. (1976): Spontaneous regression of hematologic cancers. *Natl. Cancer Inst. Monogr., 44*:35–8.

387. Witek, R., Zembala, M., and Machaj, A. (1978): Regression of gallbladder carcinoma in a 54-year-old female. *Wiad. Lek., 31*:259–61.

388. Wolter, J. R. (1976): Thrombosis of the central retinal artery in retinoblastoma. *J. Pediatr. Ophthalmol., 13*:99–102.

389. Wood, G. W. (1976): Suppression of Moloney sarcoma virus immunity following sensitization with attenuated virus. *Cancer Res., 36*:4552–7.

390. Woodruff, J. M. (1976): Pathology of malignant melanoma—Part II. *Clin. Bull., 6*:52–9.

391. Woodruff, M. (1971/72): Residual cancer. *Harvey Lect., 66*:161–76.

392. Woodruff, M. F., and Warner, N. L. (1977): Effect of *Corynebacterium parvum* on tumor growth in normal and athymic (nude) mice. *J. Natl. Cancer Inst., 58*:111–6.

393. Woods, J. E. (1975): The influence of immunologic responsiveness on head and neck cancer. Therapeutic implications. *Plast. Reconst. Surg., 56*:77–80.

394. Yamazaki, M., Ohkuma, S., and Mizuno, D. (1974): Humoral anti-Ehrlich carcinoma factor found in mice with tumor resistance acquired by intradermal lipopolysaccharide administration. *GANN, 65*:337–44.

395. Yoshikawa, Y., Yamanouchi, K., Takahashi, R., and Fujiwara, K. (1973): Histopathological observations of spontaneous regression of Rous sarcomas in Japanese quails. *Jpn. J. Med. Sci. Biol., 28*:189–200.

396. Zbytniewski, Z., and Kanclerz, A. (1978): Probable mechanisms of regression of malignant neoplasm. *Pol Tyg. Lek., 33*:865–8.

397. Ziegler, J. L. (1976): Spontaneous remission in Burkitt's lymphoma. *Natl. Cancer Inst. Monogr., 44*:61–5.

398. A clinical atlas of hemangiopathies. J. (1978): *J. Dermatol. Surg. Oncol., 4*:829–43.

399. Feasible surgical management of selected hemangiomas in emergencies, in progressive enlargement, and in termination requiring plastic reconstruction. (1978): *J. Dermatol. Surg. Oncol., 4*:859–61.

400. Immunity against cancer. (1974): Use of spontaneous tumors of domestic animals as models for research: 2. *Bull. W.H.O., 50*:549–58.

401. Intraoral, laryngeal, and pharyngeal hemangiomas. (1978): *J. Dermatol. Surg. Oncol., 4*:863.

402. The natural course of untreated, uncomplicated, cutaneous hemangiomas. (1978): *J. Dermatol. Surg. Oncol., 4*:851–3.

40

The Prevention of Metastases as the Central Problem of Future Cancer Therapy

Ernst Krokowski

Today, cancer therapy concerned with early cases is directed exclusively against the primary tumor. Its removal or destruction is the most important and speediest task of curative cancer treatment. This goal can be reached in most cases almost without any problem, thanks to the advanced state of narcosis, surgical, and radiological technology; nevertheless, a complete cure can be achieved only in a fraction of the clinically treated early cases. In addition, we are faced with the disappointing fact that, despite the advances in modern therapeutic methods, we have not succeeded during the past 25 years in improving significantly the quota of complete cures achieved for solid tumors, as related to equal tumor stages (27)! There have been intermittent reports of tremendous successes, but they could not be reproduced elsewhere. Thus, for the mammary cancer, for example, 5-year survival rates of 57% and more have been reported (39, 43), but in other hospitals, the 5-year survival rate amounted only to 25% (42). The explanation for these considerably divergent results was provided by the investigation of Benninghoff and Tsien (4). They investigated and analyzed the progress of the mammary cancer in a total of 25,879 patients in 15 different hospitals. The result was that the differences in the 5-year survival rates were due exclusively to the variations in the composition of the groups of patients. If the group of patients contains many early cases, then the results of the treatment appear favorable; if, however, the group contains more patients from a more progressed state, then the results of the treatment remain

exceedingly unsatisfactory. The success quota is therefore not determined by the type and extent of the treatment, but solely by the proportion of early cases present (Fig. 40.1). The statistics show further that the average 5-yr survival rate amounted to 44% which means that there has been no improvement in the results since 1937, that is, in 40 years (Fig. 40.2). Equivalent results were found by Enstrom and Austin (11) for lung and rectum carcinoma, as well as other tumors. Junghanns and Ott (20) found that the results for stomach cancer have changed only a little over the past 50 years! Recent investigations by Heilmann et al. (19) and Becker et al. (3) on the results of the radiological and surgical treatment of bronchial carcinoma showed that no improvement in the success quota occurred over the past 25 years when compared to the results obtained in 1954 (35). Von Elmendorff and Albsmeier (10) found on the basis of statistics covering 8000 cancer patients that an average of 90% of these patients died before they reached the 5-yr term. Oeser (36) agrees with these results, but he excludes the mastocarcinoma. It must be added that these statements refer to solid malignant tumors in adults, not to diseases of the systems or malignant diseases of the hematological and lymphatical system.

If we consider that for some types of tumors, recognizable small increases in the success rate could be explained by the fact that because of increased health education and improved diagnosis more patients come for early treatment than did before, then we must conclude that the improvements in radiological and surgical treat-

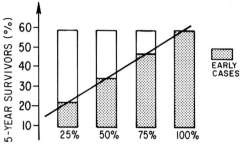

Figure 40.1. According to the cumulative statistics of Benninghoff and Tsien (4), the 5-year survival rate for mamma carcinoma depends exclusively on the percentage of early cases present in the total number of patients.

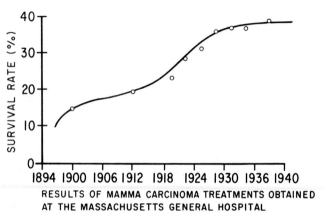

RESULTS OF MAMMA CARCINOMA TREATMENTS OBTAINED AT THE MASSACHUSETTS GENERAL HOSPITAL

Figure 40.2. Development of the average 5-year survival rate for mamma carcinoma from 1900 to 1940. Five-year survival rate: 1959, Benninghoff and Tsien, 44%; 1976, Krokowski, 42%.

ment techniques have not contributed significantly to an increase in the cure results. A confirmation to this conclusion is supplied by a study done in Berlin on the bladder carcinoma (Fig. 40.3). As far as the curative results are concerned, no differences could be found between the use of conventional x-ray, telecobalt, or betatron irradiation. Unquestioned, however, has been the progress in palliative treatment and in the reduction of the side effects of the treatment, but nothing could be changed in the decisive factor: the percentage cured. Based on this fact we must assume that our approach to cancer treatment is perhaps wrong, that it has to be analyzed and possibly revised.

This assumption seems to be supported by another observation which is generally known and has been described repeatedly (18, 40) but has not been further analyzed: In a number of tumor patients which had been classified clinically as early cases and when, after the surgical removal of the tumor, one had expected to have achieved complete cure, metastases appeared after a certain time which then decided the fate of these patients in an unfavorable way. The formation of metastases in the case of tumors which had originally been classified as early cases occurs preferably after a certain time interval (computed from the time of the surgery) as, for example, in mammary carcinoma patients, especially 1½ to 2½ years after surgery. The time required for the formation of metastases following treatment was determined for

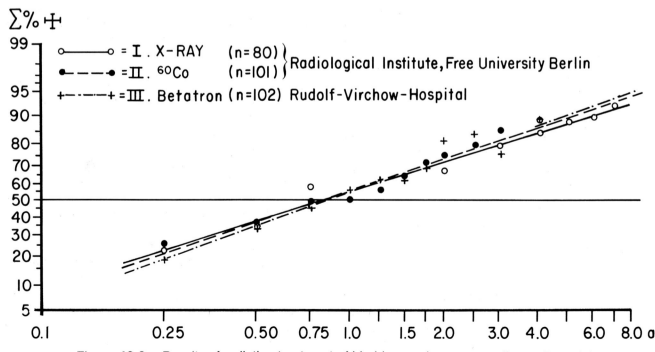

Figure 40.3. Results of radiation treatment of bladder carcinoma according to Boag (5).

other types of tumors and shown in Figure 40.4. The diagram shows that the time interval between the surgical removal of the primary tumor and the diagnosis of intrapulmonary metastases is shorter the faster the tumor grows. As a measure of growth velocity, we may use the time (t_D) required by the tumor to double; it is the time needed by the tumor to double in volume. We have recorded the appropriate ranges of the time required for the tumor to double for the seven types of tumor under investigation. A comparison of the two diagrams gives a correlation between the time interval described and the time required for the tumor to double for each type of tumor (Fig. 40.5). However, if the metastases of fast-growing tumors reach the "goal-line," i.e., if they reach the limit, where they can be rec-

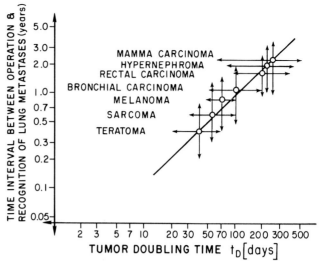

Figure 40.5. Relationship between the time intervals: Operation on lung metastases formation and tumor doubling time.

ognized earlier than the slow-growing and with respect to their growth velocity, then we must assume that the metastases "got their start" at the same time. However, what was the time, when the metastases "started" on their fateful course?

To elucidate this question, we have tried to analyze the course of growth of lung metastases. We determined the changes in diameter of a metastasis as a function of time through x-ray photographs of the thoracic organs (Fig. 40.6). Generally, this can be done much easier and more precisely with metastases than with primary tumors in the lung, because they are generally more delineated and round, they stand out well against the air-filled lung, and grow faster than their original tumors—thus, they are less subject to interfering influences. Error considerations were established for such measurements of lung metastases and the radiological determination of their changes in size as a function of time by Welin *et al.*, Wolff *et al.*, and Keller and Kallert (21, 47, 48). The results of these investigations can be summarized as follows.

The limit where lung metastases can be recognized lies, generally, at a diameter of 8–10 mm (under favorable conditions and at retrospective observation, at 4–5 mm).

The error range for the individual measurements of the metastatic diameters, which is a function of the deviations from the round form, of the blur at the edges, of the quality of the x-ray picture, and of the precision of the measurement itself, is, according to Wolff (48), at 11.1% in the case of small tumors and 3% for larger

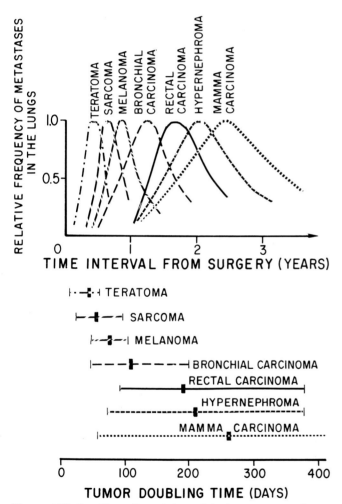

Figure 40.4. *Top*, time interval between operation and diagnosis of lung metastases for seven different types of tumors. *Bottom*, tumor doubling time for the same types of tumor.*

---

* Measured teratomas indicated in Figures 40.4, 40.5, 40.10, 40.14, 40.19, and 40.24, as well as in Tables 40.1 and 40.2 were testicular teratomas.

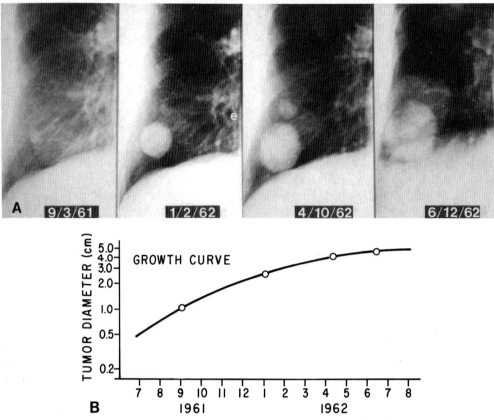

Figure 40.6. *A* and *B*, determination of the growth curves for lung metastases.

ones. The relative standard error for a determination of the time required for a tumor to double amounts to from 4 to 10% according to Wolff *et al.* (48), from 6 to 11% according to Brenner *et al.* (6). Based on this, we can derive the following guidelines for the analysis described: The differences for the evaluation should amount to at least 3 mm during the observation period. Further, observation times of more than two volume-doubling periods should be available, while changes in larger circular foci can be evaluated within shorter time spans than in smaller ones.

Consideration of these data permits us to determine growth progress and tumor doubling times with sufficient exactness over long observation periods. However, it is more difficult to extrapolate the growth curves measured to the prehospital period. In order to show the difficulties as well as the possibilities of such an extrapolation of the measured curves, we went back to a study by Welin *et al.* (47) on that aspect, which we then continued. Welin studied the growth of a tumor while it was subject to an error in the determination of the diameter of 2 mm. He then attempted to show the changes in size as a function of time graphically. It became apparent that the observed range of tumor

growth can be represented by various curves. This example demonstrates that an extrapolation of the growth curves to the preclinical phase is possible only under two conditions if satisfactory reliability is to be achieved: For singular cases, very long periods of metastatic growth have to be observed to permit the interpretation of the individual observation, and very many growth progresses have to be analyzed to permit a recognition of the basic progress of growth.

We tried to fulfill these requirements by investigating 2893 metastatic growth progresses associated with 568 primary tumors of various types and localizations. The key can be found in Table 40.1. An extrapolation to the start of the growth curve requires that two conditions be observed which are known from animal experiments: the so-called critical tumor cell number and the implantation period.

In animal tests, the transmitting of a single tumor cell is generally not enough to start injection tumors. This is possible only in exceptional cases, such as certain inbred animal strains and selected types of tumors. Generally, several thousand or million tumor cells are required to initiate tumor growth. The initiation rate increases with the number of injected cells. We

Table 40.1
Metastatic Growth Progress Associated with 568 Primary Tumors

Type of tumor	No. of Patients	No. of Metastases Measured
Mamma carcinoma	191	955
Hypernephroma	112	238
Sarcoma	92	736
Seminoma and teratoma	78	498
Melanoma	59	421
Bronchial carcinoma	28	31
Rectal carcinoma	8	14

have designated the number of tumor cells required to initiate an injected tumor or a metastasis as the critical cell number (Z_c), its volume as the critical volume (V_c), and the corresponding diameter as critical diameter (D_c). The magnitude of these critical values depends on the type of tumor, *i.e.*, on its capabilities of being transplanted and the defensive strength of the place of settlement. The variations in the defensive strengths of the various organs of the host were demonstrated by Schmähl's experiment (41) (Fig. 40.7). Rats were given an intravenous injection of tumor cells. One hr later, tumor cells could be found in the blood, the spleen, the liver, the kidneys, and the lungs. Two hr after the tumor cell injection, they still could be found everywhere, except in the spleen. A day later, the tumor cells had disappeared from the blood, the liver, and the kidneys; they apparently had been killed off, and only in the lung could the existence of living tumor cells be demonstrated—the same was true after 10 days—and these are the ones which grew into lung metastases. This animal experiment shows very clearly that the defensive strength in the individual organs shows very strong differences and that it establishes in this way a definite localization pattern for metastases development for a definite type of tumor. The localization distribution of the metastases was investigated extensively by Walther (46) and Schmähl (41). The experiment shows, further, that the growth into a metastasis does not begin immediately after the injection but after a time delay. The time period from implantation to growth is called the implantation period. It is the time required by the displaced tumor cells to overcome the local defense. Quite frequently, the number of tumor cells decreases so far during this implantation period that this tumor cell population will gradually perish after a few cell divisions. In the other cases, following an initial cell reduction,

the tumor cells will begin to multiply; they have overcome the defense of the host and start to grow to a metastasis. If in the animal experiment the number of injected tumor cells is increased, then the implantation period is shortened, and growth starts quickly because the local tissue defense is quickly overcome by the relatively high number of tumor cells. It is during this labile phase of the implantation period that the decision is made as to whether the tumor cells or the defensive power of the organs is going to win, whether the patient will recover, or whether his fate will be determined by the metastases. Since the duration of the implantation period is a function of the interaction between the deposited tumor cell embolus and the defensive power of the place of settlement, it becomes apparent that a relationship can be established between implantation time and the tumor doubling period, despite the very wide scatter range.

Taking into account the critical tumor cell number and implantation time, the measured growth curves were extrapolated back to their point of origin. An example is shown in Figure 40.8. Figure 40.8*A* shows the growth curves measured, Figure 40.8*B* the extrapolation, and Figure 40.8*C* the transformation into a double logarithmic matrix. In the second example (Fig. 40.9) one can already recognize in the representation of the growth curves two lung metastases which were already present at the time when the diagnosis was made, but which could not yet be demonstrated clinically, as well as a second metastatic attack which was released later. Figure 40.10*A*–*F* shows the metastases formation in the lungs for several patients for a particular tumor at a particular time as a function of the observation period. To guarantee greater clarity,

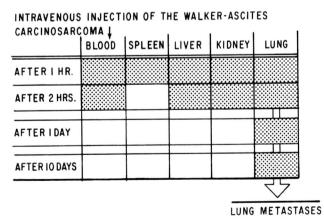

Figure 40.7. Animal experiments by Schmähl (41) disclosing the reactions of different organs to injected tumor cells.

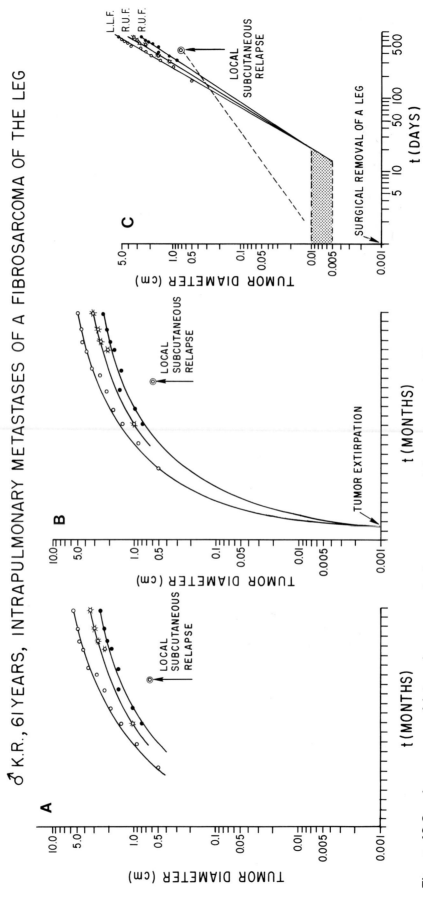

Figure 40.8. *A*, progress of intrapulmonary metastases measured from x-rays of a fibrosarcoma of the leg in a 61-year-old patient; *Inset (A)*, mathematical formula; *B*, extrapolation of the measured curves; *C*, transposition of the measured extrapolated curve into a double-logarithmic matrix.

$$\boxed{D = ct^2 \ln(bt) + D_K}$$

with $D_K = 0.005 \text{ cm}$

$$\ln b = \frac{\begin{vmatrix} t_1^2 \ln t_1 & t_2^2 \ln t_2 \\ D_1 & D_2 \end{vmatrix}}{\begin{vmatrix} D_1 & D_2 \\ t_1^2 & t_2^2 \end{vmatrix}} = \frac{D_2 t_1^2 \ln t_1 - D_1 t_2^2 \ln t_2}{D_1 t_2^2 - D_2 t_1^2}$$

$$c = \frac{D_1}{t_1^2(\ln b - \ln t_1)} = \frac{D_1}{t_1^2\left(\frac{D_2 t_1^2 \ln t_1 - D_1 t_2^2 \ln t_2}{D_1 t_2^2 - D_2 t_1^2} + \ln t_1\right)}$$

$$\boxed{D = \frac{D_1}{t_1^2(\ln b + \ln t_1)} \cdot t^2 \left[\left(\frac{D_2 t_1^2 \ln t_1 - D_1 t_2^2 \ln t_2}{D_1 t_2^2 - D_2 t_1^2}\right) + \ln t\right] + D_K}$$

$$c = f(b)$$

we have shown in these graphs only a portion of the metastatic growth processes investigated. The next step, then, was to develop a growth formula for the growth curves.

The starting point for devising a formula for metastatic growth is the fact that isolated tumor cells, which are not subject to being influenced by a host, grow exponentially, *i.e.*, they double at a constant rate. On the other hand, for a tumor growing in an organism, a slowing down of the tumor growth rate could be observed as time went on. Thus, as the tumor ages, the doubling time increases. Alexander (1) found that the isolated cells of a tumor, which show a doubling time of 60 days in the organism, in the isolated state had a doubling time of only 1 day. The exponential growth of isolated tumor cells which can be described by an e-function thus is interfered with by a host. This interference factor changes the original exponential growth formula into a new growth equation.

Uninterfered growth formula
$$D = c \cdot e^{bt}$$

Interfered growth formula
$$D = c \cdot e^{bt} \cdot a \ln(t + 1)$$

Approximation
$$D = c \cdot t^2 \cdot \ln(bt)$$

In addition, the analysis of the approximately 3000 growth curves of lung metastases produced the following.

First Fact

Metastases grow faster than their prime tumors. This statement holds true even for late metastases, the appearance of which is being explained by two different theses. One reduces late metastases to "sleeping tumor cells" which start their growth only after many years. Oeser (36) on the other hand accepted the theory of Collins *et al.* (7) of the consistency of the tumor doubling time and explains that for large tumor doubling periods, that is, for very slow growth, the assumption of "sleeping tumor cells" is superfluous because the metastases transgress the diagnostic threshold only many years after their coming into existence. Through our own observations we could disprove Oeser's theory. It became apparent, that even late metastases grow with their own tumor-specific speed and thus faster than their prime tumors, but that they start their growth only after many years. This confirms the assumption of "sleeping tumor cells." For the first time we succeeded with the growth equation developed by us to give a formal explanation for the preferred occurrence of late metastases at specific types of tumors and also for the "resting time interval" and its duration (28).

Second Fact

Metastases originate only from prime tumors, generally in one or only a few attacks. That metastases do not come from metastases can be shown also statistically. Even if a prime tumor produces only two metastases, which would then scatter again, then, after 7–8 tumor doubling times, we could expect at least several hundred metastases. However, Denoix (8) found only 15–25 metastases on the average in a tumor carrier who had died.

Third Fact

Metastases in the lymph node have to be evaluated differently from a biological aspect than metastases of the organs. This statement is supported by the following arguments.

In the cases we investigated, there was not a single indication that pulmonary metastases have started from lymph node metastases.

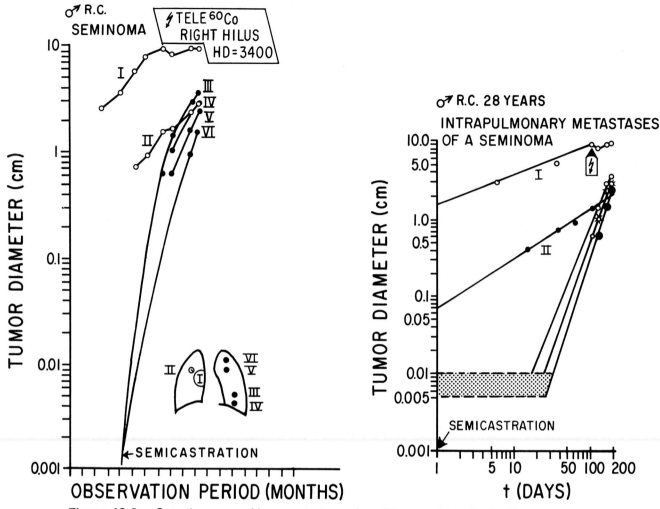

Figure 40.9. Growth curves of lung metastases in a 28-year-old patient with seminoma.

Animal experiments have shown that tumor cells which have penetrated into lymph nodes can be destroyed. This should also be the case in man.

Final cures are possible despite the presence and the remaining of so-called lymph node metastases.

Fourth Fact

The extrapolation of the growth curve shows that the date of origin of the metastases in very many cases coincides with the time of the first treatment. This then gives rise to the serious question: Does tumor therapy perhaps produce metastases itself under certain conditions? Are metastases caused by diagnostic (biopsy, exploratory excision) or therapeutic (tumor extirpation, radical operation) measures? Does our cancer therapy lead to cure in certain cases, but to

metastases formation and thus worsening of the total course of the disease in others? Do we have a cancer therapy with two faces? Do we have a new Semmelweis phenomenon?

However, before we discuss these questions and their consequences, let us investigate whether further observations, clues, and experiments will support the correctness of the growth curves shown and document the interpretation of provoked metastases formation.

Proofs for the Growth Curves Developed by the Author

Numerous growth progresses of animal tumors were measured and recorded on a double-logarithmic graph paper (Fig. 40.11). In principle, this resulted in the same type of curve as those based on our measurements of pulmonary metastases from cancer patients.

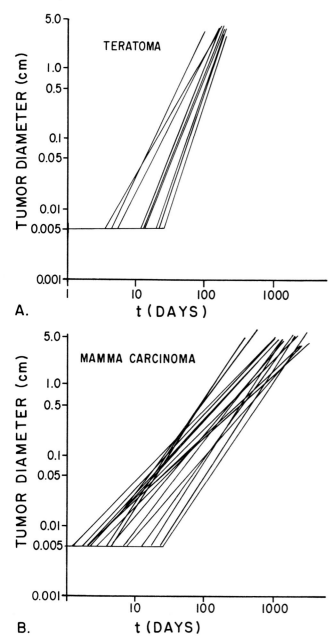

Figure 40.10. Growth curves of lung metastases of various patients. *A*, primary tumor, teratoma; *B*, primary tumor, mamma carcinoma.

Various authors described growth processes (but for primary tumors) which can be represented without constraint and even much better by our growth equations. We shall support this statement with two examples.

Spratt *et al.* (44) followed the growth of an adenocarcinoma in the transverse colon of a 67-year-old patient through nine investigations of the intestine over a period of 7½ years. During this time span, the (calculated) tumor volume increased from 232 mm³ to 6750 mm³. If we

assume a constant tumor doubling time of 636.5 days, then we can compute that 56.9 years have elapsed since the tumor came into being. Since the patient was only 67 years old, however, such a tumor duration seems unrealistic. However, if we use the growth formula that we developed, then the total tumor duration time would amount to only 14 years (Fig. 40.12).

The growth of an untreated, undifferentiated bronchial carcinoma was observed by Garland *et al.* (13) over a period of 13 years in a 68-year-old patient. If we assume a constant tumor doubling time, then the preclinical tumor duration can be calculated as 46 years. Using our growth equation, the total tumor duration amounts to 22 years—this gives a much better interpretation to the course of the disease (Fig. 40.13).

In numerous cases, the computed tumor time exceeds the total life-span of the patient; this makes the validity of the assumption of a constant tumor doubling time most unlikely.

The time interval (t′) between surgery and the diagnosable (about 2 cm large) lung metastases as computed from the growth equation corresponds well with the actually observed values t″ (Fig. 40.14).

Cytokinetic results agree with the growth curves. Mendelsohn (32) found a growth fraction of 0.66 through experiments. Cell multiplication having such a growth fraction produces a growth curve of the type we described.

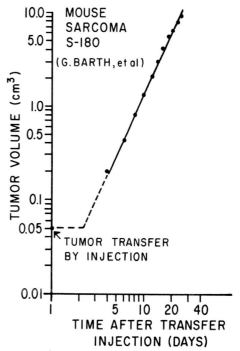

Figure 40.11. Example of growth curves for animal tumors. Growth of a mouse sarcoma S 180 (2).

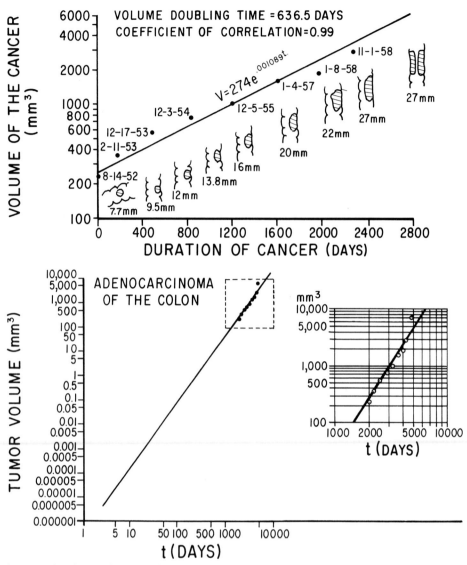

Figure 40.12. *A*, growth of an adenocarcinoma of the colon transversum observed by Spratt *et al.* (44) over a period of 7½ yr. *B*, interpretation of the measurements using our growth dynamic concept.

Facts Confirming the Time of Metastases Formation

Formation of metastases due to surgery has been known from animal experiments for a long time. Druckrey and coworkers (9) reported on their experiments with animals in 1939: The experiments show "that surgical removal of a tumor cannot be regarded as a local operation, but that it has decisive general effects. One result can be cure with total resistance, the other the feared worsening, the creation of metastases." They continue: "Extirpation of the regional glands favored the generalized dispersion in our experiments." Another quotation from the same publication states: "After the operation most animals contracted metastases; under these circumstances they perished sooner than the animals which had not been operated on their prime tumors." Because of the importance of these statements, let us quote another: "In rats with benzopyrene-tumors the extirpation of the primary tumor was very frequently followed by the extensive formation of metastases; those rats who had not been operated on the other hand never developed metastases." Such a behavior, the surgically released metastases formation, does not appear in all animal species and races and certainly not for all types of tumors but, because of the research results available today concerning tumors in man, the results obtained by Druckrey seem to have special importance. However, it is apparent that no consequences

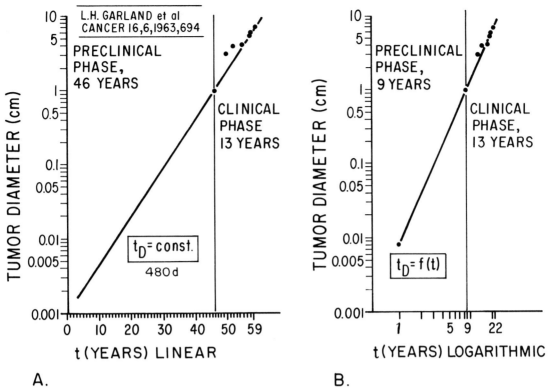

Figure 40.13. Observation of the growth of an undifferentiated bronchial carcinoma in a 68-year-old patient over a period of 13 years (13). *Left*, interpretation based on the assumption of a constant tumor doubling time of 480 days (13). *Right*, interpretation based on the growth dynamic concept developed by the author.

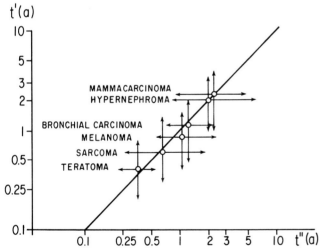

Figure 40.14. Relationship between the time intervals: operation on lung metastases formation t', calculated from the growth formula and the time interval, t'', actually observed.

were drawn for the clinical treatment of cancer from the results of animal studies published in 1939. However, since the quantitative evaluation of metastatic growth has demonstrated the high probability of metastases provocation through surgery even in man, we can no longer avoid the

appropriate therapeutic consequences. The research results presented by this author have demonstrated that the results obtained in animals by Druckrey and coworkers almost four decades ago do have validity also for man.

Almost in harmony with the quota from Druckrey's publication is the clinical observation of Gregl (17) that old women with untreated breast cancer will live longer than women of the same age who had undergone palliative or radical therapy; this prompted his coworker Müller (33) to conclude that old women with breast cancer should not be subjected to therapy.

A very impressive confirmation of metastases formation caused by surgery was provided by the animal experiments of Fisher and Fisher (12): If cancer cells were injected into rats intraperitoneally, tumor growth could not be detected even after a long period of time. However, if these animals were operated 3 months after the injection, then tumors appeared in all animals within a few weeks (Fig. 40.15). These results were interpreted by the authors to mean that the tumor cells remain in a dormant state after the injection, but that they do not lose their ability to grow. It is the surgical trauma and the subsequent metabolic changes which start growth and thus the origin of tumors.

An additional confirmation of the release of metastases through surgery is provided by the following observation (Fig. 40.16). A 67-year-old patient had a tumor at the right shoulder joint which could be removed only incompletely surgically. The histological tests showed it to be a reticuloendothelial sarcoma. Three hundred seventy days after the operation, a lung metastasis having a diameter of about 3 mm was observed. Its growth was followed for more than a year until it reached 5.3 cm. Ninety days after the

first operation, a local recurrence appeared which also caused a lung metastasis which was noticed 300 days after the second operation. Its diameter was 1.5 cm, and it was observed for about 200 days. During this period its diameter increased to 2.8 cm. One hundred thirty-five days after the first treatment, a third operation became necessary, again because of a local recurrence. This third operation also caused a lung metastasis which, 310 days after the third operation, had a diameter of 1 cm; after 150 days, the diameter had increased to 1.6 cm. Local recurrence of this unfavorably located tumor forced a fourth and a fifth local operation, 245 and 345 days after the first operation respectively. Each operation, was responsible for the formation of a new metastasis in the lung. Two hundred fifty days after both the fourth and fifth operation, the corresponding lung metastases had diameters of 1.5 and 2.0 cm, respectively. All during this observation time up to the time of the patient's death, the various lung metastases, their origin, and development could be observed through thorax radiography. This impressive series shows that each of the five operations at the prime tumor caused a lung metastasis and that all metastases had the same growth velocity when it was related to the respective surgically caused release time.

In order to disprove the idea of metastasis

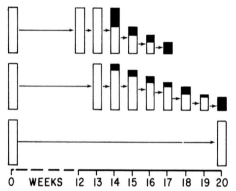

Figure 40.15. Experiments of Fisher and Fisher (12) show that following intraportal injection of 50 tumor cells into Sprague-Dawley rats, tumors (*closed bars*) will appear only if a test operation has preceded the injection. Without the operation all animals survive (*lower open bar*).

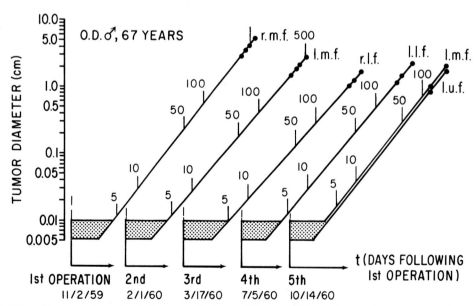

Figure 40.16. Observed metastatic growth in a 67-year-old patient with a retothelial sarcoma at the right shoulder joint. The operation of the prime tumor and each of its local relapses caused the foundation of a pulmonary metastasis. Related to the point of metastases release, every one of the daughter tumors has the same growth velocity and approximately the same implantation time.

formation due to surgery, Oeser (37) introduced the case of a 65-year-old patient with bladder cancer (Fig. 40.17). However, this case proves especially well my thesis of provoked metastasis formation. The diagnosis of the bladder cancer was secured by way of a test excision on June 6, 1961; but if we consider the implantation period, that is the date to which the growth curve is extrapolated.

The facts just cited prove and reinforce the statement that under certain conditions manipulation at the tumor will provoke the formation of metastases. One biological explanation may be that the tumor cells which are constantly circulating in the blood and which can be proven to exist in a large percentage of patients, without permitting a prognostic statement, increase suddenly during tumor manipulation. However, an increase in the number of circulating tumor cells increases the possibility of metastatic settlement. In some cases, however, we can observe the beginning of metastases formation through an operation not related to and removed from a tumor. This shows that it was not an increased tumor cell release from the primary tumor, but a reduction in defensive power which led to metastases formation.

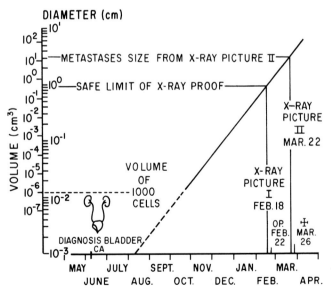

Figure 40.17. Course of a lung metastases formation due to bladder carcinoma is being used by Oeser (37) as "proof" against the concept of metastasis formation provoked by surgery. Exact evaluation of anamnesis shows, however, that it was not the bladder operation itself but the test excision made to aid in the diagnosis that initiated metastases formation. Thus, this example becomes a proof for the theory advanced here.

Wood *et al.* (50, 51) and Gastpar (14–16) have demonstrated how tumor cells aggregated to thrombocytes or in the company of leukocytes cling to the wall of vessels, how they penetrate these by following the blood cells, how they get into lymphatic clefts and are carried on, or how they settle at the point of wall penetration to multiply; however, unexplained in this connection, at least until now, is the critical tumor cell number. We do not know yet whether at the place where the tumor cell has penetrated the capillary wall other tumor cells from the circulating blood assemble until the critical number is reached, or whether in individual cases tumor cell emboli of about 500–1000 tumor cells are released from the primary tumor to settle at a place of lower resistance. It is certain, however, that the settling of tumor cells and their growth into metastases depend on the prime tumor and on the general defensive condition of the host. In addition to the operation as the release factor, it requires predisposing factors before a tumor cell resettlement or release can form a metastasis. These factors are inherent first in the tumor itself and then in the tumor carrier. Contributing partial factors of the prime tumor are its histological structure and its rate of growth, but especially its size and capability of being transplanted. Important partial factors inherent in the tumor carrier are his general and local defensive condition, as reported in detail by Schmähl (41). The general defensive effort depends on age, the seasonal and bioclimatologic fluctuations, blood viscosity, local blood circulation rate, and other factors. On the local resistance, we have reported above in connection with the tumor cell transmission experiment of Schmähl. The relationship between stickiness and aggressivity of the tumor cells on the one hand and the defensive power of the host on the other determines the magnitude of the critical cell number for the development of a metastasis. Therefore, the value of the critical cell number fluctuates as a function of the type of tumor and the organ under attack. The fact that the size of the primary tumor is of special importance for the possibility of the appearance of metastases can be derived from simple mathematical considerations. If we consider that metastases in general originate through a single push and that according to Denoix (8) on the average 20 metastases were present in cancer patients who had died but that for the development of a single metastasis 500–1000 tumor cells were required (9), then we arrive at a total number of tumor cells between 10,000 and 20,000. This quantity of cells corresponds to a volume of about 1 mm^3, which was released at a certain point in time from the primary tumor. It can be seen quite readily that such a relatively high scatter volume can be released from a primary tumor easier, the larger its own volume. This explains why after an operation metastases originate earlier, the larger the primary tumor (Fig. 40.18), and also why metastases are not released after every operation. However, since there is no possibility for testing in advance the influence of the predisposing or realizing factors on metastasis formation, we have to proceed in practice as if the danger of provoked metastases formation due to an operation were present in each case.

Basically, we have to differentiate between a metastasis originating spontaneously, that is, from unknown causes, and that provoked by surgery (25, 26). To avoid the latter should be the prime therapeutic goal. This now leads us to the question of the percentage of spontaneous and provoked metastases. We counted the quantitatively evaluated metastatic cases from the total of our patients. This gave us the percentage, the growth curves of which could be extrapolated back to the date of the first treatment, that is, to metastases which were already present at that time in a preclinical phase but could not yet be diagnosed. This relationship varies according to the type of tumor (Table 40.2). This means that

the percentage of metastases provoked by surgery varies between 30 and 90% (Fig. 40.19).

We now have to investigate whether we can explain these large differences in the relative frequency of provoked metastases. Two factors are of decisive importance: the average size of the primary tumor at the time of the diagnosis and the transplantability (the readiness to form metastases) of the individual tumors. We shall investigate the influence of these two factors in greater detail for three types of tumor: the bronchial carcinoma, the mamma carcinoma, and the hypernephroid carcinoma. The average size of the tumors at the time of diagnosis was a diameter of 2.5 cm for both the bronchial and the mamma carcinoma and at 8- and 10-cm diameter, respectively, for hypernephroma. The willingness to form metastases in the three types of carcinoma mentioned is shown in Figure 40.20. It can be seen that the bronchial carcinoma, on the average, is about the same size as the mamma carcinoma at the time of diagnosis, but because of their ability to form metastases, al-

Table 40.2
Differentiation Rates of Spontaneous versus Provoked Metastases

	Spontaneous Metastases (%)	Provoked Metastases (%)
Hypernephroma	70	30
Mamma carcinoma	46	54
Bronchial carcinoma	41	59
Seminoma and teratoma	18	82
Sarcoma	12	88

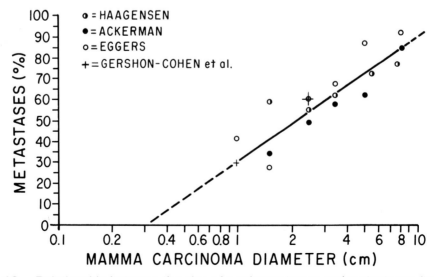

Figure 40.18. Relationship between the size of a primary tumor and metastases frequency (18).

most all bronchial carcinomas have at that point already begun to form metastases, a fact which reduces the chances for a cure to only a few percent. Despite the same size, the mamma carcinoma has a lower rate of metastases formation and, consequently, a higher success rate for therapy. The hypernephroma, despite its large size at the point of diagnosis, has a low tendency towards metastases formation so that cures can be obtained despite the size of the diagnosed

hypernephroma.

It becomes quite clear from what we have first said that the ability to form metastases depends on a number of factors. Consequently, the therapeutic fulcrum has to be applied to these factors.

The New Concept of Cancer Therapy

The importance of earlier cancer diagnosis and therefore of cancer prophylaxis becomes apparent, if we consider the fundamental role played by the size of the primary tumor in the formation of metastases. However, it doesn't make much sense to try to expand cancer prophylaxis examinations universally to all types of cancer. Rather, cancer prophylaxis examinations should be used only in a differentiated way, directed at certain central points. Cancer prophylaxis should be directed in a concentrated way at those types of tumors which belong to the most frequently occurring cancer diseases for which, basically, an early diagnosis can be made and therapy promises some kind of cure, and the examination process is financially and technically feasible. The importance of an early diagnosis in this sense can be demonstrated most clearly in a mamma carcinoma (Fig. 40.21). The sooner the tumor is diagnosed, that is, the smaller its diameter, the greater is the chance

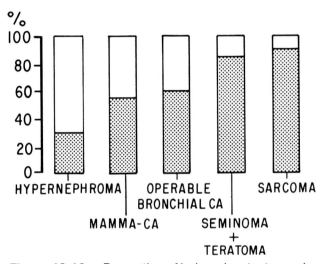

Figure 40.19. Proportion of induced metastases due to provoked intervention as a function of the total number of lung metastases diagnosed, corresponding to equal tumor stages.

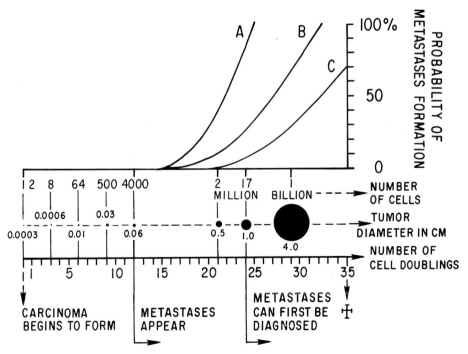

Figure 40.20. Schematic representation of the course of a tumor in the various stages of the preclinical and clinical phase with tumor growth (cell number, tumor diameter, number of doublings) and the tendency towards formation of metastases for bronchial carcinoma (*A*), mamma carcinoma (*B*), and hypernephroid carcinoma (*C*).

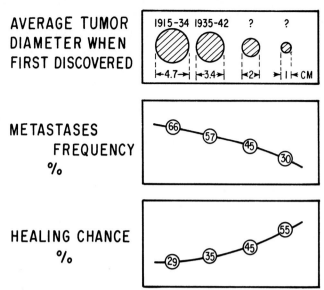

Figure 40.21. Relationship between the size of the primary tumor, the tendency towards metastases formation, and chance for cure for the mamma carcinoma.

for cure. In other words: the rate of metastases formation and cure are inversely proportional (24). These examples show quite impressively how important cancer prophylaxis and early diagnosis are, especially for breast cancer.

Furthermore, during the diagnosis of tumors one should see to it that all those diagnostic possibilities have been taken into consideration which permit a diagnosis without an alteration of the tumor itself. Only if these means do not lead to a reliable, therapy-deciding diagnosis should one use diagnostic methods like test excision or tumor puncture, which touch the tumor itself. However, then the process should be the same as for an operation itself.

From the investigations presented here, we can derive the following conclusions as far as tumor therapy is concerned: The removal of the primary tumor still remains a primary goal, firstly to eliminate the space demands, secondly to eliminate the primary tumor as a source of metastases, and finally to influence the immunity defense in a positive way. However, the operation should not be done as radically as possible but as radically as necessary. The spatial expansion of the area to be operated on has not had any favorable influence on the final recovery rate, and an extension of the remission period can be achieved in many cases by different, less incisive methods. As something fundamentally new in the therapy concept, we recommend the insertion of a metastasis prophylaxis before each diagnostic or therapeutic attack of the tumor. Up to now, we have a choice

of four possibilities, the effectiveness of which has to be established through further research:

1. Immunotherapy of tumors
2. Use of anticoagulants or fibrinolytica or aggregation retardants
3. Use of the so-called radiogenic protection effect
4. Application of special drugs

Let us elaborate on these points.

As far as immunotherapy of the cancer patient is concerned, we must consider today the non-specific immunotherapy using stimulants, bacillus Calmette-Guerin, or levamisol, or possibly the specific active immunotherapy with tumor vaccines or the adoptive immunotherapy.

The facility of tumor cells to attach at the endothel of a capillary depends on two factors: (a) *the tendency of tumor cells to attach themselves, or the cancer cell stickiness.* The capability of cancer cells to adhere is a tumor-specific, determined, physicochemical property of the cell surface, which is conditioned essentially through thromboplastic activities which are cell-specific and preformed in the tumor tissue. Tumor cells with a high thromboplastic activity have a correspondingly high stickiness (which correlates with the adhesive tendency at the capillary endothelium) and a transplantation rate and metastases formation frequency which are directly proportional (22, 23). (b) *The coagulation conditions of the blood and the behavior of the thrombocytes* are the other factors which influence the process of tumor adhesion at the capillary endothelium. Animal experiments and *in vivo* microscopical experiments have proved that an anticoagulation therapy will reduce the adhesive tendency of the tumor cells and that fibrinolytica will bring about a release of the tumor cell clots adhering to the capillary walls and recirculate them. In this, the aggregation inhibitors are of special interest. In animal experiments, this type of treatment caused a significant reduction in the rate of metastasis formation.

In 1966, the author showed, through a number of animal experiments (29–31), that whole body irradiation, as expected, will cause a more or less distinct intensity of the irradiation effect if the second irradiation was applied a short time after the first one with a corresponding delay in the time creating a protective effect against the second irradiation (Fig. 40.22). This radiologically induced increase in tolerance can be so pronounced that a second lethal dosis can be tolerated without pronounced damage (31). It can be shown that this protective effect exists

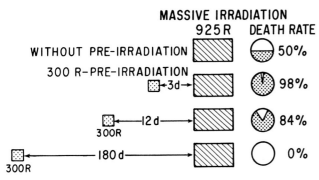

Figure 40.22. Time interval between pre- and massive irradiation periods; principle of application and result of the radiogenic protective effect (29–31). *Br.-Ca*, bronchial carcinoma.

also in large animals, such as goats, pigs, and sheep (38). Further, it was found that the protective effect can be transmitted by blood and that it does not relate only to a secondary irradiation following whole body irradiation, but that it includes many biological effects, such as the tumor initiation rate as shown first by Stutz (45). After whole body or sectional irradiation, the tumor initiation rate decreases after the injection of tumor cells, if one permits a time interval of at least 4 wk to pass following irradiation. We have applied this principle to tumor therapy. We used a sectional irradiation of 150–250 rads from the gammatron 4 wk prior to tumor removal as metastasis prophylaxis in tumor patients. The results are shown in Fig. 40.23. The number of patients treated by this ray is still small—a fact which does not yet permit generalizations—but we were using tumors which form metastases relatively early and very frequently. We did not expect any successes for bronchial carcinoma following this irradiation treatment because this type of tumor, as indicated above, generally has already spontaneously formed metastases by the time the diagnosis has been done.

As to the studies on the effectiveness of drugs as metastases prophylaxis which we have initiated at this institute, we are not able at this point to give definitive results.

Without any doubt, the four possibilities of metastases prophylaxis which we have mentioned above have to be retested, selected, or supplemented. The fundamental path, however, the insertion of a metastases prophylaxis before the actual removal of the tumor, appears absolutely necessary for the therapeutic approach. On the basis of the animal experiments and the metastatic growth analysis described above, there can no longer be any doubt that surgical interventions can release metastases. The provoking of metastases formation through surgical

activities gives us also an explanation for the fact that no improvements in the rate of actual cures have been achieved in the last 25 years despite the enormous improvements made in all therapeutic processes. Further, with the present concepts in therapeutic procedures, we can not even expect a substantial improvement in therapeutic successes in the future.

The time when metastases prophylaxis should be used can be found through analysis of the metastases growth curves: it has to occur during or before the regular first treatment so that it can become effective during the range of the implantation period. We have shown above that a decisive battle takes place during the implantation period: the tumor cells, once settled, try to expand their bridgehead. If they are repulsed by the tissue defense, which differs in strength from organ to organ, then they will eventually perish. However, if they succeed in gaining a foothold, then the further invasion cannot be stopped. Metastatic growth starts unnoticed and unnoticeable until the time when the diagnostic threshold has been reached or symptoms have become apparent. However, once this stage has been reached, all curative therapy is too late. During the implantation stage, which has to be regarded as relatively unstable for the just attached metastases, the number of tumor cells which have settled is still relatively small. An effective metastases prophylaxis, by effecting a reduction of tumor cells, can cause the newly formed metastases to regress because their sizes have shrunk below the critical cell number. This means that it is not even necessary that all the

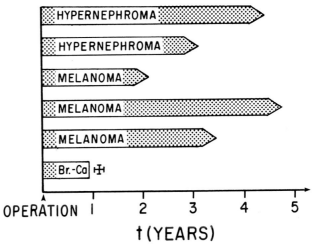

Figure 40.23. Results of treatment obtained thus far following the use of the radiogenic protective effect as a metastatic prophylaxis: 4 wk prior to the operation, the patient was subjected to sectional irradiation with a gammatron at doses of 150–250 rads.

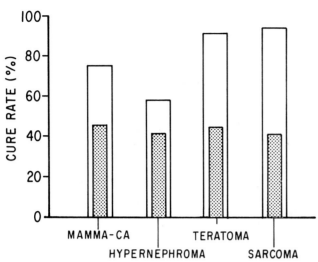

Figure 40.24. Possible increase in the cure rate, provided that an effective metastases prophylaxis can be developed. *Gray bars*, expected increase in the cure rate if we can succeed in avoiding provoked metastases or in destroying them in the implantation phase.

tumor cells which have settled be destroyed; this has been demonstrated unequivocally and successfully through the animal experiments of Mundinger *et al.* (34). It is at this point, at the time of the first treatment, that the fate of very many tumor patients who come as so-called early cases is being decided. If we could succeed during this formation period in forcing the provoked metastases into regression by one of the four methods mentioned above, then the number of cures for these early clinical cases would increase tremendously. The expected increases in successful cures are shown in Figure 40.24, but the chance occurs only once in the course of cancer treatment: during the implantation phase or the time of the first treatment. Once the metastases have grown, that is, once they are big enough, then they cannot be forced to regress with the methods known today. However, a successful metastases prophylaxis could result in greater success in tumor treatment than at any time since the start of a systematic attack on cancer!

Summary

Despite the great advances in surgical and radiological technology, we have not succeeded in improving the rate of cures for cancer treatment during the last 25 years. A small increase in the number of successful cures is due solely to improved diagnosis and an early recognition of the tumors. The removal of the primary tumor is the most important goal of present-day cancer therapy, but the primary tumor generally is only of low clinical importance; it is the formation of metastases that is decisive. The rate of cure and the formation of metastases have a complimentary relationship with respect to each other. Metastases appear after an operation in definite time intervals, depending on the type of tumor. The duration of this time interval is closely related to the rate of growth of the tumor in question. The quantitative analysis of the growth of 2893 metastases has shown that, according to the type of tumor, metastases are caused by operation with a frequency of 30–90%. Thus, our present-day tumor therapy of early cases will bring about either cure and resistance or the formation of metastases and a worsening of the disease. It is recommended that a metastases prophylaxis be inserted before each diagnostic or therapeutic-surgical intervention as a therapeutic consequence.

References

1. Alexander, P.: Personal communication, 1962.
2. Barth, G., Graebner, H., and Strössenreuther, H. (1960): On the effect of organ extract increasing cell breathing on the mouse carcinoma S 180 subjected to radiation therapy following paratumoral and intramuscular injection. *Strahlentherapie*, 113(4):2.
3. Becker, H., Borst, H. G., Brieler, H. S., Dahm, P., Dalichau, H., Donhöfer, A., Hegemann, G., Junginger, T., Kessler, E., Kümmerle, F., Mühe, E., Pichlmaier, H., Riedemeister, I. C., Reusch, G., Satter, P., Savic, B., Sommerwerck, D., Schotte, I. F., Schwaiger, R., Stöhr, U., Strothmann, A., Träger, B., Timm, D., Ungeheuer, E., Viereck, R., Wache, H., Wassner, U. J., and Zierott, E. (1976): Results of the surgical treatment of bronchial carcinoma. *Deutsch. Med. Wochenschr.*, 43(101): 1553.
4. Benninghoff, D., and Tsien, J. (1959): Treatment and survival in breast cancer; a review of results. *Br. J. Radiol.*, 32:450.
5. Boag, I. W. (1948): The presentation and analysis of the results of radiotherapy. *Br. J. Radiol.*, 21:128 and 189.
6. Brenner, M. W., Holst, L. R., and Perttala, Y. (1967): The study by graphical analysis of the growth of human tumors and metastases of the lung. *Br. J. Cancer*, 21(1):1.
7. Collins, V. P., Loeffler, R. K., and Tivey, H. (1955): Observation on growth rates of human tumors. *Am. J. Roentgenol.*, 76:988.
8. Denoix, P. (1970): *Treatment of Malignant Breast Tumors.* Springer, Berlin.
9. Druckrey, H., Hamperl, H., Herken, H., and Ravei, B. (1939): Surgical treatment of animal tumors. *Z. Krebsforsch.*, 48:451.
10. von Elmendorff, H., and Albsmeier F., (1969): The cause of death in cancer patients after 5-year cure. *Münch. Med. Wochenschr.*, 111:1027.
11. Enstrom, J. E., and Austin, D. F. (1977): Interpreting cancer survival rates. *Science*, 195:847.
12. Fisher, B., and Fisher, E. R. (1959): Experimental evidence in support of the Dovmant tumor cell. *Science*, 130:981.
13. Garland, H., Coulson, W., and Wollin, E. (1963): The rate of growth and apparent duration of untreated primary bronchial carcinoma. *Cancer*, 16(6):694.
14. Gastpar, H. (1970): Stickiness of platelets and tumor cells influenced by drugs. In *Platelet Adhesion and Aggregation in Thrombosis: Countermeasures*, edited by E. F. Mammen, G. F. Anderson, and M. I. Bernhart. F. K. Schattauer Verlag, Stuttgart.
15. Gastpar, H. (1976): Preliminary results of a long-time metastases prophylaxis using the pyrimido-pyrimidine derivate RA 233 in patients with primary sarcoma and malignant lymphoma in the head-throat region. In *Onkohämostaseologie*, edited by H. Gastpar. F. K. Schattauer Verlag, Stuttgart.
16. Gastpar, H. (1977): Platelet cancer cell interaction in metastasis formation. *I. Med.*, 8:2.
17. Gregl, A. (1963): Life expectancy of the untreated mamma carcinoma. *Klin. Wochenschr.*, 41:676.

18. Haagensen, C. D. (1971): *Diseases of the Breast.* Saunders, Philadelphia.
19. Heilmann, H.-P. *et al.* (1976): Results of the radiological treatment of the bronchial carcinoma. *Deutsch. Med. Wochenschr., 43* (101):1557.
20. Junghanns, K., and Ott, G. (1971): Early diagnosis and preliminary examination in stomach cancer. *Med. Welt., 22*(9):319.
21. Keller, H. L., and Kallert, S. (1966): The roentgenological determination of the growth rate for metastatic circular aggregations in the lung. *Fortschr. Roentgenstr., 104*(4):504.
22. Koike, A. (1964): Mechanism of blood borne metastasis. *Cancer, 17*:450.
23. Kojima, K., and Sakai, J. (1964): On the role of stickiness of tumor cells in the formation of metastasis. *Cancer Res., 24*:1887.
24. Krokowski, E. (1964): The dynamics of tumor growth. *Strahlentherapie, 57*:189.
25. Krokowski, E. (1965): The doubling time of malignant tumors. *Wien Klin. Wochenschr., 77*(15):258.
26. Krokowski, E. (1967): Tumor growth and prognosis. *Strahlentherapie, 64*:87.
27. Krokowski, E. (1978): Does tumor therapy also program its failures? *Strahlentherapie,* 154.
28. Krokowski, E.: Krebsbekämpfung in der Krise (Cancer fight in the crisis.)
29. Krokowski, E., and Taenzer, V. (1966): The radiogenic protective effect. *Strahlentherapie, 130*(1):139.
30. Krokowski, E., and Taenzer, V. (1967): Radiation protection through x-rays. *Deutsch. Med. Wochenschr., 92*(16):737.
31. Krokowski, E., and Taenzer, V. (1968): Increased radiation tolerance after whole-body irradiation. *Strahlenschutz Forsch. Prax., 8*:171.
32. Mendelsohn, M. L. (1961): Autoradiographic analysis of cell proliferation in spontaneous breast cancer of C3H mouse. *J.N.C.I., 22*:1015.
33. Müller, J. (1976): The untreated mamma carcinoma in the mammogram. Inaugural. Dissertation, Göttingen.
34. Mundinger, F., Vogt, P., Jakobi, C., Fischer, H. V., Ostertag, C. (1972): Clinical and experimental results of the interstitial Brachy-Curie-therapy in combination with radiosensors in infiltrating brain tumors. *Strahlentherapie, 143*(3):318.
35. Oeser, H. (1954): *Radiation Treatment of Tumors.* Urban and Schwarzenberg, Munich.
36. Oeser, H. (1974): *Cancer Treatment: Hope and Reality.* Thieme, Stuttgart.
37. Oeser, H., Krokowski, E., and Gerstenberg, E. (1964): The importance of the tumor-doubling time for cancer treatment. *Münch. Med. Wochenschr., 106*(14):675.
38. Page, N. P. *et al.* (1965): Recovery from radiation injury in sheep, swine and dogs as evaluated by the split-dose technique. In *13th Annual Radiation Research Society Meeting,* Philadelphia, 24.05.
39. Prudente, A. (1950): Ciba Chin. Symposium, 299.
40. Schermuly, W., Solth, K., and Weber, R., (1961): The sequence of metastases formation in mamma carcinoma. *Strahlentherapie, 115*:265.
41. Schmähl, D. (1970): *Origin, Growth and Chemotherapy of Malignant Tumors.* Canter K. G., Aulendorf/Wurttemberg.
42. Seeber, S. (1977): Internal therapy of the metastases-forming mamma carcinoma. *Klinikarzt, 6*(7):569.
43. Spiessl, B. (1976): Uniform classification of malignant tumors according to the TNM-system. *Z. Allgemeine Med., 22*:1133.
44. Spratt, J. S., Spjut, H. H., and Roper, C. L. (1963): The frequency distribution of the rates of growth and the estimated duration of primary pulmonary carcinomas. *Cancer, 16*(6):687.
45. Stutz, E. (1966): Effect of x-ray treatment on the progress of the Yoshida-Ascites sarcoma in white rats. *Strahlentherapie, 130*:440.
46. Walther, H. E. (1948): *Cancer Metastases.* Schwabe, Basel.
47. Welin, S. *et al.* (1963): The rate and patterns of growth of 375 tumors of the large intestine and rectum observed cervically by double contrast enema study. *Am. J. Roentgenol., 90*(4):673.
48. Wolff, G. (1967): The growth of human tumors. *Arch. Geschwulstforsch., 29*:98.
49. Wolff, G., Schwarz, H., and Bohn, K.-J. (1964): On the growth of benign lung tumors and lung metastases. *Med. Klin., 59*(46):1817.
50. Wood, S., Jr. (1974): Experimental studies of the spread of cancer, with special reference to fibrinolytic agents and anti-coagulants. *I. Med., 5*:7.
51. Wood, S., Jr., Holyoke, E. D., and Yardley, I. H. (1961): Mechanism of metastasis production from blood-born cancer cells. *Can. Cancer Conf., 4*:167.

41

Contribution of Experimental Comparative Pathology to Research on Metastasis

Hans E. Kaiser

The preceding chapter has clearly indicated the significance of metastatic growth for the patient concerned and suggested that certain revisions in cancer treatment may be necessary.

The question then naturally arises: What contribution can be made by experimental comparative pathology?

Lima-de-Faria and Smith were able to implant plant plastids successfully in human HeLa cells (see the chapters by Lima-de-Faria and Ames). As set forth by Butenandt, Krokowski, and others, approximately 1000 tumor cells are needed to initiate a primary tumor, a fact which also holds true for the stimulation of metastatic growth, a development highly dependent upon the defense mechanisms of the tumor host. We know from experience that after surgical removal of the primary tumor, patients often show marked improvement in their general health. This improvement continues until the remaining tumor cells and consequent metastatic growth regain their vigor, influencing again the metabolism of the host. The primary neoplasm itself is considered as the result of possibly years of damage to metabolism and the breakdown of the immunity system. It is the author's belief that important contributions by experimental tumor pathology can be made; these are possible through vertebrate as well as invertebrate studies.

More extensive studies are needed on the immunologic and defensive condition of the body at specified time intervals and in different vertebrate species, following removal of metastatic growth. Particularly important are investigations on how the fast-growing and the slow-growing tumors, with varying metastatic potential, differ among different species, and why they differ.

If the immunity requirements for implantation are met, invertebrates provide us with the means of studying the survival of experimentally inoculated tumor cells of neoplasms growing at different rates.

Invertebrates should be used for these studies because of the different possibilities for metastatic growth. Two general modes of metastatic cell spread are known: (a) hematogenic and (b) lymphatic. Invertebrates offer a vast array of different systems of body fluids not known to occur in vertebrates. Among these are highly specialized members, such as the cephalopods, which may therefore offer new avenues of research. Extrapolation of these data to conditions in vertebrates may enrich our knowledge of the metastatic spread of human neoplasms. Such studies as these not only may make it possible to learn about species-specific immune reactions and several species-specific modes of metastatic distribution, but more importantly, may inform us on species-specific organ resistance to metastatic invasion. The results thus obtained could later be broadened and deepened by comparative studies of defense mechanisms in the bodies and organs of a number of different species, without overlooking species-specific tumor susceptibility, be it with primary or metastatic growth. Such an approach is warranted by experimental knowledge already acquired on certain tumors in laboratory rodents and the experience of spontaneous tumors in man, dog, cat, some birds, and fishes.

42

Applicability of Comparative Oncology to Therapy

Hans E. Kaiser

Chapters 12–41, especially, were devoted to the different aspects and viewpoints of comparative oncology. The next step now is to ask whether these findings will have a new impact on human therapy. The topic of this book deals with comparative aspects of abnormal growth. However, man, in this whole spectrum of comparison, is only one species among many others. Thus therapy, as far as humans are concerned, is only one aspect among many. Nevertheless, comparative oncology has a wide applicability to therapy involving humans. We do not intend to give a detailed description of all the facts; rather, in the form of a summary, we will review those subfields discussed previously in these chapters, which may be especially concerned with human therapy of neoplastic diseases (Table 42.1).

Finally, in this section we can say that the future fight against neoplasms or cancers will have to concentrate on the steps depicted in XAF 42.1.

References

1. Fortner, J. (1978): The present status and future possibilities of organ transplantation in cancer surgery. XII. International Cancer Congress Symposium, Vol. 24, p. 70, program.
2. Raven, R. W. (1978): Surgical oncology as a specialty, the making of the surgical oncologist. XII. International Cancer Congress Symposium, Vol. 24, p. 69, program (abstract symposia, p. 78).

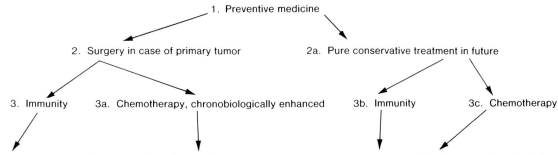

1. Preventive medicine
2. Surgery in case of primary tumor
2a. Pure conservative treatment in future
3. Immunity
3a. Chemotherapy, chronobiologically enhanced
3b. Immunity
3c. Chemotherapy
4. In any case curtailment of metastatic growth and possible improvement of patient's condition by organ transplantation.

**Table 42.1
Subfields of Comparative Oncology Which May Have a Special Impact on Human Therapy**

Subfield	Based on Reason	New Studies Required	Contribution of Comparative Oncology/Why	Envisaged Accomplishments	Reference to Chapter	References
Subcellular biochemical, biophysical, & ultrastructure	Species-specific differences in biochemical, biophysical, and ultrastructural makeup of neoplastic cells	To complete the uniting and diversified picture	Comparison of various subcellular patterns	Comparison of variations in different species may lead to a better understanding of basic principles involved	Trump, Weisburger, E. K. Pitot, Wallach	
Species-specific and organ-specific biochemical pathways	Metabolic differences in chain reaction initiated by carcinogenic compounds: (1) direct acting; (2) reaction of metabolites	For better understanding of species-specific pathways and chain reactions of similar carcinogenic compounds	The comparison may give a profound understanding of important factors of chain reactions in neoplastic cell transformation	Splitting of metabolic chain reactions of certain carcinogens in humans	E. K. Weisburger	
Chronooncology	Species-specific and organ-specific rhythmic differences	To elucidate the best approach to application of chemotherapeutical agents	To prevent unwarranted assumptions among species	Rhythmic most powerful approach of chemotherapy and immunology	Halberg, Scheving, Herberman	
Species-specific aspects of immunity	Findings on regression of neoplasms	For a better understanding of normal and artificial regression of neoplasms	To understand regression of neoplasms better through a species-specific comparison	Immunologic methods to enhance antineoplastic regression by strengthening the immunological defense; better understanding through comparative approach in finding these methods	Herberman, Kaiser	
Epidemiology Veterinary	Findings in pets, especially dogs, which may lead to an expectation of future happenings in man	With animal models, especially the dog (similar food and environment), normal death as in man	Using the dog as a model under comparative conditions with man but with a much shorter life-span	Participation of preventive medicine	Hayes, Boonyanit	

Theoretical and basic

Medical	Epidemiologic experience with regard to racial and geographic differences	Using the racial (anthropologic) differences as a parameter (differences of female breast)			
Chemotherapy	Tumor hampering or destruction by several chemotherapeutica	Better understanding of mechanisms to cope with side effects by species-specific research due to biochemical (especially enzymatic differences), but also through those differences in the distribution of chemical compounds in the organisms	Improvement of understanding in the possibilities of enhancing antitumorigenic effects and coping with side effects	E. K. Weisburger	
Prevention and treatment of metastatic (secondary neoplastic) growth	Clinical findings of metastatic growth in cancer patients	Species-specific understanding of metastatic spreading	Prevention or slowing down of metastatic initiation and recovery	Korkowski, (Kaiser)	
Rehabilitation	Experience with organ transplantation in the clinic	More studies are needed, to gain insight into the metabolic/immunologic conditions in the patients' primary tumors but especially with metastasis and cachexia, regarding implant rejection	Species-specific aspects of organ transplantation may result in new insights for the clinical work	Prevention or slowing down of general metabolic damage (cachexia)	1, 2

V

Comparative Aspects of Neoplastic Growth

43

The Species-specific Spectrum of Neoplasms

Hans E. Kaiser

In this chapter the neoplasms of the organisms are arranged histologically and are compared; the neoplasms of man are used as parameters. It is the purpose of this chapter to show where in the organismic world the different types of neoplasms can be expected and where they have been found to exist.

COMPARABILITY OF NEOPLASMS IN THE DIFFERENT ORGANISMS

To deal with general and specific findings, a comparison of neoplasms must be placed within the framework of a comparison of abnormal growth. General facts must be based on an understanding of subcellular structure because neoplasms are composed of cells; their true nature can be comprehended only when the transformation of normal into neoplastic cells is understood. Complicated processes are involved in these changes. The diagnoses depend on pathohistology and the knowledge of normal tissues is a preliminary condition.

A neoplasm in the sense of human pathology is composed either of parenchyma and stroma, or rarely only of parenchyma. It consists of a number of cells which may be malignant from the start, as is now believed to be the case, judging from the initial stages of oat cell carcinoma of the lung (457). Benign neoplasms grow expansively and crowd out but do not invade the tissues about them; often, they are surrounded by a stroma capsule, whereas malignant neoplasms grow and infiltrate the underlying or surrounding tissues in man and animals also by metastasis. Two important facts should be noted: (a) in general, neoplasms display in their cells, which are of less value, some remnants of the characteristics of the parent tissue or tissues; and (b) neoplasms are composed of a

number of cells. It was stated once that a neoplasm may start perhaps with 1500 cells. A neoplasm therefore consists of a number of parenchyma cells and mostly of stroma, with the exception of such cases as the leukemias, the experimental ascites tumor of the mouse, and the choriocarcinoma. Thus, one may speak of the neoplastic tissue in contrast to the surrounding, normal, or pathological (metaplastic, scar, granulation) and other tissues. This relationship in contrast with normal tissue prevents us from considering a single cell or a few abnormal cells found as a cell accumulation, or in a cell accumulation as a neoplasm. The next step in tissue relationships can be found in cell accumulations in which a normal cell population can be distinguished from a pathological one which is not unconditionally equal to a neoplastic form. This cannot happen in cell accumulations as, for example, in most algae when all cells are alike, but more highly developed ones where the beginning of true tissues already produce galls. Within the framework of pathological growth, these aspects should be considered as preliminary conditions of neoplastic growth, either phylogenetically or ontogenetically.

DIFFERENCES IN TISSUE DISTRIBUTION AMONG PHYLA

In the two-kingdom approach, the greatest differences in tissue distribution exist between the kingdoms, but variations in tissue distribution are also found among the phyla of the animal kingdom and are not as diversified as among plant phyla. The comparative distribution of neoplasms is correlated in two ways: (a) the distribution in time, that is, the phylogenetic distribution of tissues and neoplasms, and (b) the parallel distribution of tissues and neoplasms in species, developed along convergent lines, at one particular time interval.

It is evident that neoplasms of epithelial tissues have occurred since pre-Cambrian time, but they do not appear with the same distribution in all phyla. Simple epithelia and the neoplasms developing from them are phylogenetically older than the stratified epithelia and their neoplasms. From a comparative point of view, rhabdomyomas and rhabdomyosarcomas must have a broader historical and species-specific distribution than leiomyomas and leiomyosarcomas because the majority of species (insects and several other phyla) is characterized by transverse striated musculature. The distribution of chordal tissue, the chordoma theoretically limited to the species of the superphylum chordata, is restricted. Simple epithelia and some stratified ones can be compared in animals and plants and, as a consequence, also the tumors developing from them.

SPONTANEOUS TUMORS IN MAN—THE MULTIPLICITY OF DESCRIBED NEOPLASMS IN A SINGLE SPECIES

The neoplasms of man are the phylogenetic ultimate. Man appeared very late in the history of the earth. Although a highly specialized mammal, he is to some degree less specialized in regard to certain adaptations.

The neoplasms of man represent the multiplicity of described types if compared to other species. There are natural, historical, and technological reasons for that. Certain types of neoplasms do not occur in man, such as those deriving from plant tissues, or from animal tissues not present in man. By the comparative method, these other neoplasms can be related to those described in man. Man's neoplasms are the focal point for a comparison with those of other species since the knowledge of their histology is the most extensive. In their usefulness as basis for comparison of spontaneous tumors, the neoplasms of man are followed by those of certain other mammals, birds, and fishes for the vertebrates: those of the molluscs and perhaps the fruit fly for the invertebrates; and, finally, those of the vascular plants, especially dicotyledones. However, for the majority of the approximately 5000 mammalian species, no tumors have been observed because our knowledge of the normal conditions of most species is inadequate. As far as experimental neoplasms have been investigated, those of the laboratory rodents play a

dominant role, followed by those of dog, cat, monkey (especially, the baboon), fish, and fruit fly.

Approximately 16% of the deaths in the United States are due to cancer, second only to cardiovascular disease. Death caused by neoplasms in animals of the Zoological Society of San Diego was 2.75% in mammals, 1.8% in birds, and 2.1% in reptiles. The comparison with domestic animals shows 5% in dogs, 1% in cats, 0.1% in cattle, and 0.1% in horses.

The most frequent mammalian tumors in a survey by the Zoological Society of San Diego in 1977 were those originating in the lung, comprising 14%. Skin cancer, in many areas the most frequent human cancer, is rare in this series. The cystic teratoma, the most common ovarian neoplasm in man, and the rarer choriocarcinoma were not found. Neoplasms of the biliary duct were again common. Lymphosarcomas were of very high frequency (132).

The neoplasms in the wild animals showed also an increase over the years. A large colony of Galapagos giant tortoises, which are able to live longer than 150 yrs, showed no neoplasms in 32 necropsies. Neoplasms in whales were rarely reported and also in the redwoods, *Sequoia* sp. It seems to be a falacious assumption that age and large body size are preconditions of neoplastic growth (see Chapter 13 of the neoplasms from tissues with embryonal potential). Two separate neoplasms were diagnosed in two reptiles, three birds, and eight mammals in the San Diego series (132). No amphibian tumors have been detected in this study.

There are two sources of neoplastic growth. In the eumetazoans, man is that species which shows a multiplicity of spontaneous neoplasms; also, these have been the most extensively investigated histologically. The other basic source of a large variety of neoplasms is the vascular plants, especially angiosperms and particularly dicotyledones.

The transformation of the normal plant tissues into neoplastic ones is discussed: Some questions are significant. Is it possible to relate certain neoplasms of plants to those in man? Can we compare neoplasms deriving from epithelia and, if malignant specified as carcinomas, to those that derived from nonepithelial or mesenchymatic tissues and, if malignant specified as sarcomas, to comparable groups in plants? This is a bold undertaking, but it must be attempted to relate the two main groups of eumetazoan and plant neoplasms to each other. This will be possible if two main viewpoints, the histological and the ontogenetic (embryonal, developmental), are used. The histologic approach, especially from a diagnostic point of view, is the more important one. The following pages present a review of the phylogenetic and species-specific tumor patterns reflecting the histologic approach.

Figure 43.1 and Table 43.1 are a review of the distribution spectrum of the tissues, either according to the phyla (a term which equals types of body plans of organisms), or according to the number of species. The graphs show only a rough approximation. The reason is twofold: (a) the real number of many taxonomic groups is not known and depends on how the taxonomist distinguishes between species and subspecies; and (b) in many species the real character of a tissue underwent different interpretation due to technology with the electron microscope; it was found that structures which were described years ago with the light microscope, such as, for example, smooth musculature, are now seen to be obliquely striated musculature. However, this change in designation could only occur in species recently reinvestigated; so for many species investigated only with the light microscope decades ago, the spectrum remains unclear. In addition to this uncertainty about the structure of normal tissues, we are uncertain about the diagnosis of many rare neoplasms of some vertebrates, but especially of invertebrates and plants diagnosed years ago, or even recently.

Certain tissue types are known which have been observed without exception in several organisms: for example, insect muscle is always transverse striated, and bone occurs only in vertebrates, with the exception of cartilaginous fishes, the mammary glands in mammals, and sweat and sebaceous glands not even in all mammals in the same diversification. These facts show the wide difference in the distribution of tissues.

The theoretical spectrum of neoplasms, *i.e.*, where they can be expected to exist according to histogenesis, varies in the distribution of the different tissues. Certain tissues of the same type, especially of the group of connective tissues, have a different value in various phyla. A mesenchymal cell in an acoelomate invertebrate cannot transform itself into cartilage, whereas one in certain arthropods may have that ability, but not the ability to produce bone, a privilege of the mesenchymal cell of vertebrates, such as mammals. The variability of invertebrate muscle is also in the assumed five types (Chapter 3) not clearly circumscribed, such as this one of simple

and striated epithelia in animals and plants or fully differentiated cell invariable tissues. This reflects itself in tumor diagnosis. Certain factors exist in addition to the comparability of tissues which make such a comparison valuable. Among similar organismic groups, such as certain species of fish, important geographic differences exist in cancer tumorigenesis. Worldwide epidemiologic studies of the flatfish (Pleuronectidae) and eels concerning papillomas and the viral lymphocystic disease have shown remarkable differences in varying geographical locations (493). Outside certain "risk" regions, flatfish and eel populations are not affected, even in areas with high rates of natural or man-made pollution.

Around the South American continent especially Argentina, those fish tumors have not been observed (for fish tumors in South America's waters; see Chapter 48). It is thought that this is due to the water streaming along the Atlantic coast of Argentina from south to north and the clean condition of the antarctic water feeding (343).

Different organisms show varying reactions to carcinogens; therefore, their susceptibility differs.

The ascidiacea or sea squirts belonging to the phylum tunicata are a class of filter-feeding marine organisms that are sessile in the adult stage. It was observed that *Ciona intestinalis,* a species frequently used for studies in embryology and development because of the determinate cleavage pattern of its eggs, grows in dock regions where oil pollution exists. Petroleum and its combustible products contain numerous polycyclic aromatic hydrocarbons, some of which induce toxicity and cancer in a number of mammalian species after metabolic activation by the organism. To determine if the ability of *Ciona intestinalis* to thrive in areas containing such hydrocarbons is due to their ability to metabolize the hydrocarbons through pathways which do not form biologically active metabolites, the metabolism of benzo(a)pyrene (BP), a widespread environmental contaminant, was examined. Large (3–4 cm in length) or small (1.5–2 cm in length) *Ciona* were placed in beakers of 50 ml seawater containing [^{3}H]BP (0.5 nmol/ml). After 24 hr, the small ascidians contained 15–25% of the BP, while the large ones contained 60–75%. Water-soluble derivatives of BP were recovered from the water and the intestine, branchial basket, and tunic of both sizes of the organism. Other than quinones, which may have formed spontaneously, no BP metabolites were detected

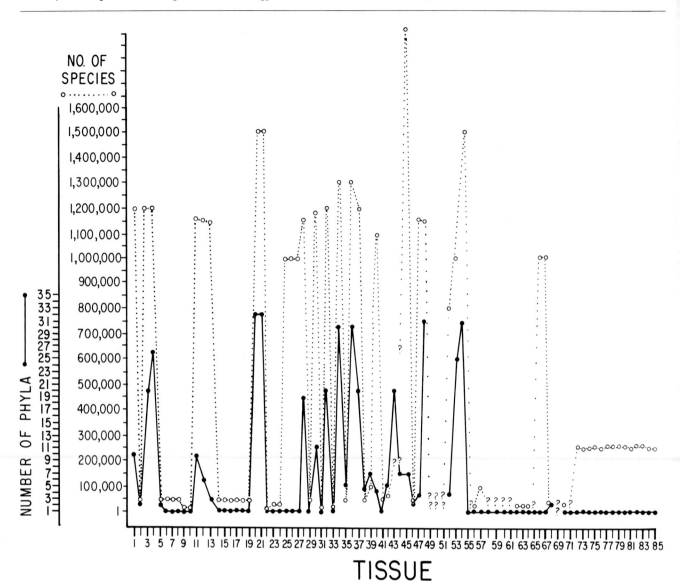

Figure 43.1. Tissue-distribution in phyla and species as a lead to the theoretical potential of tumor formation. See Table 43.1, which further describes this figure.

by high-pressure liquid chromatography of organic solvent extracts of the water or tissue samples. The amount of BP converted to quinones and water-soluble derivatives in 24 hr was low, approximately 0.1–0.15 nmol/organism. However, some BP appears to become covalently bound to the protein of several tissues.

We conclude that *Ciona intestinalis* is able to concentrate BP from the water; a major portion is found in the branchial basket and intestine. An unidentified water-soluble derivative of BP is formed in the organism and can be recovered from the seawater. Thus, *Ciona intestinalis* may be protected from deleterious effects of polycyclic hydrocarbons by the low rate of metabolism, or by not forming free primary oxidation products such as dihydrodiols (which have been found to lead to the induction of biological effects in several mammalian species) or by a

combination of both of these mechanisms (25, 26).

Other taxonomically widely separated species such as mammals and fungi exhibit the same chemical pathways of carcinogens such as BP. In the case of oxidation of polynuclear aromatic hydrocarbons, such as benzo(a)pyrene, in which process the active carcinogenic metabolics are found, fundamental biochemical differences exist in prokaryotic and eukaryotic cells. Cis dihydrodiols are the oxidation products in bacteria; areneoxides are the first detectable products in mammals leading to dihydrodiols.

However, the fungus *Cunninghamella elegans* oxidizes benzo(a)pyrene similar to the oxidization of mammalian microsomes (188). These findings show species-specific variables and the wide range of comparability in which the aspects of biochemistry, cytology, histology, and

Table 43.1
Distribution of Tissues by Number of Phyla and Species

Type of Tissue	Number of Phyla	Approximate No. of Species
1. Simple squamous epithelium	10	1,200,000*
2. Stratified squamous epithelium	2	45,000
3. Simple cuboidal epithelium	20	1,200,000**
4. Simple columnar epithelium	26	1,203,000**
5. Pseudostratified columnar epithelium	2	45,250
6. Stratified cuboidal epithelium	1	45,000
7. Stratified columnar epithelium	1	45,000
8. Transitional epithelium	1	45,000
9. Sebaceous and sweat glands	1	5,000
10. Mammary glands	1	5,000
11. Salivary glands	10	1,154,000
12. Liver and hepatic portion of hepatopancreas	6	1,151,000
13. Exocrine portion of pancreas and pancreatic portion of hepatopancreas	3	1,145,000
14. Islets of Langerhans	1	less than 45,000
15. Pineal gland	1	less than 45,000
16. Pituitary gland	1	less than 45,000
17. Thyroid gland	1	less than 45,000
18. Parathyroid/ultimobranchial gland	1	less than 45,000
19. Adrenal cortex and medulla	1	less than 45,000
20. Testis	32	1,500,000
21. Ovary	32	1,500,000
22. Optic gland (cephalopoda)	1	600
23. Y-organs (crustacea)	1	20,000
24. Androgenic glands (0 crustacea)	1	20,000
25. Corpora allata (insecta)	1	1,000,000
26. Thoracic glands (insecta)	1	1,000,000
27. Ventral glands (insecta)	1	1,000,000
28. Desmal epithelium	19	1,167,000
29. Desmal epithelia/synovial origin	1	45,000
30. Mesenchyme	11	1,185,000
31. Spinocellular connective tissue	1	10,000
32. Reticular connective tissue	20?	1,200,000
33. Gelatinous connective tissue	1+	10,000+
34. Loose connective tissue	30	1,300,000
35. Fibrous connective tissue	5+	50,000+
36. Melanogenic system	30	1,300,000
37. Adipose tissue	20	1,200,000
38. Chordal tissue	4	50,000
39. Chondroid tissue	7+	100,000?
40. Cartilage	4+	1,100,000
41. Bone	1	45,000
42. Myoepithelial tissue	5	59,400
43. Smooth musculature	20	?
44. Helically striated musculature	7+	?
45. Transverse striated musculature	7	1,000,000– 7,000,000
46. Cardiac musculature	2	50,000
47. Neurons of the central nervous system	4	1,154,000
48. Neurons of the peripheral nervous system	31	1,500,000?
49. Autonomous nervous system and chromaffin tissue	?	?
50. Meninges	?	?
51. Choroid tissue	?	?
52. Central glia	4	+800,000?
53. Peripheral glia	±25	+1,000,000?
54. Neurosecretory cells/tissue	31	1,500,000
55. Neurohemal structures of nemertinea	1	?
56. Cerebrovascular complex (annelida)	1	9,000
57. Neural perineum (mollusca)	1	100,000
58. Organ juxtacomissural (amphineura polyplacophora)	1	?
59. Organesjuxtaganglionaires (proso- and opisthobranchia)	1	?
60. Dorsal bodies and comparative structures (pulmonata)	1	?
61. Neurohemal organs of arachnida	1	?
62. Sinus glands (crustacea)	1	20,000
63. Postcommissural organs (crustacea)	1	20,000
64. Pericardial organs (crustacea)	1	20,000
65. Cerebral glands (chilopoda, diplopoda)	1	
66. Corpora cardiaca of insecta	1	1,000,000
67. Perisympathetic organs of insecta	1	(1,000,000)
68. Plectenchymata	2	20,000±
69. Pseudoparenchymata	?	
70. Phylloid, cauloid, or rhizoid true tissues	1	20,000±
71. True tissues of bryophyta	1	
72. Apical meristems	1	251,000+
73. Lateral meristem	1	250,000+
74. Meristemoids	1	250,000+
75. Succeeding meristems	1	251,000+
76. Phellogen	1	250,000+
77. Phytoepidermis	1	251,000+
78. Rhizodermis	1	251,000+
79. Collenchyma	1	251,000+
80. Sclerenchyma	1	250,000+
81. Xylem	1	251,000+
82. Phloem	1	251,000+
83. Periderm	1	250,000+
84. Secretory structures	1	250,000+

disciplines complement each other. This similarity or variability must be seen on the diagnostically irreplaceable background of the comparability of cells and tissues as experimentally proven by the cell fusion of animal and plant cells (see Chapters 28 and 33).

Spontaneous and experimental (artificially spontaneous) neoplasms have been described in nearly the same sequence in domesticated mammals as in man. Certain areas are rare, such as the transitional cancer in the cat.

The first basis are the tissue types: A specific tissue type may vary according to (a) taxonomic and phylogenetic level (connective tissues); (b) topographical differences (circulatory systems); (c) species-specific biochemistry; (d) biophysical species specificity; (e) nutritional and environmental species specificity such as different food intake, which may be influenced by the acidity of rain pollution.

Newest literature on the electron microscopy of human and other neoplasms has been included and, concerning mammals, especially domesticated ones, a selection only of the newest literature, besides some basic texts, is given due to the enormous amount of material available.

Three topics seem to be significant: the theoretical expectance according to tissue types to be dealt with; the appearance of spontaneous neoplasms; and the evaluation of experimental neoplasms.

NEOPLASMS ARISING FROM SIMPLE SQUAMOUS EPITHELIUM

Proceeding from the condition in man, we distinguish the simple squamous epithelium proper (as in portions of uriniferous tubule, parietal layer of Bowman's capsule, portions of rete testis), the mesenchymal epithelium[1] (as in subarachnoid and subdural spaces, perilymphatic spaces of the inner ear, chambers of the eyeball), the mesothelium[2] (as in peritoneum, pleura, pericard), and the endothelium[3] (as in the inner layer of blood vessels, inner layer of lymph vessels, and the endocard). The neoplasms of man are the benign papilloma and the malignant squamous cell cancer. The papilloma is a noninvasive tumor with evidence of squamous diferentiation which occurs rarely in man. The squamous cell cancer is invasive with evidence of squamous differentiation. Variation is pronounced, infiltration into underlying tissues is common, and the tumor progresses with extensions like roots of a tree into the underlying tissues. Variable cells occur in wall-like fashion; prominent nuclei and mitotic figures are characteristic. The normal distribution of the tissue in the animal phyla or subgroups is as follows: integuments of simple squamous epithelium occur in porifera, cnidaria, ctenophora, platyhelminthes, mollusca, tardigrada, arthropoda, chae-

---

[1] Cells exhibit fibroblast characteristics and form no continuous sheet.

[2] See section on neoplasms arising from desmal epithelium of serous membranes (coelomic epithelium) and pseudoepithelia of vessels.

[3] See section on neoplasms arising from desmal epithelia of synovial origin.

tognatha, tunicata. This type of epithelium is found in the digestive systems of ctenophora and structures of gaseous exchange in mollusca and vertebrata and structures dealing with excretion in vertebrata.

Depending on the species, the epithelium is restricted to certain locations in one case and to wide distribution in another. Tumor cases in several vertebrates have been observed. Regarding invertebrates, our knowledge is rather meager. Neoplasms deriving from cells of body fluids in certain invertebrates belong to epithelia of coelomic surfaces if the normal precursors of these hemocytic neoplasms derive from the peritoneum, as is believed to be the case in amebocytes in annelida (polychaeta). The typical plant epidermis and the inner sheaths of the plant body (vascular plants) are comparable (see pp. 90, 91).

For convenience, epithelial thymoma observed in *Hemitragus jemlahicus jemlahicus* (132) is placed here between the sections of simple and stratified squamous cell epithelum.

NEOPLASMS ARISING FROM STRATIFIED SQUAMOUS EPITHELIUM[4]

The stratified squamous epithelium is widely distributed in man and is found in the skin, the external auditory canal, conjunctiva, cornea, mouth, esophagus, portion of the larynx, vagina, vestibule, labia majora, portions of urethra, and penis. Several epidermal papillomas are known from human skin and exhibit a papillary pattern, prickle cells, basal cells, and sometimes keratinization. The subtypes of these papillomas show varying characteristics.

The squamous papilloma exhibits a thickened hyperplastic epidermis with keratinizing material on top. A regularly arranged granular layer of cells is typical; the basal cell layer is undisturbed.

The seborrheic keratosis shows a papillary appearance of epithelial cells around dermal papillae and hyperkeratosis. The basal cell layer is seldom disturbed.

In the case of senile keratosis, parakeratosis, cell disorganization, mitotic activity, large pleomorphic nuclei, and downgrowth into the corium are found. The progression may lead to squamous cell carcinoma.

Xeroderma pigmentosum presents dry, rough

---

[4] Variation of benign and malignant can hardly be separated.

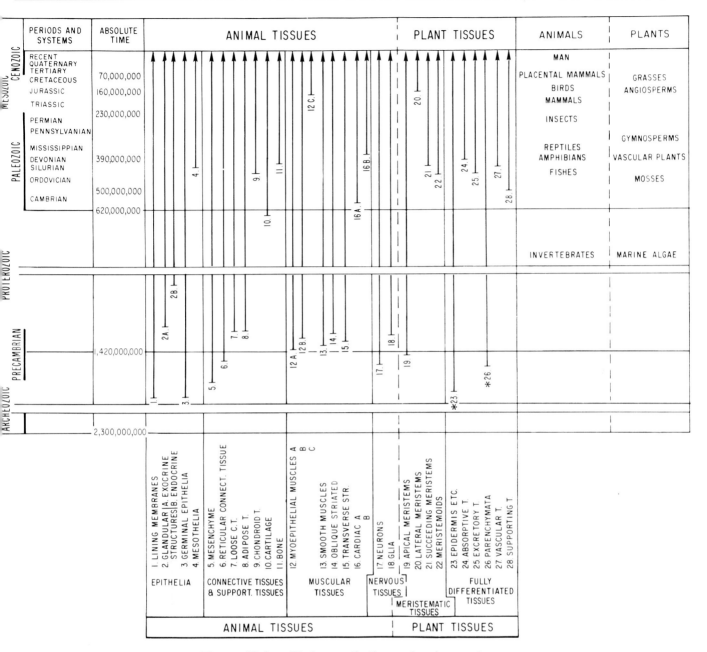

Figure 43.2.   Phylogenetic tissue development.

scalding hyperpigmentation and telangectic lesions.

The kerato-acanthoma consists of craters of keratin and a surrounding epidermal lip, upward and downward growing atypical cells which form cornification with horny pearls. The keratinization is stronger than in the squamous cell carcinoma. The lateral activity is more extensive than downward spreading. For clinicohistological aspects in the mongoloid race group, see Uyeno et al. (568), and for experiments in the rabbit see Harms et al. (214).

The sebaceous adenoma, a benign tumor, is well circumscribed, mostly encapsulated, composed of sebaceous cells, irregular and larger than in normal sebaceous glands and basal cells. The change of this benign neoplasm to basal cell carcinoma has been reported.

Sebaceous carcinoma is characterized by sebaceous and atypical cells. The cell variation is pronounced. The tumor may be seen as a variation of basal cell carcinoma.

The benign calcifying epithelioma shows dead stratified epithelium, shadow cells, basal cells, calcification, and metaplastic ossification.

The biochemistry of preneoplasia in skin

needs further investigation concerning the variation in different phyla and subgroups. For mouse skin, see Boutwell (58).

The basal cell carcinoma is a multicentric infiltrative growth of basal cells. The locally invasive tumor spreads slowly, nearly never metastasizing. The peripheral cells mimic the basal cells of the epidermis. The superficial multicentric type, the morphea type, and the fibroepithelial type are distinguished (546). Tongue-like processes, cell nests, and connected strands of cells with basophil large nuclei and scanty cytoplasm are present. Keratinization occurs, and horny pearls may be found; the supporting tissue is plentiful or scanty. The ultrastructural differences between basal cell carcinoma and human skin showed a decrease in hemidesmosomes and an increase in actin-like microfilaments in cells at the tumor margins (347, 368).

In the case of the squamous cell carcinoma with squamous differentiation, the epidermal thickness has increased. The tumor is an invasive growing neoplasm which rarely metastasizes; the adenoid squamous cell carcinoma and the spindle cell type are subtypes (12). Root-like prolongations proceed into the underlying tissue. Inflammatory reaction occurs; cells are differentiated and undifferentiated. Horny pearls of prickle cells are found. Nuclear pleomorphism and lack of prickle cells characterize the undifferentiated variation. Mitotic activity and giant cells are present. Primary mucinous carcinoma of skin is a rare variation of squamous cell cancer, the ultrastructure of which reveals a highly differentiated character with mucin secretion (26). Concerning the ultrastructure, see also about the oral squamous cell carcinoma (pp. 657 and 658).

The metatypical or basosquamous cell carcinoma is a mixed type between the aforementioned ones.

The normal distribution of the body covering of stratified squamous epithelium is found in the rostral body region of highest chaetognatha concerning the invertebrata and the vertebrata. Comparable to this type of epithelium are certain covering membranes of the vascular plants, such as the stratified lining of the body in xerophyta (plants adapted to the desert).

One of the most frequently observed tumors occurring on a wide range of species is the epidermal papilloma. The most often used experimental animals in research of papillomas are hamsters, rats, mice, and primates. The kinetics of regression were observed in the mouse

(74) and rabbit (503), with reference to the induction of new hair follicles by promoters in mouse tail epidermis (495). Epidermal (skin) papillomas are known from the following species: *Carassius auratus, Catostomus commersoni, Proterorhinus marmaratus, Anthogobius flavimanus, Anabas testudineus, Colias labius, Genyonemus lineatus, Glyptocephalus cynoglossus, Glyptocephalus stelleri, Glyptocephalus zachirus, Hippoglossoides dubius, Hippoglossoides elassodon, Limanda herzensteiri, Limanda limanda, Paravetulus sp., Platichthys stellatus, Pleuronectes platessa, Psettichthys melanostictus, Pseudopleuronectes herzensteiri, Electrophorus electricus, Salmo trutta* regarding fishes; in the reptiles *Chelonia midas, Lacerta agilis, Pseudechis porphyriacus, Crocodilus sp.;* the bird *Neophena splendida* and the mammal *Sarcophilus harrisii.* For additional cases, see Chapter 48. (It is self-explanatory that these selected cases give no attempt at a statistical evaluation of species-specific tumor distribution.) It is appropriate to discuss details of some of the newest studies. Papillomas in Atlantic salmon (*Salmo salar*) were investigated concerning immunology and ultrastructure. Histology and immunology indicated that a cellular immune response led the tumors to be sloughed. The ultrastructure of the nuclei of the papillomas was unusually regular in shape, and the chromatin was slumped near the nucleic margins (81–83). Atwell and Summers (19) reported concerning the congenital disease in the fowl. Papillomas or papilloma-like lesions have been seen in black and white colobus monkeys (*Colobus polykomus*), dogfish (*Mustelus canis*) by Wolke and Murchelano (604), racing greyhound by Davis *et al.* (115), and the black rhinoceros by Boever (54).

For geographic variations of papilloma occurrence in flatfish, see Stich *et al.* (529), Wellings *et al.* (591), and Stich and Acton (528). For viral investigations concerning other fish in Japanese waters, see Ito *et al.* (263).

The stratified squamous epithelium at body openings such as the mouth and anus changes from a keratinized to a more or less nonkeratinized epithelium. For convenience the neoplasms of stratified squamous cell epithelium and especially the papillomas of these regions are discussed here. Certain papillomas as types of papillomatous diseases of human skin and mucous membranes are transmitted by a virus of the papova group (15). There exist different contagious papillomatous diseases such as the one described above (e.g., 81), or virus (herpes, reo, and papova)-associated lesions in the dorsal body's skin region in the green lizard (*Lacerta viridis*) (449), or papillomatosis in nutrias (*Myocastor coypus*), recorded for the first time in Czechoslovakia in 1975 (266) and with papillomas on the extremities, tail, head, and in oral and nasal cavities. The electron microscopic examination of the virus revealed structures corresponding to papillomatous viruses. The eel virus (Berlin) is found in the blood of eels (*Anguilla anguilla*) with skin papilloma (494), and also in Japanese serow (*Capricornis crispens*).

Oral neoplasms papillomas and others such as ameloblastomas are known for cunners (*Tautogolabrus adspersus*) (218), and oral papillomas from white croakers (*Genyonemus lineatus*) (428). A papilloma of the lip was seen in *Equus asinus* (132).

Oral papillomatosis, a widely distributed condition with surely varying etiology, was observed in coyotes (*Canis latrans*) and wolves (*Canis lupus*) ranging from mild to severe affection, nearly covering the surface of lips, tongue, and buccal cavity (478.) For cultivation of canine papilloma cells, see Tokita *et al.* (551). Tweedle and White (564) reported anal fibropapillomatosis in cows from Australia. A papilloma from the orbit *Anatolichthys* sp. has been found (132). The conversion of Shope papillomas connected with serum changes was reported by Seto *et al.* (502) for domesticated rabbits; see also Sundberg *et al.* (535) for horses and Pour *et al.* (434–437) for hamsters.

The kerato-acanthoma of vertebrates has been observed in such species as *Poecilobrycon harrison*, *Siredon mexacanum*, *Rana temporaria*, *Mastomys natalensis* (469), *Chimpansee troglodytes*, and *Macaca mulatta*. The tumor or a comparable equivalent is also known from the bivalve mollusc, *Crassostrea gigas*.

Sebaceous adenomas and sebaceous carcinomas are restricted to the class of mammals in which they are not infrequently found. It is impossible to review all the cases in detail.

Basal cell carcinoma is also frequent and, for example, known from *Macaca mulatta* and *Lagotheri humboldti*.

Squamous cell carcinoma has been described from *Myxine glutinosa*, *Scyliorhinus caniculus*, *Salmo salar*, *Barbus barbus*, *Carassius auratus*, *Chondrostoma soetta*, *Cyprinus carpio*, *Ictalurus catus*, *Leuciscus idus*, *Xiphophorus helleri*, *Gadus virens*, *Theragra chalcogramma*, *Spinachia spinachia*, *Bathygobius soporator*, *Triturus alpestris*, *Geomyda trijuga*, the birds *Himanto-*

pus himantopus leucolophus and *Neophema elegans elegans*; and the mammals *Macaca mulatta*, *Trichechus senegalensis*, and *Antilocapra americana* americana.

Neoplasms of the integument of this type of epithelium may theoretically occur in many vertebrates, but they have not been described in all species in which they may have appeared. The tissue types from which the neoplasms derive can only give us a guide to the theoretical possibilities, and here, as in the other tissues with a particular location, only selected examples can be given. The ultrastructure of moderately differentiated human squamous cell carcinoma of the oral cavity revealed nuclear bodies, clustered ribosomes, many lysosomal bodies, cell residues in other cells, absence and multilayering of basal lamina, pseudopodal structures and other abnormalities which were related to the hyperactivity, and differentiation of the cancer cells (91).

A 15-year-old, white, female cat showed a neoplasm probably originating in the external auditory canal, with intraocular and orbital metastases (222).

Cancer of the lip in man is mainly of the squamous cell type and is well differentiated. It was also described of *Tinca tinca* and *Pogonias chromis*.

Cancer of the tongue in man occurs for two-thirds in the anterior end and is mainly a squamous cell growth. The squamous cell cancer shows a variation in degree of differentiation and keratinization as well as the occurrence of undifferentiated types. Theoretically, the tumor may be found from fishes to mammals but cannot occur in invertebrates; it is incomparable to plant tumors. A squamous papilloma of the tongue was found in the whale *Balaenoptera musculus*.

Most cancers of cheek and floor of mouth are moderately well-differentiated epidermoid cancers. These neoplasms occur just in vertebrates. Man's intraalveolar epidermoid cancer of the jaw composed of glycogen, rich clear cells, is sometimes an undifferentiated squamous cell cancer. Theoretically, it can be found in every class from reptiles to mammals. It has been described in *Macaca mulatta* and other species, especially domesticated and laboratory mammals.

Cancer of the pharynx is rare in man. It is poorly differentiated, with the exception of squamous types. The poorly differentiated lesions show small, round, closely packed cells, reminding us of sarcomas. Comparison to other groups is possible, at least theoretically, in highly developed coelomates. Squamous papilloma, which can be considered as a preliminary condition was, for example, described in the pharynx of *Hylobetes* sp.

The postcricoid, or squamous cell cancer of hypopharynx, in man is composed of squamous cells. It can be compared with vertebrates, especially mammals, but species-specific distribution in the sexes needs clarification.

The epidermoid esophageal cancer accounts for 95% of neoplasms of the esophagus in man. Oat-like cells are common in the more undifferentiated form. The circadian influence on mitotic frequency was studied in stratified squamous epithelium of mouse esophagus (75). Well-formed squamous cells may be mixed with pleomorphic cells. Sometimes, the differentiation goes in the direction of basal cell cancer. The lesion is exclusive to vertebrates.

Squamous cell cancer as the most common type of cancer in the esophagus has also been detected in other vertebrates, such as the Lama vicugna (132); for the horse, see Moore and Kintner (384). The first simian or human cell line (816A) of a spontaneous esophageal carcinoma of the rhesus monkey, *Macaca mulatta*, was established by Rabin *et al.* (445).

The benign papillomas of the larynx are predunculated warty epithelial lesions in man and occur in the vertebrates with different frequency.

A squamous cell carcinoma of the cervix was seen in *Thylogale parma*, an adenocarcinoma of cervix from *Aepyceros melampus rendilis* (132), and a benign vaginal polyp in *Equus asinus*.

Cancer of the vagina, in the human an everting or ulcerative lesion, is mostly squamous. The cell lesion is similar to that of the cervix. Sometimes keratinization and pearl formation occur. Occasionally, it is also similar to the adeno-acanthoma. For the verrucous carcinoma of the vagina, as a continuously growing, destructive, generally not metastasizing neoplasm of this tissue type, see Wood *et al.* (605). Squamous cell carcinoma of the vagina was observed in *Arctocephalus ursinus* (132).

A papillomatous tumor of the vulva is known from *Elephas maximus indicus* (132).

The intra-epidermal cancer of the vulva is a collective term for the following types. Bowen's disease of the labia majora in man is similar to lesions of the same disease in other regions. Paget's disease of the labia majora in man is characterized by ulcers, large pale cells with granular or vacuolated cytoplasm. The epidermoid cancer of the vulva exhibits well-differentiated forms with keratinization and horny pearl formation (see integument).

Squamous cancer of the urethra shows squamous characteristics as keratinization and horny pearls. Most cases are undifferentiated. Root-like extensions invade the adjacent tissue.

Squamous cell cancer of the penis in man is well differentiated, exhibiting root-like extensions, narrow stroma, covered by the squamous epithelium. Variations are in regard to infiltrating capacity, differentiation, keratinization, and horny pearl formation. These types of tumors have been described in different vertebrates. They do not occur in invertebrates and are incomparable to plants with respect to organ topography and location.

The benign Queyrat's erythroplacia is a dyskaryotic proliferation of the epithelium. The cells are often large and clear; distortion of the basal layer occurs.

The benign condyloma in man is a papillary growth of squamous epithelium; well-differentiated prickle cells and a peripheral basal cell layer characterize it. Infiltration has not been observed. Effron *et al.* (132) observed an adenocarcinoma.

NEOPLASMS ARISING FROM SIMPLE CUBOIDAL EPITHELIUM

In man this type of tissue is found at the inner surface of the lens capsule, portions of the labyrinth, the choroid plexus, in glands, glandular secretory ducts, the kidney, and the free surface of the ovary. As a neoplasm of the cuboidal pigment epithelium of the eye, the very rare pigmented epithelioma should be mentioned.

As far as the portions of the labyrinth with simple cuboidal epithelium are concerned, tumors of the inner ear are quite rare; generally, the squamous cell cancer (metaplastic?) is the most common tumor in this area. (The malignant melanoma of the choroid is the most common of the interocular malignant tumors in man.

With respect to the lining of the ventricles and the choroid plexus in man, two types of tumors should be discussed here which show simple cuboidal epithelial lining, the ependymoma and the choroid plexus papilloma. The glandular epithelium of both tumors is closely related; they show varying degrees of differentiation and malignancy, theoretically and practically. The lining of the spaces in the ependymoma consists of typical ependymal cuboidal or columnar epithelium.

The presence of cell rosettes is of diagnostic value. The subependymoma with dominating astrocytes and those in the region of the cauda equina occur with the following variants: myxopapillary ependymomas (with mucinous change of collagenous stroma. The ultrastructure shows: few cilia, cellular interdigitations, abundant material of basement membrane). Malignant versions have been observed, such as in the fish *Xiphophorus helleri*. Renal cortical adenomas are known from the reptiles *Pituophis melanoleucas annectens*, *Bitis arietans* (scirrhous), *Eclectus roratus* solomnensis (bilateral), the Prairie dog *Cynomys ludovicianus*; renal tubular adenoma are known from *Tadorna cana* and tubular adenoma of renal medulla of *Gymnorhyna tibicen tibicen*; renal adenocarcinoma are known from *Gallus sonneratii*, *Melopsittacus undulatus*, *Brotogeris versicolorus versicolorus*, and the monkey *Macaca mulatta*.

The destructive adenoma (35), or malignant cyst adenoma (184), is a malignant tumor of man's kidney. Certain cases of classical or hypernephroid kidney cancer belong in this category. The histological structure is similar to that of the benign adenoma, but the growth of this malignant tumor is destructive, occasionally metastasizing. A benign tumor of this group in the human ovary is the surface papilloma; the malignant version is the surface papillary carcinoma.

The normal distribution of this tissue type in the animal phyla or subgroups includes: Cnidaria (integument), ctenophora (integument), platyhelminthes (integument, excretory structures), entoprocta (integument, digestive structures), gastrotricha (digestive structures), kinorhyncha (digestive structures), nematoda (digestive structures), nematomorpha (integument), pentastomida (digestive structures), arthropoda (integuments, digestive and excretory structures), phoronida (digestive structures), brachiopoda (integument), echinodermata (integument, digestive, respiratory structures), chaetognatha (integument and digestive structures), hemichordata (integument, respiratory structures), tunicata (integument), cephalochordata (integument), vertebrata (digestive, respiratory, excretory structures and those of propagation and sensitivity). This summary shows that at least

theoretically this type of tissue, as a parent tissue of neoplasms, has a wide range of distribution. A comparison with certain lining membranes to plants is also possible. According to location and organ, papillomas not present in man have been described from fish gills as in *Salmo trutta*.

NEOPLASMS ARISING FROM SIMPLE COLUMNAR EPITHELIUM

The distribution of this tissue extends in man from the cardia of the stomach to the anus. It is also found in the excretory ducts of many glands. A ciliary variation is known to exist in a portion of the paranasal sinus, the small bronchi and the central canal.

The papilloma of the choroid plexus, accounting for only 0.4–0.6% of all intracranial neoplasms in man, is characterized by a lining of simple cuboidal or, more often, columnar epithelium. The other components of the tumor are thin-walled vessels of the pia surrounded by loose connective tissues.

A choroid plexus papilloma was seen in the elasmobranch, *Squalus acanthias*, with columnar epithelium. (442). Ultrastructural features are: apical-basal polarity, uncommon cilia and varying number of microvilli, basement membrane and, in specimens from infancy or childhood, abundant glycogen granules (85, 468).

A third tumor type is the colloid cyst of the third ventricle, showing in most cases cuboidal or columnar lining.

The neoplasms of glandular ducts with single cuboidal epithelium include certain mixed tumors, as well as tubular adenomas of the salivary glands. As for the mammary gland, extraductal carcinomas with tubular structure are adenocarcinomatous in character. The glandular elements are characterized by a flat, cuboidal, or columnar, either simple or multilayered, epithelium. Therefore, some metaplasia takes place in the case of flat or columnar neoplastic epithelium.

The neoplasms (adenomas or carcinomas) which develop from septal bile ducts or terminal ductules and larger ducts are another group (see pp. 670 and 671, liver). The characteristic epithelial cells are of the cubic form. The nucleus is hyperchromatic, the cytoplasm eosinophilic. They account for only 1% of all primary liver cancers.

The neoplasms deriving from the ducts of the pancreas tend more to columnar cells in their epithelium.

The extremely rare tubulary and papillary adenoma of the human kidney, a benign tumor, occur frequently in mixed forms composed of glandular tubes; the epithelium is simple cuboidal to columnar. For cases in domestic and laboratory animals, see Baskin and De Paoli (34) on the dog, and Coleman et al. (101) on the rat. Tumors were also described from other vertebrates: of the spinal cord, the oviduct, and the uterus. The bird *Kakatoe galerita galerita* exhibited a mucinous cystadenoma of the oviduct.

Polyps of the intestinal tract in man, which are benign tumors, are of nodular or mainly papillary makeup. Glandular tissue is comparable to the mucous membrane and composed of simple cuboidal or cylindrical epithelium. Adenoma-like polyps have been observed in the stomach of hatchery-grown salmonids and other fishes (295). They are common in domesticated animals such as the dog (212) and laboratory animals, for example, *Paromys (Mastomis) natalensis* (477). The birds *Loriculus vernalis phileticus* and *Pavo cristatus* exhibited an adenoma of the ventriculus and adenomatous polyps of the duodenum, respectively; the mammal *Arctictis binturong* exhibited an adenoma of the colon (132).

In man, the pattern of stomach cancer permits the distinction of the following subtypes: adenocarcinoma (see Patnaik et al. (418) on the dog), adenopapillary carcinoma, signet ring cell carcinoma, gelatinous carcinoma, undifferentiated carcinoma, scirrhous carcinoma, Linitis plastica, adeno-acanthoma, and squamous cell carcinoma. These subtypes have not been distinguished with exactness described in other species, aside from veterinary cases, a circumstance which hampers a species-specific comparison. These types are patterns of stomach cancer, with heterogenous differentiation of well-formed to atypical structures, lined by cuboidal or columnar cells. Goblet cells may occur. The stroma varies greatly, is well formed in the case of tubular structures, and is scanty in undifferentiated regions. Patches of squamous elements occur in the pattern of the adeno-acanthoma due to metaplastic change. In man the relatively rare villous adenoma of the intestine has a mostly pseudostratified or stratified epithelium. Adenocarcinoma of the stomach is known from the Prairie dog, *Cynomys ludovicianus*, and the adenocarcinoma from the guanaco *Lama guanicoe* (132).

Spontaneous gastrointestinal carcinomas have been seen in dogs (187), cats (268), horses (235), and Meuten et al. (372), to cite only a few species. For spontaneous intestinal neoplasms in other species, see Chapter 48. Experimentally, the rat (565, 566), the European hamster, the Syrian golden hamster, the Chinese hamster, mice (72), dogs, and miniature pigs have been the mammalian species most often investigated.

Carcinoma of the Appendix

In man the tumors of this type are mostly well-differentiated adenocarcinomas, but undifferentiated and mucinous cases have been also observed.

Cancer of Colon and Rectum in Man

The pattern is adenocarcinomatous in most cases with varying differentiation. The cells are columnar cuboidal or polygonal; the well-differentiated specimens mimic normal mucosa. The tubules are irregular in the case of medial differentiation; few or no adenoid structures occur in cases of poor differentiation. The epithelium of the tumors is tall and stains darker than normal mucosa. The nuclei are somewhat hyperchromatic. The neoplasms with less advanced differentiation stain darkly and exhibit centrally located nuclei which are hyperchromatic. Pseudostratification and karyokinesis are typical. An adenocarcinoma of the intestine is known from the bird *Larus atricilla* (132).

The immogenicity of spontaneous murine colonic adenocarcinoma has been investigated by Avdeev et al. (21).

The cancer of the anal canal is uncommon in man. In the upper position the neoplasms are less differentiated; in the lower position keratinization is stronger. They resemble the squamous cell cancer of the lip.

Duodenal Carcinoma in Man

In general glandular, they are most common in the duodenal papilla, where they arise from duodenal epithelium, the crypts of Lieberkuehn, or glands of Brunner. They arise also from the tall columnar cells of Wirsung's duct or the terminal portion of the bile duct.

Carcinoid Tumor of Argentaffin Cells

The histogenesis of carcinoid tumor is still unclear, even in man; they may derive from the mucosa. However, fat-forming cells are not present in normal mucosa. The cells are uniformly arranged in nests and islets.

Polyps in Man

They may show no full differentiation (these being benign), may exhibit organoid occurrence with fully differentiated epithelium, and they may be limited benign or without organic makeup with pronounced parenchyma and full differentiation. The growth inside the polyp is destructive. The small neoplasms are particularly malignant (492). Benign juvenile polyps should not be considered as being neoplasms. The adenomatous polyps of the large bowel are benign. These tumors exhibit glandular structures composed of simple columnar epithelium and stroma. The nucleus is hyperchromatic; the cytoplasm stains darker.

The papilloma of the gall bladder in man exhibits a columnar epithelium with Paneth cells, interspersed goblet cells and not many argentaffin cells. Nuclei are dark staining, located at the cell base near the stroma. Occurring mitoses produce a pseudostratified appearance of epithelium. A benign polyp of gallbladder epithelium was diagnosed in the bird *Trichoglossus haematodus moluccanus* (132).

The adenoma of the gall bladder is of tubular or glandular structure, and the stroma is sparse. In the majority of the cases, the carcinoma of the gallbladder is an adenocarcinoma. The same holds true for the carcinoma of the extrahepatic ducts. Metastatic adenocarcinoma of the renal pelvis is rare.

Extremely rare in man is the carcinoma of the oviduct. There have been reports of papillary adenomas or papillomas, but these reports are uncertain and the carcinomas are mostly considered to be well-differentiated ones. This adenocarcinoma, originating from tubal epithelium, exhibits a papillary and/or glandular pattern. These lesions are papillary structures with extremely atypical cuboidal, rarely cylindrical, cells building a simple to stratified layer. The cords of the neoplasm may be solid or glandular; islets of squamous cells occur. (Mixed tumors have been observed.) The cells of the cancer are nonciliated and uniform or pleomorphic, with nuclei often dividing.

Polyps of the corpus uteri, very common in man (?), are glandular, with columnar epithelium and stroma. The latter is rich in collagenic fibers.

Polyps of the cervix, also common, are glandular with tall columnar epithelium, which may produce mucus. Variable development of stroma is exhibited which may be undifferentiated mesenchyme characterized most often by rich collagen fibrils and vessels with strong walls. Difficulties in diagnosis occur when squamous cell epithelium of the portio occurs also in the tumor (especially in ducts of cervical glands).

Cancer *in situ* of the uterus exhibits glandular structures of bizarre pattern with sparse stroma.

Frequently, the endometrial adenocarcinoma is well differentiated, but it occurs also in moderately or poorly differentiated form (three types). The epithelium is simple or multilayered and shows glandular pattern; the staining of cells is pale, eosinophilic or vasophilic with H & E. The cells are tall and columnar, sometimes cuboidal; the stroma is generally scanty.

The granulosa cell tumor resembling the histologic pattern as observed in the granulosa cell tumors of the ovary is a variation.

The clear cell-mesonephroid adenocarcinoma of the uterus has cells with clear cytoplasm ± cells of hobnail type and tubular or papillary pattern; the nucleus is located at the cell base. This variety of tumor simulates the clear cell carcinoma of the kidney.

The adenoacanthoma, also malignant, shows considerable squamous change, as a variation of the former type by developing metaplasia. Horny pearl formation may occur.

The rare squamous cancer (squamous cell carcinoma) of the uterus is characterized by increased squamous elements (metaplasia).

In the adenosquamous (mucoepidermoid) cancer, intermingled adenocarcinomatous and squamous carcinomatous components are found.

The undifferentiated carcinoma must be regarded as the poorly differentiated form which cannot be assigned to any other because of its poor differentiation.

Relatively rare in man is stromal endometriosis which shows an uncertain histogenesis. The tumor behaves malignantly; the cells are round or oval but uniform in type. Generally, the hyperchromatic, spherical, oval nuclei sit in a narrow cytoplasm; reticulin fibrils are present.

The carcinosarcoma of the uterus consists of

spindle-shaped epithelial and stromal sarcomatous cells.

The tumor pattern of neoplasms arising from simple columnar epithelium changes frequently into more cuboidal sections or even into a squamous type of cell. This is a condition which the tumors mimic from variations in the parent tissues. Nevertheless, a comparison requires exactness of the wide distribution of this type of tissue in the animal phyla. It can be found in the following: Cnidaria (integuments, digestive structures), ctenophora (integuments), platyhelminthes (integuments and digestive structures), nemertina (integuments, digestive structures), entoprocta (integuments and digestive structures), gastrotricha (digestive structures), kinorhyncha (digestive structures), nematoda (digestive structures), mollusca (integuments, digestive structures), sipunculida (integuments, digestive structures), annelida (integuments, digestive structures), pentastomida (integuments, digestive structures), tardigrada (digestive structures), arthropoda (integuments, digestive structures), phoronida (integuments, digestive structures), ectoprocta (digestive structures), brachiopoda (integuments, digestive structures), echinodermata (integuments, digestive structures), chaetognatha (integument, digestive structure), pogonophora (integument), hemichordata (digestive and respiratory structures), tunicata (digestive structures), cephalochordata (digestive structures), vertebrata (digestive, respiratory, and excretory structures and those of propagation and sensitivity).

Neoplasms of this type of epithelium can also be compared to relevant structures of, for example, the inner and outer lining membranes in members of plant phyla. The tumors principally observed in vertebrates are too numerous to list, especially if we consider the great number of species investigated regularly. That they occur also in species not so frequently observed becomes evident, so the presence of squamous cell cancers has been established in the stomach of the lion, *Leo leo,* or colon cancer in *Molliniesia velifera.* New efforts at registration are urgently needed.

Uterine carcinomas are frequently observed in domesticated animals such as adenocarcinoma in the dog (301) or the pig (594) (see also ref. 142 on cats, ref. 44 on laboratory animals such as the Chinese hamster, and ref. 162 on the baboon *Papio doguera*). For more details, see Chapter 48. Experimentally, rat and mouse are the species most frequently used for the investigation of uterine tumors.

NEOPLASMS ARISING FROM PSEUDOSTRATIFIED COLUMNAR EPITHELIUM

This type of tissue is found in man in a portion of the tympanic cavity, the lacrimal sac, the large ducts of glands, and the excretory passages of the male reproductive system, such as the vas deferens, the epididymis, and the male urethra. The ciliated variation occurs in a large portion of the respiratory passages, such as the respiratory part of the nasal cavity, nasopharynx, part of the larynx (with exception of the anterior surface and one-third to one-half of the posterior surface of epiglottis, aryepiglottic folds, and the vocal cords), trachea and bronchi, and the eustachian tube. Approximately 50% of tumors of the lacrimal sac belong to the papilloma-carcinoma group comparable to the neoplasms arising from the epithelium of nasal and paranasal cavities (18, 475).

The rare cancer of the male urethra originates in columnar cells.

The benign adenomatoid tumor of the epididymis in man has a questionable histogenesis. Cell cords, hollow acini of low columnar or cuboidal cells, and irregular channels lined by flattened cells are characteristic. Connective tissue and, occasionally, smooth muscle fibers compose the stroma.

The rare carcinoma of the same organs is similar in appearance but exhibits signs of malignancy.

NEOPLASMS ORIGINATING FROM THE CILIATED VARIETY OF PSEUDOSTRATIFIED COLUMNAR EPITHELIUM IN MAN

Nasal Cavity

Papillomas with transitional or columnar epithelium are rare; the same is the case with columnar-cell adenocarcinomas.

Nasopharynx

Papillomas and carcinomas arise infrequently from this region and type of epithelium.

Cancers of this epithelium in the larynx is also an exception. In the trachea we find the so-called cylindromas and columnar cell cancer of the adenomatous type.

Lung/Bronchus

The histological classification of lung tumors by the WHO was recently revised and will be published shortly (517). The different types of adenomas appear as benign neoplasms.

Squamous cell (epidermoid) carcinoma is a metaplastic neoplasm (278). Flat, polygonal pavement-type cells are characteristic; they are arranged in whorls and show keratinization and intercellular bridges.

Three degrees of histological differentiation can be distinguished.

Small cell carcinoma, as the name implies, is composed of small anaplastic cells. The most important subtype is the oat cell carcinoma, of richly cellular consistency, of more or less regular cells, with dark staining nuclei and scanty, almost invisible cytoplasm, recalling oat grains (name!); the nuclei lack nucleoli; the cells are closely packed; the connective tissue, the stroma, is delicate.

Electron Microscopy

A second subtype includes the carcinomas with intermediate cell types, such as polygonal or fusiform.

A third subtype is composed of the oat cell carcinomas which contain portions of squamous cell and/or adenocarcinomas.

Adenocarcinoma

Four subtypes may be distinguished: acinar, papillary, bronchioalveolar, and solid carcinomas with mucus formation.

Undifferentiated or Large Cell Carcinoma of the Lung

The following cases have been observed on the premises of the Zoological Society of San Diego from 1964 to 1976 (132): Bronchiogenic adenoma is *Didelphis marsupialis virginianus*,

Erinaceus pruneri hinder, Chrysocyon aureus syriacus, Lama guanicoe guanicoe; adenoma of lung in *Panthera tigris longipitis*; multiple adenomas of lung and Citellus leucurus, Aepyceros melampus rendilis (all mammals); bronchogenic adenocarcinoma in the Cape cobra *Naja nivea*, in the painted quail (*Coturnix chinensis lineata*), in the snow leopard *Panthera uncia*, and in the Cretan goat, *Capra aegagrus cretica*; scirrhous bronchogenic adenocarcinoma in the East African eland (*Taurotragus oryx pattersonianus*); an undifferentiated adenocarcinoma of the lung in the Angolan springbok, *Antidorcas marsupialis angolensis*; and mixed epithelial and connective tissue tumor of the lung in the red and green macaw, *Arachloroptera*.

The normal distribution of the tissues in animal phyla or subgroups shows the occurrence in brachiopoda (digestive structures) and vertebrata (digestive, respiratory, and excretory structures and those of propagation).

The tumor distribution in vertebrates is extensive; a case comparable to bronchial adenoma has been found in *Haplochromis multicolor* concerning vertebrates in addition to the many cases known to exist in domestic and laboratory animals. In invertebrates an adenoma was described from *Bombus terrestris*, a rare case indeed.

The comparison of the tissue for tumor transformation extends into the plant kingdom according to the old approach first proposed by Aristotle.

NEOPLASMS ARISING FROM STRATIFIED CUBOIDAL EPITHELIUM

The normal distribution of the tissue in man is as follows: fornix of conjunctiva, ducts of sweat glands, sebaceous glands, cavernous portion of urethra, seminiferous tubules, lining of outer ovarian follicle, and portion of anal mucous membrane. Neoplasms of the glands will be discussed in the sections dealing with glands; those dealing with the portion of the urethra and of the anal mucous membrane have already been discussed on pp. 660 and 662. An extremely rare tumor in man is the carcinoma of the seminiferous tubule.

The squamous cell carcinoma of the conjunctiva and the basal cell carcinoma are the important tumors of the conjunctival epithelium, appearing in a ratio of 10 to 1 (259).

The cavernous portion of the urethra is the side favored by the rare squamous cell carcinoma of the urethra. The tumor may originate from both cuboidal or squamous cell epithelium, or from both together because of the change in the epithelium of this body region. A high mortality results from the cases of this tumor. This type of tissue is restricted to vertebrates (integuments, digestive and excretory structures, and those of propagation and sensitivity). No close comparison to invertebrates or plants is possible.

NEOPLASMS ORIGINATING IN STRATIFIED COLUMNAR EPITHELIUM

The normal tissues in man are distributed in enamel, epiglottis, pharynx, and large excretory ducts of some glands, such as the mammary and prostate glands. The ciliated variety is found in the nasal surface of the soft palate, the larynx, and the fetal esophagus, and at other places of developmental stages.

NEOPLASMS ARISING FROM ODONTOGENIC EPITHELIUM (430)

Phylogenetically, the earliest development of teeth occurred on the skin of fish-like creatures in the Silurian period. From this time on they improved in their development until the condition was reached which appears today in the mammalian body. In man the teeth are confined to the mouth cavity; remnants of the epithelial as well as the mesenchymal elements of this development can provide the basis for the development of neoplasms. The mesenchymal neoplasm, *i.e.,* those with only mesenchymal components, are discussed in the sections on connective tissues as, for example, certain fibromas. The tumors of the area with epithelial components having simple cuboidal or columnar character belong in this section.

During general tooth development a ridge of the oral epithelium is formed during the seventh week of embryonal life. Subsequently, it sinks into the tissue below. Bud-like structures appear as the precursors of the milk teeth; they are converted into bell-like organs forming the enamel where the single-layered inner and outer dental epithelium change from one into the other. The inner epithelium is a simple columnar

layer and the outer a simple cuboidal one. It is for this reason that a discussion of these odontogenetic epithelia was placed after a discussion of these two types of epithelia. It is not always possible to establish clearly whether a tumor derives from remnant tissues composed of cuboidal or columnar cells.

The adamantinoma in man varies from being benign to malignant. Histologically, it is comparable to the enamel organ. Microscopically, the appearance varies. There are islets of stellate cells covered by a layer of cylindrical cells, and mature connective stroma. The nuclei of the tall columnar cells located at the upper portion of cells, are rich in chromatin, sometimes mitotically active.

The ameloblastoma is a benign tumor which shows local invasion and is composed of ontogenic epithelium surrounded by fibrous stroma. Different patterns such as the follicular, plexiform, acanthomatous, basal cell-like, granular cell-like, and others are known.

Also, the calcifying epithelial odontogenic tumor, which arises from the intraepithelial structures, is locally invasive.

In ameloblastic fibroma the odontogenic epithelium is embedded in mesodermal tissue comparable to that of dental papilla, but odontoblasts are missing.

As the name implies, the adenomatoid odontogenic tumor has duct-like structures of the odontogenic epithelium with a variable pattern of connective tissue.

The very rare dentinoma again exhibits odontogenic epithelium and immature connective tissue, and forms displastic dentin. The ameloblastic fibro-odontoma is similar in structure to an ameloblastic fibroma, but dentin and enamel are present. The very rare odonto-ameloblastoma exhibits enamel dentin and odontogenic epithelium similar in structure and function to the ameloblastoma.

The malignant variations of these tumors form the odontogenic carcinomas. The signs of malignancy in the malignant ameloblastoma are expressed by primary growth in the jaw and metastatic growth. The primary intraosseous carcinoma develops inside the jaw bone; it is assumed that it arises from the odontogenic epithelium because a connection with surrounding epithelial structures is absent. The pattern is squamous cell type. Other types of carcinomas which arise from the odontogenic epithelium are possible but need not be discussed here.

The carcinoma of the outer larynx is extremely rare in man. The undifferentiated carcinoma of the pharynx arises from the cylindrical epithelium in man. For a discussion of the tumors of the large excretory ducts of glands, see pp.

Cancer of the nasal cavity is pseudostratified, and is sometimes composed of ciliated epithelium. In the larynx, papillomas occur, and cancer of the larynx is extremely rare.

The normal distribution of this type of tissue is restricted to the vertebrates (integuments, digestive and respiratory structures, and those of propagation). Adamantinomas have been described in *Melanogrammus aeglefinus*, *Scyliorhinus caniculus*, *Salmo trutta*, *Micropogon undulatus*, and *Cyprinodon variegatus*. An adenocarcinoma of the biliary duct was observed in *Homalopsis buccata*.

NEOPLASMS ARISING FROM TRANSITIONAL EPITHELIUM

This type of epithelium in man and the vertebrates is restricted to the renal calyces, the ureters, the bladder, and the urethra and urachus. For example, transitional cell papillomas of this type of epithelium occur in the bladder where the transitional cell papilloma, made up by not more than six layers of the epithelium and tender stroma, as well as the inverted type, with endophytic growth pattern, can be distinguished. In addition to these papillomas, squamous cell papilloma occur with regular squamous epithelium and tender stroma. The distribution in the pelvis of the kidney is generally diffuse, but several varieties are also found in the bladder. For this reason, we speak of papillomatosis.

The transitional cell carcinoma has transitional epithelium which shows malignancy, either by anaplasia or invasion. Sometimes, regions of squamous and glandular arrangement, or both occur, in which case the tumors are known as transitional cell carcinoma with squamous metaplasia or transitional cell carcinoma with squamous and glandular metaplasia.

The metaplastic squamous cell cancer of the renal pelvis shows a predomination of squamous cell epithelium and may be partially papillary in character. Keratinization and horny pearls may occur.

The squamous cell carcinoma of the bladder which contains keratin and intercellular bridges, is composed of only one type of similar cells,

and frequently has a nodular appearance and infiltrates.

The adenocarcinoma of the bladder in man has epithelial components composed of columnar to cuboidal cells. Sometimes, the cells are filled with mucin; signet cells may be present. The pattern is glandular and tubular, and may produce mucus.

The adenocarcinoma of the renal pelvis is predominantly a columnar cell carcinoma.

The undifferentiated carcinoma in man, sometimes considered an undifferentiated variant of papillary carcinoma, is a malignant neoplasm, less differentiated, which makes it impossible to put these neoplasms in any of the aforementioned groups.

The Metaplastic Epidermal Cancer of the Human Bladder

The more species are investigated, the more types of neoplasms are found which, so far had been undetected as, for example, the transitional carcinoma which involves the urethra in the cat (33). Other cases reported involved the dog (543), the cynomolgus monkey (*Macaca fascicularis*) (90), and cattle (413). It is of interest to know that in the same type of transitional epithelium, tumors are rarely found in certain locations, such as in the transitional portion of the male urethra of the cat. This leads to the question as to why this abberration occurs.

Adenomas of the urachus are compact tumor masses which may occur with inner degenerative changes. The lining epithelium is transitional or mucinous, with the cystadenomas as a variation.

The carcinoma of the urachus is primarily a mucinous adenocarcinoma, with a different arrangement of columnar and goblet cells.

The papillary carcinoma was described in *Anguilla anguilla*, *Barbus tetrazona*, *Rana pipiens*, *Constrictor constrictor*, *Meleagris* sp.

NEOPLASMS ORIGINATING FROM EXOCRINE APPENDAGE GLANDS OF SKIN. I. SEBACEOUS AND SWEAT GLANDS

The normal distribution in man is restricted to the subaceous glands as far as this first type of tissue is concerned. Sebaceous gland neoplasms are frequently observed in dogs (208, 532, 533). The benign neoplasm is the rare sebaceous adenoma composed of polylobular sebaceous components; basal cells may be poorly or not at all developed, but they are generally present. Connective tissue may be the outer border. The sebaceous adenoma may undergo a malignant change which generally will result not in a sebaceous but a basal cell carcinoma. Electron microscopic investigations were performed by Niizuma (397, 398), who distinguishes three cell types similar to the normal sebaceous gland in sebaceous epithelioma. Reports have appeared of transplantable adenomas in the mouse with virus particles perhaps similar to those of leukemia or mammary tumors, or even of a new type (470). Adenomas are also known to exist in other animals such as the Tasmanian devil (Sarcophilus harrisii) (132) or Speke's gazelle (56).

The malignant tumor is the sebaceous carcinoma, a variation of the basal cell carcinoma. The distribution of these tumors agrees with the normal tissue distribution; it is restricted to the mammals and known, for example, in the rabbit (433) and the horse (367). An investigation of the ultrastructure of lipid droplets of sebaceous carcinoma (Meibomian gland carcinoma) showed the presence of whirled lamellar structures at their outer portion and a homogeneous interior (398). The ceruminous gland adenocarcinoma (ceruminoma) is rarely found in man (376).

The tissue distribution of the second type is found in the sweat glands.

Electron microscopic studies indicate that the cylindroma is a derivative of the sweat glands and most likely of the apocrine ones. The hyaline substance originates from both parenchyma and stroma of the neoplasm (120). The sweat gland origin was indicated before by Sutherland (537), whereas Ronchese (462) and Traenkle (555) evaluated the tumor as originating from sebaceous glands. The neoplasm is relatively benign.

The first benign tumor in man is the syringocystadenoma papilifferum. The tumor is composed of sweat gland ducts which possess a lining of a two-layered epithelium composed of basic columnar and upper cuboidal cells.

The eccrine spiradenoma, which is benign also, is composed of undifferentiated cell masses, arranged in whorls, bands, and cords. Cuboidal or columnar cells line the ducts; myoepithelial cells are also present.

The "mixed" skin tumor shows the following composition: epithelial tissue is mixed with cartilage, chondroid, and myxoid tissue; it is followed by two rows of epithelial cells; squamous metaplasia exists occasionally.

The malignant clear cell hidradenoma is composed of small spindle cells and oval, clear, glycogen-rich cells. Portions are glandular in appearance; keratinization may occur.

The benign hidradenoma of the vulva contains cyst scanty stroma, double columnar epithelium, and a not well-developed layer of myoepithelial cells.

The adenocarcinoma of Bartholin's gland is comparable to salivary gland tumors and produces mucus. The squamous cell cancer of Bartholin's glands arises from the ducts; undifferentiated varieties have been observed. The epidermoid cancer of Bartholin's gland develops from squamous epithelium.

The possibility that these tumors may appear is highly limited because the glands do not exist in all mammals. In some, the appearance is already limited theoretically to the pads of the feet, as in certain carnivora, in the dog, for example; it is totally lacking in some rodents, rabbits, whales, sea cows, and the scaly anteater.

A papillary sweat gland adenoma is known from *Taurotragus oryx pattersonianus* (132).

The occurrence of a perineal adenocarcinoma is known from the black-footed ferret (*Mustela nigripes*) (84) (see also Chapter 46); the papillary carcinoma of apocrine sweat glands was first reported to exist in nonhuman primates, such as the capuchin monkey *Cebus albifrons*, in 1976 (79).

NEOPLASMS ORIGINATING FROM EPITHELIA OF EXOCRINE GLANDS. II. MAMMARY GLANDS

The normal distribution in man is self-explanatory.

The benign fibroadenoma is very common in women from 15 to 35 years of age. The connective tissue covers the ducts and ductules, which have two layers of polygonal cuboidal or columnar cells. New glandular structures are built in a more irregular way. The stroma shows different patterns.

The giant fibroadenoma occurs commonly in older women; it is characterized by the presence of abundant connective tissue and columnar and cuboidal cells of the epithelium.

Adenoma of the nipple, also benign, is most common in women from 40 to 45 years of age. Adenomatous or pseudopapillary appearance, like in sweat gland tumors (columnar epithelium and myoepithelium) is characteristic. Columnar cells may be present.

The intraduct papilloma is also benign; it is common in women. The neoplasm is composed of ductal epithelium and inner fibrous stroma. The epithelium consists of a basal layer of round cells and an inner layer of columnar cells; uniform nuclei are placed in an orderly manner. The intraductal cystadenoma which is benign also resembles the normal epithelium (579).

The human mammary cancers display a wide variety of types which can be diagnosed either as infiltrating or noninfiltrating carcinomas. The noninfiltrating carcinomas are either intraductal or interlobular and opposed to the infiltrating carcinomas which show a general group ranging from the high differentiation of adenocarcinomas to totally undifferentiated forms, as well as a number of special histological subtypes such as the medullary carcinoma, the papillary carcinoma, the cribriform carcinoma, the mucous carcinoma, the lobular carcinoma, the squamous cell carcinoma, and Paget's disease of the breast (386).

The intraductal carcinoma starts at different locations simultaneously; large, hyperchromatic cells of variable size are typical.

The human lobular carcinoma is located in the ducts of lobules and consists of disorderly arranged epithelial cells which obliterate the ducts. They have large uniform nuclei and few mitoses.

Extraductal carcinoma in man starts multicentrically and occurs as different subtypes, such as the scirrhous structure characterized by rich, hard hyaline stroma. The malignant epithelial cells occur in small clusters and nests. The neoplastic cells are flat or cuboidal. The nuclei are of different sizes; the tubular structure is adenocarcinomatous in pattern, with flat, cuboidal, or columnar epithelial cells.

The Papillary Adenocarcinoma Starts from Ducts:

The papillary pattern is characteristic but may appear obscured. Uniform hyperchromatic nuclei and common mitoses are present.

Medullary carcinoma is highly cellular and composed of large oval cells. The nuclei contain one or two nucleoli and basophilic cytoplasm; necrotic foci are common.

The colloid carcinoma exhibits extensive mu-

cin production in which the darkly staining neoplastic cells are located.

The cylindroma has a honeycombed pattern. The epithelial cells are uniform.

The sweat gland carcinoma originates in the ducts or ductules and is characterized by large cells of pale, pink appearance with glandular and tubular arrangements (this tumor is commonly known as sweat gland cancer, but this is a misnomer).

Paget's disease of the nipple exhibits large and vacuolated Paget cells.

Two cases of a rare type of carcinoma of the human breast, where the light and electron microscopic studies indicated the presence of reactive stroma giant cells, were described by Factor et al. (145). The neoplasms were reminiscent of giant cell tumors of the bone. The giant cells were found to be benign; there was also a strong inflammatory reaction in these tumors. A review of the research on the ultrastructure of the human breast under normal and pathological conditions is given by Fisher (156), and reports of metastatic mammary neoplasms are presented by Radnot (447) and Legrand and Pariente (331). For a discussion of an electron microscopic study of a human breast carcinoma cell lining (MCF-7), see Russo et al. (474).

Cribriform carcinomas are those tumors which are also described as adenoid cystic carcinoma or as cylindromas. The term seems to be unwarranted to the author.

Squamous cell carcinoma with characteristics such as spine cells or keratinization is uncommon in the breast of the human female.

Cubilla (110) described the primary carcinoid tumor of the breast as a new type of mammary cancer, characterized by small cells appearing in solid nests which are separated by fibrous tissue. The arrangement resembles this one of carcinoids in other locations of the body. The role of myoepithelial cells in human breast carcinoma (30 infiltrating ductal carcinomas, five infiltrating lobular carcinomas, five lobular carcinomas in situ and four ductal carcinomas in situ, and 10 tissue samples from dysplasia and 10 samples from patients with normal conditions) was studied by Ghosh et al. (186). The light microscopic investigation showed no remarkable changes, but the electron microscopic investigation revealed slightly swollen myoepithelium in carcinoma in situ and large size of myoepithelium in infiltrating carcinoma with an increased endoplasmic reticulum, swollen mitochondria, increased density of the chromatin membrane, and abundant microfilaments.

The angiogenic capacity and neoplastic transformation in the rat mammary gland were recently studied by Maiorana and Gullino (354) using tissue transplanted onto the rabbit iris and observed through the transparent cornea.

Whether the presence of estrogen receptors in benign or malignant tumors indicates hormonal dependence as reported in man seems to be questionable in the dog (209). For reports on the dog, see also Warner (587) and Harvey and Gilbertson (219); for reports on the cat, see Hayes (223). Malignant mammary tumors of the cat can also contain an endogenous virus different from RD-114 virus (77). Comparable studies in the mouse are reported by Kemmer et al. (288), Goldfeder (1976), Calberg-Bacq et al. (78), Nair and Gangal (391), Hakim (204), Stock et al. (530), Braunschweiger et al. (61), on the rat, studies were reported by Braunschweiger and Schiffer (59, 60). The species specificity of virus tumors in laboratory animals with respect to rarely observed species is of great interest because it allows a comparison between these specific tumors in mammals and the more general picture involving a wider range of species for leukemias and related disorders (see Chapter 25 by Fischinger and Frankel).

The mammal, distinguished by the presence of the mammary gland, appears phylogenetically, for the first time during the Triassic period. There exist a number of virus tumors which have been described as being characteristic of this class.

Several types of these tumors have not been observed, even in the well-known species of mammals; it should not be overlooked that as far as the number of mammalian species is concerned, the majority of these tumors is very characteristic and surely not restricted to the mammals which have been observed.

On the other hand, we find neoplastic diseases of the body liquids and the organs, which are caused by viruses, producing them, like bone marrow, lymphatic glands, spleen, etc. Within the framework of the vertebrates, the bone marrow is much more widely distributed than the mammary gland. These tissues are derived from the reticular connective tissue, which appears either in hemoreticular or lymphoreticular form.

Today, we suspect that various cells of the body liquids in invertebrates are not derived from reticular connective tissue but, even if mesodermal, from the pseudoepithelia of the coelom. This is the case in the peritoneum of certain annelids, which is the point of origin of the blood cells of these animals. As explained in

Chapter 25 by Fischinger and Frankel, certain oncornaviruses show very characteristic phylogenetical correlations with their hosts. Viruses and genes are related—the first may split off from the second. The degree of distribution of these conditions, derived phylogenetically on the basis of the histogenetic principle, may supply us with new insights in the area of comparative oncology, provided we are willing to pursue them.

The intraductal papillary mammary adenoma is known from *Camelus ferus arabicus*; the adenocarcinoma of the mammary gland is known from *Sarcophilus harrisi, Tupaia belangeri, Dipodomis merriami,* and *Arectictis binturong* (132); and the adenocarcinoma of mammary ducts is known from *Mus musculus* (see laboratory animals).

NEOPLASMS ARISING FROM EPITHELIA OF EXOCRINE GLANDS. III. SALIVARY GLANDS

The normal tissues in man are represented by the glandula parotis, glandula submaxillaris, and glandula sublingualis. The histogenesis of salivary gland neoplasms must be considered from two cell types, the excretory duct reserve cell and the intercalated duct reserve cell. It is believed that the former develops into squamous cells and mucoepidermoid carcinomas and the latter into all others (454). For a report on the electron microscopy of parotid tumors, see Kessoku (291).

Mixed tumors (pleomorphic adenomas) are common in man. The histochemistry of the epithelial cells and the solid and ductal portion of the tumor show a variable reaction for both ATPase and IDPase. The capsule, epithelial and myoepithelial components of different pattern and a stroma, which may be abundant or scanty and may show fibrous chondroid tissue cartilage or bone, can be distinguished. The salivary gland nature is proven by the presence of an inner layer of cuboidal or columnar cells and an outer layer of myoepithelial elements lining the ducts. Cysts and horny pearls may occur.

Monomorphic adenomas (oxyphilic adenomas) exhibit very regular epithelia in glandular arrangement, but without connective tissue components as a pleomorphic adenoma. There exist other rare types of monomorphic adenomas with different cellular patterns of epithelial cells (tubular, alveolar, trabecular, basal-like, clear and varying participation of myoepithelial cells. The ultrastructure of the basal cell adenoma of the parotis revealed four types of cells: the squamous epithelial cells with tonofilaments and prominent desmosomes, mainly in the center of the neoplasm; basally located secretory cells with granules; less numerous intermediate cells with scanty cytoplasmic microfilaments; and peripherally located myoepithelial cells (265). In other cases of the same tumor, the fine structure was characterized by numerous desmosomes, large secretory granules, and a replication of the basal lamina. In contrast, myoepithelial cells were not observed (345). Carcinoma in pleomorphic adenomas, also known as malignant mixed tumor, is composed of areas showing the characteristics of malignancy and simultaneously those of pleomorphic adenoma.

Adenocarcinoma exhibits a tubular or papillary glandular pattern without remnants of the pleomorphic adenoma. The histochemistry and ultrastructure of the neoplasm reveals large amounts of cytoplasmic microfilaments (114). Adenocarcinoma of the glandular epithelium of the oral cavity is known from *Protemnodon rufogrisea* and *Chrysocyon aureus syriacus* (132).

For carcinoma in the horse, see Stackhouse *et al.* (523), and for metastases of this type of tumor in the dog, see Grevel *et al.* (199).

The oncocytoma (oxyphilic adenoma), which is also benign, is rare in humans and shows lobes and lobules with separated fibroconnective tissue. Large oval cells with granular eosinophilic cytoplasm and pycnotic nuclei with marked nucleolus can be observed. The malignant oncocytoma is rare and is characterized by mitotic activity, pleomorphism, and an increased number of closely packed mitochondria (327).

The benign adenolymphoma occurring most commonly in men older than 40 years comprises 6% of the epithelial tumors of salivary glands. The tumor starts from epithelial nests in lymph nodes. Epithelial and lymphatic components are characteristic.

The acinic carcinoma is rare in man. Capsule, glandular elements, and scanty stroma can be distinguished. Glandular elements are serous cells, with ample bluish cytoplasm; small dark-staining eccentric nuclei are characteristic.

The adenocystic carcinoma represents 7% of all epithelial salivary gland neoplasms in man. Cords of basal cells, arranged in two layers, can be found around cavities. A wide variation in patterns occurs. Acidic mucosubstances with varying histochemical properties were present

in different structures of the neoplasm, such as chondroitin 4- and/or 6-sulfate, polysaccharides of relatively low degree of sulfation, and nonsulfated acid mucin (52).

The mucoepidermoid cancer is composed of squamous cells, mucin-secreting cells, clear epidermoid, basal, columnar, and oxyphilic cells. A variation in pattern occurs.

The epidermoid cancer represents 3% of all epithelial salivary gland tumors in man. Epidermoid squamous cells and fibrous stroma are characteristic.

Undifferentiated carcinoma shows mainly cells which are spherical in form or spindle-like but are also epithelial in character. The cells of these tumors are not sufficiently differentiated to be categorized with the other cell types and therefore with cancers of salivary glands.

Neoplasms of salivary glands are theoretically possible in vertebrates and invertebrates as well as in plants. In invertebrates, the phyla affected are the rotifera (only in juvenile stages because of cell invariability), gastrotricha, kinorhyncha, nematoda, mollusca, annelida, onychophora, tardigrada (possibly only in juvenile stages, according to the unexplained question of cell invariability), and arthropoda.

Vertebrate salivary glands show the following picture: Often, they are considered to be oral glands. Aquatic mammals have poorly developed salivary glands; herbivorous mammals have the best developed ones. Edentata have a small parotid gland, the submaxillary (submandibulary in man) are the largest in these animals. Seven sets of salivary glands are found in birds (Patt and Patt (422, p. 167). The structure of reptilian salivary glands is diffuse or compact as in the lizard, but is generally comparable to the condition in amphibians (ref. 422), (p. 163). In amphibians lingual intermaxillary and pharyngeal glands can be distinguished (ref. 422, p. 160). Oral glands are practically not present in fishes or aquatic amphibians (ref. 290, p. 315).

Glands in plants which are to a certain degree comparable are those of the carnivorous plants, belonging to the dicotyledones; 1st order Polycariacae, 15th family nepenthaceae, such as *Nepenthes* sp.; 16th family Cephalotoceae, genus *Cephalotus*; 17th family Sarraceniaceae, with the genera *Sarracenia* and the related *Darlingtonia*; the 7th order of Parietales with the 3rd family Droseracea with the genera *Drosera* (*Drosera rotundifolia*), *Dionaea*, *Aldrovanda*, and *Drosophyllum*; the 34th order Personatae, 4th family Lentibulariaceae, and the genera *Utricularia* and *Pinguicula*. The glandular structures on flowers or leaves of these plants secrete digestive juices to extract primarily nitrogen from their animal victims. The secretions contain the same digestive compounds as those from the comparable glands of animals, but these plant species are at the same time autotrophic. These glands can also be compared to glandular structures from the digestive tract of animals. New experiments such as feeding these plants with animals or meat pieces contaminated with carcinogens, especially water-soluble carcinogens, could result in highly interesting discoveries (see Chapters 3 and 4).

NEOPLASMS ARISING FROM EPITHELIA OF EXOCRINE GLANDS. IV. LIVER[5] (HEPATIC PORTION OF HEPATOPANCREAS)

The organ in man of concern is the liver. It is questionable whether the extremely rare cyst-adenoma is a true benign neoplasm in man. It is a papillary structure of cysts filled with mucinous material and lined by one or more layers of cuboidal or columnar cells. Embryonic tumors of the liver, either benign or malignant, are also rare in man. they are characterized by embryonal cells, differentiated or undifferentiated epithelial and mesenchymal components.

An embryonic type of hepatocyte at the ultrastructural level was seen in a mixed hamartoma of human liver by Rhodes et al. (455).

Also extremely rare in man is the benign adenoma, composed of well-differentiated cells, which may be vacuolated; some are atypical. Portal ducts, bile ducts and central vessels are absent. Human primary cancers of the liver exhibit remarkable race and geographic differences. Some are uncommon, for example, in caucasians but common in negroid and mongoloid races (see Chapter 36). Different types of cancers can be distinguished in the liver. The qualitative formation of benzo(a)pyrene metabolites by salamander hepatic microsomes was similar to that in other species. The animals of the species *Ambystoma tigrinum* found in a sewage-polluted pond had a high rate of spontaneous cancer (Busbee et al. (76)).

Liver cell cancer shows massive or nodular

distribution. The growth of the eosinophilic neoplastic cells occurs in cordlike fashion, the outer cells may be low columnar, cystlike spaces occur, the stroma is scanty and the differentiation varies. Thirty-two percent (20 of 62) of the English sole (*Parophys vetulus*) from the Duvamish river estuary, Seattle, Washington showed hepatomas; 92 percent of the fish had some form of liver abnormalities (Pierce et al. (429)). Spontaneous hepatocellular cancer in sand rats (*Psammomys obesus*) range from nodules in which the hepatocytes showed hyperbasophilin, glycogen-accumulation, eosinophilic cytoplasm in different cellular mixture at the age of 6 months, which changed in animals of 25 months to hepatocellular cancer. A chemically carcinogenic influence could be secured and the identity, so claim the authors of this gerbil and the laboratory rat support the assumption of a general law of carcinogenesis (Ungar and Adler (567)). The assumption concerning rodents may be true but if it is the case in liver carcinogenesis in a species specific view generally cannot be answered positively or negatively before more species of more orders are investigated under similar circumstances.

The kinetic patterns of L-threonine and L-serine dehydratosis from mouse hepatomas were distinct from normal liver tissue of the mouse, strain CBA (Akopov et al. (3)).

Recent studies on hepatoma of the liver have shown that the internal organization of hepatoma mitochondria, as determined by stereological analysis of electron micrographs of cross sections through cells and by measuring the surface areas of the mitochondrial envelope and cristae membranes differs distinctly from that of normal liver mitochondria (Volman (578)). Other studies involving human hepatoma cells were performed by Kendrey and Laszlo (289) who located coat and core of a hepatitis B virus in parenchymal cells of a liver biopsy; by MacNab and co-workers (350) who found a hepatitis B surface antigen and the association between this antigen and primary liver cancer. The relationship between hepatic tumors and oral contraceptives was studied by Balazs (28) and Fechner (152). Undulating membranous structures associated with the endoplastic reticulum in tumor cells were investigated by Schaff et al. (482). Other studies of interest include the following. Reddy et al (450) have reported on the induction of liver tumors by aflatoxin B1 in the tree shrew (*Tupaia glis*), a non-human primate. Bryant et al. (68) have studied ultrastructural and metabolic determinants of resistance to azo-

---

[5] A precise quantitative analysis of DNA repair in cultured rat hepatocytes after different exposures was given in 1978 (610).

dye susceptibility to nitrosamine carcinogenesis of the guinea pig. Strombeck and co-workers (534) have reported on hypoglycemia and hypoinsulinemia associated with hepatoma in a dog. Bucana and others (69) have searched for morphological evidence for the translocation of lysosomal organelles from cytotoxic macrophages into the cytoplasm of tumor target cells.

Studies involving mice and rats include those of Becker et al. (40) on serum α-fetoprotein in a mouse strain with spontaneous hepatocellular carcinomas; Novi (402) of liver carcinogenesis following aflatoxin B1 administration; Helyer and Petrelli (233) of cytoplasmic inclusions in spontaneous hepatomas of mice; Ishihara *et al.* (260) on ultrastructural changes of intercellular junctions in rat ascites hepatoma cells with calcium depletion; Hanaoka *et al* (211) have performed a biochemical and morphological comparison of two tumour-cell-aggregation factors; Katsuya *et al.* (281) have investigated dissociation of rat ascites hepatoma cells under activation of neutral protease and calcium depletion.

Bannasch (29) on studying the cytology and cytogenesis of neoplastic (hyperplastic) hepatic nodules has found that at least four different types of altered hepatocytes can be distinguished: (a) "clear" glycogen storage cells with a dislocation and relative reduction of the granular endoplasmic reticulum; (b) "acidophilic" glycogen storage cells with a hypertrophy of the agranular endoplasmic reticulum; (c) fat-storing cells; and (d) basophilic cells poor in glycogen and rich in ribosomes. In addition, Bannasch found diverse intermediate cell types. Also, it was seen that the clear and the acidophilic cells precede the development of the neoplastic nocules by weeks and months (preneoplastic lesions?). During the formation of neoplastic nodules and hepatocellular carcinomas originating from foci the glycogen of the clear and the acidophilic cells is progressively reduced, whereas the number of ribosomes (basophilia) increases. Neoplastic nodules in which basophilic cells prevail may already be carcinomas. Although the neoplastic nodules seem to be a frequent precursor of hepatocellular carcinomas, the latter may also develop without going through the nodule stage.

An extensive treatise on viral hepatitis was published by Krugman and Gocke (310).

Cholangiocarcinoma in man accounts for approximately 10–22% of primary epithelial neoplasms of the organ. The neoplasm is a well-differentiated adenocarcinoma with fibrous stroma. Different patterns (tubular, papillar) oc-

cur and the lining is simple and composed of cuboidal or columnar cells. Clear cytoplasms and small and round or oval nuclei characterize the cells. Signet-ring cells may occur.

Cholangiocellular carcinoma is extremely rare in man, and composed of neoplastic variants of the smallest bile ducts. A cordlike appearance is characteristic. The cells are small, faintly eosinophilic, cuboidal, flattened or irregular.

Cholangiohepatocarcinoma can be seen as a variant of the liver cell cancer. Liver cell and cholangiocarcinomatous and bridging elements are typical.

The carcinoid tumor of the liver is composed of argentaffin cells of bile duct epithelium.

Because of tissue distribution, neoplasms of this tissue type are theoretically possible in mollusca, arthropoda, echinodermata, tunicata, cephalochordata and vertebrata. On a limited basis, a comparison to glandular structures of carnivorous plants (see pp. 90 and 91) is also possible. Some cases of occurrence in vertebrates shall be mentioned: cystadenoma has been described in *Salmo gairdneri*; the adenoma has been described in *Prionace glauca*, *Salmo gairdneri*, *Salmo trutta*; and the liver has been described in the hagfish, *Myxine glutinosa*, and the river lamprey, *Lampetra fluviatilis* (146).

Adenomatous proliferation in intrahepatic bile ducts may be considered as a preneoplastic condition and was observed in the reptile *Malacocherus tornieri*; in the birds *Coturnix chinensis lineata*, *Platycercus eximius eximius*, *Agapornis nigrigenis*, and *Pharmomachrus mocinno costaricensis*; and in mammals *Protemnodon agilis jardani* and *Cercopithecus diana roloway*.

Biliary adenoma occurred in the reptiles *Dispholidus typus* and *Cyclura ricordi*; biliary adenocarcinoma occurred in the reptile *Agkistrodon halys brevicaudus*; in the birds *Anser caerulescens caerulescens*, *Lophophorus impejanus*, *Agapornis lilianae*, *Agriocharis ocellata*, and *Pitta erythrogaster macklotti*; and the mammal *Cervus axis axis*.

The hepatoma is known from the bird Cissa chinensis and Lemur macaco macaco (132). A scirrhous biliary adenocarcinoma was seen in the Gaboon viper *Bitis gabonica gabonica*.

Other studies of nonhuman liver neoplasms include those of Patnaik *et al.* (417) on extraskeletal osteosarcomas of the liver in a dog, those of Jurgelski *et al.* (275) of embryonal neoplasms in the opossum, those of Koppang and Rimesl-Atten (302) on toxic and carcinogenic effects of nitrosodimethylamine in mink, those of Hasler and Van den Ingh on malignant mastocytosis and duodenal ulceration in a cat, those of Pour et al. (434–437) in Syrian hamsters, and those of Adler et al. (1) in sand rats.

NEOPLASMS ARISING FROM EPITHELIA OF EXOCRINE GLANDS. V. EXOCRINE PORTION OF PANCREAS AND PANCREATIC PORTION OF HEPATOPANCREAS

The organ in man of concern is the exocrine pancreas and tissue nests in accessory position.

The epithelial exocrine tumors of the pancreas, as of other big glands, in vertebrates and invertebrates can be divided into neoplasms arising from the epithelium of the ducts and those arising from the glandular epithelium. Of course, there are intermediate or indistinguishable cases! The neoplasms found in invertebrates especially are not diagnosed exactly enough at this time to be compared to man. The reason for this lies in the difficulty of direct comparison and lack of experience, and less in insufficient work.

Neoplasia arising from the epithelia of the ducts are the benign adenomas which are tubular in character. They are distinguished from the non-neoplastic cysts by their epithelial lining. The epithelium is simple columnar; it may also be flat in the adenomas per se and cuboidal in cystadenomas. Frequently, papillary processes with cuboidal or columnar epithelium occur, and the stroma may become myxomatous. The distinction between cystadenomas and cystadenocarcinomas is often hard to make, especially when the epithelium becomes more developed and pseudostratified.

The malignant neoplasms of this group are the carcinomas of the ducts or the adenocarcinomas; they exhibit cuboidal or columnar cells, and are the most frequent type of human pancreatic cancers. Ducts and tubules are usually irregular but may be well developed; goblet cells may be present. Subtypes are: the colloidal (gelatinous) uncommon cancers originating from goblet cells of the larger ducts; the adenocancroids; the squamous cell cancers (adenoacanthomatous cancers or mucoepidermoid cancers) characterized by squamous cell epithelial features, derived by metaplasia; and the anaplastic forms, which may resemble sarcomas.

Because of their tissue origin, these ductular

neoplasms actually belong into the sections on cuboidal or columnar epithelia, but they have been discussed here because they often intermingle with forms arising from the glandular epithelia (parenchyma) of the exocrine gland. They are also the most frequent neoplasms of this organ in man; these in turn account for approximately 1% of all the neoplasms found in all organs.

Adenomatous proliferation of intrapancreatic ducts occurs comparable to the liver and ducts in other glands and was seen in *Macropus robustus erubescens*, an adenoma in the bird *Balbopsittacus lunulatus lunulatus*; a biliary adenoma in the head of the pancreas of the Giant pitta, *Pitta caerulea caerulea*; the adenoma of intrapancreatic ducts in Felis chaus furax; the adenocarcinoma of intrapancreatic ducts in *Zalophus californianus*; the scirrhous adenocarcinoma of intrapancreatic ducts in *Bothrops atrax*, a reptile; the adenocarcinoma of pancreatic ducts in the Tiger rat snake, *Spilotes pullatus* and the Southwestern speckled rattlesnake, *Crotalus mitchelli phyrrhus* and in the bird *Geopelia striata striata* (132). A discussion at this point results in an easier comparison of the invertebrate analogs to the vertebrate tumors.

The islets in areas of exocrine cancers remain normal for a considerable time; this is important to know if we compare the exocrine neoplasms of the vertebrate pancreas to corresponding components of the invertebrate hepatopancreas, because invertebrates have no islands of Langerhans. Additionally, it must be understood that in a comparison between mammalian pancreas and liver on the one side and the hepatopancreas of invertebrates on the other, the parenchymata can be compared exactly, but fewer the epithelia of the ducts; however, this must be done not on the basis of the organs but exclusively on the basis of the epithelial ductular lining from which the pathologic lesion derives. It is of phylogenetic importance that Frantz (167) and Sommers and Meissner (518) described a ciliated type of adenocarcinoma of the human pancreas, when we remember that ciliated cells occur normally in the hepatopancreas of molluscs. The lower vertebrates may comprise intermediate positions.

The neoplasia of the exocrine epithelia of the mammalian (human) pancreas and perhaps of corresponding parenchyma (glandular epithelia) of the hepatopancreas of invertebrates are the benign exocrine acinous adenomas and the parenchymal pancreatic cancers of this type in the acinous gland. These benign adenomas are extremely rare, but their postulation is theoretically justified. Priesel described such benign adenoma in 1928 (439).

The malignant form of the acinar cell carcinomas occurs infrequently. The cells are polygonal and well-distinguished borders or small roundish cells with mainly undistinguishable borders.

The normal distribution and therefore the theoretical possibility of neoplasms is given in mollusca, arthropoda, and vertebrata. A comparison with the glands in carnivorous plants is possible.

As to recent investigations of interest, the following deserve to be mentioned: Occurrences of neoplasms with at least partial involvement of the hepatopancreas (pancreatic portion) and related structures in invertebrates have been observed. Cases of mollusca have been reported in bivalves by Rosenfield (465), Mix (382), Farley (148), Cooper (104), Wolf (603), Frierman and Andrews (169), and Lowe and Moore (344); they have been reported in aquatic pulmonate snails by Michelson and Richards (377). Several of these described cases involved proliferative atypical hemocytes, as in the cases of Lowe and Moore in which the terminal stage of the pathologic lesion in *Mytilus edulis* showed a replacement of connective tissue and necrosis of the cells of the digestive gland. Cooper commented in 1976 that the neoplasms in these animals, the molluscs, resemble certain cancers in vertebrates, but that it is not clear whether a relationship exists between the invertebrate immune system and the development of neoplasia. There are surely certain comparabilities between the neoplasms with an involvement in pancreas and hepatopancreas, even if only partially involved, which need further intensive investigation.

Of interest also are the studies dealing with neoplastic lesions in *Drosophila melanogaster* by Gateff (179, 180), in the roach by Bucke (71), in the tiger salamander by Rose (463), and in reptiles by Elkan and Cooper (133). Studies concerning zoo animals have been described by Ermoshchenkov and Khudolei (139), Effron *et al.* (132), and by Barahona *et al.* in the owl monkey (*Aotus trivirgatus*) (30). Studies dealing with spontaneous pancreatic neoplasms in laboratory rodents are numerous (see refs. 10, 73, 388, 542, and 549 for the rat, refs. 421 and 466 for the mouse, ref. 293 for the hamster, and ref. 339 for arvicoline rodents).

Reports concerning other animals deal with the Indian water buffalo (201), horses and cattle (273), goats (618), dogs and cats (308), and monkeys (311).

NEOPLASMS ARISING FROM EPITHELIA OF ENDOCRINE GLANDS. I. ISLETS OF LANGERHANS

The tissue occurs in the islets of Langerhans or the endocrine pancreas. In man the benign neoplasm is the adenoma or benign nesidioblastoma, composed of abundant vessels, with parenchymatic cells arranged in a cord-like manner, or in one to three rows of cells if measured crosswise. The cells are of cuboidal or columnar form.

The endocrine cells of the gastrointestinal tract and the neoplasms arising from them are reviewed by Dawson (116).

The insulinoma is known from the hagfish *Myxine glutinosa* and the river lamprey, *Lampetra fluviatalis* (146); from domesticated and laboratory animals such as the dog (269, 361, 373, 374); from the rat, arising from B-cells as diagnosed by electron microscopy (304); and from the hamster (504). See also Chapter 48.[6]

The malignant neoplasm is the islet cell cancer or malignant nesidioblastoma. The neoplasms are larger and less well separated from the surrounding tissues than the benign counterparts, and they show more disorganization. Abundant regular and irregular mitoses, large nucleoli, and necroses are present. Malignant islet cell tumors are, according to Hess (237), who considered only 26 cases in 1950, as proof, very rare. Nizze (401) reports that a medullary island cell carcinoma of the pancreas with liver and peritoneal metastases which may have been derived from A1 (D) islet cells was found in a 10-year-old girl.

The occurrence of the epithelium and therefore the possibility of growth of those tumors is restricted to the vertebrata. This tumor is also well known in dogs (272, 373, 374) and the rat (73).

NEOPLASMS ARISING FROM EPITHELIA OF ENDOCRINE GLANDS. II. PINEAL GLAND

The pinealoma, an extremely rare tumor in man, of which some variations may be considered gliomas, is composed of parenchymal cells

---

[6] The islet cell adenomatosis of the pancreas is known from the spider monkey, *Ateles geoffroyi,* and the islet cell adenoma of pancreas from *Hystrix brachyura javanicum* (132).

of the pineal. It is more or less possible to distinguish among three subtypes, with the pinealoma or atypical teratoma of the pineal body, the most common tumor of this group, occurring in benign and malignant variations. Inner large epithelioid and outer small lymphocytoid cells which stain darkly are responsible for the mosaic-like appearance. Virus-like particles, perhaps from the herpes, leuro, or arena groups, have been seen in a human pinealoma (313). The second variation, occurring either in benign or malignant form, is the pinealocytoma, which is composed of pineal cells and fibrovascular stroma. The pinealoblastoma is the undifferentiated variation of the former subtype. The normal distribution of the tissue and the theoretical expectance of these tumors is restricted to the vertebrates.

NEOPLASMS ARISING FROM EPITHELIA OF ENDOCRINE GLANDS. III. PITUITARY GLAND

The neoplasms of the pituitary gland have to be differentiated into those from the anterior lobe and those from the neurohypophysis.

The craniopharyngioma, a benign tumor, comprises 3% of all intercranial tumors in man. A thin capsule, abundant stroma, epithelial columns with cylindrical cells at the outside, and stellate cells in the center can be distinguished. Cystic spaces are abundant. It simulates an adamantinoma.

Another benign tumor in man is the adenoma which lacks a capsule. The chromophobe adenoma has cylindrical, polygonal, or spindle-like cells arranged in a sinusoidal or diffuse pattern. The *eosinophil (acidophil) adenoma* has large encapsulated strumas and shows cysts. It generally occurs as a diffuse structure with islands and fibrovascular stroma; some cells have giant nuclei, with different granules present in the cells. *Basophil adenomas* are characterized by polygonal basophilic cells and granulation.

ACTH-secreting tumors are of interest in relation to the Cushing syndrome after adrenalectomy.

The malignant tumor in man is the carcinoma of the adenohypophysis, which accounts for 3–4% of pituitary tumors. Most cells lack specific granules, they are strongly pleomorphic, and they appear in different patterns around vessels.

The neoplasms of the neurohypophysis include, on one hand, some rare gliomas and, on the other, some questionable forms as well as the extremely rare teratoma with subtypes also known as ectopic pinealomas.

A chromophobe adenoma of the pituitary was observed in *Ovis ammon musimon.*

An adenoma of the anterior lobe of *Equus burchelli* was described, but it must be recognized that in cases where the taxonomy of the human neoplasms is still debated, the taxonomy in other species is not secured.

Pituitary neoplasms have been seen in dogs (614), including the basophil adenoma (285); the acidophilic adenoma in the cat (183) and the pituitary carcinoma with metastasis in a cow (438); in the sheep (151), and of course in different strains of the rat (11, 257, 305, 306, 388, 541).

NEOPLASMS ARISING FROM EPITHELIA OF ENDOCRINE GLANDS. IV. THYROID GLAND

The benign tumor in man is the adenoma characterized by a capsule, a uniform structure differing from healthy tissue by the lack of colloid.

The follicles of autonomous adenomas are small or normal sized; the lining is columnar, and the cells are partly vacuolated with eosinophilic cytoplasm. The thyroid globulin content, which is high, parallels the rough endoplasmic reticulum. The electron microscope reveals a well-developed network of cavities of the cells and generally apically located lysosomes. The Golgi area is prominent and characterized by vesicles and vacuoles. In contrast to nonfunctioning adenomas the cell surface shows long microvilli and basally deep infoldings in the apical region ((126), see also (414)).

With regard to malignant tumors in man the comparison to other species is difficult due to the large variety of histological patterns. This difficulty is proven by the special classifications of malignant thyroid tumors (131, 218, 334, 540). For example, poorly differentiated follicular carcinoma exhibited during ultrastructural analysis simultaneously features of papillary carcinoma, follicular adenoma, anaplastic carcinoma, and through the presence of secretory granules a medullary carcinoma (284). The carcinoma of the thyroid exhibits infiltrative capabilities and pleomorph or atypical cells. The differentiated adenocarcinoma and the undifferentiated carcinoma with subtypes can be distinguished.

Differentiated Adenocarcinoma

The first subtype is the papillary adenocarcinoma characterized by semicystic to firm consistency, lack of colloid, cuboidal or columnar epithelium which lines the connective tissue axes in simple rows. The occult sclerosing carcinoma in turn is a subtype of the former exhibiting no capsule and calcification and comprising small tumors of stellate pattern. The ultrastructure of the neoplastic cells of the papillary carcinoma shows large pleomorphic cysternae, irregularly shaped mitochondria, dense bodies, phagolysosomes and lamellar or multivesicular structures (97). The second subtype of the differentiated adenocarcinoma is the follicular (acinar) adenocarcinoma composed of microfollicular structure and scanty cytoplasm.

The ultrastructural relief of follicular carcinomas is irregular containing follicles of different sizes and shapes. The irregularities also apply to the internal surface of the neoplastic follicles. Abundant microvilli occur at the apical region of the follicular cells. Cells of cylindrical or high columnar form with the abundant microvilli, the well-developed ergastic plasmic reticulum, and the hypertrophic Golgi complexes predominate (97).

Peroxidase activity in the epithelial cells of follicular and papillary carcinomas is mainly found in the membrane of the rough endoplasmic reticulum, the perinuclear space, and the outer membrane of the microvilli (96).

The last subtype of the differentiated adenocarcinoma is the solid alveolar (medullary) adenocarcinoma. It lacks follicular pattern, sheetlike parenchyma, and stroma. The cell forms are round to bizarre.

Cellular degeneration of particulate and fibrillar matters is considered to be the precursor of ameloid deposits in the medullary carcinoma of the thyroid. The ultrastructure of the stored granules shows heterogenicity and contains immunoreactive calcitonin (250).

The tumor cells representing a diverse picture exhibit a strong activity of oxidative and hydrolytic enzymes. Specific endocrine types of secretory granules are present (45); for a discussion of the familial appearance, see Schürch et al. (492) as well as Metz and Levine (371) concerning the reaction of active peptides and amines.

The squamous carcinoma is very rare in the thyroid of man; it is metaplastic in origin and may show even keratinization and whorls.

In addition to the differentiated adenocarcinoma, the second main group of thyroid carcinoma in man, the undifferentiated carcinoma, comprises about 15–20% of the primary neoplasms. The cells exhibit the characteristic after which the following neoplasms are named: round cell cancer, spindle cell cancer, pleomorphic cancer, giant cell cancer, and small cell cancer.

During transformation to malignancy the enzyme pattern in the mitochondria of the thyroid changes, and a remarkable decrease in enzyme activity seems to characterize the qualitative changes of the mitochondria, which changes also morphologically (122). Receptor techniques may be valuable to distinguish anaplastic thyroid tumors from malignant lymphoma (348).

Rare Miscellaneous Tumors

They are somewhat problematic and mentioned here only with the greatest of reservation for the sake of completeness. They may contain epithelial elements of the thyroid, or may be mixed in character, such as the Hürtle cell tumor.

With respect to epithelial neoplasms, this organ also contains the hemangioendothelioma, the teratomas, and the mixed tumors. Certain elements in these tumors may have a relationship to thyroid parenchyma. Cytology is an accurate and reliable method also in preoperative diagnostic procedure (446).

Woodhead et al. (607) studied the appearance of thyroid neoplasia in aged amazon mollies, *Poecilia formosa*, and the same group of researchers used this fish as a model to study DNA damage (501). The pretumorous thyroid gland was studied in the teleost, *Poecilia formosa* as well as other species of the same group of fishes (606).

The neoplasms of this tissue type, due to the normal distribution of it, are restricted to the vertebrates. Adenomas of the thyroid have been reported in *Xiphophorus helleri*, *Ovis ammon musimon* (thyroid medullary adenoma), *Echidna sp.*, *Sarcophilus harrisii*, and *Lycaon lupinus*.

Carcinoma of the thyroid was described in *Geomyda trijuga* and *Iguana iguana*. The differentiated adenocarcinoma (without mentioning the subtypes) was studied in *Salmo trutta*, *Salmo sp.*, *Rutilus rutilus*(?), and *Angelichthys isabelita*.

In the Andean goose, *Chloeophaga melanoptera*, an adenocarcinoma of thyroid, was seen.

In domesticated and laboratory animals, thyroid neoplasms have been observed in the dog (615); cow (577); goat (467); horse (274); rat (10,

11, 73, 206, 388, 588); and the Syrian hamster (434–437).

NEOPLASMS ARISING FROM EPITHELIA OF ENDOCRINE GLANDS. V. PARATHYROID GLAND AND ULTIMOBRANCHIAL GLAND, RESPECTIVELY

The normal tissue in man occurs in the form of the parenchyma of the parathyroid gland. The benign neoplasm is the adenoma: a capsule and cystic cavities may be present. The tumor inside and the normal tissue outside the capsule are separated. The stroma divides the parenchymal tissue of the tumor. Cuboidal and columnar cells, some transitional (clusters), and oxyphilic cells occur. Cell composition differs. The nonfunctional adenoma is considered to be a variation of the neoplasm.

The carcinoma of the parathyroid is rare in man. The histologic and cellular pattern is similar to the adenoma. Invasion, recurrence, and metastasis are the criteria of malignancy. The distribution of the normal tissues and the possibility of tumorigenesis are restricted to vertebrates. The ultrastructure of abnormal hyperfunction was studied from hyperplasia, adenoma, and carcinoma of the parathyroid to correlate with the ultrastructure of hormone secretion (93). The tissue of adenoma shows a sparsity of secretory granules; see also Murayama et al. (389), Nilsson (399), and Yamaguchi (612). The morphologic changes of parathyroid adenomas permit us to distinguish between adenomas of main cells, oxyphilic, and C-cells (403).

A parathyroid adenocarcinoma in a German short-haired pointer consisted of clear cells with well-established boundaries against a tender stroma. The cells contained few organelles, irregularly distributed glycogen, clear cytosole, prominent infoldings of the plasma membranes, and desmosomes (419); see also Legendre et al. (329) for data on the dog and Wegiel et al. (588) for data on the rat.

The ultimobranchial body is the equivalent of the parathyroid in fishes, composed of epithelioid cells and delicate connective tissues capsule, located between the ventral wall of the esophagus and aorta or sinus venosus (422). Neoplasms are not known to the author.

NEOPLASMS ARISING FROM EPITHELIA OF ENDOCRINE GLANDS. VI AND VII. ADRENAL CORTEX AND MEDULLA (INTERRENAL AND CHROMAFFIN TISSUES)

Adrenal cortex and medulla are the characteristic tissues in man. In the cortex, the benign neoplasm of the tissue in man is the struma suprarenalis. It is a tumor with adenomatous characteristics which mimics zona fasciculata and, in regions, also zona glomerulosa. The carcinoma shows anastomosing columns or solid alveoli or sheets of compact and clear cells, multiple nuclei, and frequent mitoses. In the medulla, the very rare benign pheochromocytoma as the benign tumor of the medulla in man exhibits large epithelial cells with very rare acidophilic cytoplasm. The stroma is rich in capillaries.

In man, the pheochromoblastoma is the rare malignant variant of the benign tumor.

The normal tissue distribution is restricted to the vertebrates and so is the possibility of tumorigenesis. Adrenal cortical adenomas are known from *Synoicus australis, Pionus senilis decoloratus* (all birds), and *Ovis ammon musimon*; a carcinoma of the adrenal cortex was described from *Meleagris* sp. Pheochromocytomas are known from the California glossy snake, *Arizona elegans occidentalis,* and *Ovis ammon musimon*. Adrenal gland neoplasms are known from domesticated animals such as the dog (phaeochromocytoma, adrenal carcinoma, and others) (89, 153, 596) and from laboratory animals such as Syrian hamster and rat (11, 189, 434–437, 589).

NEOPLASMS ARISING FROM GERMINAL EPITHELIUM[7] AND ORGAN-RELATED STRUCTURES (ENDOCRINE GLANDS). VIII. TESTES

Testical tumors can always be considered as being malignant in man.

---

[7] In the vertebrate, for example, the mammal, the germinal glands with the germinal parenchyma (epithelium) are also endocrine structures. This is not the case in all animal phyla. In contrast, they perform no endocrine function, for example, in insects. As we have chosen to take the neoplasms of man according to the tissues they originate from as the focal arrangement of discussion for animal neoplasms, the sex glands are described concerning their neoplasms with the endocrine glands.

The seminoma is a monstrous structure, the cells of which are round, with columnar arrangement, uniform and 15 to 20 μm in ϕ. For a report on the ultrastructure in the dog, see ref. 581.

Teratoma shows a mixed pattern, differentiated and undifferentiated elements, nests of squamous epithelium, and tooth buds; horny pearls may occur. Mixed tissue derivatives (three germ layers) can be found with glandular epithelium and undifferentiated components.

The embryonal cancer is characterized by large pleomorphic cells, large nuclei, connective tissue, stroma, and giant cells.

In the choriocarcinoma, trophoblastic elements occur; necrosis and hemorrhage are very prominent.

The testicular adenocarcinoma in infancy shows undifferentiated and differentiated epithelium and mesenchymal structures, vacuolated cells, and adenopapillary appearance of nonvacuolated cells. The stroma is loose, myxomatous, or fibroblastic.

The interstitial cell tumor comprises 1.2–2% of all neoplasms found in the testes of man. According to von Albertini (579), until 1949 not more than approximately 30 cases had been described. On the other hand, the occurrence of spontaneous neoplasms in the rat strain CHBB: THOM (SPF), observed over a period of almost 3 years by Tilov et al. (549), showed the highest tumor rate of 34.5% for this tumor in the male animals. The tumor originating from Leydig and/or gonadal cells is encapsulated. The cells are large and polygonal; the cytoplasm is eosinophilic, containing lipochrome or lipids. Vacuolizations are possible. The nuclei are well defined, with chromatin and nucleolus. Giant nuclei may occur; the stroma is tender.

The tubular adenoma arises from Sertoli cells and is composed of tubules of pseudostratified epithelium. They resemble the mesenchymal stroma of the testes (?) and contain epithelial and mesenchymal elements.

The male germinal tissues have a wide distribution occurring in invertebrates, in the majority of species in metazoans (diffuse or organoid), in vertebrates, and also in the form of male germ cells (isogamous and unisogamous) and tissues in plants. The variation occurring in the organisms concerned is tremendous, and it must be realized that to undertake a review of their comparability is a bold beginning. This last fact can be kept well in mind if we start to think about the different hormonal relationships of these tissue structures in the various organisms. Teratomas have been found in *Lumbricus terrestris*

and *Cyprinus carpio* as well as *Cryptobranchus allegheniesis*. For observations in other, especially more common species, see Chapters 13 and 48.

Seminomas in birds have been described in *Threskiornis aethiopicus, Anas platyrhynchos laysanensis* (three cases, one metastatic), *Coturnix lineata* (bilateral), *Aratinga holochlora holochlora,* and *Psittacula cyanocephala bengalensi.*

Two types of Sertoli cell tumors (one with abundant Sertoli cells with little or no lipid content and small numbers of germinal cells, and the other with abundant spermatogonia and Sertoli cells with large amounts of lipids and smooth endoplasmic reticulum) are found in Lake Ontario carp (*Cyprinus carpio*) and goldfish (*Carassius auratus*) and their F_1 hybrids (323). The same authors (520) compared the state of the pituitary in such tumor-bearing fish with that in normal fish.

In birds, Sertoli's cell tumors are known from *Dendrocygna viduata,* and the white face tree duck *Gallus gallus murghi,* as well as from the clouded leopard *Neofelis nebulosa nebulosa.* In domestic and laboratory animals, Sertoli cell tumor, interstitial cell tumor, and seminoma are found to be approximately equal to the dog, but the cellular origin of testicular tumors varies in different breeds (224; see also refs. 65 and 526). The boxer is known as the most tumor-prone breed of dogs. In one case, nine simultaneously occurring primary tumors have been described, including an interstitial cell tumor and seminoma (441); see for other breeds, refs. 67, 287, 330, 338. The Brown-Pearse carcinoma in rabbits shows a high proliferation activity of cells (to 1%), high chromosome variability (to 34%), and a high genome variability (to 60%). Concerning the presence of Sertoli cell tumors in other species, see ref. 315 for the bull, see ref. 10 for data on the rat, and see ref. 220 for data on cell-free systems.

NEOPLASMS ARISING FROM GERMINAL EPITHELIUM AND ORGAN-RELATED STRUCTURES (ENDOCRINE GLANDS. IX) OVARIES

The ovaries are the organs of concern in humans. From a comparative point of view, cell structures with ovarial functions occur as female sex organs in a compact or diffuse version in the different animal phyla. The topographic structure of the sex organs, including outer sexual organs, vagina, uterus, and oviduct of the human female, permits even a comparison with the topographic arrangement of such angiosperms as the snowdrop. The cell type of chief central concern is the female sex cell, the ovum, in all its various stages of development. Therefore, the germ cell tumors must be the center of discussion in this section. Sernov and Scully list the main tumor groups of this category as follows: dysgerminoma, endodermal sinus tumor, embryonal carcinoma, polyembryoma, choriocarcinoma, teratomas, and mixed forms. We may add the gonadoblastoma because this tumor may be mixed in one version with the dysgerminoma or other types of germ cell tumors. When we mention the teratomas, we touch on the question of mixed type tumor and the combination of different tissue types which is so characteristic for ovarian tumors. We are aware of the fact that the epithelial tumors, for example, those developing from the surface epithelium of the ovary, can be assigned to the lining membrane with cuboidal cells, or to the pseudoepithelia of the coelomic surface also known as mesothelium. Within this group belong either the benign, low malignant, or malignant serous and mucinous tumors; the endometric tumors, the clear cell tumors, the Brenner tumors, and the mixed epithelial tumors; the undifferentiated carcinomas; and the unclassified epithelial tumors. Like other organs, the ovary has a stroma; therefore, we find the sex cord stromal tumors, which can be divided into granulosastroma cell tumors, the arrhenoblastoma, the Sertoli-Leydig cell tumors, the gynandroblastoma, and the unclassified tumors.

The germ cell tumors are a diversified group with varying differentiation which is explained once we recall that they can originate from any or all of the three germinal layers.

The malignant dysgerminoma is solitary, composed of nests with irregular patterns of uniform ovoid cells of the parenchyma, with delicate or coarse stroma. The parenchymal cells have a light eosinophilic granular cytoplasm and a round nucleus with marked nucleolus.

The endodermal sinus tumor is made up of a loose network of embryonal cells and perivascular structures with hyaline lobules sharing a positive periodic acid-Schiff reaction.

In accordance with its name, the embryonal carcinoma has anaplastic embryonal cells of the epithelium which grow in acinar, tubular, papillar, and solid patterns.

The polyembryoma is composed of embryonic bodies, and the choriocarcinoma is composed of cytotrophoblast and syncytiotrophoblast.

The teratoma is very common, totally differ-
entiated, and mainly ectodermal, but may also arise from other germ layers. In humans, dermoid cysts comprise 10% of the ovarian tumors which are limited by a thick wall. Fatty material, Rokitansky's protuberances, hair, sweat, and sebaceous glands occur. The epithelium may be squamous, columnar, cuboidal or transitional, branchial, or gastrointestinal mucosa. Teeth, cartilage, bone, even undeveloped extremities may be found. Different subtypes of teratomas are distinguished, such as the immature teratoma containing immature structures and the mature teratoma, which may be solid or cystic. In the latter case, the dermoid cyst shows a lining of epidermis with appendages whereas in the case of a malignant transformation, we find mainly a squamous cell carcinoma and sometimes an adenocarcinoma or sarcoma and, very rarely, a melanoma. Highly specialized teratomas are the struma ovarii, the carcinoid, and such forms of tumors as the epidermoid cyst, the sebaceous gland tumor, and the tumor of the retinal system.

Struma ovarii

In this tumor, thyroid tissue dominates the cyst. The tumor comprises 2.7% of the ovarian teratomas and varies from being benign to malignant. The malignant variation is reminiscent of thyroid cancer.

The solid teratoma which is generally malignant but very rare in humans has no complete capsule but exhibits an abundant mixture of tissues from all three germ layers. The same is true of the polycystic teratoma, which is also very rare.

The gonadoblastoma has large germ cells and small supporting cells such as immature granulosa and Sertoli cells. The epithelial tumors have a simple cuboidal epithelium if they originate from the free surface of the ovary and a simple columnar epithelium if they resemble the oviduct or uterine lining. The serous tumors, for example, resemble the epithelium of the Fallopian tube or the ovarian surface. In the case of mucinous tumors, mucous-filled cells are found, and the epithelium looks similar to endocervical or enteric epithelium. The endometrioid tumors have the appearance of neoplasia of the endometrial tissue described before. The clear cell tumors exhibit clear cells with glycogen, and similar cells such as the renal cell carcinoma and the Brenner tumors contain transitional epithelial cells and ovarian stroma. The ultrastructure of the clear cell carcinoma shows large nuclei, much glycogen, and lamellated rough endoplasmic reticulum, sparse lipid droplets, and also sparse but well-developed microvilli. In the tubular type of the neoplasm, which can be distinguished from the solid type, basophilic dark cells are found. The tumor is similar to clear cell carcinoma of the endocervix, and both may have a Muellerian origin (405). For a discussion of the ultrastructure of endometrioid carcinomas, see Fenoglio et al. (154). The mixed epithelial tumors consist of at least two or more components of the previously described types whereas the undifferentiated carcinoma because its poor differentiation cannot be diagnosed otherwise; this condition leads to the unclassified epithelial tumors which have to be regarded as being intermediate cases.

Argentaffin Carcinoma

The cytoplasm of carcinoid cells is strongly argentaffin. The rare choriocarcinoma develops from trophoblastic tissue.

Extreme variations occur in the granulosa cell tumor. The neoplasm is encapsulated; the cells resemble follicle cells, where atypical variants occur. The tumor cells are uniform, pear-shaped, cuboidal, or columnar, often with a roundish mitotic inactive nucleus (?). The stroma is composed of theca cells and fibroblasts. A tubercular structure is characteristic.

The thecoma is very rare in humans. The derivation from stroma and the condition of the capsule differ. We find plump oval cells, and the cytoplasmic processes are well developed. As for hemangioma, it is an unanswered question as to whether this is a true neoplasm or a malformation. The lesions are composed of vessel-like structures or only reticular connective tissue. Masson (translation by Kobernick, ref. 358) considered these adenoma-like structures as vegetant intravascular hemangio-endothelioma, the main component of which is given by the abnormally growing endothelial cells. Spindle-shaped nuclei are found in varying cell patterns of islands, sheets, or whorls. The intercellular substance exhibits argyrophilic fibrils. Malignant variants occur.

Ovarial structures of different development occur in all animal phyla, either diffuse or organoid, and the same holds true for female germ cells in plants. However, the hormonal relationship and the control of these structures is totally different among several groups and similar in others. The human ovarian tumors are not classified satisfactorily, so that a proper comparison and division according to the tissues involved can only be considered as a hopeful beginning for the future.

The teratoma has been described in *Poecilia reticulata* and the argentaffin carcinoma in *Rana esculenta* (?) (see Chapters 13 and 48).

The granulosa cell tumor is known from reptiles such as *Eunectes murinus* the anaconda; from birds such as *Caloenas nicobarica nicobarica*; from mammals such as *Ailurus fulgens* and *Procavia capensis capensis*; granulosa-theca cell tumor from the green tree viper *Trimeresiurus albolabui*; malignant infiltrating granulosa cell tumor from *Gallus gallus murghi*; metastatic granulosa cell tumor from the bonneted langur *Presbytis pileatus*; papillary cystadenoma from *Lycaon pictus lupinus*; and a bilateral papillary cystadenoma of the ovary from the bird *Melopsittacus undulatus*. A papillary ovarial carcinoma is known from the Syrian golden jackal *Chrysocyon aureus syriacus* (132).

NEOPLASMS OF EPITHELIAL ENDOCRINE GLANDS OF INVERTEBRATES

To date, nothing has been reported in the literature on this type of neoplasm.

NEOPLASMS OF NEUROHEMAL ORGANS OF INVERTEBRATES

Secured cases have not been reported.

NEOPLASMS ARISING FROM THE DESMAL EPITHELIUM OF SEROUS MEMBRANES (COELOMIC EPITHELIUM) AND PSEUDOEPITHELIA OF VESSELS

The tissues in man lining the serous cavity are the mesothelium, and the mesothelioma, varying from benign to malignant, is the respective neoplasm. It is composed of spindle cells to epithelial-like structures. Theoretically, and according to tissue distribution, the tumor is possible in coelomate phyla in general, including the vertebrates. There are no comparable representatives in plants.

Endothelial cells of blood and lymph vessels compose the pseudoepithelia of vessels found also in man.

Kaposi's disease is a sarcoma of multicentric origin, characterized by spindle cells which arise from fibroblasts or smooth muscle cells.

The hemangio-endothelioma (angiosarcoma) is composed of anastomosing channels and increased and atypical endothelium. Variations in structure occur; layers of single lining of round polygonal or fusiform cells with hyperchromatic nuclei or spindle-form may be present. Infiltration by bud-like invaginations is found, and intermediate tumors of the hemangioma-lymphangioma type exist. The neoplasm is commonly observed in dogs (109, 124, 328, 424 and others), also in cats, as well as spontaneously in laboratory rodents such as the mouse, rat, and hamster. The frog, duck, dog, hamster, guinea pig, rat, and mouse have been used as experimental animals.

Hemangiopericytoma

The neoplasm exhibits abundant endothelial channels and round ovoid or fusiform cells with prominent nuclei. Vessels, parenchymal cells, and reticulum fibrils are the main portions of the tumor.

The benign glomangioma has a fibrous capsule, vessels, and glomus cells as the three main components. The cells are round to fusiform, with large nucleus and pale cytoplasm. Reticulin fibers are surrounding the cells. The vessels dominate the picture.

Lymphangioendothelioma: the existence of benign and malignant variations, is not secured. It is comparable to hemangioma and is composed of large channels and flat to cuboidal epithelium. The contained fluid is lymph-like and includes some lymphocytes.

The tumor of the carotid body and allied structures such as glomus jugulare, gl. intervagale is the malignant nonchromaffin paraganglioma. Glomus cells and vascular channels produce a framework of vessels and epithelioid parenchyma. The variation of cellular patterns is remarkable, also by shape and size. The tumor of the carotid body or chemodectoma is known from the dog (177) and from bovines at high sea levels, where it effects especially the chief cells. This tumor starts with severe hyperplasia which can be considered as a reaction to changed environmental condition (14). The rat was used for comparable studies (317). Chemodectoma-like neoplasms have been described in the cod (*Gadus morrhua*, see Chapter 48).

Primary tumors of coelomic surfaces or mesotheliomas, which are also benign or malignant, are composed of spindle cells or epithelial-like structures with nests and cords of cuboidal or polygonal cells or pseudoglandular structures of columnar cells. Different transitional structures may be observed. Infiltrative growth may reach and penetrate the underlying tissues.

Pseudoepithelia of vessels are found in phyla with closed and mixed circulatory systems and in portions of open circulatory systems in which tumorigenesis is theoretically possible. No comparison with plants can be made. The hemangioendothelioma was observed in *Conger conger*, *Plecoglossus altevelis*, and *Salvelinus namaycush*. The hemangioma was found in *Raja maculata*, *Chilodus punctatus*, *Gadus morhua*, *Gadus virens*, *Gasterosteus aculeatus*, *Pungitius pungitius*, and *Scomber scombrus*, all fishes; in the reptiles *Dispholidus typus* (liver) and *Sistrurus catenatus catenatus* (ovary); in the birds *D. arborea* (spleen), *Syrmaticus soemmeringii ijimae*, and *Centropus sinensis bubatus* (cavernous hemangioma of liver); and the mammals *Cubiculus paca* (bladder), *Acionyx jubatus jubatus* (tongue), and *Hippotragus niger roseveltii* (spleen).

Hemangiosarcomas appeared in the Indian blue peafowl *Pavo cristata* and the mammals *Chrysocyon mesomelas* (neck) and *Lycaon pictus lupinus*.

The lymphangioendothelioma was diagnosed in *Pomatus saltatrix*.

NEOPLASMS ARISING FROM DESMAL EPITHELIA (SYNOVIAL ORIGIN)

Desmal epithelia in man are found in joints, tendon sheaths, ligaments, and bursae. The benign neoplam is the giant cell synovioma composed of small oval or spindle cells, and connective tissue of collagenic quality.

The malignant synovioma is composed of pleomorphic, spindle, and pseudoepithelial cells. The tissues are distributed in vertebrates, and the distribution of comparable structures in invertebrates such as bivalve molluscs, arthropods, or echinoderms is questionable. No comparison with plant tissues is possible. The benign tumor of these tissues was observed in *Blennius* sp.

NEOPLASMS ARISING FROM CONNECTIVE TISSUE (RICH IN CELLS— 1. MESENCHYME)

The normal tissue in man is the mesenchyme, a tissue remnant from embryonal time (?) and reverted adult connective tissue. The myxomas of man are benign and develop most often in superficial tissues such as the skin of fingertips and in the jaw. They mimic mucoid connective tissue of the umbilical cord. Also benign is the (mixed embryonal) mesenchymoma, of which malignant variations have been described; they recall embryonal mesenchyme. The highly undifferentiated sarcomas, the round cell, the spindle cell and the giant cell sarcomas, which exhibit no reticulum fibers but have a characteristic cell network are malignant. Mesenchyme is found in porifera, cnidaria, ctenophora, entoprocta, nematoda, mollusca, pentastomida, arthropoda, echinodermata, and chaetognatha, vertebrata and may surely have even a wider distribution as well as tumorigenesis. Mesenchymal cells exhibit a varying phylogenetic potential determining which cell types may derive from them (see Chapter 3).

Myxomas were diagnosed in *Cacajo rubicundus* (eyelid), *Papio hamadryas hamadryas* (skin), and *Helactos malayanus malayanus* (conjunctiva).

NEOPLASMS ARISING FROM CONNECTIVE TISSUE (RICH IN CELLS— 2. SPINOCELLULAR CONNECTIVE TISSUE)

This type of tissue occurs in man in the form of stroma ovarii and theca cells, and in the uterus (lamina propria). In the first case, the benign neoplasm is the thecoma composed of plump, oval, fusiform, or stellate cells, with prominent cytoplasmatic processes. Vesicular, broad, or spindle-shaped nuclei are arranged in different patterns as islets or sheets; delicate or coarse stroma is present. The neoplasm is rare.

The stromal endometriosis may be benign to malignant and should best be considered semimalignant. It is composed of nodules and islands of bundles and cords. It has been observed in monkeys (118, 119). Round to elongated uniform small cells are typical, and the nuclei are prominent, oval, and hyperchromatic. The cytoplasm is scanty, and the stroma contains reticulin fibers. The thecoma occurs in invertebrates and vertebrates and has been found in *Crassostrea gigas* (comparable with reservations), but no comparison with plants is possible.

NEOPLASMS ARISING FROM CONNECTIVE TISSUE (RICH IN CELLS— 3. RETICULAR CONNECTIVE TISSUE) AND FREE CONNECTIVE TISSUE CELLS

Reticular connective tissue in man appears in two versions: the hematopoietic connective tissue which is considered to be hematopoietic-reticular and the lymphoreticular connective tissue (583). In this review, some cells known as free cells of connective tissue are included, as well as certain cells of body fluids of invertebrates which may be related, although they develop from the mesoderm but in a somewhat distant position.

CLASSIFICATION OF NEOPLASTIC DISEASES OF THE HEMATOPOIETIC AND LYMPHOID TISSUES OF MAN (359) WITH CELL TYPES INVOLVED

I. *Systemic Diseases* — Characteristic Cells

A. *Acute Leukemias and Related Diseases*
  1. Acute lymphoid leukemia — Lymphoid cells
  2. Acute myeloid leukemia — Immature granulocytes
  3. Acute monocytoid (monocytic) leukemia — Immature monocytes
  4. Malignant histiocytosis — Atypical histiocytes or mononuclear phagocytes
  5. Acute erythremia (di Guglielmo) — Erythroblasts
  6. Erythroleukemia — Erythroid and granulocytic cells
  7. Megacaryocytoid (megacaryocytic) leukemia — Megacaryocytic cells
  8. Acute panmyelosis — All three components of bone marrow
  9. Acute leukemia, unclassified — Highly unclassified cells

B. *Chronic Lymphoid Leukemia and Other Lymphoproliferative Diseases*
  1. Chronic lymphoid leukemia — Small lymphocytes (B cells)

Systemic Diseases (cont.)	Characteristic Cells (cont.)
2. Primary macroglobulinemia (Waldenstroem)	Lymphocytes with immunoglobulin proliferation
3. Myeloma	Plasmacells
4. Plasma-cell leukemia	Plasmacells, immunoglobulin production
5. Heavy-chain disease	Plasmacytoid cells in bone marrow
6. Sezary's disease	Sezary cells
7. Chronic lymphoproliferative disease, unclassified	Unclassified lymphocytes

C. *Chronic Myeloid Leukemia and Other Myeloproliferative Diseases*

Systemic Diseases (cont.)	Characteristic Cells (cont.)
1. Chronic myeloid leukemia	Cells of granulocyte series
2. Variants of chronic myeloid leukemia	
(a) Neutrophilic leukemia	Mature neutrophilic granulocytes
(b) Eosinophilic leukemia	Mature eosinophilic granulocytes
(c) Basophilic leukemia	Mature basophilic granulocytes
3. Chronic erythremia (Heilmeyer-Schoener)	Cells of erythroid series
4. Polycythemia vera (Vaquez-Osler)	Erythrocytosis, leucocytosis, thrombocytosis, and normoblastic, granulocytic, megacaryocytic cells
5. Idiopathic thrombocythemia	Megacaryocytes, thrombocytes
6. Myelosclerosis with myeloid metaplasis	Megacaryocytes and all three types of myeloid cells
7. Chronic myeloproliferative diseases, unclassified	Unclassified myeloid cells

D. Chronic Monocytoid Leukemia and Systemic Histiocytoid Diseases

1. Chronic monocytoid (monocytic leukemia	
2. Histiocytosis X	Histiocytes

E. *Unclassified Leukemia*

1. Hairy cell leukemia	Cells with hair-like projections

F. *Others*

1. Malignant mastocytosis	Tissue mast cells

II. *Tumors*

A. *Lymphosarcomas*

Systemic Diseases (cont.)	Characteristic Cells (cont.)
1. Nodular lymphosarcoma	Lymphoid cells
2. Diffuse lymphosarcoma	Lymphoid cells
(a) Lymphocytic	Lymphocytes
(b) Lymphoplasmacytic	Lymphocytes and plasma cells
(c) Prolymphocytic	Intermediates of lymphocytes and lymphoblasts
(d) Lymphoblastic	Lymphoblastic cells
(e) Immunoblastic	Large lymphoid cells with basophil cytoplasm
(f) Burkitt's tumor	Lymphoid cells (B-cell type), macrophages

B. *Mycosis fungoides*	Lymphoid, pleomorphic cells, infiltrated
C. *Plasmacytoma*	Atypical plasma cells
D. *Reticulosarcoma*	Reticulum cells, histiocytes, or mononuclear phagocytes
E. *Unclassified Malignant Lymphomas*	Lymphoid or histiocyte cells
F. *Hodgkin's Disease*	Sternberg-Reed cells
1. With lymphocyte predominance	Mature lymphocytes
2. With nodular sclerosis	Sternberg-Reed cells, lymphocytes, eosinophilic and neutrophilic mature granulocytes, histiocytes, plasma cells, and lacunar cells

Tumors (cont.)	Characteristic Cells (cont.)
3. With mixed cellularity	Lymphocytes, histiocytes, Sternberg-Red and mononuclear cells
4. With lymphocyte depletion	Paucity of lymphocytes
G. Others	
1. Eosinophilic granuloma	Histiocytes, eosinophilic granulocytes
2. Mastocytoma	Tissue mast cells

The neoplasms of hematopoietic and lymphoid tissues, including the so-called systemic diseases, are not arranged according to the two parameters, whether they are acute or chronic. Such a chracterization for these groups of diseases is necessary for clinical use, but it does not provide a satisfactory arrangement which can be used in comparative pathology. For this purpose, it is useful to arrange the diseases according to cell arrangement, as we have done for other tissue types.

Human hematopoietic and lymphoid tissues are derivatives of reticular connective tissue. Not even under normal conditions do all of these tissues necessarily form organs as in the lymph nodes, spleen, or bone marrow. Leukemias, which in this case make up the group of systemic diseases, can be considered as being neoplasms without stroma. This seems unusual, for neoplastic diseases, but neoplasms without stroma occur also in the group of epithelial neoplasms, as, for example, in the relatively rare choriocarcinoma. This seems to be the only known case of an epithelial neoplasm without stroma. The intercellular substance and fibers, typical for connective tissues, become apparent when the blood, the main fluid-like tissue, coagulates. Lymph is also a fluid-like tissue. We distinguish further between a medullary, and especially during embryogenesis under normal conditions, a nonmedullary production of the freely movable body fluid cells.

As far as the invertebrates are concerned, the unifying character of the hemocytes, amebocytes, and other body fluid cells must not be overestimated when they are compared to the so-called hemocytic neoplasms as described from lamellibranches such as the oyster. Not only are the reticular connective tissues mesodermal in origin, but this holds true also for the pseudoepithelia of coelomic surfaces. The question arises now as to how closely we are able to compare cells of body fluids which arise from reticular connective tissue in the vertebrates with those, for example, which originate from the peritoneal lining of the coelomic cavity in annelid worms. The only way out of the confusion at present is to arrange the neoplasms according to the precursor cells from which they derive. This seems to become even more important when looking at the biochemical background of neoplastic cells. The main respiratory pigment in vertebrate cells is the hemoglobin whereas the comparable structures to erythrocytes in the invertebrate exhibit mostly hemerythrine as respiratory pigment. The cancerization of any normal cell is characterized by some metabolic change in the cells via the pathways of certain components. Therefore, it is important to know which components are characteristic for the precursors of neoplastic cells in different phyla. If the disease is characterized by abnormally produced neoplastic cells in a systematic manner, then it is proper to speak of systematic diseases. These are like an army of anarchistic cells of a special type. If the cells are arranged in a sessile form and are of a special type, we usually speak of neoplasms or tumors. In a comparative sense, it is not possible today to characterize these lesions efficiently, based on the character of cells, especially with respect to the invertebrates with the tremendous varieties of cellular stages belonging to the different body fluids. It is not yet known how many of these cell types are real and how many are only normal intermediate stages. The system used here is based on the conditions found in man which will have to be expanded and revised in the future. A comparison to plant diseases is not possible, because plants lack floating, freely movable cells (cell wall).

In man, the reticular connective tissue occurs in the myeloid and the lymphoid versions and in hematopoietic organs. It is a part of the reticuloendothelial system. In the adult, this most primitive of the connective tissues is found in two versions, the hematopoietic-reticular connective tissue and the lymphoreticular connective tissue. It occurs as red bone marrow only in the sternum, ilium, hipbone, diploe, vertebra, sacrum, and phalanges. In other bones, it is transformed under normal conditions into the yellow bone marrow, but it may reoccur under pathologic conditions such as leukemia, the systemic neoplastic disease of this organ. The lymphoreticular connective tissue is found in spleen, lymph nodes, tonsils, and lamina propria of the intestinal mucosa. According to the fixed components, two types of neoplasms, the leukemias and the sarcomas, can be distinguished. Hematopoietic tissues and wandering cells, as stated before, occur also in invertebrates.

The only possible basis for comparability is given by the involvement of different cell types. The most frequent leukemias in man are the myeloid, lymphoid and monocytic ones. The same distinction is possible for sarcomas. The hematopoietic tumors, which have either been found or can be postulated in comparison to the precursor cells of vertebrates have been included where the comparison of the normal cells seems to be most appropriate.

This somewhat artificial classification of the hematogenic cells of vertebrates and invertebrates is justified because today we still do not know enough about the functional histology of the cells especially in the invertebrates.

Free cells
Plasma cells, immature and mature

    a. Plasmoblasts: heavy chain disease
    b. Proplasmocytes
    c. Plasma cells

Early stages of plasma cells are important in the heavy chain disease, characterized by special abnormal protein (immunoglobulin) and intermedullary plasmacytoid cells. The diseases of this group are the alpha heavy chain disease (alpha chain disease), the gamma heavy chain disease (gamma chain disease), and the mu heavy chain disease (mu chain disease). The first version, especially, is related to mediterranean lymphoma. The lamina propria and the submucosa of the jejunum are infiltrated by plasma cells. The lymph nodes also are affected. For proteins, see ref. 359.

For lymphoplasmacytic sarcoma, the characteristic cells are lymphocytes and plasma cells.

Plasmacytoma. The tumor, which is oriented locally, exhibits atypical and probably neoplastic plasma cells. Atypical glycogen deposits have been observed in a plasmacytoma by use of electron microscopy (185). The tumor is also known from an East Indian water lizard, *Hydrosaurus amboinensis*, which involved stomach, liver, and lung. The diagnosis for plasma cell tumor was based on histological and ultrastructural findings (489).

Myeloma. This systemic disease is characterized by a neoplastic proliferation of plasma cells, often producing tumors in many bones, also fractures and infiltration and tumors in bone marrow and viscera. An extramedullary myeloma is known from the dog, as described by Funderburg (171). Thirty-two elements were de-

termined in a myeloliposarcoma of a 15-year-old female *Perodicticus potto* (108).

Plasma Cell Leukemia. This systemic neoplastic disease of plasma cells shows diffuse infiltration of the bone marrow and monoclonal immunoglobulin production.

Lymphoplasmacytic Diffuse Lymphosarcoma. The cells are lymphoblastic, resembling either macro- or microlymphoblasts.

Macrophages

Burkitt's tumor (+). "Starry sky pattern" of large pale or vacuolated macrophages is characteristic among the tumor cells of this neoplastic disease.

Mast Cells

Malignant Mastocytosis. Atypical tissue mast cells of this systemic disease are characteristic in hematopoietic organs and many other tissues. Mastocytomas are known from the dog, as in the case of a mast cell sarcoma of the larynx (36), or concerning the lymph nodes (346), as well as the cat (590). Long-term survival of two cats with mastocytosis was reported by Confer *et al.* (103).

Histiocytes (Clasmatocytes, Adventitial Cells)

When loaded with ingested material, histiocytes are called: melanophages, siderophages, lipophages.

Malignant Histiocytosis (+) and Similar Diseases. The characteristic cells of this progressive and neoplastic disease, called malignant histiocytosis, are atypical histiocytes or other mononuclear phagocytes. Letterer-Siwe disease, characterized by proliferation of reticulum cells in children replacing the normal cells of lymph nodes, spleen, and bone marrow, belongs also in this group. The theoretical restriction of this type of disease to the mammals can be explained by the involvement of the organs (lymph nodes).[8] Another rare disease occurring in the lung of

---

[8] Perhaps in primitive form in crocodiles and birds (mesenteric lymph nodes).

adults of this group is Turiaf's disease. The species-specific distribution may vary to the former one according to the organ involvement, but this is unknown.

Histiocytosis X. This neoplastic proliferation of differentiated histiocytes involves bone, viscera, and skin. Another disease of related character is the Hand-Schüller-Christian disease affecting bone but also lung, thyroid, lymph nodes, spleen, liver, skin, and vagina in older childhood as well as the eosinophilic granulomatosis of bone in the adult. The typical histiocytes of these diseases show a foamy appearance. Eosinophilic granulomatosis of bone in adults must also be mentioned.

Unclassified malignant Lymphomas (+). Multiple cell groups with pleomorphic and anaplastic characters occur in these lymphomas.

Hodgkin's disease with mixed cellularity is the classic type of the disease. These are unclassifiable malignant tumors of lymphoid or histiocytoid cells: dominating abnormal reticulum cells, lymphocytes and Sternberg-Reed cells, eosinophils, neutrophils, plasma cells, and fibroblasts occur. Mitotic figures are abundant. Varying reticulin meshworks are found.

Eosinophilic Granuloma (+) The tumor-like growth shows well-differentiated histiocytes often intermingled with mature eosinophilic granulocytes. It is the third type of histiocytosis X.

NEOPLASMS AND SYSTEMIC DISEASES OF HEMATOPOIETIC TISSUES (197)

Lymphoid or Lymphatic Tissue

Lymphoblasts

Acute Lymphoid Leukemia. The proliferating cells are blastic and lymphoid, exhibiting a high nuclear-cytoplasmic ratio. The cytoplasm is basophilic and lacks granules, the (?) nucleolus is singular. Prolymphoblastic, macro-, and micro-lymphoblastic prolymphocytic variants occur.

Nodular Lymphosarcoma. According to the name of the disease, the lymphoid cells of this malignant tumor are arranged in nodular pattern. The disease is also known as Brill-Symmers disease.

Prolymphocytic Diffuse Lymphosarcoma. The cells are prolymphocytic in type, like a transitional stage of lymphoblasts and lymphocytes.

Lymphoblastic diffuse Lymphosarcoma with Lymphoblastic cells

Mycosis fungoides (+)

It always starts in the upper dermis, is a cellular infiltrate, is pleomorphic in character, is composed of T-cells, large cells with round or ovoid nucleus, and scanty cytoplasm.

Unclassified malignant lymphomas (+) are composed of anaplastic cells. Multiple cell groups with pleomorphic and anaplastic characters occur in these lymphomas. Hodgkin's disease with mixed cellularity is the classic type of the disease composed of unclassifiable malignant tumors of lymphoid or histiocytoid cells. Dominating abnormal reticulum cells, lymphocytes, and Sternberg-Reed cells, eosinophils, neutrophils, plasma cells and fibroblasts occur. Mitotic figures are abundant. Varying reticulin meshworks are found.

Lymphocytes

Small lymphocytes. *Chronic Lymphoid Leukemia.* The characteristic cells of this disseminated neoplastic disease are of the type of small lymphocytes (mostly B cell type, but also T cell type).

Medium Lymphocytes. *Lymphatic Diffuse Lymphosarcoma.* Hodgkin's disease with lymphocyte predominance, the characteristic picture reveals an abundance of mature lymphocytes. Well differentiated histiocytes may be proliferating, leading to the lymphocytic and/or histiocytic type of the disease. A sparse, abnormal reticulin-fiber-network is present.

In Hodgkin's disease with lymphocyte depletion, the scarcity of lymphocytes is characteristic.

Large Lymphocytes. In immunoblastic diffuse lymphosarcoma, diffuse pattern of lymphoid cells with basophilic cytoplasm containing vacuoles.

Other Lymphocytes. *Acute Leukemia (unclassified).* Highly unclassified blast cells close to stem cells.

Primary Macroglobulinemia (Waldenstroem). Obliteration of small darkly stained cells (atypical B lymphocytes related to plasma cells)—cytoplasm is more abundant than normal. Atypical lymphocytes invade the area around the lymph node. In addition, mitotic figures are rare, but mature plasma cells are abundant, in addition to lymphocytes.

Sezary Disease. Large mononuclear cells, so-called Sezary or Lutzner cells in blood and dermis, characterize this chronic progressive dermatosis. A cerebriform nucleus, a resemblance to mature lymphocytes, an association with small lymphocytes, plasma cells, and histiocytes are seen.

Chronic Lymphoproliferative Disease (Unclassified) The name derives from the fact that no distinction can be made between a chronic lymphoid leukemia and a lymphocytic lymphosarcoma. Lymphomas have been described from the northern pike, *Esox lucius* L. (238) and from fowl (48), and lymphosarcomas are known from northern pike, *Esox lucius* (415), from the northern fur seal, *Callorhinus ursinus*, characterized by monomorphic lymphoid cells of the mesenteric lymph nodes (525), from the nude mouse (556), from the New Zealand white rabbit (100), from the dog (411), from the horse (164, 198), from the swine (262), and in bovine twin calves (88); for zoo animals, see Effron *et al.* (132).

As pointed out by the author, the relationship of the cells in the circulatory sytems of invertebrates and vertebrates is comparatively not well enough established for the determination of an exact comparison; this even holds true for the vertebrate classes themselves, as pointed out by Effron *et al.* Therefore, the very frequent lymphosarcomas of reptiles, birds, and mammals are listed taxonomically (see also Chapter 48 for additional cases).

Concerning reptiles, lymphosarcomas have been observed in: *Naja nigricollis nigricollis*, *Acanthophis antarcticus* (leukemic), *Bitis arietans* (leukemic), *Bitis nasicornis* (leukemic), *Bitis nasicornis*, *Crotalus horridus horridus* (leukemic), *Uromastix acanthurinus*.

The following bird species exhibited lymphosarcomas: *Branta nigricans*, *Anas castanea* (neural and visceral), *Alectura lathami* (visceral), *Coturnix coturnix japonica* (visceral, including thymus), *Rollulus roulroul*, *Ptermistes leucoscepus infuscatus* (visceral), *Gallus gallus murghi* (visceral, leukemic), *Gallus lafayetti* (visceral), *Gallus lafayetti* (visceral and skin), *Gallus sonneratii* (visceral), *Gallus varius* (visceral), *Lophura diardi* (visceral), *Argusianus argus grayi* (visceral), *Phasianus versicolor versicolor* (visceral), *Pavo cristatus* (visceral; fibrosarcoma), *Pavo cristatus* (visceral); *Pavo cristatus* (visceral, leukemic), *Pavo muticus imperator* (visceral), *Numida meleagris* (visceral, skin), *Num-*

ida meleagris (visceral), *Agriocharis ocellata* (mandible, liver; fibroma), *Agriocharis ocellata* (visceral), *Meleagris domestica* (visceral), *Platycercus adscitus palliceps* (visceral, lumen of brain, lung and vessels), *Polytelis swainsonii* (visceral), and *Gracula religiosa intermedia* (visceral).

Lymphosarcomas of mammals have been found in such species as: *Ursus rctus sheldoni*, *Panthera leo*, *Acinonyx jubatus obergi*, *Phoca vitulina geronimensis* (leukemic), *Cervus nippon talouanus*, *Oryx leucoryx*, and *Bubalus bubalus* (leukemia).

Myeloid Tissue

Myeloblasts. *Chronic Myeloid Leukemia.* Typical are cells of varying maturity belonging to the granulocyte series. Three subtypes exist: chronic myeloid leukemia, Ph'-positive, chronic myeloid leukemia, Ph' negative; atypical chronic myeloid leukemia, Ph' negative. They can be distinguished due to the abnormality of the Philadelphia chromosome (Ph'). No other neoplastic disease has a cytogenetic abnormality.

Heterophilic (Neutrophilic) Myelocyte. *Acute Myeloid Leukemia.* The neoplastic cells of this systemic proliferation correspond to early stages of the cells of the granulocyte series. In general, the nuclear chromatin exhibits tender reticulation, several nucleoli are present, and the cytoplasm is abundant.

Myelomonocytic leukemia in an orangutan, *Pongo pygmaeus* (178), led to the establishment of a cell line and isolation of an Epstein-Barr virus like herpesvirus as the first herpesvirus from this species.

Eosinophil Myelocytes.
Basophil Myelocytes.
Heterophil (Neutrophil) Granulocytes.
Neutrophilic Chronic Myeloid Leukemia. The cells from all stages of development belonging to the neutrophilic granulocytes are characteristic and show a predominance of mature neutrophils in the blood.

Polycythemia vera (Vaquez-Osler). Erythrocytosis, leukocytosis, thrombocytosis with medullary hyperplasia exhibiting cells of the normoblastic, granulocytic, and megakaryocytic development are present here.

Eosinophilic Granulocytes. *Eosinophilic Chronic Myeloid Leukemia.* In this subtype of myeloid leukemia, the eoinophilic granulocytes dominate; in cases of acute forms, the more immature cells prevail.

Myelosclerosis with Myeloid Metaplasia (+). This panmyelosis exhibits myeloid metaplasia of all three types of myeloid cells, atypical megakaryocytic proliferation, and intermedullary fibrosis.

Eosinophilic Granuloma (+). Neoplasm-like growth processes are composed of nonmalignant well-differentiated histiocytes and generally mature eosinophils.

Basophilic Granulocytes. *Basophilic (Chronic myeloid) leukemia.* Basophils dominate in this subtype of chronic myeloid leukemia.

Granulocytes of Merostomata. The granular material in these invertebrate cells seems to be hemocyanin. No systemic or neoplastic diseases involving these cells have been described to date.

Granulocytes of Decapod Crustacea Appear in Three Developmental Stages. (a) hyaline cell with smooth endoplasmic reticulum; (b) half-granular hemocytes with granules, lysosomes, and 1–2 Golgi apparatuses; and (c) granulocytes abundant and electron dense-granules, which contain copper.

Series of Body Fluid Cells in Insects Which Are Considered as Being Ontogenetic or Functional Stages. *Prohemocytes.* The cells are small, round, or oval; the granular cytoplasm is scarce.

Plasmatocytes. Motile cells, with functional pseudopodia, central nucleus, and abundant granules are present. The cells are round, oval, or spindle-shaped.

Granular Cells. The cells are round or oval, have a central nucleus and cytoplasmic granules, and are able to extend fine processes.

Spherule Cells. These spindle-shaped or oval cells contain large granules.

Cystocytes. The cells are round with granular material, which may be released for precipitation.

Onocytoids. These cells are comparable to erythrocytes of vertebrates. The nucleus of these large cells is small, and granular and membranous organelles are scarce; they have abundant ribosomes and tender particles in the cytoplasm.

Thrombocytoids. Thrombocytoids of the fly *Calliphora* (see ref. 593) are a particular type of body fluid cell and due to the tendency toward fragmentation (comparable to the mammalian megakaryocytes) are involved in the formation of blood clotting. During the fragmentation, more or less naked nuclei with a very narrow rim of cytoplasms and the split-off fragments of fusiform shape, comparable to mammalian

thrombocytes, remain. The nonnuclear cell fragments are the ones involved in blood clotting.

Erythrocytes of *Lingula* (Brachiopoda-Hemerythrin). The brachiopod *Lingula*, one of the phylogenetically very old invertebrates which has as type endured hundreds of millions of years from the Paleozoicum (Cambrian), has a cell type in the body fluid; the respiratory pigment of *Lingula* is hemerythrin, and of course, it is different from the hemoglobin of the body fluid of vertebrates.

Erythrocytes. Erythrocytes without nucleus from the polychaete *Magelona* are the only erythrocytes in invertebrates which lack a nucleus and organelles. They contain hemerythrin also. Neoplasms of these "blood" corpuscles have been described particularly in molluscs and insects. However, it is questionable how close a comparison may be drawn. The closest comparison would be between vertebrates and insect larvae where the body fluid contains hemoglobin. However, even then the question of cellular binding or dilution of the body fluid makes an exact comparison difficult. New studies are urgently needed.

Basophilic Erythroblast. *Acute Erythremia (Di Guglielmo).* Also known as erythremic myelosis is a malignant neoplasm in which many nucleated erythrocytes occur in the blood in addition to splenomegaly, with irregular size and type of these primitive cells of the erythropoietic series. Chronic versions of this disease are also known.

Erythroleukemia (+). This neoplastic lesion is characterized by atypical cells of the erythroid and granulocyte series.

Chronic Erythremia (Heilmeyer-Schoener). The cells of this rare, chronic disease belong to the erythroid series, and the bone marrow is generally involved.

Polychromatophilic Erythroblasts See above. Normoblasts See above.

Erythrocytes. *Erythroleukemia.* Atypical cells of the erythroid and granulocytic series characterize the disease.

Chronic Erythremia. see on p. ——.

Polycythemia vera. Erythrocytosis, leukocytosis, and thrombocytosis are persistent, and cells of the normoblastic, granulocytic, and megakaryocytic series are seen in the bone marrow.

Megakaryocytes. *Megakaryocytoid (Megakaryocytic) Leukemia.* The poorly differentiated atypical cells of this rapidly progressing disease belong to the megakaryocytic series.

Polycythemia vera. See above.

Idiopathic Thrombocythemia. In addition to abundant megakaryocytes and platelets, the pronounced thrombocytosis is a remarkable characteristic.

Myelosclerosis with Myeloid Metaplasia. Fibrosis of the bone marrow, atypical megakaryocytosis, and myeloid metaplasia of all three cell types are characteristic.

Thrombocytes. *Polycythemia vera (+).* See above.

Idiopathic Thrombocythemia (+). See above.

Monocytes. *Chronic Monocytoid Leukemia.* The typical neoplastic cells are monocytes in spleen, liver, and bone marrow but rarely in the blood.

Acute Monocytoid (Monocytic) Leukemia. The monoblastic, promonocytic, or promonoblastic cells show all monocytic features, and one or the other type may dominate in this acute disease.

Diseases with Multiple Cells. *Acute Panmyelosis.* All three components of the bone marrow, those of the megakaryocytic series, are especially abundant and are involved in this fast-progressing disease.

Hairy Cell Leukemia. The cells of this chronic disease show leukemic cells with hair-like extensions.

Hodgkin's Disease with Nodular Sclerosis. Broad bands of collagen separate eyelets of Sternberg-Reed cells, lymphocytes, mature eosinophils and neutrophils, and histiocytes and plasma cells.

Reticulum Cells. *Reticulosarcoma (+).* The newly applied term (473) is immunoblastic sarcomas, because the main cells are considered to be immunoblasts as transformed lymphocytes. The cells are large; much cytoplasm occurs; and the outline is irregular. The large, mostly oval nucleus and the nucleolus or the nucleoli are prominent.

Amoebocytes. *Amoebocytes in Pulmonate Molluscs.* Neoplasms with involvement of these cells, just as with the involvement of hemocytes in insects, have been described, especially in pelacypods such as *Ostrea* sp. The neoplastic character of these invertebrate lesions cannot be denied, but in the author's opinion, histogenetic comparison among the different invertebrate groups and the vertebrates needs further clarification (see also Chapter 48).

Amoebocytes in Annelida, Originating from Peritoneum.

Eleocytes. *Eleocytes in Annelida.*

Eleocytes in Echinodermata.

Sixteen of 994 *Mytilus edulis* mussels from the River Lynher showed infiltration and replacement of the connective tissue by enlarged atypical, mitotically active, basophilic hemocyte-like cells. Two cell types characterize the disorder. The exact relationship of these cells differing from hemocytes could not be established (344). This report indicates that despite exact scientific work and methodology, a tremendous emphasis will still have to be placed in the comparative investigation of those findings described here.

NEOPLASMS ARISING FROM CONNECTIVE TISSUE (RICH IN FIBERS. 1. GELATINOUS CONNECTIVE TISSUE

Gelatinous connective tissue in man occurs in the pulp of the tooth, the villi of the placenta, and the umbilical cord. The benign neoplasm is the myxofibroma composed of a network of anastomosing star-like cells, gelatinous ground-substance with mucin-positive reaction, and collagenic fibers.

The myxosarcoma is richer in cell content than the myxofibroma with atypic and polymorphic cells.

The tissue is known to exist in vertebrates, but new investigations are necessary to determine which comparable tissues occur in invertebrates. A comparison with plants is not possible. Myxosarcomas have been described for the following species: *Plecoglossus altevelis, Phenecogrammus interruptus, Tinca tinca, Pleuronectes platessa, Scophthalmus maximus,* and *Rana clamitans* and, recently, in a pet hamster (457), to name only a few.

NEOPLASMS ARISING FROM CONNECTIVE TISSUE (RICH IN FIBERS. 2. LOOSE CONNECTIVE TISSUE)

In man, loose connective tissue is found in mucus membranes, in the subcutis, and as packing material nearly everywhere in the body, between organs such as individual muscles, nerves, arteries, and veins.

The fibroma mole is composed of a few cells (fibrocytes) and loose curled collagen fibers. The lipofibroma mole as a related type is built like the above tumor but has additional adipose cells. The lipofibroma myxoides also is composed similar to the above but shows mucinous degener- the above but shows mucinous degeneration.

The undifferentiated round cell sarcoma is a malignant variant of fibroma mole of the mesenchymal type without intercellular substance. The undifferentiated spindle cell sarcoma is another variation with spindle cells, and the undifferentiated polymorphic cellular sarcoma is again another one with polymorphic cells.

Loose connective tissue is widely distributed in invertebrates and vertebrates alike, but whether it can be compared to certain parenchymata in plants is questionable. Fibroma mole has been found in the bivalve mollusc *Andonta implicata* and in quite a number of vertebrates such as: *Sardinia pilchardus, Esox lucius, Oncorhynchus kisutch, Salvelinus fontinalis, Abramis brama, Carassius auratus, Poecilia reticulata, Rasbora daniconius, Gadus virens, Gasterosteus aculeatus, Caranx hippos, Scorpaena inermis, Stizostedion vitreum, Hippoglossus hippoglossus, Hippoglossus stenolepis, Pleuronectiformes, Scophthalmus maximus, Megalobatrachus maximus, Triturus taeniatus, Bufo bufo japonicus, Rana esculenta, Xenopus laevis, Chelonia mydas, Agkistrodon piscivorus, Elaphe obsoleta, Anser anser, Balaenoptera borealis,* and domestic and laboratory animals.

NEOPLASMS ARISING FROM CONNECTIVE TISSUE (RICH IN FIBERS. 3. FIBROUS OR FIBRILLAR CONNECTIVE TISSUE)

In man the tissue occurs in such structures as fasciae and others.

Desmoid Tumor

The lesion (questionable if a true tumor) occurs in the fascia of rectus abdominis anterior in multiparous females, but it is questionable as to whether it is a true tumor. Hypocellular, avascular bands of fibrous tissue are typical, in addition to orderly fibroblasts with uniform nuclei and abundant collagen fibers.

The calcifying fibroma is a lesion which occurs in the palm of children less than 10 years old. The cells are oat shaped; the nuclei, arranged in one direction, are clumpy. Collagenous fibers and reticular fibers are a sign of infiltrative growth. Depositions of calcium salts occur.

In the case of the palmar or plantar fibromatosis, fasciae and dermis are involved. Spindle cells and collagen occur, and large atypical fibroblasts may show mitosis.

The congenital, generalized fibromitosis is an extremely rare lesion, and it is questionable as to whether this "malignant" condition is neoplastic rather than systemic.

Benign elastofibroma dorsi is composed of cords of collagen with elastic fibers and adipose cells. It is extremely rare in man.

The malignant intramural fibroma of the heart comprises a distinct group of primary myocardial tissues.

The benign histiocytoma comprises lesions which are either true neoplasms or only granulomas. Their growth may be limited in time and extent, but it is believed that they originate from histiocytes. The main cells may be large atypical, sometimes vacuolated, pale-staining, eosinophilic or modified histiocytes. The nucleus is round or ovoid; some nuclei may be large and hyperchromatic.

The dermatofibrosarcoma protuberans is a clinical and not a histologically characterized entity. The ultrastructure suggests the origin from histiocytes (412) or fibroblasts (407). The duration of the tumor may extend to up to 20 years (303).

The Fibrosarcoma

The tumors with widespread distribution originate from fibroblasts. We distinguish: (a) differentiated fibrosarcoma in which the texture is characterized by bundles and cells and is of an interwoven pattern. Nuclei of the elongated cells surrounded by scanty cytoplasm appear prolonged and rarely show mitosis. The cells are reticulin-wrapped, and collagen is abundantly present; (b) undifferentiated fibrosarcoma in which the undifferentiated cells are more abundant, and the intercellular matrix is diminished. The general ultrastructure of fibrosarcoma was used to distinguish between the ultrastructure of normal cells, and that of neoplasms. Iagubow (254) pointed out the different relationships between the protein-synthesizing and energetic apparatuses. It was also found that neoplastic cells were less differentiated than normal ones, and the more malignant tumors showed no less differentiation than the more benign ones. Shin and Abramson (506) discussed the practical value of electron-microscopy for diagnosis of fibrosarcoma of the larynx, and Woods and Papadimitriou (608) the effect of inflammatory stimuli on the stroma of neoplasms. A primary fibrosarcoma of the human heart was described by Kissler (296). The ultrastructure of fibrosarcoma revealed histiocyte-like, fibroblast-like, and little differentiated cells. In some of the latter ones, the same macrophage differentiation was evident (175). Fibroblast-like cells are contained in the cytoplasmic fragments of collagenic fibrils and crystalloid formations in the small canals of the granular endoplasmic reticulum (176). Investigations by Smith et al. (515) suggest that the human fibrosarcoma cell line HT 1080 is expressing an antigen related to the P 30 protein of RD 114 baboon endogenous virus group oncornaviruses without producing complete virions.

Fibrillar connective tissue is widely distributed in vertebrates and in invertebrates, but a direct comparison to plant parenchymata is not possible. Neoplasms of this type have been reported as existing abundantly in captive wild, domesticated, and laboratory animals. These are summarized in the tables of Chapter 48. We have reported here on one case of fibroma of the heart which occurred in Poecilia reticulata, a fibroma at the intercostal region in the African rock python, Python sebae; in a fibroma of the thoracic inlet in the painted quail Coturnix lineata; in a fibroma of the dermis of the thick-billed parrot Rhynchopsitta pachyrhyncha pachyrhyncha and a fibroma of the uterus of the Eurasian brown bear Ursus arctos.

Fibrosarcomas have been described in diverse species: Raja macrorhynchus, Carcharchinus leucas, Anguilla anguilla, Conger conger, Esox lucius, Hucho hucho, Oncorhynchus keta, Oncorhynchus gorbuscha, Salmo gairdneri, S. trutta, Leuciscus leuciscus, Phoxinus phoxinus, Xiphophorus helleri, Xiphophorus masculatus, Gadus morrhua, Gadus virens, Melanogrammus aeglefinus, Theragra chalcogramma, Lateolabrax japonicus, Leopdotrigla alata, Pogonias chromis, Scorpaena porcus, Stizostedion vitreum, Crotalus viridus, Cerytophrys ornata, Ambystoma tigrinum, Scophthalmus maximus, Pleuronectes platessa, Hippoglossus hippoglossus. Other observations, from fish to mammals, include the trout and salmon (540), Vipera russelli; birds, Chenonetta jubata, Axis galericulata,

Coturnix chinensis lineata, Gallus gallus murghi, Pavo cristatus (skin), Pavo muticus imperator, Pavo cristatus (35,124, 298, 299, 556), the cat (140); the white-tailed deer (135); and monkeys (66, 496).[9] The most frequently used experimental species are the chicken, Japanese quail, mouse, guinea pig, rat, and monkeys.

NEOPLASMS ARISING FROM MELANIN-CONTAINING CELLS (MELANOCYTES)—FROM MELANOGENIC SYSTEMS AND OTHER PIGMENT CELLS, SUCH AS GUANOPHORES

The melanophores in man occur in the skin but also other tissue types, such as the connective and nervous tissues. All are seastar- or spindle-like cells with a high melanin content of the cytoplasm.

The melanin content characterizes cells of animals and plants as well as fungi. A table reviewing the situation is given in Chapter 38. The melanin-containing cells offer an excellent model for the study of carcinogenesis in the widest sense of tumorigenesis, bridging the gap between animals and plants in the old Aristotelian two-kingdom approach.

The metabolism of highly carcinogenic compounds such as BP in mammalian microsomes is similar to the one in fungal cells as stated by Gibson and mentioned at the beginning of the chapter. BP is an external compound which enters the metabolism of organisms which are taxonomically as far apart as fungi and mammals, whereas the pigment melanin is an endogenous pigment or, chemically speaking, a group of compounds characterizing the cells of different organisms and groups of tissues. Melanin is unifying on one hand and is the characteristic of highly malignant neoplasms on the other.

The benign tumor in man is the naevus bleu or melanoma which is a lesion of dopa-positive connective tissues.

Giant melanosomes were present in two cases of eruptive naevi when investigated with light and electron microscopy (130), and there were multiple layers of basement membrane around myelinated and unmyelinated fibers in cellular blue nevus (49).

---

[9] A neurofibrosarcoma of the spine was diagnosed in Agkistrodon halys brevicaudis.

The malignant tumors are the melanosarcomas. The cells of the tumors which may be dormant in a benign fashion for years and finally start to grow and metastasize very rapidly act in a totally unpredictable manner. The characteristic cell in all melanomas is the melanin-producing melanocyte. The ability to produce melanin is characteristic for certain cells in man, animals (including invertebrates), vascular plants, and fungi. The characteristic cells in the animal (vertebrate) derive from the neuroectoderm, but they derive their particular origin not from the same tissue, as carcinomas or sarcomas do in general, but from the aforementioned transitional embryonal structure. Main characteristics are the pigment production and the wide distribution in kingdoms, phyla, species, organs, and tissues. As pointed out by Sancho and Cesarini (479), the accuracy of the histological staging of primary malignant melanoma is still unsatisfying. The rodents used most often in experiments are the mouse, rat, Syrian and golden hamsters, and the guinea pig.

Electron microscopy: Hunter et al. (252) used the fine structure in invasive nodules of different histogenetic types of malignant melanoma to establish their distinction. Melanosomes spread superficially, and nodular melanomas are generally spheroidal and abnormal in appearance whereas those lentigo malignant melanomas are generally ellipsoidal and look like those in normal melanocytes (251). Melanosome polymorphism is expressed in a wide spectrum of melanosomal morphology (253). Human melanoma cells in vitro kept the characteristics of the melanoma cells in vivo from which they were derived (147). Investigations of melanosome formation in a cultured cell line showed that the mitochondria seem to be involved in the process of melanosome formation (486). Achromatic skin examined with the electron microscope shows that in the case of malignant melanoma, abnormalities of melanocytes and perhaps immunologic factors occur also in the normal skin of patients with malignant melanoma (427). An observation by Szekeres and Orfanos (539) has confirmed that in the case of malignant melanoma, changes in the melanocytes occur even outside the tumor region (see also Hach et al. (203) and Aubert et al. (20)). Schieferstein (485) investigated the immunology of malignant melanomas. The occurrence of tyrosinase in transplantable amelanotic melanoma was studied in the Syrian hamster by Bomirski and Wrzolkowa (57).

The growth of the pigment epithelium of the retina in different regions such as the posterior pole, the equator region, and the ora region shows a varying pattern and number of layers (335). Nucleoli, chromatin, and cytoplasmic structures varied extensively in four malignant melanomas of spindle cell type in the iris (342). The phosphorylase system in choroidal melanoma of the spindle B and epithelioid cell types exhibited two patterns of synthesized polyglucose particles: fine granular, or amorphous. The same holds true for melanophages. These two types of melanoma cells showed no difference in glycolysis (7). Pülhorn and Winter (443) reported about the histology of a malignant melanoma of the choroid, type "Knapp-Rönne", in 1976. Studies by Spence et al. in 1976 (521) reconfirmed the opinion of Pierrre Masson (358) that neoplastic nerve sheath cells are capable of melanogenesis. Smooth membranes are important for the formation of premelanosomes and melanosome microtubules for melaninisation concerning in vitro cultivation of human uveal melanomas (70). Melanomas as well as tumors of neural origin and sarcomas in tissue culture investigated by scanning and transmission electron microscopy do not exhibit desmosomes (193).

A possible melanoma in invertebrates has been observed in the echinoderm, Ophiurus sp. (?). Some species in which melanosarcomas have been observed are: Raja clavata; Oncorhynchus tshawytscha; Anoptichthys jordani; eye; Carassius auratus, orbit; Poecilia reticulata x P. sphenops; Poecilia reticulata x P. sphenops, skin; Xiphophorus variatus xiphidium, skin; X. masculatus; X. helleri; skin; X. pygmaeus, eye; X. spp.; Lophius piscatorius, skin; Epinephelus gauza; Menidea beryllina, skin; Micropterus salmoides; Pterophyllum eimekei; Pterophyllum scalare; Anser anser; Brachydania rerio; Xiphophorus masculatus, eye; Xiphophorus spp.; Gadus morhua; Scomber colias, skin; and Canis sp.

Neoplasms in fish have brought a new aspect to the study of genetics, as related to the origin of cancer (2, 493, 509, 571–575). Melanomas have of course been observed in domesticated animals such as dogs, cats, horses, and cattle (125). See also Betton and Owen (47) and Betton (46), Gwin et al. (202), Kraft and Frese (307), Brodey et al. (65) for the dog; Cardy (80) and Peiffer et al. (425) for the cat; Traver et al. (557) and others for the horse; Mangkoewidjojo and Kimb (355) for the hamster; Hu et al. (249) for cell lines of rhesus monkey and mouse; and Thirloway *et al.* (548) for duroc boar.

Bellotti *et al.* (43) reported about the histological variance of cutaneous malignant melanoma in relation to prognosis.

A malignant melanoma of a ground squirrel, *Spermophilus tridecemlineatus*, revealed ultrastructurally oval cells, spindle-shaped cells, and spindle-shaped cells with electron-dense cytoplasmic granules. The cell culture showed a virus belonging to the herpes group whose buoyant density was 1.298 g/cm³ and whose diameter of the enveloped virus particles was 146 nm (129). A malignant melanoma (of the eye) was seen in *Zalophus californianus*, and another one was seen in *Ovis ammon aries* (132).

Another pigment cell not present in man but in the skin of teleosts is the guanophore. The tumor is the guanophorama, which was described in such fish as *Ctenobrycon spilurus*, *Archosargus probatocephaulus*, and *Hexagrammos otakii*.

NEOPLASMS ARISING FROM SPECIALIZED CONNECTIVE TISSUES. I. ADIPOSE TISSUE

The adipose cells have a wide distribution in the human body, where they occur for support and storage.

The most common benign lesion is the lipoma, which is a tumor composed of adipose cells, generally well circumscribed and often encapsulated.

The infiltrating lipoma or intramuscular lipoma is a benign tumor, which can be considered as a variation of the lipoma and which infiltrates striated muscle but lacks any sign of atypia. The lipoma includes also such versions as fibrolipoma, angiolipoma, and others.

The benign hibernoma is a brown, lipoid-rich encapsulated tumor with large, lipid-rich (brown) fat cells. Certain fibrolipomas can be considered a subtype. Other versions which may be considered as benign tumors or hamartomas are the angiomyolipoma, which derives from the renal cortex and exhibits adipose tissue, vascular structures, and smooth musculature but generally no capsule, and the myelolipoma consisting of hematopoietic tissue and adipose tissue. This rare tumor is most often found in the adrenal gland. Finally, the lipoblastomatosis or fetal lipoma and the diffuse lipomatosis have to be mentioned.

The liposarcoma exhibits a variable, uniform, or differing structure. Different subtypes can be distinguished according to the predominant character of the lesion under investigation: well-differentiated, myxoid (embryonal), containing round cells, pleomorphic or poorly differentiated and mixed in character. This distinction is clinically very important because of differing prognoses paralleling the histologic character. However, this distinction is also essential for comparative pathology for the sake of the accuracy of the comparative diagnosis and to make the results reliable, especially regarding metabolism.

The myxosarcoma presents a primitive, indifferent mesenchymatic appearance, like mucoid connective tissue. It may be considered as being a subtype or a single unit. The electron microscopy of the myxoid sarcoma shows immature fat cells with active pinocytosis and some signet ring cells (159). Lipid-containing neoplastic cells with other mesenchymal cells lacking adipose characteristics were seen in cystosarcoma phyllodes with liposarcomatous stroma (444). Adipose tissue occurs in different variations, the best known of which in the invertebrates is that of insects (the so-called fat body) and the regular or white adipose tissue and the brown adipose tissue in vertebrates. No comparison to plants is possible. A fibrolipoma was described of *Hippoglossus stenolepis* and in invertebrates, and lipomas have been found in *Esox lucius*, subcutaneously; *Plecoglossus altevelis*, subcutaneously; *Salvelinus namaycush*; *Abramis brama*; *Leuciscus leuciscus*, coelom; *Gadus virens*, liver; *Micropterus salmoides*; *Pomixix nigromaculatus*; *Sebastes diploproa*; *Trachurus trachurus*; *Hippoglossus hippoglossus*; *Paralichthys oblivaceus*; *Pleuronectes platessa*; *Xenopus laevis laevis*, integument; *Crocodilus acutus*; *Melopsittacus undulatus*; monkey (body wall), monkey (uterus); *Balaenoptera musculus*, liver surface; *Megaptera novaengliae*, cerebral; *Lama guanicoe glama*; *Leo pardus*.

Lipomas have also been observed in the dog (547); the cat (498); the neonatal calf (256); and the horse (106). The liposarcoma is known from *Panthera tigris tigris* (132) (see Chapter 48).

NEOPLASMS ARISING FROM SPECIALIZED CONNECTIVE AND SUPPORTING TISSUES. II. CHORDAL TISSUE

Chordal tissue in man is restricted in the adult to the nucleus pulposus of the intervertebral disk.

The chordoma occurs in benign or malignant variants which are characterized by pleomorphic lobulated appearance. According to the parent tissue, the tumors of chordal tissue can theoretically only appear in the chordate phyla (hemichordata, urochordata, cephalochordata, and vertebrata). The rat is mainly used as experimental animal. Organ culture of a human sacral chordoma revealed one type of basic cell which was small and polygonal and exhibited a large central spherical nucleus, abundant endoplasmic reticulum, Golgi apparatus, and vacuoles (244). For the ultrastructure, biochemistry, and cytophotometry, see also Mikuz et al. (379).

NEOPLASMS ARISING FROM CONNECTIVE AND SUPPORTING TISSUES. III. CHONDROID TISSUE

Menisci and tendons represent this type of tissue in man.

The fibroma, either benign or malignant, is the tumor of concern. Islets of spindle cells resemble the characteristics of a benign fibroma. Special fibromas of tendons are the benign giant cell tumors (see the section on reticular connective tissue, p. 681), composed of spindle and multinucleated giant cells. A high amount of collagen fibers may be present, as well as infiltration with lipoids.

The malignant forms are characterized by atypical, somewhat smaller giant cells with bizarre contours.

Until now the tissue is known only from vertebrates but it may also occur in certain invertebrates, perhaps in the tendinous insertions of echinoderm muscles. A comparison to plants is not possible.

NEOPLASMS ARISING FROM SPECIALIZED CONNECTIVE AND SUPPORTING TISSUES. IV. CARTILAGE

Cartilage comprises the cartilaginous portion of the skeleton in man. The chondroma is a solitary benign cartilaginous tumor in endochondral bone. Chung and Enzinger (98) reviewed 104 cases of chondroma of the soft parts. The general age of the patients was in the third and fourth decade of which 61% were male patients; 64% of the neoplasms occurred in the hand and

20% in the soft tissues in the feet. The well-demarcated tumors showed a lobulated appearance and a size of 1–2 cm. The main tissue composing the neoplasms was mature hyaline cartilage often undergoing calcification but there occurred also histologic variations with giant cells or chondroblastic activity. But these variations produced no other behavior of the neoplasms than the general type. Electronmicroscopy of chondroma is described by Winkelmann and Becker (602).

The enchondroma is also benign and occurs in two subtypes; the first one is the solitary enchondroma composed of hyaline cartilage. It is more cellular than the chondroma. The cells often look like normal chondrocytes. They lie frequently in well-prepared lacunae. The cells and the nucleus are round. The cytoplasm, which may be vacuolated, is eosinophilic. Some cartilaginous tissues may also be formed by the periosteum. The lesion is more cellular than the solitary enchondroma, and the nuclei of the cells are larger. The second subtype is the multiple enchondromatosis. Some cartilaginous tissues may likewise be formed by the periosteum. The lesion is more cellular than the solitary enchondroma, and the nuclei of the cells are larger.

Solitary Osteochondroma

The tumor-like lesion occurs as a sessile or stalked protuberance of the epiphyseal region of the endochondral bone. A cap of cartilage over a bony protuberance and a fibrous layer as perichondrium are the characteristics in well-developed cases.

The multiple osteochondromatosis is an infrequent (genetic) disorder in man, of skeletal growth which may change to malignancy with development of pleomorphism, especially large cartilage cells with bizarre nuclei.

The chondroblastoma is a malignant tumor related to the chondromyxoid fibroma.

The chondromyxoid fibroma, rare and benign in man, is composed of chondroid material, sometimes also hyaline cartilage, a myxoid substance, and fibrous components.

Only one case of chondromyxoid fibroma of the pterygopalatine space is known and described by Toremalm et al. (554). However, the extraskeletal myxoid chondrosarcoma is also a very rare tumor with only 42 cases reported (516).

Chondrosarcomas of different subtypes are fundamental neoplasms of osteogenous tissue. Dense cellular pattern, large nuclei, quite a number of binucleated cells, cells with multiple nuclei and irregular nuclear size, and hyperchromatism are characteristic. The mesenchymal chondrosarcoma arises from mesenchyme which forms cartilage, and the extraosseous chondrosarcoma arises outside the bone.

The comparison and ultrastructure of chondrosarcoma of high differentiation (dedifferentiated foci) and a poorly differentiated chondrosarcoma with spindle cells showed similarities between both tumors. The endoplasmic reticulum was abundant, and the cell membrane showed microvilli. The cells of the differentiated tumor (276) variety were compared with the poorly differentiated sarcoma with spindle cells.

Cartilage occurs in mollusca, annelida, arthropoda, and vertebrata. No comparison is possible to plants. The potential in regard to succeeding tissues in cartilage varies in taxonomic groups. This is a problem with connective tissues generally. Chondromas have been observed in *Scyliorhinus caniculus* (right flank); *Squalus fernandinus* (lumbar); *Barbus barbus* and *Phoxinus phoxinus* (mandible); *Gadus virens* (head); and *Triturus vulgaris* (integument). An endochondroma is known from *Varanus draconea*.

Cases found in domesticated laboratory and zoo animals include osteochondromatosis of cervical vertebrae in the dog (5), the tracheal osteochondroma in the dog (246), and the osteochondroma in a lioness (545). Chondrosarcoma of the dog was light- and electron microscopically investigated by Halliwell and Kinden (207), and biochemically the chondrosarcoma of the swarm rat was investigated by Oegema et al. (404).

NEOPLASMS ARISING FROM SPECIALIZED CONNECTIVE AND SUPPORTING TISSUE. V. BONE

Bone is the major tissue of the human skeleton, but at the same time bone is the peak of connective tissue development in the vertebrates for which (with exceptions—agnatha, chondrichthyes, carangidae) it is characteristic. Phylogenetically, bone is also the youngest major type of animal tissue, and it stands at the end of phylogenetic development which began with mesenchymatic cells, perhaps comparable to those occurring today in acoelomate animals such as flatworms far back in Precambrian time, more than a billion years ago. The tumor pattern in human bone, as an example of vertebrate bone, reflects this development like a mirror. This can be easily seen when we look at the different types of neoplasms occurring in bone seen as an organ.

First, there are the unclassified neoplasms which cannot be included in any other group of mesenchymatic or other tissues because their cells are too anaplastic. Tumors are known which can be considered as being remnants of the intermediate stages from the mesenchymatic stem cell to the osteoblast in the convergent lines of tissue development. To this group belong such neoplasms as certain fibromas, lipomas, fibrosarcomas, liposarcomas, or malignant mesenchymomas which appear in bone, but to the same group belong neoplasms like the chordoma, neurolemmoma, and neurofibroma. These neoplasms are somewhat distinct from the other because the chorda tissue already belongs to a specialized type of supporting tissues and the cells of the neurilemmoma to the glial series of the peripheral nerves. The organ bone also contains vessels from which neoplasms may arrive which cannot be directly included in bone as a tissue: these are hemangiomomas, lymphangiomas, glomangiomas, hemangioendotheliomas, hemangiopericytomas, and angiosarcomas. In addition to the intramembranous bone formation, the endochondral or intracartilaginous bone formation occurs and is characterized by a replacement of cartilage through bone. Cartilage-forming tumors in bone as an organ have been in general described with the neoplasms of the tissue groups known as cartilage. In this presentation only those tumors which form or are involved in the growth of bone tissue are discussed. These are the benign osteoma, the benign osteoid osteoma, the benign osteoblastoma, and the osteosarcoma, either osteogenic or parosteal. The neoplasms of bone marrow have been evaluated together with the hematogenic tissues. For practical purposes a discussion of the Ewing sarcoma has been added. On account of practical relationship and topographical position, the tumors of the other "hard tissues" of the body, the teeth, the adamantinomas, ameloblastomas, and adontomas are included. Bone is the tissue of the human skeleton; from it originate tumors which belong in the osteogenic series of connective tissues but are not directly characteristic for bone tissue; one example is the benign fibroma. Also benign is the chondroblastoma.

The osteoma is a term which has been applied to several different lesions, of which not many can be considered as neoplastic because they are more or less initiated by trauma or infection.

Comparative evaluation has to be done, therefore, with utmost care.

The fibroosteoma is composed of neoplastic osteoblasts in abundant fibrous stroma.

Osteoid osteoma is an entity for which it is questionable whether it can be distinguished from other osteogenic tumors. It is a rare lesion.

The osteosarcoma is the most important, most common, and most aggressive of the malignant bone tumors. The pattern is highly variable and shows a mimicry from spindle cells to osteoblast or osteoblast-like cells. Malignant spindle cells show hyperchromatic nuclei. Pleomorphism may occur, as well as an increased number of nuclei.

For the classification of osteosarcomas, see Le Charpentier et al. (324), and for the osteogenesis and chondrogenesis in osteoma cell cultures, see Hanamura and Urist (210).

In the sarcoma of Paget's bone disease, all types of skeletal tissue differentiation may be seen. The parosteal osteosarcoma is a slow-growing highly differentiated version which grows from the external bone surface. The osteoclastoma, which makes up 5% of all primary bone tumors in man, exhibits stromal cells (spindle, ovoid, or round mononuclear cells) and interspersed multinucleated giant cells with from 10 to more than 200 distinct nuclei. The fibrosarcoma is a nontypical malignant tumor of the osteogenic series of connective tissues. The same is the case with the liposarcoma of bone, which is extremely rare.

Ewing's sarcoma has small cells characterized by round nuclei, prominent nucleoli, and well-delineated cytoplasmic outlines. In this malignant tumor the tissue may be divided by fibrous septa, but reticulin fibers are not visible. In its histology, reticulum cell sarcoma of the bone simulates the reticlum cell sarcoma of lymph nodes. It is composed of round or oval cells with generally round or somewhat indented horseshoe-shaped pronounced nuclei and relatively poor cytoplasm. Reticulin fibrils surround cells or cell groups uniformly. Extraosseous sarcoma is composed of giant cells and fibrosarcomatous tissue.

Bone tissue is characteristic of and restricted to the vertebrates, with the exception of cartilaginous fish and those teleosts exhibiting the osteoid substance of Koelliker. The following cases were observed and described: A fibroosteoma was seen in *Hypoglossus stenolepis* and osteomas in *Scyliorhinus caniculus* (trunk); *Esox lucius* (mandible); *Oncorchynchus keta*; *Salvelinus fontinalis*; *Cyprinus carpio* (skull); *Gadus morhua* (maxilla); *Gadus morhua* (vertebra);

Theragra chalcogramma (fin); *Chaetodipterus faber* (vertebra); *Chrysophrys major* (multiple); *Lepidopus spp.* (fin); *Micropogon opercularis*; *Pongonias chromis* (vertebra); *Sciaenida spp.* (multiple cases); and *Gallirallus australis greyi*.

Osteosarcomas are known from *Esox lucius* (fin); *Oncorhynchus kisutch* (osteogenic); *Chimpanzee troglodytes* (skin), and *Chrysocyon brachyurus* (osteogenic). The hamster and the rat are the most often used laboratory animals for osteosarcoma research. Foremost among domesticated animals are the cat and the dog, but the latter especially exhibits a multiplicity of cases. An osteoma spongiosum in the cat was reported by Papmahl-Hollenberg (416), and an osteoma in the zygomatic arch of a cat by Knecht and Greene (297). Primary and secondary bone tumors in the dog were reviewed by Dorfman et al. (124); primary neoplasms of the nasal cavity, paranasal sinuses, and nasopharynx in the dog by Confer and Depaoli (102); musculoskeletal tumors in dogs by Knecht and Priester (298, 299); Brodey and Abt (64) in 1976 reported about the surgical treatment of 65 dogs with osteosarcoma. For osteosarcoma in the dog, see also Owen (410) and Wilson and Alsaker (600), and for osteosarcoma in the canine skull, Johnson (271), for osteosarcoma of the hard palate Howard et al. (247), and for osteosarcoma of the axial skeleton in the dog (490). The frequency of osteosarcoma among first degree relatives of St. Bernard dogs was investigated by Bach-Nielsen et al. (24); for extraskeletal osteosarcomas in the dog, see Patnaik et al. (417) and Eckerlin et al. (131). Osteogenic sarcoma occurs frequently in chronic nonunion fractures in dogs (see Madewell et al. (351)). The osteogenic sarcoma appears also spontaneously in mice (392) and the rat (349); for experiments and related questions, see Siniakov (510), Ash and Loutit (17), Sinibaldi et al. (511), and also Wandera (586). An osteosarcoma in a squirrel monkey was reported by Reed and Garman (451).

NEOPLASMS ARISING FROM SPECIALIZED CONNECTIVE AND SUPPORTING TISSUE. VI. OSTEOID TISSUE

The tissue does not occur in man. Real neoplasms have not been described to date, but phylogenetic, type-specific conditions known as pachystoses have been described in such species as carangid fish (277).

NEOPLASMS ARISING FROM MYOEPITHELIAL TISSUES (BASKET CELLS IN MAMMALS)

Only one of the three subtypes, subtype C, is present in man as the basket cells in salivary and mammary glands. The incident of myoepithelial cells in the formation of spindle cells of mixed mammary gland tumors in bitches was investigated by von Bomhard and Sandersleben (580). For reports of the normal myoepithelial cell in this topographical area, see Schlotke (487) (see also Ghosh et al. (186)). The benign lymphoepithelial lesions in salivary glands are somewhat similar to but also different from Sjögren's syndrome. The apocrine myoepithelioma, which is also benign, is composed of cuboidal cells and myoepithelial cells. It has sheet proliferation.

The malignant clear cell hidradenoma is made up of glycogen rich, large clear cells. Also malignant is the myoepithelial tumor (hidradenoma) of the vulva, which is composed of mixed myoepithelial cells.

The three types of myoepithelial tissue (A, B, and C) have to be separated according to their phylogenetic appearance: Subtype A occurs in low eumetazoans such as cnidaria, ctenophora, and entoprocta; subtype B in forms like the ectoprocta; and subtype C in mammals. There is no comparability to plant tissues, and it does not occur in other muscle tissues.

Neoplasms involving myoepithelial musculature have been observed only in mammals, but they are theoretically possible in other groups mentioned before.

NEOPLASMS ARISING FROM SMOOTH (UNSTRIPED) MUSCULATURE

In man this type of tissue is found in the alimentary tract from the middle of the esophagus to the internal anal sphincter; the ducts of alimentary glands; respiratory passages; urinary and genital ducts; walls of arteries; veins and lymphatic vessels; the skin, as in the arrectores pillorum; and the eye, as in the ciliary body.

The benign neoplasm is the leiomyoma composed of smooth muscle cells. It may originate from vascular origin at different locations, such as the choroid (264).

The malignant neoplasm of this type of tissue is the leiomyosarcoma, which occurs either in a typical or atypical variety and which is made up of smooth muscle cells (uniform or variable, according to cell content), similar to leiomyoma. The fine structure of leiomyosarcoma is characterized by radial cisternae, composed of numerous short cisternae, as a variant of annulate lamellae and numerous spherical particles (394).

The semimalignant congenital mesoblastic nephroma must be distinguished from Wilms' tumor and occurs usually at birth. The cells are spindle cells with uniform nuclei and regular mitosis, collagen fibers between the neoplastic cells, an angiomatous marginal zone without tumor capsule, hematopoietic foci, and displastic glomeruli and tubuli which characterize the area where the neoplastic parenchyma intermingles with that of the normal kidney. Small myxomatous regions appear in the tumor, and no invasion of blood vessels or pelvis takes place. In the case when this fibroleiomyomatous kidney tumor occurs in the newborn, it can be considered as an embryonal tumor (53).

Vascular tumors are another type of smooth muscle tumor in which neoplastic smooth muscle cells are a typical component. The neoplasm can be considered as a type of mixed tumor (282).

An investigation of the ultrastructure of the ciliary body leiomyoma reveals several cell types: Small immature myoblasts, large differentiated myoblasts, dystrophic muscle cells with lipofuscin inclusions, and fibroblast-like cells (617).

Light microscope investigation of a leiomyosarcoma of the scrotum showed interlacing fascicles of neoplastic cells with eccentric cigarshaped nuclei. A study of the ultrastructure confirmed the origin of the neoplastic cells from smooth musculature (270).

Annulate lamellae have been found in cases of leiomyoma, leiomyosarcoma, rhabdomyosarcoma, and malignant melanoma whereas radical cisternae occur only in leiomyosarcoma (394).

A vulvar leiomyosarcoma was metastatic to the spinal cord in a dog (232).

An evaluation of the distribution of this tissue type is somewhat problematical because it is generally believed that many invertebrates which we assume exhibit this tissue type, if viewed with the electron microscope, may exhibit obliquely striated musculature. The distribution, according to mainly older light microscope studies, looks as follows: platyhelminthes, nemertinea, rotifera, and other nemathelminth phyla, annelida, mollusca, echinodermata, and chordate phyla, including the vertebrates. This tissue type proves once more why we should start with man and other mammals in the evaluation of animal tumors because the diagnosis, including ultrastructure, is best developed in these species. These facts are also important for comparative oncology where a knowledge of the ultrastructure is essential for proper diagnosis. Leiomyomas have been described in invertebrates such as the bivalve mollusc *Mya arenara*, and in vertebrates like *Clupea harengus harengus* (?), *Salmo gairdneri* (mouth and stomach), *Alburnus alburnus* (trunk), *Carassius arratus*; *Mystus seenghala*; *Arripis trutta*; *Morone saxatilis* (?); *Columbia* sp. (liver); monkey (uterus); *Macaca silenus* (uterus); *Allenopithecus nigroviridis* (uterus); *Dasypus novemcinctus* (stomach); *Myocaster coypus coypus* (uterus).

A cutaneous leiomyosarcoma was seen in *Myxine glutinosa*.

NEOPLASMS ORIGINATING FROM OBLIQUE (HELICALLY, LONGITUDINALLY) STRIATED MUSCULATURE

This type of tissue is not present in man; it is composed of helically striated muscle cells. To date, the tissue has been found in turbellarian platyhelminthes, nematodes, molluscs, and polychaete and oligochaete annelids. Spontaneous neoplasms have not been observed. Experimental proliferations were observed in oligochaeta.

NEOPLASMS ARISING FROM TRANSVERSE STRIATED OR SKELETAL MUSCULATURE

The transverse striated musculature in man is the somatic musculature, composing the active portion of the locomotory system, the skeletal muscles. The cytoplasm exhibits in its ultrastructure two types of fibrillar bundles of 40–60 Å and 100–150 Å and regular C-like bands (ref. 92; see also Galil-Ogly et al. (174)).

Leiomyomas of skin arteries and ecophagus and leiomyosarcomas and rhabdomyosarcomas were compared recently by Galil-Ogly et al. (174) to establish a comparative histogenetic approach. Two types of filaments (40–60 Å and 100–150 Å) can be used as a diagnostic tool in the case of myogenic neoplasms using electron microscopy (92).

The rare rhabdomyoma composed of immature (Misch), well-striated muscle cells and the granular cell myoblastoma composed of undifferentiated muscle cells and a well-organized border of neoplasm are the benign tumors in man. The cells in fetal rhabdomyoma, of which only nine fetal and 35 adult cases have been described until 1976, are characterized by myoblastic or myotubular differentiation of the neoplastic cells (585).

Fetal rhabdomyoma is a very rare lesion, with only 10 cases reported. They are nearly exclusively restricted to the musculature of mouth and neck. About the findings of the ultrastructure with the cells showing myoblastic or myotubular differentiation, it is believed that the tumor is a different stage in the life history of rhabdomyoma. It is questionable as to whether it should be considered a hamartoma or a neoplasm (585).

The rhabdomyosarcoma, which is rhabdomyomatous, poorly demarcated, partially very destructive, and characterized by cellular pleomorphism, is the main malignant neoplasm, occurring in man in three subtypes: these are pleomorphic in adults, characterized by large and small spindle cells; embryonic, which is characterized by an indifferent blastema with long spindles and a variation of striation; and finally the juvenile alveolar subtype with multinucleated alveolar pattern. The ultrastructure of embryonal rhabdomyoma exhibits rhabdomyoblasts (105). Electron microscopy revealed rhabdomyoblasts in three cases of the rare orbital, embryonal rhabdomyosarcomas (105).

The main portion of an alveolar rhabdomyosarcoma consisted of small polygonal cells with polyribosomes, a short strand of rough endoplasmic reticulum, and varying amounts of glycogen. In addition, small desmosome-like structures were observed. Next to similar cells, larger ones appeared also along the septa; they seem to have derived from small cells. These forms exhibited copious cytoplasm and rarely developed myofilaments. The third type was composed of giant cells. The septa were built of collagen and fibroblasts. The histogenesis of the tumor organization may represent a cellular pattern, as at the stage of somite differentiation (99). Concerning ophthalmic rhabdomyosarcoma, which has to be regarded as the most common primary malignant tumor in the orbita of childhood, Knowles et al. (300) arrived at results similar to those of Churg and Ringus (99). The neoplastic cells of the tumor are rhabdomyoblasts in different stages and in differentiation comparable to the embryogenesis of normal muscle. They seem to start from pluripotential embryonal mesenchyme, and these childhood tumors are nearly always of the embryonal type; 162 cases had been described until 1976. Ultrastructural studies of experimental rhabdomyosarcomas by Riede et al. (458) confirmed the earlier reports.

Two other types of neoplasms should also be mentioned: the sarcoma botryoides of the cervix and the very rare and varying mesodermal mixed tumors of the uterus.

The tissue distribution of striated musculature, and therefore the theoretical neoplastic potential of this tissue is very wide because it has been found in rotifera, mollusca, arthropoda, entoprocta, echinodermata, chaetognatha, and vertebrata, comprising, therefore, as the characteristic musculature of the insects in addition to others, the majority of animal species. There exists no comparability to plants. The rhabdomyoma has been found in *Clupea harengus harengus*; *Osmerus eperlanus* (trunk); *Salmo clarki*; *Salmo gairdneri*; *Labrus mixtus*; *Perca fluviatilis*; *Scophtalmus maximus* (trunk); and *Sternothaerus niger* (heart).

Myoblastomas have been found in *Lumbricus terrestris* (body wall), concerning invertebrates and in *Catostomus macrocheilus*, to name just one vertebrate.

NEOPLASMS ARISING FROM CARDIAC MUSCULATURE

Cardiac musculature occurs in man in the heart as well as the roots of the ascending aorta, the pulmonary trunk and arteries, the roots of venae cavae, and the pulmonary veins.

The two types of striated musculature are often treated together as far as the tumors originating from striated muscle cells, their precursors, and developmental stages are concerned. The benign and malignant tumors, rhabdomy-

omas and rhabdomyosarcomas, even have the same name; no attention is paid as to whether they derive from skeletal striated musculature or cardiac-striated musculature. However, in the field of comparative pathology, it is absolutely necessary that we distinguish between these two types and furthermore even between subtypes. This fact can be easily understood if we consider the distribution of these tissue variations as shown in Table 43.1. Skeletal cross-striated musculature is one of the most widely distributed tissues because it is characteristic of the musculature of insects. Nevertheless, subtypes of lesser magnitude may be present. In contrast, striated cardiac musculature is of a much more narrow, species-specific distribution. The major type is known from vertebrates, another subtype from crustaceous decapod arthropods, such as the American crayfish *Homarus*. It is questionable as to whether some variations may occur in different molluscs. Therefore, cardiac rhabdomyomas and rhabdomyosarcomas have a much more limited general distribution. Theoretically, it is even more restricted through the presence of subtypes. Neoplasms of these tissue types have not been found in invertebrates to date.

The benign neoplasm is the rhabdomyoma, rare in man, and composed of long, striated anastomizing muscle cells with fibrils.

Cardiac rhabdomyomas are rare tumors of childhood. (In a series of 36 patients investigated by Fenoglio et al. (154), 78% were under 1 yr of age, and only one patient was over 15 years old.) The generally multiple lesions, which could therefore also be considered hamartomas, showed typical spider cells. The ultrastructure was characterized by scattered bundles of myofibrils, free glycogen in cytoplasm and mitochondria, and intercellular junctions with well-defined desmosomes, and many cells contained leptofibrils.

The malignant neoplasm is the rhabdomyosarcoma of the heart, similar in texture to the rhabdolytic sarcoma.

Light microscope studies have shown that the tissue occurs equally in arthropods (decapod crustaceans) and vertebrates, but that electron microscopy and functional characteristics (innervation) required distinction between subtype A in arthropods and subtype B in chordate phyla. The two show differences in nerve supply and phylogenic appearance.

Rats, mice, Syrian hamsters, and cats were used as experimental animals. See Hirano et al. (239) for tumor enhancement in rats, and for the ultrastructure in the dog, Meyvisch *et al.* (375); for mixed glioma combined with the rhabdomyosarcoma in the brain of a wild deer, see Holscher *et al.* (243).

NEOPLASMS OF NEUROENDOCRINE TISSUES

Neoplasms of neuroendocrine tissues, despite the cell consistency of neurons, could be evaluated on the basis of the neuroendocrine action due to juvenile precursors of the invariable cells; however, to the knowledge of the author, they have never been evaluated in this way. The possible distribution in the phyla and, concomitantly, the theoretical tumor potential show the following picture as described in Chapter 4, p. 93. Due to these functional aspects, this section was placed here (Fig. 43.3).

NEOPLASMS OF THE NERVOUS SYSTEM (168).

The tumors of the nervous tissues are arranged in this section, starting with maldeformations. The two main groups are those arising from cells of the neurone series (precursors because of cell invariability) and those of the glial series and related structures. According to species-specific distribution, the neoplasms arising from the peripheral neurone series have, at least theoretically, the widest distribution, in contrast to those of the neurons of the CNS. The position of those deriving from the glial series seems to be medial. However, new comparative investigations are urgently needed because of this relationship, and because studies of the CNS are most restricted. (This is especially true if we consider that a real CNS with developed brain exists only in molluscs, arthropods, and vertebrates, and perhaps in annelids.) However, this is more or less a matter of opinion (see Bullock and Horridge, Chapter 3).

In human pathology the neoplasms of the nervous system are divided into primary intramedullary neurogenic tumors and primary extramedullary neurogenic tumors. Both groups contain neoplasms of nerve cells and of sup-

porting, glial cells, and they differ in their cell content.

Maldeformations may occur in all stages, with the exception of the cell invariable ones.

From the standpoint of comparative pathology, it is useful to distinguish first between neoplasms of the neuron series and the glial series. Both groups can be again divided into those of the CNS and parasympathetic nervous system (PNS). This is important because not all invertebrates have a CNS or glial elements.

This consideration results in the following list for the main types of neoplasms of the nervous systems:

1. Neoplasms of the neurogenic series
   a. Neoplasms of the CNS (primary intramedullary nerve cell tumors)
      medulloblastoma
      neurocytoma (ganglioneuroma)
      neuroblastoma
      retinoblastoma (neuroepithelioma of retina)
   b. Neoplasms of the PNS (primary extramedullary nerve cell tumors)
      ganglioneuroma
2. Neoplasms of the supporting cell series
   a. Neoplasms of the CNS (primary intramedullary supporting cell tumors)
      the gliomas
      ependymoma
      oligodendroglioma
      astrocytoma
      astroblastoma
      glioblastoma multiforme
   b. Neoplasms of the PNS (primary extramedullary supporting cell tumors)
      schwannoma (neurilemmoma)
      neurofibroma
      malignant schwannoma

In man, and especially other mammals, intercranial neoplasms exhibit certain peculiarities resulting from the topographic position and the nature of the cells they originate from. The intracranial neoplasms, through their growth, contribute to the pressure in the rigid bony box of the cranium. (The benign ones are a good example of histologically benign neoplasms, which may become practically malignant.) Edema and obstruction of the pathways of cerebrospinal fluid may worsen the situation.

In the invertebrates, a continuous series of developments can be followed. In the annelids the brain is surrounded by soft tissues, including connective tissues. The best investigated brain in invertebrates, and one of the most highly developed, is that of the cephalopods (molluscs), such as squids, which is not enclosed in a rigid

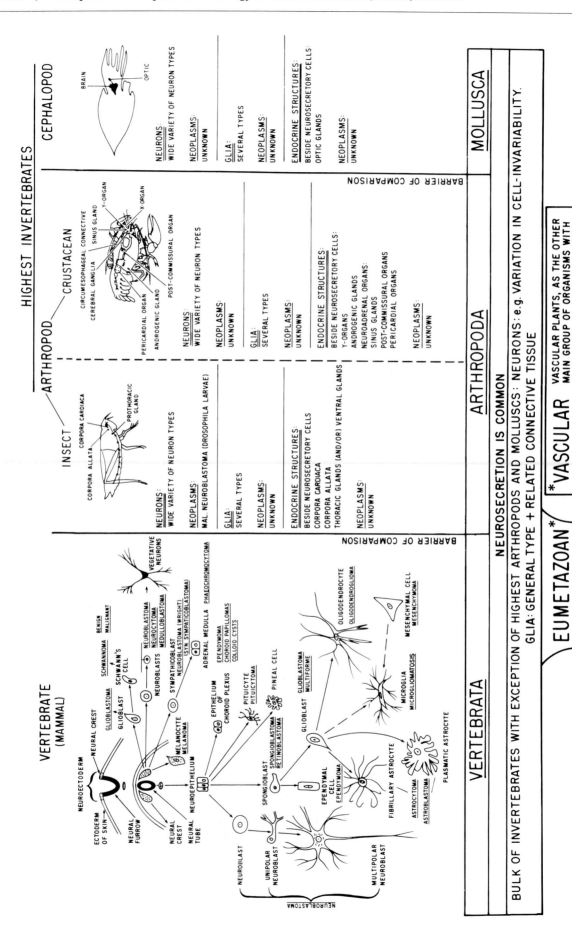

Figure 43.3 Nervous and endocrine system with detected neoplasms in vertebrates, insects, crustaceans, and cephalopods.

capsule. Cartilage is the most important surrounding tissue.

The adult fully differentiated eye of the cephalopods resembles completely, in its arrangement, that found in humans; only the development is different.

In arthropods the brain is enclosed in the exoskeleton but not in a separate rigid capsule applied more or less directly, as in the brain capsule of vertebrates (Fig. 43.4).

This short review shows that the relationship between the brain and other topographical areas is totally different in these species than in mammals. The rigidity of the bone in the vertebrates is an important factor in the development of the neoplasms of their CNS, as contrasted to that of the invertebrates. A different evaluation of these neoplasms from the standpoint of comparative pathology is required because pressure differences in vertebrate and invertebrate brains through tumor growth will reflect on further tumor development in the individuals of these different species.

These differences are not as variable as far as the spinal cord and the other cords are concerned. Nowhere else in the vertebrate trunk is there such a rigid surrounding as for the spinal cord, but even it is interrupted by metamerization and foramina. The dura proper is separated from the inside of the vertebral column and gives space for adipose and areolar tissues (473). Neoplasms belonging to the nervous system by topographical relationship, such as lipomas and others deriving from non-nervous tissue types are not included in the present review.

CONGENITAL TUMORS OF MALDEVELOPMENTAL ORIGIN

These neoplasms are attributed to misplaced cell rests in the sense of the Cohnheim theory.

Ectopic meningiomas occur because of misplaced inclusions of arachnoid cells.

Olfactory neuroblastoma concerning the embryonal elements of the nasal cavity ranges from benign to malignant. This rare neoplasm is composed of undifferentiated neuroblasts and a highly vascular stroma and exhibits a convoluted pattern, which surrounds the blood vessels. The neuroblasts of the richly cellular neoplasm exhibit a round or oval nucleus, without mitoses. The cytoplasm is only a narrow rim.

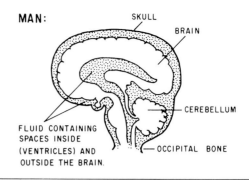

MAN:

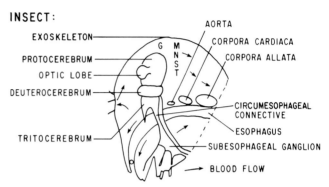

INSECT:

G=GLANDS; M=MUSCULATURE; N=NERVES; S=SINUSES; T=TRACHEAE ARE OTHER STRUCTURES PRESENT IN THE HEAD.

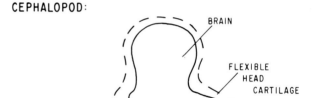

CEPHALOPOD:

Figure 43.4. Conditions of the CNS surroundings in arthropod, mollusc, and vertebrate in relation to glioma development—a theoretical consideration.

The ultrastructure shows a neuronal nature with cytoplasmic filaments, microtubules, and dense vesicles.

Extraspinal gliomas are ectopias or hamartomas of neural origin composed of extracranial and extraspinal tissues and mostly appearing in the area of the nose or pharynx of young people. There are several lesions of which the demarcation between true neoplasms and hamartomas cannot be easily established.

Lindau's syndrome is one of the syndromes connected with tumor formation and first described in 1926 by Lindau. It is known as Lindau-von Hippel disease. Hemangiomas are found in the brain (especially the cerebellum) and retina. Additional commonly observed visceral lesions occur, for example, in liver and pancreas.

Tuberose sclerosis is heredofamilial disease of childhood which also exhibits skin tumors comparable to sebaceous adenomas.

With von Recklinghausen's neurofibromatosis, dominant heredity is established. The tumors of the nervous system which belong to this disease show as their most characteristic phenomenon, multiplicity. In the nerves (cranial, spinal, and peripheral), the sheath elements are affected, in brain and spinal cord glia and meninges can be involved; harmartomas can be added, and sarcomatous changes may occur.

NEOPLASMS ARISING FROM THE NEURON SERIES

These are the one big category of neoplasms of the nervous system.

NEOPLASMS ARISING FROM THE NEURON SERIES OF THE CNS AND RETINA

The retina is included with the neurons of the CNS because optic tract and retina can be considered as a portion of the brain. The organs of concern here in man are the brain and the spinal cord. This is also the case for the other vertebrates. A CNS is most pronounced in the annelida, the mollusca with the highest development in the cephalopods, and the arthropods with the highest development in decapod crustaceans and insects.

Medulloblastoma

The medulloblastoma occurs in benign and malignant variations and is composed of cells of spongioblastic and neuroblastic development. It is a poorly differentiated tumor rich in cells. The cells are round, parashaped, or a spindle in form. Mitoses are usually abundant. The cytoplasm is scanty and lacks structure. The ultrastructure unravels the very primitive cell character (see also Arseni and Nereantiu, ref. 16).

Medulloepithelioma

The histological makeup of this very primitive tumor shows a papillary and tubullary pattern of columnar cells reminiscent of the primitive medullary epithelium.

Neuroblastoma

Neuroblastomas in areas other than the cerebellum of the nervous system are very rare. They occur also in the adrenal medulla and the sympathetic ganglia. High cellular density, some variations in pattern, and small round or oval cells are characteristic. Mitoses are numerous. Mature neurons may occur.

The malignant neuroblastoma is made up of differently arranged, closely stacked cells. Cell rosettes and neurofibrillary processes are important for diagnosis. The most frequently used experimental animals are chicken, mouse, rat, and hamster. Recently, comparative neoplasms have been seen in the fruitfly, *Drosophila melanogaster* (180). For the dog, see Zaki (614).

A neuroblastoma with Homer Wright rosettes in a 10½-year-old boy exhibited foci of immature neoplastic neurons, many mitoses, necrotic areas, and tumor vessels with endothelial proliferation. Electron microscopy revealed cellular characters of early fetal neuroblasts (455); see also Azzarelli et al. (23), especially because of catecholamine determinations. A diagnosis of metastases of the so-called small round cell tumors of childhood, neuroblastoma, Ewing's sarcoma, lymphoma, and rhabdomyosarcoma is difficult. Generally, Ewing's sarcoma contains glycogen, and neuroblastoma does not, but glycogen alone is diagnostically unreliable due to its presence in several neoplasms other than Ewing's sarcoma, including neuroblastoma on one hand and its absence in some cases of Ewing's sarcoma on the other (558). For the comparison of neoplastic cells from parent and hybrid lines of C1300 mouse neuroblastoma and C6 rat glioma, see Anzil et al. (12). Nonspecific cell surface phenomena are considered responsible for the tumor cell differentiation *in vivo* of murine neuroblastoma rather than neuromuscular interactions. The neuroblastoma which was implanted with injured muscle underwent partial neuronal differentiation, during which the tumor cells lost their round appearance and developed many cytoplasmic processes. The microtubules in the neuritic processes increased. Glia-like processes occurred with abundant microfilaments as well as growth vesicles (558).

For antibody formation in mice with neuroblastoma tumors, see Farraggiana *et al.* (150).

Ganglioneuroma and Ganglioglioma

More or less pronounced transitions exist between these two extremes. Neoplasms with mature ganglion cells are more common in the PNS than in the CNS. A pure ganglioneuroma or gangliocytoma is composed of mature ganglion cells and a stroma of spindle cells. Gangliogliomas are mixed versions of neoplasms with mature ganglion cells and mature glial cells. Remarkable variations may occur based on different neoplastic evolution, and this is the reason why both types are treated together.

In the pure ganglioneuroma, composed of many cells from neuronal origin, giant to small cells with bizarre processes may be recognized. Binuclear cells particularly are frequent. The stroma contains spindle cells.

In gangliogliomas the glial elements show astrocytic proliferation. However, oligodendroglial elements also may be seen. Small spheroidal, or spindle-shaped cells, with round or oval small darkly staining nuclei considered as being precursors of neurons appear also. The existence of these cells has been interpreted in different ways. Electron microscopy reveals dense core vesicles in the neuronal cell. Concentrically laminated bodies occur. A change to malignancy is very rare.[10]

Retinoblastoma

The retinoblastomas, ranging from benign to malignant occur, in the latter case, with or without stephanocytes. Cells are closely packed without a special pattern; immature elements remind us of the retina in the embryo. The stroma is tender and highly vascular. An undifferentiated variant is composed of round, oval, or polygonal retinoblasts. The nuclei of these cells, 7–8 μm in diameter, stain deeply. Cyto-

plasm is sparse. The majority of the cells are uniform, but multinucleated and cytoplasma-rich cells occur also. Mitoses may be numerous.

Photoreceptor differentiation was found in developmental direction by electron microscopy. The tumor cells are grouped like flowers; 9+0 pattern cilia, abundant cytoplasmic microtubules, and dense core vesicles occur. The normal distribution of the tissue types and the theoretical tumor spectrum shows that the tissue type is present with variations, of course, in mollusca, annelida, arthropoda, and vertebrata.

The retinoblastoma was described in *Macaca mulatta* and the olfactory neuroblastoma in *Coregonus hoyi* and *Sparus auratus*, in addition to other species (see Chapter 48).

NEOPLASMS ARISING FROM THE NEURON SERIES OF THE PNS (PERIPHERAL TUMORS OF THE NEURONE SERIES)

Neoplasms Arising from Neurons of the Peripheral Nervous System

The tissue type in man occurs in the form of the peripheral ganglia. The benign neoplasm is the ganglioneuroma; the neurosarcomas are the primary malignant tumors of the peripheral nerves, which have been described above as far as their histology and cytology are concerned. The normal distribution spectrum of this tissue type and the theoretical tumor spectrum comprise all eumetazoan phyla. Neurosarcomas have been described in the bivalve mollusc *Crassostrea gigas* and, e.g., in the vertebrates *Lepidorhombus whiffiagonis* and *Pseudopleuronectes* sp.

Neuroblastoma is composed of small regular cells. The spheroidal, ovoid nuclei stain darkly, and cytoplasm is scanty. Rosettes of Homer Wright are present in varying frequency. There is also a large variation in the amount of mitoses. A vascular connective tissue stroma, quite often necrosis, and hemorrhage are typical. Immature neurons appear also. Electron microscopy (EM) reveals cell forms of transition from immature to mature neurons.

Olfactory neuroblastoma is composed of undifferentiated neuroblasts and a highly vascular stroma. The fine structure of this neuronal neoplasm is characterized by cytoplasmic filaments, microtubules, vesicles, and synapses.

---

[10] Different types of pyruvate kinase isoenzymes have been found and compared in normal brain tissue and meningiomas and malignant gliomas (569).

Neuroepithelioma or medulloepithelioma of peripheral nerves is an exceedingly rare malignant neoplasm, whose structure is comparable to the primitive neoplasms with the same name in the CNS. Cell rosets have been observed.

Ganglioneuroblastoma is composed of neuroblasts, transitional cells, and mature neurons. The neuroblastoma is highly malignant, the ganglioneuroma more or less benign. This type of neoplasm is of intermediate character; an imperfect and an immature stage are distinguished. EM reveals similarity of the neoplastic cells with the neurons of the autonomic nervous system.

Ganglioneuromas of the PNS differ from those in the CNS with the same name by the appearance of capsular cells, abundant Schwann cells, and connective tissue elements. EM exhibits rich, rough endoplasmic reticulum (ER) of the ganglion cells, neurofilaments, microtubules, vesicles, and synapses.

With pheochromocytoma, compact alveolar cell groups are separated by a tender connective tissue stroma. The neoplastic structure shows variations. Its cells are polygonal or spheroidal, similar to the cells of the adrenal medulla. The nuclei exhibit different sizes and forms. Nucleoli may be enlarged; the neoplasm is highly vascular. EM shows no neuronal processes or synapses. Experimentally, the rat is the preferred animal. Spontaneous tumors occur in the rat and the dog, in addition to other mammals.

NEOPLASMS ORIGINATING IN THE GLIAL SERIES AND RELATED STRUCTURES

Glial elements are widely distributed throughout the animal phyla but not as widely as the elements of the neuron series. Too little is known from invertebrates to give an exact picture. New experimental research using species with different neuron-glial pattern is urgently needed, and it will be rewarding if we succeed in clarifying certain questions of tumor composition on a comparative basis. The spectrum for these studies in invertebrates is much larger than in vertebrates. Practically and important questions such as the lack of a rigid bony capsule around the CNS may also play a significant role in such considerations.

Neoplasms Arising from Meninges

The normal tissues in man are the meninges. The tumors are the meningiomas, accounting for one-fifth of all intracranial neoplasms in man and occurring in benign to malignant variants. In the case of the pure arachnoid meningiomas, the tumors are composed of capillaries, around which thick collagenous structures occur, and the neoplastic cells simulate arachnoid villi. The main components of the mixed arachnoid and subarachnoid meningiomas are meningiocytes, fibroblastic, and mixed structures. Secondary components are fibrous, angiomatous, lipomatous, osseous, and chondrous. Subarachnoid meningiomas can be wet, lacunar, dry, and lamellar. There occur also pigmented meningiomas. Distribution and neoplastic spectrum include the fact that in cyclostomes and fishes, a single membrane, the meninx primitiva, exists; in amphibians, reptiles, and birds, two structures occur, the inner leptomeninx and the outer pachymenix or dura mater; in mammals, the pachymeninx is again composed of two layers, the inner pia mater and the outer arachnoid which, together with the dura mater, amount to three layers (394). To a certain degree comparable structures exist in invertebrates (see Chapter 3). Due to the species number and anatomic differences of the CNS of higher invertebrates, utmost care must be applied to a comparison of structures in invertebrates which surround the ganglia of higher invertebrates and the cords. The glial surrounding of the larger nerves should, in the author's impression, not be included in such a comparison of vertebrates and invertebrates because only the brain and the spinal cord comprise the CNS in vertebrates. In the invertebrates a strong outer sheath covers ganglia, cords, and larger nerves in the higher types (Bullock and H., Chapter 3). Whether the so-called outer sheath in the invertebrates can be compared to meninges in the vertebrate is questionable today and deserves new studies with more species of higher invertebrates, in the author's opinion especially of the CNS of cephalopods because of their wide range in size from the giant squid *Architheutis* sp. (body length 6.6 m, with arms 18 m long), to the pigmy squid *Idiosepus* sp. (total length, 15–20 mm).

In man and the other mammals, the picture becomes complicated as the situation changes from the skull at the foramen magnum to the spinal cord (vertebrate column). The differences of pressure and surrounding and connecting structures around the two portions of the mammalian CNS cannot be underestimated. The penetration deep into the CNS by meningeal structures is important for neoplastic development. The pia mater penetrates the CNS in relation to the nutrient blood vessels (473). Looking again at invertebrates, the situation of the glial cells in an insect ganglion, as investigated in *Rhodnius* (Hemiptera) by Wigglesworth in 1959 (597), offers the source for a comparison also in the case of the vertebrate meninges if the differences of invertebrate and vertebrate glia are observed. The pressure conditions in the vertebrate skull surrounding the brain (and reflected in the aforementioned different conditions of the meninges in the vertebrate classes), the surrounding cartilaginous structures of the cerebral ganglion in cephalopods and, finally, the conditions of the exoskeleton surrounding the arthropod brain cannot be without influence of disease development originating from neurons and glia.

Meningioma

Cushing and Eisenhardt (112) described nine types with 21 subtypes in 1938. According to tissue culture, the meningiomas can be divided into the following five groups (51):

1. Endotheliomatous
2. Fibroblastic
3. Angioblastic
4. Xanthomatous
5. Myxomatous

In 1945, Courville (107) established the following classification

Type of meningioma	Histologic characteristic
1. Syncytial ⎫	Polygonal, poorly defined cells, arranged in sheets
2. Transitional ⎬ benign	Cell are arranged in whorls.
3. Fibrous ⎪	Spindle cells arranged in interlacing bundles
4. Angioblastic ⎭	Prominent capillary and related structures
5. Sarcomatous malignant	Spindle cells

The picture is further complicated by the appearance of melanin, bone and cartilage, myxomatous nature, giant cells, plasma cells, and lymphoid follicles. Especially for the first groups, the EM exhibits surface specialization and intracytoplasmic filaments, as well as whorled cytoplasmic filaments. There are also eosinophilic inclusions. The cells of type 4 are plump with blunt cytoplasmic edges. Surface specializations are lacking, but hemidesmosomes have been described (432). In group 5, the following subgroups can be distinguished: fi-

brous, spindle-celled, and polymorphocellular with increasing malignancy.

Neoplasms Arising from the Glia of the Central Nervous System

The central glia is the tissue of interest in man. The gliomas are the neoplasms occurring in benign to malignant variations in the vertebrates. The neuroglia and the distribution of their types in phyla are the basis for an understanding of the comparability of the tumors which derive from glial elements. The neuroglia are the non-nervous cells of the nervous system, with the exception of certain cells of blood vessels and other structures more or less connected with the nervous system. The neuroglial elements have not only supporting functions. Glia are considered a special type of connective tissue in vertebrates, but certain types, such as astrocytes, are excluded from this consideration. Again, the comparison of tumors in the different phyla in regard to the glia has to be undertaken with great care because there exist different types of glia in invertebrates; astrocytes (important with regard to the tumors deriving from them in man) do not occur in invertebrates according to some authors.

Astrocytic Group

Astrocytoma. The astrocytoma is composed of glial fibrils in varying abundance and osteocyte-like cells; round to elongated cells without processes are also present. Fasciculated, reticulated, and intermediate variants occur. From a histological basis, Russell and Rubinstein (473) suggested five types of neoplasms originating in astrocytes: (a) protoplasmatic (evenly distributed cells, the cell body is swollen, the processes are short). (b) Fibrillary, diffuse, or circumscribed (the cell bodies are uneven, different looking; criss-crossing neuroglial fibrils are present. EM stresses these variations; glial bipolar fibrils run parallel. The cell processes contain compact bundles of glial filaments, as revealed by EM). (c) Gemistocytic (large closely packed cells are typical with globoid cell bodies and short cell processes. The lesion known as tuberose sclerosis may be included in this group.); (d) Anaplastic (increased cellularity, pronounced polymorphism with mitoses, architectural alteration, and secondary changes are characteristic). Astrocytomas have been observed in the raccoon, *Procyon lotor* (121), and domestic animals such as dogs, less often in cats (168) and pigs (158).

Astroblastoma

Sometimes, the neoplastic cells contain more than one nucleus; the perikaryon is angulated. The tumor cells are clustered in pseudorosets around the abundant vessels.

Polar Spongioblastoma

Compact cell groups, arranged in parallel fashion and palisading (?) nuclei, are separated and supported by vascular-connective tissue stroma. The cells are thin, uni- or bipolar with tender neuroglial fibrils.

Oligodendroglioma is an uncommon neoplasm; the cells resemble oligodendrocytes. These nests of pale cells exist with scanty or no fibrillary material. The neoplasm consists of a compact arrangement of swollen cells, separated by scarce and tender stroma of blood vessels and collagen. Mitoses range from rare to numerous. EM studies reported by different authors revealed abundant, sometimes abnormally enlarged mitochondria, cytoplasmic protogliafibrils, and an overlapping of glial cell processes.

Ependymoma and Homologues

These neoplasms have perivascular pseudorosets, cell rosets in differentiated variations, no special feature, few supporting stroma, and blepharoblasts. EM studies exhibit a mosaic of cell bodies and processes in pavement-like arrangement, and intracellular microrosets. A thalamic ependymoma in a white-tailed deer, *Odocoileus virginianus*, was described recently (396) but it is also known from other mammals, such as the dog (86).

Subependymoma is a variant with fibrillary subependymal astrocytes.

Glioblastoma Multiforme

This neoplasm is characterized by a variety of cell forms. Giant-celled glioblastomas are characterized by multinucleate giant cells.

Neoplasms Arising from the Glia of the Peripheral Nervous System (Tumors of the Nerve Sheath)

The Schwann cells and/or fibroblasts (143), p. 360) give rise to tumors especially of peripheral nerves such as the neurilemmoma (schwannoma), neurofibroma/neurofibromatosis and malignant schwannoma (143, 358, 473). The schwannoma is known from the German shepherd dog (499), congenital neurofibromatosis from the skin of calves (513) and other animals (see also Chapter 48). For a discussion of tissue and organ culture, see (521).

ABNORMAL GROWTH IN HIGHER AND LOWER PLANTS

Abnormal Growth Processes Arising from Plectenchymata[11]

Plectenchymata are not present in angiosperms but occur instead in rhodophyta and basidiomycetes belonging to the eumycetes. They are especially highly developed in the sporophores of higher fungi. The occurrence is quite common, and the pathologic structures are represented by nodular and irregular outgrowth. They are built by the interweaving of the cellular threads. These structures are known as galls and have been found in the following rhodophyta: *Chantransia* sp., *Chondrus* sp., *Furcellaria* sp., and *Gracilaria confervoides*. From fungi, galls have been described in: *Boletus grannulatus*, *Clitocybe* sp., *Tricholoma* sp., *Fomes salicinus*, and *Ganoderma applanatum*. There is no comparison to neoplasms in vertebrates, including man, but perhaps to a certain degree, at least theoretically, to abnormal growth processes in lower porifera.

Abnormal Growth Processes Arising from Pseudoparenchymata

Pseudotissue produced by postgenital coalescence of fiber systems is not present in angiosperms but occurs in Rhodophyta, Phaeophyta,

---

[11] The galls of plants are reviewed by Mani (356) and recently by Beiderbeck (42); see also Chapter 49.

Chlorophyta, and Fungi. Galls of those tissues have been observed in *Urospora mirabilis* (chlorophyta) and *Sphacelaria* sp., *Desemarestia aculeata* of the Phaeophyta. Galls of pseudoparenchymata have also been described in lichens. No comparison is possible to structures in animals.

Abnormal Growth Processes Arising from Phylloid, Cauloid, or Rhizoid Tissues of Algae

These tissues are not present in angiosperms but at least partially comparable to angiosperm tissues and also to true tissues in vertebrates and invertebrates, similar to the true tissues of vascular plants. Cases of galls belonging in these groups of tissues have been found in different species of algae as, for example, highest phaeophyta. These true tissues of algae originate from single vegetation crowns.

Abnormal Growth Processes/Neoplasms Arising from True Tissues of Bryophyta

These tissues are not present in angiosperms but are comparable to their tissues in a certain degree; they are less well developed than the tissues in vascular plants. Concluding tissues such as the epidermis are functionally not as effective as the epidermis in vascular plants such as angiosperms. Roots are still missing. These tissues are comparable to the tissues of vertebrates and invertebrates just as those of the vascular plants but are somewhat restricted. The galls occur as swellings. From Europe alone more than 30 genera of leafy mosses with galls have been described. Bryophyta with cases of abnormal growth include the following genera: *Blasia pusilla, Lophocolea bidentata, Cephalozia connivens laxa, Pottia* sp., *Dicranium longifolium, Cephalozia* sp., and *Lophozia* sp.

Abnormal Growth Processes/Neoplasms Arising from Succeeding Meristems ("Folgemeristeme")

The normal tissues in angiosperms are the succeeding meristems. Many of the galls deriving from fully differentiated tissues and of limited and unlimited growth belong in this group occurring in vascular plants. They are characterized by the participation of newly formed gall meristems initiating increased inhibition of fully differentiated gall tissues. They are very common in vascular plants and are comparable to certain larval tissues and their abnormal growth processes in invertebrates.

Abnormal Growth Processes/Neoplasms Arising from Meristemoids

The normal tissues in angiosperms and other vascular plants are the meristemoids; the abnormal growth processes are the leaf galls (epidermal gall) which are very common abnormalities of stomata and trichomes. There exist no direct comparison to abnormal growth processes in vertebrates or invertebrates.

Abnormal Growth Processes/Neoplasms with the Involvement of Apical Meristems

The normal tissue in angiosperm is the apical meristem. The abnormal growth is characterized by bud galls and galls on the shoot axis. Some show arrest of the growth of the tip; they are common in Tracheophyta (vascular plants) and to a certain theoretical degree, comparable to abnormal growth processes of some larval tissues.

Abnormal Growth Processes/Neoplasms Arising from Lateral Meristem (Cambium)

The normal tissue of origin in angiosperms is the cambium, and the galls of concern appear at shoot and root axis. They are common, comparable to certain larval tissues in invertebrates but not to those of vertebrates. Reports of a comparability to tissues of gills in lamellibranchiata are interesting and need further investigation (332, 387).[12] Galls of the roots of leguminosae belong in this category.

Abnormal Growth Processes/Neoplasms Arising from Phellogen

The tissue occurs in the tracheophyta and galls at the shoot and root axis. The abnormal growth is mainly located in the subepidermal layer, in the area of the axis outside the vascular cambium. There is no comparison possible to vertebrates or invertebrates.

---

[12] In medicine the term cambium is also used for structures in the kidney which should not get confused with the term in botany (113).

Abnormal Growth Processes/Neoplasms Arising from Phytoepidermis

The abnormal growth processes or galls are widely distributed and show different subgroups. They are common in occurrence. An increased size of the cells is typical. In some cases a remarkable heterogeneity of the cells which derive from the epidermis or subepidermal tissue has been observed. The involved epidermis may become stratified. Galls of trichomes, as appendages of the epidermis, are characterized by changes into glands and show a diversity in size, shape, and structure.

Hypertrophy with hairy outgrowth, a decrease of stomata, or even their absence is also characteristic for leaf margin roll galls. Lenticula galls have thickened epidermal cells. "Epidermal galls" exhibit hairy outgrowth, and fleshy emergences. The epidermal cells are highly enlarged. To observed cases belong those of *Synchytrium* sp. and *Ulmus* sp. Comparability exists to invertebrates and vertebrates.

Abnormal Growth Processes/Neoplasms Arising from Rhizodermis

The normal tissue occurs at the root of tracheophyta; the common galls show cytologic and histologic characteristics as in the epidermis. The tissue of the tracheophyta is comparable to that of the phytoepidermis.

Abnormal Growth Processes/Neoplasms Arising from Phytoparenchymata

Phytoparenchymata in angiosperms occurs as tissue or as cell nests in other tissues: in stem and root—pith and cortex, leaves, mesophyll; in fruits, flesh; and in seeds, endosperm. The most common galls with the involvement of phytoparenchymata are the leaf galls. Phytoparenchymata can be compared to the connective tissues in the animal body. The tissue occurs in highest rhodophyta, phaeophyta, bryophyta, and tracheophyta. Observed cases are: Hieracium spp. (pocken-gall); *Maerua arenaria* (fold gall); *Quercus* (lenticular gall); *Machilus* sp. (mark gall); *Acacia leucophloea* (leaf gall); and *Acacia suma* (cylinder-piston gall).

Abnormal Growth Processes/Neoplasms Arising from Collenchyma

The tissue occupies the axes of tracheophyta, and observed cases are those such as the petiole gall on *Populus* sp. No comparability exists to invertebrates or vertebrates.

Abnormal Growth Processes/Neoplasms Arising from Sclerenchyma

Normally the tissue is distributed in tracheophyta and is involved in the formation of root galls, shoot axis galls, leaf galls, and galls on flowers. Sclerotic cells occur in certain galls, such as the lenticular one in *Quercus* sp., but also, in the same species whole sclerenchyma zones have been found. This is also the case in leaf galls of *Fagus silvatica* or in the flower galls of *Indigofera gerardiana*. These structures are relatively common but are incomparable to abnormal growth processes in invertebrates or vertebrates.

Abnormal Growth Processes/Neoplasms Arising from Xylem

The normal tissue occurs in plant axes of ferns, gymnosperms, and angiosperms. The regions of galls of this tissue, which are common, develop from the living cells or precursors of nonliving cells. A partial comparison to invertebrates and vertebrates is possible. The tissue is distributed in tracheophyta, and as an observed case the gall of *Glechoma hederacea* may be mentioned.

Abnormal Growth Processes/Neoplasms Arising from Phloem

The tissue distributed in tracheophyta, for example, in the plant axes of the angiosperms, takes part in the formation of common galls, which are histologically characterized by suppression or excessive development. Partial comparability to vertebrates and invertebrates is possible. Observed cases are the galls on *Epilobium* sp., *Zea mays*, and *Pistacia* sp.

Abnormal Growth Processes/Neoplasms with the Involvement of Secretory Structures

External, internal structures, and lactifers occur in angiosperms (tracheophyta). A comparability to vertebrates and invertebrates is possible. The tissue plays a role in galls of flowers and fruits, to name only those.

Abnormal Growth Processes/Neoplasms with the Involvement of Periderm

The tissue present in tracheophyta contributes to the development of common galls and is normally distributed in the bark of the plants. No comparability to animal structures is possible, and typical examples are the galls on *Quercus robur*.

Tissue and Species-specific Patterns of Neoplasms Reviewed from a Phylogenetic and Species-specific Point of View

Neoplasms always originate from one or more normal tissues (the parent tissue or tissues).

Among the various organisms, the mammalian tissues are the most widely specialized but also are the most extensively studied.

Human neoplasms are those spontaneous neoplasms with which we are most familiar with respect to their histologic characteristics and appearance. The second basic groups comprise the more than 14,000 types of recorded plant neoplasms. The best known experimental neoplasms are those of the laboratory animals.

The neoplasms of man can be considered a phylogenetic ultimate.

The different types of normal tissues are not of the same phylogenetic age nor do they exhibit the same distribution in recent species.

The number of species affected by certain tissues varies greatly.

The phylogenetic age of neoplasms is at least theoretically different.

The number of species affected by certain tumors varies at least theoretically.

The number of individuals of a species affected by a neoplasm varies in subspecies and races.

The malignancy of the same tumor type in different species varies also with the similar tissue types which may be involved.

Other differences of species-specificity could be listed, but we should not forget the general character of neoplastic growth.

From the above we may conclude that every tumor type will exhibit, at least theoretically, a characteristic distribution pattern and phylogenetic age, based on recent distribution and the phylogenetic age of normal tissues.

It was the purpose of this chapter to demonstrate the theoretical and practical patterns of all neoplasms, as classified both from human experience and on the basis of occurrence among the angiosperms.

Meristems Lacking in Animals

Meristematic tissues of plants, with at least theoretically unlimited embryonal potential (see Romberger, Chapter 9) are not present in animals. More than 100 years ago, Virchow's most important student, Cohnheim, postulated the embryonal cell theory which stated that embryonal tissue remnants maintaining the embryonal potential in the adult may be the initiators of neoplastic growth. In the mammalian body no embryonal tissues exhibit an unlimited duration. We could consider the embryonal connective tissue as the best comparative structure with remarkable limitations.

The picture changes, however, when we consider the invertebrates in which embryonal tissues remain during the often numerous stages of larval or pupal life. Such tissues may persist for 90% of the duration of the life, for example, of the 17-yr locust. These embryonal tissues, with a tremendous growth potential, occupy a little space in the body of the animal, just as do the meristems in the body of the plants. Hence, the comparison is valid.

Plants Lack Muscle and Nerve Tissues

The tumors associated with these types of tissue are consequently limited to the eumetazoan animal phyla. The cardiac musculature to certain authors as well as the neurons of the nervous system are cell invariable in most species (see Chapter 3). This finding demonstrates that the comparable limitations by the absence of muscular and nervous tissues in plants are of lesser importance, because cell invariable structures cannot produce neoplasms. The only exceptions to the above are the precursors of cells of cell invariable tissues. It should be emphasized that this limitation on comparability is applicable only to the mesenchymal tumor if seen from the animal kingdom, from those known as sarcomas, if malignant.

Not all plant tissues can develop tumors in their functionally fully active stages because they are nonliving when they reach full functional maturity. In addition to the functionally more limited diversity of plant tissues resulting from their vital requirements (photosynthesis nutrition) and their phylogenetic age, this fact helps explain the simpler character of normal plant tissues, as well as that of plant neoplasms.

Malignant neoplasms of vascular plants are unable to metastasize because the body of the plants does not contain the prerequisites for floating cells as do the body fluids of animals. Floating cells in plants that originate from cuts or other injury cannot survive.

No floating cells occur in the body fluids and therefore in the vessels of plants. There are also plant vessels whose walls in functional condition are composed of nonliving cells.

It is well known that the multipotential mesenchymal cell is the precursor of connective tissue cells and of muscle cells by metaplasia. The potential of the theoretically assumed mesenchymal cell will differ, depending upon the cells' phylogenetic and taxonomic position. In a platyhelminth, it will be able to produce only smooth, or, as the case may be, obliquely striated muscle in addition to connective tissue, but never cartilage, chordal tissue, or bone. In an arthropod, it can produce cross-striated muscle, cardiac muscle (type I), connective tissue, and cartilage, but never chordal tissue or bone. In an ascidian, the mesenchymal cell will be able to create smooth muscle, connective tissue, cartilage, and chordal tissue, but never bone. Finally, in the vertebrate, this cell may produce connective tissue, smooth muscle, basket cells (myoepithelial muscle), cross-striated muscle, cardiac muscle (type II), cartilage, chordal tissue, and bone, along with the tumors associated with these tissues.

If a tumor originates from the tissue and retains in its structure the original structure of the mother tissue, this tumor must be considered as being of primary character. For example, if a tumor derives from a squamous cell epithelium and exhibits itself as a squamous cell cancer, it is a tumor of primary character. With respect to its function, such a tumor will be more closely related to the mother tissue than a tumor deriving from another tissue and assuming the same structure by metaplasia.

The epithelial neoplasms, if malignant, are carcinomas. In animals, they may derive from the lining membrane or from the glandular, the germinative, or the desmal epithelia. The latter are represented by the mesothel of joints, tendinous vaginae, and bursae as well as the desmal epithelium of the coelom. In the plants neoplasms of the first three types of epithelia cited above also exist, at least theoretically. The question of the presence of the last group, the desmal epithelia, is unresolved, but it must be kept in mind that linings of internal cavities and inner membranes also occur in the plants. These last groups of epithelia are also less common among the lower animals. As regards the mesenchymal neoplasms in animals (sarcomas, if malignant), a much greater variation occurs in the animal than in the plant kingdom. The parenchyma of plants, of course, is comparable to the connective tissues in general. The parenchyma is not to be confused, however, with the parenchymata as the term generally used in medicine (e.g., liver parenchyme) but can be compared to the structures for which the term is used in zoology (parenchymata, e.g., in flatworms).

Considering the specialized connective tissues, such as cartilage, chordal tissue, and bone, the limits of comparability are perceived. From a metaplastic point of view, the muscle tissue does not possess comparable counterpart in the plant. The same holds true for the nerve tissues, including the glia. Many nonliving tissues are characteristic of plants. It is apparent that the epithelial tissues and neoplasms of animals and plants can be compared on a much broader basis than the nonepithelial tissues and neoplasms.

Other Principles of Comparability

Since nervous tissues do not occur in plants and nonliving tissue do not occur in animals, it appears that these two types of tissues have nothing in common. However, the precursors of animal cell invariable tissues and the precursors of nonliving plant tissues are able, at least theoretically, to produce neoplasms, whereas the adult functional tissues in both cases do not. A common similar principle becomes apparent.

References

1. Adler, J. H., Roderig, H., and Ungar, H. (1976): Neoplastic liver nodules of unknown cause in a colony of sand rats (*Psammomys obesus*). *Isr. J. Med. Sci.*, 12(10):1212-1215.
2. Ahuja, M. R., and Anders, F. (1976): A genetic concept of the origin of cancer, based in part upon studies of neoplasms in fishes. *Prog. Exp. Tumor Res.*, 20:380-397.
3. Akopov, M. A., Berezov, T. T., and Kagan, Z. S. (1978): Characteristics of L-threonine- and L-serine dehydratases from mouse liver and spontaneous hepatomas. *Vopr. Med. Kim.*, (3):394-401.
4. Al-Dahash, S. Y., and David, J. S. (1977): The incidence of ovarian activity. Pregnancy and bovine genital abnormalities shown by an abattoir survey. *Vet. Rec.*, 101(15):296-299.
5. Alden, C. L., and Dickerson, T. V. (1976): Osteochondromatosis of the cervical vertebrae in a dog. *J. Am. Vet. Med. Assoc.*, 168(2):142-144.
6. Alderman, D. J., Van Banning, P. and Perez-Colomer, A. (1977): Two European oyster (*Ostrea edulis*) mortalities associated with an abnormal haemocytic condition. *Aquaculture*, 10:335-340.
7. Amemiya, T. (1977): Electron histochemical study of phosphorylase system in choroidal melanoma. *Acta Histochem.* (Jena), 58(1):58-62.
8. Anderson, W. A. D., and Scotti, T. M. (1976): *Synopsis of Pathology.* Ed. 9. C. V. Mosby, St. Louis.
9. Andrews, E. J. (1976): Mammary neoplasia in the guinea pig (*Cavia porcellus*). *Cornell Vet*, 66(1):82-96.
10. Anisimov, V. N. (1976): Spontaneous tumors in rats of different lines. *Vopr. Onkol.*, 22(8):98-110.
11. Anisimov, V. N., Aleksandrov, V. A., Klimashevskii, V. F., Kolodin, V. I., and Likhachev, A. I. (1978): Spontaneous tumors in rats from the Rappolovo Breeding Nursery of the Academy of Medical Sciences of the USSR. *Vopr. Onkol.*, 24(1):64-70.
12. Anzil, A. P., Stavrou, D., Blinzinger, K., Herrlinger, H., and Dahme, E. (1977): Ultrastructural comparison between the parenchymal cells of tumors derived from parent and hybrid lines of C1300 mouse neuroblastoma and C6 rat glioma. *Cancer Res.*, 37(7, Part 1):2236-2245.
13. Appleby, E. C., Hayward, A. H., and Douce, G. (1978): German shepherds and splenic tumors (letter). *Vet. Rec.*, 102(20):449.
14. Arias-Stella, J., and Bustos, F. (1976): Chronic hypoxia and chemodectomas in bovines at high altitudes. *Arch. Pathol. Lab. Med.*, 100(12):636-639.
15. Arnold, W., Ganzer, U., and Nasemann, T. (1977): Pathogenesis and clinical observations of papillomatous diseases of the skin and of the mucous membranes. *Arch. Otorhinolaryngol.*, 214(3):221-239.
16. Arseni, C., and Nereantiu, F. (1977): Ultrastructural aspects of medulloblastoma. *Neurol. Psychiatr.* (Bucur.), 15(3):207-210.
17. Ash, P., and Loutit, J. F. (1977): The ultrastructure or skeletal haemangiosarcomas induced in mice by strontium-90. *J. Pathol.*, 122(4):209-218.
18. Ashton, N., Choyce, D. P., and Fison, L. G. (1951): Carcinoma of the lacrimal sac. *Br. J. Ophthalmol.*, 35:366-376.
19. Atwell, R. B., and Summers, P. M. (1977): Congenital papilloma in a foal (letter). *Aust. Vet. J.*, 53(6):299.
20. Aubert, C., Rosengren, E., Rorsman, H., Rouge, F., Foa, C., and Lipcey, C. (1977): 5-S-cysteinyldopa in diagnosis and treatment of human malignant melanomas and ultrastructural observations. *Eur. J. Cancer*, 13(11):1299-1308.
21. Avdeev, G. I., Svet-Moldavskaya, I. A., Khatuntseva, N. I., and Kovaleva, L. P. (1978): The immunogenicity of a spontaneous murine colonic adenocarcinoma. Program, XIIth International Cancer Congress, Buenos Aires, p. 255.
22. Awwad, H. K., El Bolkaini, N., Hegazy, M., Ezzat, S., and Burgers, M. V. (1978): Workshop 51(9), Abstracts, Vol. 3, pp. 106-197. XXIIth International Cancer Congress, Buenos Aires.
23. Azzarelli, B., Richards, D. E., Anton, A. H., and Roessman, U. (1977): Central neuroblastoma. Electron microscopic observations and catecholamine determinations. *J. Neuropathol. Exp. Neurol.*, 36(2):384-397.
24. Bach-Nielsen, S., Haskins, M. E., Reif, J. S., Brodey, R. S., Patterson, D. F., and Spielman, R. (1978): Frequency of osteosarcoma among first-degree relatives of St. Bernard dogs. *J. Natl. Cancer Inst.*, 60(2):349-353.
25. Baird, W. M.: Personal communication.
26. Baird, W. M., Chemerys, R. A., Meedel, T. H., Whittaker, J. R., and Diamond, L. (1978): Metabolism of benzo(a)pyrene by *Ciona intestinalis*. Symp. on Carcinogenic Polynuclear Aromatic Hydrocarbons in the Marine Environment, U.S. EPA, Environmental Res. Lab., Gulf Breeze, Fla. p. 13.
27. Baker, J. R., Neal, P. A., and Wyn-Jones, G. (1978): Equine sarcoids letter. *Vet. Rec.*, 102(8):179-180.
28. Balazs, M. (1976): Electron microscopic study of benign hepatoma in a patient on oral contraceptives. *Beitr. Pathol.*, 159(3):299-306.
29. Bannasch, P. (1976): Cytology and cytogenesis of neoplastic (hyperplastic) hepatic nodules. *Cancer Res.*, 36(7, Part 2):2555-2562.
30. Barahona, H., Melendez, L. V., Hunt, R. D., and Daniel, M. D. (1976): The owl monkey (*Aotus trivirgatus*) as an animal model for viral diseases and oncologic studies. *Lab. Anim. Sci.*, 26(6, Part 2):1104-1112.
31. Barcos, M., Kim, U., Pickren, J., Reese, P., Freeman, A., and Stutzman, L. (1978): Survival of non Hodgkin's malignant lymphomas according to two histopathologic classifications. Program, XIIth Internat'l Cancer Congress, Buenos Aires, p. 241.
32. Barranco, S. C., Haenelt, B. R., and Gee, E. L. (1978): Differential sensitivities of five rat hepatoma cell lines to anticancer drugs. *Cancer Res.*, 38(3):656-660.
33. Barrett, R. A., and Nobel, T. A. (1976): Transitional cell carcinoma of the urethra in a cat. *Cornell Vet.*, 66(1):14-26.
34. Baskin, G. B., and De Paoli, A. (1977): Primary renal neoplasms of the dog. *Vet. Pathol.*, 14(6):591-605.
35. Battaglia, P. (1924): Über Carcinoma adenomatodes ("Adenoma destruens") der Niere. *Virchows Arch. Pathol. Anat.*, 250:555.
36. Beaumont, P. R., O'Brien, J. B., Allen, H. L., and Tucker, J. A. (1979): Mast cell sarcoma of the larynx in a dog; a case report. *J. Small Anim. Pract.*, 20(1):19-25.
37. Becci, P. J., McDowell, E. M., and Trump, B. F. (1978): The respiratory epithelium. II. Hamster trachea, bronchus, and bronchioles. *J. Natl. Cancer Inst.*, 61:551-561.
38. Becci, P. J., McDowell, E. M., and Trump, B. F. (1978): The respiratory epithelium. IV. Histogenesis of epidermoid metaplasia and carcinoma in situ in the hamster. *J. Natl. Cancer Inst.*, 61:577-586.
39. Becci, P. J., McDowell, E. M., and Trump, B. F. (1978): The respiratory epithelium. VI. Histogenesis of lung tumors induced by benzo(a)pyrene-ferric oxide.
40. Becker, F. F., Stillman, D., and Sell, S. (1977): Serum alpha-fetoprotein in a mouse strain (C3H-AVY FB) with spontaneous hepatocellular carcinomas. *Cancer Res.*, 37(3):850-856.
41. Becker, F. F. (1976): Sequential phenotypic and biochemical alterations during chemical hepatocarcinogenesis. *Cancer Res.*, 36(7, Part 2):2563-2566.
42. Beiderbeck, R. (1977): *Pflanzentumoren.* Eugen Ulmer Verlag, Stuttgart.
43. Bellotti, M. S., Elsner, B., Curutchet, H. P., Oria, H., and Marcos, F. G. (1978): Histological variants of cutaneous malignant melanoma and their prognostic value. XIIth International Cancer Congress, Buenos Aires, p. 235.
44. Benjamin, S. A., and Brooks, A. L. (1977): Spontaneous lesions in Chinese hamsters. *Vet. Pathol.*, 14(5):449-462.
45. Beskic, M., Dabska, M., Klos, R., Majdecki, T. (1977): Histochemical features of C-cell thyroid carcinoma. *Acta Histochem. (Jena)*, 58(2):210-218.
46. Betton, G. R. (1976): Agglutination reactions of spontaneous canine tumour cells, induced by concanavalin A., demonstrated by an isotopic assay. *Int. J. Cancer*, 18(5):687-696.
47. Betton, G. R., and Owen, L. N. (1976): Allogeneic grafts of spontaneous canine melanomas and their cell culture strains in neonatal immunosuppressed dogs. *Br. J. Cancer*, 34(4):374-380.
48. Beyer, J. (1978): Comparative pathology and etiology of lymphatic tumors in fowl. *Arch. Exp. Vet. Med.*, 32(3):441-448.
49. Bhawan, J., DeGirolami, U., and Edelstein, L. M. (1977): Multiple layers of basement membrane around myelinated and unmyelinated fibers in cellular blue nevus. *Acta Neuropathol.* (Berl.), 38(3):243-245.
50. Birkmayer, G. D., Lubitz, W., Hammer, C., Eberhard, H., Tichmann, I., Chaussy, C., and Brendel, W. (1976): Biochemical and immunological evidence for oncorna viral features in human melanoma, glioblastoma and leukemia. In *Molecular Base of Malignancy*, pp. 197-204. Edited by E. Deutsch et al. Thieme, Stuttgart.
51. Bland, J. O. W., and Russell, D. S. (1938): Histological types of meningiomata and a comparison of their behaviour in tissue culture with that of certain normal human tissues. *J. Pathol. Bacteriol.*, 47:491.
52. Bloom, G. D., Carlsö, O. B., Gustavsson, H., and Henriksson, R. (1977): Distribution of mucosubstances in adenoid cystic carcinoma. *Virchows Arach. [Pathol. Anat.]*, 375(1):1-12.
53. Böhm, N., and Riede, U. N. (1976): Congenital mesoblastic nephroma—a semimalignant fibroleiomyomatous kidney tumor of the newborn. *Beitr. Pathol.*, 159(1):80-93.
54. Boever, W. J. (1976): Interdigital corns in a black rhinoceros. *Vet. Med. Small Anim. Clin.*, 71(6):827-830.
55. Boever, W. J., and Kern, T. (1976): Papillomas in black and white Colobus monkeys (*Colobus polykomus*). *J. Wildl. Dis.*, 12(2):180-181.
56. Boever, W. J., and Herbers, H. (1977): Congenital sebaceous gland adenoma in a Speke's gazelle. *Vet. Med. Small Anim. Clin.*, 72(2):268-269.
57. Bomirski, A., and Wrzolkowa, T. (1976): Ultrastructural studies of the occurrence of tyrosinase in transplantable amelanotic melanoma in Syrian hamster. *Przegl. Dermatol.*, 63(1):11-18.
58. Boutwell, R. K. (1976): The biochemistry of preneoplasia in mouse skin. *Cancer Res.*, 36(7, Part 2):2631-2635.
59. Braunschweiger, P. G., and Schiffer, L. M. (1978): Therapeutic implications of cell kinetic changes after cyclophosphamide treatment in spontaneous and transplantable mammary tumors. *Cancer Treat Rep.*, 62(5):727-736.
60. Braunschweiger, P. G., and Schiffer, L. M. (1978): Cell kinetics after

vincristine treatment of C3H/He spontaneous mammary tumors; implications for therapy. *J. Natl. Cancer Inst.,* 60(5):1043–1048.

61. Braunschweiger, P. G., Poulakos, L., and Schiffer, L. M. (1977): Cell kinetics in vivo and in vitro for C3H/He spontaneous mammary tumors. *J. Natl. Cancer Inst.,* 59(4):1197–1204.

62. Brill, E., Radomski, J. L., and MacDonald, W. E. (1977): Failure of the N-oxydized metabolites of some carcinogenic amines to induce tumors in normal and wounded rat skin. *Res. Commun. Chem. Pathol. Pharmacol.,* 18(2):353–360.

63. Briones, H., Dabancens, A., and Chianale, M. (1978): Intraepithelial carcinoma of the vulva. Program, XIIth International Cancer Congress, Buenos Aires, p. 246.

64. Brodey, R. S., and Abt, D. A. (1976): Results of surgical treatment in 65 dogs with osteosarcoma. *J. Am. Vet. Med. Assoc.,* 168(11):1032–1035.

65. Brodey, R. S., Pflugfelder, C., Mikkilineni, S., and Twitchell, M. J. (1978): Clinico-pathologic conference; a 6-year-old German shepherd dog with a rapid growing mass in the left popliteal fossa. *J. Am. Vet. Med., Assoc.,* 172(7):837–841.

66. Brown, R. J., Kessler, M. J., and Kupper, J. L. (1977): Myocardial fibrosarcoma in rhesus monkey. *Lab. Anim. Sci.,* 27(4):524–525.

67. Brown, T. T., Burek, J. D., and McEntee, K. (1976): Male pseudohermaphroditism, cryptorchism, and sertoli cell neoplasia in three miniature schnauzers. *J. Am. Vet. Med. Assoc.,* 169(8):821–825.

68. Bryant, G. M., Sohal, R. S., Argus, M. F., and Arcos, J. C. (1977): Ultrastructural and metabolic determinants of resistance to azo-dye susceptibility in nitrosamine carcinogenesis of the guinea-pig. *Br. J. Cancer,* 36(6):687–691.

69. Bucana, C., Hoyer, L. C., Hobbs, B., Breesman, S., McDaniel, M., and Hanna, M. G., Jr. (1976): Morphological evidence for the translocation of lysosomal organelles from cytotoxic macrophages into the cytoplasm of tumor target cells. *Cancer Res.,* 36(12):444–458.

70. Bucek, J., and Vrba, M. (1976): Ultrastructure of human uveal melanomas cultivated *in vitro. Neoplasma,* 23(1):109–118.

71. Bucke, D. (1976): Neoplasia in roach (*Rutilus rutilus* L.) from a polluted environment. *Prog. Exp. Tumor Res.,* 20:205–211.

72. Bulay, O., Urman, H., Clayson, D. B., and Shubik, P. (1977): Carcinogenic effects of niridazole on rodents infected with *Schistosoma mansoni. J. Natl. Cancer Inst.,* 59(6):1625–1630.

73. Burek, J. D., and Hollander, C. F. (1977): Incidence patterns of spontaneous tumors in BN/BI rats. *J. Natl. Cancer Inst.,* 58(1):99–105.

74. Burns, F. J., Vanderlaan, M., Sivak, A., and Albert, R. E. (1976): Regression kinetics of mouse skin papillomas. *Cancer Res.,* 36(4):1422–1427.

75. Burns, E. R., Scheving, L. E., Fawcett, D. F., Gibbs, W. M., and Galatzan, R. E. (1976): Circadian influence on the frequency of labeled mitoses method in the stratified squamous epithelium of the mouse esophagus and tongue. *Anat. Rec.,* 184(3):265–273.

76. Busbee, D. L., Guyden, J., Kingston, T., Rose, F. L., and Cantrell, E. T. (1978): Metabolism of benzo(a)pyrene in animals with high aryl hydrocarbon hydroxylase levels and high rates of spontaneous cancer. *Cancer Lett.,* 4(2):61–67.

77. Calafat, J., Weijer, K., and Daams, H. (1977): Feline malignant mammary tumors. III. Presence of C-particles and intracisternal A-particles and their relationship with feline leukemia virus antigens and RD-114 virus antigens. *Int. J. Cancer,* 20(5):759–767.

78. Calberg-Bacq, C. M., Francois, C., Gosselin, L., Osterrieth, P. M., Rentier and Delrue, F. (1976): Comparative study of the milk fat globule membrane and the mouse mammary tumour virus prepared from the milk of an infected stain of Swiss albino mice. *Biochim. Biophys. Acta,* 419(3):458–478.

79. Cameron, A. M., and Conroy, J. D. (1976): Papillary carcinoma of apocrine sweat glands in capuchin monkeys (*Cebus albifrons*). *J. Med. Primatol.,* 5(1):56–59.

80. Cardy, R. H. (1977): Primary intraocular malignant melanoma in a Siamese cat. *Vet. Pathol.,* 14(6):648–649.

81. Carlisle, J. C. (1976): A study of epithelioma in the Atlantic salmon (*S. salar*). In *Wildlife Diseases,* pp. 443–444, edited by L. A. Page, Plenum Press, New York.

82. Carlisle, J. C. (1977): An epidermal papilloma of the Atlantic salmon. II. Ultrastructure and etiology. *J. Wildl. Dis.,* 13(3):235–239.

83. Carlisle, J. C., and Roberts, R. J. (1977): An epidermal papilloma of the Atlantic salmon I: Epizootiology, pathology and immunology. *J. Wildl. Dis.,* 13(3):230–234.

84. Carpenter, J. W., and Novilla, M. N. (1977): Diabetes mellitus in a black-footed ferret. *J. Am. Vet. Med. Assoc.,* 171:(9):890–893.

85. Carter, L. P., Beggs, J., and Waggener, J. D. (1972): Ultrastructure of three choroid plexus papillomas. *Cancer,* 30:1130.

86. Chaffee, V. W. (1977): Spinal cord ependymoma in a dog. *Vet. Med. Small Anim. Clin.* 72(12):1854–1857.

87. Challa, V. R., and Jona, J. (1977): Eccrine angiomatous hamartoma; a rare skin lesion with diverse histological features. *Dermatologica,* 155(4):206–209.

88. Chander, S., Whitt, L. A., Greig, A. S., and Hare, W. C. (1977): Bovine lymphosarcoma in twin calves. *Can. J. Comp. Med.,* 41(3):274–278.

89. Chastain, C. B., Mitten, R. W., and Kluge, J. P. (1978): An ACTH-hyper-

responsive adrenal carcinoma in a dog. *J. Am. Vet. Med. Assoc.,* 172(5):586–588.

90. Cheever, A. W., Kuntz, R. E., Moore, J. A., and Huang, T. C. (1976): Proliferative epithelial lesions of the urinary bladder in cynomolgus monkeys (*Macaca fascicularis*) infected with *Schistosoma intercalatum. Cancer Res.,* 36(8):2928–2931.

91. Chen, S. Y., and Harwick, R. D. (1977): Ultrastructure of oral squamous-cell carcinoma. *Oral Surg.,* 44(5):744–753.

92. Chernina, L. A. (1976): The ultrastructure of human rhabdomyosarcomas. *Vopr. Onkol.,* 22(5):37–43.

93. Chertow, B. S., Manke, D. J., Williams, G. A., Baker, G. R., Hargis, G. K., and Buschmann, R. J. (1977): Secretory and ultrastructural responses of hyperfunctioning human parathyroid tissues to varying calcium concentration and vinblastine. *Lab. Invest.,* 36(2):198–205.

94. Chihaya, Y., Ohshima, K., Miura, S., and Numakunai, S. (1976): Pathological study on cutaneous papillomatosis in a Japanese serow (*Capricornis crispus*). *Jpn. J. Vet. Sci.,* 38:327–328.

95. Cho, S. Y., and Choi, H. Y. (1978): Causes of death in patient with breast cancer ten years autopsy study. Program, XIIth International Cancer Congress, Buenos Aires, p. 218.

96. Christov, K., and Stoichkova, N. (1977): Histochemical localization of peroxidase activity in normal, proliferating and neoplastic thyroid tissues of rats. An ultrastructural study. *Acta Histochem.* (Jena), 58(2):275–289.

97. Christov, K., Sugihara, T., Lindenfelser, R., Haubert, P., Thomas, C., and Sandritter, W. (1976): Transmission and scanning electron microscopy of experimentally induced thyroid tumors in rats. *Exp. Pathol.* (Jena), 12(6):315–325.

98. Chung, E. B., and Enzinger, F. M. (1978): Chondroma of soft parts. *Cancer,* 41(4):1414–1424.

99. Churg, A., and Ringus, J. (1978): Ultrastructural observations on the histogenesis of alveolar rhabdomyosarcoma. *Cancer,* 41(4):1355–1361.

100. Cloyd, G. G., and Johnson, G. R. (1978): Lymphosarcoma with lymphoblastic leukemia in a New Zealand white rabbit. *Lab. Anim. Sci.,* 28.(1):66–69.

101. Coleman, G. L., Barthold, W., Osbaldiston, G. W., Foster, S. J., and Jonas, A. M. (1977): Pathological changes during aging in Barrier-reared Fischer 344 male rats. *J. Gerontol.,* 32(3):258–278.

102. Confer, A. W., and Depaoli, A. (1978): Primary neoplasms of the nasal cavity, paranasal sinuses and nasopharynx in the dog. A report of 16 cases from the files of the AFIP. *Vet. Pathol.,* 15(1):18–30.

103. Confer, A. W., Langloss, J. M., and Cashell, I. G. (1978): Long-term survival of two cats with mastocytosis. *J. Am. Vet. Med. Assoc.,* 172(2):160–161.

104. Cooper, E. L. (1976): Immunity and neoplasia in mollusks. *Isr. J. Med. Sci.,* 12(4–5):479–494.

105. Cori, G., Farraggiana, T., Grandi, C., and Nardi, F. (1977): The diagnostic usefulness of electron microscopy investigation of orbital embryonal rhabdomyosarcomas. *Tumori,* 63(2):205–213.

106. Cotchin, E. (1977): A general survey of tumours in the horse. *Equine Vet. J.,* 9(1):16–21.

107. Courville, C. B. (1945): *Pathology of the Central Nervous System,* Ed. 2. Pacific Press, Mountain View, Calif.

108. Cowgill, U. M. (1977): A myeloliposarcoma in a female *Perodicticus potto;* mineralogical and elemental chemical analysis. *J. Med. Primatol.,* 6(2):114–118.

109. Crow, S. E. (1977): Primary hemangiosarcoma of the femur in a dog. *Mod. Vet. Pract.,* 58(4):343–346.

110. Cubilla, A. L. (1978): Primary carcinoid tumor of the breast; a new type of mammary cancer. Program, XIIth International Cancer Congress, Buenos Aires, p. 218.

111. Cubilla, A. L., and Fitzgerald, P. (1978): Differential diagnosis of adenocarcinoma of the pancreaticoduodenal region. Program, XIIth International Cancer Congress, Buenos Aires, p. 201.

112. Cushing, H., and Eisenhardt, L. (1938): *The Meningiomas.* Charles C Thomas, Springfield, Ill.

113. Darovski, B. P. (1975): Intertubular cells and their relationship to renal cambium. *Bull. Exp. Biol. Med.,* 79(6):705–707.

114. David, R., and Buchner, A. (1978): Amyloid stroma in a tubular carcinoma of palatal salivary gland; a histochemical and ultrastructural study. *Cancer,* 41(5):1836–1844.

115. Davis, P. E., Huxtable, R. R., and Sabine, M. (1976): Dermal papillomas in the racing greyhound. *Australas J. Dermatol.,* 17(1):13–16.

116. Dawson, I. M. (1976): The endocrine cells of the gastro-intestinal tract and the neoplasms which arise from them. *Curr. Top. Pathol.,* 63:221–258.

117. Deys, B. F. (1976): Atlantic eels and cauliflower disease (orocutaneous papillomatosis). *Prog. Exp. Tumor. Res.,* 20:94–100.

118. DiGiacomo, R. F. (1977): Gynecologic pathology in the rhesus monkey (*Macaca mulatta*). II. Findings in laboratory and free-ranging monkeys. *Vet. Pathol.,* 14(6):539–548.

119. DiGiacomo, R. F., Hooks, J. O., Suliman, M. R., Gibbs, C. J., Jr., and Gajdoser, D. C. (1977): Pelvic endometriosis and simian foamy virus infection in a pigtailed macaque. *J. Am. Vet. Med. Assoc.,* 171(9):859–

861.

120. Dikshtein, E. A., Torsuev, N. A., Romanenko, V. N., Shevchenko, N. I., and Merezhko, V. A. Morphology of multiple cylindroma of the skin (histochemical and electron-microscopic study). *Cancer Res.*, 37(11): 3957-3963.

121. Diters, R. A., Kircher, C. H., and Nielsen, S. W. (1978): Astrocytoma in a raccoon. *J. Am. Vet. Med. Assoc.*, 173(9):1152-1153.

122. Dmitrieva, N. P., Stefanov, S. B., and Amirkhanian, E. A. (1977): Electron-cytochemical and morphometric study of the activity of several enzymes in thyrocyte mitochondria during malignant degeneration. *Biull. Eksp. Biol. Med.*, 83(4):432-435.

123. Dome, S. H., and Staton, J. F. (1976): German shepherds and splenic tumours [Letter]. *Vet. Rec.*, 102(10):224.

124. Dorfman, S. K., Hurvitz, A. I., and Patnaik, A. K. (1977): Primary and secondary bone tumours in the dog. *J. Small Anim. Pract.*, 18(5):313-326.

125. Dorn, C. R., and Priester, W. A. (1976): Epidemiologic analysis of oral and pharyngeal cancer in dogs, cats, horses, and cattle. *J. Am. Vet. Med. Assoc.*, 169(11):1202-1206.

126. Dralle, H., and Böcker, W. (1977): Immunohistochemical and electron microscope analysis of adenomas of the thyroid gland. I. A comparative investigation of hot and cold nodules. *Virchows Arch. [Pathol. Anat.]*, 374(4):285-301.

127. Dronova, L. M., Belich, L. I., and Erokhin, V. N. (1977): Critical phenomena during the first transplantations of spontaneous mammary gland tumors in mouse strain A. *Dokl. Akad. Nauk. SSSR*, 232(6):127-129.

128. Dutra, F. R. (1978): Common neoplasms of pet animals. *West J. Med.*, 128(1):50-51.

129. Dutta, S. K., Gorgacz, E. J., Albert, T. F., and Ingling, A. L. (1977): Isolation of a herpesvirus from the cell culture of a malignant melanoma of a ground squirrel (*Spermophilus tridecemlineatus*). *Am. J. Vet. Res.*, 38(5):591-595.

130. Eady, R. A., Gilkes, J. J., and Jones, E. W. (1977): Eruptive nevi; report of two cases, with enzyme histochemical, light and electron microscopical findings. *Br. J. Dermatol.*, 97(3):267-278.

131. Eckerlin, R. H., Garman, R. H., and Fowler, E. H. (1976): Chondroblastic osteosarcoma in the jejunum of a dog. *J. Am. Vet. Med. Assoc.*, 168(8): 691-693.

132. Effron, M., Griner, L., and Benirschke, K. (1977): Nature and rate of neoplasia found in captive wild mammals, birds, and reptiles at necropsy. *J. Natl. Cancer Inst.*, 59(1):185-198.

133. Elkan, E., and Cooper, J. E. (1976): Tumours and pseudotumours in some reptiles. *J. Comp. Pathol.*, 86(3):337-348.

134. Elsner, B., Curutchet, P., Bellotti, M. S., Blanco, G., Marcos, F. G., Degrossi, O. J., and Niepomniszcze, H. (1978): Value of histological classification of thyroid cancer; a study of 134 cases. Program, XIIth International Cancer Congress, Buenos Aires, p. 186.

135. Elwell, M. R., Burger, G. T., Moe, J. B., White, J. D., and Stookey, J. L. (1977): Fibrosarcoma in a white-tailed deer. *J. Wildl. Dis.*, 13(3):279-289.

136. Enzinger, F. M. (1969): *Histological Typing of Soft Tissue Tumours*, No. 3. WHO, Geneva.

137. Enzinger, F. M. (1978): Classification of soft tissue tumors. Program XIIth International Cancer Congress, Buenos Aires, p. 91.

138. Ermin, R. (1954): On an ocular tumor with exophthalmia in an interspecific hybrid of *Anatolichthys*. *Istanb. Univ. Fen. Fak. Mecm.*, 19: 203-211.

139. Ermoshchenkov, V. S., and Khudolei, V. V. (1976): Tumors in Leningrad zoo animals. *Vopr. Onkol.*, 22(5):78-84.

140. Essex, M. (1977): Immunity to leukemia, lymphoma, and fibrosarcoma in cats; a case for immunosurveillance. *Contemp. Top Immunobiol.*, 6: 71-106.

141. Evans, B. A., Borthwick, G., Wilson, D. W., and Pierrepoint, C. G. (1978): Steroid metabolism and oestradiol-17-beta binding in canine mammary tumours (proceedings). *J. Endocrinol.*, 77(2):64P-65P.

142. Evans, J. G., and Grant, D. I. (1977): A mixed mesodermal tumour in the uterus of a cat. *J. Comp. Pathol.*, 87(4):635-638.

143. Evans, R. W. (1966): *Histological Appearances of Tumours*, Ed. 2. Williams & Wilkins, Baltimore.

144. Ezdanian, B. A., Manvelian, K. R., Khachaturova, T. S., and Arzakanian, A. A. (1976): Cytomorphological characteristics and the features of growth *in vitro* of spontaneous mammary gland tumors in C3HA mice. *Zh. Eksp. Klin. Med.*, 16(3):3-7.

145. Factor, S. M., Biempica, L., Ratner, I., Ahuja, K. K., and Biempica, S. (1977): Carcinoma of the breast with multinucleated reactive stromal giant cells. A light and electron microscopic study of two cases. *Virchows Arch. [Pathol. Anat.]*, 374(1):1-12.

146. Falkmer, S., Emdin, S. O., Ostberg, Y., Mattisson, A., Sjobeck, M. L., and Fange, R. (1976): Tumor pathology of the hagfish, myxine glutinosa, and the river lamprey, *Lampetra fluviatilis*. A light-microscopical study with particular reference to the occurrence of primary liver carcinoma, islet-cell tumors, and epidermoid cysts of the skin. *Prog. Exp. Tumor Res.*, 20:217-250.

147. Farley, C. A., and Sparks, A. K. (1970): Proliferative diseases of hemocyte thelial cells, and connective tissue cells in mollusks. *Bibl. Haematol.*, 36:610-617.

148. Farley, C. A. (1976): Ultrastructural observations on epizootic neoplasia and lytic virus infection in bivalve mollusks. *Prog. Exp. Tumor Res.*, 20:283-294.

149. Farley, C. A. (1977): Neoplasms in estuarine mollusks and approaches to ascertain causes. *Ann. N. Y. Acad. Sci.*, 298:225-232.

150. Farraggiana, T., Biasio, L., Marinozzi, V., Butler, R., Bertolini, L., and Revoltella, R. (1978): Antibody formation and transient immune complex glomerulopathy in A-strain mice with C1300 neuroblastoma tumors. *Virchows Arch. [Cell Pathol.]*, 27(1):23-38.

151. Fatzer, R., and Fankhauser, R. (1977): Contributions to the neuropathology of ruminants. II. Neoplasms. *Schweiz. Arch. Tierheilkd.*, 119(2): 67-78.

152. Fechner, R. E. (1977): Hepatic tumors and oral contraceptives. *Pathol. Annu.* (Part 2), 1:293-310.

153. Feldman, E. C., Tyrrell, J. B., and Ettinger, S. J. (1977): Cushing's syndrome in a dog. *Mod. Vet. Pract.*, 58(12):995-999.

154. Fenoglio, C. M., Puri, S., and Richart, R. M. (1978): The ultrastructure of endometrioid carcinomas of the ovary. *Gynecol. Oncol.*, 6(2):152-164.

155. Fenoglio, J. J., Jr., McAllister, H. A., Jr., and Ferrans, V. J. (1976): Cardiac rhabdomyoma; a clinicopathologic and electron microscopic study. *Am. J. Cardiol.*, 38(2):241-251.

156. Fisher, E. R. (1976): Ultrastructure of the human breast and its disorders. *Am. J. Clin. Pathol.*, 66(2):361-375.

157. Fisher, L. F., and Robinson, F. R. (1976): Basal cell tumor in a debrazza monkey. *Vet. Pathol.*, 13(6):449-450.

158. Fisher, L. F., and Olander, H. J. (1978): Spontaneous neoplasms of pigs—a study of 31 cases. *J. Comp. Pathol.*, 88(4):505-517.

159. Flenker, H. (1976): Myxoid liposarcoma. Light and electron microscopic investigation. *Virchows Arch. [Pathol. Anat.]*, 371(2):171-176.

160. Foa, C., and Aubert, C. (1977): Ultrastructural comparison between cultured and tumor cells of human malignant melanoma. *Cancer Res.*, 37(11):3957-3963.

161. Foley, R. H. (1977): A selection of cutaneous and related tumors of cats (A photographic essay). *Vet. Med. Small Anim. Clin.*, 72(1):43-45.

162. Folse, D. S., and Stout, L. C. (1978): Endometriosis in a baboon (*Papio doguera*). *Lab. Anim. Sci.*, 28(2):217-219.

163. Frangione, B., and Franklin, E. C. (1973): Heavy chain diseases; clinical features and molecular significance of the disordered immunoglobulin structure. *Semin. Hematol.*, 10(1):53-64.

164. Frankhauser, R., Bestetti, G., Fatzer, R., Straub, R., and von Tscharner, C. (1977): Lymphosarcoma of the horse with involvement of the peripheral nerves. *Deutsch. Tieraerztl. Woechenschr.*, 84(3):85-89.

165. Frankman, O., and Kabulski, Z. (1978): Histologic malignancy grading in invasive squamous cell carcinoma of the vulva. Program, XIIth International Cancer Congress, Buenos Aires, p. 228.

166. Franks, L. M., and Knowles, M. A. (1978): The structure of tumours derived from mouse submandibular gland epithelium transformed in vitro. *Br. J. Cancer*, 37(2):240-247.

167. Frantz, V. K. (1959): Tumors of the pancreas. *Atlast of Tumor Pathology*, Section VII, Fascicles 27 and 18. Washington, Armed Forces Institute.

168. Frauchiger, E., and Frankhauser, R. (1957): *Vergleichende Neuropathologie*. Springer-Verlag, Berlin.

169. Frierman, E. M., and Andrews, J. D. (1976): Occurrence of hematopoietic neoplasms in Virginia oysters (*Crassostrea virginica*). *J. Natl. Cancer Inst.*, 56(2):319-324.

170. Frisk, C. S., Wagner, J. E., and Doyle, R. E. (1978): An ovarian teratoma in a guinea pig. *Lab. Anim. Sci.*, 28(2):199-201.

171. Funderburg, M. R. (1977): Adenocarcinoma subsequent to extramedullary myeloma in a German shepherd dog. *Vet. Med. Small Anim. Clin.*, 72(7):1185-1188.

172. Gabbiani, G., Osank-Brassert, J., Schneeberger, J. C., Kapanci, Y., Trenchev, P., and Holborow, E. J. (1976): Contractile proteins in human cancer cells. Immunofluorescent and electron microscopic study. *Am. J. Pathol.*, 83(3):457-474.

173. Gad, A., Rowlatt, C., and Sheriff, M. U. (1977): Spontaneous mammary carcinoma in C57Bl and C3H mice; a histochemical study. *Acta Pathol. Microbiol. Scand.* [A], 85(3):311-318.

174. Galil-Ogly, G. A., Krylov, L. M., and Poroshin, K. K. (1978): Electron-microscopic study of myogenic neoplasms. *Arkh. Pathol.*, 40(2):19-25.

175. Galil-Ogly, G. A., Krylov, L. M., and Poroshin, K. K. (1977): Ultrastructure of malignant fibrosarcoma. *Arkh. Pathol.*, 39(6):42-48.

176. Galil-Ogly, G. A., Krylov, L. M., and Poroshin, K. K. (1977): Ultrastructural features of fibrosarcoma. *Arkh. Patol.*, 39(3):51-56.

177. Garand, M. (1977): Malignant chemodectoma of the carotid body in a basset hound bitch. *Can. Vet. J.*, 18(8):228-231.

178. Gardner, M. B., Esra, G., Cain, M. J., Rossman, S., and Johnson, C. (1978): Myelomonocytic leukemia in an orangutan. *Vet. Pathol.*, 15(5): 667-670.

179. Gateff, E. (1977): Malignant neoplasms of the hematopoietic system in three mutants of *Drosophila melanogaster*. *Ann. Parasitol. Hum. Comp.*, 52(1):81-83.

180. Gateff, E. (1978): Malignant neoplasms of genetic origin in *Drosophila melanogaster*. *Science*, 200(4349):1448-1459.

181. Gautam, S., and Aikat, B. K. (1976): Effect of syngeneic sensitized lymphoid cells on incidence and growth of methyl cholanthrene-induced and spontaneous tumors in mice. *Indian J. Med. Res.*, 64(3):494-503.

182. Gebhart, W., and Niebauer, G. W. (1977): Comparative investigations of depigmented and melanomatous lesions in gray horses of the Lipizzaner breed. *Arch. Dermatol. Res.*, 259(1):29-42.

183. Gemhardt, C., and Loppnow, H. (1976): Pathogenesis of spontaneous diabetes mellitus in the cat; II. Acidophilic adenoma of the pituitary gland and diabetes mellitus in two cases. *Berl. Münch. Tierärztl. Wochenschr.*, 89(17):336-340.

184. Geschickter, C. F., and Widenhorn, H. (1934): Nephrogenic tumors. *Am. J. Cancer*, 22:620.

185. Ghadially, F. N., Lowes, N. R., and Mesfin, G. M. (1977): Atypical glycogen deposits in a plasmacytoma; an ultrastructural study. *J. Pathol.*, 22(3):157-162.

186. Ghosh, L., Ghosh, B. C., and Das Gupta, T. K. (1978): Myo epithelial cells in human breast cancer. Program, XIIth International Cancer Congress, Buenos Aires, p. 217.

187. Gialamus, J., and Schaffraneck, E. (1977): Three gastrointestinal neoplasms in the dog. *DTW*, 84(10):386-388.

188. Gibson, D. T., and Cerniglia, C. E. (1978): Microbial oxidation of polynuclear aromatic hydrocarbons. Symposium on Carcinogenic Polynuclear Aromatic Hydrocarbons in the Marine Environment, U.S. Environmental Protection Agency, Gulf Breeze, Fla. p 11.

189. Glaister, J. R., Samuels, D. M., and Tucker, M. J. (1977): Ganglioneuroma-containing tumours of the adrenal medulla in Alderly-Park rats. *Lab. Anim.*, 11(1):35-37.

190. Glockner, A. (1905): Beiträge zur Kenntnis der soliden Ovarialtumoren. *Arch. Gynaekol.*, 75:49.

191. Goldfeder, A. (1976): Induction of type B virions to bud into cytoplasmic vacuoles in a mammary tumor of an X-ray- and urethan-treated X-GF mouse. *Cancer Res.*, 36(11, Part, 1):4190-4194.

192. Gomez Rueda, N. (1978): Pathology; sex cord stromal tumours, soft tissue tumours and secondary tumours. Program, XIIth International Cancer Congress, Buenos Aires, p. 103.

193. Gonda, M. A., Aaronson, S. A., Ellmore, N., Zeve, V. H., and Nagashima, K. (1976): Ultrastructural studies of surface features of human normal and tumor cells in tissue culture by scanning and transmission electron microscopy. *J. Natl. Cancer Inst.*, 56(2):245-263.

194. Graham, C. E., and McClure, H. M. (1976): Sertoli-Leydig cell tumor in a chimpanzee. *Lab. Anim. Sci.*, 26(6, Part 1):948-950.

195. Graham, C. E., and McClure, H. M. (1977): Ovarian tumors and related lesions in aged chimpanzees. *Vet. Pathol.*, 14(4):380-386.

196. Greager, J. A., and Baldwin, R. W. (1978): Influence of immunotherapeutic agents on the progression of spontaneously arising, metastasizing rat mammary adenocarcinomas of varying immunogenicities. *Cancer Res.*, 38(1):69-73.

197. Greaves, M., and Janossy, G. (1978): Patterns of gene expression and the cellular origins of human leukaemias. *Biochim. Biophys. Acta*, 516(2):193-230.

198. Green, P. D., and Donovan, L. A. (1977): Lymphosarcoma in a horse. *Can. Vet. J.*, 18(9):257-258.

199. Grevel, V., Schmidt, S., and Mettler, F. (1978): Multiple bone metastases of a salivary-gland carcinoma in a dog. *Schweiz. Arch. Tierheilkd.*, 120(1):13-22.

200. Gruys, E., and Van Dijk, J. E. (1976): Four canine ovarian teratomas and a nonovarian feline teratoma. *Vet. Pathol.*, 13(6):455-459.

201. Gupta, P. P., Singh, B., and Gill, B. S. (1977): Some uncommon neoplasms of Indian water buffaloes (*Bubalus bubalis*). *Zentralbl. Vet. (A)*, 24(6):511-519.

202. Gwin, R. M., Alsaker, R. D., and Gelatt, K. N. (1976): Melanoma of the lower eyelid of a dog. *Vet. Med. Small Anim. Clin.*, 71(7):929-931.

203. Hach, P., Borovansky, J., and Duchon, J. (1977): Tumourous melanosomes under the electron microscope. *Sb. Lek.*, 79(11-12):326-328.

204. Hakim, A. A. (1977): Antigenicity of a spontaneous murine mammary adenocarcinoma during *in vitro* cultivation. *Tumori*, 63(5):415-427.

205. Hakim, A. A. (1978): Modification of the immunologic properties of the cell surface. *Immunol. Commun.*, 7(1):25-39.

206. Haley, T. J. (1978): Retrospective analysis of control animal data—the rat. *Clin. Toxicol.*, 12(2):249-263.

207. Halliwell, W. H., and Kinden, D. A. (1977): Chondrosarcoma; a light and electron microscopic study of a case in a dog. *Am. J. Vet. Res.*, 38(10):1647-1652.

208. Halouzka, R., and Nevole, M. (1976): Sebaceous gland tumors in dogs. *Vet. Med. (Praha)*, 21(9):565-572.

209. Hamilton, J. M., Else, R. W., and Forshaw, P. (1977): Oestrogen receptors in canine mammary tumours. *Vet. Rec.*, 101(13):258-260.

210. Hanamura, H., and Urist, M. R. (1978): Osteogenesis and chondrogenesis in transplants of Dunn and Ridgway osteosarcoma cell cultures. *Am. J. Pathol.*, 91(2):277-298.

211. Hanaoka, Y., Kudo, K., Ishimaru, Y., and Hayashi, H. (1978): Biochemical and morphological comparison of two tumour-cell-aggregation factors from rat ascites hepatoma cells. *Br. J. Cancer*, 37(4):536-544.

212. Happe, R. P., Van der Gaag, I., Wolvekamp, W. T., and Van Toorenburg, J. (1977): Multiple polyps of the gastric mucosa in two dogs. *J. Small Anim. Pract.*, 18(3):179-189.

213. Hargis, A. M., Thomassen, R. W., and Phemister, R. D. (1977): Chronic dermatosis and cutaneous squamous cell carcinoma in the beagle dog. *Vet. Pathol.*, 14(3):218-228.

214. Harms, M., Olmos, L., Hunziker, N., and Laugier, P. (1976): Experimental keratoacanthoma. *Arch. Dermatol. Res.*, 257(2):131-142.

215. Harris, C. C., Autrup, H., Stoner, G. D., McDowell, E. M., Trump, B. F., and Schafer, P. (1977): Metabolism of dimethylnitrosamine and 1,2-dimethylhydrazine in cultured human bronchi. *Cancer Res.*, 37(7, Part 1):2309-2311.

216. Harris, C. C., Autrup, H., Stoner, G. D., McDowell, E. M., Trump, B. F., and Schafer, P. (1977): Metabolism of acyclic and cyclic N-nitrosamines in cultured human bronchi. *J. Natl. Cancer Inst.*, 59(5):1401-1406.

217. Harris, C. C., Hsu, I. C., Stoner, G. D., Trump, B. F., and Selkirk, J. K. (1978): Human pulmonary alveolar macrophages metabolise benzo(a)pyrene to proximate and ultimate mutagens. *Nature*, 272(5654):633-634.

218. Harshbarger, J. C., Shumway, S. E., and Bane, G. W. (1976): Variably differentiating oral neoplasms, ranging from epidermal papilloma to odontogenic ameloblastoma, in cunners (*Tautogolabrus adspersus*) Osteichthyes; Perciformes: Labridae. *Prog. Exp. Tumor Res.*, 20:113-128.

219. Harvey, H. J., and Gilbertson, S. R. (1977): Canine mammary gland tumors. *Vet. Clin. North Am.*, 7(1):213-219.

220. Haselbacher, G. K., and Eisenfeld, A. J. (1976): Macromolecular binding of estradiol by nuclei in a cell-free system. *Biochem. Pharmacol.*, 25(23):2571-2581.

221. Hasler, U. C., and Van den Ingh, T. S. (1978): Malignant mastocytosis and duodenal ulceration in a cat. *Schweiz. Arch. Tierheilkd.*, 120(5):63-68.

222. Hayden, D. W. (1976): Squamous cell carcinoma in a cat with intraocular and orbital metastases. *Vet. Pathol.*, 13(5):332-336.

223. Hayes, A. (1977): Feline mammary gland tumors. *Vet. Clin. North Am.*, 7(1):205-212.

224. Hayes, H. M., Jr., and Pendergrass, T. W. (1976): Canine testicular tumors; epidemiologic features of 410 dogs. *Int. J. Cancer*, 18(4):482-487.

225. Hayes, H. M., Jr., and Wilson, G. P. (1977): Hormone-dependent neoplasms of the canine perianal gland. *Cancer Res.*, 37(7, Part 1):2068-2071.

226. Headington, J. T. (1977): Primary mucinous carcinoma of skin: Histochemistry and electron microscopy. *Cancer*, 39(3):1055-1063.

227. Heavner, J. E., and Dice, P. F., II (1977): Pituitary tumor as a cause of blindness in a dog. *Vet. Med. Small Anim. Clin.*, 72(5):873-876.

228. Hedinger, C. (1974): *Histological Typing of Thyroid Tumours*. No. 11. WHO, Geneva.

229. Heine, H., and Schaeg, G. (1976): Ultrastructural investigations on the pathogenesis of hyperplasias and tumors of skin connective tissue. *Arch. Dermatol. Res.*, 257:67-77.

230. Heine, H., Schaeg, G., and Nasemann, T. (1977): Annulate nexus and "virus like particles." *Arch. Dermatol. Res.*, 260(3):241-246.

231. Helpap, B. (1978): The proliferative pattern of the prostatic carcinoma. Program, XIIth International Cancer Congress, Buenos Aires, p. 220.

232. Helphrey, M. L., and Meierhenry, E. F. (1978): Vulvar leiomyosarcoma metastatic to the spinal cord in a dog. *J. Am. Vet. Med. Assoc.*, 172(5):583-584.

233. Helyer, B. J., and Petrelli, M. (1978): Cytoplasmic inclusions in spontaneous hematomas of CBA/H-T6T6 mice. Histochemistry and electron microscopy. *J. Natl. Cancer Inst.*, 60(4):861-869.

234. Henson, D. (1978): The international classification of disease for oncology (ICD-O). Program, XIIth International Cancer Congress, Buenos Aires, p. 182.

235. Hertsch, B., and Eidt, E. (1976): Clinical diagnosis of gastric carcinoma in horses. *Deutsch. Tieraerztl. Wochenschr.*, 83(3):92-96.

236. Hess, P. W. (1977): Canine mast cell tumors. *Vet. Clin. North Am.*, 7(1):133-143.

237. Hess, W. (1950): Chirurgie des Pankreas, Schwabe, Basel.

238. Hiraki, S., Mulcahy, M. F., and Dmochowski, L. (1978): "Particle-filament complex" in tumor cells of northern pike, *Esox lucius* L. *Tex. Rep. Biol. Med.*, 36:111-120.

239. Hirano, T., Miyajima, H., Watanabe, T., Tsukuda, R., and Shimamoto, K. (1977): Enhancement of tumor induction in rats with moloney murine sarcoma virus by a "new method based on direct injection into fetuses. *J. Natl. Cancer Inst.*, 58(1):73-82.

240. Hirone, T., Eryu, Y., Otsuki, N., and Fukushiro, R. (1976): Light and electron microscopic studies of trichoepithelioma papulosum multiplex. In *Biology and Disease of the Hair*, pp. 397-407, edited by K. Toda *et al*. University Park Press, Baltimore.

241. Hollmann, K. H., and Verley, J. M. (1978): Mammotropic and somatotropic pituitary cells in spontaneous mammary tumor bearing C3H female mice. A quantitative electron microscope study. *Experientia*, 34(1):98-100.

242. Holmberg, C. A., Sesline, D., and Osburn, B. (1978): Dysgerminoma in a rhesus monkey; morphologic and biological features. *J. Med. Prima-

tol., 7(1):53-58.

243. Holscher. M. A., Page, D. L., Netsky, M. G., and Powell, H. S. (1977): Mixed glioma and rhabdomyosarcoma in brain of a wild deer. Vet. Pathol., 14(6):643-647.

244. Horten, B. C., and Montague, S. R. (1976): In vitro characteristics of a sacrococcygeal chordoma maintained in tissue and organ culture systems. Acta Neuropathol. (Berl.), 35(1):13-25.

245. Horvath, Z., Tury, E., and Sellyei, M. (1976): A case of cutaneous bovine leucosis in Hungary. Acta Vet. Acad. Sci., Hung., 26(2):131-147.

246. Hough, J. D., Krahwinkel, D. J., Evans, A. T., Caprig, C. B., Tvedten, H. W., and Schirmer, R. G. (1977): Tracheal osteochondroma in a dog. J. Am. Vet. Med., 170(12):1416-1418.

247. Howard, D. R., Lammerding, J. J., Merkley, D. F., and Bloomberg, M. S. (1976): Osteosarcoma of the hard palate in a dog. Vet. Med. Small Anim. Clin., 71(1):59-61.

248. Hsu, L., and Trupin, G. L. (1978): The in vivo differentiation of murine neuroblastoma. Virchows Arch. [Cell Pathol.], 27(1):49-61.

249. Hui, F., Pasztor, L. M., and Teramura, D. J. (1977): Somatic cell hybrids derived from terminally differentiated rhesus cells and established mouse cell lines. Mech. Aging Dev., 6(4):305-318.

250. Huang, S. N., and Goltzman, D. (1978): Electron and immunoelectron microscopic study of thyroidal medullary carcinoma. Cancer, 41(6): 2226-2235.

251. Hunter, J. A., Paterson, W. D., and Fairley, D. J. (1978): Human malignant melanoma. Melanosomal polymorphism and the ultrastructural dopa reaction. Br. J. Dermatol., 98(4):381-390.

252. Hunter, J. A., Zaynoun, S., Patterson, W. D., MacKie, R. M., Cochran, A. J., and Bleehen, S. S. (1976): Proceedings; malignant melanoma. A comparison of cellular fine structure in invasive nodules of different histogenetic type. Br. J. Dermatol., 95 (Suppl.), 14:13-14.

253. Hunter, J. A., Zaynoun, S., Patterson, W. D., Bleehen, S. S., Mackie, R., and Cochran, A. J. (1978): Cellular fine structure in the invasive nodules of different histogenetic types of malignant melanoma. Br. J. Dermatol., 98(3):255-272.

254. Iagubov, A. S., and Kats, V. A. (1976): Tumor cell ultrastructure. Vopr. Onkol., 22(3):64-67.

255. Idowu, L. (1977): The chromosomes of the transmissible venereal tumour of dogs in Ibadan, Nigeria. Res. Vet. Sci., 22(3):271-273.

256. Ikede, B. O. (1976): Bilateral retroperitoneal lipomata in a neonatal calf. Vet. Rec., 98(14):280.

257. Ilse, G., Kovacs, K., Horvath, E., Ilse, R., and Ilse, D. (1976): Lysosomal disposal of secretory granules and their transformation into pigment particles in spontaneous prolactin cell adenomas of the rat pituitary. Z. Mikrosk. Anat. Forsch., 90(5):876-882.

258. Innes, D. J., Jr., and Cutler, L. S. (1977): Phosphatase enzymes. Cytochemical study of pleomorphic adenoma and normal human salivary glands. Arch. Pathol. Lab. Med., 102(2):90-94.

259. Irvine, R. A., Jr. (1967): Diffuse epibulbar squamous-cell epithelioma. Am. J. Ophthalmol., 64:550-554.

260. Ishihara, H., Ishimaru, Y., and Hayashi, H. (1977): Ultrastructural changes of intercellular junctions in rat ascites hepatoma cells with calcium depletion. Br. J. Cancer, 35(5):643-656.

261. Ishikawa, T., Kuwabara, N., and Takayama, S. (1976): Spontaneous ovarian tumors in domestic carp (Cyprinus carpio); light and electron microscopy. J. Natl. Cancer Inst., 57(3):579-584.

262. Ito, T., and Fujita, N. (1977): Pathological studies on lymphosarcoma in swine. Nippon Juigaku Zasshi, 39(6):599-608.

263. Ito, Y., Kimura, I., and Miyake, T. (1976): Histopathological and virological investigations of papillomas in soles and gobies in coastal waters of Japan. Prog. Exp. Tumor Res., 20:86-93.

264. Jakobiec, F. A., Witschel, H., and Zimmerman, L. E. (1976): Choroidal leiomyoma of vascular origin. Am. J. Ophthalmol., 82(2):205-212.

265. Jao, W., Keh, P. C., and Swerdlow, M. A. (1976): Ultrastructure of the basal cell adenoma of parotid gland. Cancer, 37(3):1322-1333.

266. Jelinek, P., Valicek, L., Smid, B., and Halouzka, R. (1978): Demonstration of papillomatosis in nutrias (Myocastor coypus Molina). Vet. Med. (Praha), 23(2):113-119.

267. Johannessen, J. V., Gould, V. E., and Jao, W. (1978): Fine structure of human thyroid cancer. Human Pathol., 9(4):385.

268. Johnson, G. F., and Twedt, D. C. (1977): Endoscopy and laparoscopy in the diagnosis and management of neoplasia in small animals. Vet. Clin. North Am., 7(1):77-92.

269. Johnson, R. K. (1977): Insulinoma in the dog. Vet. Clin. North Am., 7(3): 629-635.

270. Johnson, S., Rundell, M., and Platt, W. (1978): Leiomyosarcoma of the scrotum; a case report with electron microscopy. Cancer, 41(5):1830-1835.

271. Johnson, T. C. (1976): Osteosarcoma of the canine skull (a case report). Vet. Med. Small Anim. Clin., 71(5):629-631.

272. Jones, B. R., Nicholls, M. R., and Badman, R. (1976): Peptic ulceration in a dog associated with an islet cell carcinoma of the pancreas and an elevated plasma gastrin level. J. Small Anim. Pract., 17(9):593-598.

273. Joyce, J. R. (1976): Cryosurgical treatment of tumors of horses and cattle. J. Am. Vet. Med. Assoc., 168(3):226-229.

274. Joyce, J. R., Thompson, R. B., Kyzar, J. R., and Hightower, D. (1976): Thyroid carcinoma in a horse. J. Am. Vet. Med. Assoc., 168(7):610-612.

275. Jurgelski, W., Jr., Hudson, P. M., Falk, H. L., and Kotin, P. (1976): Embryonal neoplasms in the opossum; a new model for solid tumors of infancy and childhood. Science, 193(4250):328-332.

276. Kahn, L. B. (1976): Chondrosarcoma with dedifferentiated foci. A comparative and ultrastructural study. Cancer, 37(3):1365-1375.

277. Kaiser, H. E. (1960): Studies in the comparative osteology of fossil and recent pachyostoses. Palaeontographica, CXIV (Abt. A):113-196.

278. Kaiser, H. E. (1964): Gedanken über die Genese des primären, epidermoiden Bronchialcarcinoms. Arch. Geschwulstforsch., 24(1):15-19.

279. Kalter, S. S., Heberling, R. L., McGill, H. C., Carey, K. D., and Smith, G. C. (1978): Isolation of baboon endogenous virus from naturally occurring lymphoproliferative disease in a baboon. Program, XIIth International Cancer Congress, Buenos Aires, p. 116.

280. Karstad, L., Thorsen, J., Davies, G., and Kaminjolo, J. S. (1977): Poxvirus fibromas on African hares. J. Wildl. Dis., 13(3):245-247.

281. Katsuya, H., Ishimaru, Y., Koono, M., and Hayashi, H. (1978): A light and electron microscopic study on complete dissociation of rat ascites hepatoma cells under activation of neutral protease and calcium depletion. Virchows Arch. (Cell Pathol.), 27(2):159-172.

282. Kats, V. A., Iagubov, A. S., and Lavnikova, G. A. (1977): Light and electron microscopy in determining the histogenesis of vascular tumors. Arkh. Patol., 39(12):34-39.

283. Kawada, K., and Ojima, A. (1978): Various epithelial and non-epithelial tumors spontaneously occurring in long-lived mice of A/St, CBA, C57Bl/6 and their hybrid mice. Acta Pathol. Jpn., 28(1):25-39.

284. Kay, S., and Terz, J. J. (1976): Ultrastructural observations on a follicular carcinoma of the thyroid gland. Am. J. Clin. Pathol., 65(3):328-336.

285. Kelly, D. F., and Darke, P. G. (1976): Cushing's syndrome in the dog. Vet. Rec., 98(2):28-30.

286. Kelly, D. F., and Watson, W. J. (1976): Epidermoid cyst of the brain in the horse. Equine Vet. J., 8(3):110-112.

287. Kelly, D. F., Long, S. E., and Strohmenger, G. D. (1976): Testicular neoplasia in an intersex dog. J. Small Anim. Pract., 17(4):247-253.

288. Kemmer, C., Müller, M., and Zotter, S. (1977): Electron microscopic investigations of intracytoplasmic A particles in mouse mammary tumours. Exp. Pathol. (Jena), 13(6):313-319.

289. Kendrey, G., and Laszlo, B. (1976): Hepatitis virus cirrhosis in primary carcinoma of the liver; an electromicroscopic study. Z. Krebsforsch. Klin. Oncol., 88(1):97-100.

290. Kent, G. C., Jr. (1954): Comparative Anatomy of the Vertebrates, p. 315. McGraw-Hill, New York.

291. Kessoku, A. (1974): Electron microscopic observations on papillary cystadenoma (lymphadenism). Warthin's tumor of the parotid. J. Otolaryngol. (Jpn.), 26:77-81.

292. Kharkovskaia, N. A., Khrustalev, S. A., and Vasileva, N. N. (1977): Spontaneous neoplasms in guinea pigs. Vopr. Onkol., 13(11):98-102.

293. Kharkovskaia, N. A., Khrustalev, S. A., and Vasileva, N. N. (1978): Spontaneous neoplasms in Syrian hamsters from the Stolbovaia Breeding nursery of the Academy of Medical Sciences of the USSR. Vopr. Onkol., 24(4):72-76.

294. Kimeto, B., and Mugera, G. M. (1974): Transmissible veneral tumour of dog in Kenya. Bull. Epizoot. Dis. Afr., 22(4):327-329.

295. Kimura, I., Miyake, T., Kubota, S., Kamata, A., and Morikawa, S. (1976): Adenomatous polyps in the stomachs of hatchery-grown salmonids and other types of fishes. Prog. Exp. Tumor. Res., 20:181-194.

296. Kissler, W. (1977): Primary fibrosarcoma of the right atrium. Zentralbl. Allg. Pathol., 121(3):235-238.

297. Knecht, C. D., and Greene, J. A. (1977): Osteoma of the zygomatic arch in a cat. J. Am. Vet. Med. Assoc., 171(10):1077-1078.

298. Knecht, C. D., and Priester, W. A. (1978): Musculoskeletal tumors in dogs. J. Am. Vet. Med. Assoc., 172(1):72-74.

299. Knecht, C. D., and Priester, W. A. (1978): Musculoskeletal tumors in dogs. Exp. Cell Res., 111(2):465-468.

300. Knowles, D. M., Jakobiec, F. A., Potter, G. D., and Jones, I. S. (1976): Ophthalmic striated muscle neoplasms. Surv. Ophthalmol., 21(3):219-261.

301. Koch, F., and Kaiser, E. (1976): Uterine cancer in a dog. Berl. Münch. Tierärztl. Wochenschr., 89(19):373-377.

302. Koppang, N., and Rimesl Atten, H. (1976): Toxic and carcinogenic effects of nitrosodimethylamine in mink. Iarc. Sci. Publ., 14:443-452.

303. Korom, I. (1976): Dermatofibrosarcoma protuberans with 20-year duration. Z. Hautkr., 51(14):583-586.

304. Kovacs, K., Horvath, E., Ilse, R. G., and Ilse, D. (1976): Spontaneous pancreatic beta cell tumor in the rat. A light and electron microscopic study. Vet. Pathol., 13(4):286-294.

305. Kovacs, R., Horvath, E., Bilbao, J. M., and Ilse, R. G. (1977): Annulate lamellae in spontaneous prolactin cell adenomas of the rat pituitary. Anat. Anz., 141(1):59-65.

306. Kovacs, R., Horvath, E., Ilse, R. G., Ezrin, C., and Ilse, D. (1977): Spontaneous pituitary adenomas in aging rats. A light microscopic, immunocytological and fine structural study. Beitr. Pathol., 161(1):1-16.

307. Kraft, I., and Frese, K. (1976): Histological studies on canine pigmented

moles. The comparative pathology of the naevus problem. *J. Comp. Pathol.*, 86(1):143–155.

308. Krahwinkel, D. J., Jr., Merkley, D. F., and Howard, D. R. (1976): Cryosurgical treatment of cancerous and noncancerous diseases of dogs, horses, and cats. *J. Am. Vet. Med. Assoc.*, 169(2):201–207.

309. Kraus, H., Knoerr-Gaertner, H., and Schuhmann, R. (1978): Early malignant transformation in mesothelial tumors of the ovary (comparative cytogenetic and histologic studies). Program, XIIth International Cancer Congress, Buenos Aires, p. 232.

310. Krugman, S., and Gocke, D. J. (1978): Viral hepatitis. *Major Probl. Intern. Med.* 15:1–147.

311. Krylova, R. I., and Lapin, B. A. (1977): Tumors of the liver, biliary tracts and pancreas in monkeys. *Arkh. Patol.*, 39(3):63–69.

312. Kthudolei, V. V. Tumor growth in amphibians. *Usp. Sovrem. Biol.*, 81(2):306–318.

313. Kurumado, K., and Mori, W. (1976): Virus-like particles in human pinealoma. *Acta Neuropathol.*, (Berl.), 35(3):273–276.

314. Kyono, Y., and Egami, N. (1977): The effect of temperature during the diethylnitrosamine treatment on liver tumorigenesis in the fish, *Oryzias latipes*. *Eur. J. Cancer*, 13(10):1191–1194.

315. Ladds, P. W., and Saunders, P. J. (1976): Sertoli cell tumours in the bull. *J. Comp. Pathol.*, 86(4):503–508.

316. Ladds, P. W., and Entwistle, K. W. (1977): Observations on squamous cell carcinomas of sheep in Queensland, Australia. *Br. J. Cancer*, 35(1):110–114.

317. Laidler, P., and Kay, J. M. (1976): The effect of combined chronic hypoxia and N-ethyl-N-nitrosourea on the carotid bodies of rats. *Experientia*, 32(7):899–900.

318. Landolfo, S., Giovarelli, M., and Forni, G. (1977): *In vitro* arming and blocking activity of sera from BALB/c mice bearing a spontaneous transplantable adenocarcinoma. *Eur. J. Cancer*, 13(11):1217–1223.

319. Lange, J., and Johannessen, J. V. (1977): Histochemical and ultrastructural studies of chemodectoma-like tumors in the cod (*Gadus morrhua* L.). *Lab. Invest.*, 37(1):96–104.

320. Larsson, L. I. (1978): Endocrine pancreatic tumors. *Human Pathol.*, 9(4):401.

321. Lavach, J. D., and Severin, G. A. (1977): Neoplasia of the equine eye, adnexa, and orbit; a review of 68 cases. *J. Am. Vet. Med. Assoc.*, 170(2):202–203.

322. Leatherland, J. F., and Sonstegard, R. A. (1977): Structure and function of the pituitary gland in gonadal tumor-bearing and normal cyprinid fish. *Cancer Res.*, 37(9):3151–3168.

323. Leatherland, J. F., and Sonstegard, R. A. (1978): Structure of normal testis and testicular tumors in cyprinids from Lake Ontario. *Cancer Res.*, 38:3164–3173.

324. Le Charpentier, Y., Forest, M., Carlioz, A., Abelanet, R., Tomeno, B., Postel, M., Maurer, P., and Kerboull, M. (1977): How to classify certain osteosarcomas (letter). *Nouv. Presse Med.*, 6(28):2524.

325. Lee, C. G., and Ladds, P. W. (1976): Vascular hamartoma of the ovary in a cow. *Aust. Vet. J.*, 52(5):236.

326. Lee, D. J., Sinnhuber, R. O., Wales, J. H., and Putnam, G. B. (1978): Effect of dietary protein on the response of rainbow trout (*Salmo gairdneri*) to aflatoxin B1. *J. Natl. Cancer Inst.*, 60(2):317–320.

327. Lee, S. C., and Roth, L. M. (1976): Malignant oncocytoma of the parotid gland. A light and electron microscopic study. *Cancer*, 37:1606–1614.

328. Legendre, A. M., and Krehbiel, J. D. (1977): Disseminated intravascular coagulation in a dog with hemothorax and hemangiosarcoma. *J. Am. Vet. Med. Assoc.*, 171(10):1070–1071.

329. Legendre, A. M., Merkley, D. F., Carrig, C. B., and Krehbirl, J. D. (1976): Primary hyperparathyroidism in a dog. *J. Am. Vet. Med. Assoc.*, 168(8):694–696.

330. Leger, L. (1977): Sertoli cell tumor in a dog. *Can. Vet. J.*, 18(9):253–256.

331. Legrand, M., and Pariente, R. (1976): Electron microscopy in the cytological examination of metastatic pleural effusions. *Thorax*, 31(4):443–449.

332. Leibson, N. L., and Movchan, O. J. (1975): Cambial zones in gills of bivalvia. *Mar. Biol.*, 31:175–180.

333. Leicher, H. (1978): The origin of malignant tumors of the upper-airways, the digestion tract and the ear. Organ-resistance and organ-disposition (organotrophy) by the origin of malignant primary tumors. *Laryngol. Rhinol. Otol.* (Stuttg.), 57(3):162–176.

334. Lema, B. (1978): Pathology: Germ cell tumors. Program, XIIth International Cancer Congress, Buenos Aires, p. 103.

335. Lerche, W., and Maslo, K. H. (1977): On the structure of the pigment epithelium proliferation over malignant melanoma of the choroid. *Klin. Monatsbl. Augenheilkd.*, 171(3):450–458.

336. Leung, B. (1978): Prolactin and estrogen dependency in human breast cancer cells. Program, XIIth International Cancer Congress, Buenos Aires, p. 215.

337. Lewis, J. C., Reardon, M. J., and Montgomery, C. A., Jr. (1976): Paraganglioma involving the spinal cord of a dog. *J. Am. Vet. Med. Assoc.*, 168(9):864–865.

338. Lindberg, R., Jonsson, O. J., and Kasstrom, H. (1976): Sertoli cell tumours associated with feminization, prostatitis and squamous metaplasia of the renal tubular epithelium in a dog. *J. Small Anim. Pract.*, 17(7):451–458.

339. Lindsay, J. W. (1976): Spontaneous occurrence of tumors in laboratory-reared arvicoline rodents. *Cancer Res.*, 36(11, Part 1):4092–4098.

340. Linna, T. J. (1976): Increased growth rate of a benzo(a)pyrene-induced transplantable tumor in bursectomized chickens. *Cancer Res.*, 36(5):1705–1709.

341. Ljungberg, O. (1977): Tumors in pike on the Swedish Baltic coast (author's transl.) *Nord. Vet. Med.*, 29(12, Suppl. 1):15–16.

342. Lommatzsch, P., and Klug, H. (1977): A contribution to the ulstrastructure of malignant melanomas of the iris. *Albrecht von Graefes Arch. Klin. Ophthalmol.*, 203(2):101–117.

343. Lopez, Dr. Personal communication.

344. Lowe, D. M., and Moore, M. N. (1978): Cytology and quantitative cytochemistry of a proliferative atypical hemocytic condition in *Mytilus edulis* (Bivalvia, mollusca). *J. Natl. Canc. Inst.*, 60(6):1455–1459.

345. Luna, M. A., and Mackay, B. (1976): Basal cell adenoma of the parotid gland. Case report with ultrastructural observations. *Cancer*, 37(3):1615–1631.

346. Lund, J. E., and Park, J. F. (1978): Focal mastocytosis in lymph nodes from a Beagle dog. *Vet. Pathol.*, 15(1):64–67.

347. Lupulescu, A., and Pinkus, H. (1976): Electron microscopic observations on rat epidermis during experimental carcinogenesis. *Oncology*, 33(1):24–28.

348. Macaulay, R. A., Dewar, A. E., Langlands, A. O., and Stuart, A. E. (1978): Cell receptor studies on six anaplastic tumours of the thyroid. *J. Clin. Pathol.*, 31(5):461–468.

349. Machado, E. A., and Beauchene, R. E. (1976): Spontaneous osteogenic sarcoma in the WI/Ten rat: a case report. *Lab. Anim. Sci.*, 26(1):98–100.

350. MacNab, G. M., Alexander, J. J., Lecatsas, G., Bey, E. M., and Urbanowicz, J. M. (1976): Hepatitis B surface antigen produced by a human hepatoma cell line. *Br. J. Cancer*, 34(5):509–515.

351. Madewell, B. R., Pool, R. R., and Leighton, R. L. (1977): Osteogenic sarcoma at the site of a chronic nonunion fracture and internal fixation device in a dog. *J. Am. Vet. Med. Assoc.*, 171(2):187–189.

352. Madewell, B. R., Nyland, T. G., and Weigel, J. E. (1978): Regression of hypertrophic osteopathy following pneumonectomy in a dog. *J. Am. Vet. Med. Assoc.*, 172(7):818–821.

353. Maeta, T., Fujiwara, Y., Ohizumi, T., Kato, E., and Kakizaki, G. (1977): Pathological study of tracheal and pulmonary lesions in autopsy cases of congenital esophageal atresia. *Tohoku J. Exp. Med.*, 123(1):23–32.

354. Maiorana, A., and Gullino, P. M. (1978): Acquisition of angiogenic capacity and neoplastic transformation in the rat mammary gland. *Cancer Res.*, 38:4409–4414.

355. Mangkoewidjojo, S., and Kimb, J. C. (1977): Malignant melanoma metastatic to the lung in a pet hamster. *Lab. Anim.*, 11(2):125–127.

356. Mani, J. S. (1964): *Ecology of Plant Galls*. W. Junk, The Hague.

357. Mareso, E. A., Glatstein, T. B., Citera, L. G., Escobar, T., and Germino, N. I. (1978): Carcinoma transicional vesical: Caracteristicas citrometricas e histoquimicas. Workshop no. 51(11), Abstracts, Vol. 3, p. 107. XIIth Congreso Internacional del Cancer, Buenos Aires.

358. Masson, P. (1970): *Human Tumors*. Ed. 2 (translated by S. D. Kobernick). Wayne State University Press, Detroit.

359. Mathe, G., and Rappaport, H. (1976): *Histological and Cytological Typing of Neoplastic Diseases of Haematopoietic and Lymphoid Tissues*. WHO, Geneva.

360. Matsuda, I., Kikuchi, H., Furuse, S., Karasawa, J., and Manabe, T. (1976): Dermoid tumor in left cerebellum—A case report. *Neurol. Surg.* (Tokyo), 4(6):597–604. (Jpn.)

361. Mattheuws, D., Rottiers, R., De Rijcke, J., De Rick, A., and De Schepper, J. (1976): Hyperinsulinism in the dog due to pancreatic islet-cell tumour; a report on three cases. *Horm. Metab. Res. (Suppl.)*, 6:26–33.

362. McDowell, E. M.: Personal communication.

363. McDowell, E. M., Barrett, L. A., Glavin, F. et al. (1978): The respiratory epithelium. I. Human bronchus. *J. Natl. Cancer Inst.*, 61:539–549.

364. McDowell, E. M., McLaughlin, J. S., Merenyi, D. K., et al. (1978): The respiratory epithelium. V. Histogenesis of lung carcinomas in the human. *J. Natl. Cancer Inst.*, 61:587–606.

365. McDowell, E. M., Becci, P. J., Schürch, W., et al. (1978): The role of mucous cells in repair and in the histogenesis of metaplastic and neoplastic change in tracheobronchial epithelium. *J. Histochem. Cytochem.*, 26:215.

366. McLennan, M. W., and Kelly, W. R. (1977): Hypertrophic osteopathy and dysgerminoma in a mare. *Aust. Vet. J.*, 53(3):144–146.

367. McMartin, D. N., and Gruhn, R. F. (1977): Sebaceous carcinoma in a horse. *Vet. Pathol.*, 14(5):532–534.

368. McNutt, N. S. (1976): Ultrastructural comparison of the interface between epithelium and stroma in basal cell carcinoma and control human skin. *Lab. Invest.*, 35(2):132–142.

369. Mearns, A. J., and Sherwood, M. J. (1976): Ocean wastewater discharge and tumors in a southern California flatfish. *Prog. Exp. Tumor Res.*, 20:75–85.

370. Mesa, C. P., and Hori, J. M. (1978): Patterns of growth and spread of carcinomas of colon and rectum as observed in giant histological

sections. A study of 250 cases. Program, XIIth International Cancer Congress, Buenos Aires, p. 198.

371. Metz, S. A., and Levine, R. J. (1977): Neuroendocrine tumours that secrete biologically active peptides and amines. *Clin. Endocrinol. Metab.*, 6(3):719–744.

372. Meuten, D. J., Price, S. M., Seiler, R. M., and Krook, L. (1978): Gastric carcinoma with pseudohyperparathyroidism in a horse. *Cornell Vet.*, 68(2):179–195.

373. Meyer, D. J. (1976): Pancreatic islet cell carcinoma in a dog treated with streptozotocin. *Am. J. Vet. Res.*, 37(10):1221–1223.

374. Meyer, D. J. (1977): Temporary remission of hypoglycemia in a dog with an insulinoma after treatment with streptozotocin. *Am. J. Vet. Res.*, 38(8):1201–1204.

375. Meyvisch, C., Thoonen, H., and Hoorens, J. (1977): The ulstrastructure of rhabdomyosarcoma in a dog. *Zentralbl. Vet. Med. A*, 24(7):542–551.

376. Michel, R. G., Woodard, B. H., Shelburne, J. D., and Bossen, E. H. (1978): Ceruminous gland adenocarcinoma; a light and electron microscopic study. *Cancer*, 41(2):545–553.

377. Michelson, E. H., and Richards, C. S. (1975): Neoplasms and tumor-like growths in the aquatic pulmonate snail *Biomphalaria glabrata*. *Ann. N. Y. Acad. Sci.*, 266:411–425.

378. Mike, V., Safai, B., Giraldo, G., and Good, R. A. (1978): Association of Kaposis sarcoma with second primary malignancies; possible etiopathogenetic implications. Program, XIIth International Cancer Congress, Buenos Aires, p. 223.

379. Mikuz, G., Myola, F., and Gütter, W. (1977): Chordoma; ultrastructural, biochemical and cytophotometric findings. *Beitr. Pathol.*, 161(2):150–165.

380. Mills, J. H., Fretz, P. B., Clark, E. G., and Ganjam, V. K. (1977): Arrhenoblastoma in a mare. *J. Am. Vet. Med. Assoc.*, 171(8):754–757.

381. Mimura, T., Ito, K., Hosoda, Y., Yakumaru, K., Harada, T., and Shimaoka, K. (1978): A study of 47 autopsied cases of thyroid carcinoma. Program, XIIth International Cancer Congress, Buenos Aires, p. 185.

382. Mix, M. C. (1976): A review of the cellular proliferative disorders of oysters (*Ostrea lurida*) from Yaquina Bay, Oregon, *Prog. Exp. Tumor Res.*, 20:275–282.

383. Monis, B., De Cejas, A. G., and Cejas, H. A. (1978): The lumenal glycocalyx as an expression of cell differentiation in transitional cell carcinomas of urinary tract of man. Workshop no. 51(3), Abstracts, Vol. 3, p. 103, XIIth Congreso Internacional del Cancer, Buenos Aires.

384. Moore, J. N., and Kintner, L. D. (1976): Recurrent esophageal obstruction due to squamous cell carcinoma in a horse. *Cornell Vet.*, 66(4):590–597.

385. Moscovici, C., Moscovici, M. G., Jimenez, H., Lat, M. M., Hayman, M. J., and Vogt, P. K. (1977): Continuous tissue culture cell lines derived from chemically induced tumors of Japanese quail. *Cell*, 11(1):95–103.

386. Mostofi, F. K. (1973): *Histological Typing of Urinary Bladder Tumours*. International Histological Classification of Tumours No. 10. WHO, Geneva.

387. Movchan, O. T. (1971): The proliferation activity in tissues of bivalves; I. The cambial zones in gills of the mussel *Crenomytilus grayanus* (Ruike). *Tsitologiya*, 13:75–181.

388. Muraoka, Y., Itch, M., Yamashita, F., and Hayashi, Y. (1977): Spontaneous tumors in aged SD-JCL rats. *Exp. Anim.* (Tokyo), 26(1):13–22.

389. Murayama, T., Kawabe, K., and Tagami, M. (1977): A case of parathyroid carcinoma concurred with hyperplasia; an electron microscopic study. *J. Urol.*, 118(1, Part 1):126–127.

390. Nagasawa, H., Yanai, R., and Azuma, I. (1978): Suppression by *Nocardia rubra* cell wall skeleton mammary DNA synthesis, plasma prolactin level, and spontaneous mammary tumorigenesis in mice. *Cancer Res.*, 38(7):2160–2162.

391. Nair, P. N., and Gangal, S. G. (1976): Studies on histocompatibility antigens in an inbred mouse strain showing spontaneous mammary tumour and leukaemia. *Indian J. Cancer*, 13(4):345–350.

392. Nakakuki, K., Shimokawa, K., Yamauchi, H., and Ojima, A. (1976): A spontaneous transplantable osteogenic sarcoma in AKR/Ms mice. *Gann*, 67(4):513–521.

393. Nakatsukasa, Y. (1977): Subcutaneous fibroma of the "Hibuna," *Carassius auratus*. (author's transl.) *Igaku Kenkyu*, 47(2):115–121.

394. Nakayama, I., Moriuchi, A., Taira, Y., Takahara, O., and Itoga, T. (1977): Fine structural study of annulate lamellae complexes in human tumors. *Acta Pathol. Jpn.*, 27(1):25–39.

395. Ndiritu, C. G., Mbogwa, S. W., and Sayer, P. D. (1977): Extragenitally located transmissible venereal tumor in dogs. *Mod. Vet. Pract.*, 58:940–946.

396. Nettles, V. F., and Vandevelde, M. (1978): Thalamic ependymoma in a white-tailed deer. *Vet. Pathol.*, 15(1):133–135.

397. Niizuma, K. (1977): An electron microscopic study of sebaceous epithelioma. A case report with two new observations on lipid droplet formation. *Dermatologica*, 154(2):98–106.

398. Niizuma, K. (1977): Lipid droplet of sebaceous carcinoma. Electron microscopic study utilizing glycol methacrylate-glutaraldehyde-urea procedure. *Arch. Dermatol. Res.*, 206(2):111–119.

399. Nilsson, O. (1977): Studies on the ultrastructure of the human parathyroid glands in various pathological conditions. *Acta Pathol. Microbiol.*

Scand. (Suppl.), 263:1–88.

400. Niman, H. L., Gardner, M. B., Stephenson, J. R., and Roy-Burman, P. (1977): Endogenous RD-114 virus genome expression in malignant tissues of domestic cats. *J. Virol.*, 23(3):578–586.

401. Nizze, H. (1976): Metastasizing islet cell carcinoma of the pancreas in a 10-year-old girl. *Zentralbl. Allg. Pathol.*, 120(6):467–472.

402. Novi, A. M. (1977): Liver carcinogenesis in rats after aflatoxin B1 administration. A light- and electron microscopic study. *Curr. Top. Pathol.*, 65:115–163.

403. Odinokova, V. A., Dmitrieva, N. P., Kalinin, A. P., and Astakhov, A. F. (1976): Morphologic changes in the parathyroid glands in primary hyperparathyroidism. *Arkh. Patol.*, 38(7):18–24.

404. Oegema, T. R., Jr., Brown, M., and Dziewiatkowski, D. D. (1977): The link protein in proteoglycan aggregates from the swarm rat chondrosarcoma. *J. Biol. Chem.*, 252(18):6470–6477.

405. Ohkawa, K., Amasaki, H., Terashima, Y., Aizawa, S., and Ishikawa, E. (1977): Clear cell carcinoma of the ovary; light and electron microscopic studies. *Cancer*, 40(6):3019–3029.

406. Okukov, V. B., Anisimov, V. N., and Azarova, M. A. (1977): Effect of epidermal chalones on the growth of transplantable tumors. *Biull. Eksp. Biol. Med.*, 84(10):466–468.

407. Ol'khovskaia, I. G., and Shubin, A. S. (1977): Histogenesis of dermatofibrosarcoma protuberans. *Arkh. Patol.*, 39(5):33–37.

408. Onderka, D. K., and Zwart, P. (1978): Granulosa cell tumor in a garter snake (*Thamnophis sirtalis*). *J. Wildl. Dis.*, 14(2):218–221.

409. Overstreet, R. M., and Van Devender, T. (1978): Implication of an environmentally-induced hamartoma in commercial shrimps. *J. Invertebr. Pathol.*, 31:234–238.

410. Owen, L. N. (1976): Osteosarcoma in the dog. *Proc. R. Soc. Med.*, 69(8):546–547.

411. Owen, L. N. (1977): Lymphosarcoma in the dog. *Proc. R. Soc. Med.*, 70(8):563–566.

412. Ozzello, L., and Hamels, J. (1976): The histiocytic nature of dermatofibrosarcoma protuberans. Tissue culture and electron microscopic study. *Am. J. Clin. Pathol.*, 65(2):136–148.

413. Pamukcu, A. M., Price, J. M., and Bryan, G. T. (1976): Naturally occurring and braken-fern-induced bovine urinary bladder tumors. Clinical and morphological characteristics. *Vet. Pathol.*, 13(2):110–122.

414. Panke, T. W., Croxson, M. S., Parker, J. W., Carriere, D. P., Rosoff, L., Sr., and Warner, N. E. (1978): Triiodothyronine-secreting (toxic) adenoma of the thyroid gland; light and electron microscopic characteristics. *Cancer*, 41(2):528–537.

415. Papas, T. S., Pry, T. W., Schafer, M. P., and Sonstegard, R. A. (1977): Presence of DNA polymerase in lymphosarcoma in northern pike (*Esox lucius*). *Cancer Res.*, 37(9):3214–3217.

416. Papmahl-Hollenberg, U. (1978): Pictorial report. Osteoma spongiosum in the cat. *Berl. Munch. Tieraerztl. Wochenschr.*, 91(7):136.

417. Patnaik, A. K., Liu, S., and Johnson, G. F. (1976): Extraskeletal osteosarcoma of the liver in a dog. *J. Small Anim. Pract.*, 17:365–370.

418. Patnaik, A. K., Hurvitz, A. I., and Johnson, G. F. (1977): Canine gastrointestinal neoplasms. *Vet. Pathol.*, 14(6):547–555.

419. Patnaik, A. K., MacEwen, E. G., Erlandson, R. A., Lieberman, P. H., and Liu, S. K. (1978): Mediastinal parathyroid adenocarinoma in a dog. *Vet. Pathol.*, 15(1):55–63.

420. Patniak, A. K., Schaer, M., Parks, J., and Liu, S. K. (1976): Metastasizing ovarian teratocarcinoma in dogs. A report of two cases and review of literature. *J. Small Anim. Pract.*, 17(4):235–246.

421. Patricio, M. B., Clode, W. H., and Ricardo, J. A. (1977): Active immunization against spontaneous tumors in mice. *J. Surg. Oncol.*, 9(2):111–115.

422. Patt, D. I., and Patt, G. R. (1969): *Comparative Vertebrate Histology*, pp. 160, 163, 167. Harper & Row, New York.

423. Pavelic Z. P., Porter, C. W., Allen, L. M., and Mihich, E. (1978): Alteration of sodium transport in mouse mammary epithelium associated with neoplastic transformation. *Cancer Res.*, 38(6):1356–1361.

424. Pearson, G. R., and Head, K. W. (1976): Malignant haemangioendothelioma (angiosarcoma) in the dog. *J. Small Anim. Pract.*, 17(11):737–745.

425. Peiffer, R. L., Jr., Seymour, W. G., and Williams, L. W. (1977): Malignant melanoma of the iris and ciliary body in a cat. *Mod. Vet. Pract.*, 58(10):854–856.

426. Peiffer, R. L., Jr., Duncan, J., and Terrell, T. (1978): Hemangioma of the nictitating membrane in a dog. *J. Am. Vet. Med. Assoc.*, 172(7):832–833.

427. Perrot, H., Ortonne, J. P., and Schmitt, D. (1977): Vitiliginous achromia with malignant melanoma. Tyrosinase activity and ultrastructural study of achromic and normal skin. *Arch. Dermatol. Res.*, 257(3):247–253.

428. Phillips, M. L., Warner, N. E., and Puffer, H. W. (1976): Oral papillomas in *Genyonemus lineatus* (white croakers). *Prog. Exp. Tumor Res.*, 20:208–212.

429. Pierce, K. V., McCain, B. B., and Wellings, S. R. (1978): Pathology of hepatomas and other liver abnormalities in English sole (*Parophrys vetulus*) from the Duwamish river estuary, Seattle, Washington. *J. Natl. Cancer Inst.*, 60(6):1445–1453.

430. Pindborg, J. J., and Kramer, I. R. H. (1971): *Histological Typing of*

Odontogenic Tumours, Jaw Cysts, and Allied Lesions. WHO, Geneva.

431. Pollet, L., Van Hove, W., and Mattheeuws, D. (1978): Blastic crisis in chronic myelogenous leukaemia in a dog. *J. Small Anim. Prac.,* 19(8):469–475.

432. Popoff, N. A., Malin, T. J., and Rosomoff, H. L. (1974): Fine structure of intracranial haemangiopericytoma and angiomatous meningioma. *Cancer,* 34:1187.

433. Port, C. D., and Sidor, M. A. (1978): A sebaceous gland carcinoma in a rabbit. *Lab. Anim. Sci.,* 28(2):215–216.

434. Pour, P., Althoff, J., Kmoch, N., Mohr, U., Cardesa, A., and Greiser, E. (1976): Spontaneous tumors and common diseases in two colonies of Syrian hamsters. Part I. Incidence and sites. *J. Natl. Cancer Inst.,* 56:931–935.

435. Pour, P., Mohr, U., Cardesa, A., Althoff, J., and Kmoch, N. (1976): Spontaneous tumors and common diseases in two colonies of Syrian hamsters. II. Respiratory tract and digestive system. *J. Natl. Cancer Inst.,* 56(5):937–948.

436. Pour, P., Mohr, U., Althoff, J., Cardesa, A., and Kmoch, N. (1976): Spontaneous tumors and common diseases in two colonies of Syrian hamsters. III. Urogenital system and endocrine glands. *J. Natl. Cancer Inst.,* 56(5):949–961.

437. Pour, P., Mohr, U., Althoff, J., Cardesa, A., and Kmoch, N. (1976): Spontaneous tumors and common diseases in two colonies of Syrian hamsters. IV. Vascular and lymphatic systems and lesions of other sites. *J. Natl. Cancer Inst.,* 56(5):963–974.

438. Powers, R. D., and Winkler, J. K. (1977): Pituitary carcinoma with extracranial metastasis in a cow. *Vet. Pathol.,* 14(5):524–526.

439. Priesel, A. (1928): Über ein ungewöhnliches Gewächs der Bauchspeicheldrüse. *Virchows Arch. Pathol. Anat.,* 267:354.

440. Priester, W. A. (1977): Multiple primary tumors in domestic animals; a preliminary view with particular emphasis on tumors in dogs. *Cancer,* 40(Suppl. 4):1845–1848.

441. Priester, W. A., Goodman, D. G., and Theilen, G. H. (1977): Nine simultaneous primary tumors in a boxer dog. *J. Am. Vet. Med. Assoc.,* 170(8):823–826.

442. Prieur, D. J., Fenstermacher, J. D., and Guarino, A. M. (1976): A choroid plexus papilloma in an elasmobranch (*Squalus acanthias*). *J. Natl. Cancer Inst.,* 56(6):1207–1209.

443. Pülhorn, G., and Winter, R. (1976): Malignant chorioidal melanoma of the "Knapp Rønne" type. *Klin. Monatsbl. Augenheilkd.,* 169(3):352–358.

444. Qizilbash, A. H. (1976): Cystosarcoma phyllodes with liposarcomatous stroma. *Am. J. Clin. Pathol.,* 65(3):321–327.

445. Rabin, H., Neubauer, R. H., Gonda, M. A., Nelson-Rees, W. A., Charman, H. P., and Valerio, M. G. (1978): Spontaneous esophageal carcinoma and epithelial cell line of an adult rhesus monkey. *Cancer Res.,* 38:3310–3314.

446. Radetic, M., Padovan, I., Jakesa, V., and Maricic, Z. (1978): Cytohistological correlations in thyroid gland tumors. Program, XIIth International Congress, p. 250, Buenos Aires.

447. Radnot, M. (1977): Metastatic epibulbar carcinoma. *Ophthalmologica,* 174(5):251–254.

448. Rasheed, S., Rongey, R. W., Bruszewski, J., Nelson-Rees, W. A., Rabin, H., Neubauer, R. H., Esra, G., and Gardner, M. B. (1977): Establishment of a cell line with associated Epstein-Barr-like virus from a leukemic orangutan. *Science,* 198(4315):407–409.

449. Raynaud, A., and Adrian, M. (1976): Cutaneous lesions with papillomatous structure associated with viruses in the green lizard (*Lacerta viridis* Laur.), *C. R. Acad. Sci. D* (Paris), 283(7):845–847.

450. Reddy, J. K., Svoboda, D. J., and Rao, M. S. (1976): Induction of liver tumors by aflatoxin B1 in the tree shrew (*Tupaia glis*) a nonhuman primate. *Cancer Res.,* 36(1):151–160.

451. Reed, C., and Garman, R. H. (1977): Osteosarcoma in a squirrel monkey. *J. Am. Vet. Med. Assoc.,* 171(9):976–979.

452. Reed, D. E., Shave, H., Bergeland, M. E., and Gates, C. E. (1976): Necropsy and laboratory findings in free-living deer in South Dakota. *J. Am. Vet. Med. Assoc.,* 169(9):975–979.

453. Reese, A. B. (1976): *Tumors of the Eye,* Ed. 3. Harper & Row, New York.

454. Regezi, J. A., and Batsakis, J. G. (1977): Histogenesis of salivary gland neoplasms. *Otolaryngol. Clin. North Am.,* 10(2):297–307.

455. Rhodes, R. H., Davis, R. O., Kassel, S. H., and Clague, B. H. (1978): Primary cerebral neuroblastoma; a light and electron microscopic study. *Acta Neuropathol.* (Berl.), 41(2):119–124.

456. Richards, R. (1977): Diseases of aquarium fish—2: Skin diseases. *Vet. Rec.,* 101(7):532–534.

457. Ridgway, R. L. (1977): Spontaneous myxoma in a pet hamster. *Vet. Med. Small Anim. Clin.,* 72(1):75.

458. Riede, U. N., Thomas, C., and Sandritter, W. (1977): Ultrastructural study on formal pathogenesis of experimentally induced rhabdomyosarcomas. *Exp. Pathol.* (Jena), 13(2–3):162–174.

459. Riley, M. G., and Forsyth, W. M. (1976): Bilateral adrenal glangioneuroblastoma in a premature calf. *Aust. Vet. J.,* 52(5):234–245.

460. Riotton, G., and Christopherson, W. M. (1973): *Cytology of the Female Genital Tract,* No. 8. WHO, Geneva.

461. Robinson, M., and Haywood, S. (1978): Equine sarcoids letter. *Vet. Rec.,* 102(11):248.

462. Ronchese, F. (1933): Multiple benign epithelioma of the scalp (turban tumours). *Am. J. Cancer,* 18:875.

463. Rose, F. L. (1976): Tumorous growths of the tiger salamander. *Ambystoma tigrinum,* associated with treated sewage effluent. *Prog. Exp. Tumor Res.,* 20:251–262.

464. Rose, F. L., and Harshbarger, J. C. (1977): Neoplastic and possibly related skin lesions in neotonic tiger salamanders from a sewage lagoon. *Science,* 197(4287):315–317.

465. Rosenfield, A. (1976): Recent environmental studies of neoplasms in marine shellfish. *Prog. Exp. Tumor Res.,* 20:263–274.

466. Rowlatt, C., Chesterman, F. C., and Sheriff, M. U. (1976): Lifespan, age changes and tumour incidence in an ageing C57BL mouse colony. *Lab. Anim.,* 10(10):419–442.

467. Roy, K. S., Saigal, R. P., Nanada, B. S., and Nagpal, S. K. (1976): Gross, histomorphological and histochemical changes in the thyroid gland of goat with age. III. Occurrence of thymic tissue. *Anat. Anz.,* 139(1–2):158–164.

468. Rubinstein, L. J., and Northfield, D. W. C. (1964): The medulloblastoma and the so-called 'archnoidal cerebellar sarcoma'. A critical re-examination of a nosological problem. *Brain,* 87:379.

469. Rudolph, R., and Thiel, W. (1976): Pathological anatomy and histology of spontaneous epithelial skin tumors in *Mastomys natalensis. Zentralbl. Vet. Med.* (A), 23(5):429–441.

470. Rühland, D., Fasske, E., Fetting, R., and Themann, H. (1976): Transplantable sebaceous adenoma of the mouse with virus particles studied by electron microscopy. *Z. Krebsforsch.,* 85(1):51–62.

471. Russel, W. O., Enzinger, F., Hajdu, S. I., Heise, H., Martin, R., Morse, I. S., Schmitz, R. L., and Suit, H. D. (1978): American Joint Committee (AJC) T N M G system for staging soft tissue sarcoma; application and use. Program, XIIth International Cancer Congress, Buenos Aires, p. 222.

472. Russell, D. S. (1950): Meningeal tumours (a review). *J. Clin. Pathol.,* 3:191.

473. Russell, D. S., and Rubinstein, L. J. (1977): *Pathology of Tumours of the Nervous System.* Ed. 4, p. 65. Williams & Wilkins, Baltimore.

474. Russo, J., Bradley, R. H., McGrath, C., and Russo, I. H. (1977): Scanning and transmission electron microscopy sutdy of a human breast carcinoma cell line (MCF-7) cultured in collagen-coated cellulose sponge. *Cancer Res.,* 37(7, Part 1):2004–2014.

475. Ryan, S. J., and Font, R. L. (1973): Primary epithelial neoplasms of the lacrimal sac. *Am. J. Ophthalmol.,* 76:73–88.

476. Sacksteder, M. R. (1976): Occurrence of spontaneous tumors in the germfree F344 rat. *J. Natl. Cancer Inst.,* 57(6):1371–1373.

477. Saito, S., Kurokawa, Y., and Sato, H. (1977): Effects of various diets on growth, longevity and incidence of spontaneous tumors of *Praomys* (*Mastomys*) *natalensis. Sci. Rep. Res. Inst. Tohoku Univ. Med.,* 24(1):33–42.

478. Samuel, W. M., Chalmers, G. A., and Gunson, J. R. (1978): Oral papillomatosis in coyotes (*Canis latrans*) and wolves (*Canis lupus*) of Alberta. *J. Wildl. Dis.,* 14(2):165–169.

479. Sancho, H., and Cesarini, J. P. (1978): Accuracy of the histological staging of primary malignant melanoma (PMM). Program, XIIth International Cancer Congress, p. 235.

480. Sass, B. (1978): NCI registry of experimental cancers and WHO collaborating centre for reference on tumours of laboratory animals. Program, XIIth International Cancer Congress, Buenos Aires, p. 182.

481. Scarff, R. W., and Torloni, H. (1968): *Histological Typing of Breast Tumours,* No. 2. WHO, Geneva.

482. Schaff et al.

483. Schajowicz, F. (1978): Classification of bone tumors. Program, XIIth International Cancer Congress, Buenos Aires, p. 92.

484. Schajowicz, F., Ackerman, L. V., and Sissons, H. E. (1972): *Histological Typing of Bone Tumours,* No. 6. WHO, Geneva.

485. Schieferstein, G. (1976): Immunology of malignant melanomas. *Fortschr. Med.,* 94(14):833–837.

486. Schjeide, Q. A., Schactschabel, D., and Molsen, D. V. (1976): On formation of melanosomes in a cultured melanoma line. *Cytobios,* 17(66):87–102.

487. Schlotke, B. (1976): Histochemical studies on the role of myoepithelial cells in the morphogenesis of mammary tumors in the bitch. 1. Staining, enzyme histochemical and immunohistochemical demonstration of myoepithelial cells in the normal mammary gland. *Zentralbl. Vet. Med.* (A), 23(8):661–669.

488. Schmidt, G. R., Cowles, R. R., and Flynn, D. V. (1976): Granulosa cell tumor in a broodmare. *J. Am. Vet. Med. Assoc.,* 169(6):635.

489. Schmidt, R. A. (1977): Plasma cell tumor in an East Indian water lizard (*Hydrosaurus amboinensis*). *J. Wildl. Dis.,* 13(1):47–48.

490. Schroder, J. (1976): Osteosarcoma of the axial skeleton in a dog. *J. S. Afr. Vet. Assoc.,* 47(4):293–294.

491. Schürch, W.: Personal communication.

492. Schürch, W., Babai, F., Boivin, Y., and Verdy, M. (1977): Light-electron microscopic and cytochemical studies on the morphogenesis of familial medullary thyroid carcinoma. *Virchows Arch. [Pathol. Anat.],* 376(1):

29–46.

493. Schwab, M., Ahuja, M. R., and Anders, F. (1976): Elevated levels of lactate dehydrogenase in genetically controlled melanoma of xiphophorin fish. *Comp. Biochem. Physiol.* (B), 54(1):197–199.

494. Schwanz-Pfitzner, I. (1976): Further studies of eel virus (Berlin) isolated from the blood of eels (*Anguilla anguilla*) with skin papilloma. *Prog. Exp. Tumor Res.,* 20:101–107.

495. Schweitzer, J., and Marks, F. (1977): Induction of the formation of new hair follicles in mouse tail epidermis by the tumor promoter. *Cancer Res.,* 37(11):4195–4201.

496. Scolnick, E. M., Williams, D., and Parks, W. P. (1976): Purification and characterisation of viral RNA of a sarcoma virus isolated from a woolly monkey. *Nature,* 264(5588):809–811.

497. Sedlacek, H. H., and Seiler, F. R. (1977): Spontaneous mammary tumors in mongrel dogs. A relevant model to demonstrate tumor therapeutical success by application of neuraminidase-treated tumor cells. *Dev. Biol. Stand.,* 38:399–412.

498. Sen, A. K. (1976): Lipomas in the cat (letter). *Vet. Rec.,* 98(17):346.

499. Sen, A. K. (1977): A large schwannoma in a German Shepherd dog. *Vet. Med. SAC,* 72(3):389–391.

500. Serov, F. S. (1978): Pathology: Common "epithelial" tumours. Program, XIIth International Cancer Congress, Buenos Aires, p. 103.

501. Setlow, R. B., Woodhead, A. D., and Hart, R. W. (1978): Identical genetic material as a source for studies of cell injury. Animal model; damage to DNA in the Amazon molly by physical and chemical agents. *Am. J. Pathol.,* 91(1):213–216.

502. Seto, A., Tokuda, H., and Ito, Y. (1978): Malignant conversion of shopee papillomas and associated changes of serum ceruloplasmin in domestic rabbits. *Proc. Soc. Exp. Biol. Med.,* 157(4):694–696.

503. Seton, A., Notake, K., Kawanishi, M., and Ito, Y. (1977): Development and regression of Shope papillomas induced in newborn domestic rabbits. *Proc. Soc. Exp. Biol. Med.,* 156(1):64–67.

504. Shapiro, S., Kaneko, Y., Baum, S. G., and Fleischer, N. (1977): The role of calcium in insulin release from hamster insulinoma cells. *Endocrinology,* 101(2):485–493.

505. Shewell, J., and Davies, R. W. (1977): Combined therapy of the spontaneous mouse mammary tumour; methotrexate and hyperbaric oxygen irradiation. *Eur. J. Cancer,* 13(9):977–984.

506. Shin, W. Y., and Abramson, A. L. (1976): The value of electron microscopy in the diagnosis of fibrosarcoma of the larynx. *Trans. Am. Acad. Ophthalmol. Otolaryngol.,* 82(5):582–587.

507. Shostak, S. (1977): Vegetative reproduction by budding in Hydra; a perspective on tumors. *Perspect. Biol. Med.,* 20(4):545–568.

508. Shubik, P. (1977): The implications of multiple tumor induction in rodent skin for the bilogic nature of neoplasia. *Cancer,* 40(Suppl. 4): 1821–1824.

509. Siciliano, M. J., and Wright, D. A. (1976): Biochemical genetics of the platyfish-swordtail hybrid melanoma system. *Prog. Exp. Tumor. Res.,* 20:398.

510. Siniakov, E. G. (1976): Role of rat age and the quantity of plutonium administered to them on the development of osteosarcoma. *Radiobiologia,* 16(4):631–634.

511. Sinibaldi, K., Rosen, H., Liu, S. K., and DeAngelis, M. (1976): Tumors associated with metallic implants in animals. *Clin. Orthop.,* 118:257–266.

512. Sinnhuber, R. O., Wales, J. H., Hendricks, J. D., Putnam, G. B., Nixon, J. E., and Pawlowski, N. E. (1977): Trout bioassay of mycotoxins. In *Mycotoxins,* pp. 731–744, edited by J. V. Rodricks. Park Forest South, Pathotox.

513. Slanina, L., Konrad, V., Vajda, V., Lojda, L. and Zibrin, M., Tomajkov, A. E., Sokol, J., Lehock, Y. J., Skarda, R., and Mad'ar, Jr. (1978): Congenital neurofibromatosis of the skin in calves. *DTW,* 85(2):41–45.

514. Smith, D. F., and Gunson, D. E. (1977): Branchial cyst in a heifer. *J. Am. Vet. Med. Assoc.,* 171(1):64–66.

515. Smith, H. S., Riggs, J. L., and Springer, E. L. (1977): Expression of antigenic crossreactivity to RD114 P 30 protein in a human fibrosarcoma cell line. *Proc. Natl. Acad. Sci. U.S.,* 74(2):744–748.

516. Smith, M. T., Farinacci, C. J., Carpenter, H. A., and Bannayan, G. A. (1976): Extraskeletal myxoid chondrosarcoma; a clinicopathological study. *Cancer,* 37(2):821–827.

517. Sobin, L. H. (1978): The WHO histological classification of lung tumours, Rev. Ed., Panel 6, XIIth International Cancer Congress, Buenos Aires, pp. 105–106.

518. Sommers, S. C., and Meissner, W. A. (1954): Unusual carcinomas of the pancreas. *Arch. Pathol.,* 58:101.

519. Sonstegard, R. A. (1977): Environmental carcinogenesis studies of fishes of the Great Lakes of North America. *Ann. N. Y. Acad. Sci.,* 298:261–269.

520. Sonstegard, R. A., Leatherland, J. F., and Dawe, C. J. (1976): Effects of gonadal tumours on the pituitary-gonadal axis in cyprinids from the Great Lakes. *Gen. Comp. Endocrinol.,* 29:269.

521. Spence, A. M., Rubinstein, L. J., Conley, F. K., and Herman, M. M. (1976): Studies on experimental malignant nerve sheath tumors maintained in tissue and organ culture systems. III. Melanin pigment and melanogenesis in experimental neurogenic tumors: a reappraisal of the histogenesis of pigmented nerve sheath tumors. *Acta Neuropathol.* (Berl.), 35(1):27–45.

522. Spitz, E. B., Shenkin, H. A., and Grant, F. C. (1947): Cerebellar medulloblastoma in adults. *Arch. Neurol. Psychiatry,* 57:417.

523. Stackhouse, L. L., Moore, J. J., and Hylton, W. E. (1978): Salivary gland adenocarcinoma in a mare. *J. Am. Vet. Med. Assoc.,* 172(3):271–273.

524. Starink, T. H., Hausman, R., Van Delden, L., and Neering, H. (1977): Atypical fibroxanthoma of the skin. Presentation of 5 cases and a review of the literature. *Br. J. Dermatol.,* 97(2):167–177.

525. Stedham, M. A., Casey, H. W., and Keyes, M. C. (1977): Lymphosarcoma in an infant northern fur seal (*Callorhinus ursinus*). *J. Wildl. Dis.,* 13(2): 176–179.

526. Steele, W. B., McNeil, P., Munro, C. D., Renton, J. P., and Douglass, T. A. Testicular tumours in dogs (letter). (1977): *Vet Rec.,* 101(7):142.

527. Stenkvist, B., Westman-Naeser, S., Holmquist, J., Nordin, B., Bengtsson, E., Vegelius, J., Eriksson, O., and Fox, C. H. (1978): Computerized nuclear morphometry as an objective method for characterizing human cancer cell populations. *Cancer Res.,* 38:4688–4697.

528. Stich, H. F., and Acton, A. B. (1976): The possible use of fish tumors in monitoring for carcinogens in the marine environment. *Prog. Exp. Tumor Res.,* 20:44–54.

529. Stich, H. F., Acton, A. B., Dunn, B. P., Oishi, K., Yamazaki, F., Harada, T., Peters, G., and Peters, N. (1977): Geographic variations in tumor prevalence among marine fish populations. *Int. J. Cancer,* 20(5):780–791.

530. Stock, C. C., Martin, D. S., Sugiura, K., Fugmann, R. A., Mountain, I. M., Stockert, E., Schmid, F. A., and Tarnowski, G. S. (1978): Antitumor tests of amygdalin in spontaneous animal tumor systems. *J. Surg. Oncol.,* 10(2):89–123.

531. Strafuss, A. C. (1976): Basal cell tumors in dogs. *J. Am. Vet. Med. Assoc.,* 169(3):322–324.

532. Strafuss, A. C. (1976): Sebaceous gland carcinoma in dogs. *J. Am. Vet. Med. Assoc.,* 169(3):325–326.

533. Strafuss, A. C. (1976): Sebaceous gland adenomas in dogs. *J. Am. Vet. Med. Assoc.,* 169(6):640–642.

534. Strombeck, D. R., Krum, S., Meyer, D., and Kappesser, R. M. (1976): Hypoglycemia and hypoinsulinemia associated with hepatoma in a dog. *J. Am. Vet. Med. Assoc.,* 169(8):811–812.

535. Sundberg, J. P., Burnstein, T., Page, E. H., Kirkham, W. W., and Robinson, F. R. (1977): Neoplasms of equidae. *J. Am. Vet. Med. Assoc.,* 170(2):150–152.

536. Sukuki, S., Miwa, Sakita, R., Nomiyama, T., Harasawa, S., Tani, N., and Miwa, T. (1978): Endoscopy stereoscopic microscopy and scanning electron microscopy of colorectal polyps as an aid for endoscopic diagnosis. Program, XIIth International Cancer Congress, Buenos Aires, p. 198.

537. Sutherland, T. W. (1956): Non-papillary hyalinising hidradenoma, sometimes forming turban tumours. *J. Path. Bacteriol.,* 72:663.

538. Symmers, W. St C. (ed.) (1978): *Systemic Pathology.* Vol. 2, Ed. 2, Churchill Livingstone, Edinburgh.

539. Szekeres, L., and Orfanos, C. E. (1978): Alterations of the clinically noninvolved skin in patients with malignant melanoma. An electron microscopic study before and after repeated application of BCG. *Dermatologica,* 156(3):142–154.

540. Takashima, F. (1976): Hepatoma and cutaneous fibrosarcoma in hatchery-reared trout and salmon related to gonadal maturation. *Prog. Exp. Tumor Res.,* 20:351–366.

541. Takizawa, S., and Miyamoto, M. (1976): Observations on spontaneous tumors in Wistar Furth strain rats. *Hiroshima. J. Med. Sci.,* 25(2–3):89–98.

542. Takizawa, S., and Miyamoto, M. (1977): Observations on spontaneous tumors in Wistar Furth strain rats. *Hiroshima J. Med. Sci.,* 25(2–3):89–98.

543. Tarvin, G., Patnaik, A., and Greene, R. (1978): Primary urethral tumors in dogs. *J. Am. Vet. Med. Assoc.,* 172(8):1931–1933.

544. Taylor, G. N., Shabestari, L., Williams, J., Mays, C. W., Angus, W., and McFarland, S. (1976): *Cancer Res.,* 36(8):2740–2743.

545. Taylor, R. F., Park, R. D., and Kollias, G. (1976): Osteochondroma in a lioness. *J. Am. Vet. Med. Assoc.,* 169(9):966–967.

546. Ten Seldam, R. E. J., and Helwig, E. B. (eds.) (1974): *Histological Typing of Skin Tumours.* WHO, Geneva.

547. Teunissen, G. H. (1977): Intrathoracic lipoma in a dog. *Tijdschr. Diergeneeskd.,* 102(2):113–116.

548. Thirloway, L., Rudolph, R., and Leipold, H. W. (1977): Malignant melanomas in a duroc boar. *J. Am. Vet. Med. Assoc.,* 130(3):345–347.

549. Tilov, T., Köllmer, H., Weisse, I., and Stötzer, H. (1976): Occurrence of spontaneous tumours in the rat strain Chbb: THOM (SPF). *Arzneim. Forsch.,* 26(1):45–50.

550. Tiniakov, G. G., and Prusak-Glotov, V. E. (1976): Cytogenetic characteristics of the growth of Brown-Pearce carcinoma in rabbits. *Tsitol. Genet.,* 10(2):144–147.

551. Tokita, H., Konishi, S., Ogata, M., Takahashi, R., and Goto, N. (1977): Studies on canine oral papillomatosis. III. Cultivation of papilloma cells

in vitro. Nippon Juigaku Zasshi, 39(6):619–626.

552. Tokuzen, R., Okabe, M., and Nakahara, L. W. (1976): Combined effect of cyclocytidine and lentinan of spontaneous mammary tumors in mice. *Gann, 67(2):327–329.*

553. Torbaghan, S. S. (1978): Histological classification of bone tumours. Program, XIIth International Cancer Congress, Buenos Aires, p. 223.

554. Toremalm, N. G., Lindström, C., and Malm, L. Chondromyxoid fibroma of the petrygo-palatine space. *J. Laryngol. Otol., 90(10):971–978.*

555. Traenkle, H. L. (1940): Epithelioma adenoides cysticum, trichoepithelioma and basal-cell cancer. Relation between these diseases, as shown by histological studies of multiple benign cystepithelioma. *Arch. Dermatol. Syph., 42:822.*

556. Tralka, T. S., Costa, J., Sindelar, W. F., Rabson, A., Gullino, P. M., Henson, E., Chu, E. W., and O'Conor, G. T. (1977): Spontaneous lymphosarcoma arising in a nude mouse; characterization *in vivo* and *in vitro. J. Natl. Cancer Inst., 58(4):977–982.*

557. Traver, D. S., Moore, J. N., Thornburg, L. P., Johnson, J. H., Coffman, Jr. (1977): Epidural melanoma causing posterior paresis in a horse. *J. Am. Vet. Med. Assoc., 170(12):1400–1403.*

558. Triche, T. J., and Ross, W. E. (1978): Glycogen-containing neuroblastoma with clinical and histopathologic features of Ewing's sarcoma. *Cancer, 41(4):1425–1432.*

559. Trump, B. F., Hinton, D. E., Dees, J. H., Heatfield, B. M., and Barrett, L. A. (1975): Renal adenocarcinomas induced by N-4-4'-fluorobiphenyl acetamide and their comparison with human renal adenocarcinomas. *Lab. Invest., 32:438.*

560. Trump, B. F., McDowell, E. M., Barrett, L. A., Frank, A. L., and Harris, C. C. (1975): Ultrastructural, cytochemical, and metabolic studies on the pathogenesis of human bronchogenic carcinoma. *Lab. Invest., 32: 50–51.*

561. Trump, B. F., and Laiho, K. U. (1975): Studies of cellular recovery from injury. I. Recovery from anoxia in Ehrlich ascites tumor cells. *Lab. Invest., 33:706–711.*

562. Trump, B. F., McDowell, E. M., Barrett, L. A., Jones, R. T., Valerio, M. G. (1976): Ultrastructural and cytochemical studies on the mechanism of chemical carcinogenesis in the human . *Microsc. Soc. Canada, 3: 142–145.*

563. Trump, B. F., McDowell, E. M., Glavin, F., Barrett, L. A., Becci, P. J., Schürch, W., and Kaiser, H. E. (1978): Respiratory epithelium. III. Histogenesis of epidermal metaplasia and carcinoma *in situ* in the human. *J. Natl Cancer Inst. 61(2):563–575.*

564. Tweddle, N. E., and White, W. E. (1977): An outbreak of anal fibropapillomatosis in cows following rectal examinations. *Aust. Vet. J., 53(10): 492–495.*

565. Uchida, Y., Schlake, W., Roessner, A., Ruhland, D., Themann, H., and Grundmann, E. (1976): Development of tumors in the glandular stomach of rats after oral administration of carcinogens. I. Histological findings. *Z. Krebsforsch., 87(2):199–212.*

566. Uchida, Y., Roessner, A., Schlake, W., Ruhland, D., Themann, H., and Grundmann, E. (1976): Development of tumors in the glandular stomach of rats after oral administration of carcinogens. II. Different cell types in antral carcinoma as revealed by electron microscopy. *Z. Krebsforsch., 87(2):213–228.*

567. Ungar, H., and Adler, J. H. (1978): The histogenesis of hepatoma occurring spontaneously in a strain of sand rats (*Psammomys obesus*). *Am. J. Pathol., 90(2):399–410.*

568. Uyeno, K., Ohmi, T., Wakashin, K., Azuma, C., and Kato, R. (1976): A clinicohistological study of keratoacanthoma in Japan with special reference to radiotherapy. In *Biology and Disease of the Hair,* pp. 337–357, edited by Toda, K. et al. University Park Press, Baltimore.

569. Van Veelen, C. W. M., Verbiest, H., Vlug, A. M. C., Rijksen, G., and Staal, G. E. J. (1978): Isozymes of pyruvate kinase from human brain, meningiomas, and malignant gliomas. *Cancer Res., 38:4681–4687.*

570. Viarengo, A., Zoncheddu, A., Cordone, A., Mancinelli, G., and Orunesu, M. (1978): DNA-dependent RNA polymerase activities in hepatopancreas nuclei from *Mytilus galloprovincialis* Lamarck. *Istanbul. Univ. Dishekim. Fak. Derg. 27(1):43–54.*

571. Vielkind, U. (1976): Genetic control of cell differentiation in platyfish-swordtail melanomas. *J. Exp. Zool., 196(2):197–204.*

572. Vielkind, U., and Eberhard, P. (1978): Normal and malignant melanin-containing pigment cells of xiphophorine fish as studied with formaldehyde-induced fluorescence. *J. Invest. Dermatol., 70(2):80–83.*

573. Vielkind, J., Haas-Andela, H., and Anders, F. T. (1976): DNA-mediated transformation in the platyfish-swordtail melanoma system. *Experientia, 32(8):1043–1045.*

574. Vielkind, U., Schlage, W., and Anders, F. (1977): Melanogenesis in genetically determined pigment cell tumors of platyfish and platyfish-swordtail hybrids; correlation between tyrosine activity and degree of malignancy. *Z. Krebsforsch., 90(3):233–239.*

575. Vielkind, U., Schlage, W., and Anders, F. (1977): Melanogenesis in genetically determined pigment cell tumors of platyfish and platyfish-swordtail hybrids; correlation between tyrosine activity and degree of malignancy. *Z. Krebsforsch., 80(3):285–299.*

576. Vijadinovic, B., Zguricas, M. J., Djordjevic, M., Dimitrijevic, A., and

577. Djordjevic, D. (1978): Clinico-morphological characteristics of islet cells tumors of the pancreas. Program, XIIth International Cancer Congress, Buenos Aires, p. 201.

577. Vitovec, J. (1976): Epithelial thyroid tumors in cows. *Vet. Pathol., 13(6): 401–408.*

578. Volman, H. (1978): A morphologic and morphometric study of the mitochondria in several hepatoma cell lines and in isolated hepatocytes. *Virchows Arch. (Cell Pathol.), 26(3):249–259.*

579. Von Albertini, A. (1974): *Histologische Geschwulstdiagnostik.* Georg Thieme, Stuttgart.

580. Von Bomhard, D., and Von Sandersleben, J. (1976): The ultrastructure of mixed mammary gland tumors in bitches. IV. The incidence of myoepithelial cells in formation of spindle cells. *Virchows Arch. [Pathol. Anat.], 371(3):219–226.*

581. Von Bomhard, D., Pukkavesa, C., and Haenichen, T. (1978): The ultrastructure of testicular tumours in the dog. I. Germinal cells and seminomas. *J. Comp. Pathol., 88(1):49–57.*

582. Von Bomhard, D. V., Schaffer, E., and Sandersleben, J. V. (1977): On the histogenesis of osseous structures in epithelial tumours. A light and electron-microscopical study illustrated at the so-called mixed tumour of the mammary gland in bitches (author's transl.). *Strahlentherapie, 153(6):362–370.*

583. Von Mayersbach, H. (1973): Grundriss der Histologie des Menschen. In *Allgemeine Histologie,* Vol. 1. Gustav Fischer, Stuttgart.

584. Wales, J. H., Sinnhuber, R. O., Hendricks, J. D., Nixon, J. E., and Eisele, T. A. (1978): Aflatoxin B1 induction of hepatocellular carcinoma in the embryos of rainbow trout (*Salmo gairdneri*). *J. Natl. Cancer Inst., 60(5): 1133–1139.*

585. Walter, P., and Guerbaoui, M. (1976): Foetal rhabdomyoma. Case report and ultrastructural study. *Virchows Arch. (Pathol. Anat.), 271(1):59–67.*

586. Wandera, J. G. (1976): Further observations on canine spirocercosis in Kenya. *Vet. Rec., 99(18):348–351.*

587. Warner, M. R. (1976): Age incidence and site distribution of mammary dysplasias in young beagle bitches. *J. Natl. Cancer Inst., 57(1):57–61.*

588. Wegiel, J., Waniewski, E., and Dumanski, Z. (1978): Spontaneous pathomorphological changes in the thyroid and parathyroid glands of rats. *Endokrynol. Pol., 29(1):11–20.*

589. Wegiel, J., Waniewski, E., and Dumanski, Z. (1978): Spontaneous pathomorphological changes in rat adrenals. *Biochem. Pharmacol., 27(5): 673–677.*

590. Weller, R. E. (1978): Systemic mastocytosis and mastocytemia in a cat. *Mod. Vet. Pract., 59(1):41–43.*

591. Wellings, S. R., McCain, B. B., and Miller, B. S. (1976): Epidermal papillomas in pleuronectidae of Puget Sound, Washington. Review of the current status of the problem. *Prog. Exp. Tumor Res., 20:55–74.*

592. Welsch, C. W. (1976): Interaction of estrogen and prolactin in spontaneous mammary tumorigenesis of the mouse. *J. Toxicol. Environ. Health (Suppl.), 1:117–129.*

593. Welsch, U., and Storch, V. (1976): *Comparative Animal Cytology and Histology.* Sidgwick & Jackson, London.

594. Werdin, R., and Wold, K. (1976): Uterine carcinoma in a sow. *Vet. Pathol., 13(6):451–452.*

595. West, J. L., and Bell, M. C. (1977): A probable radiation-induced epidermal carcinoma in a sheep. *Health Phys., 32(1):32–35.*

596. White, R. A., and Cheyne, I. A. (1977): Bone metastases from a phaeochromocytoma in the dog. *J. Small Anim. Pract., 18(9):579–584.*

597. Wigglesworth, V. B. (1959): The histology of the nervous system of an insect *Rhodnius prolixus* (Hemiptera). II. The central ganglia. *Quart J. Micr. Sci., 100:299–314.*

598. Willis, R. A. (1961): *The Principles of Pathology.* Ed. 2. Butterworths, Washington, D. C.

599. Willis, R. A. (1973): *The Spread of Tumours in the Human Body.* Ed. 3. Butterworths, London.

600. Wilson, J. W., and Alsaker, R. D. (1977): Osteosarcoma in an 11-month-old dog. *J. Am. Vet. Med. Assoc., 170(5):513–515.*

601. Windsor, J. R., Jr., LaFlamme, R. E., and Hites, R. A. (1977): Neoplastic skin lesions in salamanders from a sewage lagoon containing perylene letter. *Science, 198(4323):1280–1281.*

602. Winkelman, W., and Becker, W. (1976): Chondroma (an electronmicroscopic study). *Z. Orthop., 114(3):364–377.*

603. Wolf, P. H. (1976): Studies on the geographical distribution, etiology, and transmission of integumentary epitheliomas in rock oysters from Australian estuaries. *Prog. Exp. Tumor Res., 20:295–303.*

604. Wolke, R. E., and Murchelano, R. A. (1976): A case report of an epidermal papilloma. *Mustelus canis. J. Wildl. Dis., 12(2):167–171.*

605. Wood, W. G., Giustini, F. G., Sohn, S., and Aranda, R. R. (1978): Verrucous carcinoma of the vagina. *South Med. J., 71(4):368–371.*

606. Woodhead, A. D., and Scully, P. M. (1977): A comparative study of the pretumorous thyroid gland of the gynogenetic teleost, *Poecilia formosa,* and that of other poeciliid fishes. *Cancer Res., 37(10):3751–3755.*

607. Woodhead, A. D., Setlow, R. B., and Hart, R. W. (1977): The development of thyroid neoplasia in old age in the Amazon molly, *Poecilia formosa. Exp. Gerontol., 12(5–6):193–200.*

608. Woods, A. E., and Papadimitriou, J. M. (1977): The effect of inflamma-

tory stimuli on the stroma of neoplasms; the involvement of mononuclear phagocytes. *J. Pathol., 123*(3):165–174.

609. Wyman, M., Rings, M. D., Tarr, M. J., and Alden, C. L. (1977): Immunotherapy in equine sarcoid; a report of two cases. *J. Am. Vet. Med. Assoc., 171*(1):87–92.

610. Yager, J. D., Jr., and Miller, J. A., Jr. (1978): DNA repair in primary cultures of rat hepatocytes. *Cancer Res., 38*:4385–4394.

611. Yamada, T. (1977): Control mechanisms in cell-type conversion in newt lens regeneration. *Monogr. Dev. Biol., 13*:1–126.

612. Yamaguchi, A. (1977): Histological and fine structural studies on the parathyroid glands in primary hyperparathyroidism. *Nippon Naibunpi Gakkai Zasshi, 53*(2):110–130.

613. Yanovich, S., Harris, K., Sallan, S. E., Schlossman, S. F., and Inbar, M. (1978): Dynamic parameters of membrane lipids in normal and leukemic human lymphocytes isolated from peripheral blood and bone marrow. *Cancer Res., 38*:4654–4661.

614. Zaki, F. A. (1977): Spontaneous central nervous system tumors in the dog. *Vet. Clin. North. Am., 7*(1):153–163.

615. Zarrin, K. (1977): Naturally occurring parafollicular cell carcinoma of the thyroid in dogs. A histological and ultrastructural study. *Vet. Pathol., 14*(6):556–566.

616. Zguricas, M. J., Vujadinovic, B., Bozovic, B., Duric, D., Micic, J., and Dordevic, M. (1978): The ultrastructure of insulinoma and correlation with clinical picture. Program, XIIth International Cancer Congress, Buenos Aires, p. 200.

617. Ziangirova, G. G., Shubin, A. S., and Raikhlin, N. T. (1977): Ultrastructure of leiomyoma of the ciliary body. *Arkh. Patol., 39*(5):37–42.

618. Zubaidy, A. J. (1976): Caprine neoplasms in Iraq; case reports and review of the literature. *Vet. Pathol., 13*(6):460–461.

VI

Systematic Review of Neoplasms

44

Phylogeny and Paleopathology of Animal and Human Noeplasms

Hans E. Kaiser

The phylogeny of neoplasms poses a challenging question. There are two approaches to this question: one is theoretical, and one is practical, based on the availability of adequate fossils showing neoplastic or related phenomena.

Only the theoretical approach is truly rewarding, as shown by tissue distribution (Figs. 43.1 and 43.2), because fossils with tumors or related disorders are so rare. This is especially the case with regard to the older period of the earth's history. The Paleozoic, Proterozoic, and Archeozoic periods are out of our range due to the limitation of distinguishable normal fossils, almost all unknown to us. The oldest relevant fossils appear in the Jurassic, in which, with the exception of man, all groups of organisms are already present. From these forms, it is impossible, however, to learn anything of real significance as, for example, with regard to the important questions of tissue evolution, with the exception of some minor animal and bone tissues and the plant tissues.

As a result, the only method open to us for reconstruction of these early conditions is the comparison of tissue distribution in recent organisms, together with their taxonomic position on the one hand, and additional application of the basic principles of oncology and geology, histogenesis, and actualism on the other. As described in Chapter 2, on malignant transformation, the principle of histogenesis holds that all neoplastic cells and tissues originate from normal cells and tissues of a particular organism. The principle of actualism maintains that experience of a condition today may be applied to explain a preexisting condition of a geological period (6).

When we evaluate the neoplasms of the geological past, the following facts should be taken into consideration (a) only a minute portion of all members of a fauna or flora becomes fossilized; (b) only a certain percentage of diseases is neoplastic in origin; (c) diseased animals fall as easy prey to their pursuers; (d) only vertebrate neoplasms and some plant galls from geologic time are known.

The invertebrates which comprise the majority of species have not contributed valuable information on neoplastic changes. This fact, however, does not simply mean that such changes are not discovered in perhaps some obscure place or that they have not been described somewhere. Neoplastic remains of invertebrates with precise diagnosis, if at all, have not been discovered.

Bone is the only tissue for which entire phylogeny of the tissue is known and presentation of fossils since the occurrence of this type of tissue.

Thus, the chief emphasis concerning animal neoplasms must be placed on the discovery of fossil or subfossil bones.

The x-ray method is a very important tool in the study of fossil bones. Fossil bones, similar to dried and naturally macerated skeletons from grave sites, lack cells; the remains are mostly inorganic. The x-ray method is preferred above cutting and grinding of the specimen which practically destroy it. Also, postmortem changes can be easily detected with the x-ray method (4).

Some theoretical considerations apply. Neoplasms of the bones, if we look at them as individual organs, are able to provide information on benign and malignant tumors, just as we

Table 44.1
Neoplasms in Fossil Vertebrates, with the Exception of Man

Type of neoplasm	Taxonomic group	Genus/species	Geologic period	Topographical area	Geographic location	Reference
Hemangioma	Dinosaurs (Saurischia, Sauropoda)	*Apatosaurus*	Jurassic	Vertebrae	U. S.	Moodie (5, 9)
Osteoma	Mosasaurs (Phytonomorpha)	Mosasaur	Cretaceous	?	U. S.	Moodie (5, 9)
Osteosarcoma	Carnivora	*Hyena spelaea*	Quaternary (Pleistocene)	Metatarsus	Germany	Kaiser (7)
Odontoma	Carnivora	*Ursus spelaeus*	Quaternary (Pleistocene)	Skull	Switzerland	Kaiser (8)
Bone-invading carcinoma	Rodentia	*Microtus* sp.	Quaternary (Pleistocene)	Left ulna	Germany	Heller and Kaiser (2)

Table 44.2
Selected Cases of Neoplasms in Prehistoric and Historic Man

Type of neoplasm	Type of human	Period	Topographic area	Geographic location	Reference
Hemangioma	Egyptian		Skull	Egypt	Brothwell (12)[a]
Hemangioma	Nubian		Vertebra	Nubia	Smith and Dawson (12)[a]
Hemangioma		VIII–X c.c.	Multiple	Altai district, USSR	Rokhlin (11)
Osteoma	Frenchman	Medieval	Skull	France	Beraud et al. (12)[a]
Osteoma	Peruvian		Skull	Peru	Moodie (9)
Button osteoma (1033 cases)	American Indian		Skull	America	Steinbock (summar.) (12)[a]
Multiple osteoma (tympanic ring)	Peruvian		Skull	Peru	Hrdlicka (12)[a]
Osteoma (1033 cases)	American Indian		Skull	America	Steinbock (summar.) (12)[a]
Osteoma (14 cases)				Eski-Kermen (5–13th century)	Rokhlin (11)
Osteoma	Californian		Skull	America	Roney, Jr. (12)[a]
Osteosarcoma	Egyptian		Pelvis	Catacombs of Kom el Shogofa	Kaiser (8)[a]
Osteosarcoma	American Indian		Multiple	America	Jarcho (3)
Enchondroma (various)		X–XII c.c. c.c.		Sarkel, USSR	Rokhlin (11)
Exchondroma (various)		Sarkel, X–XII c.c.		USSR	Rokhlin (11)
Osteochondroma		XV–V cc., B.C.		Krasnoyarsk district, USSR	Rokhlin (11)
Osteochondroma	Egyptian	V. Dynasty	Femur	Egypt	Smith and Dawson (12)[a] Rowling (12)[a]
Osteochondromatosis		X–XII c.c.	Joint (?)	Sarkel, USSR	Rokhlin (11)
Myelomatous lesions	Nomad	VIII–X c.c.	Skull, multiple	Altai district, USSR	Rokhlin (11)
Multiple myeloma (8 cases)	New world		Skull, femur	America	Steinbock (12)[a]
Osteosarcoma	European	Medeival	Ilium	Europe	Gejvall (12)[a]
Meningioma	Egyptian	3400 B.C.	Skull	Egypt	Rogers (12)[a]
Meningioma	Egyptian	1200 B.C.	Skull	Egypt	Steinbock (12)[a]
Meningioma	Romano-British		Skull		Brothwell (12)[a]
Meningioma	Peruvian	Pre-Hispanic	Skull	Paucarcancha	MacCurdy (12)[a], Moodie (12)[a], Zariquiey (12)[a]
Meningioma	Peruvian		Skull	Chavina	Moodie (12)[a], Abbott and Courville (12)[a]
Meningioma	Californian		Skull	? island,	Abbott and Courville (12)[a]

Table 44.2—*continued*

Type of neoplasm	Type of human	Period	Topographic area	Geographic location	Reference
Eosinophilic granu-loma	Mississippian cul-ture	1000–1600 A.D.	Vertebrae and il-ium	Illinois	Morse (12)[a]
Eosinophilic granu-loma		1200 A.D.	General	New York State	Williams et al. (12)[a]
Metastases		Bronze age	Vertebral bodies	N. Kazakhstan XV. B.C.	Rokhlin (11)
Metastases		VII c.c. B.C.		Krasnoyarsk dis-trict, USSR	Rokhlin (11)
Metastases		III c. B.C.		Tuvinsky, USSR	Rokhlin (11)
Metastases		I c. B.C.		Barrow, near Biysk, USSR	Rokhlin (11)
Metastases		X–XII c.c.		Sarkel, USSR	Rokhlin (11)
Metastat. CA	Egyptian	3000 B.C.	Skull	Egypt	Wells (12)[a]
Metastat. CA	British	425–850 A.D.	Skull and skeleton	Britain	Brothwell (12)[a]
Metastat. CA	Danish	1200–1500 A.D.	Skull	Denmark	Møller and Møller-Christensen (12)[a]
Metastat. CA	Swedish	1100–1400 A.D.	Skull	Sweden	Gejvall (12)[a]
Metastat. CA	New Mexican	500–900 A.D.	Ulna, radius (verte-brae)	Pecos Pueblo, N. M.	Steinbock (12)
Metastat. CA	New Mexican	1000–1300 A.D.	Humerus, ulna (thoracic v.)	Pecos Pueblo, N. M.	Steinbock (12)
Metastat. CA	Peruvian	Before 1500	Skull	Llactashica	Steinbock (12)
Metastat. CA	Peruvian	Before 1500	Skull, skeleton	Huacho	Steinbock (12)
Metastat. CA	American Indian	500–1500 A.D.	Skull, skeleton	Hooper Bay, Alaska	Steinbock (12)
Metastat. CA	American Indian	500–1500 A.D.	Skull	St. Lawrence Is-land	Steinbock (12)

[a] The original literature is cited in this particular publication.

are able to see carcinomas and sarcomas. The reason for this is that the single bone is composed of the periosteum, the bone itself, the marrow, the joints (at best, partially), blood vessels, and nerves, and back differentiation to mesenchyma is possible. Second, we have the tumor infiltrating into bone. Third, we have the metastasizing bone tumors. There are certain tumors which metastasize, especially frequently into skeletal tissues. This group includes, in topographic sequence, the tumors of the thyroid gland, lung, breast, kidney, prostate, testes, and ovary. As far as frequency is concerned, the order would be: hypernephroma of kidney, prostate cancers, and those of lung, ovary, breast, testes, and thyroid. A large number of metastatic bone tumors originate from bronchiogenic tumors. The transport takes place via the circulatory system; the most frequent locations of settlement are the spine, pelvis, femur, skull, ribs, and humerus.

The metastatic tumors which are often multiple are either osteolytic, destroying the bone (the majority of cases), or bone-forming (osteosclerotic), as is often the case in metastases of prostatic or well-differentiated mammary carcinoma. Mixed cases occur also.

Undifferentiated bronchiogenic carcinoma often cause no reaction in bone. Hypercalcemia

may accompany the metastatic neoplasms in bone as a side reaction.

Lesions simulating bone tumors are *myositis ossificans, osteoperiostitis, osteitis fibrosa,* and *bone cysts* (1, 10).

Another group of tumors besides the bone tumors detectable in paleopathological material is the odontogenic tumors, such as odontomas, ameloblastomas, craniopharyngiomas, and mesodermal odontogenic tumors.

Table 44.1 reviews the few really proven bone and ondotogenic neoplasms of animals which are known in the paleopathological literature.

Table 44.2 gives a general review of the subfossil neoplasms of man.

(Chapter 45 deals with plant galls from earlier periods, whereas Chapter 46 discusses in detail archeological specimens of human bone tumors, and in Chapter 47 the probable extinction of the black-footed ferret as a typical sample of the effect of diseases of an endangered species is investigated. These four chapters are therefore combined by their phylogenetic approach.)

References

1. Anderson, W. A. D., and Scotti, T. M. (1976): *Synopsis of Pathology,* Ed. 9. C. V. Mosby, St. Louis.
2. Heller, F., and Kaiser, H. E. (1955): Observations on the pathology of fossil rodents and other mammals. *Zentrabl. Pathol.,* 93:383–395.
3. Jarcho, S. (1966): *Human Paleopathology.* Yale University Press, New Haven.

4. Kaiser, H. E. (1954): Analysis of intravital fractures in paleopathology. *Mh. Vet. Med., 9*(2):60–61.

5. Kaiser, H. E. (1954): Pathological conditions of bones of saurishian and ornithishian dinosaurs. *Zenthalbl. Pathol., 91*:196–213.

6. Kaiser, H. E. (1962): Examples for the use and the limitations of actualism in geology. *Acta Biotheor.* (Leiden), XIV:3–4.

7. Kaiser, H. E. (1962). Comparative bone and joint pathology of fossil and recent animals. *Frankf. Z. Pathol., 72*:276–282.

8. Kaiser, H. E. (1970): *Abnormalities in Evolution.* Brill, Leiden.

9. Moodie, R. L. (1923): *Paleopathology, An Introduction to the Study of Ancient Disease.* University of Illinois Press, Urbana, Ill.

10. Pales, L. (1930): *Paleopathologie et Pathologie Comparative.* Masson et Cie, Paris.

11. Rokhlin, D. G. (1965): *Diseases of Ancient Men.* Nauka, Moscow.

12. Steinbock, R. T. (1976): *Paleopathological Diagnosis and Interpretation.* Charles C Thomas, Springfield, Ill.

45

Fossil Plant Galls

E. B. Wittlake

Plant galls have aroused the curiosity of man from the early Christian era. Since galls were used primarily for medicinal purposes in ancient times, little was known of their use in tanning and the production of ink. The Roman naturalist and philosopher Pliny knew that flies emerged from galls but did not associate the insect with the growth of the gall.

Malpighi observed, late in the 17th century, that the puncture of the tissues of the plant by an insect is subsequently followed by the gradual development of a gall (19).

Present-day galls are produced by the physiological activities of a plant, as well as by insects or other organisms which invade the plant tissues. Fungi, bacteria, viruses, mites, and nematodes are also gall-makers. It seems that in the modern flora, the plant family *Fagaceae*, according to Hutchins (16), holds the distinction of being afflicted by the greatest number of galls. Salicaceae (Willow family) is fourth in the number of galls produced, and the remaining groups in which galls are produced are herbs. The principal insect orders involved in gall formation are the Homoptera (aphids), Lepidoptera (moths), Diptera (flies, midges), and the Hymenoptera (sawflies).

Fossil galls occur on impressions of fossil vegetation in sand, sandstone, lignite, coal, clay, shale, and even in chert nodules. They occur in a great variety of geologic formations. Fossil galls compared to the numbers of modern galls are rather small in number. Hoffman (15) reported fossil insect gall impressions on an imperfectly preserved leaf specimen of *Quercus cognatus* Knowlton. Brown (7) changed the name of this species to Q. *payettensis* Knowlton, a species established by Knowlton previously. These impressions resemble present-day galls of the Cynipids, namely, *Dryophanta, Neuroteus,* or *Cecidomyia,* and are found in the late Micocene shales.

Another group of insects causing galls on fossil leaves is the Phylloxerids. They belong to insect order *Homoptera,* generally known as plant lice or aphids. In the subfamily *Phylloxeridinae,* aphids form galls on the leaves and roots of modern varieties of *Vitis* (grapes). Berry (5) studied the vegetation of the Lower Lance Formation in Harding County, South Dakota. Many fossil leaves showed galls resembling those produced by *Phylloxera.* The galls were 2 mm in diameter and were located away from the veins of the leaf. They occurred primarily on *Vitis dakotana.* Other leaves of the same formation were sent to Cockerell for evaluation. On some leaves, the latter observed small roundish perforations (2–4 mm in diameter) which greatly resembled the activity of the larvae of *Incurvaria,* a member of the *Lepidoptera.* The Lower Lance is an Upper Cretaceous formation.

Brown (8) published a monograph on the Paleocene Flora of the Rocky Mountains and the Great Plains in which he illustrates a leaf of *Rhamnus goldiana* on which there are gall-like impressions, possibly of *Phylloxera.* Although he makes no comment about this, they appear to be old galls produced by this genus.

Wittlake (20) reported, in an investigation of the flora of the Upper Wilcox formation in Arkansas, fossil galls in a fresh water deposit composed of very fine buff-colored-to-whitish sandstone. These galls were rather large but were similar to those produced by aphids. The galls in question lie well within the limits of shape and other characteristics exhibited by present-day phylloxerid galls that occur on genera of the *Juglandaceae,* specifically the genus *Carya.*

They are similar to modern galls produced by *Phylloxera rimosalis* Perg. described and illustrated by Felt (13).

The mature fossil galls average 9 mm long and 6 to 7 mm wide. The conical body of the gall is 2–3 mm in height. Young and older galls range in length from 2 to 12 mm. Three or four large galls show a raised margin with compressions of equally spaced spires or bristles (14 in number) attached at their bases to the flange-like rim of the gall. The orifice at the summit of the cone of the gall ranges in diameter from 0.75 to 2.5 mm. The galls cluster as in present-day galls.

Brooks (6) observed and described healed wounds and insect galls found on fossil leaves from the Wilcox Formation of Western Tennessee. Kinsey (17) studied the fossil *Cynipidae*, many of which were found in amber in various geologic formations.

None of the fossil fungi has been found that cause strictly true galls. However, they do form gall-like injuries. The fossil fungi are represented by many major groups plus those of uncertain position. Berry (3) published an article on the fossil fungi. The fungi are quite old geologically and hardly distinguishable from our modern *Phycomycetes*, having been seen in the tissues of our oldest land plants in the Devonian and Carboniferous periods.

Berry (2) cited *Caenomyces cassiae* on *Cassia emarginata* and *C. pestalizzites* on *Sabalites grayanus*. Knowlton (18) reported *C. eucalyptae* on the leaves of *Eucalyptus* and *C. spindicola* on the leaves of *Sapindus*. Berry (4) reported *C. jacksonensis*, a spot fungus on *Combretum petraflumense*. *Caenomyces* is a fungal genus classified in the Ascomycetes and found to date in the Eocene and Upper Cretaceous. However, Pia placed Caenomyces in the "Fungi incertae sedis" (19).

Ball (1) studying the Eocene Flora of Texas reported *Sphaerites gloeoporoides* on the leaves of *Malopaenna texensis* and found that it had many characteristics of our modern species. Nearly 100 species are cited in geologic record. A few have been challenged as not being gall-like perithecia but merely fossil spiny spores. *Sphaerites* is placed in the Ascomycetes.

Many fossil fungi have fructifications which simulate microgalls. Two examples in our modern species which have large gall-like structures are the aecial heads of the White Pine Blister Rust and Cedar Apple gall which is the telium on cedar trees. Another quite spectacular gall is Crown Gall, which is the work of a bacterium, *Agrobacterium tumefaciens*. Crown Gall pro-

duces huge growths on stems and roots of plants. Yet another huge gall caused by a virus, similar in form to Crown Gall, is produced on various species of trees (16).

Dilcher (11) illustrated and reported genera in the families Microthyriaceae and Meliolaceae that had never been reported from fossil deposits in the United States. He illustrated several fruiting bodies, possibly of the genus *Phragmothyrites*, which he does not identify. Edwards (12) reported the same genus from Eocene deposits from Mull, Scotland. The fruiting bodies or ascocarps could be interpreted as flat microgalls.

In conclusion, it appears in the fossil record that insects and fungi are the chief makers of galls and gall-like structures. Bacteria remain a question mark and all other organisms as well. The difficulty lies in the fact that the paleontologist's or the paleobotanist's only reference for comparison is in modern galls and injuries. One cannot isolate the causal organism in the case of bacteria and fungi. In the case in which the fossil has the cuticle intact, one can use transfer techniques, as described by Dilcher (11). When dealing with fossil insect galls, the form, size, and shape of modern galls is paramount in arriving at a decision associating a certain gall with an insect. It appears to some that scientists describing malformations on fossil plants are taking liberties with our scientific method of naming organisms. At least if we name an object in the fossil record, it has a name to which we may refer and we can wonder, discuss, and investigate until the proper identity can be achieved. This can be accomplished by studying fossil cuticles or fossils that are exceptionally well preserved. Scientific names can be changed in the fossil record and have been many times before when additional evidence is brought to light.

In fact the comments of Knowlton (18) are interesting from the standpoint of this problem. We quote: "The presence of spots on fossil leaves is exceedingly common. The identification of these fossil forms obviously rest on very insecure foundation especially when it is recalled that scale insects and a great variety of insect galls would represent epiphyllous fungi when preserved on impressions of fossil leaves. Nevertheless, large numbers of undoubted fungi are preserved in this manner and it is the legitimate duty of the paleobotanist to describe and illustrate them. In order to accomplish this work without unwarranted definiteness in generic classification, I propose the term *Caenomyces* as a form genus for leaf spot fungi for the Cenozoic age whose precise botanic affinities cannot be determined."

A statement was made earlier that gall formation is due to the physiological activities of plants as well as the substances which the insect injects. The insect injects the cortical parenchyma of the plant. Parenchymal tissue, when mature, has the ability to divide and convert into meristematic tissue. It responds to wounding by restoring the phellogen or cork cambium and the production of more parenchyma. The insect usually injects the plant when young, and at this time plant hormones are at an optimum concentration for normal growth of the cells. The question arises as to what is the response of auxins to the substances injected by the insect? We know a mRNA, carbohydrates, proteins, and other substances are introduced by the insect. Could it be that mRNA translates the formation of substances which act as hormones controlling the size and shape of the gall? Or could these substances interact with plant hormones, together with constant irritation by the substance emitted by the insect egg or constant mechanical irritation in the form of destruction of cell tissue by the larvae of the insect?

The growth of insect galls remains an avenue of investigation and notable scientific interest. Perhaps someday we will know why a particular type of gall involves a particular species of insect.

References

1. Ball, O. M. (1931): A contribution to the paleobotany of the Eocene of Texas. *Bull. Agric. Mech. Coll Tex.* (Fourth Ser.), 2(5):31, plate 46.
2. Berry, E. W. (1916a): The Lower Eocene Flora of southeastern North America. *U. S. Geol. Surv.*, Prof. Paper 91, Plate IX, Figs. 2 and 3.
3. Berry, E. W. (1916b): Remarkable fossil fungi. *Mycologia*, 8:73.
4. Berry, E. W. (1924): The Middle and Upper Eocene floras of southeastern America. *U. S. Geol. Surv.*, Prof. Paper 92, Plate VII, p. 52.
5. Berry, E. W. (1934): The Lower Lance Florale from Harding Co., South Dakota. *U. S. Geol. Surv.*, Prof. Paper 185-F, Plate 26, Fig. 4.
6. Brooks, H. K. (1955): Healed wounds and galls of the territory of Florissant, Colorado. *Bull. Museum Comp. Zool.*, 54:1–25.
7. Brown, R. W. (1937): Additions to some fossil floras of the western United States. *U. S. Geol. Surv.*, Prof. Paper 186-J, p. 166.
8. Brown, R. W. (1962): Paleocene flora of the Rocky Mountains and Great Plains. *U. S. Geol. Surv.*, Prof. Paper 375, Plate 48, Fig. 5.
9. Cockerell, T. D. A. (1908): Fossil insects from Florissant, Colorado. *Am. Mus. Nat. Hist.*, 24:59–69.
10. Comstock, J. H. (1949): *An Introduction to Entomology.* Comstock, New York.
11. Dilcher, D. L. (1963): Eocene epiphyllous fungi. *Science,* 142(3593):667–669.
12. Edwards, W. N. (1922): An Eocene microthyriacous Fungus from Mull, Scotland. *Trans. Br. Mycol. Soc.,* 8:66. Cambridge.
13. Felt, E. P. (1940: *Plant and Gall Makers.* Comstock, New York.
14. Hirmer, M. (1927): *Handbuch der Paläobotanik, mit Beiträgen von Julius Pia und Wilhelm Troll,* Vol. I, p. 119. Oldenbourg, München.
15. Hoffman, A. D. (1932): Miocene insect gall impressions. Bot. Gazette, 93: 341–344.
16. Hutchins, R. E. (1969): *Galls and Gall Insects.* Dodd, Mead and Co., New York.
17. Kinsey, A. C. (1919): Fossil Cynipidae. *Psyche,* 26:44–49.
18. Knowlton, F. W. (1922): Revision of the flora of the Green River Formation. *U. S. Geol. Surv.*, Prof. Paper 131-F, Plate 39, p. 148.
19. Lutz, F. E. (1948): *Field Book of Insects,* revised 12th impression.
20. Wittlake, E. B. (1969): Fossil phylloxerid plant galls from the Lower Eocene. *Proc. Arkansas Acad. Sci.,* 23:164–167, Figs. 1–4.

46

Bone Tumors in Archeological Human Skeletons (Paleopathology of Human Bone Tumors)

Donald J. Ortner

In reviewing the paleopathology of human tumors, one needs to keep in mind the fundamental difference between modern clinical experience and conditions associated with ancient populations. Most important are differences in average age at death. Populations on which much of modern clinical experience with tumors is based live at least twice as long as populations studied by paleopathologists. Since primary malignant tumors of bone usually occur or arise during the growth period, their frequency should be the same in ancient skeletons as in modern. However, secondary tumors of bone are associated with the older age categories and are thus less likely to be found in archeological skeletons since individuals in archeological times died of other causes before secondary tumors became a serious factor in morbidity and mortality.

Another factor is the well-known environmental effect on the types and incidence of cancer. Squamous cell, oat cell, and undifferentiated carcinomas of the lung, for example, are (but adenocarcinomas and alveolar cell carcinomas are not) associated with smoking and air pollution (6, 7). Metastases to the skeleton from this type of cancer may be minimal where such environmental problems do not exist. Wells (15) has noted the relatively high incidence of nasopharyngeal tumors of bone in paleopathological specimens. Today, this condition is rare in the western world but is rather common in Africa.

Of the several primary benign tumors of bone known in modern medical practice, few have been identified in archeological specimens. This may be due partly to the lack of knowledge by paleopathologists of the gross morphological features associated with these tumors but also may be due to the problems in identifying a tumor in a dry bone specimen. However, two types of primary benign tumor are fairly common in archeological specimens and have been described by several authors. The first of these is the small button osteoma which occurs primarily on the skull vault. Many examples of this tumor are found in the human skeletal collections of the National Museum of Natural History in Washington, D.C. Typically, the button osteoma is no larger than 1 cm in diameter. It is solitary and dense, with little relief but with a slight degree of undercutting at the boundary with normal bone. Large osteomas also occur. One such tumor is found on a skull from Peru (NMNH No. 242462) and measures 2.0 cm in diameter and almost 4 mm high at the center.

The second common type of tumor seen in archeological specimens is the small bony growth which may partially to completely fill the external auditory meatus. Hrdlička (9) was unable to reach any firm conclusion regarding cause of these ear exostoses. He did not feel that they were infectious or malignant diseases and suggested chemical or mechanical irritation as a possibility. Hrdlička observed sex variation, with males far more subject to the disease. His report of racial variation suggests a genetic component but environmental or cultural conditions cannot be ruled out. Hrdlička did find that the incidence increased with age. Other scholars, including Adis-Castro and Neumann (2) and Gregg and McGrew (8), have described cases of this tumor in archeological populations.

There are numerous examples of this condition in the National Museum of Natural History collections. Only two will be described here. The first of these is an adolescent skull from Chicama, Peru (NMNH No. 264345), illustrating what appears to be the incipient stage of this condition. All adult teeth have erupted; however, the basio-occipital synchondrosis is still not fused, indicating an age of around 18 years at the time of death. Sex is thought to be female. Both auditory canals exhibit narrowing; however, the right auditory meatus has a slight hypertrophic ridge and may represent the early stage of tumor development.

The second skull is from Illinois (U.S.A.) (NMNH 243180). The skull is that of a fully adult male, although the third molars are unerupted due to impaction. The mandible is missing; however, the maxilla has slight development of bony tumors in the buccal region of both sides. As in the previous specimen, the auditory canals are abnormally narrow. This condition is compounded by the presence of large bony tumors in both meatus with the most pronounced development on the left side. Both tumors arise from the posterior portion of the canal.

Beraud et al. (3) describe an osteoma of the ethnofrontal region in a skull from France. The specimen is from the medieval cemetery of St. Hermentaire and is dated to the 11th century. The authors estimate the age at death to be 22–25. The tumor encroaches on the endocranium.

An archeological example of multiple cartilaginous exostoses is located in the Winchester-Saxon, skeletal-pathology collections of the British Museum (Natural History) in London. This specimen (Catalog No. G932, CG 69, TR XL 1085) includes most of the major postcranial bones. The age estimate based on femur length is around 4 years; sex is unknown. Prominent bony projections can be seen on the distal metaphyses of the left humerus, and both femora. The left scapula and both iliac bones are affected as well. Other bones, including the ribs, vertebrae, and tarsals, are normal. Since this tumor is usually benign, it is unlikely to have been the cause of death, particularly in view of the young age at death.

Primary malignant tumors of bone are very rare in modern medical practice and are equally rare in archeological specimens. Ruffer and Willmore (13) report a tumor of the pelvis from Egypt dated about 250 A.D. The tumor appears to have started in the cancellous tissue of the pelvis and is slightly expansive in nature, producing a deformation of the obturator foramen and encroaching on the acetabulum. The authors rule out secondary carcinoma and infection and suggest osteosarcoma, adding that they cannot determine if the tumor was primary or secondary. The illustration of the lesion is of little value but does not show the active irregular growth of bone usually seen in osteoblastic osteosarcoma. The lesion appears to be chronic rather than acute, suggesting that a relatively slow-developing metastatic carcinoma or chronic infection would be more probable.

Dastugue (5) describes a tumor of the right maxilla and malar on a skull from a medieval site associated with the town of Caen in France. The tumor measures 60 mm wide and 40 mm high and encroaches both on the nasal passage and the right orbit. The surface of the tumor is very irregular with relatively large coalescing spicules. There are three inferior projections. Curiously, there is antemortem damage to the right malar adjacent to the tumor, and the author suggests the possibility of surgical intervention to explain this defect. The tumor appeared malignant to Dastugue, and he expresses the opinion that it caused the death of the individual. The morphology of the lesion is compatible with a primary malignant tumor of bone, but other possibilities, such as myositis ossificans following trauma to the face, seem more probable in my opinion, particularly in view of the injury to the malar for which trauma rather than surgical intervention is more probable.

A tumor of the mandible was found in an American Indian skeleton excavated in the state of West Virginia (10). The authors date the specimen to the mid-17th century. The lesion is rather large, measuring about 24 mm in diameter and 19 mm in depth. The mandible is probably from a female about 20 years of age. The authors suggest several possible neoplastic conditions, including osteoma and osteosarcoma, as the cause of the lesion. The position of the tumor near the symphysis and the young age of the individual are compatible with a diagnosis of primary malignant tumor. However, again the chin is prone to trauma and infection, so that myositis ossificans or infection appear more likely.

An umambiguous example of a primary malignant tumor of bone is found in the skeletal collections of the Natural History Museum in Bern, Switzerland. This specimen (Museum No. A95) is the left humerus from a Celtic warrior tomb dated to approximately 800–600 B.C. and found near the town of Muensingen in Canton Bern. Although damaged by postmortem erosion, the humerus is complete except for the distal epiphysis, which was lost post-mortem. The lesion extends completely around the proximal humerus but is least developed on the medial aspect. The bone associated with the lesion is approximately 7 cm in maximum diameter, and abnormal tissue extends slightly more than one-third the length of the humerus. The tumor overlies the insertion of the joint capsule but does not involve the joint surface itself. The gross morphology of the tumor consists of large coalescing bony projections which have a coarse coral-like appearance. While the age at death of the individual cannot be determined, the humeral head appears to be fused, indicating an age in excess of 15 years.

An x-ray film of this specimen was obtained through the courtesy of Dr. Walter Huber, director of the Natural History Museum in Bern. The film reveals a lytic process extending 2–3 c into the grossly normal cortex distal to the lesion. The location of the tumor, as well as its gross and x-ray film appearance, is compatible with the diagnosis of primary osteosarcoma or chondrosarcoma.

Secondary tumors of bone are by definition malignant; although bone may react to an adjacent tumor such as a meningioma without being part of the neoplastic process. These types of tumors are much more common than primary malignant tumors of bone. Thus, even though they are associated with the older age categories, they are more common in archeological skeletons. However, like primary malignant tumors, they pose problems in differential diagnosis in gross specimens, particularly with infectious diseases.

As we have noted earlier in this chapter malignant secondary tumors of the skeleton may produce blastic, lytic, or mixed lesions. Abbot and Courville (1) attribute a periosteal osteoblastic lesion seen in two skulls located in the San Diego, California Museum (U.S.A.) to periosteal reactions to underlying tumors of the dura (meningiomas). One skull was from Peru and had a large lesion of the skull vault consisting of fused spicules of bone which radiate out perpendicular to the skull surface. The abnormal bone is loosely attached to the underlying outer table, which is largely intact. The second skull is from San Nicolas Island off the coast of southern California. The lesion is similar to the Peruvian specimen. Meningiomas are known to produce

lytic lesions in early stages of the tumor development (14), but blastic lesions are more common (Cushing (4).

Rogers (12) briefly describes two skulls from Egypt having lesions which he attributes to meningiomas. The first of these is from the 1st Dynasty and shows a hyperostotic lesion of the right parietal involving both the inner and outer table. The second specimen is from the 20th Dynasty and exhibits a large honeycomb lesion with a focus in the right parietal, but involving the left parietal and the frontal bone. The lesion is large, including most of the right parietal. It is not clear whether the inner table was involved. The first of these two cases differs from the two cases of Abbot and Courville in involving both tables of the skull.

MacCurdy (11) describes an adult male skull from Paucarcancha with a large tumor of the left parietal and frontal bones. The coalescing osteophytes extend outward from the skull about 4.5 cm. The tables of the skull have been destroyed beneath the tumor. MacCurdy attributes this tumor to osteosarcoma, but a secondary tumor of bone seems more probable, such as hemangioma. Another possibility would be a bony reaction to meningioma.

A skeletal specimen from the cemetery at Dubendorf, Canton Zurich, Switzerland, dated between the 11th and 15th centuries, exhibits a diffuse osteoblastic reaction. The specimen is an adult male, probably in excess of 50 years of age at death, and is currently stored in the Anthropological Institute of the University of Zurich, Switzerland (Catalog No. 7757). The right innominate contains a lesion largely limited to the periosteal surfaces of the ilium. The lesion consists of extensive, fine, porous, bony buildup. There is no obvious destruction of underlying bone or evidence of abscess or cloacas. There is a similar bony reaction on the right, anterior, proximal femur. Two of the ribs in this specimen also show periosteal lesions. The disseminated nature of the disease, as well as the morphology of the lesions, is compatible with metastatic tumor. The extensive involvement of the innominate and the sex of the case suggest prostate cancer.

Osteolytic metastatic cancer of the skeleton is probably the most common type of cancerous lesion seen in archeological specimens. The major problem in diagnosis is to distinguish between metastatic carcinoma from tissue such as breast or lung and multiple myeloma.

An example of osteolytic metastatic cancer is seen in a female skeleton (NMNH No. 290064) from the Indian Knoll site in Kentucky, U.S.A. Most of the artifacts in the site are dated in the Late Archaic Period (ca. 3000–1000 B.C.); however, some components date to the Late Woodland Period (ca. 800–1700 A.D.). Thus, the archeological age of this specimen remains obscure but with a strong probability of being Archaic. The precise age at death is not known; however, judging from tooth wear and the condition of the joints, it is certainly fully adult but probably not older than 40 years.

The disease process consists of multifocal, mostly lytic lesions distributed in the skull, mandible, axial skeleton, and the proximal end of the left femur (the right femur is missing). The bones of the hands and feet are unaffected, except for a slight superficial osteoporosis of the superior surface of the calcanei. The gross lesions vary in size from being barely detectable to about 1 cm in diameter. Most of the gross lesions penetrate both tables, with no clear pattern as to which table is most extensively involved. The lytic process is more extensive in the diploë, suggesting that the marrow was the focal point for the disease process. The roentgen films of the skull and long bones reveal many lytic foci which are not seen grossly.

The scapulae are present, and both show multiple lytic foci. However, unlike lesions elsewhere in the skeleton, there is a slight osteo-

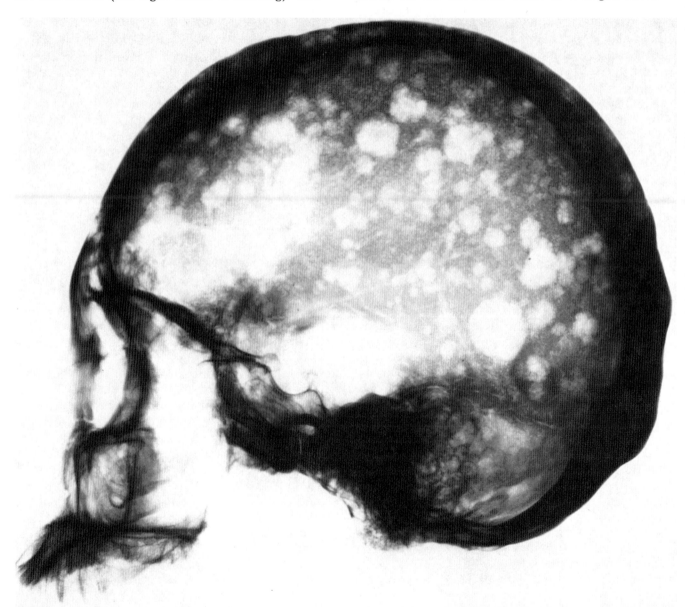

Figure 46.1. Roentgen film of an archeological skull from Caudivilla, Peru (NMNH No. 242559), showing multifocal, lytic lesions. Multiple myeloma or metastatic carcinoma are possible diseases involved in this lytic process.

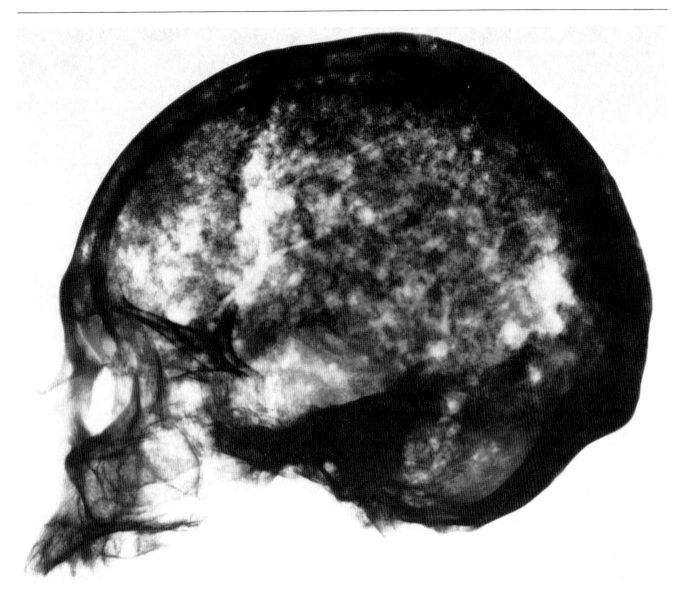

Figure 46.2. Roentgen film of an archeological skull from Cuzco, Peru (NMNH No. 242578), showing multifocal lytic lesions having poorly defined borders. Either multiple myeloma or metastatic carcinoma could be implicated in this case.

blastic response associated with several of the lytic foci. With this exception, there is no osteoblastic response adjacent to the lesion and no osteoblastic circumscription of the lytic focus. This suggests a rather acute disease process.

The age and sex of the specimen are compatible with both myeloma and metastatic carcinoma such as breast cancer. The variation in the size of the lytic foci, the acute nature of the disease process, and the probability of death in young adulthood rather than old age are, however, more compatible with metastatic carcinoma.

Two cases of multifocal lytic lesions of the skull from Peru were collected in the late 19th century and are currently in the Smithsonian collections. Unfortunately, archeological pro-

venience is poorly documented. One of these skulls (Fig. 46.1) was collected in the region of Caudivilla, Peru (NMNH No. 242559). It is fully adult and probably in the 30–40 year age range, with all teeth missing, mostly due to postmortem loss. The entire skull is involved in the disease process, except for the bones of the face. The occipital bone is only slightly affected.

The lesions vary in size up to 1.5 cm in diameter. Both tables are affected with no apparent predilection for either table. The diploë is more extensively involved than the tables. The lytic process has created a loculate appearance in the remaining bone of each lesion, suggesting multiple small coalescing lytic foci. There is no gross evidence of osteoblastic circumscription in the lesion. This case from Peru is very similar to the

Indian Knoll specimen described earlier, and again both myeloma and metastatic carcinoma are possible diseases, with the morphological evidence slightly in favor of the latter cause.

The second skull (Fig. 46.2) from Peru is from the region around Cuzco (NMNH No. 242578). The skull is probably that of a female in the 35–45 year age range. Grossly, there are multiple, small, lytic foci concentrated on the skull vault but also found on the facial bones and the occiput. The greater wings of the sphenoid and the region around the basi-occipital synchondrosis are markedly affected, with the latter totally destroyed.

Unlike the other skull from Peru, lytic involvement is more extensive on the inner table. However, the major focus again is the diploë. There is no evidence of any osteoblastic reaction in any of the lesions. A typical lesion itself consists of a lytic cavity ranging in diameter up to 2 cm, with lysis concentrated in the diploë. The remaining portion of the tables is delicate and morphologically similar to lace. In this case the distinction between metastatic carcinoma and myeloma is even more difficult. However, the coalescing nature and the more uniform size of the lesions would favor myeloma.

The last example of a lytic process which could be caused by a tumor occurs in an Eskimo skull from St. Lawrence Island, Alaska (NMNH No. 280091). The archeological provenience is obscure. The skull is male and fully adult, probably in the 45–65 year age category. The mandible is missing, as are all the postcranial bones. There is a diffuse porosity of the external table of the vault which is also seen to a more limited degree on the nasal bones and maxilla. There has been some postmortem erosion which obscures the surface texture somewhat, but the remaining surface has a pumice-like quality. The most dramatic feature is a large lytic lesion on the posterior portion of the left parietal which is confluent with a smaller lytic lesion encroaching on the right parietal. The larger of the two lytic components has a maximal diameter of 4 cm and has a slightly scalloped but well-circumscribed appearance, with the inner table somewhat more affected than the outer. The smaller lytic component is similar in appearance but less

well circumscribed, suggesting lytic activity at the time of death. Other smaller lesions occur primarily on the left side of the skull, with one moderately large lesion measuring 1.5 cm in diameter in the right temporal bone and also involving the sphenoid bone. The skull is somewhat thicker than normal, measuring 13 mm near the edge of the major lytic foci.

There are several conditions which could give rise to the pattern seen in the skull. Eosinophilic granuloma is a syndrome for which the disease process is still unknown but which produces lesions similar to that seen in the Eskimo skull. Metastatic carcinoma, meningioma, and cancerous hemangioma are also possibilities.

Representatives of all the clinical varieties of bone neoplasm known in modern clinical experience are not yet described in archeological specimens. However, the general categories such as primary and secondary and benign and malignant have been identified. This demonstrates the general principle that while the incidence of various neoplasms may change, the basic problem probably has considerable antiquity in human populations.

References

1. Abbot, K. H., and Courville, C. B. (1939): Historical notes on the meningiomas. I. A study of hyperostoses in prehistoric skulls. Bull. Los Angeles Neurol. Soc., 4:101.
2. Adis-Castro, E., and Neumann, G. (1948): The incidence of ear exostosis in the Hopewell people of Illinois valley. Proc. Indiana Acad. Sci., 57: 33–36.
3. Beraud, C., Morel, P., and Boyer, A. (1961): Osteome geant Frontoethmoidal Decouver sur un Crane medieval du var. J. Radiol. Electrol. Med. Nucl. (Paris), 42:45–47.
4. Cushing, H. (1922): The cranial hyperostoses produced by meningeal endotheliomas. Arch. Neurol. Psychiatry, 8:139–152.
5. Dastugue, J. (1965): Tumeur maxillaire sur un Crane du Moyen-age. Bull. Assoc. Franc. Étude Cancer, 52:69–72.
6. Doll, R., and Hill, A. B. (1964): Mortality in relation to smoking. Ten years' observation on British doctors. Brit. Med. J., 1:1397, 1460.
7. Doll, R., Hill, A. B., and Kreyberg, L. (1957): The significance of cell type in relation to the aetiology of lung cancer. Br. J. Cancer, 11:43.
8. Gregg, J. B., and McGrew, R. N. (1970): Hrdlička revisited (external auditory canal exostosis). Am. J. Phys. Anthropol., 33(1):37–40.
9. Hrdlička, A. (1935): Ear exostoses. Smithsonian Misc. Collect., 93:1–100.
10. Kelln, E. E., et al. (1967): A seventeenth century mandibular tumor in a North American Indian. Oral Surg., Oral Med., Oral Pathol., 23:78–81.
11. MacCurdy, G. G. (1923): Human skeletal remains from the highlands of Peru. Am. J. Phys. Anthropol., 6:217–329.
12. Rogers, L. (1949): Meningiomas in Pharaoh's people; hyperostosis in ancient Egyptian skulls. Br. J. Surg., 36:423–424.
13. Ruffer, M. A., and Willmore, J. G. (1914): Note on a tumor of the pelvis dating from Roman times (250 A.D.) and found in Egypt. J. Pathol. Bacteriol., 18:480–484.
14. Schinz, H. R., Baensch, W. E., Fredl, E., and Uehlinger, E. (1951): Roentgen-Diagnostics, Vols. 1 and 2. Grune & Stratton, New York.
15. Wells, C. (1964): Bones, Bodies and Disease. Thames & Hudson, London.

47

Neoplasia and Other Disease Problems in Black-footed Ferrets: Implications for an Endangered Species

James W. Carpenter, Meliton N. Novilla, and Hans E. Kaiser

Extinction, a natural process, is one of the most conspicuous of all evolutionary events. A number of factors (acting alone or in concert), including habitat modification and destruction, overharvesting by man or newly introduced predators, competition with more successful species, and, possibly, exposure to new diseases and parasites have been identified in causing extinctions among species (4, 9, 15, 17, 23, 24, 26).*

For any species, extinction occurs when existing genotypes are unable to adapt to environmental change. Inability to adapt in the face of environmental change can be due to small population size and limited genetic variability, to the rapidity of environmental change, or to a combination of these factors. Insular populations seem to be particularly vulnerable to extinction because of their relatively small population sizes, inbreeding, habitat specialization, small gene pools, and reduced competitive abilities (2, 16). However, even widely distributed species are vulnerable when environmental change is extremely rapid.

The black-footed ferret (*Mustela nigripes*), the only ferret native to North America, is one of the rarest mammals in North America, with few verified sightings reported in over 5 years. Although once widely distributed from Saskatchewan and Alberta to Texas, New Mexico, and Arizona, the range of this endangered species has been reduced considerably, due to reduction and local eradication of prairie dogs, loss of habitat, and possibly secondary poisoning (10, 22). It is clear that the species is now reduced to small disjunct populations. As an adjunct to field studies, habitat preservation, and legal protection, a captive propagation program for this species was initiated by the Endangered Wildlife Research Program of the Patuxent Wildlife Research Center in 1971 (6).

This chapter examines neoplasia and some concurrent disease conditions in the world's last five captive black-footed ferrets and suggests that their origin is associated with genetic homozygosity resulting from inbreeding. Although it is difficult to extend implications from the study of five captive ferrets to wild ferrets, it is conceivable that any small, remnant population existing in the wild may be experiencing attrition from similar pathological processes.

TUMORS IN BLACK-FOOTED FERRETS

Between 1976 and 1978, all five of the black-footed ferrets maintained at the Patuxent Wildlife Research Center developed adnexal tumors in the caudal area (Table 47.1). Despite intensive care and supportive treatment, two ferrets have died as a result of metastases to internal organs.

Sweat gland carcinomas developed on the tail of ferrets 1 and 5 and the perineum of ferret 3.

* See also reference 8 of Capter 44.

Table 47.1
Neoplasia and Concurrent Pathology in Black-footed Ferrets at the Patuxent Wildlife Research Center

	Ferret No.				
	1	2	3	4	5
Sex	Male	Female	Male	Female	Male
Age (years) at which primary neoplasia was detected	6	6	6 (approx.)	12–13 (approx.)	12–13 (approx.)
Neoplasms	Adenocarcinoma (sweat gland origin) of tail; cystadenoma; tumor metastases in lungs	Adenocarcinoma (sebaceous gland origin) of tail; no metastasis (?)	Adenocarcinoma (sweat gland origin) in perineal area; tumor metastases to an internal iliac lymph node; interstitial cell tumor in undescended testis	Basal cell carcinoma (basosquamous variety) of tail; no recurrence; a metastatic, papillary, cystadenocarcinoma of the mammary gland	Adenocarcinoma (sebaceous and sweat gland origin) of tail; no recurrence
Status[a]	Dead at 7 mo	Dead at 6 mo	Dead at 1 mo	Dead 6 mo after basal cell carcinoma and 2 wk after cystadenocarcinoma	Dead at 11 mo
Concurrent pathology	Arteriosclerosis	Mild, focal granulomatous hepatitis; mild atherosclerosis	Diabetes mellitus; arteriosclerosis; intestinal coccidiosis	Arteriosclerosis; renal infarcts; multiple thrombi in right atrium	Arteriosclerosis; hepatitis
Reproductive disorders	No detectable interest in females in estrus	Abnormal estrus cycle	Monorchid; no detectable interest in females in estrus	Produced two litters containing 80% stillbirths	Normal libido (?)

[a] Indicates time interval from first observation of neoplasia to death of animal.

In addition, a papillary cystadenoma and a sebaceous gland carcinoma also occurred in ferrets 1 and 5, respectively. Histologically, the adenocarcinoma from the tail of ferret 1 consisted of irregular tubules and solid cords of cells with a fibrous stroma (Fig. 47.1). The tumor cells were cuboidal or low columnar, and poorly oriented. The nuclei were hyperchromatic, and the mitotic index was high. The covering epithelium was ulcerated, hyperkeratotic, and acanthotic. Neutrophilic infiltration was prominent in the dermis, particularly around the sebaceous glands and the dilated ducts of sweat glands. Tumor metastases (0.5–1.0 mm) consisting of irregular tubular structures associated with marked fibrosis were found in the lung (Fig. 47.2).

The tail adenoma of ferret 1 was a well-circumscribed mass consisting of cysts lined by a single layer of cuboidal or low columnar epithelium. Brownish-yellow secretions and intracystic papillary infoldings of the lining epithelium were seen in some cysts. Morphologic features of the sweat gland carcinoma in ferret 5 were similar to those of ferret 1, although in one mass there were more discernible ducts and multilayered intraluminal papillae.

In ferret 3, the carcinomatous cells were generally cuboidal and hyperchromatic and were forming ducts, and there was one area of cartilaginous metaplasia (Fig. 47.3). Tumor metastases were observed in an internal iliac lymph node and were obliterating a large section of the parenchyma (Fig. 47.4). The mass was composed of cords and lobules of cells separated by collagenous stroma. Mitotic figures were abundant, and large areas of necrosis were present.

Due to metastases, these adenocarcinomas of sweat gland origin were the primary cause of death in ferret 1 and a contributing mortality factor in ferret 3. There was no recurrence of the tail tumor in ferret 5. Although this appears to be the first report of this neoplasm in a mustelid, sweat gland adenocarcinomas in the canine also metastasize commonly to the regional lymph nodes and lungs (18).

Sebaceous gland carcinomas occurred as a firm growth (1.0 × 0.6 cm) on the ventrolateral aspect of the tail of ferret 2 and as multiple growths on the tail of ferret 5. Histological examination of the excised tumors revealed multiple packets of cells separated by thin collagenous septae (Fig. 47.5). Tumor cells were pleo-

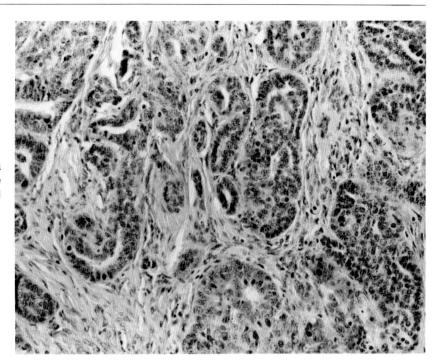

Figure 47.1. Photomicrograph of a sweat gland adenocarcinoma on the caudal area of a black-footed ferret (H & E stain, ×160).

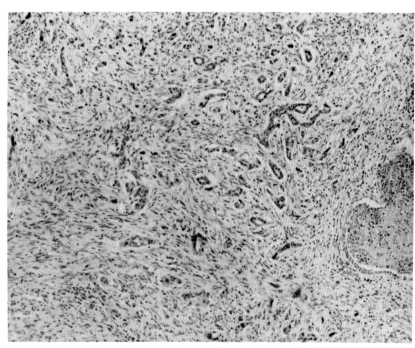

Figure 47.2. Pulmonary metastases of a sweat gland adenocarcinoma in a black-footed ferret. Note extensive fibrosis (H & E stain, ×63).

morphic, although most were large and polyhedral with large nuclei and prominent nucleoli. The cytoplasm was abundant and finely granular with discernible vacuoles in some packets. Mitotic figures and a few bizarre multinucleated cells were also present.

Small, darker-staining cells proliferating around tumor lobules were observed in ferret 2. Cystic ducts, associated with hair follicles and normal sebaceous glands, were present in ferret

5. In both animals, the tumor masses contained necrotic foci and a neutrophilic infiltrate. The covering epithelium was intact in both ferrets, but there was a mild follicular keratosis in ferret 5. The histological findings of these tumors are compatible with adenocarcinomas of the sebaceous glands reported in other species (18, 20, 25).

Ferret 4 had a firm reddish-white nodule, 1 cm in diameter, excised from the dorsum of the tail,

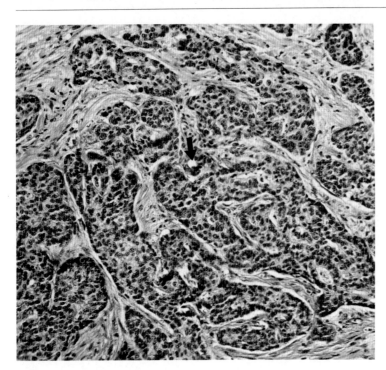

Figure 47.3. Section of a perineal mass from a diabetic ferret consisting of lobules and cords of carcinomatous cells. A few duct-like structures (*arrow*) are in some of the lobules (H & E stain, ×180).

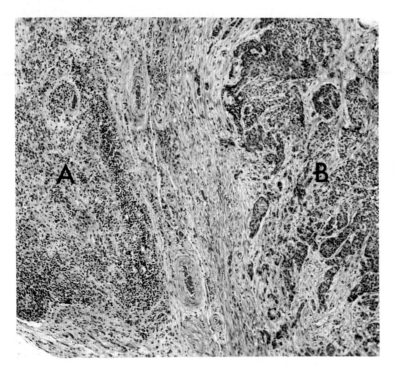

Figure 47.4. Photomicrograph of an internal iliac lymph node (*A*) of a diabetic ferret that is invaded by a perineal adenocarcinoma (*B*) of sweat gland origin (H & E stain, ×180).

3 cm from the tail head. Microscopically, the mass was composed of lobules and sheets of basosquamous cells (Fig. 47.6). Mitotic figures and large coalescing areas of necrosis were prominent. Unequivocal differentiation of tumor cells toward adnexal glands was not evident. Skin tumors forming solid epithelial lobules without lumens have been classified recently as basal cell tumors (21). These tumors are considered benign in all respects, but they may recur

following incomplete excision.

In addition, a simple, papillary cystic adenocarcinoma of the mammary gland with metastases to the internal iliac and mesenteric lymph nodes, liver, and spleen was observed in black-footed ferret (4). Histopathologically, the tumor was aggressive, and evidence of lymphatic invasion was found. The tumor was considered a reflection of the old age (about 12–13 years) of the animal; attempts at virus isolation were negative. Bilateral infarcts were observed in the kidneys, apparently resulting in acute renal shutdown and death of the ferret.

OTHER PATHOLOGIC OBSERVATIONS

Diabetes Mellitus

In addition to the tumors observed in these captive ferrets, other pathologic conditions were identified in this population (Table 47.1). Diabetes mellitus was tentatively diagnosed in black-footed ferret 3 with polyuria, polydipsia, polyphagia, dehydration, and weight loss (3). Laboratory findings (marked hyperglycemia (724 mg/100 ml), glycosuria, and ketonuria) and the subsequent favorable response to insulin therapy confirmed the diagnosis. Although lesions were not observed in the pancreas, gross and histologic findings concomitant with diabetes mellitus included arteriosclerosis, mild proliferative glomerulonephritis, and mild necrotiz-

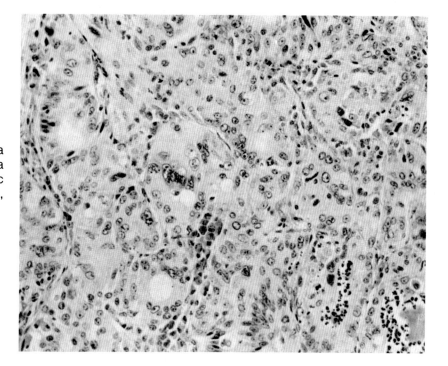

Figure 47.5. Photomicrograph of a sebaceous gland adenocarcinoma in a black-footed ferret. Note pleomorphic tumor cells in lobules (H & E stain, ×160).

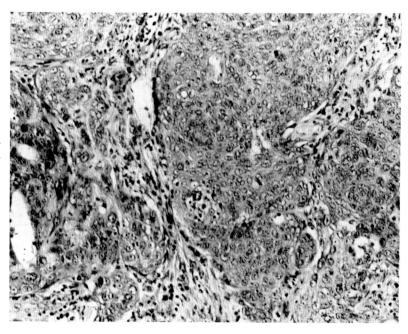

Figure 47.6. Section of a tail mass excised from a black-footed ferret. Note lobules of basosquamous cells (H & E stain, ×63).

ing hepatitis, the latter of which (and possibly the renal lesions as well) is frequently associated with diabetes, probably as a result of ketosis (12, 19).

Special stains demonstrated adequate numbers of β-cell granules in the islets of Langerhans. Thus, the diabetes was apparently due to a lack of release of the synthesized insulin or to the diminished effectiveness of the secreted insulin. The other lesions concomitant with the diabetes, therefore, were probably responsible for the ferret's death. The difficulty in accurately assessing the insulin requirement of the ferret probably contributed to the patient's debilitated condition.

Although this is apparently the first report of diabetes mellitus in a mustelid, this disease has been reported in other groups of exotic animals. Diabetes is a chronic, multisystem disorder due to either a deficient secretion of insulin by beta cells of the pancreatic islets or to diminished effectiveness of the secreted insulin (12, 14). Various extrapancreatic factors, including neurogenic disturbance, stress, trauma, diet, obesity, infection, certain drugs, hormones, and heredity may also influence the development of diabetes (1, 7).

Arteriosclerosis

Postmortem examination of black-footed ferrets 1, 3, 4, and 5 revealed moderate-to-severe arteriosclerosis. The aorta and proximal portion of the carotid arteries contained a series of firm, roughened rings of pale yellow mineral deposits (Fig. 47.7). The rings were generally 2 to 3 mm apart, becoming more widely spaced in the distal portion of the aorta. Several arteries branching off the aorta also had mineralized rings extending 0.5 to 1 cm from the base of the artery.

Widespread arteriosclerosis with calcification was evident on the histopathologic examination of ferrets 1, 3, and 5 in the aorta, pulmonary arteries, and carotid arteries. Arteriosclerosis in ferret 4 was apparently present only in the aorta. The calcified plaques emanated from the tunica media (Fig. 47.8).

Arteriosclerosis apparently occurs in many captive wild animals (8). Although the nature of the insult to the vessel walls that results in sclerosis is not known, hemodynamic factors probably contribute to the development of plaques about the orifices of arterial branches (11). The sclerotic vessels are usually not accompanied by significant disturbances of blood flow, although ischemic changes, especially of the heart and brain, have been reported (11). Lesions in the ferret, however, were generally restricted to the aorta and, to some degree, some of the major vessels emanating from the aorta. The predilection of sclerosis for the abdominal aorta and points of arterial branching (11) are compatible with the findings in this case.

Calcification as a dystrophic or metastatic process occurs frequently in the arteries of many animals, generally accompanying other degenerative changes. The complete encirclement of the large elastic arteries in this ferret, however, appears to be a rare finding. The causes of

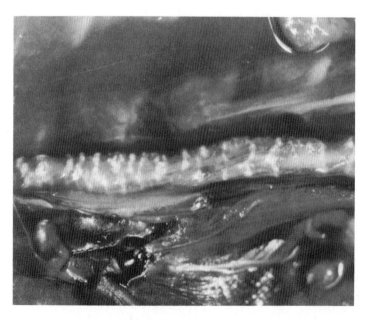

Figure 47.7. Calcified rings in the thoracic portion of the aorta of a black-footed ferret.

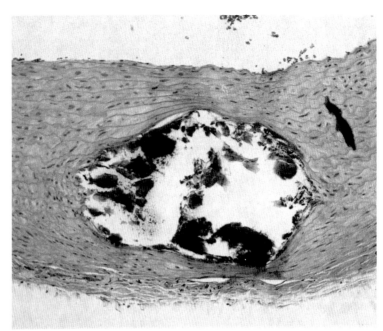

Figure 47.8. Arteriosclerotic plaque in the tunica media of the aorta from a diabetic black-footed ferret (H & E stain, ×130).

medial calcification are unknown and are probably nonspecific, although it more commonly occurs in animals of advancing age and is frequently associated with a variety of debilitating diseases (11).

Reproductive Disorders

Although one of the three wild-caught male ferrets was a monorchid, a condition frequently considered to be hereditary, most of the reproductive problems were associated with the two females. One female produced five young in each of two litters; four in each were stillborn. Histopathologic examination of the stillborn kits did not reveal the cause of their deaths. Apparently, whatever condition had resulted in the stillbirths also weakened the two remaining kits because they both died 36–48 hr postpartum. The second female entered estrus during at least three seasons, but was not receptive to any of the three males with which she was placed and never bred. During the 1978 season, she entered proestrus for only a few days, then became anestrus.

DISCUSSION

The role of disease in causing species extinction is unknown. Since diseased wild animals are more susceptible to mortality factors such as predation, accidents, and malnutrition, the etiology of a population decline in a species with low numbers is difficult to determine. However, it does seem reasonable to assume that a species with extremely low numbers, and one already impaired (weakened) by other factors, might become extinct through some pathological mechanism.

The occurrence, therefore, of the adenocarcinomas in five black-footed ferrets has important implications. Since this colony represents the entire world's captive population, any disease or condition affecting these individuals may adversely influence their successful breeding and the subsequent reintroduction of their offspring into the wild. In addition, the diseases encountered in captivity may actually be a reflection of pathological processes occurring in the wild population—and these processes may actually be partly responsible for the recent decrease in the number of wild ferrets.

It should be noted, however, that all of the ferrets in this study were captured within a fairly restricted area of several adjoining ranches in Mellette County, South Dakota, where the possibility of obtaining closely related animals would be likely. Therefore, this colony may not be characteristic of the species as a whole but rather may be a reflection of problems in other localized populations of ferrets. Also, the magnitude of the pathologic problems may be magnified in captivity, during which the stress and density of the hosts generally are increased.

The etiology of the neoplasms resulting in the death of three individuals is undetermined. Viral inclusion bodies have not yet been identified in the neoplastic tissues, and results of virus isolation in one ferret were negative. Although the husbandry and the nutrition of these animals is similar to that for the numerous European ferrets (*Mustela putorius*) and Siberian polecats (*Mustela eversmanni*) maintained in a separate facility at the Patuxent Wildlife Research Center as research surrogates, the pathological conditions observed in the black-foots have not occurred in any of these 200 or more surrogates.

The site predilection for the neoplasms in the black-footed ferret is also intriguing. Although the adnexal tumors occurred on the anterior part of the tail or perineum of all five ferrets, most adnexal tumors in the dog and cat are more frequent in the head and neck than in the caudal area (21).

Although the tumors in these ferrets may be a reflection of age, it is possible that a genetic predisposition towards these tumors may in fact exist, enhanced by a high inbreeding coefficient. Since many species are generally heterozygous carriers of deleterious recessive traits, the traits have a greater probability of becoming homozygous in species with low localized populations in which inbreeding occurs (5).

The concurrent pathologic conditions, including the diabetes mellitus and the monorchidism in one individual, also may have implications for any remnant ferret population that still exists in the wild, because both conditions may be heritable (1, 11–13). In addition, the breeding disorders observed in the two captive females are also suggestive of inbreeding difficulties. If the pathologic processes and disorders observed in these ferrets are in fact a reflection of an inbreeding problem, black-footed ferrets may be having difficulty coping with their present environment due to a decrease in genetic variability and, correspondingly, due to a decrease in species adaptability. If these circumstances apply, survival of the black-footed ferret in the wild, and the procurement of suitable stock with which to produce animals in captivity to bolster the wild population, appear to face more formidable obstacles than previously envisioned.

References

1. Bloom, F. (1968): Diseases of endocrine glands. In *Canine Medicine*, pp. 419–454, edited by E. J. Catcott. American Veterinary Publications, Inc., Wheaton, Ill.
2. Bonnell, M. L., and Selander, R. K. (1974): Elephant seals; genetic variation and near extinction. *Science*, 184:908–909.
3. Carpenter, J. W., and Novilla, M. N. (1977): Diabetes mellitus in a black-footed ferret. *J. Am. Vet. Med. Assoc.*, 171(9):890–893.
4. Curry-Lindahl, K. (1972): *Let Them Live*. Murrow, New York.
5. Dobzhansky, T. (1970): *Genetics of the Evolutionary Process*. Columbia University Press, New York.
6. Erickson, R. C. (1968): A federal research program for endangered wildlife. *Trans. North Am. Wildlife Natl. Resource Conf.*, 33:418–433.
7. Feldman, E. C. (1977): Diabetes mellitus. In *Current Veterinary Therapy*, pp. 1001–1009, edited by R. W. Kirk. W. B. Saunders, Philadelphia.
8. Fiennes, R. N. T-W. (1965). *Comparative Atherosclerosis*, pp. 113–126, edited by J. Roberts, Jr., and R. Straus, Harper & Row, New York.
9. Fisher, J., Simon, N., and Vincent, J. (1969): *Wildlife in Danger*. Viking Press, New York.
10. Hall, E. R., and Kelson, K. R. (1959): *The Mammals of North America*. Ronald Press, New York.
11. Jubb, K. V. F., and Kennedy, P. C. (1970): *Pathology of Domestic Animals*. Vol. 1. Academic Press, New York.
12. Jubb, K. V. F., and Kennedy, P. C. (1970): *Pathology of Domestic Animals*, Vol. 2. Academic Press, New York.
13. Keen, H. (1960): Spontaneous diabetes in man and animals. *Vet. Rec.*, 72:555–557.
14. Ling, G. V. (1974): Diabetes mellitus. In *Current Veterinary Therapy*, pp. 814–818, edited by R. W. Kirk. W. B. Saunders, Philadelphia.
15. Martin, P. S. (1967): Prehistoric overkill. In *Pleistocene Extinctions: The Search for a Cause*, pp. 75–120, edited by P. S. Martin and H. E. Wright. Princeton University Press, Princeton.
16. Mayr, E. (1965): The nature of colonization in birds. In *The Genetics of Colonizing Species*, edited by H. G. Baker and G. L. Stebbins. Academic Press, New York.
17. Mayr, E. (1970): *Populations, Species, and Evolution*. The Belknap Press, Cambridge, Mass.
18. Moulton, J. E. (1962): *Tumors of the Domestic Animals*. University of California Press, Berkeley.
19. Smith, H. A., Jones, T. C., and Hunt, R. D. (1972): *Veterinary Pathology*. Lea & Febiger, Philadelphia.
20. Squire, R. A., Goodman, D. G., Valerio, M. G., Frederickson, T., Strandberg, J. D., Levitt, M. H., Lingeman, C. H., Harshbarger, J. C., and Dawe, C. J. (1978): Tumors. In *Pathology of Laboratory Animals*, pp. 1051–1283, edited by K. Bernischke, F. M. Garner, and T. C. Jones. Springer-Verlag, New York.
21. Stannard, A. A., and Pulley, L. T. (1978): Tumors of the skin and soft tissues. In *Tumors of the Domestic Animals*, pp. 16–74, edited by J. E. Moulton. University of California Press, Berkeley.
22. U.S. Department of the Interior (1973): *Threatened Wildlife of the United States*, Publ. 114. U.S. Govt. Print. Off., Washington, D.C.
23. Uetz, G., and Johnson, D. L. (1974): Breaking the web. *Environment*, 16(10):31–39.
24. Warner, R. E. (1968): The role of introduced diseases in the extinction of the endemic Hawaiian avifauna. *Condor*, 70(2): 101–120.
25. Weiss, E., and Frese, K. (1974): VII. Tumors of the skin. *Bull. World Health Org.*, 50:79–100.
26. Ziswiler, V. (1967): *Extinct and Vanishing Animals*. Springer, New York.

48

Animal Neoplasms—A Systematic Review

Hans E. Kaiser

Intensive studies of the tissues of vertebrates, invertebrates, and plants show clearly that a more or less defined comparability of the structures exists as shown in Chapter 43. What was missing in all the summaries concerning the neoplasms of different animal species published until today was the histological and comparative biochemical background which is so important for a comparative pathology. It must be pointed out that it is especially the knowledge of the normal conditions (histologically as well as biochemically) that forms the preliminary condition for such an understanding. Otherwise, such a study will remain only a poor recounting of single cases or a literary exercise. Until now we have demonstrated that the histological comparison results in a species-specific special biological pattern for the tissues. Species-specific morphological results are supported by biochemistry and biophysics (see Chapters 17, 18, and 21 by Weisburger, Pitot, and Wallach). This chapter is devoted to a review of the spontaneous tumors; it will lead later to a review of plant tumors (Chapter 49) and a more detailed description of the most important autonomic growth in plants, so-called crown gall disease (Chapters 50–52). We shall not neglect to mention fossil cases of neoplasms and some tumors which have been produced experimentally in the different animal phyla. Table 48.1 shows the species number in relation to the described spontaneous tumors in all eumetazoans from which it is possible to fix the location of a particular tumor, together with the application of its taxonomic position. But the differences in the same tissue coming from organisms of the various hierarchical orders, with regard to their taxonomic position, should not

be overlooked. Our knowledge of the species-specific differences of tumor development is based on facts known from the biochemical pathways within the different organisms, the biophysical differences, etc. These findings are supported by epidemiology based on the facts of comparative morphology. They lead to the distinction of immunological and other aspects of species-specific particularities in tumors. The morphological particularities of species specificity can therefore be explained by biochemical and biophysical facts. But we cannot say that neoplastic growth is simply a universal biological phenomenon, because not all organisms can produce true neoplastic growth. In these, the concluding chapters of our comparison, we must look for the reason. It was shown in the discussion of the phylogenetical aspects of neoplastic growth that the preliminary conditions for such growth have developed throughout geological history (Table 48.2); but neoplastic growth per se could not occur before the phylogenetic appearance of the various types of true tissues. Even the same histological tissue can vary within different species because of its interrelationship with the whole organism and certain particularities found in its own framework (see Chapter 13 and Tables 48.3 and 48.4). It must be remembered that a large number of organisms without true tissues cannot attain the prerequisites for developing neoplastic growth. Of course there exist only a few such organisms in the animal kingdom as compared to the plant kingdom, especially when considered relatively. Unicellular organisms cannot produce true neoplastic growth by definition, but they do develop preliminary neoplastic conditions (Table 48.4).

Table 48.1
Comparison of Species Number of Phyla to Species Number and Estimated Individual Numbers in Which Neoplasms Have Been Described

Phylum	No. of species	Estimated Species No.	No. of Species with Described Neoplasms	Approximate Individual Cases
Protozoa	20,000 (Kaestner) 30,000 (Mayer)		5	
Mesozoa	50		0	0
Porifera	5,000 (Kaestner) 4,500 (Mayer)		0	0
Cnidaria	9,000 (Kaestner) 8,900 (Mayer)			
Platyhelminthes	12,400 (Kaestner) 6,000 (Mayer)		3	less than 100
Nemertinea	800 (Kaestner) 750 (Mayer)		0	0
Gnathostomulida	100		0	0
Entoprocta	60		0	
				0
Acanthocephala	800		0	0
Rotifera	2,000		0	0
Gastrotricha	100		0	0
Kinorhyncha	100		0	0
Nematoda	10,000	500,0000 (Hyman)	1	100
Nematomorpha	230		0	0
Priapulida	8		0	0
Mollusca	128,000 (Kaestner) 80,000 (Mayer)		32	more than 100
Sipunculida	250		2	less than 10
Echiurida	150 (Kaestner) 60 (Mayer)		0	0
Annelida	8,700 (Kaestner) 7,000 (Mayer)		4	10 to 100
Onychophora	70 (Kaestner) 65 (Mayer)		0	0
Pentastomida	60 (Kaestner) 70 (Mayer)		0	0
Tardigrada	200 (Kaestner) 180 (Mayer)		0	0
Arthropoda	850,000 (Kaestner) 910,000 (Mayer)	5–7 million (J Briggs)	24	More than 1,000
Phoronida	4 (Mayer)		0	0
Ectoprocta	5,300 (Kaestner)		0	0
Brachiopoda	250 (Kaestner)		0	0
Echinodermata	6,000 (Kaestner) 4,000 (Mayer)		Less than 10	Less than 10
Chaetognatha	50 (Kaestner) 30 (Mayer)		0	0
Hemichordata	80		0	0
Cephalochordata	3		0	0
Tunicata	2,000		1?	
Vertebrata	43,000 (Kaestner) 37,390 (Mayer)		400	Countless

The capability for developing true neoplasms can thus be ascribed generally to the histonia animalia, mainly the eumetazoans, and the histonia plantae, mainly the tracheophyta or vascular plants. Certain neoplasms may also develop in sponges and the highest rhodophyta, phaeophyta, and bryophyta. Before we list the neoplasms of the animals in systemic order, it must be understood that the comparison, based on histology opens the way to a general, thorough comparability, but it also shows that certain differences based mainly on the different

Table 48.2

Comparative Phylogenetic Histogenesis of Neoplasms: Attempt to See Phylogenetic Development of Neoplastic Principles as Multistep Process

PHYLOGENETIC DEVELOPMENT OF NEOPLASTIC CHARACTERISTICS
(in convergent lines)

	Restrictions in nonliving plant tissues	
	Restriction through adult cell invariability affecting the mammalian neurons	*Paleozoic Era*
	Restriction through adult cell invariability affecting whole organisms (e.g., rotifers)	Silurian/Devonian (borderline)
	Restriction of tumor development through high regeneration (autotomy)	Period (390,000,000 years)
		Permanent plant tissues
Cambrian Period (620,000,000 years)	Large potential of youth forms of neoplasms, such as embryomas, certain teratomas in both kingdoms—most malignant when less differentiated	Fully differentiated plant tissues
		Meristems
Proterozoic Era	No metastasis in plant malignancies	Plants with true tissues since the borderline between Silurian/Devonian period
Nerve tissues	Metastasis in animal malignancies	
Muscle tissues	Decrease of differentiation, increase of malignancy	
Connective tissues	Increase of tumor-producing potential in phylogeny, running parallel specialization	
Epithelia tissues		
Animals with true tissues since Precambrian	Possibility of transplantability	
1,500,000 (7,000,000) recent species	Possibility of tissue invasion with the first appearance of epithelia	Multicellular plants with beginning of true tissues in highest forms since Precambrian; 25,000 recent species
Multicellular animals with beginning of true tissues in highest forms since Precambrian, 5,000 recent species	Remaining autonomous growth in multicellular organisms without tissues—cell anomalies	
	Nuclear anomalies in unicellular eukaryotes	Multicellular plants without true tissues since Precambrian, 80,000 recent species
	RNA and DNA anomalies in prokaryotic cells	
Multicellular animals without true tissues since	Eukaryotic cells	
Precambrian (?)		
50 recent species	Prokaryotic cells	

UNICELLULAR ORGANISMS

Table 48.3
Tissue and Growth Characteristics of Animals

Characteristics	Group
Animals without true tissues	Protozoa, mesozoa, low porifera
Animals with cell-invariable tissues	
1. *in toto*	Adult rotifera, adult tardigrada
2. Partial	e.g., acanthocephala and other members of the superphylum aschelminthes, as adult kinorhyncha or gnathostomulida
Animals with high regenerative powers, where asexual reproduction occurs	
1. high power of regeneration	Porifera, cnidaria, echinodermata especially asteroidea, holothuroidea
2. fragmentation, fission	Certain annelida

Table 48.4
Animal Phyla in Which Neoplasms Have and Have Not Been Observed

Phyla without Spontaneous Neoplasms		Phyla with Spontaneous Neoplasms
Porifera	Linguatulida	Cnidaria (?)[a]
Ctenophora	Tardigrada	Platyhelminthes
Nemertinea	Phoronida	Mollusca
Gnathostomulida	Ectoprocta	Sipunculida
Entoprocta	Brachiopoda	Annelida
Acanthocephala	Chaetognatha	Arthropoda
Rotifera	Pogonophora	Echinodermata (?)[a]
Gastrotricha	Hemichordata	Vertebrata
Nematoda	Cephalochordata	
Nematomorpha	Urochordata	
Priapulida	Onychophora	
Echiurida		

[a] It cannot be decided from the information currently available whether the changes observed do satisfy the criteria established for considering the lesions observed as being true neoplasms.

patterns of normal growth, must be included. These differences derive from a controlled growth and from the way of growth exhibited by different organisms, manifested in the appearance of larval forms, placentae, cell invariability, capacity for regeneration, alteration of generations, etc. It must be emphasized, however, that it would be totally misleading if we said that the neoplasms in invertebrates, are microscopically, clearly distinguishable from those in the vertebrates (591). This only appears to be the case because our knowledge of the oncology of invertebrates is so limited. The principle of histogenesis has not been pursued consistently, and to date there exists no easily available review of comparative histology covering both animals and plants. Thus we must ask that if the tissues of organisms can be compared meaningfully, how is it that the tumors of these tissues can be held to be noncomparable?

At the beginning of this book it was stated that human neoplasms provided us with the basis of a pathological background so that we might acquire an understanding from the histological point of view. The adult human body has only one type of tissue which is of the cell-invariable type, the neurons, which are the principle cell group of the nervous tissue. Cardiac musculature is considered cell invariable by some authors. Fully differentiated neurons are incapable of developing neoplasms, but their differentiating precursors, the neuroblasts, are able to do so even when we consider the neuroblastoma alone. Hence, even if we consider the basic statements of Harms' theory (201), it must nonetheless be asserted that in cell-invariable animals the not fully differentiated life stages must at least theoretically contain the potential for development of neoplasms.

The exceptions to normal growth, which disallow the development of neoplastic growth in the adult stage, at least theoretically, are summarized as follows: (a) tissues, organs, the whole organism, within an individual species with cell invariability in animals (eumetazoans); (b) certain cases of autotomy and regeneration in animals (eumetazoans); and (c) permanent, nonliving plant tissues, when functioning.

We do not yet have enough knowledge to decide whether highly regenerative animals will also develop neoplasms, but it does not seem improper to assume that this capability varies from case to case and should be possible in one phase of development. It is wrong to assume that certain animal groups in which no, or almost no, neoplasms have been found will not be able to support neoplastic growth. Until recently it was believed that whales were immune to malignant neoplasms because those found were benign and well encapsulated. In recent years malignant neoplasms have been observed occasionally, which leads us to question the earlier statement. But because of the many whales slaughtered and examined by veterinarians we must assume that they provide us with more information than most other species of wild mammals. Thus we are able to compare them on the basis of the number observed with domesticated animals, especially the dog and cat.

Based on the law of actuality (see Chapter 44), we can well imagine that the living animal species of our time reflect the stages of neoplastic development like a mirror. This holds true when we consider the spontaneous tumors found in the various groups of organisms and their preliminary stages. These stages include nucleic or cytoplasmic anomalies, comparable to certain galls of lower plants. Additionally, experimentally produced neoplasms may shed some light on tissue reaction to neoplastic stimuli, because the described neoplasms of the majority of the phyla are so rare that we can only imagine or guess at their significance. It must be realized that the phyla with the majority of species, although smaller in number, are those of which spontaneous neoplasms have been described. Table 48.5 presents a review of the known preneoplastic conditions and known neoplasms according to taxonomic position. As far as vertebrates are concerned we can give only a general pattern of the tumor distribution because of the enormous number of cases described.

A special condition of mimicry of tumor development exists in the cases of osteomas such as described in fishes e.g. *Chaetodon* sp. These conditions, the so-called pachyostoses, are genus-specific, phylogenetic particularities and not neoplasms (276). Pachyostoses are also seen in such recent mammals as sea cows and the insectivore *Scutisorex* sp. and many fossil forms, including reptiles. All these cases are pachyostotic conditions which are phylogenetic and genus-specific but nonpathologic.

Table 48.5 gives a selected review of the tumors of all eumetazoans described, including mammalian orders such as artiodactyla, carnivora, and perissodactyla which include our domesticated animals such as cattle, swine, sheep, horse, dog, and cat, as well as their nondomesticated species. The facts for the domesticated species have been summarized in Tables 48.6 and 48.7 and Figure 48.1. As far as the laboratory

Table 48.5
Preneoplastic Conditions and Neoplasms According to Taxonomic Position

(*Note:* It is impossible to list all animal neoplasms which have been reported. In this selection it was necessary to limit the quotations frequently to review articles or book chapters which sometimes are marked "see," sometimes not. If the name of the author differs from the reference, the original author is listed in that review article.)

	PHYLUM: CNIDARIA	
Chlorhydra viridissima	Abnormal heterocytes	Filosa, 1962 (143)
Obelia sp.		Hammette and Reinmann, 1935 (190)
Syncoryna sp.	Abnormal growth	Korschelt, 1924 (300), Pflugfelder, 1954 (434)
Coral[+]	Abnormal skeleton	Squires, 1965 (524)
	PHYLUM: PLATYHELMINTHES Class: Turbellaria	
Dugesia tigrina	Epithelial lesions, perhaps benign to malignant neoplasms	Goldsmith, 1939 (175) Goldsmith, 1941 (176) Stephan, 1962 (526, Tar and Tarock, 1964 (568, Lange, 1966 (315)
	Cell inclusions	Dawe, 1968 (95)
Dugesia dorotocephala	Swelling and cell proliferations	Kenk, 1967 (see 205) Kenk, 1971 (see 205)
	PHYLUM: MOLLUSCA Class: Gastropoda	
Arion rufus	Growth anomalies	Froemming, et al., 1960 (153)
Cepea hortensis	Growth anomaly	Krieg, 1970 (307)
Helix aspersa	Marked epithelial and connective tissue proliferations	Moretti and Bellini, 1951 (see 95)
Helix pomatia		Krieg, 1970 (307)
	Lymphosarcoma (?)	Gersch, 1950 (164), Krieg, 1973 (308), Nolte, 1962 (405), Pauley, 1969 (423)
Limax flavus	Glandular and connective tissue proliferation	Szabo and Szabo (1934 (565)
Polinices lewisii	Oedomatous swelling (foot)	Smith and Taylor, 1968 (510)
Pleurobranchus plumula	Fibropapilloma	Fischer, 1954 (147)
	Class: Bivalvia	
Anodonta californiensis	Adenomyomas Polypose adenomas Polypose tumors	Pauley, 1967 (421), Pauley, 1967, 1969 (421,423) Pauley, 1967 (421)
Anodonta cygnea	Adenomyomas	Williams, 1890 (631) Collinge, 1891 (84)
Anodonta implicata	Fibromas	Butros, 1948 (61)

Table 48.5—Continued

Anodonta oregonesis	Polypose adenomas	Pauley, 1969 (423)
Crassostrea commercialis	Adenocarcinoma	Wolf, 1969 (634)
	Papilloma	Pauley, 1967 (420)
	Papilloma, mantle	Wolf, 1977 (exp.) (212)
Crassostrea gigas	Epitheliomas	Pauley and Sayce, 1968 (205)
	Fibroadenoma	Pauley and Sayce, 1968 (205)
	Fibrous tumors	Pauley, 1967 (205, 427)
	undiff. sarcomas	Otto, 1977 (212)
	Ganglioneuromas	Wolf, 1967 (205)
	Hematopoietic tumors	Farley 1969 (134)
	Hematopoietic neoplasms	Farley and Sparks, 1970 (136)
	Mesenchymal tumors	Pauley, 1967 (205); Wolf, 1967 (205)
	Neurinomas	Pauley et al., 1968 (205)
	Tumors	Sparks et al., 1964, 1969 (521, 520); Pauley and Sayce, 1968 (427)
Crassostrea virginica	Benign mesenchymal tumors	Ryder 1887 (468)
	Hematopoietic tumors	Farley 1969 (134); Otto, 1977 (212); Couch, 1977 (212); Wolf, 1977 (212)
	Mesenchymal tumors	Smith, 1934 (511)
	Polypoid vesicular tumor with inflammation	Otto, 1969 (205)
	Reticulum-cell sarcomas	Couch, 1969 (91)
	Reticulum-cell sarcomas ?	Pauly, 1967 (205)
	Sarcomas	Newman, 1971 (205)
	Germinoma	Otto, 1977 (212)
	Tumorlike proliferations	Galtsoff, 1967 (205)
	Hyperplasias	Otto, 1977 (212)
	Cytoplasmic inclusions	Otto, 1977 (212)
	Rickettsia-like inclusions	Otto, 1969 (205)
	Virus-infections of germ cells	Farley, 1976 (135)
Gonidea angulata	Polyp-like adenomas	Pauley, 1969 (423)
Macoma balthica	Neoplasm	Farley, 1976 (135)
Margaritifera marg.	Polyp	Pauley, 1968 (422)
	Polyp-like adenoma	Pauley, 1969 (423)
	Polyp-like tumor	Pauley, 1967 (205)
Mercenaria mercenaria	Polyp	Yevich and Berry, 1969 (639)
	Chlamydia inclusions	Otto et al., 1975 (209)
	Intracellular inclusions	Otto, 1975 (209)
Modiolus modiolus	Benign neoplasm of vesicular connective tissue	Robert, 1975 (209)
Mya arenaria	Papillomas	Shumwav, 1975 (209)
	Benign mesenchymal tumors	Pauley and Cheng, 1968 (426)
	Leiomyoma (?)	Barry et al., 1971 (24)
	Leiomyoma	Potter & Kuff, 1967 [++]
	Germinomas	Yevich, 1975 (209)
	Gonadal neoplasms	Yevich, 1977 (212)

Table 48.5—Continued

<u>Mya arenaria</u>	Hematopoietic neoplasms	Yevich, 1977 (212)
	Atypical hyperplasias	Pauley, 1977 (212)
	Rickettsia-like inclusions	Otto, 1975 (209)
	Cytoplasmic inclusions	Otto, 1977 (212)
<u>Mytilus californianus</u>	Inclusions	Yevich and Barszcz, 1977 (212)
<u>Mytilus edulis</u>	Fibroma	Wolf, 1975 (209)
	Hematopoietic tumors	Farley and Sparks, 1970 (136)
	Lymphomas	Farley, 1969 (205)
<u>Ostrea edulis</u>	Polyps	Katkansky, 1968 (281)
	Hematopoietic neoplasms	Alderman et al., 1977 (212)
<u>Ostrea lurida</u>	Hematopoietic tumor	Farley and Sparks, 1970 (136)
	Multilobed polypoid neoplasm of pericardial mesothelium associated with a marked proliferation of connective tissue differentiating into heart muscle	Mix, 1976 (375)
	Diffuse sarcoma of possible amebocyte stem cell origin	Yevich, 1970 (205)
	Hematopoietic neoplasms	Alderman et al., 1977 (212)
<u>Pinctata margarit.</u>	Polyps	Dix, 1971 (205)
<u>Saxidomus giganteus</u>	Adenomyomas	Pauley, 1967, 1969 (205,423)
	Polyp-like tumors	Pauley, 1967 (205)
<u>Spisula solidissima</u>	Multiple polypoid myomas of the foot	Leibovitz, 1975 (209)
<u>Tresus nutalli</u>	Papillomas	Desvoigne, et al., 1970 (104)
	Class: Cephalopoda	
<u>Sepia eledone</u>	Inflammation	Jacquemain, 1947 (243)
		Jullien, 1940 (269)
	Tumor, under skin of visceral sac	Jacquemain et al., 1947 (243)
<u>Sepia officinalis</u>	Growth anomalies	Jullien, 1928 (268)
		Gersch, 1951 (comments)
	Nodules on visceral sac (connective tissue, vascularizations, granulation tissue)	Jullien et al, 1952 (271)
	PHYLUM: SIPUNCULIDA	
<u>Sipunculus nudus</u>	Defense reactions (tumors ?)	Herubel, 1906 (223)

Table 48.5—Continued

<u>Sipunculus</u> sp.	Hypertrophies of Polish channels	Ladreyt, 1922 (311) cited in: Thomas, 1932 (585); Pflugfelder, 1954 (434); Scharrer and Lochhead, 1950 (486); Krieg, 1973 (308)
	PHYLUM: ANNELIDA	
<u>Eisenia foetida</u>	Aberrant regeneration	Andrews, 1974 (8)
<u>Lumbricus terrestris</u>	Epithelial (hyperplastic changes)	Cooper, 1969 (87); Gersch, 1954, 1957 (166, 167); Hancock, 1961 (191, 192)
	Epithelial proliferation of pharynx	Stolk, 1961 (557)
	Myoblastomas (body wall)	Hancock, 1961 (191, 192); Cooper, 1968 (86)
	Seminoma	Hancock, 1965 (194-196)
<u>Nereis diversicolor</u>	Inflammatory reaction with cell proliferation	Thomas, 1930 (572-575); Needham, 1942 (388); Gersch, 1931 (165); Thomas, 1930 (591)
<u>Potamilla</u> sp.	Pseudotumors	Mesnill and Caullery, 1911 (367)
	PHYLUM: ARTHROPODA Class: Merostomata	
<u>Limulus polyphemus</u> L.	Ectodermal lesion with articular enlargement	Hanstrom, 1926 (199); Krieg, 1973 (comments) (308)
	Class: Arachnida	
<u>Phalangium opilio</u>	Expansive growing neoplasms	Kolosvary, 1934 (299)
	Class: Crustacea	
<u>Mitella polymerus</u>		Shimkin, Koe, Zechmeister, 1951 (505)
<u>Tetraclita squamosa rubescens</u>		Shimkin, Koe, Zechmeister, 1951 (505)
<u>Lernaenicus radiatus</u>	Parasitic fungi	Meyers, 1975 (209)
Crab ? (Brachiura) [+]	Cellular growth	Fischer, 1928 (146); Krieg, 1973 (308)
<u>Gigantocypris mueller</u>	Physical injury (?)	Kornicker, 1975 (209)
<u>Homarus vulgaris</u>	Parasitic fungi	Alderman, 1977 (212)
<u>Homarus</u> sp.	Stomach neoplasm	McIntosh, 1884, 1885 (361)

Table 48.5—Continued

<u>Penaeus aztecus</u>	Hamartomas	Overstreet and van Devender, 1977 (212)
	Epidermal hyperplasia	Lightner, 1977 (212)
	Class: Insecta	
	Lesions of larvae	
<u>Pygaera curtula</u>	Neoplasms of trachea, rectum, hypoganglion, musculature, testis and coelomic fluid	White, 1921 (626)
<u>Drosophila</u> sp.	Malignant neuroblastoma	Gateff, 1978 (155)
	Semi-malignant and malignant imaginal disk neoplasms	Gateff, 1978 (155)
	Malignant neoplasms of larval hematopoietic system	Gateff, 1978 (155)
	Embryonal neoplasms	Gateff, 1978 (155)*
<u>Gilpinia hercyniae</u>	Proliferation of midintestinal epithelium	Bird, 1949 (36)
<u>Gryllotalpa</u> sp.	Cell proliferation in area of corpus	Palm, 1948 (415); Scharrer and Lochhead, 1950 (486) (comments)
	Lesions of imagines	
	Order: Orthoptera	
<u>Blatella germanica</u>	Intestinal neoplasms	Schreiner and Johannson, 1966 (494)
<u>Leucophaea maderae</u>	Intestinal neoplasms (Cells with enlarged nuclei and abnormal mitoses (exp.))	Scharrer, 1953 (485) Matz, 1961 (343)
<u>Locusta migratoria</u>	Intestinal neoplasms	Matz, 1961 (343); Harshbarger and Taylor, 1968 (213) review
<u>Orygia pseudotsugata</u>	Developmental anomaly	Mattignoni and Iwai, 1977 (212) (AR)
<u>Periplaneta americana</u>	Tumorlike growth	Llewellyn et al., 1976 (324)
	Large genital tumors	O'Farell and Stock, 1964 (407)
	Aggregation of hemocytes	Schlumberger, 1952 (489)
	Unspecific changes	Sutherland, 1969 (561, 562, 563)
	Proliferation	Baerwald and Boush, 1969 (15)

*See also Chapter 30 by Burdette.

Table 48.5—Continued

Order: Hymenoptera

Apis mellifera	Connective tissue growth near second thoracic ganglion	Federlay, 1935, 1936 (137, 138) ?
	Growth of vacuolized giant cells	Orösi-Pal, 1937 (411)
Bombus terrestris	Adenoma-like growth of pharyngeal glands with hypersecretion and regressive changes	Palm, 1949 (416)

Order: Coeloptera

Phydecta variabilis	Abnormal growth of prothorax	Kirby and Spencer, 1826 (292) Balazuc, 1948 (17)
Other species of coeloptera	Developmental abnormalities	Kraatz, 1881 (301); Pantel, 1898 (417); Balazuc, 1948 (17); Krieg, 1973 (308) (review)

Order: Diptera

Musca domestica	Melanotic tumors with sclerotizations	Bodnaryk, 1968 (38) (exp.)
Drosophila sp.	Benign neoplasms in the sclerotizations	Gateff, 1978 (155)*

PHYLUM: ECHINODERMATA
Class: Asteroidea

Asterias forbesi	Abnormal growth	Bang, 1977 (212)

Class: Ophiuroidea

Ophiocomina nigra	Melanoma (?) (Accumulation of pigment cells)	Fontaine, 1962 (148)

PHYLUM: TUNICATA

Ascidiella sp.	Multiple cysts containing protozoa	Laird, 1975 (209)

PHYLUM: VERTEBRATA
Superclass: Pisces
Class: Agnatha

Superorder: Cyclostomata
O.: Petromyzontiformes

Lampetra fluviatilis	Well-differentiated hepatocellular neoplasm	Falkmer, 1975 (209), 1976 (132)

*See also Chapter 30 by Burdette.

Table 48.5—Continued

<table>
<tr><td></td><td colspan="2">O.: Myxiniformes</td></tr>
<tr><td><u>Myxine glutinosa</u></td><td>Adenocarcinoma - solid tumor (mucus granuloma)</td><td>Falkmer, 1975 (209); 1976 (132)</td></tr>
<tr><td></td><td>Adenocarcinoma - solid tumor</td><td>Falkmer, 1975 (209); 1976 (132)</td></tr>
<tr><td></td><td>Cholangioma</td><td>Falkmer, 1975 (209)</td></tr>
<tr><td></td><td>Cholangiocellular carinoma</td><td>Falkmer, 1975 (209); 1976 (132)</td></tr>
<tr><td></td><td>Cholangiohyperplasia</td><td>Falkmer, 1975 (209); 1976 (132)</td></tr>
<tr><td></td><td>Cutaneous leiomyosarcoma</td><td>Falkmer, 1975 (209); 1976 (132)</td></tr>
<tr><td></td><td>Cutaneous leiomyosarcoma - fibroma (?) sarcoma</td><td>Falkmer, 1975 (209); 1976 (132)</td></tr>
<tr><td></td><td>Cutaneous leiomyosarcoma, sessile skin polyp containing ganglion cells (?), myelomeningocoele (?) "myxoma"</td><td>Falkmer, 1975 (209); 1976 (132)</td></tr>
<tr><td></td><td>Epidermoid cyst</td><td>Falkmer, 1975 (209); 1976 (132)</td></tr>
<tr><td></td><td>Non-neoplastic cysts</td><td>Falkmer, 1975 (209); 1976 (132)</td></tr>
<tr><td></td><td>Hamartoma (?) highly differentiated insuloma</td><td>Falkmer, 1975 (209); 1976 (132)</td></tr>
<tr><td></td><td>Hamartoma (?), insuloma-hamartoma</td><td>Falkmer, 1975 (209); 1976 (132)</td></tr>
<tr><td></td><td>Hemorrhage</td><td>Falkmer, 1975 (209); 1976 (132)</td></tr>
<tr><td></td><td>Hepatocellular carcinoma</td><td>Falkmer, 1975 (209); 1976 (132)</td></tr>
<tr><td></td><td>Hepatocellular and cholangiocellular (cholangiocellular carcinoma and nodular hyperplasia (?))</td><td>Falkmer, 1975 (209); 1976 (132)</td></tr>
<tr><td></td><td>Hepatocellular and cholangiocellular adenomas</td><td></td></tr>
<tr><td></td><td>Hepatocellular and cholangiocellular bleedings</td><td>Falkmer, 1975 (209); 1976 (132)</td></tr>
<tr><td></td><td>Hepatocellular and cholangiocellular carcinomas</td><td>Falkmer, 1975 (209); 1976 (132)</td></tr>
<tr><td></td><td>Hepatocellular hyperplasia (nodular) vs. adenoma</td><td>Falkmer, 1975 (209); 1976 (132)</td></tr>
<tr><td></td><td>Hepatocellular neoplasm; granuloma (well-differentiated)</td><td>Falkmer, 1975 (209); 1976 (132)</td></tr>
<tr><td></td><td>Hepatocellular neoplasm; incipient</td><td>Falkmer, 1975 (209); 1976 (132)</td></tr>
<tr><td></td><td>Hepatocellular neoplasm (multiple) and cholangiohyperplasias</td><td>Falkmer, 1975 (209); 1976 (132)</td></tr>
<tr><td></td><td>Hepatocellular neoplasm (multiple nodules, well-differentiated)</td><td>Falkmer, 1975 (209); 1976 (132)</td></tr>
</table>

Table 48.5—Continued

Class: Chondrychthyes

O.: Squaliformes

Carcharhinus leucas	Fibrosarcoma	Harshbarger, 1973 (204)
Carcharhinus milberti	Reticulum cell sarcoma	Harshbarger, 1973 (204)
Ginglymostoma cirratum	Adenoma or follicular hyperplasia possibly of thyroid origin	Gruber et al., 1977 (212)
Prionace glauca	Adenoma, liver	Schroeders, 1908 (496)
Scyliorhinus caniculus	Chondroma, right flank	Thomas, 1933 (see 482)
	Epidermoid carcinoma, oral	Stolk, 1956 (349)
	Odontoma	Ladreyt, 1929 (312)
	Osteoma, trunk	Thomas, 1933 (see 482)
Squalus acanthias	Choroid plexus papilloma	Prieur, 1976 (209)
	Fibroepithelial polyps, oral	Wellings, 1969 (617)
Squalus fernandinus	Chondroma, lumbar vertebrae	Takahashi, 1929 (567)
	Thyroid tumor	Cameron and Vincent, 1915 (62)
Raja batis	Malignant melanoma, posterior fin	Johnstone, 1911-1912 (247, 248)
	Malignant melanoma	Johnstone, 1913 (249)
Raja clavata	Malignant melanoma, head	Johnstone, 1910-1911 (246)
	Malignant melanoma, head	Johnstone, 1911-12 (247, 248)
	Melanomas	Haddow and Blake, 1933 (186)
Raja macrorhynchus	Fibrosarcoma	Drew, 1912 (115)
Raja maculata		Drew, 1912 (115)

Class: Osteichthyes
O.: Elopiformes

Elops saurus	Chondroma, subcutaneous	Surbeck, 1921 (560)

O.: Acipenseriformes
(Anguilliformes)

Acepenser oxyrhynchus	Normal hematopoietic tissue peripheral to heart	Meyers, 1975 (209)
Anguilla anguilla	Adenocarcinoma	Plehn, 1924 (444)
	Adenocarcinoma, kidney	Schmey, 1911 (492)
	Fibrosarcoma, coelom	Wolff, 1912 (635)
	Fibrosarcoma, coelom	Plehn, 1924 (444)
	Papilloma	Thomas and Oxner, 1930 (588)
	Papilloma	Christiansen and Jensen, 1947 (77)
	Papilloma	Schaeperclaus, 1953 (481)
	Papilloma	Luemann and Mann, 1956 (332)
	Papilloma	Mattheis, 1964 (342)
	Papilloma, oral	Deys, 1969 (105)

Table 48.5—Continued

	Papilloma	Mann et al., 1970 (335)
	Hepatoma	Hine, 1975 (209)
	Hyperblastic epidermis with hypertrophic goblet cells	Hine, 1975 (209)
	Tissue with cyst-like structure	Hine, Boustead, 1975 (209)

O.: Clupeiformes

Bevoortia sp.	Double fracture of fin spine, associated with parasitic granulomas	Kandrashoff (?) (212)
Bevoortia gunteri	Lipoma	Johnson, 1977 (212)
Clupea harengus harengus	Leiomyoma (?)	Thomas, 1933 (586)
	Lymphosarcoma	Johnstone, 1926 (263)
	Rhabdomyoma	Williams, 1931 (630)
	Rhabdomyoma	Mawdesley-Thomas, 1972 (348)
Conger conger	Fibrosarcoma, subcutaneus	Johnstone, 1920 (254)
	Hemangioepithelioma	Drew, 1912 (115)
	Lymphosarcoma, kidney	Williams, 1931 (630)
Electrophorus electricus	Papilloma, trunk	Coates et al., 1938 (81)
Muraena helena	Adenocarcinoma, oral	Ladreyt, 1935 (314)
Sardinia pilchardus	Fibroma	Johnstone, 1911-12 (see 349)
	Fibroma	Johnstone, 1924-25 (259)
	Fibroma	Biavati and Mancini, 1967 (35)
Coregonus hoyi	Olfactory neuroepithelioma	Harshbarger, 1973 (204)
Esox lucius	Adenocarcinoma, ovary	Haddow and Blake, 1933 (186)
	Fibrosarcoma, kidney	Plehn, 1906 (440)
	Fibrosarcoma, trunk	Ohlmacher, 1898 (408)
	Fibroma, trunk	Plehn, 1906 (440)
	Lipoma, subcutaneous	Bergman, 1921 (32)
	Lymphosarcoma, general	Mulcahy, 1963 (381)
	Lymphosarcoma, general	Mulcahy and O'Rourke, 1964 (383, 384)
	Lymphosarcoma, kidney	Nigrelli, 1947 (392)
	Lymphosarcoma, subcutaneous	Haddow and Blake, 1933 (186)
	Osteoma, fin	Plehn, 1906 (440)
	Osteoma, mandible	Bland-Sutton, 1885 (564)
	Osteosarcoma, fin	Wahlgren, 1876 (613)
	Sarcoma	Ljungberg and Lange, 1968 (322)
	Thyroid tumor (?)	Marine and Lenhart, 1910 (337)
Hucho hucho	Fibrosarcoma, liver	Plehn, 1909 (441)
Hypomesus	Sarcoma	Hoshina, 1950 (234)
Oncorhynchus gorbuscha	Fibrosarcoma	Takahashi, 1929 (567)

Table 48.5—Continued

Oncorhynchus keta	Fibrosarcoma	Takahashi, 1929 (567)
	Lymphosarcoma	Honma and Hirosaki, 1966 (233)
	Osteoma	Bell, 1975 (209)
Oncorhynchus kisutch	Glochidia from Margaritifera margaritifera producing epithelial and stromal hyperplasia of host	Meyers, 1975 (209)
	Ependymoblastoma	Hoskins, 1977 (212)
	Ependymoblastoma	Hendricks, 1977 (212)
	Nephroblastoma	Hoskins and Bell, 1975 (212)
	Fibroma, back	Milleman, 1968 (370)
	Fibroma	Milleman, 1968 (370)
	Lymphosarcoma, stomach	Ashley et al., 1973 (205)
	Osteogenic sarcoma	Harshbarger, 1973 (204)
Oncorhynchus nerka	Rhabdomyosarcoma	Harshbarger, 1973 (204)
	Teratoid anomaly	Bell, 1977 (212)
Oncorhynchus rodurus	Hepatoma	Harshbarger, 1973 (204)
	Polyps, stomach	Harshbarger, 1973 (204)
Oncorhynchus tshawytscha	Glochidia from Margaritifera margaritifera producing epithelial and stromal hyperplasia of host	Meyers, 1975 (209)
	Melanoma	Hoskins and Bell, 1977 (212)
	Partial reduplication of the digestive tract: developmental anomaly	
	Undifferentiated spindle cell sarcoma; possibly an embryonal rhabdomyoma	Stevenson, 1977 (212)
Osmerus eperlanus	Squamous cell carcinoma, oral	Breslauer, 1916 (41)
	Rhabdomyoma, trunk	Bergman, 1921 (32)
Osmerus mordax	Neurilemmoma	Logan and Odense, 1975 (209)
Plecoglossus altevelis	Adrenal tumor	Honma, 1966 (230)
	Hemangioendothelioma	Honma, 1966 (230)
	Lipoma, subcutaneous	Takahashi, 1929 (567)
	Lymphosarcoma, ovary	Honma, 1966 (230)
	Myxoma	Honma, 1965 (229)
Salmo aguabonita	Renal vs. thyroid adenocarcinoma	Smith, 1975 (209)
	Rhabdomyosarcoma	Adami, 1908 (2)
Salmo clarki	Carcinoma (? of ultimobranchial gland)	Smith, 1977 (212)
	Rhabdomyoma, trunk	Hine, 1975 (209)
Salmo gairdneri	Adenoma, liver	Haddow and Blake, 1933 (186)

Table 48.5 — Continued

	Adenoma, thyroid	Leger, 1925 (318)
	Cavernous hemangioma	Stevenson, 1977 (212)
	Cholangiocystadenoma	Honma and Shirai, 1959 (231)
	Cystadenoma, liver	Honma and Shirai, 1959 (231)
	Fibrosarcoma	Leger, 1925 (318)
	Fibrosarcoma, trunk	Mawdesley-Thomas, 1971 (345, 346)
	Hepatoma	Bucke, 1975 (209)
	Hyperplasia, thyroid	Robertson and Chaney, 1953 (460)
	Leiomyoma, oral	Kubota, 1955 (349)
	Leiomyoma, stomach	Plehn, 1906 (440)
	Lymphoma (?)	Hine, 1975 (209)
	Malignant lymphoma, diffuse and poorly differentiated	Smith, 1975 (209)
	Nephroblastoma	Hnath, 1975 (209)
	Nephroblastoma	Wolf, 1977 (212)
	Neurilemmoma	Wolf, 1977 (212)
	Neurilemmoma	Stevenson, 1977 (212)
	Rhabdomyoma	Mawdesley-Thomas and Jolly, 1968 (354)
	Rhabdomyoma	Mawdesley-Thomas, 1969 (see 349)
Salmo mykis	Adenoma, gut	Thomas, 1931 (582)
Salmo salar	Leiomyosarcoma of swim bladder	McKnight, 1978 (212)
	Lymphosarcoma, kidney	Haddow and Blake, 1933 (186)
	Pseudocysts of possible parasitic origin in the liver	Smith, 1975 (209)
	Thyroid tumor (?)	Gilruth, 1902 (173)
	Thyroid tumor (?)	Wilkie, 1891 (627)
	Teratoid anomaly	Hnath, 1977 (212)
Salmo trutta	Adenoma, gill	Sarkar and Dutta Chaudhuri, 1964 (473)
	Adenoma, liver	Plehn, 1909 (441)
	Adenocarcinoma, thyroid	Smith, 1909 (516)
	Fibroma, coelom	Kreyberg, 1937 (304)
	Fibroma, subcutaneous	Eberth, 1878 (120)
	Leiomyoma, stomach	Pesce, 1907 (431)
	Leiomyoma, viscera	Stevenson, 1977 (212)
	Myxofibrosarcoma	Hine, 1975 (209)
	Odontoma	Plehn, 1915 (443)
	Papilloma, skin	Thomas, 1932 (585)
	Thyroid tumor (?)	Bonnet, 1883 (39)
	Thyroid tumor	Ayson, 1896 (12)
	Thyroid tumor	Ayson, 1898 (13)
	Thyroid tumor	Ayson, 1902 (14)
Salmo spp.	Adenocarcinoma, thyroid	Gilruth, 1902 (173)

Table 48.5—Continued

<u>Salmo</u> spp.	Adenocarcinoma, thyroid	Jaboulay, 1908 (241)
	Adenocarcinoma, thyroid	Jaboulay, 1908 (242)
	Erythrophoroma, skin	Thomas, 1931 [++]
	Thyroid tumor (?)	Plehn, 1902 (439)
	Thyroid tumor (?)	Pick, 1905 (436)
	Thyroid tumor (?)	Marine and Lenhart, 1910 (336, 337)
	Thyroid tumor (?)	Gaylord and Marsh, 1912 (163)
	Thyroid tumor (?)	Gaylord and Marsh, 1912 (163)
	Thyroid tumor (?)	Peyron and Thomas, 1930 (432)
<u>Salvelinus fontinalis</u>	Lymphosarcoma	Dunbar, 1969 (117)
	Osteoma	Thomas, 1932 (584)
	Sarcoma, trunk	Plehn, 1906 (440)
	Thyroid tumor (?)	Scott, 1891 (499)
<u>Salvelinus fontinalis</u> X <u>S. miyabe</u>	Fibrosarcoma	Harshbarger, 1973 (204)
<u>Salvelinus namaycush</u>	Fibroma	Broughton and Choquette, 1971 (see 349)
	Hemangioendothelioma arising from blood vessels in the liver	Smith, 1977 (212)
	Lipoma, well differentiated	Bell, 1975 (209)
	Lymphosarcoma	Dunbar, 1969 (117)
<u>Abramis brama</u>	Fibroma, coelom	Plehn, 1906 (440)
	Lipoma, subcutaneous	Mawdesley-Thomas and Bucke, 1968 (352)
	Lymphosarcoma	Bucke, 1975 (209)
<u>Alburnus alburnus</u>	Leiomyoma, trunk	Plehn, 1906 (440)
<u>Anoptichthys jordani</u>	Melanoma, eye	Stolk, 1959 (see 349)
<u>Astyanax mexicanus</u>	Lymphosarcoma, head	Nigrelli, 1947 (392)
<u>Barbus barbus</u>	Chondroma, mandible	Surbeck, 1921 (560)
	Squamous cell carcinoma, lip	Keysselitz, 1908 (288)
	Squamous cell carcinoma, lip	Clunet, 1910 (80)
	Tumor, thyroid	Stolk, 1957 (see 349)
<u>Barbus tetrazona</u>	Adenocarcinoma, kidney	Stolk, 1957 (541)
<u>Brachydania rerio</u>	Liver cell tumor	Stanton, 1965 (205)
	Melanosarcoma	Stolk, 1953 (532)
<u>Carassius auratus</u>	Carcinoma, generalized	Ceretto, 1968 (70)
	Carcinoma, transitional cell, urinary bladder	Plehn, 1909 (441)
	Fibroma, orbit	Guglianetti, 1910 (185)
	Fibroma, skin	Sagawa, 1925 (470)
	Fibroma, subcutaneous	Eguchi and Oota, 1926 (121)
	Fibroma, subcutaneous	Wago, 1922 (611)
	Fibrosarcoma, fin	Dominguez, 1928 (112)

Table 48.5—Continued

Carassius auratus	Fibrosarcoma, fin	Sutton, 1885 (564)
	Fibrosarcoma, skin	Montpellier and Dieuziede, 1932 (377)
	Fibrosarcoma, skin	Schamberg and Lucke, 1922 (482)
	Fibrosarcoma, subcutaneous	Johnstone, 1923 (257)
	Fibrosarcoma, subcutaneous	Roffo, 1924 (462)
	Fibrosarcoma, subcutaneous	Lucke et al., 1948 (331)
	Fibrosarcoma, urinary tract	Semer, 1888 (501)
	Leiomyoma	Lucke et al., 1948 (331)
	Lymphosarcoma, kidney	Plehn, 1924 (444)
	Melanoma, orbit	Mawdesley-Thomas, 1972 (347, 348)
	Neurofibroma/neurolemmoma	Roberts, 1975 (209)
	Neurofibroma, subcutaneous	Picchi, 1933 (435)
	Neurilemmomas	Schlumberger, 1951 (488)
	Neurilemmomas	Schlumberger, 1952 (see 349)
	Neurilemmomas	Mawdesley-Thomas, 1972 (347, 348)
	Neurilemmomas (two cases)	Wolf, 1977 (212)
	Papilloma, skin (?)	Sagawa, 1925 (470)
	Ichthyematoma (fish scale tumor)	Herwig, 1977 (212)
Carassius carassius	Nephroblastoma metastatic to pancreas	Bucke, 1975 (209)
	Polycystic kidney	Bucke, 1975 (209)
Catostomus commersoni	Cholangiosarcoma	Dawe et al,,1964 (see 349)
	Papilloma, skin	Schlumberger and Lucke, 1948 (491)
Catostomus macrocheilus	Myoblastoma	Becker, 1975 (209)
Chilodus punctatus	Hemangioma	Stolk, 1958 (see 349)
Chondrostoma nasus	Fibrosarcoma, trunk	Plehn, 1906 (440)
Chondrostoma soetta	Squamous cell carcinoma, lip	Mazzarelli, 1910 (356)
	Squamous cell carcinoma lip	Stolk, 1959 (see 349)
Clarias dumerilii	Thyroid tumor (?)	Schreitmueller, 1924 (495)

O.: Cypriniformes

Ctenobrycon spilurus	Guanophoroma	Stolk, 1959 (551)
Cyprinus carpio	Fibromyxoma vs. inflammatory polyp	Migaki, 1975 (209)
	Focal spermatocytoma/early seminoma	Bucke, 1975 (209)
	Fibroma, coelom	Crips, 1854 (93)
	Fibroma, coelom	Ronca, 1914 (465)
	Nephroblastoma	Blasiola, Jr., 1977 (212)
	Neurilemmal sarcomas	Blasiola, Jr., 1977 (212)
	Olfactory neuroepithelioma, well differentiated	Prince Hitachi, 1975 (209)

Table 48.5 — Continued

Cyprinus carpio	Neurilemmoma	Harshbarger, 1973 (204)
	Osteoma, skull	Fiebiger, 1909 (140)
	Squamous cell carcinoma	Bashford et al., 1905 (26)
	Squamous cell carcinoma, operculum	Fiebiger, 1909 (140)
	Squamous cell carcinoma, skin	Dauwe and Penneman, 1904 (94)
Danio albolineatus	Thyroid tumor (?)	Klemm, 1927 (295)
Gobio gobio	Squamous cell carcinoma	Mawdesley-Thomas and Bucke, 1967 (350)
Gobio spp.	Papilloma, skin	Schroeders, 1908 (496)
Heteradandria formosa	Thyroid tumor (?)	Smith et al., 1936 (515)
Ictalurus catus	Adenoma, kidney	Schlumberger et Lucke, 1948 (491)
	Squamous cell carcinoma	McFarland, 1901 (360)
Ictalurus natalis	Papilloma, skin	Harshbarger, 1973 (204)
Ictalurus nebulosus	Liver cell tumor	Dawe et al., 1964 [++]
	Papilloma, skin	Steeves, 1969 (525)
Ictalurus sp.	Papilloma, skin	Harshbarger, 1973 (204)
Leuciscus idus	Fibrosarcoma, trunk	Plehn, 1906 (440)
	Squamous cell carcinoma	Mawdesley-Thomas, 1972 (348)
Leuciscus leuciscus	Lipoma, coelom	Mawdesley-Thomas, 1972 (348)
Mesogobius migroratatus	Papilloma, skin	Anitschkow and Pavlowsky, 1923 (9)
Mollienesia velifera	Adenocarcinoma, coelom	Raabe, 1939 (450)
Mystus seenghala	Leiomyoma	Sarkar et al., 1955 (474)
	Kidney tumor	Sathyanesan, 1966 (478)
Mystus vittatus	Pituitary tumor	Sathyanesan, 1962 (476)
Phenecogrammus interruptus	Epidermal carcinoma, well differentiated	Hicks, 1977 (212)
Phoxinus phoxinus	Chondroma, mandible	Andre, 1927 (7)
	Fibrosarcoma, tail	Bugnion, 1875 (57)
	Fibrosarcoma, trunk	Plehn, 1906 (440)
Poecilia reticulata	Adenoma (?), Carcinoma (?)	Vivian and Ruhland-Gaiser, 1954 (606)
	Carcinoma, pharynx	Stolk, 1955 (see 349)
	Fibroma, heart	Stolk, 1957 (see 349)
	Fibroma, gut	Stolk, 1957 (see 349)
	Pituitary chromophobe adenoma	Stolk, 1953 (see 349)
	Sarcoma, undifferentiated	Wessing, 1959 (624)
	Sarcoma, generalized	Wessing and von Bargen, 1959 (625)
	Teratoma	Stolk, 1955 (see 349)
	Teratoma	Hisaoka, 1961 (226)

Table 48.5—Continued

Poecilia reticulata	Teratoma, ovary	Stolk, 1953 (see 349)
	Thyroid adenoma	Stolk, 1955 (see 349)
	Thyroid (?) tumor	Woodhead and Ellett, 1967 (205)
Poecilia reticulata X P. sphenops	Melanoma	Ghadially and Gordon, 1957 (170)
	Melanoma, skin	Stolk, 1958 (see 349)
Poecilobrycon harrison	Anal epithelioma	Harshbarger, 1973 (204)
Pristella riddlei	Sarcomas	Wessing, 1959 (624, 625)
	Sarcomas	Wessing and von Bargen, 1959 (624, 625)
Proterorhinus maratus	Papilloma, skin	Anitschkow and Pavlowsky, 1923 (9)
Rasbora daniconius	Fibroma, dorsal fin	Smith et al., 1936 (515)
Rasbora lateristriata	Lymphosarcoma	Smith et al., 1936 (515)
	Lymphosarcoma, coelom	Smith et al., 1936 (515)
	Thyroid tumor (?)	Smith et al., 1936 (515)
	Thyroid tumor (?)	Smith and Coates, 1937 (513)
Rasbora trilineata	Adenocarcinoma	Blasiola, 1975 (209)
Rhodeus ocellatus	Nephroblastoma	Prince Hitachi, 1975 (209)
Rutilus rutilus	Early bile duct adeno-fibrosis	Bucke, 1977 (212)
	Probable thyroid adenocarcinoma	Bucke, 1975 (209)
Semotilus atromaculatus	Protozoan cyst	Bucke, 1975 (209)
Tanichthys albonubes	Thyroid tumor (?)	Stolk, 1953 (see 349)
Thayeria obliqua	Adenocarcinoma, kidney	Stolk, 1957 (see 349)
Tinca tinca	Myxoma, orbit	Plehn, 1906 (440)
	Rhabdomyosarcoma, trunk	Kolmer, 1928 (298)
	Rhabdomyosarcoma, well-differentiated	Bucke, 1975 (209)
	Squamous cell carcinoma, lip	Fiebiger, 1909 (139)
Wallago attu	Osteogenic fibroma	Sarkar and Dutta-Chaudhuri, 1958 (see 349)
Xiphophorus helleri	Adenoma, kidney	Jahnel, 1939 (244)
	Adenoma, kidney	Stolk, 1955 (see 349)
	Adenoma, thyroid	Jahnel, 1939 (244)
	Adenoma, thyroid	Stolk, 1955 (see 349)
	Fibrosarcoma, eye	Jahnel, 1939 (244)
	Squamous cell carcinoma	Stolk 1953 (see 349)
	Teratoma	Hisaoka, 1963 (227)
Xiphophorus maculatus	Erythrophoroma	Ghadially and Whiteley, 1951 (169)
	Fibrosarcoma, head	Stolk, 1954 (see 349)

Table 48.5—Continued

Xiphophorus maculatus	Melanosarcoma, eye	Levine and Gordon, 1946 (319)
	Teratoma, ovary	Stolk, 1959 (see 349)
	Thyroid tumor (?)	Baker et al., 1955 (see 349)
	Xanthoerythrophoroma	Ermin, 1953 (130)
Xiphophorus maculatus X X. helleri	Erythrophoroma, skin	Smith et al., 1936 (515)
	Melanoma, eye	Levine and Gordon, 1946 (319)
	Melanoma, skin	Haeussler, 1928 (187)
	Melanoma, skin	Haeussler, 1929 (591)
	Melanoma, skin	Haeussler, 1934 (188)
	Melanoma, skin	Gordon, 1937 (180)
	Xanthoerythrophoroma (exp.)	Nigrelli et al., 1951 (400)
Xiphophorus montezumae	Thyroid tumor (?)	Gorbman and Gordon, 1951 (179)
	Thyroid tumor (?)	Berg et al., 1953 (31)
Xiphophorus pigmaeus	Melanoma, eye	Levine and Gordon, 1946 (319)
Xiphophorus variatus	Thyroid hyperplasia	Aronowitz et al., 1951 (11)
Xiphophorus variatus xiphidium	Melanoma, skin	MacIntyre and Baker-Cohen 1961 (334)
	Thyroid tumor (?)	MacIntyre and Baker-Cohen 1961 (334)
Xiphophorus spp. *	Adenocarcinoma, pancreas	Nigrelli and Gordon, 1951 (398)
	Erythromelanoma	Nigrelli et al., 1950 (399)
	Melanoma	Vielkind et al., 1971 (604, 605)
	Melanoma	Siciliano et al., 1971 (507)
	Melanosarcoma	Weissenfels et al., 1970 (616)
	O.: Lophiformes	
Acentrophyrne longidens	Fibrosarcoma	Nigrelli, 1946-47 (see 349)
Lophius piscatorius	Melanoma, skin	Ingleby, 1929 (237)
	O.: Gadiformes	
Gadus macrocephalus	Adenoma, pectoral gland	Takahashi, 1929 (567)
	Adenoma, parabranchial	Takahashi, 1929 (567)
	Neurofibroma, head	Wellings, 1969 (205)
	Neurofibroma	Wellings, 1969 (205)

---

* See chapter 29 by Schwab, Anders.

Table 48.5—Continued

<u>Gadus morhua</u>	Fibroma, esophagus	Williamson, 1911 (632)
	Fibroma, gut	Thomas, 1931 (581)
	Fibroma, orbit	Johnstone, 1914 (250, 251)
	Fibroma, stomach	Hunter, 1782 (235)
	Fibroma, stomach	Sutton, 1885 (564)
	Fibroma, stomach	Johnstone, 1923-25 (258)
	Fibroma, stomach	Johnstone, 1924-25 (259)
	Fibroma, subcutaneous	Sutton, 1885 (564)
	Fibrosarcoma, oral	Johnstone, 1920 (254)
	Fibrosarcoma, ovary	Thomas, 1927 (579)
	Fibrosarcoma, subcutaneous	Thomas, 1927 (579)
	Fibrosarcoma, subcutaneous	Johnstone, 1911-1912 (see 349)
	Fibrosarcoma, trunk	Williams, 1931 (630)
	Ganglioneuroma, trunk	Thomas, 1927 (579)
	Hemangioma, pectoral region	Murray, 1908 (387)
	Hemangioma, swim bladder	Johnstone, 1923-25 (258)
	Hemangioma, swim bladder	Johnstone, 1924-25 (259)
	Lymphosarcoma, orbit	Wolke and Wyand, 1969 (636)
	Melanosarcoma	Mawdesley-Thomas, 1971 (345, 346)
	Osteoma, maxilla	Sutton, 1885 (564)
	Osteoma, maxilla	Williams, 1929 (629)
	Osteoma, vertebra	Sutton, 1885 (564)
	Osteoma, vertebra	Williamson, 1911 (632)
	Osteosarcoma, operculum	Murray, 1908 (387)
	Osteosarcoma, pectoral fin	Thomas, 1932 (584)
	Sarcoma, swim bladder	Bashford and Murray, 1904 (25)
<u>Gadus virens</u>	Chondroma, head	Thomas, 1932 (584)
	Fibroma	Lawrence, 1895 (316)
	Fibroma, oral	Fiebiger, 1909 (139)
	Fibrosarcoma, mandible	Johnstone, 1926 (263)
	Fibrosarcoma, skin	Fiebiger, 1912 (142)
	Fibrosarcoma, subcutaneous	Johnstone, 1926 (263)
	Hemangioma, trunk	Johnstone, 1926 (263)
	Lipoma, liver	Thomas, 1933 (587)
	Rhabdomyoma, gut	Fiebiger, 1909 (141)
	Squamous cell carcinoma	Williams, 1929 (629)
<u>Melanogrammus aglefinus</u>	Adamantinoma, maxilla	Thomas, 1926 (578)
	Fibroma, subcutaneous	Johnstone, 1923-25 (258)
	Fibroma, subcutaneous	Johnstone, 1924 (260)
	Fibroma, subcutaneous	Johnstone, 1924-25 (259)
	Fibroma, subcutaneous	Johnstone, 1910-11 (246)

Table 48.5—Continued

	Fibroma, subcutaneous	Johnstone, 1911-12[++]
	Fibroma, trunk	Mawdesley-Thomas, 1971 (345, 346)
	Fibrosarcoma, head	Johnstone, 1922 (256)
	Melanoma, skin	Prince, 1891
Merlangus merlangus	Fibroma	Mawdesley-Thomas, 1971 (345, 346)
	Hamartoma, gut	Labbe, 1930 (310)
	Squamous cell carcinoma, oral	Johnstone, 1923-25 (258)
Merlucius merlucius	Hemangioma, gut	Johnstone, 1926 (263)
Molva molva	Adenoma, ovary	Johnstone, 1915 (253)
	Hemangioma, trunk	Johnstone, 1923-25 (258)
	Hemangioma, trunk	Johnstone, 1924 (260)
	Hemangioma, trunk	Johnstone, 1924-25 (259)
Therargra chalcogramma	Adenoma, parabranchial body	Takahashi, 1929 (567)
	Fibroma, trunk	Takahashi, 1929 (567)
	Fibrosarcoma, subcutaneous	Takahashi, 1929 (567)
	Fibrosarcoma, trunk	Takahashi, 1929 (567)
	Melanoma, skin	Takahashi, 1929 (567)
	Osteoma, fin	Takahashi, 1929 (567)
	Sarcoma	Nishikawa, 1954 (402)
	Squamous cell carcinoma, oral	Takahashi, 1929 (567)
Zoarces viviparus	Melanoma, skin	Bergman, 1921 (32)
	O.: Cypridontiformes	
Anatolichtys sp.	Carcinoma of orbit	Ermin, 1954 (131)
Cyprinodon variegatus	Ameloblastoma, jaw	Stolk, 1957 (see 349)
	Thyroid adenoma	Nigrelli, 1952 (see 349)
Epiplatys chaperi	Thyroid tumor (?)	Klemm, 1927 (295)
Fundulus heteroclitus	Thyroid adenoma	Nigrelli, 1952 (see 349)
Girardinus falcutus	Thyroid tumor (?)	MacIntyre, 1960 (333)
Jordanella floridae	Thyroid tumor (?)	Schreitmueller 1924 (495)
Nothobranchius guentheri	Erythrophoroma	Stolk, 1959 (see 349)
Rivulvus xanthonotus	Xanthophoroma	Stolk, 1959 (see 349)
Various species	Sarcomas	Breider, 1939 (40)
	O.: Gasterosteiformes	
Gasterosteus aculeatus	Fibroma, tail	Mawdesley-Thomas, 1972 (348)
	Hemangioma, head	Plehn, 1906 (440)
Pungitius pungitius	Hemangioma, eye	Johnstone, 1915 (253)

Table 48.5—Continued

Spinachia spinachia	Squamous cell carcinoma, skin	Murray, 1908 (387)
	O.: Perciformes	
Acanthogobius flavimanus	Papilloma (?)	Oata, 1952 (409)
	Papilloma, skin	Nishikawa, 1954 (402)
	Papilloma, skin	Oata, 1952 (409)
	Papilloma, skin	Imai and Fujiwara, 1959 (236)
	Papilloma, skin	Kimura et al., 1967 (290)
	Papilloma, skin	Harshbarger, 1973 (204)
	Sarcoma, undifferentiated	Nishikawa, 1955 (403)
Aequidens maronii	Malignant lymphoma	Harshbarger, 1973 (204)
Anabas testudineus	Papilloma, skin	Fiebiger, 1909 (139)
Angelichthys isabelita	Adenocarcinoma, thyroid	Nigrelli, 1952 (395)
	Adenocarcinoma, thyroid	Nigrelli, 1952 (393)
Archosargus probatocephalus	Guanophoroma, skin	Mawdesley-Thomas, 1972 (347, 348)
Arripis trutta	Leiomyoma	Hine, 1975 (209)
Bathygobius soporator	Squamous cell carcinoma	Tavolga, 1951 (570)
Betta anabantoides	Adenocarcinoma, pharyngeal	Stolk, 1962 (see 349)
Blennius spp.	Xanthoma, skin	Schroeders, 1908 (496)
Boops boops	Thyroid tumor (?)	Johnstone, 1923-25 (258)
	Thyroid tumor (?)	Johnstone, 1924 (260)
	Thyroid tumor (?)	Johnstone, 1924-25 (259)
Callionymus lyra	Lipoma	Williams, 1929 (629)
Caranx hippos	Fibroma	Schwartz, 1975 (209)
Caranx lutescens	Melanocytic neurilemmoma (blue nevus)	Stevenson, 1977 (212)
Chaetodipterus faber	Osteoma, vertebrae	Schlumberger and Lucke, 1948 (491)
Chelidonichtys kumu	Allophoroma, subcutaneous	Takahashi, 1929 (567)
Chrysophris major	Adenocarcinoma, coelom	Takahashi, 1929 (567)
	Osteomas	Kazama, 1924 (282)
	Osteomas	Sagawa, 1925 (470)
Cichlasoma biocellatum	Thyroid tumor (?)	Stolk, 1956 (see 349)
Cichlasoma tetracanthus	Squamous cell carcinoma, skin	Puente-Duany, 1930 (449)
Colias labius	Papilloma, skin	Nigrelli, 1952 (see 349)
Cottus gobio	Neurilemmoma	Swinney, 1975 (209)
Cynoscion regalis	Ganglioneuroma	Zwerner and Ruddell, 1977 (see 212)

Table 48.5—Continued

Diodon hystrix	Lymphocystis	Cubit, 1977 (see 212)
Echeneis naucrates	Thyroid tumor (?)	Schlumberger and Lucke, 1948 (491)
Epinepheles guaza	Melanoma	Dollfuss et al., 1938 (111)
Epinepheles itajara	Mesotheliomas; rodlet cells	Shields, 1977 (see 212)
Etroplus maculatus	Squamous cell carcinoma	Stolk, 1960 (553)
Euthynnus alletteratus	Erythrophoroma, skin	Thomas 1931 (see 349)
Genyonemus lineatus	Epidermal papillomas	Chamberlain, 1975 (209)
	Papilloma	Russel and Kotin, 1957 (467)
Girella nigricans	Thyroid adenoma	Herman, 1975 (209)
Haplochromis multicolor	Adenoma, pharyngeal gland	Stolk, 1957 (see 349)
Hemichromis bimaculatus	Osteochondroma	Nigrelli and Gordon, 1946 (see 349)
Hexagrammos otakii	Guanophoroma, skin	Takahashi, 1929 (567)
Lateolabrax japonicus	Fibrosarcoma, subcutaneous	Takahashi, 1929 (567)
	Fibrosarcoma, pharynx	Takahashi, 1929 (567)
Labrus mixtus	Rhabdomyoma	Ladreyt, 1930 (313)
Leistomus xanthurus	(1) Thyroid hyperplasia in all fish; (2) gill hyperplasia in one fish	Cosgrove, 1975 (209)
Lepidopus, spp.	Osteoma, fin	Gervais, 1875 (168)
Lepidotrigla alata	Fibrosarcoma, subcutaneous	Takahashi, 1929 (567)
Lepomis megalotis	Thyroid hyperplasia	Schlumberger, 1955 (see 349)
Lumpenus sagitta	Neurofibroma	McArn and Wellings, 1967 (357)
Lutianus apodus	Neurofibroma	Lucke, 1942 (330)
Lutianus griseus	Neurofibroma	Lucke, 1942 (330)
	Neurofibroma	Harshbarger, 1973 (204)
Lutianus jocu	Neurofibroma	Lucke, 1942 (330)
Menidea beryllina	Melanoma, skin	Nigrelli and Gordon, 1944 (397)
Micropogon opercularis	Osteoma	Bertullo and Traibel, 1955 (34)
Micropogon undulatus	Odontoma, mouth	Roffo, 1925 (463)
	Sarcoma, subcutaneous	Roffo, 1926 (464)

Table 48.5—Continued

Micropterus salmoides	Lipoma	Mawdesley-Thomas, 1972 (348)
	Melanoma	Erdman, 1968 (128)
Mojarra (? member fam. Geridae) +	Lipoma	Kandrashoff, 1977 (see 212)
Morone americana	Bile duct adenofibrosis	Beckerman and Morgan, 1975 (209)
	Bile duct adenofibrosis	Beckerman and Morgan, 1975 (209)
	Hyperplasia of dermis	Beckerman and Morgan, 1975 (209)
Morone saxatalis	Leiomyoma (?)	Smith, 1975 (209)
	Nephroblastoma	Helmboldt and Wyand, 1971 (219)
Mugil cephalus	Dermal fibroma with areas of ossification	Overstreet, 1975 (209)
Myxocephalus octodecemspinosus	Renal cystadenoma	Harshbarger, 1973 (204)
	Teratocarcinoma	Harshbarger, 1973 (204)
Ophiodon elongatus	Lymphocystis	Bell and Hoskins, 1975 (209)
Perca flavescens	Testicular tumor	Budd, Schroeder, Dukes, 1975 (56)
Perca fluviatalis	Malignant schwannoma (?)	Finkelstein and Dancheno-Ryzchkova, 1965 (144)
	Rhabdomyoma	Finkelstein and Dancheno-Ryzchkova, 1965 (144)
Pogonias chromis	Fibrolipoma	Johnson, 1977 (212)
	Fibrosarcoma, subcutaneous	Beatti, 1916 (29)
	Osteoma, vertebra	Beatti, 1916 (29)
	Squamous cell carcinoma, mouth	Beatti, 1916 (29)
Pomatomus saltatrix	Lymphangioepithelioma	Harshbarger, 1973 (204)
Pomoxix nigromaculatus	Lipoma	Harshbarger, 1973 (204)
Porgy (Pagrus pagrus ? - member fam. Sparidae) +	Lipoma	Kandrashoff, 1977 (212)
Platyglossus bivattus	Papilloma	Lucke, 1937-38 (329)
Pseudotropheus tropheops	Neurilemmal sarcoma	Blasiola, 1975 (209)
Pterogobius elapoides	Adenoma	Prince Hitachi, 1977 (212)
Pterophyllum eimekei	Melanoma	Mawdesley-Thomas, 1971 (346)
Pterophyllum scalare	Melanoma	Stolk, 1960 (554)

Table 48.5—Continued

Sciaenida spp.	Osteomas	Chabanaud, 1926 (71)
Scomber colias	Melanosarcoma, skin	Takahashi, 1929 (567)
Scomber scombrus	Hamartoma, pineal	Charlton, 1929 (75)
	Hemangioma, trunk	Johnstone, 1923-25 (258)
	Hemangioma, trunk	Johnstone, 1924 (260)
	Hemangioma, trunk	Johnstone, 1924-25 (259)
Scorpaena inermis	Fibroma, subcutaneous	Takahashi, 1929 (567)
Scorpaena porcus	Fibrosarcoma, subcutaneous	Schroeders, 1908 (496)
Sebastes crameri	Thyroid carcinoma	Harshberger, 1973 (204)
Sebastes diploproa	Lipoma	Harshbarger, 1973 (204)
Sebastes sp.	Parabranchial body adenoma	Hoskins, 1975 (209)
Seranus cabrilla	Thyroid tumor (?)	Marsh and Vonwiller, 1916 (338)
Serranus scrila	Thyroid tumor (?)	Marsh and Vonwiler, 1916 (338)
Snapper (member of fam. Lutjanidae)+	Neurilemmoma	Sigel, 1975 (209)
Sparus auratus	Neuroepithelioma, olfactory plate	Thomas, 1932 (see 349)
Stizostediion vitreum	Fibroma and fibrosarcoma	Walker, 1958 (614)
Tautoglabrus	Papilloma	Harshberger, 1973 (204)
Trachurus trachurus	Lipoma, trunk	Anadon, 1956 (5)
	O.: Pleuronectiformes	
Glyptocephalus cynoglossus	Papilloma, skin	Honma and Kon, 1968 (232)
Glyptocephalus stelleri	Papilloma, skin	Honma and Kon, 1968 (232)
Glyptocephalus zachirus	Papilloma, skin	Wellings et al., 1965 (619)
Hippoglossoides dubius	Papilloma, skin	Kimura et al., 1967 (290)
Hippoglossoides elassodon	Papilloma, skin	Wellings et al., 1964 (618)
Hippoglossus hippoglossus	Fibroma, coelom	Johnstone, 1913 (249)
	Fibroma, trunk	Johnstone, 1914 (250, 251)
	Fibroma, subcutaneous	Johnstone, 1926 (263)

Table 48.5—Continued

<u>Hippoglossus hippoglossus</u>	Fibrosarcoma, trunk	Johnstone, 1926 (263)
	Lipoma, trunk	Williams, 1929 (629)
	Melanoma, skin	Johnstone, 1915 (253)
	Papilloma, snout	Johnstone, 1911-12 (349)
	Rhabdomyoma, trunk	Thomas, 1932 (583)
<u>Hippoglossus stenolepis</u>	Fibroma, mandible	Wellings, 1969 (617)
	Fibroma, trunk	Wellings, 1969 (617)
	Fibrolipoma, tail	Wellings, 1969 (617)
	Fibroosteoma	Wellings, 1969 (617)
	Lipoosteoma	Wellings, 1969 (617)
<u>Isopsetta isolepis</u>	Papilloma, skin	McArn, et al., 1968 (358)
<u>Lepidopsetta bilineata</u>	Epidermal papilloma	Bell, 1975 (209)
	Papilloma, skin	Nigrelli, et al., 1965 (401)
	Papilloma, skin	Wellings, 1969 (617)
<u>Lepidorhombus whiffiagonis</u>	Ganglioneuroma	Haddow and Blake, 1933 (186)
<u>Limanda herzensteiri</u>	Papilloma, skin	Kimura et al., 1967 (290)
<u>Limanda limanda</u>	Papilloma, skin	Johnstone, 1923-25 (258)
	Papilloma, skin	Johnstone, 1924-25 (259)
<u>Microstomus pacificus</u>	Papillomas, epidermal	Chamberlain, 1975 (209)
	Papillomas epidermal	Chamberlain, 1975 (209)
	Papilloma, skin	Harshbarger, 1973 (204)
	Papilloma, skin	Wellings, 1969 (205)
	Papilloma, skin	Young, 1964 (641)
<u>Paralichthys lethostigma</u>	Subcutaneous fibroma	Overstreet, 1975 (209)
<u>Paralichthys olivaceus</u>	Lipoma, trunk	Kazama, 1924 (282)
	Osteoma, vertebra	Takahashi, 1929 (567)
<u>Paraphrys vetulus</u>	Papilloma, skin	Cooper and Keller, 1969 (88)
	Papilloma, skin	Good, 1940 (177)
	Papilloma, skin	McArn, et al., 1968 (358)
	Papilloma, skin	Pacis, 1932 (414)
	Papilloma, skin	Wellings et al., 1966 (620)
<u>Platichthys flesus</u>	Lymphosarcoma, orbit	Johnstone, 1911-12 (349)
	Papilloma, skin	Sandeman, 1893 (471)
<u>Platichthys stellatus</u>	Papilloma, skin	Ketchen, 1953 (287)
	Papilloma, skin	McArn et al. (1968 (358)
	Papilloma, skin	Wellings et al. 1966 (620)
<u>Pleuronectes platessa</u>	Fibroma, fin	Johnstone, 1922 (255,256)
	Fibroma, fin	Johnstone, 1926 (263)
	Fibrosarcoma, subcutaneous	Drew, 1912 (115)
	Hemangioma, trunk	Johnstone, 1923-25 (258)
	Hemangioma, trunk	Johnstone, 1924-25 (259)
	Lipoma, trunk	Bergman, 1921 (32)
	Melanoma, skin	Johnstone, 1923-25 (258)
	Melanoma, skin	Johnstone, 1924-25 (259)

Table 48.5—Continued

Pleuronectes platessa	Myxoma, trunk	McIntosh, 1908 (365)
	Papilloma, skin	Chuinard, et al. 1966 (79)
	Papilloma, skin	Johnstone, 1923-25 (258)
	Papilloma, skin	Johnstone, 1924-25 (259)
	Papilloma, skin	Sandeman, 1893 (471)
	Papilloma, skin	Wellings and Chuinard, 1964 (618)
	Papilloma, skin	Wellings et al., 1963 (622)
	Papilloma, skin	Wellings et al., 1965 (619)
	Papilloma, skin	Wellings et al., 1966 (620)
	Papilloma, skin	Wellings et al., 1967 (621)
Psettichthys melanostictus	Papilloma, skin	Ketchen, 1953 (287)
	Papilloma, skin	Wellings et al., 1965 (619)
	Papilloma, skin	Nigrelli et al., 1965 (401)
	Papilloma, skin	McArn et al., 1968 (358)
Pseudopleuronectes americanus	Erythrophoroma	Smith, 1934 (512)
Pseudopleuronectes herzensteiri	Papilloma, skin	Kimura et al., 1967 (290)
Pseudopleuronectes yokohamae	Ganglioneuroma	Takahashi, 1929 (567)
Scophthalmus maeoticus	Fibrosarcoma, subcutaneous	Schroeders, 1908 (496)
	Myxoma, head	Schroeders, 1908 (496)
	Myxoma, trunk	Schroeders, 1908 (496)
	Osteoma, vertebra	Schroeders, 1908 (496)
Scophthalmus maximus	Fibroma, dorsal fin	Johnstone, 1924 (260)
	Fibrosarcoma, trunk	Johnstone, 1927 (264)
	Fibrosarcoma, subcutaneous	Johnstone, 1923 (257)
	Myxoma, trunk	Williams, 1929 (629)
	Rhabdomyoma, trunk	Young, 1925 (640)
Solea solea	Myxoma, coelom	Johnstone, 1926 (263)
	Papilloma, skin	Thomas, 1930 (580)

O.: Tetraodontiformes

Aluterus schoepfi	Osteoma	Schlumberger and Lucke, 1948 (491)

O.: Labyrinthici

Anabas testudineus	Epidermal papilloma	Pal, 1977 (212)

O.: Siluriformes

Corydoras sp.	Malignant melanophoroma	Herrin, 1977 (212)
Heteropneustes fossilis	Lipoma	Pal, 1977 (212)

O.:Atheriniformes

Cynolebias nigripinnis	Malignant lymphoma	Blasiola, 1977 (212)

Table 48.5—Continued

Class: Amphibia

O.: Caudata

Ambystoma mexicanum	Adenoma	DeLanney, 1977 (212)
	Lymphoma, lymph nodes	DeLanney, 1971 (205)
	Intradermal melanophoroma	DeLanney, 1977 (212)
	Mast cell tumors (?)	DeLanney, 1977 (212)
Ambystoma tigrinum	Fibrosarcoma	Rose, 1975 (209)
	Metastatic pancreatic carcinoma	Rose, 1975 (209)
Cryptobranchus allegheniesis	(Sertoli cell tumor, testes)	Cosgrove, 1968 (205)
Cynops pyrrhogaster	Neophroblastoma, kidney	Zwart, 1968 (205)
	Papilloma, integument	Duryee, 1971 (205)
	Papilloma, integument	Duryee, 1971 (205)
	Papilloma, integument	Duryee, 1971 (205)
Diemictylus viridescens	Mes. musculature	Burns and White, 1971 (59)
Megalobatrachus maximus	Adenocarcinoma, testes	Pick and Poll, 1903 (437)
	Fibroma, integument	Vaillant and Petit, 1902 (597)
	Fibroma, integument	Schwarz, 1923 (497)
Necturus maculatus	Undifferentiated tumor, kidney	Naumann, 1967 (205)
Necturus maculosus	Adenocarcinoma, kidney	Schlumberger, 1958 (490)
Notophthalmus viridescens	Neural neoplasm	Counts III, 1975 (209)
Siredon maxicanum	Epithelioma, integument	Sheremetieva, 1953 (502)
	Melanosarcoma, integument	Krontowsky, 1916 (309)
	Melanosarcoma, integument	Teutschlander, 1920 (571)
	Melanosarcoma, integument	Sheremetieva
	Neuroepithelioma, mouth	Brunst and Roque, 1967 (54)
Triturus alpestris	Adenocarcinoma, integument	Champy and Champy, 1935 (72)
	Carcinoma, integument	Rickenbacher, 1950 (458)
Triturus cristatus	Adenocarcinoma, integument	Murray, 1908 (387)
Triturus pyrrhogaster	Lymphosarcoma (?) abdomen	Inoue, 1954 (238)
	Nephroblastoma, kidney	Zwart, 1970 (643)
	Sarcoma, liver	Mori, 1954 (378)
	Sarcoma, liver	Inoue and Singer, 1963 (239)
Triturus taeniatus	Fibroma, integument	Stolk, 1958 (591)
Triturus vulgaris	Chondroma, integument	Broz, 1947 (51)

O.: Anura

Bufo americanus	Xanthosis (?)	Counts III, 1975 (209)

Table 48.5—Continued

Bufo bufo	Encapsulated tumor, kidney	Stolk, 1950 (591)
Bufo bufo japonicus	Fibroma, integument	Stolk, 1961 (591)
Bufo calamita	Adenocarcinoma, lungs	Elkan, 1960 (122)
Bufo marinus	Adenoma, parotis	Stolk, 1957 (591)
Ceratophryx ornata	Carcinoma, lungs	Ratcliffe, 1960 (454)
Cerytophrys ornata	Fibrosarcoma, appendage	Volterra, 1928 (607)
Dendrobates typographicus	Erythrophoroma, integument	Stolk, 1959 (591)
Diemictylus viridescens	Neoplasm of mesenchymal cells	Burns and White, 1971 (59)
Hyla arborea	Guanophoroma, integument	Stolk, 1959 (591)
	Xanthophoroma, integument	Stolk, 1959 (591)
	Hemangioma, heart	Stolk, 1958 (591)
Hyla regilla	Chondromyxoma	Frye, 1975 (209)
Rana arvalis	Adenoma, integument	Stolk, 1957 (591)
Rana catesbyana	Adenocarcinoma, integument	Duany, 1932 (116)
	Adenoma, integument	Llambles and Garcia, 1949 (323)
	Neurosarcoma	Schlumberger and Lucke, 1948 (491)
Rana calmitans	Myxosarcoma, tail	Schlumberger and Lucke, 1948 (491)
Rana esculenta	Adenoma, integument	Sechser, 1919 (500)
	Adenocarcinoma, integument	Masson and Schwarz, 1923 (341)
	Carcinoma, ovaries	Plehn, 1906 (440)
	Fibroma, mouth	Vaillant and Petit, 1902 (597)
	Hepatoma, liver	Willis, 1948 (633)
	Hypernephrotic carcinoma, kidney	Carl, 1913 (68)
	Sarcoma, appendage	Gheorhiu, 1930 (172)
Rana fusca	Myxochondrofibroma, appendage	Pirlot and Welsch, 1934 (438)
	Adenoma, integument	Pirlot and Welsch, 1934 (438)
Rana pipiens	Adenocarcinoma, kidney	Smallwood, 1905 (509)
	Adenocarcinoma, kidney	Downs, 1932 (114)
	Adenocarcinoma, kidney	Lucke, 1934 (327, 328)
	Adenocarcinoma, ovaries	Abrams, 1969 (1)
	Cutaneous neoplasms	Van Der Steen et al., 1972 (600)
	Hepatoma, liver	Abrams, 1969 (1)
	Liposarcoma	Duryee, 1965 (119)
	Lymphosarcoma, integument	Duryee, 1965 (119)
	Lymphosarcoma, lungs	Duryee, 1965 (119)
	Carcinoma, lungs	Rose, 1952[++]
	Mesothelioma, pleural sac	Duryee, 1965 (119)
	Papilloma, integument	Duryee, 1971 (205)

Table 48.5—Continued

<u>Rana temporaria</u>	Epithelioma, integument	Elkan, 1963 (123)
	Melanoma, integument	Rostand, 1958 (466)
<u>Rana virescens</u>	Osteogenic tumor, femur	Ohlmacher, 1898 (408)
<u>Rana</u> spp.	Adenoma, integument	Ebert, 1968 (591)
	Adenoma, integument	Pawlowsky, 1912 (429)
	Adenoma, integument	Pentimalli, 1914 (430)
	Adenocarcinoma, integument	Murray, 1908 (387)
	Adenocarcinoma, integument	Pawlowsky, 1912 (429)
<u>Triturus</u> sp.	Visceral tumor	Inoue et al., 1965 (591)
<u>Xenopus fraseri</u>	Lymphosarcoma, viscera	Balls, 1962 (20)
	Lymphosarcoma, viscera	Balls, 1962 (20)
<u>Xenopus laevis</u>	Adenocarcinoma, kidney	Elkan, 1960 (122)
	Adenocarcinoma, stomach	Elkan, 1970 (125)
	Fibroma, integument	Elkan, 1960 (122)
	Fibroma, pelvis	Elkan, 1960 (122)
	Hyperplasia (?) pancreatic islet	Cosgrove, 1977 (212)
	Lymphosarcoma, multiple	Cosgrove, 1977 (212)
	Lymphosarcoma, viscera	Balls, 1962 (20)
	Lymphosarcoma, viscera	Balls, 1962 (20)
	Lymphosarcoma, viscera	Balls, 1962 (20)
	Melanocarcinoma, integument	Elkan, 1963 (124)
	Nephroblastoma, kidney	Elkan, 1963 (124)
	Virus tumor	Balls, 1965 (22)
<u>Xenopus laevis laevis</u>	Lipoma, integument	Balls, 1962 (20)

Class: Reptilia

O.: Chelonia

<u>Chelonia mydas</u>	Fibroma, integument (?)	Smith, 1970 (205)
	Fibropapilloma, integument (?)	Waddell, 1966 (205)
	Fibropapillomas, integument	Balazs, 1977 (212)
	Fibropapillomas, integument	Balazs, 1977 (212)
	Papilloma, gallbladder	Smith, Coates, Nigrelli, 1941 (591)
	Papilloma, integument	Lucke, 1938 (329)
	Papilloma, integument	Smith and Coates, 1938 (514)
	Papilloma, integument	Nigrelli and Smith, 1938 (591)
	Papilloma, integument	Cantwell et al., 1968 (66)
<u>Chrysemis ornata callirostris</u>	Multiple granulomas, spleen	Elkan, 1975 (209)
<u>Emys orbicularis</u>	Fibroadenoma, lung	Bresler, 1963 (42)
<u>Eretmochelys imbricata</u>	Granuloma	Balazs, 1977 (212)
<u>Geomyda trijuga</u>	Carcinoma, integument	Cowan, 1968 (92)
	Carcinoma, thyroid	Cowan, 1968 (92)

Table 48.5—Continued

Malacocherus tornieri	Adenomatous proliferation of intrahepatic bile ducts	Effron et al.,1977 (132/43)*
Pelomedusa subruta	Myelogenous leukemia	Gorman, 1975 (212)
Pelusios subniger	Carcinoma, stomach Carcinoma, stomach	Plimmer, 1912 (446) Cowan, 1908 (92)
Platemys geoffroyana	Adenoma	Pick and Poll, 1903 (437)
Sternothaerus niger	Rhabdomyoma, heart	Plimmer, 1913 (447)
Sternothaerus odoratus	Papilloma, integument	Schlumberger and Lucke, 1948 (491)
Testudo elephantina	Adenocarcinoma, stomach	Plimmer, 1912 (446)
Testudo horsfeldi	Fibroadenoma, lung	Tsvetaeva, 1941 (592)

O.: Squamata

Acanthophis antarctieus	Lymphosarcoma, leukemic	Effron et al.,1977 (132/43)*
Agkistrodon halys brevicaudus	Biliary adenocarcinoma	Effron et al.,1977 (132/43)*
	Neurofibrosarcoma of spine	Effron et al.,1977 (132/43)*
Agkistrodon piscivorus	Fibroma, ovaries	Ippen, 1965 (240)
	Plasma cell tumor which was leukemic in the terminal phase	Finne, 1975 (209)
	Sarcoma, stomach	Cowan, 1968 (290)
Arizona elegans occidentalis	Pheochromocytoma	Effron et al.,1977 (132/43)*
Bitis arietans	Lymphosarcoma, leukemic	Effron et al.,1977 (132/43)*
	Scirrhous renal cortical adenoma	Effron et al.,1977 (132/43)*
Bitis gabonica gabonica	Scirrhous biliary adenocarcinoma	Effron et al.,1977 (132/43)*
Bitis nasicornis	Lymphosarcoma	Effron et al.,1977 (132/43)*
	Lymphosarcoma, leukemic	Effron et al.,1977 (132/43)*
Boa constrictor	Lymphocytic thyroiditis resembling Hashimoto's disease	Cowan, 1975 (209)
	Anitschkow myocyte tumor (?)	Elkan, 1975 (209)
	Lymphosarcoma, liver	Cowan, 1968 (290)
	Lipoma	Frye, 1977 (212)
	Renal adenocarcinoma	Montali, 1975 (209)
Bothrop atrax	Scirrhous adenocarcinoma of intrapancreatic ducts	Effron et al.,1977 (132/43)*

Table 48.5—Continued

<u>Coluber flagellum</u>	Adenocarcinoma, abdominal cavity	Ball, 1956, see also Wadsworth, 1956 (609)
<u>Crotalus horridus</u>	Adenoma, intestines	Wadsworth, 1956 (609)
	Adenocarcinoma, intestines	Wadsworth, 1956 (609)
<u>Crotalus horridus horridus</u>	Lymphosarcoma, leukemic	Effron et al., 1977 (132/43)*
<u>Crotalus mitchelli pyrrhus</u>	Adenocarcinoma of pancreatic duct	Effron et al., 1977 (132/43)*
<u>Crotalus viridus</u>	Fibrosarcoma	Ball, see Wadsworth, 1956 (609)
<u>Cyclura cornuta</u>	Osteochondrofibroma	Ippen, 1965 (240)
<u>Cyclura ricordi</u>	Biliary adenoma	Effron et al., 1977 (132/43)*
<u>Dispholidus typus</u>	Biliary adenoma	Effron et al., 1977 (132/43)*
	Hemangioma of liver	Effron et al., 1977 (132/43)*
<u>Elaphe guttata guttata</u>	Low grade granulocytic leukemia	Jacobson and Brannian, 1977 (212)
<u>Elaphe obsoleta</u>	Adenocarcinoma, intestines	Wadsworth, 1954 (608)
	Fibroma	Wadsworth, 1956 (609)
<u>Eunectes murinus</u>	Adenoma (polyps), stomach	Wadsworth, 1956 (609)
	Lymphosarcoma, liver	Frank & Schepky, 1969 (151)
	Granulosa cell tumor	Effron et al., 1977 (132/43)*
<u>Heterodon nasicus</u>	Lipo(?)sarcoma, cloaca	Wadsworth, 1954 (608)
<u>Heterodon platyrhinos</u>	Lymphosarcoma, liver	Cowan, 1968 (92)
<u>Homalopsis buccata</u>	Adenocarcinoma, biliary duct	Bergmann, 1941 (33)
<u>Hydrosaurus amboiensis</u>	Malignant lymphoma	Zwart and Harshbarger, 1972 (643)
<u>Iugana iugana</u>	Carcinoma, thyroid gland	Ippen, 1965 (240)
	Adenocarcinoma, in teratoma	Zwart, 1971 (205)
	Hepatoma, liver	Bland-Sutton, 1885 (564)
	Hepatoma, liver	Stolk, 1964 (591)
<u>Lacerta agilis</u>	Papilloma, integument	Koch, 1904 (296)
	Squamous cell cancer	Stolk, 1953 (591)
	Rhabdomyoma, heart	Stolk, 1958 (591)
<u>Lacerta muralis fiumensis</u>	Papilloma, integument	Heller, 1906 (218)
	Papilloma, integument	Schwarz, 1923 (497)

Table 48.5 — Continued

Lacerta viridis	Epidermal papilloma with intranuclear virus-like inclusions	Elkan, 1977 (212)
	Fibromatosis, integument	Ippen, 1965 (240)
	Osteoma	Stolk, 1958 (591)
	Papilloma, integument	Blanchard, 1890 (37)
	Papilloma, integument	Plehn, 1910 (442)
	Papilloma, integument	Klein, 1952 (294)
	Papilloma, integument	Schnabel, 1954 (493)
	Papilloma, integument	Potel, 1960 (448)
	Papilloma, integument	Elkan, 1963 (123,124)
	Papilloma, integument	Kridler, 1971 (205)
Lampropeltis getulus	Squamous, possibly mucoepidermoid carcinoma, salivary gland (?)	Hill, 1977 (212)
Naja naja	Lymphosarcoma, liver	Cowan, 1968 (92)
Naja melanoleucea	Adenocarcinoma, salivary gland	Hill, 1952 (225)
Matrix matrix	Rhabdomyoma, musculature	Stolk, 1958 (591)
Naja nigricollis	Adenoma, biliary duct	Cowan, 1968 (92)
Naja nigricollis nigricollis	Lymphosarcoma	Effron et al., 1977 (132/43)*
Naja nivea	Bronchogenic adenocarcinoma	Effron et al., 1977 (132/43)*
Naja sp.	Osteochondrosarcoma, vertebral column	Wadsworth, 1954 (608)
Pituophis catenifer	Adenocarcinoma, intestines	Cowan, 1968 (92)
Pituophis melanogaster	Sarcoma, serosa	Ratcliffe, 1953 (609)
Pituophis melanoleucas	Melanotic tumor, integument	Ball, 1946 (18)
	Melanotic tumor, lip	Ball, 1946 (18)
	Sarcoma, abdomen	Cowan, 1968 (92)
Pituophis melanoleucas annectens	Renal cortical adenoma	Effron et al., 1977 (132/43)*
Pituophis sp.	Intestinal polyposes/ intestinal papillomatoses	Frye. 1975 (209)
Pseudechis porphyriacus	Papillomas of skin; adenomatous proliferation of intrahepatic bile ducts	Effron et al. 1977 (132/43)*
Pseudoboa cloelia	Hepatoma, liver	Cowan, 1968 (92)
Python molorus	Malignant lymphoma	Robinson, 1977 (212)

Table 48.5—Continued

<u>Python reticulatus</u>	Melanotic tumor, integument	Schlumberger and Lucke, 1948 (491)
	Melanotic tumor, integument	Schlumberger and Lucke, 1948 (491)
<u>Python sebae</u>	Adenocarcinoma, ovaries	Sutton, 1885 (564)
	Adenoma, stomach	Vaillant and Pettit, 1902 (598)
	Fibroma at intercostal region	Effron et al., 1977 (132/43)*
<u>Sistrurus catenatus catenatus</u>	Hemangioma of ovary	Effron et al., 1977 (132/43)*
<u>Spilotes pullatus</u>	Adenocarcinoma of pancreatic ducts	Effron et al., 1977 (132/43)*
	Reticulosarcoma (?), orbit	Wadsworth, 1960 (610)
<u>Trimeresurius albolabui</u>	Granulosa-theca cell tumor of ovary	Effron et al., 1977 (132/43)*
<u>Tropidonotus natrix</u>	Adenocarcinoma, kidney	Patay, 1933 (418)
<u>Tubinambis teguixin</u>	Squamous cell cancer, integument	Schwarz, 1923 (497)
	Liver cell cancer	Ippen, 1965 (240)
<u>Uromastix acanthurinus</u>	Lymphosarcoma	Effron et al., 1977 (132/43)*
<u>Varanus draconea</u>	Enchondroma	Rodhain, 1949 (591)
	Osteochondroma	Zwart, 1971 (205)
<u>Varanus komodoensis</u>	Toe-ancient encapsulated hematoma; pancreas-islet cell tumor; colon carcinoma; spleen-metastatic mucinous adenocarcinoma; adrenal-pheochromocytoma; thyroid-multiple follicular adenomas; testiscystic interstitial cell tumor	Ross and Montali, 1975
<u>Varanus salvator</u>	Lymphosarcoma	Zwart, 1971 (205)
	Lymphosarcoma	Zwart and Harshbarger, 1972 (643)
<u>Vipera russelli</u>	Myxofibroma	Zeigel and Clark, 1969 (591)

Table 48.5 — Continued

	Class; Aves	
	O.: Struthioniformes	
Struthio sp. [++]	Epiphyseal, cartilagi-nous tumor of metatar-salia	
	Epithelial ependyoma kidney	
	Tumors of metatarsal	
	O.: Pelecaniformes [++]	
Pelecanus sp.	Liver cancer	Hamerton and Rewell, 1947
	Metastasizing liver carcinoma	Fox, 1930
	Ovarial tumor	Goss, 1949
Morus bassanus	Papillary tumors of gallbladder,multiple	Hamerton, 1939
	O.: Ciconiformes	
Threskiornis aethiopicus	Seminoma	Effron et al., 1977 (132/43)[*]
	O.: Anseriformes	
Anas castanea	Lymphosarcoma, neural and visceral	Effron et al.,1977 (132/43)*
Anas platyrhynchos laysanensis	Semimoma Semimoma, metastatic	Effron et al.,1977 (132/43)*
Aix galericulata	Fibrosarcoma	Effron et al.,1977 (132/43)*
Anser anser	Adenocarcinoma, intes-tine	
	Adenocarcinoma	Kelly, 1949 [++]
	Abdominal carcinoma	Rajan et al., 1968 [++]
	Primary pulmonary cys-tic adenocarcinoma	Mehrotra et al., 1969 [++] (366)
	Fibroma	Mawdesley-Thomas & Hague, 1968 (353)
	Fibroma	Chang et al., 1969 (73)
	Fibrosarcoma, skin of head	
	Kidney, diffuse cancer	Seligman, 1907 [++]
	Lymphoma, malignant, thymus	Ratcliffe, 1928 [++]
	Marek's disease	Baxendale, 1969 (27)
	Melanoma, two teratomas	Rigdon, 1967 (459)
	Osteogenic sarcoma	Mawdesley-Thomas & Solden, 1967 (351)
	Sarcoma, neck muscles	Lucas, 1922[++]
	Sarcoma, wing	
	Seminoma, malignant	Rewell, 1948[++]
	Seminoma, testicle	Ratcliffe, 1942 [++]
	Skin carcinoma	Rewell, 1948 [++]
		Seligman, 1907 [++]
	Squamous cell carcinoma of esophagus	Kelly, 1949 [++]

Table 48.5—Continued

<u>Anser caerulescens caerulescens</u>	Biliary adenocarcinoma	Effron et al., 1977 (132/43)[*]
<u>Branta nigricans</u>	Lymphosarcoma,	Effron et al., 1977 (132/43)[*]
<u>Chenonetta jubata</u>	Fibrosarcoma	Effron et al., 1977 (132/43)[*]
<u>Chloephaga melanoptera</u>	Adenocarcinoma of thyroid	Effron et al., 1977 (132/43)[*]
<u>Dendrocygna arborea</u>	Hemangioma of spleen	Effron et al., 1977 (132/43)[*]
<u>Dendrocygna javanica</u>	Fibrosarcoma	Effron et al., 1977 (132/43)[*]
<u>Dendrocygna viduata</u>	Sertoli's cell tumor	Effron et al., 1977 (132/43)[*]
<u>Tadorna cana</u>	Renal tubular adenoma	Effron et al., 1977 (132/43)[*]
	O.: Falconiformes	
<u>Cathartes</u> sp.	Sarcoma of liver, heart, pericardium	Plimmer, 1912 (446)
	Lung carcinoma	Ratcliffe, 1952 [++]
	O.: Galliformes	
<u>Agriocharis ocellata</u>	Biliary adenocarcinoma Lymphosarcoma, mandible and liver; fibroma Lymphosarcoma, visceral	Effron et al., 1977 (132/43)[*]
<u>Alectura lathami</u>	Lymphosarcoma, visceral	Effron et al., 1977 (132/43)[*]
<u>Argusianus argus grayi</u>	Lymphosarcoma, visceral	Effron et al., 1977 (132/43)*
<u>Coturnix chinensis lineata</u>	Adenomatous proliferation of intrahepatic bile duct Bronchiogenic adenocarcinoma Fibroma at thoracic inlet Fibrosarcoma Seminoma, bilateral	Effron et al., 1977 (132/43)*
<u>Coturnix coturnix japonica</u>	Epizootic reticulum cell sarcoma in a sequestered colony	Nishimura et al., 1970 (404)
	Lymphoid cell leucosis	Löliger et al., 1967 (325)
	Lymphoid leucosis	Wight, 1963
	Lymphosarcoma, visceral including thymus	Effron et al., 1977 (132/43)*
	Marek's disease	Busch & Williams, 1970 (60)
	Mixed cell sarcoma	Henderson et al., 1969 (222)
	Unidentified ovarian tumor	Effron et al., 1977 (132/43)*
<u>Gallus gallus</u>	Diseases of the leucosis/sarcoma group; Marek's disease; tumors of unknown etiology	Hofstad et al., 1978[+]
	Peritoneal carcinomatosis; myosarcomas; leiomyomas; hemangiopericytomas	Sokkar et al., 1979 (647)

Table 48.5—Continued

<u>Gallus gallus murghi</u>	Fibrosarcoma Granulosa cell tumor, malignant (infil- trating) Lymphosarcoma, visceral; leukemic, rhabdomyo- sarcoma Sertoli's cell tumor	Effron et al., 1977 (132/43)*
<u>Gallus lafayetti</u>	Lymphosarcoma, visceral Lymphosarcoma, visceral, skin	Effron et al., 1977 (132/43)*
<u>Gallus sonneratii</u>	Lymphosarcoma, visceral	Effron et al., 1977 (132/43)*
<u>Gallus varius</u>	Lymphosarcoma, visceral	Effron et al., 1977 (132/43)*
<u>Lophophoris impejanus</u>	Biliary adenocarcinoma	Effron et al., 1977 (132/43)*
<u>Lophura diardi</u>	Lymphosarcoma, visceral	Effron et al., 1977 (132/43)*
<u>Meleagris domestica</u>	Lymphosarcoma, visceral	Effron et al., 1977 (132/43)*
	Diseases of the leuco- sis/sarcoma group; Marek's disease; tumors of unknown etiology	Hofstad, et al., 1978+
<u>Meleagris</u> sp.	Adenocarcinoma of adrenal	Fox, 1934 (150)
	Adenocarcinoma of kidney	Fox, 1928 (150)
	Cystadenoma of cloaca	Fox, 1912 (150)
	Hypernephroma, kidney Lymphosarcoma, general- ized	
	Visceral lymphomatosis	Campbell, 1972 (65)
<u>Numida meleagris</u>	Lymphosarcoma, visceral, skin Lymphosarcoma, visceral	Effron et al., 1977 (132/43)*
<u>Odontophorus gujanensis</u>	Neoplasia of intrahe- patic bile duct, pos- sible myoepithelioma	Effron et al., 1977 (132/43)*
<u>Pavo cristatus</u>	Adenomatous polyps of duodenum Fibrosarcoma Fibrosarcoma of skin Hemangiosarcoma Lymphosarcoma, visceral; fibrosarcoma Lymphosarcoma, visceral Lymphosarcoma, visceral, leukemic	Effron et al., 1977 (132/43)*

+/Hofstad, M. S. et al. (1978): <u>Diseases of Poultry.</u>(7th ed.). Ames, Iowa:
  Iowa State University Press.

Table 48.5—Continued

<u>Pavo muticus imperator</u>	Fibrosarcoma Lymphosarcoma, visceral	Effron et al., 1977 (132/43)*
<u>Phasianus versicolor versicolor</u>	Lymphosarcoma, visceral	Effron et al., 1977 (132/43)*
<u>Phasianus</u> sp.	Parasitic neoplasia	Helmboldt & Wyand, 1972 (220)
<u>Pternistes leucoscepus infuscatus</u>	Lymphosarcoma, visceral	Effron et al., 1977 (132/43)*
<u>Rollulus roulroul</u>	Lymphosarcoma	Effron et al., 1977 (132/43)*
<u>Synoicus australis</u>	Adrenal cortical adenoma	Effron et al., 1977 (132/43)*
<u>Syrmaticus soemmeringii ijimae</u>	Hemangioma	Effron et al., 1977 (132/43)*

O.: Gruiformes

<u>Gallirallus australis greyi</u>	Osteoma	Effron et al., 1977 (132/43)*

O.: Charadriformes

<u>Himantopus himantopus leucolophus</u>	Squamous cell carcinoma of skin	Effron et al., 1977 (132/43)*
<u>Larus atricilla</u>	Adenocarcinoma of intestine	Effron et al., 1977 (132/43)*
<u>Pluvialis apricaria apricaria</u>	Hemangioma of kidney	Effron et al., 1977 (132/43)*

O.: Columbiformes

<u>Caloenas nicobarica nicobarica</u>	Granulosa cell tumor	Effron et al., 1977 (132/43)*
<u>Columba</u> sp.	Bile duct carcinomas Liver leiomyoma Neoplasm, eyelid and cornea and others	
<u>Geopelia striata striata</u>	Adenocarcinoma of pan- creatic ducts	Effron et al., 1977 (132/43)*
<u>Scaradefella inca</u>	Fibrosarcoma	Effron et al., 1977 (132/43)*

O.: Psittaciformes

<u>Agapornis lilianae</u>	Biliary adenocarcinoma	Effron et al., 1977 (132/43)*
<u>Agapornis nigrigenis</u>	Adenomatous prolifera- tion of intrahepatic bile ducts	Effron et al., 1977 (132/43)*
<u>Ara chloropetra</u>	Mixed epithelial and connective tissue tumor of lung	Effron et al., 1977 (132/43)*
<u>Aratinga holochlora holochlora</u>	Seminoma	Effron et al., 1977 (132/43)*

Table 48.5 — Continued

<u>Barnardius zonarius</u> <u>zonarius</u>	Biliary adenoma	Effron et al., 1977 (132/43)*
<u>Bolbopsittacus lunulatus</u> <u>lunulatus</u>	Adenoma of intrapancre-atic ducts	Effron et al., 1977 (132/43)*
<u>Brotogeris versicolorus</u> <u>versicolorus</u>	Renal adenocarcinoma	Effron et al., 1977 (132/43)*
<u>Cacatua galerita galeri-ta</u>	Mucinous cystadenoma of oviduct	Effron et al., 1977 (132/43)*
<u>Eclectus roratus solo-monensis</u>	Renal cortical adenoma, bilateral	Effron et al., 1977 (132/43)*
<u>Loriculus vernalis</u> <u>phileticus</u>	Adenoma of ventriculus	Effron et al., 1977 (132/43)*
<u>Lorius lory erythro-thorax</u>	Adenocarcinoma of cloaca	Effron et al., 1977 (132/43)*
<u>Melopsittacus undulatus</u>	Papillary cystadenoma of ovary, bilateral Renal adenocarcinoma Lipoma Benign basaloid cell tumor ("trichoepithelioma ") of eyelid.	Effron et al., 1977 (132/43)* Brightman and Burke, 1978 (42a)
<u>Neophema elegans elegans</u>	Squamous cell carcinoma of skin	Effron et al., 1977 (132/43)*
<u>Neophema splendida</u>	Papilloma of skin	Effron et al., 1977 (132/43)*
<u>Pionus senilis decolora-tus</u>	Adrenal cortical adenoma	Effron et al., 1977 (132/43)*
<u>Platycercus adscitus</u> <u>palliceps</u>	Lymphosarcoma, visceral, lumen of brain, and lung vessels	Effron et al., 1977 (132/43)*
<u>Platycercus eximius</u> <u>eximius</u>	Adenomatous prolifera-tion of intrahepatic bile ducts	Effron et al., 1977 (132/43)*
<u>Polytelis swainsonii</u>	Lymphosarcoma, visceral	Effron et al., 1977 (132/43)*
<u>Psephotus varius</u>	Fibrosarcoma	Effron et al., 1977 (132/43)*
<u>Psittacula cyanocephala</u> <u>bengalensi</u>	Seminoma	Effron et al., 1977 (132/43)*
<u>Psittacula krameri</u> <u>manillensis</u>	Hemangioma of spleen	Effron et al., 1977 (132/43)*
<u>Rhynchopsitta pachy-rhyncha pachyrhyncha</u>	Fibroma of dermis	Effron et al., 1977 (132/43)*
<u>Trichoglossus haematodus</u> <u>moluccanus</u>	Benign polyp of gall-bladder epithelium	Effron et al., 1977 (132/43)*
	O.: Cuculiformes	
<u>Centropus sinensis</u> <u>bubutas</u>	Cavernous hemangioma of liver	Effron et al., 1977 (132/43)*

Table 48.5 — Continued

	O.: Apodiformes	
Pharomachrus mocinno costaricensis	Adenomatous prolifera- tion of intrahepatic bile ducts	Effron et al., 1977 (132/43)*
	O.: Passeriformes	
Amandina fasciata	Fibrosarcoma	Effron et al., 1977 (132/43)*
Cissa chinensis	Hepatoma	Effron et al., 1977 (132/43)*
Gracula religiosa inter- media	Lymphosarcoma, visceral	Effron et al., 1977 (132/43)*
Gymnorhina tibicen tibicen	Tubular adenoma of renal medulla	Effron et al., 1977 (132/43)*
Pitta caerulea caerulea	Biliary adenoma of head of pancreas	Effron et al., 1977 (132/43)*
Pitta erythrogaster macklotii	Biliary adenocarcinoma	Effron et al., 1977 (132/43)*
	Class: Mammalia	
	O.: Monotremata	
Tachyglossus aculeatus	Adenoma (cystic), thyroid	Hamerton, 1944 (591)
	O.: Marsupialia	
Dasyrus viverrinus	Adenocarcinoma intes- tinal tract Medullary cancer of rectum Multiple tumors of liver	Scott, 1927 (591)
Didelphis marsupialis virginianus	Bronchogenic adenoma	Effron et al., 1977 (132/43)*
Didelphis virginiana	Adenocarcinoma of bile duct, mixosarcoma of peritoneum, lung and mesentery	AFIP 1 3013/8 (10)
	Adenomatosis,pulmonary	Sherwood et al., 1969 (504)
	Bone tumor starting from jaw	Hamerton, 1921 (591)
	Bronchiolar adenoma of lung	AFIP 1 410521 (10)
	Hepatocellular carci- noma, solitary bron- chiolar adenoma of lung	AFIP 1 410518 (10)
	Lymphosarcoma mesentery node and stomach	AFIP 202373 (10)
	Multiple hepatomas	AFIP 1 410517 (10)
	Osteosarcoma, ribs and face	Hamerton, 1921 (591)

Table 48.5—Continued

Didelphis virginiana	Primary tumor of bladder	Fox, 1923 (150)
	Squamous cell carcinoma of esophagus	AFIP 638224 (10)
	Tubular adenoma of kidney	AFIP 1410516 (10)
Macropus robustus erubescens	Adenomatous proliferation of intrapancreatic ducts	Effron et al., 1977 (132/43)*
Malabar rat	Cancer of the lung	
	Primary cancer of lung	Campbell, (591)
Phalanger cuscus	Cancer	Crisp, 1860 (150)
Phasolarctus cinereus	Stem cell leukemic lymphoma	AFIP 978624 (10)
Protemnodon agilis jardini	Adenomatous proliferation of intrahepatic bile ducts	Effron et al., 1977 (132/43)*
Protemnodon rufogrisea	Adenocarcinoma of oral cavity glandular epithelium	Effron et al., 1977 (132/43)*
Sarcophilus harrisii	Adenoma of thyroid, adenocarcinoma of mammary gland	Effron et al., 1977 (132/43)*
	Adenoma of thyroid, adenoma of sebaceous gland	
	Papillomas of skin	
	Multiple neurofibroma, skin, lung, spleen, kidney	AFIP 1 250369 (10)
	Squamous cell ca at anal region, lymphosarcoma of skin, granulating seroma of skin	
Thylogale parma	Carcinoma of cervix	AFIP 1529252 (10)
	Squamous cell carcinoma of cervix	Effron et al., 1977 (132/43)*
	O.: Insectivora	
Crocidura sp. (?)	Adrenal neoplasm	AFIP 217511 (10)
Erinaceus europaeus	Pituitary adenoma	Campbell and Smith, 1966 (64)
	Tumor of intestine and musculature	Murray, 1919 (150)
Erinaceus pruneri hinder	Bronchiogenic adenoma	Effron et al., 1977 (132/43)*
Tenrec ecaudatus	Fibrosarcoma of abdominal wall with lung and lymph node metastases	AFIP 1 312550 (10)

Table 48.5 — Continued

	O.: Chiroptera	
Plecotus townsendii virginianus	Leiomyosarcoma, cutaneous	Conrad et al., 1965 (85)
	O.: Primates	
Allenopithecus nigrovirdis	Leiomyoma of uterus	Effron et al., 1977 (132/43)*
Alonatta sp.	Spontaneous tumors	Newberne and Johnson, 1960 (389)
Aotus trivirgatus	Renal carcinoma	Lund et al., 1970 (591)
Ateles geoffroyi	Islet cell adenomatosis of pancreas	Effron et al., 1977 (132/43)*
Cacajo rubicundus	Myxoma of eyelid	Effron et al., 1977 (132/43)*
Cercopithecus diana roloway	Adenomatous proliferation of intrahepatic bile ducts, multiple adenomas of lung	Effron et al., 1977 (132/43)*
Chimpanzee troglodytes	Epithelioma Fibromyxoma Osteogenic sarcoma, skin	
Gorilla gorilla	Bilateral osteoma, skull	Hartwell, 1951, 1957 (461)
Hylobetes sp.	Squamous cell cancer, stomach Squamous cell papilloma of pharynx Tumor, breast	
Lagotheri humboldti	Atypical basal cell cancer at upper arm	Meyer-Holzapfel, 1961 (461)
Lemur macaco macaco	Hepatoma	Effron et al., 1977 (132/43)*
Macaca mulatta	Adenocarcinoma	Mason et al., 1972 (340)
	Adenocarcinoma of the large intestine	Plentl et al., 1968 (445)
	Ameloblastic odontoma	Splitter et al., 1972 (523)
	Basal cell tumour	Schiller et al., 1969 (487)
	Carcinoma in situ, cervix	Sternberg, 1961 (527)
	Disseminated endometriosis	McClure et al., 1971 (359)
	Endometrial adenocarcinoma	Strozier et al., 1972 (559)
	Hepatic hemangioendothelioma	Woodruff and Johnson, 1968 (638)
	Infiltrating duct carcinoma of mammary gland	Kirschstein et al., 1972 (293)
	Intracerebral angioma cavernosum	Unterharnscheidt, 1964 (595, 596)

Table 48.5 — Continued

<u>Macaca mulatta</u>	Intrauterine chorio-carcinoma	Lindsey et al., 1969 (320)
	Leukemia	Siegal et al., 1968 (508)
	Liver cell carcinoma	Williams, 1970 (628)
	Lymphoblastoid cell line with myelogenous leukemia	Dunkel and Myers, 1972 (118)
	Malignant lymphoma	Brown et al., 1971 (48)
	Multiple neoplasia	Chapman and Allen, 1968 (74)
	Multiple tumors	Allen et al., 1970 (3)
	Oral cancer	Bonnet et al., 1901 (591)
	Ovarian tumors	Martin et al., 1970 (339)
	Serous cystadenoma of ovary	Flinn, 1967 (461)
	Spontaneous carcinoid tumor	Kimbrough, 1966 (289)
	Spontaneous carcinoma of the cervix uteri	Hisaw and Hisaw 1958 (228)
	Spontaneous and irra-diation induced tumors	Kent and Pickering, 1958 (284)
	Spontaneous mammary tumor	Chopra and Mason, 1970 (461)
	Spontaneous mammary tumor	Jensen et al., 1970 (254)
	Spontaneous primary carcinoma	Engle and Stout, 1940 (127)
	Spontaneous squamous cell carcinoma of lower jaw	Sasaki et al., 1961 (475)
	Squamous cell carcinoma	Migaki et al., 1971 (396)
	Subcutaneous tumor	Bearcroft and Jamison, 1958 (28)
<u>Macaca silenus</u>	Leiomyoma of uterus	Effron et al., 1977 (132/43)*
<u>Papio hamadryas hamadryas</u>	Myxoma of skin	Effron et al., 1977 (132/43)*
<u>Papio papio</u>	Cancer, lung	Hartwell, 1951, 1957 (461)
<u>Papio</u> sp.	Adenoma of mucous mem-brane, stomach Adenocarcinoma, pancreas Sarcoma, giant cell, wrist	Robinson et al., 1974 (461)
<u>Presbytis pileatus</u>	Granulosa cell tumor, metastatic	Effron et al., 1977 (132/43)*
<u>Theropithecus</u> sp.	Squamous cell cancer, gum	Robinson et al., 1974 (461)
<u>Tupaia belangeri</u>	Adenocarcinoma of mammary gland	Effron et al., 1977 (132/43)*
	O.: Edentata	
<u>Dasypus novemcinctus</u>	Bronchiolar carcinoma	Effron et al., 1977 (132/43)*
	Leiomyoma of stomach	Effron et al., 1977 (132/43)*

Table 48.5 — Continued

	O.: Lagomorpha*	
Lepus sp.	Sarcoma undifferentiated, leiomyosarcoma fibrosarcoma	AFIP 1 102667 (10)
	O.: Rodentia**	
Citellus leucurus	Multiple adenomas of lung	Effron et al., 1977 (132/43)*
Cuniculus paca	Hemangioma of bladder	Effron et al., 1977 (132/43)*
Cynomys ludovicianus	Adenocarcinoma of stomach	Effron et al., 1977 (132/43)*
	Renal cortical adenoma	Effron et al., 1977 (132/43)*
Dicrostonyx groenlandicus	Mammary gland tumors	Van Pelt and Dietrich, 1972 (601)
Dipodomys merriami	Adenocarcinoma of mammary gland	Effron et al., 1977 (132/43)*
Hystrix brachyura	Islet cell adenoma of pancreas	Effron et al., 1977 (132/43)*
Hystrix galeate	Lymphosarcoma (leukosis)	Nobel and Klopfer, 1971 (461)
Marmota sp.	Hepatoma	Bond, 1970 (461)
Mus musculus	Adenocarcinoma of mammary ducts	Effron et al., 1977 (132/43)*
Myocaster coypus coypus	Endometrial polyp, benign; leiomyoma of uterus	Effron et al., 1977 (132/43)*
Ondatra sp.	Osteogenic sarcoma, tibiofibular	AFIP 861016 (10)
	Osteosarcoma of tibia and fibula, secondary in lung and kidney	AFIP 647263 (10)
Ondatra sp.	Primary osteosarcoma of rib, diaphragm and secondary in lung, pericard and myocard	AFIP 207868 (10)
Spermophilus undulatus	Renal adenocarcinoma	Casey et al., 1972 (69)
	O.: Cetacea*	
Balaenoptera musculus	Cystadenoma, mucinous	Cockrill, 1960 (82)
	Cystadenoma, mucinous	Cockrill, 1960 (82)
	Fibrolipoma from serous surface, liver	Cockrill, 1960 (82)
	Ganglioneuroma of mediastinum	Cockrill, 1960 (82)
	Granulosa cell tumor, ovary	Cockrill, 1960 (82)

Table 48.5—Continued

<u>Balaenoptera musculus</u>	Lipoma from serous surface of liver	Cockrill, 1960 (82)
	Papilloma of tongue (squamous cell)	
<u>Balaenoptera physalus</u>	Fibroma, skin	Stolk, 1953 (82)
	Fibroma, tongue	Stolk, 1952 (82)
	Fibroma	Cockrill, 1960 (82)
	Granulosa cell tumor, ovary	Cockrill, 1960 (82)
	Ovarial carcinoma	Stolk, 1952 (82)
	Poorly differentiated lymphosarcoma of kidney	AFIP 1 470245 (10)
	Warty tumor	Stolk, 1952 (82)
<u>Megaptera novaengliae</u>	Cerebral lipoma	Pillery, 1966 (82)
	Fibroma, skin (lower jaw)	Stolk, 1953 (82)
	Fibroma, tongue	Stolk, 1952 (82)
<u>Physeter catodon</u>	Haemangioma in liver	Stolk, 1953 (82)
	Skin fibroma near blow hole	Stolk, 1953 (82)
	Skin fibroma of lower jaw	Stolk, 1952 (82)
	Verruca between eyes	Stolk, 1953 (82)
Undefined species	Fibroma of tonsil	AFIP 1 458684 (10)
	O.: Carnivora	
<u>Acinonyx jubatus</u>	Myeloma in liver	AFIP 1 164573 (10)
	O.: Carnivora	
<u>Acinonyx jubatus jubatus</u>	Hemangioma of tongue	Effron et al., 1977 (132/43)*
<u>Acinonyx jubatus obergi</u>	Lymphosarcoma	Effron et al., 1977 (132/43)*
<u>Ailurus fulgens</u>	Granulosa cell tumor	Effron et al., 1977 (132/43)*
<u>Arctictis binturong</u>	Adenocarcinoma of mammary gland	Effron et al., 1977 (132/43)*
	Adenoma of colon	Effron et al., 1977 (132/43)*
<u>Canis dingo</u>	Melanotic skin cancer	
	Sarcoma, pharyngeal region	
	Sarcoma, testis	
Canis familiaris**		
<u>Canis latrans</u>	Hypernephroma of kidney with metastasis in lung and throat	
	Oral papillomatosis	Broughton et al., 1970 (45)
<u>Canis lupus</u>	Adenocarcinoma of thyroid	

Table 48.5—Continued

Canis lupus	Adenocarcinoma of thyroid, generalized	
	Adenocarcinoma of thyroid, generalized	AFIP 202376 (10)
	Chondrosarcoma (primary) of neck and chodrosarcoma (secondary) of liver	AFIP 202382 (10)
	Chondrosarcoma (primary) neck	
	Epithelioma, neck, liver metastases	Plimmer, 1915 (150)
	Osteosarcoma, neck	AFIP 202366 (10)
	Sarcoma, testis	
	Tumors, diffuse	Plimmer, 1915 (150)
Chrysocyon aureus syriacus	Adenocarcinoma of oral cavity glandular epithelium	Effron et al., 1977 (132/43)*
	Bronchogenic adenoma	Effron et al., 1977 (132/43)*
	Papillary carcinoma of ovary; scirrhous adenocarcinoma of the merocrine gland	Effron et al., 1977 (132/43)*
Chrysocyon brachyurus	Osteogenic sarcoma	Effron et al., 1977 (132/43)*
Chrysocyon mesomelas	Hemangiosarcoma of neck	Effron et al., 1977 (132/43)*
Felis chaus	Adenocarcinoma of stomach and thyroid, adenoma of kidney, sertoli cell tumor of testis	AFIP 739228 (10)
Felis chaus furax	Adenoma of intrapancreatic ducts	Effron et al., 1977 (132/43)*
Felis concolor	Adenocarcinoma of thyroid, metastatic to lung	AFIP 991791 (10)
	Adenoma of thyroid	AFIP 938733 (10)
	Transitional cancer, bladder	AFIP 762811 (10)
Felis lynx canadensis	Squamous cell carcinoma of oral cavity	Effron et al., 1977 (132/43)*
Felis temmincki	Adenoma of adrenal cortex	AFIP 1 219343 (10)
Galictis vittata	Adrenocortical carcinoma, lung carcinoma, kidney carcinoma	AFIP 1 259312 (10)
Helarctos malayanus malayanus	Myxoma of conjunctiva	Effron et al., 1977 (132/43)*
Herpestes sp.	Fibroma, skin of ear	AFIP 1 238745 (10)

Table 48.5—Continued

Hyaena sp.	Adenocarcinoma of mamma and leiomyoma of uterus	AFIP 1 003009 (10)
	Adenoma of thyroid	AFIP 960664 (10)
Leo leo	Adenocarcinoma of thyroid metastatic to lung	AFIP 991791 (10)
	Adenoma, multiple papillary in lung, leiomyomata of uterus and ovary	AFIP 1 294982 (10)
	Adenomatosis in lung	AFIP 1 416695 (10)
Leo tigris	Bileduct cancer	AFIP 125489 (10)
Lycaon pictus lupinus	Hemangiosarcoma of liver	Effron et al., 1977 (132/43)*
	Papillary cystadenoma of ovary; adenoma of thyroid	Effron et al., 1977 (132/43)*
Martes pennanti	Adenocarcinoma of right parotid, metastases to right mandibular lymph node	AFIP 1 378909 (10)
Meles meles (Taxidea taxus)	Hepatic angioma	Paget, 1979 (414a)
Mustela lutreola	Malignant myeloma	AFIP 264617 (10)
Mustela nigripes*		
Mustela vison	Adenomata, bile duct	AFIP 306113 (10)
	Hemangiosarcoma of spleen and liver	AFIP 1 143501 (10)
	Myeloma, multiple: spleen, liver, kidney	AFIP 287745 (10)
	Neurofibroma, skin and subcutis	AFIP 337895 (10)
	Primary osteosarcoma of rib, metastasis to lung and liver	AFIP 587610 (10)
	Psomma bodies in pineal meninges	AFIP 1 232805 (10)
Mustela sp.	Theca cell tumor ovary, arrhenoblastoma ovary	AFIP 177249 (10)
Neofelis nebulosa nebulosa	Sertoli's cell tumor	Effron et al., 1977 (132/43)*
Panthera leo	Lymphosarcoma	Effron et al., 1977 (132/43)*
Panthera tigris longipitis	Adenoma of lung	Effron et al., 1977 (132/43)*
Panthera tigris tigris	Adenoma of merocrine gland	Effron et al., 1977 (132/43)*
	Liposarcoma	Effron et al., 1977 (132/43)*

Table 48.5—Continued

<u>Panthera uncia</u>	Bronchogenic adeno-carcinoma	Effron et al., 1977 (132/43)*
<u>Procyon lotor</u>	Adenocarcinoma, granular cell type of kidney and granular cell carcinoma of kidney	AFIP 338080 (10)
	Chondroma in rib	AFIP 1 172384 (10)
	Hemangiosarcoma of nasal orifice	AFIP 1 291740 (10)
	Pyogenic granuloma of omentum	AFIP 898100 (10)
<u>Selenarctos thibethanus</u>	Malignant lymphoma, kidney, lymph node, small intestine	AFIP 1 327518 (10)
<u>Ursus arctos</u>	Adenocarcinoma, kidney	AFIP 202379 (10)
	Adenocarcinoma of lung and pancreatic node of liver which started primary from pancreas	AFIP 202441 (10)
	Hepatoma, leiomyoma of colon	AFIP 1 071285 (10)
	Leiomyoma, uterus	AFIP 1 137509 (10)
	Malignant lymphoma, generalized	AFIP 79477 (10)
	Fibroma of uterus	Effron et al., 1977 (132/43)*
<u>Ursus arctos sheldoni</u>	Lymphosarcoma	Effron et al., 1977 (132/43)*
<u>Ursus arctos X Thalarctos maritimus</u>	Acinar carcinoma of pancreas and liver	AFIP 1 439210 (10)
<u>Vulpes vulpes</u>	Adenocarcinoma, metastatic in lung and hepatoma	AFIP 1 009508 (10)
	Aortic body tumor of heart with extension to lung	AFIP 965632 (10)
	Leukemic lymphosarcoma	AFIP 124529 (10)
	Lymphosarcoma in kidney	AFIP 190266 (10)
	O.: Pinnipedia	
<u>Arctocephalus ursinus</u>	Squamous cell carcinoma	Effron et al., 1977 (132/43)*
<u>Callorhinus ursinus</u>	Squamous cell carcinoma, lymphosarcoma (?), multiple: lymph nodes, tonsils, colon	AFIP 1 521720 (10)
<u>Eumetopas jubatus</u> (?)	Lymphoblastic multifocal lymphosarcoma of myocard	AFIP 1 591120 (10)
<u>Halichoerus gripus</u>	Uterine tumors	Mawdesley-Thomas; Bonner, 1971 (355)
<u>Mirounga leonina</u>	Ovarian tumor	Mawdesley-Thomas, 1971a (346)

Table 48.5—Continued

Pagophilus groenlandicus	Histicytic malignant lymphoma of duodenum	AFIP 1 426257 (10)
Phoca vitulina	Lymphosarcoma, liver lymph nodes, spleen	AFIP 1 594509 (10)
Phoca vitulina geronimen-sis	Malignant leukemic lymphoma	Griner, 1971 (183)
	Lymphosarcoma,leukemic	Effron et al., 1977 (132/43)*
	Lymphosarcoma,leukemic	Effron et al., 1977 (132/43)*
Zalophus californianus	Adenocarcinoma of intrapancreatic ducts	Effron et al., 1977 (132/43)*
	Hypernephroma	Effron et al., 1977 (132/43)*
	Malignant melanoma of eye	Effron et al., 1977 (132/43)*
	Clear cell carcinoma of urogenital origin, with metastases in kidneys, adrenals, lungs, lymph nodes, uterus, ovaries, pancreas	AFIP 1 548063 (10)
	Malignant melanoma of eye and brain	AFIP 1 422939 (10)
	Multifocal epidermal inclusion cysts	AFIP 1 496516 (10)
	Papilloma of skin	AFIP 1 568968 (10)
	Squamous cell carci-noma	AFIP 1 428552 (10)
	Squamous cell carci-noma, metastases in lung, liver,pancreas, spleen, lymph nodes; carcinoma of cortex of adrenal	AFIP 1 590150 (10)

O.: Proboscidea

Elephas maximus	Carcinoid	Werle et al., 1968 (623)
	Fibrosarcoma of sub-cutis, locally inva-sive	AFIP 1 429198 (10)
	Leiomyoma of stomach	AFIP 935865 (10)
	Leiomyomata of myme-trium	AFIP 697204 (10)
	Multifocal hyalinisa-tion of Bowman's capsule	AFIP 1 510142 (10)
Elephas maximus indicus	Papillomatous tumor of vulva	Effron et al., 1977 (132/43)*

O.: Hyracoidea

Procavia capensis capen-sis	Granulosa cell tumor	Effron et al., 1977 (132/43)

Table 48.5—Continued

	O.: Sirenia	
Trichechus manatus sene- galensis	Cancer of skin	Kaiser (unpubl.) (279)
	O.: Perissodactyla	
Equus asinus	Benign vaginal polyp Papilloma of lip	Effron et al., 1977 (132/43)* Effron et al., 1977 (132/43)*
Equus caballus*		
Equus hemionus onager	Granulosa cell tumor of ovary	AFIP 769986 (10)
Equus sp.	Pituitary adenoma	Kennedy, Trevino, 1970 (283)
	O.: Artiodactyla	
Aepyceras melampus rendilis	Adenocarcinoma of cervix Multiple adenomas of lung	Effron et al., 1977 (132/43)* Effron et al., 1977 (132/43)*
Antidorcas marsupialis angelensis	Undifferentiated ade- nocarcinoma of lung	Effron et al., 1977 (132/43)*
Antidorcas marsupialis	Congenital hamartoma and adenoma of iris pigment epithelium	AFIP 1496981 (10)
Antilocapra americana americana	Squamous cell carci- noma of skin	Effron et al., 1977 (132/43)*
Bos indicus	Adenoma, adrenal cortex	AFIP 202372 (10)
Bubalus bubalis	Hemangioma in vertebra Multiple lipomatosis Lymphosarcoma, leukemia	AFIP 202372 (10) AFIP 798336 (10) Effron et al., 1977 (132/43)*
Camelus ferus arabicus	Intraductal papillary mammary adenoma	Effron et al., 1977 (132/43)*
Capra aegagrus cretica	Bronchogenic adeno- carcinoma	Effron et al., 1977 (132/43)*
Cervus axis axis	Biliary adenocarcinoma	Effron et al., 1977 (132/43)*
Cervus nippon talouanus	Lymphosarcoma	Effron et al., 1977 (132/43)*
Cervus sp.	Adenocarcinoma, bile duct and liver Fibroma, back Fibroma, eyelid Fibroma, foot possible viral etiology Fibroma, subcutaneous of head, leg, abdomen (viral) Fibroma, neck Fibroma, skin Fibrosarcoma, skin	AFIP 286314 (10) AFIP 317224 (10) AFIP 125131 (10) AFIP 1 301131 (10) AFIP 1151763 (10) AFIP 158317 (10) AFIP 197660 (10) AFIP 1 264329 (10)

Table 48.5—Continued

Cervus sp.	Malignant lymphocytic lymphoma of heart, lymph node, salivary gland, stomach, liver, kidney, adrenal, brain, spinal cord	AFIP 1 2957799 (10)
	Pheochromocytoma and metastases	AFIP 1 094175 (10)
	Skin tumors	Friend and Kistner, 1967 (461)
Giraffa camelopardalis	Carcinoma, undifferentiated, metastases	AFIP 797982 (10)
	Osteosarcoma	Kaiser (unpubl.) (279)
Hemitragus jemlahicus jemlahicus	Epithelial thymoma	Effron et al., 1977 (132/43)*
Hippotragus niger roosevelti	Hemangioma of spleen	Effron et al., 1977 (132/43)*
Lama guianicoe glama	Lipoma	Effron et al., 1977 (132/43)*
Lama guanicoe guanicoe	Adenocarcinoma of abomasum	Effron et al., 1977 (132/43)*
	Bronchogenic adenoma	Effron et al., 1977 (132/43)*
Lama vicugna	Squamous cell carcinoma of esophagus	Effron et al., 1977 (132/43)*
Odocoileus virginiamus	Dermatofibroma of abdomen and thigh, multiple	AFIP 566998 (10)
	Fibroma, skin and ear	AFIP 335120 (10)
	Fibroma of skin of	AFIP 1529534 (10)
	Fibromatosis of skin in axillary, inguinal and periorbital areas	AFIP 1499659 (10)
	Lymphosarcoma	Debbie and Friend, 1967 (461)
	Malignant lymphoma of pelvic peritoneum, lung and heart	AFIP 1 227864 (10)
	Sarcoma	Hayes, 1971 (461)
	Sarcoma, undifferentiated, left rear leg	AFIP 1 332961 (10)
Oryx leucoryx	Lymphosarcoma	Effron et al., 1977 (132/43)*
Oryx sp.	Malignant lymphoma	AFIP 202380 (10)
Ovis ammon aries	Malignant melanoma	Effron et al., 1977 (132/43)*
Ovis ammon musimon	Chromophobe adenoma of pituitary; adrenal cortical adenoma	Effron et al., 1977 (132/43)*
	Pheochromocytoma; thyroid medullary adenoma	Effron et al., 1977 (132/43)*

Table 48.5—Continued

Sus scrofa*	Carcinomatosis	Lyhs, 1967 (461)
Taurotragus oryx patter- sonianus	Papillary adenoma of sweat gland	Effron et al., 1977 (132/43)*
	Scirrhous bronchogenic adenocarcinoma	Effron et al., 1977 (132/43)*
Tragelaphus sp.	Adenocarcinoma of uterus, ovary, lung, lymph node, leiomyoma of uterus	AFIP 1 466430 (10)

+This species could not be exactly classified due to insufficient information.

++In a few cases the source is condensed if the author published many articles in short sequence on related topics and if taken from general sources. This was done to avoid an overextended reference list.

rodents are concerned only a few spontaneous tumors have been included. For additional spontaneous and experimental tumors, see the Refs. 30, 278, 461, 591, 593, 594, and 602.

For the sake of usefulness, the species of the lowest taxonomic unit mentioned in Table 48.5 have been arranged alphabetically; the neoplasms of given species also have been listed in alphabetical order.

For the phylogeny of neoplasms, see Table 48.2. Smaller taxonomic units have been omitted for classes in which few cases of neoplasms have been found. For a statistical evaluation of basic oncology, we have to consider three groups:

1. Spontaneous neoplasms in an undisturbed environment. These are the ones which are able to give us real information for basic cancer research. Only from these are we able to learn about species differences useful for primary concepts of variation. They should be the cornerstone for basic cancer research. It is realized of course that the group mentioned here is diminishing more and more from our earth.

2. The second aspect of species-specific basic oncology is given by the spontaneous tumors in a more or less "contaminated" natural environment, a source in which we can study the gradual changes of neoplastic development due to several factors acting mainly locally. Man himself belongs to this group of creatures.

3. The third source of information is provided by experimental work using laboratory animals and the extrapolation to, and proof by, work with human organ cultures from immediate autopsy or biopsy.

But from the comparative standpoint, based on normal histology and on the cases mentioned in the large table we can derive a group-specific pattern of neoplasms only.

Not only does the distribution of normal tissues in different taxonomic units such as phyla, etc., vary, but so does the potential of primary cell types, e.g., the mesenchymal cell as a precursor of glial cells in different phyla varying in taxonomic value. The mesenchymal cell of a flatworm or of another lower organism will not have the same potential as the mesenchymal cell of a mammal or a bird. Secondly, cells of tissues from animals with partial cell invariability such as Acanthocephala may differ in their tumorigenic or regenerating potential from cells with syncytial character in taxonomically different organisms.

Finally, tumors of the same tissue, e.g., in fishes and mammals may vary according to their metastatic potential. We have already mentioned the nephroblastoma as an example.

Basically we are able to say that the normal tissue pattern in the organisms is reflected in the pattern of neoplasms theoretically possible, spontaneously found, or experimentally produced. It is essential to take a look at the spontaneous neoplasms of the domesticated mam-

Table 48.6
Relative Frequency of Tumors in Dogs, Cats, Horse, and Cattle: Most Frequent Sites[a]

Dogs

No.	% of all tumors	Site	Cell type
2440	20.7	Skin	Adenoma
1394	11.8	Mammae	Adenocarcinoma
1051	8.9	Soft tissue	Lipoma
943	8.0	Lymph nodes	Lymphoma
677	5.7	Oral cavity[c]	Melanosarcoma
657	5.6	Bones, joints	Osteosarcoma
562	4.8	Perianal	Adenoma
487	4.1	Testes	Sertoli cell tumor
324	2.7	Nose, paranasal sinuses	Adenocarcinoma
301	2.6	Blood, spleen, marrow	Hemangiosarcoma
252	2.1	Eyelid[d]	Adenoma
202	1.7	Brain, meninges	Glioma
176	1.5	Trachea, bronchus	Carcinoma
160	1.4	Thyroid	Adenocarcinoma
158	1.3	General	Mastosarcoma
137	1.2	Liver, biliary	Adenocarcinoma
121	1.0	Adrenal	Adenoma

Cats

No.	% of all tumors	Site	Cell type
432	31.5	Lymph node	Lymphoma
224	16.3	Hematopoietic	Leukemia
102	7.4	Skin	Basal cell ca.
70	5.1	Mammae	Adenocarcinoma
51	3.7	Nose[b]	Squamous cell ca.
50	3.6	Soft tissue	Fibrosarcoma
49	3.6	Oral cavity	Squamous cell ca.
40	2.9	Bone, joint	Osteosarcoma
30	2.2	External ear	Squamous cell ca.
27	2.0	Kidney	Lymphoma
26	1.9	Liver, biliary	Lymphoma
20	1.5	Pancreas	Adenocarcinoma
18	1.3	General	Fibrosarcoma
17	1.2	Eyelid[d]	Squamous cell ca.
17	1.2	Intestine	Adenocarcinoma
17	1.2	Small intestine	Adenocarcinoma
15	1.1	Brain, meninges	Benign meningioma
15	1.1	Oropharynx	Squamous cell ca.

Horses

No.	% of all tumors	Site	Cell type
406	27.9	Skin	Papilloma
234	16.1	Soft tiss.	Fibroma
151	10.4	Eyelid, etc.	Squamous cell ca.
123	8.5	Eye, orbit	Squamous cell ca.
92	6.3	Penis	Squamous cell ca.
54	3.7	Ovary	Granulosa cell tumor
41	2.8	Bone, joint	Benign (?)
35	2.4	Lymph node	Lymphoma
28	1.9	Nasal cavity accessory sinuses	Squamous cell ca.
23	1.6	Vulva	Squamous cell ca.
21	1.4	Peripheral nerve	Neuroma
20	1.4	Thyroid	Adenoma
16	1.1	Gum, teeth	Malignant odontogenic tumor

Cattle

No.	% of all tumors	Site	Cell type
381	36.1	Eye, orbit	Squamous cell ca.
212	20.1	Lymph node	Lymphoma
151	14.3	Eyelid, etc.	Squamous cell ca.
57	5.4	Penis	Papilloma
50	4.7	Skin	Papilloma
34	3.2	Soft tissue	Fibroma
12	1.1	Stomach	Lymphoma
—			

[a] Source: W. A. Priester: Theiler and McDonald Veterinary Oncology. Lee & Febiger, Philadelphia, 1980.
[b] Nose, paranasal sinuses.
[c] Oral cavity, lips, gums, tongue, teeth.
[d] Eyelid, conjunctiva, lacrimal gland.
[e] Trachea, bronchus, lung.

Table 48.7
Relative Frequency of Tumors in Dogs, Cats, Horse and Cattle: Most Frequent Histologic Type[a]

	Dogs				Cats				Horses				Cattle		
No.	% of all tumors	Cell type	Site	No.	% of all tumors	Cell type	Site	No.	% of all tumors	Cell type	Site	No.	% of all tumors	Cell type	Site
1208	10.3	Adenocarcinoma	Mammae	525	38.3	Lymphoma[b]	Lymph node	367	25.2	Squamous cell ca.	Eye, orbit	515	48.8	Squamous cell ca.	Eye, orbit
1099	9.3	Adenoma	Skin	276	20.1	Leukemias	Hematopoietic system	327	23.5	Papilloma	Skin	281	26.6	Leukemia, lymphoma	Lymph node
919	7.8	Lymphoma	Lymph node	134	9.8	Squamous cell ca.	Nose[c]	154	10.6	Fibroma	Skin	109	10.3	Papilloma	Penis
552	4.7	Lipoma	Soft Tissue	128	9.3	Adenocarcinoma	Mammae	132	9.1	Fibroma	Forelimb	18	1.7	Adenocarcinoma	Multiple
431	3.7	Osteosarcoma	Bones, joints	57	4.2	Fibrosarcoma	Skin	41	2.8	Lymphoma	Lymph node				
434	3.7	Hemangiosteoma	Skin	40	2.9	Reticulum cell sarcoma	Lymph node	33	2.3	Fibrosarcoma	Eyelid[d]				
428	3.6	Squamous cell ca.	Skin	39	2.8	Carcinoma	Mammae	32	2.2	Lipoma	Intraabdominal				
410	3.5	Carcinoma	Mammae	33	2.4	Adenoma	Skin	31	2.1	Melanosarcoma	Skin				
396	3.4	Mastosarcoma	Skin	21	1.5	Mastosarcoma	Skin	30	2.1	Adenoma	Thyroid				
381	3.2	Papilloma	Skin	19	1.4	Basal cell ca.	Skin	30	2.1	Neuroma	Peripheral nerve				
351	3.0	Fibrosarcoma	Mouth	19	1.4	Fibroma	Skin	21	1.4	Adenocarcinoma	Thyroid				
301	2.6	Histiocytoma	Skin	14	1.0	Osteosarcoma	Bone, joint	18	1.2	Neuroma	Skin				
276	2.3	Fibroma	Mouth	14	1.0	Sarcoma	Skin	17	1.2	Melanoma	Skin				
205	1.7	Benign mixed mammary tumor	Mammae					15	1.0	Carcinoma	Nasal cavity[c]				
204	1.7	Malignant mixed mammary tumor	Mammae												
199	1.7	Hemangioma	Skin												
190	1.6	Sarcoma	Skin												
131	1.1	Mastocytoma	Skin												
124	1.1	Mastocytoma	Skin												
124	1.1	Adenoma	Perianal												
119	1.0	Reticulum cell sarcoma	Lymph node												

[a] Source: W. A. Priester: Theiler and McDonald Veterinary Oncology, Lee & Febiger, Philadelphia, 1980.
[b] And lymphatic leukemia.
[c] And paranasal sinuses.
[d] And conjunctiva, lacrimal gland.

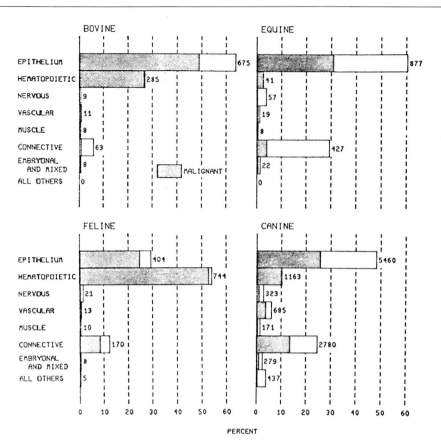

Figure 48.1. Distribution of all microscopically confirmed primary tumors and all confirmed primary malignant tumors by tissue type in the bovine, equine, feline, and canine species. Total number of tumors for each tissue type is given beside each bar.

mals (the canine, feline, equine, and bovine species) and the laboratory mammals (mainly lagomorphs and rodents), but also the rhesus monkey as the primate used most often experimentally.

In the limelight we find dog and cat, man's dearest pets, of which we have a good population; in their food and housing, they are closely related to us. They are good indicators in that they are shorter lived compared to man in a particular environment. The epidemiology of dogs and cats has been discussed by Hayes. It must be underlined that the dog, especially, almost always dies a normal death.

The dog shows the highest tumor frequency. Nearly all the tumors found in man have also been found in the dog. According to Dobberstein (109) the tumor frequency is as follows: thyroid gland (41.5%), mammary glands (14%), and testis (12%). Cats show a tumor frequency less than that of horses, but the incidence of the leukoses (lymphadenoses) is somewhat higher in cats than in dogs. Cancers of many glands, of the tongue, and of the esophagus are relatively common.

The horse has tumors of the paranasal sinus

(13.5%), the oral cavity (14%), the penis (14%), the digestive tract (12.6%), and the conjunctiva (12%). According to Lombard white horses often have melanogenic tumors (see Chapter 38).

Malignant tumors are less frequent in cattle than in the dog or horse: stomach (13.5%), skin (12.5%), conjunctiva (9%), urogenital tract (11%), and liver (8%).

The tumor frequency in sheep is low. According to Priester and Mantel the frequency is as follows: adenocarcinoma of nose and paranasal sinuses, benign neoplasms of pituitary, lymphoma of lymph nodes.

As for swine we find lymphoma of lymph nodes, fibroma of pleura, mediastinum and thoracic cavity, benign melanoma of skin, and equally malignant melanoma of skin.

The spectrum of cell types was narrowest in cattle; the widest was found in dogs. As far as sex is concerned, higher risk for tumors was observed in cows only. An increased age-dependent risk was seen in all four species, dog, cat, horse, and cattle, but it was most pronounced in the horse. One bovine, 2 equine, and 14 canine breeds had an increased tumor risk over the other breeds in their species.

References

1. Abrams, G. D. (1969): Disease in an amphibian colony, in *Biology of Amphibian Tumors*, pp. 419–428, edited by Mizell. Springer, New York.
2. Adami, J. G. (1908): On a giant-celled rhabdomyosarcoma from the trout. *Montreal Med. J., 37*:163–165. (Cited by Schlumberger and Lucké (491).)
3. Allen, J.R., Hauser, W. C., and Carstens, L. A. (1970): Multiple tumors in a *Macaca mulatta* monkey. *Arch Pathol., 90*:167–175.
4. Altman, N. H., Small, J. D., and Squire, R. A. (1974): Squamous cell carcinoma of the rumen and thymic amyloidosis in a guanaco. *J. Am. Vet. Med. Assoc., 165*:820–822.
5. Anadon, E. (1956): Nota sobre un tumor en *Trachurus trachurus* L. *Invest. Pesq., 5*:13–15.
6. An der Lan, H. (1962): Histopathologische Auswirkungen von Insektiziden (DDT und Sevin) bei Wirbellosen und ihre cancerogene Beurteilung. *Mikroskopie, 17*:85–112.
7. André, E. (1927): Sur un chondrome du vairon. *Bull. Suisse Pêche Pisciculture, 28*:177–178.
8. Andrews, E. J. (1974): Aberrant regeneration in carcinogen-treated earthworms (*Eisenia foetida*). *J. Exp. Zool., 189*:333–338.
9. Anitschkov, N., and Pavlovsky, E. N. (1923): Über die Hautpapillome bei Gobius und ihre Beziehung zur normalen Structur der Fischhaut. *Z. Krebsforsch., 20*:128–147.
10. Armed Forces Institute of Pathology (AFIP): *The Registry of Veterinary Pathology.*, Washington, D.C.
11. Aronowitz, O., Nigrelli, R. F., and Gordon, M. (1951): A spontaneous epithelioma in the platyfish, *Xiphophorus* (Platypeocilus) *variatus*. *Zool. N.Y., 36*:239–241.
12. Ayson, L. F. (1896): Carcinoma of the thyroid gland in *Salmo levensis*. (Cited by Schmey (492).)
13. Ayson, L. F. (1898): Carcinoma of the thyroid gland in *Salmo levensis*. (Cited by Schmey (492).)
14. Ayson, L. F. (1902): Carcinoma of the thyroid gland in *Salmo levensis*. (Cited by Schmey (492).)
15. Baerwald, R. J., and Boush, G. M. (1969): Abnormal cellular responses in *Periplaneta americana* L. Resulting from intracoelomic injections of benzopyrene. *Natl. Cancer Inst. Monogr., 31*:447–451.
16. Baker, K. F., Berg, O., Nigrelli, R. F., Gorbman, A., and Gordon, M. (1954): Thyroid cell origin of spontaneous adenocarcinomas of the kidneys in fishes. *Proc. Am. Assoc. Cancer Res., 1*:3 (Abstr.).
17. Balazuc, J. (1948): La tératologie des coleopteres. *Mém. Mus. Nat. Hist. Nat., 25*:1–2.
18. Ball, H. A. (1946): Melanosarcoma and rhabdomyoma in two pine snakes, *Pituophis melanoleucous*. 6:134–138.
19. Ball, H. A.: Unpublished data. (Cited by Wadsworth (608, 609).)
20. Balls, M. (1962): Spontaneous neoplasms in amphibia; a review and descriptions of six new cases. *Cancer Res., 22*:1142–1154.
21. Balls, M. (1965): The incidence of pathologic abnormalities, including spontaneous lymphosarcomas, in a laboratory stock of *Xenopus* (the South African clawed toad). *Cancer Res., 25*:3–6.
22. Balls, M. (1965): Lymphosarcoma in the South African clawed toad, *Xenopus laevis*, a virus tumor. *Ann. N.Y. Acad. Sci., 126*:256–273.
23. Baroche, C. (1968): Actions de la thalidomide chez la drosophile; developpement et tumorigenic comparison avec le phtlate de potassium et quelques composes non phtaliques. *Bull. Cancer, 55*:413–428.
24. Barry, M. M., Yevich, P. P., and Thayer, H. H. (1971): Atypical hyperplasia in the soft-shell clam *Mya arenaria*. *J. Invertebr. Pathol., 17*:17–27.
25. Bashford, E. F., and Murray, J. A. (1904): Spindle cell sarcoma of the swim bladder in a cod (*Gadus morhua*, L.) (Cited by Schmey (492).)
26. Bashford, E. F., Murray, J. A., and Cramer, W. (1905): Transplantation of malignant new growths. *Imp. Cancer Res. Fund Sci. Rep., 2*:13–17.
27. Baxendale, W. (1969): Preliminary observations on Marek's disease in ducks and other avian species. *Vet. Rec., 85*:341–342.
28. Bearcroft, W. G. C., and Jamison, M. F. (1958): An outbreak of subcutaneous tumor in rhesus monkeys. *Nature, 182*:195–196.
29. Beatti, M. (1916): Geschwülste bei Tiersen. *Z. Krebsforsch. 15*:452–491.
30. Bernirschke, K. (1972): *Comparative Pathophysiology*,
31. Berg, O., Edgar, M., and Gordon, M. (1953): Progressive growth stages in the development of spontaneous thyroid tumors in inbred swordtails, *Xiphophorus montezumae*. *Cancer Res., 13*:1–8.
32. Bergman, A. M. (1921): Einige Geschwülste bei Fischen; Rhabdomyom, Lipome und Melanom. *Z. Krebsforsch., 18*:292–302.
33. Bergmann, R. A. M. (1941): Tumoren bij Slangen. *Geneesk. T. Ned. Ind., 81*:571–577.
34. Bertullo, V. H., and Traibel, R. M. (1955): Neoplasm in fish of the Uruguayan coastal waters; I. Osteoma of the pleural rib of the sea-bass, *Micropogen opercularis*. *An. Fac. Vet. Urug., 3*:55–59.
35. Biavati, S. T., and Mancini, L. (1967): A case of fibroma in the sardine. *Nuova Vet., 43*:11–14.
36. Bird, F. T. (1949): Tumors associated with a virus infection in an insect. *Nature, 163*:777–778.
37. Blanchard, R. (1890): Sur une remarquable dermatose causee chez le lezard vert par un champignon du genre *Selenosporium*. *Mêm. Soc. Zool. Fr., 3*:241–255.
38. Bodnaryk, R. P. (1968): Dietary amino acid and nucleic acid imbalance leading to altered tumor frequency in the adult housefly *Musca domestica*. *J. Insect Physiol., 14*:223–242.
39. Bonnet, R. (1883): Studien zur Physiologie und Pathologie der Fische. *Bayer. Fischerei Z., 6*:79. (Cited by Schlumberger and Lucké (491).)
40. Breider, H. (1939): Über die Vorgänge der Kernvermehrung und -degeneration in sarkomatösen Makromelanophoren. *Z. Wiss. Zool., 152*:89.
41. Breslauer, T. (1916): Zur Kenntnis der Epidermoidalgeschwülste von Kaltblütern. *Arch. Mikrosk. Anat., 87*:200–264.
42. Bresler, V. M. (1963): A lung tumor in a turtle, *Emys orbicularis*. *Vop. Onokol., 9*:87–91.
42a. Brightman, A. H., II, and Burke, T. J. (1978): Eyelid tumor in a parakeet. *Mod. Vet. Pract., 59*:683.
43. Brodey, R. S. (1970): Canine and feline neoplasia. *Adv. Vet. Sci. Comp. Med., 14*:309–354.
44. Broughton, E., Miller, F. L., and Choquette, L. P. (1972): Cutaneous fibropapillomas in migratory barren-ground caribou. *J. Wildlife Dis., 8*:138–140.
45. Broughton, E., Graesser, F. E., Carbyn, L. N., and Choquette, L. P. E. (1970): Oral papillomatosis in the coyote in western Canada. *J. Wildlife Dis., 6*:180–181. (*Vet. Bull., 41*:816, 1971.)
46. Brown, R. J., and Kupper, J. L. (1972): Parovarian cyst (hydatid cyst of Morgagni) in a squirrel monkey (*Saimiri sciureus*). *Lab. Anim. Sci., 22*:741–742.
47. Brown, R. J., Smith, A. W., and Keyes, M. C. (1975): Renal fibrosarcoma in the northern fur seal. *J. Wildlife Dis., 11*:23–25.
48. Brown, R. J., Kupper, J. L., Trevethan, W. P., and Britz, W. E. (1971): Malignant lymphoma in a rhesus monkey. *Vet. Pathol., 8*:289–291.
49. Brown, R. J., Davis, R. D., Trevethan, W. P., and Johnson, N. L. (1972): Basal cell tumor in an Indian leopard. *J. Wildlife Dis., 8*:237–238.
50. Brown, R. J., Kupper, J. L., Trevethan, W. P., and Johnston, N. L. (1973): Fibrosarcoma in an African elephant. *J. Wildlife Dis., 9*:227–228.
51. Broz, O. (1947): Multiple "Chondrome" in der Haut von *Triton taeniatus* Vestnik. *Esl. Zool. Spolecnosti, 11*:89.
52. Brun, H. (1925–26): Ein Fall von Hirntumor bei einer Ameise. *Schweiz. Arch. Neurol. Psychiat., 16*:86–99.
53. Brunst, V. V. (1969): Structures of Spontaneous and Transplanted Tumors in the Axolotl (*Siredon mexicanum*), in *Biology of Amphibian Tumors*, pp. 215–219. Springer, New York.
54. Brunst, V. V., and Roque, A. L. (1967): Tumors in amphibians; I. Histology of a neuroepithelioma in *Siredon mexicanum*. *J.N.C.I., 38*:193–204.
55. Budd, J., and Schröder, J. D. (1969): Testicular tumors of yellow perch, *Perca flavescens* (Mitchill). *Bull. Wildlife Dis. Assoc., 5*:315–318.
56. Budd, J., Schröder, J. D., and Dukes, K. D. (1975): Tumors of the yellow perch, in *The Pathology of Fishes*, pp. 895–906, edited by W. E. Ribelin and G. Migaki. The University of Wisconsin Press, Madison, Wisc.
57. Bugnion, E. (1875): Ein Fall von Sarcoma beim Fisch [A case of sarcoma in the fish]. *Dtsch. Z. Tiermed. Vergl. Pathol., 1*:132–134.
58. Burke, T. J. (1969): Multiple lipomas in a spotted leopard (*Panthera pardus*). *J. Am. Vet. Med. Assoc., 155*:1099–1100.
59. Burns, E. R., and White, H. J. (1971): A spontaneous mesenchymal cell neoplasm in the adult newt *Diemictylus viridescens*. *Cancer Res., 31*:826–829.
60. Busch, R. H., and Williams, L. E., Jr. (1970): Case report. A Marek's disease-like condition in Florida turkeys. *Avian Dis., 14*:550–554.
61. Butros, J. M. (1948): A tumor in a fresh-water mussel. *Cancer Res., 8*:270–271.
62. Cameron, A. T., and Vincent, S. (1915): Notes on an enlarged thyroid occurring in an elasmobranch fish (*Squalus suckleyi*). *J. Med. Res., 27*:251–256.
63. Campbell, J. G. (1969): *Tumour of the Fowl*. William Heinemann, London. (*Vet. Bull., 41*:501, 1971.)
64. Campbell, D. J., and Smith, W. T. (1966): A pituitary adenoma in a hedgehog (*Erinaceus europaeus*). *Endocrinology, 79*:842–844.
65. Campbell, G. (1972): Visceral lymphomatosis in a turkey flock. *Ir. Vet. J., 26*:28–30. (*Vet. Bull., 42*:4114, 1972.)
66. Cantwell, G. E., Harshbarger, J. C., Taylor, R. L., Kenton, C., Slatick, M. S., and Dawe, C. J.: A bibliography of the literature on neoplasms of invertebrate animals. *GANN Monogr. 5: Experimental Animals in Cancer Research*, pp. 57–84. Maruzen Co., Ltd., Tokyo.
67. Cantwell, G. E., Shortino, T. J., and Robbins, W. E. (1966): The histopathological effects of certain carcinogenic 2-fluorenamine derivatives on larvae of the house fly. *J. Invertebr. Pathol., 8*:167–174.
68. Carl, W. (1913): Ein Hypernephron beim Frosch. *Zentrabbl. Allg. Pathol. Anat., 24*:436–438.
69. Casey, H. W., Simmonds, R. C., and Butcher, W. I. (1972): Renal adenocarcinoma with intranuclear inclusions in an arctic ground squirrel. *Can. J. Comp. Med., 26*:79–82.
70. Ceretto, F. (1968): Carcinoma di tipo psammomatoso in *Carassius auratus* [Carcinoma of the psammoma type in the goldfish]. *Riv. Ital. Piscis. Ittiopat. (A.), 3*:37–40.

71. Chabanaud, P. (1926): Fréquence, symetrie et constance spécifique d'hyperostoses externes chez divers poissons de la famille des sciaenides. C. R. Acad. Sci., 182:1647-1649.

72. Champy, C., and Champy, G. (1935): Sur un epithelioma transmissible chez le triton. Bull. Assoc. Fr. Cancer, 118:861-863.

73. Chang, P. W., Perry, M. C., and Jasty, V. (1969): Fibroma in a mute swan. J. Am. Vet. Med. Assoc., 155:1039.

74. Chapman, W. L., Jr., and Allen, J. R. (1968): Multiple neoplasia in a rhesus monkey Macaca mulatta. Pathol. Vet., 5:342-352.

75. Charlton, H. H. (1929): A tumor of the pineal organ with cartilage formation in the mackerel, Scomber scombrus. Anat. Rec., 43:271-276.

76. Chesterman, F. C., and Pomerance, A. (1965): Cirrhosis and liver tumours in a closed colony of golden hamsters. Br. J. Cancer, 19:802-811.

77. Christiansen, M., and Jensen, A. J. C. (1947): On a recent and frequently occurring tumor disease in eel; 1. Occurrence of the disease in the various years and its distribution (Jensen). 2. Investigations of the tumors (Christiansen). Rep. Danish Biol. Sta., 50:29-44.

78. Christopher, J., Rao, P. R., and Narayanna, J. V. (1965): A case of leiomyoma in the liver of a pigeon. Ind. Vet. J., 42:753-756.

79. Chuinard, R. G., Berkson, H. and Wellings, S. R. (1966): Surface tumors of starry flounders and English sole from Puget Sound, Washington. Fed. Proc., 25:661.

80. Clunet, J. (1910): Recherches Experimentales sur les Tumeurs Malignes [Experimenal Research on Malignant Tumors]. G. Steinbeil, Paris.

81. Coates, C. W., Cox, R. T., and Smith, G. M. (1938): Papilloma of the skin occurring in an electric eel, Electrophorus electricus (L.). Zool. N. Y. Zool. Soc., 23:248-251.

82. Cockrill, W. R. (1960): Pathology of the cetacea—a veterinary study on whales. Br. Vet. J., 116:1-28.

83. Cohrs, P., Jaffe, R., and Meessen, H. (eds.) (1958): Pathologie der Laboratoriumstiere. Springer, New York.

84. Collinge, W. E. (1890/91): Note on a tumour in Anodonta cygnaea L. J. Anat. Physiol. (Lond.), 25:154.

85. Conrad, L. G., Conrad, G. M., and Dawe, C. J. (1965): Cutaneous leiomyosarcoma in a long-eared Plecotus townsendii virgianus Handley. J.N.C.I., 35:95-101.

86. Cooper, E. L. (1968): Multinucleate giant cells, granulomata and "myoblastomas" in annelid worms. J. Invertebr. Pathol., 11:123-131.

87. Cooper, E. L. (1969): Neoplasia and transplantation immunity in annelids. Natl. Cancer Inst. Monogr., 31:655-669.

88. Cooper, R. C., and Keller, C. A. (1969): Epizootiology of papillomas in English sole, Parophrys vetulus: Neoplasms and related disorders of invertebrate and lower vertebrate animals. Natl. Cancer Inst. Monogr., 31:173-186.

89. Corley, G. J. (1975): Melanomas in platy/swordtail hybrids, in The Pathology of Fishes, pp. 945-982, edited by W. E. Ribelin and G. Migaki. The University of Wisconsin Press, Madison, Wisc.

90. Cosgrove, G. E., Lushbaugh, W. B., Humason, G., et al. (1968): Synhimantus (Nematoda) associated with gastric squamous tumors in muskrats. Wildlife Dis., 4:54-57.

91. Couch, J. A. (1969): An unusual lesion in the mantle of the American oyster, Crassostrea virginica. Nat. Cancer Inst. Monogr., 31:557-562.

92. Cowan, D. F. (1968): Diseases of captive reptiles. J. Am. Vet. Med. Assoc., 153:848-859.

93. Crisp, E. (1854): Large fungoid tumor in carp. Trans. Pathol. Soc. (Lond.), 5:347-348.

94. Dauwe, F., and Pennemann, G. (1904): Contributions a l'etude du cancer chez les poissons. Ann. Soc. Med. Gand., 84:81-90.

95. Dawe, C. J. (1968): Invertebrate Animals in Cancer Research. GANN Monograph 5: Experimental Animals in Cancer Research. Maruzen Co., Ltd. Tokyo.

96. Dawe, C. J. (1968): Neoplasms of blood cell origin in poikilothermic animals—A review. Natl. Cancer Inst. Monogr., 32:7-28.

97. Dawe, C. J. (1968): Differentiation in relation to neoplasia in old and new organisms. In Vitro, 3:57-62.

98. Dawe, C. J. (1969): Phylogeny and oncogeny. Natl. Cancer Inst. Monogr., 31:1-39.

99. Dawe, C. J. (1969): Neoplasms of blood cell origin in poikilothermic animals—a review. (Symposium on Comparative Morphology of Hematopoietic Neoplasms. Natl. Cancer. Inst. Monogr., 32:7-28.

100. Dawe, C. J. (1970): Neoplasms of blood cell origin in poikilothermic animals. A status summary. Bibl. Haematol., 36:634-637.

101. Dawe, C. J., and Harshbarger, J. C. (Eds.) (1969): Neoplasms and related disorders of invertebrate and lower vertebrate animals. Natl. Cancer. Inst. Monogr., 31.

102. Dawe, C. J., and Berard, C. W. (1971): Highlights; workshop on comparative pathology of hemopoietic and lymphoreticular neoplasms. J.N.C.I., 47:1365.

103. Dawe, C. J., and Harshbarger, J. C. (1975): Neoplasms in feral fishes; their significance to cancer research, in The Pathology of Fishes, pp. 871-906, edited by W. E. Ribelin and G. Migaki. The University of Wisconsin Press, Madison, Wisc.

104. Desvoigne, D. M., Mix, M. C., and Pauley, G. B. (1970): A papilloma-like growth on the siphon of the horse clam, Tresus nuttalli. J. Invertebr. Pathol., 15:262-267.

105. Deys, B. F. (1969): Papillomas in the Atlantic eel, Anguilla vulgaris. (Neoplasms and related disorders of invertebrate and lower extremity animals). Natl. Cancer Inst. Monogr., 31:187-194.

106. DiGiacomo, R. F. (1967): Burkitt's lymphoma in white-handed gibbon (Hylobates lar). Cancer Res., 27:1178-1179.

107. Dobberstein, J. (1937): Der Krebs der Haussäugetiere. Tierärztl. Wochenschr. Berlin, p. 100.

108. Dobberstein, J. (1949): Die Geschwülste der Tiere. Arch. Geschwulstforsch., 1:54.

109. Dobberstein, J. (1953): Vergleichende Pathologie der Geschwülste. Z. Krebsforsch., 59:600.

110. Dobberstein, J. (1955): Der Krebs der Tiere im Vergleich zum Krebs der Menschen. Strahlentherapie, 96:259-265.

111. Dollfus, R. P., Timon-David, J., and Mosinger, M. (1938): À propos des tumeurs mélanique des poissons. Bull. Assoc. Fr. Cancer, 27:37-50.

112. Dominguez, A. G. (1928): Fibroblastic sarcoma in a goldfish. Clin. Med., 35:256-257.

113. Dorn, C. R. (1964): Biliary and hepatic carcinomas in bears at the San Diego Zoological Gardens. Nature, 202:513-514.

114. Downs, A. W. (1932): An epithelial tumour of the intestine of a frog. Nature, 130:778.

115. Drew, G. H. (1912): Some cases of new growths in fish. J. Mar. Biol. Assoc., 9:281-287.

116. Duany, J. (1932): Un epithelioma glandular en una rana. Arch. Soc. Estud. Clin. Habano, 29:186.

117. Dunbar, D. E. (1969): Lymphosarcoma of possible thymic origin in salmonid fishes. Natl. Cancer Inst. Monogr., 31:167-171.

118. Dunkel, V. C., and Myers, S. L. (1972): Continuous lymphoblastoid cell line from a rhesus monkey with myelogenous leukemia. J.N.C.I., 48: 777-782.

119. Duryee, W. R. (1965): Factors influencing development of tumors in frogs. Ann. N.Y. Acad. Sci., 126:59-85.

120. Eberth, C. (1878): Fibrosarkom der Kopfhaut einer Forelle. Virchows Arch. Pathol. Anat., 72:107-108.

121. Eguchi, S., and Oota, J. (1926): Of a tumor in a fish. (Jap.). Aichi Igakkwai Zasshi, 33. (Biol. Abstracts 5: Item #20406, 1931.)

122. Elkan, E. (1960): Some interesting pathological cases in amphibians. Proc. Zbl. (Lond.), 134:375-396.

123. Elkan, E. (1963): The principle diseases of lower vertebrates, pp. 186-187. In: Lehrbuch der Erkrankungen der Amphibien und Reptilien by H. Reichenbach-Klinke, and E. Elkan. Academic Press, London.

124. Elkan, E. (1963): Three different types of tumors in Salientia. Cancer Res., 23:1641-1645.

125. Elkan, E. (1970): A spontaneous anaplastic intestinal metastasizing carcinoma in a South African clawed toad (Xenopus laevis Daudin). J. Pathol., 100:205-207.

126. El-Sergany, M. (1966): Carcinoma of the stomach in a lion. Berl. Münch. Tierärztl. Wochenschr., 79:410-412.

127. Engle, E. T., and Stout, A. P. (1940): Spontaneous primary carcinoma of the prostate in a monkey (M. mulatta). Am. J. Cancer, 39:334-337.

128. Erdman, D. S. (1968): Melanotic tumours in Micropterus salmoides (personal communication).

129. Erdman, D. S. (1968): Ovarian tumours in Coryphaena hippurus (personal communication).

130. Ermin, R. (1953): Platypoecilus maculatus var. fuliginosus da Ksantoiritroforoma Tesekkulu Hakkinda [On a case of xanthoerythrophoroma formation in Platypoecilus maculatus var. fuliginosus]. Istanb. Univ. Fen. Fak. Mecm. (B), 18:301-314.

131. Ermin, R. (1954): On an ocular tumor with exophthalmia in an interspecific hybrid of anatolichthys (Turk.). Istanb. Univ. Fen. Fak. Mecm., 19:203-211.

132. Falkmer, S., Emdin, S. O., Ostberg, Y., Mattisson, A., Johansson, M., Sjobeck, L., and Fange, R. (1976): Tumor pathology of the hagfish, Myxine glutinosa, and the river lamprey Lampetra fluviatilis. Prog. Exp. Tumor Res., 20:217-250.

133. Fankhauser, R., and Luginbuhl, H. (1968): Tumoren des Zentralnervensystems, in Handbuch der speziellen pathologischen Anatomie der Haustiere, Vol. 3, Ed. 3, pp. 366-423, edited by Joest. Parey, Berlin.

134. Farley, C. A. (1969): Probable neoplastic diseaes of the hematopoietic system in oysters, Crassostrea virginica and Crassostrea gigas: Neoplasms and related disorders of invertebrate and lower vertebrate animals. Natl. Cancer Inst. Monogr., 31:541-556.

135. Farley, C. A. (1976): Ultrastructural observations on epizootic neoplasia and lytic virus infection in bivalve mollusks. Prog. Exp. Tumor Res., 20:283-294.

136. Farley, C. A., and Sparks, A. K. (1969/1970): Proliferative diseases of hemocytes, endothelial cells and connective tissue cells in molluscs. Comp. Leukemia Res., 1969, Bibl. Haematol., 36:610-617, 1970.

137. Federley, H. (1935): Ett egendomligt fall av konsbegransad hereditar kancer. Finska Lak. Sallask. Hdl., 78.

138. Federley, H. (1936): Sex-limited hereditary cancer in lepidopterous larvae. Hereditas, 22:193-216.

139. Fiebiger, J., (1909): Über Hautgeschwülste bei Fischen nebst Bemerkungen über die Pockenkrankheit der Karpfen. Z. Krebsforsch., 7:165-179.

140. Fiebiger, J. (1909): Ein Osteochondrom bei einem Karpfen. Z. Krebs-

forsch., 7:371–381.

141. Fiebiger, J. (1909): Ein Rhabdomyom bei einem Kabeljau. Z. Krebsforsch.,, 7:382–388.

142. Fiebiger, J. (1912): Bösartige Neubildung (Fibrosarkom) bei einem Seefisch. Ost. Fisch. Zt., 9:308.

143. Filosa, M. F. (1962): Hetercytosis in cellular slime molds. Am. Naturalist, 96:79–91.

144. Finkelstein, E. A., and Danchenko-Ryzchokova, L. K. (1965): Neurinoma in the perch Perca fluviatilis. Arkh. Patol., 27:81–84.

145. Firminger, H. I., Antoine, S., and Adams, E. (1969): Epithelioma-like lesions in Lumbricus terrestris after cold injury: Neoplasms and related disorders of invertebrate and lower vertebrate animals. Natl. Cancer Inst. Monogr., 31:645–653.

146. Fischer, E. (1928): A sociation chez le crabe d'un tissu parasite et d'une trame conjonctive, analogue a certains processus tumoraux. Bull. Assoc. Fr. Cancer, 17:468–470.

147. Fischer, P. H. (1954): Tumeur fibreuse chez un pleurobranche. J. Conchiliol., 94:99–101.

148. Fontaine, A. R. (1962): The colours of Ophiocomina nigra (Abildgaard); II. The occurrence of melania and fluorescent pigments. J. Mar. Biol. Assoc. (U.K.), 42:9–31.

149. Foster, J. A. (1969): Malformations and lethal growths in planaria treated with carcinogens: Neoplasms and related disorders of invertebrate and lower vertebrate animals. Natl. Cancer Inst. Monogr., 31:683–692.

150. Fox, H. (1923): Disease in Captive Wild Mammals and Birds. J. B. Lippincott, Philadelphia.

151. Frank, W., and Schepky A. (1969): Metastasizing lymphosarcoma in a giant snake, Eunectes murinus L. Pathol. Vet. (Basel), 6:437–443.

152. Frauchiger, E., O'Hara, P. J., and Shortridge, E. H. (1966): Pincaloma in animals. Schweiz. Arch. Tierheilkd., 108:368–372.

153. Frömming, E., Peter, H., and Reichmuth, W. (1960): Beitrag zur Frage der pathologischen Gestaltsveränderung und der Geschwülste bei unseren Nacktschnecken. Zool. Anz., 166:139–147.

154. Galtsoff, P. S. (1969): Anomalies and malformations in the shells of Crassostrea virginica (Neoplasms and related disorders of invertebrate and lower vertebrate animals). Natl. Cancer Inst. Monogr., 31:575–580.

155. Gateff, E. A. Fr. (1972): Developmental and histological studies of wild-type and mutant tissues of Drosophila melanogaster. Ph.D. thesis, University of California, Irvine.

156. Gateff, E. A. F. (1975): Animal models of human disease: Neuroblastoma of genetic origin. Comp. Pathol. Bull., 7:3–4.

157. Gateff, E. (1976): Neoplasms of genetic origin in Drosophila melanogaster. Proceedings of the First International Colloquium on Invertebrate Pathology and IXth Annual Meeting, Society for Invertebrate Pathology, Queen's University at Kingston, Canada, pp. 142–146.

158. Gateff, E. (1976): Malignant blood cell neoplasms of genetic origin in Drosophila melanogaster. J. Cell Biol., 70:6a.

159. Gateff, E., and Schneiderman, H. A. (1967): Developmental studies of a new mutant of Drosophila melanogaster; lethal malignant brain tumor (abstr). Am. Zool., 7:760.

160. Gateff, E., and Schneiderman, H. A. (1969): Neoplasms in mutant and cultured wild-type tissues of Drosophila. Natl. Cancer Inst. Monogr., 31:365–397.

161. Gateff, E., and Schneiderman, H. A. (1974): Developmental capacities of benign and malignant neoplasms of Drosophila. Wilhelm Roux Arch. Entwicklungsmech. Org., 176:23–65.

162. Gateff, E., Akai, H., and Schneiderman, H. A. (1974): Correlations between developmental capacity and structure of tissue sublines derived from the eye-antennal imaginal disc of Drosophila melanogaster. Wilhelm Roux Arch. Entwicklungsmech. Org., 176:89–123.

163. Gaylord, H. R., and Marsh, M. C. (1912): Relation of feeding to thyroid hyperplasia in salmonidae. Z. Krebsforsch., 12:436–438.

164. Gersch, M. (1950): Über Zellwucherungen und Geschwulstbildung in der Lunge von Helix; II. Beitrag zur Frage der Zellentartung bei Wirbellosen. Biol. Zbl., 69:500–507.

165. Gersch, M. (1951): Untersuchungen über Zellentartung bei Enchytraeen. Zool. Anz., 146:201–222.

166. Gersch, M. (1954): Einwirkung von kanzerogenen Kohlenwasserstoffen auf die Haut von Regenwürmern. Naturwissenschaften, 41:337.

167. Gersch, M. (1957): Zellentartung und Zellwucherung bei Regenwürmern nach Behandlung mit kanzerogenen Kohlenwasserstoffen. Arch. Geschwulstforsch., 10:101–118.

168. Gervais, P. (1875): De l'hyperostose chez l'homme et chez les animaux. J. Zool., 4:272–284. (Cited by Schlumberger and Lucké (491).)

169. Ghadially, F. N., and Whiteley, H. J. (1951): Hormonally induced epithelial hyperplasia in the goldfish (Carassius auratus). Br. J. Cancer, 6:246–248.

170. Ghadially, F. N., and Gordon, M. D. (1957): A localized melanoma in a hybrid fish Lebistes X mollienesia. Cancer Res., 17:597–599.

171. Ghelelovitch, S. (1969): Melanotic tumors in Drosophila melanogaster: Neoplasms and related disorders of invertebrate and lower vertebrate animals. Natl. Cancer Inst. Monogr., 31:263–276.

172. Gheorghieu, J. (1930): Contribution a l'etude du cancer de la grenouille. C. R. Soc. Biol., 103:280–281.

173. Gilruth, J. A. (1902): Epithelioma affecting the branchial arches of salmon and trout. Rep. New Zealand Dept. Agric. Vet. Div., 1901/1902: 312–315.

174. Goldsmith, E. D. (1937): Production of supernumerary outgrowths in planarians by the application of ethyl alcohol, aniline oil, and coal tar. Anat. Rec., 70:134–135.

175. Goldsmith, E. D. (1939): Spontaneous outgrowths in Dugesia tigrina (Syn. Planaria macula). Anat. Rec. (Suppl.), 75:158–159.

176. Goldsmith, E. D. (1941): Further observations of supernumerary structures in individuals of an artificially produced clone of Dugesia tigrina. Anta. Rec., 81:108–109.

177. Good, H. V. (1940): A study of an epithelial tumor of Parophyrus vetulus. Unpublished master's dissertation, University of Washington, Seattle.

178. Gorbman, A. (1964): Comparative pathology of the thyroid, in The Thyroid, pp. 32–48, edited by J. Beach Hazard and D. E. Smith. Williams & Wilkins, Baltimore.

179. Gorbman, A., and Gordon, M. (1951): Spontaneous thyroidal tumors in a swordtail fish species (Xiphophorus montezumae). Cancer Res., 11:184–187.

180. Gordon, M. (1937): The production of spontaneous melanotic neoplasms in fishes by selective matings; II. Neoplasms with macromelanophores only; III. Neoplasms in day old fish. Am. J. Cancer, 30:362–375.

181. Graffi, A. (1967): Untersuchungen zur Frage der Bedeutung der Mitochondrien bei der Kanzerisierung. Dtsch. Ges. Wesen, 22:2305–2312.

182. Granados, R. R., and Meehan, D. J. (1973): Morphology and differential counts of hemocytes of healthy and wound tumor virus-infected Agallia constricta. J. Invest. Pathol., 22:60–69.

183. Griner, L. A. (1971): Malignant leukemic lymphoma in two harbor seals (Phoca vitulina geronimensis). Am. J. Vet. Res., 32:827–830.

184. Gross, L. J. (1940): The incidence and classification of avian tumors. Cornell Vet., 30:75–88.

185. Guglianetti, L. (1910): Fibroma dell'orbita in un ciprino [Orbital fibroma in a cyprinid]. Archo Ottal., 17:289–297.

186. Haddow, A., and Blake, I. (1933): Neoplasms in fish: a report of six cases with a summary of the literature. J. Pathol. Bacteriol., 36:41–47.

187. Häussler, C. (1928): Über Melanombildungen bei Bastarden von Xiphophorum hellerii und Platypoecilus maculatus var. rubra. Klin. Wochenschr., 7:1561–1562.

188. Häussler, G. (1934): Uber die Melanome der Xiphophorus-Platypoecilus Bastarde. Z. Krebsforsch., 40:280–292.

189. Hammett, F. S. (1933): The influence of sulfhydryl and its suboxidize derivatives on the developmental cycle of hydranths of the genus Obelia. Protoplasms, 19:510–540.

190. Hammett, F. S., and Reimann, S. P. (1935): Effect of methylcholanthrene on developmental growth of Obelia geniculata. Am. J. Cancer, 25:807–808.

191. Hancock, R. L. (1961): Giant nuclei in the earthworm Lumbricus. Nature, 189:685.

192. Hancock, R. L. (1961): Neoplasms in Lumbricus terrestris L. Experientia, 17:547–549.

193. Hancock, R. L. (1962): Lethal doses of irradiation for Lumbricus. Life Sci., 11:625–628.

194. Hancock, R. L. (1965): Irradiation induced neoplastic and giant cells in earthworms. Experientia, 21:33–34.

195. Hancock, R. L. (1965): An unusual neoplasm in Lumbricus terrestris. Experientia, 21:280–283.

196. Hancock, R. L. (1965): Giant chromocentres and nucleoli in Lumbricus. Nature, 206:1337–1338.

197. Hancock, R. L. (1969): Cytological and comparative biochemical studies on normal and neoplastic earthworm tissues: Neoplasms and related disorders of invertebrate and lower vertebrate animals. Natl. Cancer Inst. Monogr., 31:593–644.

198. Hansemann, J. D., v. (1906): Diskussionsbemerkung. Verh. Berl. Med. Ges., 39:231.

199. Hanström, B. (1926): Über einen Fall von pathologischer Chitinbildung im Inneren des Körpers von Limulus polyphemus. Zool. Ann., 66:213–219.

200. Harker, J. E. (1963): Tumors, in Insect Pathology, Vol. 1, pp. 191–213, edited by E. A. Steinhaus. Academic Press, New York.

201. Harms, J. W. (1955): Biologie des Wachstums, in Handbuch der Allgemeinen Pathologie (Biology of Growth), Vol. VI (Pt. 1), pp. 139–179. Springer, Berlin.

202. Harshbarger, J. C. (1967): Responses of invertebrates to vertebrate carcinogens. Fed. Proc., 26:1693–1697.

203. Harshbarger, J. C. (1969): The registry of tumors in lower animals. Natl. Cancer Inst. Monogr., 31:11–16.

204. Harshbarger, J. C. (1973): Invertebrate animals—what can they contribute to cancer research? Fed. Proc., 32:2224–2227.

205. Harshbarger, J. C. (1965–1973): Activities Report Registry of Tumors in Lower Animals. Smithsonian Institution, Washington, D.C.

206. Harshbarger, J. C. (1974): Activities Report Registry of Tumors in Lower Animals (Suppl.). Smithsonian Institution, Washington, D.C.

207. Harshbarger, J. C. (1974): Radiation, neoplasms, carcinogenic chemicals, and insects, in Insect Diseases, pp. 377–416, edited by G. E. Cantwell.

Marcel Dekker, New York.

208. Harshbarger, J. C. (1974): Integumentary papilloma and carcinomas in fish, Symp. No. 41: Environmental carcinogens in feral aquatic animals, in Abstracts: XIth International Cancer Congress, Florence (Italy), Vol. 1, pp. 218–219.

209. Harshbarger, J. C. (1975): *Activities Report Registry of Tumors in Lower Animals* (Suppl.). Smithsonian Institution, Washington, D.C.

210. Harshbarger, J. C. (1976): Description of polyps and epidermal papillomas in three bivalve mollusk species. *Mar. Fish. Rev.*, 38:25–29.

211. Harshbarger, J. C. (1976): *Activities Report Registry of Tumors in Lower Animals* (Suppl.). Smithsonian Institution, Washington, D.C.

212. Harshbarger, J. C. (1977): *Activities Report Registry of Tumors in Lower Animals* (Suppl.). Smithsonian Institution, Washington, D.C.

213. Harshbarger, J. C., and Taylor, R. L. (1968): Neoplasms of insects. *Annual Rev. Entomol.*, 13:159–189.

214. Harshbarger, J. C., and Bane, G. W. (1969): Case report of a fibrolipoma on a rockfish, *Sebastodes diploproa. Natl. Cancer Inst. Monogr.*, 31: 219–221.

215. Harshbarger, J. C., and Dawe, C. J. (1973): Hematopoietic neoplasms in invertebrate and poikilothermic vertebrate animals: Unifying concepts of leukemia. *Bibl. Haemtol.*, 39:1–25.

216. Harshbarger, J. C., Cantwell, G. E., and Stanton, M. F. (1970): Effects of N-nitrosodimethylamine on the crayfish, *Procambarus clarkii*, in Proceedings IVth International Colloquium on Insect Pathology, pp. 425–430.

217. Harshbarger, J. C., Shumway, S. E., and Bane, G. W. (1976): Variably differentiating oral neoplasms, ranging from epidermal papilloma to odontogenic ameloblastoma, in cunners *Tautogolabrus adspersus* (Osteichthyes; Perciformes; Labridae). *Prog. Exp. Tumor Res.*, 20:113–128.

218. Heller, J. (1906): Diskussionsbemerkung. *Verh. Berl. Med. Ges.*, 36:230–231.

219. Helmboldt, C. F., and Wyand, D. S. (1971): Nephroblastoma in a striped bass. *J. Wildlife Dis.*, 7:162–165. (Biol. Abstr. 52, No. 126110.)

220. Helmboldt, C. F., and Wyand, D. S. (1972): Parasitic neoplasia in the golden pheasant. *J. Wildlife Dis.*, 8:3–6.

221. Henderson, T. R., and Eakin, R. (1961): Irreversible alteration of differentiated tissues in Planaria by purine analogues. *J. Exp. Zool.*, 146:253–264.

222. Henderson, J. D., Jr., Bullock, B. C., and Clarkson, T. B. (1969): Naturally occurring mixed-cell sarcoma in a quail (*Coturnix coturnix japonica*). *Am. J. Vet. Res.*, 30:2245–2248.

223. Herubel, M. A. (1906): Sur une tumeur chez un invertebré (*Sipunculus nudus*). *C. R. Acad. Sci.*, 143:979–981.

224. Hill, J. R. (1977): Oral squamous cell carcinoma in a California king snake. *J. Am. Vet. Med. Assoc.*, 171:982.

225. Hill, W. C. O. (1952): Report of the society's prosector for the year 1951. *Proc. Zool. Soc. (Lond.)*, 112:513.

226. Hisaoka, K. K. (1961): Congenital teratomata in the guppy, *Lebistes reticulatus. J. Morphol.*, 109:93–113.

227. Hisaoka, K. K. (1963): A congenital teratoma in the swordtail, *Xiphophorus helleri. Copeia*, 1:189–191.

228. Hisaw, F. L., and Hisaw, F. L., Jr. (1958): Spontaneous carcinoma of the cervix uteri in a monkey (*Macaca mulatta*). *Cancer*, 11:810–816.

229. Honma, Y. (1965): A case of the myxoma developed in the head of the salmonoid fish, the auy, *Plecoglossus altivelis* Temminck et Schlegel. *Bull. Jpn. Soc. Sci. Fish.*, 31:192–197.

230. Honma, Y. (1966): Studies on the endocrine glands of the salmonoid fish, the auy, *Plecoglossus altivelis* Temminck et Schlegel; VI. Effect of artificially controlled light on the endocrines of the pond-cultured fish. *Bull. Jpn. Soc. Sci. Fish.*, 32:32–40.

231. Honma, Y., and Shirai, K. (1959): Cystoma found in the liver of rainbow trout (*Salmo gairdnerii irideus* Gibbons). *Bull. Jpn. Soc. Sci. Fish.*, 24: 966–970.

232. Honma, Y., and Kon, T. (1968): A case of the epidermal papilloma in the witch flounder from the Sea of Japan. *Bull. Jpn. Soc. Sci. Fish.*, 34: 1–5.

233. Honma, Y., and Hirosaki, Y. (1966): Histopathology on the tumors and endocrine glands of the immature chum salmon, *Onchorhynchus keta*, reared in the Enoshima aquarium (Jpn. with Eng. summary). *Jpn. J. Ichthyol.*, 14:74–83.

234. Hoshina, T. (1950): A case of fibroblastic sarcoma developed in *Hypomesus olidus* (Pallas). *Jpn. J. Ichthyol.*, 1:53–56.

235. Hunter, J. (1782): An account of the organ of hearing in fish. *Phil. Trans. R. Soc.*, 72:379–383.

236. Imai, T., and Fujiwara, N. (1959): An electron microscopic study of a papilloma-like hyperplastic growth in a goby, *Acanthogobium flavimanus. Kyushu J. Med. Sci.*, 10:135–147.

237. Ingleby, M. (1929): Melanotic tumor in *Lophius piscatorius. Arch. Pathol.*, 1016–1017.

238. Inoue, S. (1954): On the transplantable spontaneous visceral tumour in the newt, *Triturus pyrrhogaster. Sci. Rep. Res. Inst. Tohoku Imp. Univ. Ser. 4 (Biol.)*, 20:226–236.

239. Inoue, S., and Singer, M. (1963): Transmissiblity and some histopathology of a spontaneously originated visceral tumor in the newt, *Triturus pyrrhogaster. Cancer Res.*, 23:1679–1684.

240. Ippen, R. (1965): Über Sektionsbefunde bei Reptilien. *Zentralbl. Allg. Pathol. Anat.*, 107:520–529.

241. Jaboulay, J. (1908): Poissons atteints de goitres malins héréditaires et contagieux. (Fish suffering from malignant, hereditary and contagious goiters.) *J. Med. Chir. Prat.*, 79:239–240.

242. Jaboulay, M. (1908b): Poissons atteints de goitres malins hereditaires et contagieux [Fish suffering from malignant, hereditary and contagious goiters]. *Lyon Med.*, 110:335–336.

243. Jacquemain, R., Jullien, A., and Noel, R. (1947): Sur l'action de certains corps cancerigens chez les cephalopodes. *C. R. Acad. Sci.*, 225:441–443.

244. Jahnel, J. (1939): Über einige Geschwülste bei Fischen, ein Beitrag zur Erblichkeitsfrage von Tumoren. [On some tumors in fish, a contribution on the question of heredity of tumors]. *Wien. Tierärztl. Monatsschr.*, 26:325–333.

245. Jensen, E. M., *et al.* (1970): Isolation and propagation of a virus from a spontaneous mammary carcinoma of a rhesus monkey. *Cancer Res.*, 30:2388–2393.

246. Johnstone, J. (1910–11): Internal parasites and diseased conditions of fishes. *Proc. Trans. Lpool. Biol. Soc.*, 25:88–122.

247. Johnstone, J. (1911): Internal parasites and diseased conditions of fishes; III. Melanotic mixed cell sarcoma. *Rep. Lancashire Sea Fish Lab.*, 19: 41–50.

248. Johnstone, J. (1912): Internal parasites and diseased conditions in fishes. *Proc. Lpool. Biol. Soc.*, 27:103–104.

249. Johnstone, J. (1913): Diseased conditions in fishes. *Proc. Lpool. Biol. Soc.*, 27:196–218.

250. Johnstone, J. (1914): Internal parasites and diseased conditions of fishes. *Rep. Lancashire Sea Fish. Lab.*, 22:37–54.

251. Johnstone, J. (1914): Diseased and abnormal conditions of marine fishes. *Rep. Lancashire Sea Fish. Lab.*, 23:18–56.

252. Johnstone, J. (1914): Internal parasites and diseased conditions in fishes. *Proc. Lpool. Biol. Soc.*, 28:127–142.

253. Johnstone, J. (1915): Diseased and abnormal conditions of marine fishes. *Proc. Trans. Lpool. Biol. Soc.*, 29:80–113. (Cited by Schlumberger and Lucké (491).)

254. Johnstone, J. (1920): On certain parasites, diseased and abnormal conditions in fishes. *Proc. Lpool. Biol. Soc.*, 34:120–129.

255. Johnstone, J. (1922): Diseases and parasites of fishes. *Proc. Trans. Lpool. Biol. Soc.*, 36:287–301.

256. Johnstone, J. (1922): On some malignant tumours in fishes. *Rep. Lancashire Sea Fish. Lab.*, 31:87–99.

257. Johnstone, J. (1923): On some malignant tumours in fishes. *Proc. Trans. Lpool. Biol. Soc.*, 37:145–157.

258. Johnstone, J. (1923–25): Malignant tumours in fishes. *J. Mar. Biol. Assoc. U.K. (N.S.)*, 13:447–471.

259. Johnstone, J. (1924–25): Malignant tumours in fishes. *Proc. Trans. Lpool. Biol. Soc.*, 19:169–200.

260. Johnstone, J. (1924): Diseased conditions in fishes. *Proc. Trans. Lpool. Biol. Soc.*, 38:183–213.

261. Johnstone, J. (1925): Diseased conditions in fishes. *Rep. Lancashire Sea Fish. Lab.*, 33:99–121.

262. Johnstone, J. (1925): Malignant tumours in fishes. *Proc. Lpool. Biol. Soc.*, 39:169–200.

263. Johnstone, J. (1926): Malignant and other tumours in marine fishes. *Proc. Lpool. Biol. Soc.*, 40:75–98.

264. Johnstone, J. (1927): Diseased conditions in fishes. *Proc. Lpool. Biol. Soc.*, 41:162–167.

265. Jones, J. C. (1969): Hemocytes and the problem of tumors in insects: Neoplasms and related disorders of invertebrate and lower vertebrate animals. *Natl. Cancer Inst. Monogr.*, 31:481–486.

266. Jullien, A. (1928): De certaines Tumeurs et Inflammations du Manteau de la Seiche. *Arch. Exp. Cell. Pen.*, 67:139–158.

267. Jullien, A (1928): Sur la transformation des cellules sanguines de la Seiche au Cours de Reactions inflammatoites aseptiques. *Acad. Sci.* 20 Fevrier, pp. 526–529.

268. Jullien, A. (1928): Sur la signification des granulations eosinophiles des cellules sanguines de la Seiche (*Sepia offic.* L.). *Acad. Sci.* de Mars, pp. 644–645.

269. Jullien, A. (1940): Sur les reactions des mollusques cephalopodes aux injections de goudron. *Acad. Sci.*, 22 Avril, pp. 608–610.

270. Jullien, A., and Jullien, A.-P. (1951): Sur un type de tumeur non provoquée Expérimentalement et observée chez la Seiche. *C. R. Acad. Sci.*, 233:1322.

271. Jullien, A., Jullien, A. P., and Ripplinger, J. (1952): Etude histologique de tumeurs naturelles d'inflammations experimentelles chez les mollusques cephalopodes. *Ann. Sci. Univ. Besancon Zool. Physiol.*, 6/7:3–39.

272. Jullien, A., Jullien, A. P., and Ripplinger, J. (1953): Sur quelques reactions inflammationes et tumorales provoquees par l'indol et le dibenzanthracene chez la seiche et le poulpe. *Ann. Sci. Univ. Besancon Zool. Physiol.*, 8:3–20.

273. Kälin, J. A. (1937): Über Skelettanomalien bei Crocodiliden. *Z. Morphol. Ökol. Tiere*, 32:327–437.

274. Kaestner, A. (1970): *Invertebrate Zoology*. Interscience Publishers, New York.

275. Kahls, O. (1932): Über ein Rhabdomyom in der Skelettmuskulatur einer Bachforelle. *Z. Fischereikd.*, 30:279.

276. Kaiser, H. E. (1965): Pre-carcinogenesis and secondary facts of carcinogenesis in different species. *Am. Zool.*, 5:150.

277. Kaiser, H. E. (1965): Artspezifische Untersuchungen über die Carcinogenese. *Arch. Geschwulstforsch.*, 25:118–121.

278. Kaiser, H. E. (1980): *Species Specific Potential of Invertebrates for Toxicological Research*. University Park Press, Baltimore.

279. Kaiser, H. E.: Unpublished data.

280. Kast, A. (1955): Die spontanen Geschwülste der Vögel [The spontaneous tumors of birds]. Inaug.-Diss., Berlin.

281. Katkansky, S. C. (1968): Intestinal growths in the European flat oyster, *Ostrea edulia. Calif. Fish. Game*, 54:203–206.

282. Kazama, Y. (1924): Einige Geschwülste bei Fischen (*Pagrus major et Paralichthys olivaceus*). *Gann*, 18:35–37.

283. Kennedy, G. A., and Trevino, G. A. (1970): A pituitary adenoma in a zebra. *Pathol. Vet.*, 7:186–189.

284. Kent, S. P., and Pickering, J. E. (1958): Neoplasms in monkeys (*Macaca mulatta*); spontaneous and irradiation induced. *Cancer*, 11:138–147.

285. Kenton, C. (1964): Tumors in invertebrates. DHEW, PHS, NIH, Library reference unit, 496–2184.

286. Kenyon, A. J., and William, R. C., Jr. (1967): Lymphatic leukemia associated with dysproteinaemia in ferrets. *Nature*, 214:1022–1024.

287. Ketchen, K. S. (1953): Tumorous infection in sand soles of Northern Hecate Strait (Brit. Columbia). Report on the survey of Hecate Strait in July. Manuscript, p. 3.

288. Keysselitz, G. (1908): Über ein Epithelioma der Barben. *Arch. Protistenkd.*, 11:326–333.

289. Kimbrough, R. (1966): Spontaneous malignant gastric tumor in a rhesus monkey (*Macaca mulatta*). *Arch. Pathol.*, 81:343–346.

290. Kimura, I., Sugiyama, T., and Ito, Y. (1967): Papillomatous growth in sole from Wakasa Bay area. *Proc. Soc. Exp. Biol. Med.*, 125:175–177.

291. Kinmont, P. D. (1965): Sea urchin sarcoidal granuloma. *Br. J. Dermatol.*, 77:335–343.

292. Kirby, W., and Spence, W. (1826): Diseases of insects, in *An Introduction to Entomology or Elements of the Natural History of Insects, Vol. 4*, pp. 197–232. Longman, New York.

293. Kirschstein, R. L., Robson, A. S., and Rusten, G. W. (1972): Infiltrating duct carcinoma of the mammary gland of a rhesus monkey after administration of an oral contraceptive; a preliminary report. *J.N.C.I.*, 48:551–556.

294. Klein, B. M. (1952): Die Borkengeschwülste der Eidechsen. *Mikrokosmos*, 42:49–52.

295. Klemm, E. (1927): Über die Schilddrüsengeschwülste bei Aquarienfischen. *Mikrokosmos*, 20:184–187.

296. Koch, M. (1904): Demonstration einiger Geschwülste bei Tieren. *Verh. Dtsch. Pathol. Ges.*, 7:136.

297. Koller, L. D., and Olson, C. (1971): Pulmonary fibroblastomas in a deer with cutaneous fibromatosis. *Cancer Res.*, 31:1373–1375.

298. Kolmer, W. (1928): Partieller Riesenwuchs in Verbindung mit grossem Rhabdomyom bei einer Schleie, *Tinca tinca* [Particular giant growth in connection with a large rhabdomyoma in a tench, *Tinca tinca*]. *Virchow's Arch. Pathol. Anat. Physiol.*, 268:574–575.

299. Kolosvary, G., von (1934): Beiträge zur Teratologie des *Phalangium opilio* L. 1-Egyetem: 2-Acta Universitatis Szegedieus: 3-Sectio scientarium naturalium: 4-Acta Biologica. *Neue Weberknecht-Studien*, 3:1–10.

300. Korschelt, E. (1924): *Lebensdauer, Altern und Tod*, Ed. 3, pp. 53–59. Gustav Fischer, Jena.

301. Kraatz, G. (1881): *Dtsch. Entomolog. Ztg.*, 25:111.

302. Kraybill, H. F. (1976): Distribution of chemical carcinogens in aquatic environments. *Prog. Exp. Res.*, 20:3–34.

303. Kraybill, H. F., Dawe, C. J., Harshbarger, J. C., and Tardiff, R. G. (1977): *Aquatic Pollutants and Biologic Effects with Emphasis on Neoplasia, Vol. 298.* The New York Academy of Sciences, New York.

304. Kreyberg, L. (1937): An intra-abdominal fibroma in a brown trout. *Am. J. Cancer*, 30:112–114.

305. Krieg, K. (1969): Experimentelle- Kanzerogenese bei Mollusken; 2. Transplantationsversuche mit einem bei der La-Plata-Apfelschnecke *Ampullarius austris* d'Orbigny (gastropods, prosobranchia) chemisch induzierten Adenopapillom. *Arch. Geschwulstforsch.*, 33:18–30.

306. Krieg, K. (1969): Experimental carcinogenesis in molluscs; 3. Further studies on tumor formation in the La-Plata apple snail *Ampullarius australis* d'Orbigny (gastropods, Prosobranchia) with special attention to methylcholanthrene. *Arch. Geschwulstforsch.*, 33:255–267.

307. Krieg, K. (1970): Experimental carcinogenesis in mollusca and comparative studies of cancerogenesis in land snails and water snails. *Arch. Geschwulstforsch.*, 35:109.

308. Krieg, K. (1973): *Invertebraten in der Geschwulstforschung. Beitr. Krebsforsch.* Steinkopff, Dresden. Includes a shorter English version of text.

309. Krontovsky, A. A. (1916): Comparative and experimental pathology of tumors. (Cited by Finkelstein and Brunst.) Kiev.

310. Labbé, A. (1930): Une tumeur complexe chez un merlan. *Bull. Assoc. Fr. Cancer*, 19:138–158.

311. Ladreyt, F. (1922): Sur une tumeur cancereuse du Siponcle. *Bull. Inst. Oceanogr. Monaco*, 405:1–8.

312. Ladreyt, F. (1929): Sur un Odontome cutane chez un *Scyllium catulus. Bull. Inst. Oceanogr. Monaco*, 539:1–4.

313. Ladreyt, F. (1930): Sur un Rhabdomyosarcome chez un *Labrus mixtus. Bull. Inst. Oceanogr. Monaco*, 550:1–4.

314. Ladreyt, F. (1935): Sur un epithelioma de la Muqueuse Palatine chez un Murene (*Muraena helena*). *Bull. Inst. Oceanogr. Monaco*, 677:1–16.

315. Lange, C. S. (1966): Observations on some tumors found in two species of planaria, *Dugesia etrusca* and *D. ilvana. J. Embryol. Exp. Morphol.*, 15:125–130.

316. Lawrence, G. (1895): Note a tumour found attached to the stomach of a saithe. *Rep. Fish. Scotl.*, 13:236.

317. Lechner, M. (1958): Spontantumoren bei Säugetieren. Ein Beitrag zur vergleichenden Geschwulstforschung. Inaug.-Diss., Munich.

318. Leger, L. (1925): Tumeurs observes chez les salmonides d'élévage. *C. R. Assoc. Fr. Avian Sci.*, 49:395–396.

319. Levine, M., and Gordon, M. (1946): Ocular tumours with exophthalmia in xiphophorin fishes. *Cancer Res.*, 6:197–204.

320. Lindsey, J. R., Wharton, L. R., Jr., and Woodruff, J. D. (1969): Intrauterine choriocarcinoma in a rhesus monkey. *Pathol. Vet. (Basel)*, 6:378–384.

321. Lingeman, C. H., and Ganner, F. M. (eds.) (1969): Symposium on comparative morphology of hematopoietic neoplasms. *Natl. Cancer Inst. Monogr.*, 32.

322. Ljungberg, O., and Lange, J. (1968): Skin tumours of northern pike (*Esox lucius* L.); I. Sarcoma in a Baltic pike population. *Bull. Off. Int. Epizoot.*, 69:1007–1022.

323. Llambes, J. J., and Garcia, J. M. (1949): Aparicion espontanea de tumores multiples en la *Rana catesbiana. Rev. Med. Cuba*, 60:26–32.

324. Llewellyn, G. C., Sherertz, P. C., and Mills, R. R. (1976): The response of dietary stressed *Periplaneta americana* to chronic intake of pure aflatoxin B. *Bull. Environ. Contam. Toxicol.*, 15:391–397.

325. Löliger, H. C., and Schubert, H. J. (1967): Aetiology and pathology of lymphoid cell leucosis in Japanese quail. *Dtsch. Tierärztl. Wochenschr.*, 74:154–158.

326. Lombard, L. S., and Witte, E. J. (1959): Frequency and type of tumors in mammals and birds of the Philadelphia Zoological Garden. *Cancer Res.*, 19:127–141.

327. Lucké, B. (1934): A neoplastic disease of the kidney of the frog, *Rana pipiens. Am. J. Cancer*, 20:352–379.

328. Lucké, B. (1934): A neoplastic disease of the kidney of the frog, *Rana pipiens*; II. On the occurrence of metastasis. *Am. J. Cancer*, 22:326–334.

329. Lucké, B. (1937–38): Studies on tumors in cold-blooded vertebrates. *Rep. Tortugas Lab. Carnegie Inst.*, Washington, D.C., pp. 92–94.

330. Lucké, (1942): Tumors of nerve sheaths in fish of the snapper family (Lutianidae). *Arch. Pathol.*, 34:133–150.

331. Lucké, B., Schlumberger, H., and Breedis, C. (1948): A common mesenchymal tumor of the corium of goldfish, *Carassius auratus. Cancer Res.*, 8:473–493.

332. Lümann, M., and Mann, H. (1956): Beobachtungen über die Blumenkohlkrankheit der Aale [Observations on "cauliflower" disease in eels]. *Arch. Pathol. Wiss.*, 3:229–239.

333. MacIntyre, P. A. (1960): Tumors of the thyroid gland in teleost fishes. *Zoologist*, 45:161–170.

334. MacIntyre, P. A., and Baker-Cohen, K. F. (1961): Melanoma, renal thyroid tumor and reticulo-endothelial hyperplasia in a non-hybrid platyfish. *Zoologist*, 46:125–131.

335. Mann, H. K. H., *et al.* (1970): The cauliflower disease of eels. *Spec. Publ. Am. Fish. Soc.*, 5:291–295.

336. Marine, D., and Lenhart, C. G. (1910): Observations and experiments on the so-called thyroid carcinoma of brook trout (*Salvelinus fontinalis*) and its relation to ordinary goiter. *J. Exp. Med.*, 12:311–337.

337. Marine, D. (1910): On the occurrence of goiter (active thyroid hyperplasia) in fish. *Bull. J. Hopkins Hosp.*, 21:95–98.

338. Marsh, M. C., and Vonwiller, P. (1916): Thyroid tumor in sea bass (*Serranus*). *J. Cancer Res.*, 1:183–196.

339. Martin, C. B., Jr., Misenhimer, H. R., and Ramsey, E. M. (1970): Ovarian tumors in rhesus monkeys (*Macaca mulatta*): Report of 3 cases. *Lab. Anim. Care*, 20:686–692. (Biol. Abstr. 1971, 52, No. 3484.)

340. Mason, M. M., Bogden, A. E., Ilievski, V., Esber, H. J., Baker, J. R., and Chopra, H. C. (1972): History of a rhesus monkey adenocarcinoma containing virus particles resembling oncogenic RNA virus particles resembling oncogenic RNA viruses. *J.N.C.I.*, 48:1323–1331.

341. Masson, P., and Schwartz, F. (1923): Un cas d'epithelioma cutané chez le granouille verte. *Bull. Assoc. Fr. Cancer*, 12:719–725.

342. Mattheis, T. (1964): Fälle von Zystenbildung und Geschwülsten bei Aalen, *Anguilla vulgaris. Z. Fisch. N.F.*, 12:709.

343. Matz, G. (1961): Étude histologique des tumeurs expérimentales chez *Leucophaea maderae* Fabr. et *Locusta migratoira* L. *Bull. Soc. Zool. Fr.*, 86:148–156.

344. Matz, G. (1961): Tumeurs experimentales chez *Leucophaea maderae* F. et *Locusta migratoria* L. *J. Insect Physiol.*, 6:309–313.

345. Mawdesley-Thomas, L. E. (1971): Neoplasia in fish: a review, in *Current Topics in Comparative Pathology*, p. 87, edited by T. C. Cheng. Academic Press, New York.

346. Mawdesley-Thomas, L. E. (1971): Neoplasia in fish—a review. *Adv. Pathobiol.*, 1:88–170.

347. Mawdesley-Thomas, L. E. (1972): Research into fish diseases. *Nature*, 235:17–19.

348. Mawdesley-Thomas, L. E. (1972): Some tumours of fish, in: *Disease of Fish*, pp. 191–284, edited by L. E. Mawdesley-Thomas. Academic Press, New York.

349. Mawdesley-Thomas, L. E. (1975): Neoplasia in fish, in *The Pathology in Fishes*, pp. 805–870, edited by W. E. Ribelin and G. Migaki. The University of Wisconsin Press, Madison, Wisc.

350. Mawdesley-Thomas, L. E., and Bucke, D. (1967): Squamous cell carcinoma in a gudgeon (*Gobio gobio* L.). *Pathol. Vet.*, 4:484–489.

351. Mawdesley-Thomas, L. E., and Solden, D. H. (1967): Osteogenic sarcoma in a domestic white goose (*Anser anser*). *Avian Dis.*, 11:365–370.

352. Mawdesley-Thomas, L. E., and Bucke, D. (1968): A lipoma in a bream (*Abramis brama* L.). *Vet. Rec.*, 82:673–674.

353. Mawdesley-Thomas, L. E., and Hague, P. H. (1968): A fibroma in a domestic white goose (*Anser anser*). *Vet. Rec.*, 82:418.

354. Mawdesley-Thomas, L. E., and Jolly, D. W. (1968): Diseases of fish; III. The trout. *J. Small Anim. Pract.*, 9:167–188.

355. Mawdesley-Thomas, L. E., and Bonner, W. N. (1971): Uterine tumours in a grey seal (*Halichoerus grypus*). *J. Pathol.*, 103:205–208.

356. Mazzarelli (1910): Epithelioma of the mouth of *Chondrostoma soetta*. (Cited by Thomas (581).

357. McArn, G., and Wellings, S. R. (1967): Neurofibroma in a telost fish, *Lumpenus sagitta*. *J. Fish Res. Bd. Can.*, 24:2007–2009.

358. McArn, G., Chuinard, R. G., Miller, B. S., Brooks, R. E., and Wellings, S. R. (1968): Pathology of skin tumors found on English sole and starry flounder from Sound, Washington. *J.N.C.I.*, 41:229–242.

359. McClure, H. M., Ridley, J. H., and Graham, C. E. (1971): Disseminated endometroisis in a rhesus monkey (*Macaca mulatta*). Histogenesis and possible relationship to irradiation exposure. *J. Med. Assoc. Ga.*, 69:11–13.

360. McFarland, J. (1901): Epithelioma of the mouth and skin of a catfish. *Proc. Pathol. Soc. Philad.*, 4:79–81.

361. McIntosh, W. C. (1884–85): Cited in Prince, E. E.: Special report on the natural history of the lobster. *29th Ann. Rep. Dept. Mar. and Fish, Canada*, Suppl. 1, I–IV (1897), pp. 1–36.

362. McIntosh, W. C. (1884/85): Multiple tumours in plaice and common flounders. *3rd and 4th Rep. Fish. Bd. Scotl.*, 66–67.

363. McIntosh, W. C. (1885): On the spawning of certain marine fishes. *Ann. Mag. Nat. Hist.* (Ser. 5), 15:429–437.

364. McIntosh, W. C. (1885): Further remarks on the multiple tumours of common flounders, etc. *Rep. Fish. Bd. Scotl.*, 4:214–215.

365. McIntosh, W. C. (1908): On a tumour in a plaice. *Ann. Mag. Nat. Hist.* (Ser. 8), 1:373–375. (Cited by Schlumberger and Lucké (491).

366. Mehrotra, R. L., Singh, M. P., and Prasad, L. N. (1969): Cystic adenocarcinoma in ducks. *Indian J. Anim. Health*, 8:181–185 (*Vet. Bull.*, 1970, 40 (4928).)

367. Mesnil, F., and Caullery, M. (1911): Neoformations papillomateuses chez un annelide (*Potamitorelli*) dues probablement á l'influence de parasites (*Halosporidie et Levure*). *Bull. Soc. Fr. Belg.*, 45:89–105.

368. Metcalf, M. M. (1928): Cancer in certain protozoa. *Am. J. Trop. Med.*, 8:545–557.

369. Migaki, G., DiGiacomo, R., and Garner, F. M. (1971): Squamous cell carcinoma of skin in a rhesus monkey (*Macaca mulatta*); Report of a case. *Lab. Anim. Sci.*, 21:410–411. (Biol. Abstr. 52 #114797, 1971.)

370. Milleman, R. E. (1968): (Cited by Wellings (617).)

371. Misdorp, W., and Elders, R. A. R. (1965): Paraganglioma in man and dog. *Tijdschr. Diergeneeskd.*, 90:205–230.

372. Misdorp, W., et al. (1965): Malignant tumors in wild animals (a metastasized tonsillar carcinoma in a panther). *Tijdschr. Diergeneeskd.*, 90:460–468.

373. Mita, T., Tokuzen, R., and Fukuoka, F. (1965): Effect of 4-nitroquinoline 1-oxide and related compounds on normally and synchronously dividing *Tetrahymena pyriformis* Gl. *Gann*, 56:293–299.

374. Mix, M. C. (1975): Proliferative characteristics of atypical cells in native oysters (*Ostrea lurida*) from Yaquina Bay, Oregon. *J. Invertebr. Pathol.*, 26:289–298.

375. Mix, M. C. (1976): A review of the cellular proliferative disorders of oysters (*Ostrea lurida*) from Yaquina Bay, Oregon. *Prog. Exp. Tumor Res.*, 20:275–282.

376. Möller, T., and Heje, N. I. (1961): Plasma-cell leucaemia in mink. *Medlemsbl. Danske Dyrlaegeforen*, 44:57–61.

377. Montpellier, J., and Diueuzeide, R. (1932): Sur une production tumeurs cutanées du cyprin (*Carassius auratus*). *Bull. Fr. Cancer*, 21:295–306.

378. Mori, H. (1954): Observation of the liver sarcoma in the newt, *Triturns pyrrhogaster*. *Sci. Rep. Res. Inst. Tohuku Univ. Ser. 4 (Biol.)*, 20:187–188.

379. Mottram, J. C. (1939): An increase in the rate of growth of *Paramecium* subjected to the blastogenic hydrocarbon 3,4-benzo(a)pyrene. *Nature*, 144:154.

380. Mottram, J. C. (1940): 3,4-Benzopyrene, Paramecium and the production of tumors. *Nature*, 145:184–185.

381. Mulcahy, M. F. (1963): Lymphosarcoma in the pike, *Esox lucius* L. (Pisces, Esocidae) in Ireland. *Proc. R. Ir. Acad. (B)*, 63:103–109.

382. Mulcahy, M. F. (1975): Fish blood changes associated with disease; a hematological study of pike lymphoma and salmon ulcerative dermal necrosis, in *The Pathology of Fishes*, pp. 925–944, edited by W. E. Ribelin and G. Migaki. The University of Wisconsin Press, Madison, Wisc.

383. Mulcahy, M. F., and O'Rourke, F. J. (1964): Cancerous pike in Ireland. *Ir. Natl. J.*, 14:312–315.

384. Mulcahy, M. F., and O'Rourke, F. J. (1964): Lymphosarcoma in the pike *Esox lucius* L. in Ireland. *Life Sci.*, 3:719–720.

385. Mulligan, R. M. (1949): *Neoplasms of the Dog*. Williams & Wilkins, Baltimore.

386. Murphy, E. D. (1966): Characteristic tumors, pp. 521–562, in *Biology of the Laboratory Mouse*, edited by E. L. Green. McGraw-Hill, New York.

387. Murray, J. A. (1908): The zoological distribution of cancer. *Sci. Rep. Cancer Res. Fd. (Lond.)*, 3:41–60.

388. Needham, J. (1942) *Biochemistry and Morphogenesis*. Cambridge University Press, Cambridge.

389. Newberne, J. W., and Robinson, V. B. (1960): Spontaneous tumors in primates—a report of two cases with notes on the apparent low incidence of neoplasms in subhuman primates. *Am. J. Vet. Res.*, 21:150–155.

390. Nigrelli, R. F. (1946): Studies on the marine resources of southern New England; V. Parasites and diseases of the ocean pout, *Macrozoarces americanus*, IV. On a fibro-epithelial growth on the snout. *Bull. Bingham Oceanogr. Coll.*, 8:218–221.

391. Nigrelli, R. F. (1947): Spontaneous neoplasms in fishes; II Fibrocarcinoma-like growth in the stomach of *Borphryne apogon Regan, a deepsea ceratioid fish*. *Zoologica*, 31:183–184.

392. Nigrelli, R. F. (1947b): Spontaneous neoplasms in fishes; III. Lymphosarcoma in Astyanax and Esox. *Zoologica*, 32:101–108.

393. Nigrelli, R. F. (1952): Spontaneous neoplasms in fishes; VI. Thyroid tumors in marine fishes. *Cancer Res.*, 12:286.

394. Nigrelli, R. F. (1952): Virus and tumors in fishes. *Ann. N.Y. Acad. Sci.*, 54:1076–1092.

395. Nigrelli, R. F. (1952): Spontaneous neoplasms in fishes; VI. Thyroid tumors in marine fishes. *Zoologica*, 37:185–189.

396. Nigrelli, R. F., and Smith, G. M. (1943): The occurrence of leeches, *Ozobranchus branchiatus* on fibroepithelial tumors of marine turtles *Chelonia mydas*. *Zoologist*, 28:107.

397. Nigrelli, R. F., and Gordon, M. (1944): A melanotic tumor in the silverside, *Menidia beryllina peninsulae* (Good and Bean). *Zoologica*, 29:45–47.

398. Nigrelli, R. F., and Gordon, M. (1951): Spontaneous neoplasms in fishes; V. Acinar adenocarcinoma of the pancreas in a hybrid platyfish. *Zoologica*, 36:121–125.

399. Nigrelli, R. F., Jakowska, S., and Gordon, M. (1950): Histological and cytological observations on hereditary erythromelanomas in platyfish-swordtail hybrids. *Cancer Res.*, 10:234.

400. Nigrelli, R. F., Jakowska, S., and Gordon, M. (1951): The invasion and cell replacement of one pigmented neoplastic growth by a second, and more malignant type in experimental fishes. *Br. J. Cancer*, 5:54–68.

401. Nigrelli, R. F., Ketchen, K. S., and Ruggieri, G. D. (1965): Studies on virus diseases of fishes. Epizootiology of epithelial tumors in the skin of flatfishes of the Pacific coast, with special reference to the sand sole (*Psettichthys melanosticus*) from northern Hectate Strait, B.C., Canada. *Zoologica*, 50:115–122.

402. Nishikawa, S. (1954): On the tumorous growth observed in two fishes. *Collecting Breed.*, Tokyo, 16:236.

403. Nishikawa, S. (1955): A case of spindle cell sarcoma developed in the Japanese common goby. *J. Shimonoseki Coll. Fish.*, 5:171–174.

404. Nishimura, E. T., Ross, E., and Leslie, G. (1970): Epizootic reticulum cell sarcoma in a sequestered colony of Japanese quails. *Cancer Res.*, 30:2119–2126.

405. Nolte, A. (1962): Eine Geschwulstbildung bei *Helix pomatia* L. [A tumor formation in *Helix pomatia* L.]. *Z. Zellforsch.*, 56:149–156.

406. Nouvel, Henri (1947): Les dicyemides; 2. Infusoriforme, teratologie, spécificité du parasitisme, affinites. *Arch. Biol.*, 59:147–221.

407. O'Farrell, A. F., and Stock, A. (1964): Some effects of farnesyl ether on regeneration and metamorphosis in the cockroach *Blattella germanica* L. *Life Sci.*, 3:491–497.

408. Ohlmacher, H. (1898): Several examples illustrating the comparative pathology of tumors. *Bull. Ohio Hosp. Epilep.*, 1:223–226.

409. Oota, K. (1952): An epidemic occurrence of tumor-like hyperplasia of epidermis in a species of fish, *Acanthogobius flavimanus*. *Gann*, 43:264–265. (Cited by Imai and Fujiwara, (236).)

410. Ord, M. J. (1965): Effect of N-methyl N-nitroso urethane on amoebae. *Nature*, 4982:413–414.

411. Orösi-Pal, Z. (1937): Pathologische Veränderungen (Geschwülste) im Dünndarm der Honigbiene. *Zentralbl. Bakteriol. II*, 96:338–340.

412. Owen, S. E., Weiss, H. A., and Prince, L. H. (1938): Carcinogenics and growth stimulation. *Science*, 87:261–262.

413. Owen, S. E., Weiss, H. A., and Prince, L. H. (1939): Carcinogens and planarian tissue regeneration. *Am. J. Cancer*, 35:424–426.

414. Pacis, M. R. (1932): An epithelial tumor of *Parophyrs vetulus*. Master's dissertation, University of Washington.

414a. Paget, R. J. (1978): A report of hepatic angioma in the badger (*Meles meles*). *J. Zool.*, 186:572–574.

415. Palm, N. B. (1948): Notes on the structure of the corpora allata in *Gryllotalpa. Kgl. Fysiogr. Saells. Foerhdl.*, 17:13.

416. Palm, N. B. (1949): The pharyngeal gland in *Bombus* Latr. and *Psithyrus* Lep. with a description of a case of pathological development of the pharyngeal gland. *Opuscul. Entomol. (Lund)*, 14:27–47.

417. Pantel, J. (1898): Le thrixion halidayanum rond; Monog. sur les caractères exterieures la biologie et anatomie d'une larve parasite du groupe des tachinaires. *La Cellule, Louvain*, 15:7–290.

418. Patay, R. (1933): Sur un cas d'epithelioma du rein chez *Tropidonotus natrix* (*Ophidien colubride*). *C.R. Soc. Biol.*, 114:865–867.

419. Pauley, G. B., and Nakatani, R. E. (1967): Histopathology of "gas-bubble" disease in salmon fingerlings. *J. Fish. Res. Bd. (Canada)*, 24:867–871.

420. Pauley, G. B. (1967): Description of some abnormal oysters (*Crassostrea gigas*) from Willapa Bay Washington. *Northwest Sci.*, 41:156–159.

421. Pauley, G. B. (1967): A tumor-like growth on the foot of a freshwater mussel (*Anodonta californiensis*). *J. Fish. Res. Bd. (Canada)*, 24:679–682.

422. Pauley, G. B. (1968): A disease in freshwater mussels (*Margaritifera margaritifera*). *J. Invertebr. Pathol.*, 12:321–328.

423. Pauley, G. B. (1969): A critical review of neoplasia and tumor-like lesions in mollusks. *Natl. Cancer Inst. Monogr.*, 31:509–539.

424. Pauley, G. B., and Sparks, A. K. (1967): Observations on experimental wound repair in the adductor muscle and the Leydig cells of the oyster *Crassostrea gigas. J. Invertebr. Pathol.*, 9:298–309.

425. Pauley, G. B., and Becker, C. D. (1968): *Aspidogaster conchicola* in mollusks of the Colombia River system with comments on the host's pathological response. *J. Parasitol.*, 54:917–920.

426. Pauley, G. B., and Cheng, T. C. (1968): A tumor on the siphons of softshell clam. *Mya arenaria. J. Invertebr. Pathol.*, 11:504–506.

427. Pauley, G. B., and Sayce, C. S. (1968): An internal fibrous tumor in a Pacific oyster, *Crassostrea gigas. J. Invert. Pathol.*, 10:1–8.

428. Pauley, G. B., and Heaton, L. H. (1969): Experimental wound repair in the freshwater mussel, *Anodonta oregonensis. J. Invert. Pathol.*, 13:241–249.

429. Pavlovsky, E. N. (1912): Zur Kasuistik der Tumoren beim Frosch. *Zentralbl. Allg. Pathol. Pathol. Anat.*, 23:94.

430. Pentimalli, F. (1914): Über die Geschwülste bei Amphibien. *Z. Krebsforsch.*, 14:623–632.

431. Pesce, P. (1948): Revista mensile di pesca. (After Schlumberger and Lucké (491).)

432. Peyron, A., and Thomas, L. (1930): Les tumeurs thyroidiennes des salmonides. *Bull. Assoc. Fr. Cancer*, 19:795–819.

433. Pflugfelder, O. (1948): Atypische Gewebsdifferenzierungen bei Stabheuschrecken nach experimenteller Störung der inneren Sekretion. *Z. Krebsforsch.*, 56:107–120.

434. Pflugfelder, O. (1954): Geschwulstbildung bei Wirbellosen und niederen Wirbeltieren. *Strahlentherapie*, 93:181–195.

435. Picchi, L. (1933): Di un non Cummune Tumore di un Pesce (Neurinoma). *Experimentale*, 86:128–130.

436. Pick, L. (1905): Der Schilddrüsenkrebs der Salmoniden (Edelfische). *Berlin Klin. Wochenschr.*, 42:1435, 1477, 1498.

437. Pick, L., and Poll, H. (1903): Über einige bemerkenswerthe Tumorbildungen aus der Thierpathologie, insbesondere über gutartige und krebsige Neubildungen bei Kaltblütern. *Berlin Klin. Wochenschr.*, 40:518, 572.

438. Pirlot, J. M., and Welsch, M. (1934): Etude anatomique et experimentale de quelques tumeurs chez la Grenouille Rousse (*Rana fusca*). *Arch. Int. Med. Exp.*, 9:341–365.

439. Plehn, M. (1902): Bösartiger Kropf (Adenocarcinoma der Thyroidea) bei Salmoniden. *Allg. Fisch. Z.*, 27:117–118.

440. Plehn, M. (1906): Über Geschwülste bei Kaltblütern. *Z. Krebsforsch.*, 4:525–564.

441. Plehn, M. (1909): Über einige bei Fischen beobachtete Geschwülste und geschwulstartige Bildungen. *Ber. Bayer. Biol. Vers. Sta.*, 2:55–76.

442. Plehn, M. (1911): Über Geschwülste bei niederen Wirbeltieren. II. Travaux de la deuxiéme Conf. Intern, p. l' étude du cancer, p. 221. Falcan, Paris.

443. Plehn, M. (1915): Fälle von multiplem Odontom bei der Bachforelle. *Z. Fisch.*, 17:197–200.

444. Plehn, M. (1924): *Praktikum der Fischkrankheiten*, [Practical Handbook of Fish Diseases], pp. 301–479. E. Schweizerbarth, Stuttgart.

445. Plentl, A. A., Dede, J. A., and Grey, R. M. (1968): Adenocarcinoma of the large intestine in a pregnant rhesus monkey (*Macaca mulatta*); report of a case. *Folia Primatol.*, 8:307–313.

446. Plimmer, H. G. (1912): Report on the deaths which occurred in the zoological gardens during 1911. *Proc. Zool. Soc. (Lond.)*, Pt. 1:235–240.

447. Plimmer, H. G. (1913): Report on the deaths which occurred in the zoological gardens during 1912, together with the blood parasites found during the year. *Proc. Zool. Soc. (Lond.)*, Pt. 1:141–149.

448. Potel, K. (1960): Über ein gehäuftes Vorkommen von multiplen kankroiden Hautneubildungen bei der Smaragdeidechse. *Mh. Vet. Med.*, 15:653.

449. Puente-Duany, N. (1930): Tumoracion Periocular en un Pescade de Rio. *Bol. Liga Contra Cancer*, 5:240. (Abstr. *Am. J. Cancer*, 15:918, 1931.)

450. Raabe, H. (1939): Cas c'épithelioma des viscères chez le poisson *Mollienisis verlifera. Reg. Arch. Zool. Exp. Gen.*, 81:1–8.

451. Rantannen, N. W., and Highman, B. (1970): Spontaneous tumors in a colony of *Mystromys albicaudatus* (African white-tailed rat). *Lab. Anim. Care*, 20:114–119.

452. Ratcliffe, H. L. (1933): Incidence and nature of tumors in captive wild mammals and birds. *Am. J. Cancer*, 17:116.

453. Ratcliffe, H. L. (1956): *Tuberculosis in Captive Wild Birds*. Report of the Penrose Research Laboratory of the Zoological Society of Philadelphia.

454. Ratcliffe, H. L. (1960): *Tuberculosis in Captive Wild Birds*. Report of the Penrose Research Laboratory of the Zoological Society of Philadelphia.

455. Reichenberg-Klinke, H.-H. (1961): *Krankheiten der Amphibien*. Fischer, Stuttgart.

456. Reichenberg-Klinke, H.-H. (1963): *Krankheiten der Reptilien*. Fischer, Jena.

457. Reichenberg-Klinke, H.-H. (1966): *Krankheiten und Schadigungen der Fische*. Fischer, Stuttgart.

458. Rickenbacher, J. (1950): Über ein spontan entstandenes Carcinom bei *Triton alpestris. Schweiz. Z. Pathol.*, 13:493.

459. Rigdon, R. H. (1967): Neoplasms in sterile hybrid ducks—a melanoma and two teratomas. *Avian Dis.*, 11:79–89.

460. Robertson, O. H., and Chaney, A. L. (1953): Thyroid hyperplasia and tissue iodine content in spawning rainbow trout; a comparative study of Lake Michigan and California sea-run trout. *Physiol. Zool.*, 26:328–340.

461. Robinson, F. R., Brown, R. J., and Casey, H. W. (1974): References on naturally occurring neoplasms in animals. *The Registry of Veterinary Pathology Armed Forces Institute of Pathology*, Washington, D.C.

462. Roffo, A. H. (1924): Le sarcome des poissons. *Neoplasmes*, 3:231–234.

463. Roffo, A. H. (1925): Sobre un tumor paradentario en la Corvina. *Bol. Inst. Med. Exp.*, 2:28.

464. Roffo, A. H. (1926): Sarcomas fusocelular de Corvina. *Bol. Inst. Med. Exp.*, 3:206–207.

465. Ronca, V. (1914): I. Tumori nei pesci [Tumors in fish]. *Tumori*, 4:61–71.

466. Rostand, J. (1958): Anomalies des amphibiens anoures. *S.E.D.E.S.*, Paris.

467. Russell, F. E., and Kotin, P. (1957): Squamous papilloma in the white croaker. *J.N.C.I.*, 18:857–861.

468. Ryder, J. A. (1887): A tumor in an oyster. *Proc. Natl. Acad. Sci. U.S.A.*, 39:25–27.

469. Sagartz, J. W., Garner, F. M., and Sauer, R. M. (1972): Multiple neoplasia in a captive jungle cat (*Felis chaus*)—thyroid adenocarcinoma, gastric adenocarcinoma, renal adenoma and Sertoli cell tumor. *J. Wildlife Dis.*, 8:375–380.

470. Sagawa, E. (1925): Zur Kenntmis der Fischgeschwülste [On the knowledge of fish tumors]. *Gann*, 19:14–15.

471. Sandeman, G. (1893): On the multiple tumours in plaice and flounders. *Rep. Fish. Bd. Scotl.*, 11:391–392.

472. Sandeman, G. (1893): On a tumour from a tunny. *Rep. Fish. Bd. Scotl.*, 11:392–394.

473. Sarkar, H. L., and Dutta-Chaudhuri, R. (1964): On the occurrence of adenoma in the gill apparatus of a trout *Salmo fario. Trans. Am. Microsc. Soc.*, 83:93–96.

474. Sarkar, H. L., Kapoor, G. B., and Dutta-Chaudhuri, R. (1955): A study of leiomyoma, a mesenchymal tumour on the fins of an Indian catfish, *Mystus* (Osteobagrus) *Gann*, 49:65–68.

475. Sasaki, T., *et al.* (1961): A spontaneous squamous cell carcinoma of the lower jaw in *Macaca mulatta. Primates*, 3:82–87.

476. Sathyanesan, A. G. (1962): On the basophilic tumor in the pituitary of the fresh water teleost *Mystus seenghala* (Sykes). *Sci. Cult.*, 28:432–433.

477. Sathyanesan, A. G. (1963): On the functional thyroid tumour in the kidney of the freshwater teleost, *Barbus stigma*, in its natural habitat. *Sci. Cult.*, 29:90–91.

478. Sathyanesan, A. G. (1966): The structure of the glomerular cystic tumor present in the tropical freshwater catfish, *Mystus vittatus* (Bloch). *Trans. Am. Microsc. Soc.*, 85:53–57.

479. Scarpelli, D. G. (1969): Comparative aspects of neoplasia in fish and other laboratory animals, in *Fish in Research*, edited by Neuhaus and Halver. Academic Press, New York.

480. Scarpelli, D. G. (1967): *Trout Hepatoma Research*, p. 60, Res. Rep. 70, edited by J. A. Halver and I. A. Mitchell. U.S. Fish & Wildlife Service, Washington, D.C.

481. Schäperclaus, W. (1953): Die Blumenkohlkrankheit der Aale und anderer Fische der Ostsee [The cauliflower disease of eels and other fish in the Baltic Sea]. *Z. Fisch. (N.S.)*, 2:105–124.

482. Schamberg, J. F., and Lucké, B. (1922): Fibrosarcoma of the skin in a goldfish (*Carassius auratus*). *J. Cancer Res.*, 7:151–161.

483. Scharrer, B. (1945): Experimental tumors in an insect. *Science*, 102:102

484. Scharrer, B. (1953): Insect tumors induced by nerve severance; inci-

dence and mortality. *Cancer Res.*, 13:73–76.

485. Scharrer, B. (1953): Metabolism and mortality in insects with gastrointestinal tumors induced by nerve severance. *J. N. C. I.*, 13:951–954.

486. Scharrer, B., and Lockhead, M. (1950): Tumors in invertebrates; a review. *Cancer Res.*, 10:403–419.

487. Schiller, A. L., Hunt, R. D., and Digiacomo, R. (1969): Basal cell tumour in a rhesus monkey (*Macaca mulatta*). *J. Pathol.*, 99:327–329.

488. Schlumberger, H. G. (1951): Limbus tumors as a manifestation of von Recklinghausen's neurofibromatosis in goldfish. *Am. J. Ophthalmol.*, 34:415–422.

489. Schlumberger, H. G. (1952): A comparative study of the reaction to injury; I. The cellular response to methylcholanthrene and to talc in the body cavity of the cockroach (*Periplaneta americana*). *Arch. Pathol.*, 54:98–113.

490. Schlumberger, H. G. (1958): Krankheiten der Fische, Amphibien und Reptilien. In: *Pathologie der Laboratoriumstiere*, pp. 714–761, edited by P. Cohrs, R. Jaffé, and H. Meesen. Springer, Berlin.

491. Schlumberger, H. G., and Lucké, B. (1948): Tumors of fishes, amphibians and reptiles. *Cancer Res.*, 8:657–753.

492. Schmey, M. (1911): Über Neubildungen bei Fischen [On new growths in fishes]. *Frkf. Z. Pathol.*, 6:230–253.

493. Schnabel, R. (1954): Papillome an einer Smaragdeidechse (*Lacerta viridis*). *Zool. Garten*, 2:270–278.

494. Schneider, B., and Johansson, A. S. (1966): Intestinal tumors in the German cockroach *Blattella germanica L. Nature Lond.* 212:845.

495. Schreitmüller, W. (1924): Schilddrüsengeschwulst (*Struma maligna*) bei *Jordanella floridae* Goode et Bean. *Bl. Aquar. Terrarienk.*, 35:83.

496. Schröders, V. D. (1908): Tumors of fishes. Diss. (Rus.) (Transl. in Army Med. Libr., Washington, D.C.), St. Petersburg. *Z. Meditsinskii Pribavleniia* 76–92:136–151, 1.

497. Schwarz, F. (1923): Über zwei Geschwülste bei Kaltblütern. *Z. Krebsforsch.*, 20:353–357.

498. Scott, H. H., and Beattie, J. (1927): Neoplasm in a porose crocodile. *J. Pathol. Bacterial.*, 30:61–66.

499. Scott, P. E. (1891): Notes on the occurrence of cancer in fish. *Trans. Proc. N.Z. Inst.*, 24:201.

500. Sechser, K. (1917/19): Kasuistische Beiträge zur Kenntnis der Geschwülste bei Tieren. *Z. Krebsforsch.*, 16:297.

501. Semer, E. (1888): Über allgemeine Carcinose u. Sarkomatose und über multiple Fibrome und Lipome bei den Haustieren. *Dtsch. Z. Tiermed. Vergl. Pathol.*, 14:245–247.

502. Sheremetieva, E. A. (1953): An epithelioma in the axolotl. *Proc. Am. Cancer Res.*, I. (1. Abstract 51).

503. Sheremetieva-Brunst, E. A., and Brunst, V. V. (1948): Origin and transplantation of a melanotic tumor in the axolotl. *Biol. Melanomas Spec. Pub. N.Y. Acad. Sci.*, 4:269–287.

504. Sherwood, B. F., Rowlands, D. T., Jr., and Hackel, D. B. (1969): Pulmonary adenomatosis in opossums (*Didelphis virginiana*). *J. Am. Vet. Med. Assoc.*, 155:1102–1107.

505. Shimkin, M. B., Koe, B. K., and Zechmeister, L. (1951): An instance of the occurrence of carcinogenic substances in certain barnacles. *Science*, 113:650–651.

506. Shortino, T. J., Cantwell, G. E., and Robbins, W. E. (1963): Effect of certain carcinogenic 2-fluorenamine derivatives on larvae of the house fly, *Musca domestica L. J. Insect Pathol.*, 5:489–492.

507. Siciliano, M. J., Perlmutter, A., and Clark, E. (1971): Effect of sex on the development of melanoma in hybrid fish of the genus *Xiphophorus. Cancer Res.*, 31:725–729.

508. Siegal, A. M., Casey, H. W., and Bowman, R. W. (1968): Leukemia in a rhesus monkey (*Macaca mulatta*) following exposure to whole-body proton irradiation. *Blood*, 32:989–996.

509. Smallwood, W. M. (1905): Adrenal tumors in the kidney of the frog. *Anat. Anz.*, 26:652–658.

510. Smith, A. C., and Taylor, R. L. (1968): Tumefactions (tumorlike swellings) on the foot of the moon snail, *Polinices lewisii. J. Invertebr. Pathol*, 10:263–268.

511. Smith, G. M. (1934): A mesenchymal tumor in an oyster (*Ostrea virginica*). *Am. J. Cancer*, 22:838–841.

512. Smith, G. M. (1934): A cutaneous red pigmented tumor (erythorophoroma) with metastases, in a flatfish, *Pseudopleuronectes americanus. Am. J. Cancer*, 21:596–599.

513. Smith, G. M., and Coates, C. W. (1937): The histological structure of the normal and hyperplastic thyroid in *Rasbora lateristriata. Zoologica*, 22: 297–302.

514. Smith, G. M., and Coates, C. W. (1938): Fibro-epithelial growths of the skin in large marine turtles, *Chelonia mydas. Zoologica*, 23:93–98.

515. Smith, G. M., Coates, C. W., and Stong, L. C. (1936): Neoplastic diseases in small tropical fishes. *Zool. N.Y. Zool. Soc.*, 21:220–224.

516. Smith, H. M. (1909): Case of epidemic carcinoma in the thyroid of fishes. *Wash. Med. Ann.*, 8:131.

516a. Sokkar, S. M., et al. (1979): Study of some non-leukotic avian neoplasms. *Avian Pathol.*, 8:69–75.

517. Sonneborn, T. M. (1959): Kappa and related particles in *Paramecia. Adv. Virus Res.*, 6:229.

518. Sonstegard, R. (1975): Lymphosarcoma in Muskellung (*Esox masquinongy*), in *The Pathology of Fishes*, pp. 907–924, edited by W. E. Ribelin and G. Migaki. The University of Wisconsin Press, Madison, Wisc.

519. Sparks, A. K. (1972): *Invertebrate Pathology*. Academic Press, New York.

520. Sparks, A. K., Pauley, G. B., and Chew, K. K. (1969): A second mesenchymal tumor from a Pacific oyster (*Crassostrea gigas*). *Natl. Shellfish. Assoc.*, 59:35–39.

521. Sparks, A. K., Pauley, G. B., Bates, R. P., and Sayce, C. S. (1964): A tumor-like fecal impaction in a Pacific oyster, *Crassostrea gigas* (Thunberg). *J. Insect Pathol.*, 6:453–456.

522. Spencer, R. R., and Melroy, M. B. (1940): Effect of carcinogens on small free-living organisms; I. *Eberthella typhia. J.N.C.I.*, 1:129–134.

523. Splitter, G. A., Rawlings, C. A., and Casey, H. W. (1972): Renal hamartoma in a dog. *Am. J. Vet. Res.*, 33:273–275.

524. Squires, D. F. (1965): Neoplasia in a coral? *Science*, 148:503.

525. Steeves, H. R. (1969): An epithelial papilloma of the brown bullhead, *Ictalurus nebulosus. Natl. Cancer Inst. Monogr.*, 31:215–218.

526. Stephan, F. (1962): Tumeurs spontanées chez la planaire *Dugesia tigrina* [Spontaneous tumors in the planarian *Dugesia tigrina*]. *C. R. Soc. Biol.*, 156:92–922.

527. Sternberg, S. S. (1961): Carcinoma in situ of the cervix in a monkey (*Macaca mulatta*). *Am. J. Obstet. Gynecol.*, 82:96–98.

528. Stewart, H. L. (1965): Comparative aspects of certain cancers, in International Conference on Lung Tumors in Animals: Proceedings of the Third Quadrennial Conference on Cancer, University of Perugia, June 24–29, 1965, edited by L. Severi.

529. Stolk, A. (1950): Enige gevallen van gezwellen en ontstreckingen bij Poikilotherme vertebraten een bijdrage tot de vergelijkende Pathologie. Thesis (Utrecht), Arnheim, Holland.

530. Stolk, A. (1953): Tumours of fishes; II. Chromophobe adenoma of the pituitary gland in the viviparous cyprinodont *Lebistes reticulatus* Peters. *Proc. K. Ned. Akad. Wet. (C)*, 56:34–38.

531. Stolk, A. (1953c): Tumours of fishes; III. Carcinoma of the epidermis in the black variety of the viviparous cyprinodont *Xiphophorus hellerii* Heckel. *Proc. K. Ned. Akad. Wet. (C)*, 56:143–148.

532. Stolk, A. (1953e): Tumours of fishes; V. Melanoma of the skin in the cyprinid *Brachydanio rerio* (Hamilton-Buchanan). *Proc. K. Ned. Akad. Wet. (C)*, 56:152–156.

533. Stolk, A. (1954): Tumours of fishes; VI. Mesenchymal tumour of the skin in the viviparous cyprinodont *Xiphophorus maculatus* Günther (red variety). *Proc. K. Ned. Akad. Wet. (C)*, 57:652–658.

534. Stolk, A. (1955): Tumours of fishes; VII. Congenital teratoma of the skin in the viviparous cyprinodonts *Xiphophorus hellerii* Heckel and *Lebistes reticulatus* (Peters) after thiouracil treatment. *Proc. K. Ned. Akad. Wet. (C)*, 58:190–194.

535. Stolk, A. (1955): Hyperplasia and hyperplastic adenoma of the thyroid gland of the viviparous cyprinodonts *Xiphophorus hellerii* Heckel and *Lebistes reticularus* (Peters) after thiouracil treatment. *Proc. K. Med. Akad. Wet. (C)*, 58:313–327.

536. Stolk, A. (1956): Changes in the pituitary gland of the cyprinid *Tanichthys albonubes* Lin. with a thyroidal tumour. *Proc. K. Ned. Akad. Wet. (C)*, 59:38–49.

537. Stolk, A. (1956): Tumours of fishes; VIII. Thyroidal tumour in the cyprinid *Tanichthys albonubes* Lin. *Proc. K. Ned. Akad. Wet. (C)*, 59: 50–60.

538. Stolk, A. (1956): Tumours of fishes; XI. Carcinoma of the skin in the anabantid *Colis labiosa* (Day). *Proc. K. Ned. Akad. Wet. (C)*, 59:624–633.

539. Stolk, A. (1957): Tumours of fishes; XII. Carcinoma of the kidneys in the characid *Thayeria obliqua* Eigenmann. *Proc. K. Ned. Akad. Wet. (C)*, 60:31–40.

540. Stolk, A. (1957): Tumours of fishes; XIV. Fibroma of the heart in the viviparous cyprinodont *Lebistes reticulatus* (Peters). *Proc. K. Ned. Akad. Wet. (C)*, 60:185–195.

541. Stolk, A. (1957): Tumours of fishes; XV. Renal adenocarcinoma in the cyprinid *Barbus tetrazona* (Bleeker). *Proc. K. Ned. Akad. Wet. (C)*, 60: 196–211.

542. Stolk, A. (1957): Tumours of fishes; XVI. Fibroma of the intestine in the viviparous cyprinodont *Lebistes reticulatus* (Peters). *Proc. K. Ned. Akad. Wet. (C)*, 60:349–363.

543. Stolk, A. (1957): Tumours of fishes; XIX. Odontogenic tumour in the oviparous cyprinodont *Cyprinodon variegatus* Lacépède. *Proc. K. Ned. Akad. Wet. (C)*, 60:658–665.

544. Stolk, A. (1958): Tumours of reptiles. Multiple osteomas in the lizard *Lacerta viridis. Beaufortia*, 7:1–9.

545. Stolk, A. (1958): Tumours of reptiles; II. Rhabdomyoma of the heart in the lizard *Lacerta agilis* L. *Proc. K. Ned. Akad. Wet. (C)*, 61:115–123.

546. Stolk, A. (1958): Tumours of amphibians; III. Haemangioma of heart in *Hyla arborea. Proc. K. Ned. Akad. Wet. (C)*, 60:124–129.

547. Stolk, A. (1958): Tumours of amphibians; IV. A/B. Development of multiple fibroma of the adepidermal reticular network in the skin of the newt *Triturus taeniatus. Proc. K. Ned. Akad. Wet. (C)*, 61:610–630.

548. Stolk, A. (1959): Tumours in amphibians; VIII. Guanophoroma in the

frog *Hyla arborea meridionalis*. *Proc. K. Ned. Akad. Wet. (C)*, 62:390–395.

549. Stolk, A. (1959): Xanthophoroma in the frog *Hyla arborea*. *Proc. K. Ned. Akad. Wet. (C)*, 62:568–575.

550. Stolk, A. (1959): Tumours of fishes; XXVI. Erythrophoroma in the oviparous cyprinodont *Nothobranchius guentheri* (Pfeffer). *Proc. K. Ned. Akad. Wet. (C)*, 62:159–167.

551. Stolk, A. (1959c): Tumours of fishes; XXVII. Guanophoroma in the characid *Ctenobrycon spilurus* (Valenciennes). *Proc. K. Ned. Akad. Wet. (C)*, 62:155–162.

552. Stolk, A. (1959): Tumours of fishes; XXVIII. Xanthophoroma in the oviparous cyprinodont *Rivulus xanthonotus* Ahl. *Proc. K. Ned. Akad. Wet. (C)*, 62:163–171.

553. Stolk, A. (1960): Tumours of fishes; XXXI. Epidermoid carcinoma in a strain of the cichlid *Etroplus maculatus* (Bloch). *Proc. K. Ned. Akad. Wet. (C)*, 63:200–219.

554. Stolk, A. (1960): Melanoma of the skin in the black angelfish *Pterophyllum scalare* Cuvier with some theoretical considerations concerning the melanoma in extremely pigmented fishes, I and II. *Proc. K. Ned. Akad. Wet. (C)*, 63:87–118.

555. Stolk, A. (1961): Tumours of amphibians; VII. Development of the cutaneous fibroma of the adepidermal reticular network in the skin of the toad *Bufo bufo japonicus*. *Acta Morph. Neerlando-Scand.*, 4:237–253.

556. Stolk, A. (1961): Chromaffinoma in Amphioxus. *Proc. K. Ned. Akad. Wet. (C)*, 64:478–488.

557. Stolk, A. (1961): Occurrence of giant nuclei and pharyngeal tumor in the earthworm *Lumbricus terrestris*. *Experientia (Basel)*, 17:306.

558. Stolk, A. (1962): Tumours of fishes; XXXII. Adenoma of the pharyngeal glands in the mouthbreeding anabantid *Betta anabantoides* Bleeker. *Proc. K. Ned. Akad. Wet. (C)*, 65:469–482.

559. Strozier, L. M., McClure, H. M., Keeling, M. E., and Cummins, L. B. (1972): Endometrial adenocarcinoma, endometriosis, and pyometra in a rhesus monkey. *J. Am. Vet. Med. Assoc.*, 161:704–706.

560. Surbeck, G. (1921): (Cited by Thomas (580).)

561. Sutherland, D. J. (1969): Nerve severance and tumor induction in *Periplaneta americana* L. *Natl. Cancer Inst. Monogr.*, 31:399–418.

562. Sutherland, D. J. (1969): Effects of certain carcinogens on *Periplaneta americana* L. *Natl. Cancer Inst. Monogr.*, 31:433–445.

563. Sutherland, D. J. (1969): Rectal tumefaciens in the cockroach, *Periplaneta americana* L. *Nat. Cancer Inst. Monogr.*, 31:453.

564. Sutton, B. J. (1885): Tumours in animals. *J. Anat. Physiol*, 19:415–475.

565. Szabo, I., and Szabo, M. (1934): Epitheliale Geschwulstbildung bei einem wirbellosen Tier, *Limax flavus* L. [An epithelial tumor in an invertebrate animal, *Limax flavus* L.]. *Z. Krebsforsch.*, 40:540–545.

566. Szczudlowska, M. (1971): Neoplasm formation after injury to the eyelid and cornea in a pigeon. *Med. Wet.*, 27:306–307.

567. Takahashi, K. (1929): Studie über die Fischgeschwülste. *Z. Krebsforsch.*, 29:1–73.

568. Tar, E., and Tarok, L. J. (1964): Investigations on somatic twin-formation, benignant and malignant tumors in the species *Dugesia tigrina* (Planariidae, Turbellaria). *Proc. 6th Meet. Hungar. Biol. Soc.*, p. 34.

569. Tarasov, S. A. (1965): Case of sarcoma in a lion. *Proc. 14th Scientific Conf.* (Leningrad Vet. Inst., 1965) Leningrad, 104. (From *Ref. Zh. Otd. Vyrusk. Vop. Patol. Onkol.*, 1965 No. 20, 53, 316: Nos. 22, 53, 281). (Biol. Abstr. 1966, 47, No. 112870).

570. Tavolga, W. N. (1951): Epidermal fin tumors of the gobiid fish, *Bathygobius soporator Zoologica*, 36:273–278.

571. Teutschländer, O. (1920): Beiträge zur vergleichenden Onkologie mit Berücksichtigung der Identitätsfrage. *Z. Krebsforsch.*, 17:285–407.

572. Thomas, J. A. (1930): Étude d'un processùs néoplasique chez *Nereis diversicolor* O.F.M. Du à la dégénérescence des coocytes et quelquefois des soires. *Arch. Anat. Microsc. Morphol. Exp.*, 25:251–333.

573. Thomas, J. A. (1930): Sur la repartition, aux environs de Roscoff d'une néoplasie de *Nereis diversicolor* O.F.M. (*Essai ecologique*). *Bull. Biol. Fr. Belg.*, 64:332–354.

574. Thomas, J. A. (1930): Sur une réaction néoplasique due à la dégénerescence des ovocytes et quelquefois des soires chez *Nereis diversicolor* O.F.M. Formation de tissue conjonctif a partir des amibocytes néoformes. *C. R. Acad. Sci.*, 190:845–846.

575. Thomas, J. A. (1930): Dégenerescence et phagocytose des soires de *Nereis diversicolor* O.F.M. *C. R. Soc. Biol.*, 103:996.

576. Thomas, J. A. (1931): Réations de deux invertebres: *Ascidia mentula* Mull. et *Nereis diversicolor* O.F.M. a l'inoculation de substances a proprietes cancerigenes. *C. R. Soc. Biol.*, 108:667–669.

577. Thomas, J. A. (1931): Sur les réactions de la tunique d'*Ascidia mentula* Mull. a l'inoculation de *Bacterium tumefaciens* Sm. *C. R. Soc. Biol.*, 108:772–774.

578. Thomas, L. (1926): Epithelioma odontoblastique des maxillaires chez une morue [Odontoblastic epithelioma in the maxilla of cod]. *Bull. Assoc. Fr. Cancer*, 15:464–470.

579. Thomas, L. (1927): Les sarcomes fibroblastiques chez la morue. *Bull. Assoc. Fr. Cancer*, 16:78–89.

580. Thomas, L. (1930): Contribution à l'étude des lésions pré-cancereuses chez les poissons. Les papillomas cutanés de la sole [Contribution to the study of precancerous lesions in fish. Cutaneous papillomas in the sole]. *Bull. Assoc. Fr. Cancer*, 19:91–97.

581. Thomas, L. (1931): Les tumeurs des poissons (étude anatomique et pathogénique [Tumors of fish (anatomical and pathological study)]. *Bull. Assoc. Fr. Cancer*, 20:703–760.

582. Thomas, L. (1931): La tumeur des salmonides. Intéret de ses données en pathologie generale. *Rev. Med. Fr. Colon.*, 8:235–246.

583. Thomas, L. (1932): Rhabdomyome chez un flet [Rhabdomyoma in a flounder]. *Bull Assoc. Fr. Cancer*, 21:225–233.

584. Thomas, L. (1932): Deux cas de tumeurs osseuses chez de téleosteens [Two cases of bone tumors in the teleosts]. *Bull. Assoc. Fr. Cancer*, 21:280–294.

585. Thomas, L. (1932): Papillome tégumentaire chez un truite. *Bull. Assoc. Fr. Cancer*. 21:547–550.

586. Thomas, L. (1933): Sur un case de léiomyome de l'estomac chez un hareng [On a case of leiomyoma in the stomach of a herring]. *Bull. Assoc. Fr. Cancer*, 22:361–376.

587. Thomas, L. (1933): Sur un lipoma abdominal chez un colin [On an abdominal lipoma in a hake]. *Bull. Assoc. Fr. Cancer*, 22:419–435.

588. Thomas, L., and Oxner, M. (1930): Papillomes de la levre, inferieure chez *Anguilla vulgaris*. *Bull. Assoc. Fr. Cancer*, 19:708–714.

589. Tittler, I. A., and Kobrin, M. (1942): Effects of carcinogenic agents on *Paramecium caudatum*. *Soc. Exp. Biol. Med. Proc.*, 50:95–96.

590. Trebbin, H. (1968): Zur Geschichte der Geschwulstforschung bei Tieren [Notes to the history of tumor research in animals] *Dtsch. Tieraerztl. Wochenschr.*, 75:463–464.

591. Trebbin, H. (1975): Spontane Tumoren der Tiere. *Hdbuch Allgem. Pathol.*, 6:1003–1062.

592. Tsvetaeva, N. P. (1941): *Trudy Mosk. Zooparka* (Rus.), 2:2. (Cited by Finkelstein.)

593. Turusov, V. S. (ed.) (1973): *Pathology of Tumours in Laboratory Animals, Part 1, Vol. 1, Tumours of the Rat*. IARC, Lyon.

594. Turusov, V. S. (ed.) (1976): *Pathology of Tumours in Laboratory Animals. Part 2, Vol. 1, Tumours of the Rat*. IARC, Lyon.

595. Unterharnscheidt, F. (1964): Über einen sysontogenetischen Prozess mit blastomastosem Einschlag (tuberöse Sklerose) beim Affen. *Acta Neuropathol.*, 3:250–254.

596. Unterharnscheidt, F. (1964): Intracerebrales Angioma cavernosum bei einem Affen (*Macacus rhesus*). *Acta Neuropathol.*, 3:295–296.

597. Vaillant, L., and Pettit, A. (1902): Fibrome observe sur un *Megalobatrachus maximus* Schlegel, a la Menagerie Schlegel du Museum. *Bull. Mus. Hist. Nat. (Paris)*, 8:301–304.

598. Vaillant, L., and Pettit, A. (1902): Lesions stomacales observees chez un Python de Seba. *Bull. Mus. Hist. Nat. (Paris)*, 8:593–595.

599. Vakilzadeh, J., Sherwood, B. F., Hackel, D. B., and Lemay, J. C. (1971): Experimental study of pulmonary adenomas in the opossum (*Didelphis virginiana*). *Lab. Anim. Sci.*, 21:224–228.

600. Van der Steen, A. B., Cohen, B. J., Ringler, D. H., Abrams, G. D., and Richards, C. M. (1972): Cutaneous neoplasms in the leopard frog *Rana pipiens*. *Lab. Anim. Sci.*, 22:216–222.

601. Van Pelt, R. W., and Dieterich, R. A. (1972): Mammary gland tumors in collared lemmings (*Dicrostonyx groenlandicus*). *Lab. Anim. Sci.*, 22:433–439.

602. Van Wagtendonk, W. J. (1969): Neoplastic equivalents of protozoa: Neoplasms and related disorders of invertebrate and lower vertebrate animals. *Natl. Cancer Inst. Monogr.*, 31:751–768.

603. Varia, M. R., Kerur, V. K., and Heranjal, D. D. (1971): Malignant melanoma in a jackal—a case report. *Gujvet. Anad.*, 5:47–48.

604. Vielkind, J., Vielkind, U., and Anders, F. (1971): Electron microscopic studies on melanotic and amelanotic melanomas in xiphophorin fish. *Z. Krebsforsch.*, 80:243–245. (Biol. Abstr. 52 No. 91204, 1971.)

605. Vielkind, J., Vielkind, U., and Anders, F. (1971): Melanotic and amelanotic melanomas in xiphophorin fish. *Cancer Res.*, 31:868–875.

606. Vivien, J., and Ruhland-Gaiser, M. (1954): Etude preliminaire de goitres envallissants spontanes recontres chez un cyprinodonte, *Lebistes reticulatus*, V [Preliminary study of spontaneous encroaching goiters found in a cyprinodont, *Lebistes reticulatus*, V]. *Ann. Endocrinol*, 15:585–594.

607. Volterra, M. (1928): Über eine bösartige Geschwulst bei einem exotischen Frosch (*Ceratophrys ornata*) [A malignant neoplasm in an exotic frog (*Ceratophrys ornata*)]. *Z. Krebsforsch.*, 27:457–466.

608. Wadsworth, J. R. (1954): Some neoplasms of captive wild animals. *J. Am. Vet. Med. Assoc.*, 124:121–123.

609. Wadsworth, J. R. (1956): Serpentine tumors. *Vet. Med.*, 51:326–328.

610. Wadsworth, J. R. (1960): Tumors and tumor-like lesions of snakes. *J. Am. Vet. Med. Assoc.,*, 137:419–420.

611. Wago, H. (1922): A case of fibroblastic myxoma in a goldfish. *Gann*, 16:11.

612. Wahlgren, F. (1876): Beiträge zur Pathologie der wilden Tiere [Contributions to the pathology of wild animals]. *Z. Tiermed. Vergl. Pathol.*, 2:232–235.

613. Wahlgren, F. (1876): Osteoid sarcoma in the anal fin of a pike. (Cited by Schmey (492).)

614. Walker, R. (1958): Lymphocystis warts and skin tumors of Walleyed

pike. *Rensselaer Rev. Grad. Stud.*, pp. 1–5.

615. Webster, W. S., Bullock, B. C., and Prichard, R. W. (1969): A report of three bile duct carcinomas occurring in pigeons. *J. Am. Vet. Med. Assoc.*, 155:1200–1205.

616. Weissenfels, N., Schaffer, D., and Bretthauer, R. (1970): Über die Entartung der Makromelanophoren und den Einfluss des infiltrierenden Melanomwachstums auf die Muskulatur von Poeciliiden-Bastarden [Studies on the degeneration of macromelanophores and the influence of infiltrating melanoma growth on the muscle system of platy-fish-swordtail hybrids]. *Virchows Arch. (Abt. B, Zellpathol.)*, 5:144–158.

617. Wellings, S. R. (1969b): Neoplasia and primitive vertebrate phylogeny; echinoderms, prevertebrates and fishes—a review. *Natl. Cancer Inst. Monogr.*, 31:59–128.

618. Wellings, S. R., and Chuinard, R. G. (1964): Epidermal papillomas with virus-like particles in flathead sole, Hippoglossoides elassodon. *Science*, 146:932–934.

619. Wellings, S. R., Chuinard, R. G., and Bens, M. (1965): A comparative study of skin neoplasms in four species of pleuronectid fishes. *Ann. N.Y. Acad. Sci.*, 126:479–501.

620. Wellings, S. R., Cooper, R. A., and Chuinard, R. G. (1966): Skin tumors of pleuronectid fishes in Puget Sound, Washington. *Bull. Wildlife Dis. Assoc.*, 2:68.

621. Wellings, S. R., Chuinard, R. G., and Cooper, R. A. (1967): Ultrastructural studies of normal skin and epidermal papillomas of the flathead sole, *Hippoglossoides elassodon*. *Z. Zellforsch. Mikrosk. Anat.*, 78:370–387.

622. Wellings, S. R., Bern, H. A., Nishioka, R. S., and Graham, J. W. (1963): Epidermal papillomas in the flathead sole (abstr.). *Proc. Am. Assoc. Cancer Res.*, 4:71.

623. Werle, E., Haendle, H., and Schmal, A. (1968): A case of a carcinoid in an elephant. *Pathol. Vet.*, 5:81–83.

624. Wessing, A. (1959): Über einen bösartigen, virusbedingten Tumor bei tropischen Zierfischen [On a malignant tumor caused by a virus in tropical fishes]. *Naturwissenschaften*, 46:517–518.

625. Wessing, A., and Von Bargen, G. (1959): Untersuchungen über einen virusbedingten Tumor bei Fischen [Studies on a tumor caused by a virus in fish]. *Arch. Ges. Virusforsch.*, 9:521–536.

626. White, P. B. (1921): Note on a case of fibroma in a honey bee. *J. Pathol. Bacteriol.*, 24:138–139.

627. Wilkie (1891): Carcinoma of the thyroid gland in two trout species (*Salvelinus fontinalis*, Mitchill and *Salmo irideus*, Richardson). (Cited by Schmey (492).)

628. Williams, A. O. (1970): Ultrastructure of liver cell carcinoma in *Macaca mulatta* monkey. *Exp. Mol. Pathol.*, 13:359–369.

629. Williams, G. (1929): Tumorous growths in fish. *Proc. Trans. Lpool. Biol. Soc.*, 43:120–148.

630. Williams, G. (1931): On various fish tumours. *Proc. Trans. Lpool. Biol. Soc.*, 45:98–109.

631. Williams, J. W. (1888–1890): A tumor in the fresh-water mussel. *J. Anat. Physiol.*, 23–24:307–308.

632. Williamson, H. C. (1911): On diseases and abnormalities in fishes of the cod (*Gadus*), flat-fish (*Pleuronectes*), salmon (*Salmo*), skate (*Raia*), etc. families. *Scient. Invest. Fish. Bd. (Scotl.)*, 11:3–39.

633. Willis, R. A. (1948): *Pathology of Tumors*, Ed. 1; Ed. 2, 1953. Butterworth, London.

634. Wolf, H. (1969): Neoplastic growth in two Sydney rock oysters, *Crassostrea commercialis* (Iredals and Roughley); neoplasms and related disorders of invertebrate and lower vertebrate animals. *Natl. Cancer Inst. Monogr.*, 31:563–574.

635. Wolff, B. (1912): Über ein Blastom bei einem Aal (*Anguilla vulgaris*), nebst Bemerkungen zur vergleichenden Pathologie der Geschwülste. *Virch. Arch. Pathol. Anat.*, 210:365–385.

636. Wolke, R. E., and Wyand, D. S. (1969): Ocular lymphosarcoma of an Atlantic cod, *Gadus morhua*. *Bull. Wildlife Dis. Assoc.*, 5:401–403.

637. Wolman, M. (1939): A proliferative effect of carcinogenic hydrocarbons upon multiplication of paramecia. *Growth*, 3:387–396.

638. Woodruff, J. M., and Johnson, D. K. (1968): Hepatic hemangioendothelioma in a rhesus monkey. *Pathol. Vet.*, 5:327–332.

639. Yevich, P. P., and Berry, M. M. (1969): Ovarian tumors in the quahog *Mercenaria mercenaria*. *J. Invertebr. Pathol.*, 14:266–267.

640. Young, M. W. (1923–25): Muscle tumours in the European turbot. *J. Mar. Biol. Assoc. U.K.*, 13:910–913.

641. Young, P. H. (1964): Some effects of sewer effluent on marine life. *Calif. Fish Game*, 50:33–41.

642. Zwart, P. (1970): A nephroblastoma in a fire-bellied newt, *Cynops pyrrhogaster*. *Cancer Res.*, 30:2691–2694.

643. Zwart, P., and Harshbarger, J. C. (1972): Hematopoietic neoplasms in lizards; report of a typical case in *Hydrosaurus amboiensis* and a probable case in *Varanus salvator*. *Int. J. Cancer*, 9:548.

49

Pathology and Distribution of Plant Tumors

Millicent Kalil and A. C. Hildebrandt

INTRODUCTION

Plant neoplasms and abnormal growths have been observed in a wide variety of plant species and have been induced by many different agents. The conditions responsible for their initiation, continuation, and inhibition suggest the importance of a vast variety of chemical and environmental balances that are generally poorly understood.

The widespread distribution of tumors in plant species has been largely underestimated. The literature on plant tumors, even including the crown gall disease, often is published in obscure journals. Table 49.1 gives some examples indicating the wide distribution of plant neoplasms. The plant galls and tumors cited here can only serve as a few examples in a vast field of material.

Plant galls may be of many origins. They may be induced by insects, mites, bacteria, fungi, nematodes, viruses, environmental conditions, and influenced by the genetics of the plant species (8, 9, 11–13, 19, 23, 28, 31, 43, 45, 58, and 67).

In most cases, the galls are obviously associated with an injury to the plant. The continued growth and development of the gall may result from hyperplasia or hypoplasia of the host cells or both. In addition, various forms of organ differentiation may be induced in the plant as the gall develops and ages. The gall is usually a part of the host plant although in certain galls the main mass of the structure may in fact consist of some stage of the inciting agent (as is seen in fungus-induced smut galls). In the latter case, the epidermal layers of the host plant provide for containment of the fungus mycelium and spores with only a scattering of host cells also contained within.

Gall induction is accomplished by various methods. Various terminologies for galls and gall inductions have been discussed by Mani (43). In most cases, the actual mechanisms of gall induction is still not clear. Insects may inject an irritant into the plant part at the time of egg laying; the egg itself may provide secretions for stimulation of cell growth and divisions; the chewing injury of adult and immature forms of insects and mites along with mouth secretions may be involved and, finally, larval activities and waste products or secretions may induce and continue to stimulate gall enlargement and deformation. Fungi, bacteria, and nematodes may similarly provide a changed chemical environment along with injury, to support the development of their respectively induced plant galls.

The mechanisms and balances of products, chemicals, and environment interacting at the cellular level for gall production offer promise of suggesting the experiments needed to provide the information to clarify the induction, development, and cessation of gall formation in plants.

No plant tumors are known to metastasize.

A most complete discussion of plant galls is that of Mani (43). His comprehensive review of the subject describes reports from a wide literature listing 5500 galls on angiosperms in Europe and America. Others list 3000 different galls from Central and North Europe, 3000 from Asia, Africa, Australia and Oceania, and 1300 from South America. The total of described galls from the whole world is noted as not less than 14,750.

A comprehensive recent review of plant tumors was given by Beiderbeck (5). It seems to be

Table 49.1 Some Representative Galls on Plants

Plant group	Host Scientific name	Host Common name	Type of Neoplasm	Tissue Involved	Incitant Scientific name	Incitant Common name	Distribution	Ref.
Alga	Rhodymenia palmata	Red alga	Gall	Thallus	Harpacticus chelifer	Copepod	U.K.	(4, 43)
Fungus	Omphalia campanelia	Mushroom	Gall	Pileus, gills	Eipterous larvae of Mycetophidae	Insect	U.S.A.	(60)
Moss	Eurhynchium swartzii	None	Gall	Antheridial branch	Anguillulae	Nematode	Not known	(17, 43)
	Porotrichum dopercurum	None	Gall	Antheridial branch	Anguillulae	Nematode	Not known	(17, 43)
	Pottia bryoides	None	Gall	Thallus	Anguillulina brenari	Nematode	U.S.A.	(25, 43)
Ferns	Cystopteria fragiles	Bladder fern	Gall	Root	Cecidomyea	Midge	Wide	(23)
Gymnosperms	Ephedra trifucco	Gnetum	Fusiform gall	Twig	Losioptera	Midge	Wide	(23)
	Juniperus	Juniper	Cedar apple gall	Stem	Gymnosporangium juniperi-virginianae	Fungus	Wide	(45)
	Picea	Spruce	Pseudo cone gall	Cone	Adelges abietis	Aphid	Wide	(13)
	Pinus scopulorum	Pine	Gall	Bud	Contarinia colorodensis	Midge	Wide	(23)
	Pyrus malus (alternate host)	Apple	Cedar apple gall	Leaf	Gymnosporangium juniperi-virginianae	Fungus	Wide	(45)
	Taxodium	Cyprus	Gall	Seed	Retinodiplosis	Midge	Wide	(23)
	Pinus	Pine	Mistletoe burl	Branch	Arceuthobium complyopodium	Flowering plant	Wide	(66)
Angiosperms Monocots:	Agropyron repens	Wheatgrass	Gall	Roots	Ditylenchus radicicolus	Nematode	U.K., Canada, Europe	(35, 61)
	Cattleya sp.	Orchid	Root gall	Roots	Parallelodiplosis cattleya	Midge	Wide	(23)
	Hordeum sp.	Barley	Gall	Roots	Ditylenchus radicicolus	Nematode	Europe, U.K., Canada	(35, 61)
	Poa annua	Bluegrass	Gall	Roots	Ditylenchus radicicolus	Nematode	Europe, U.K., Canada	(35, 61)
	Secale sp.	Rye	Gall	Roots	Ditylenchus radicicolus	Nematode	Europe, U.K., Canada	(35, 61)
	Saccharum sp.	Sugar cane	Fiji disease	Cane	None	Virus	Wide	(42)
	Secale sp.	Rye	Ergot	Seed	Claviceps purpurea	Fungus	Wide	(66)
	Secale sp.	Rye	Gall	Seeds, leaves	Anguina tritici	Nematode	Wide	(35)
	Triticum sp.	Wheat	Smut gall	Seed	Tilletia foetida	Fungus	Wide	(66)
	Zea mays	Corn	Smut gall	Seed	Ustilago maydis	Fungus	Wide	(66)
	Zea mays	Corn	Wallaby ear	Seed	None	Virus	Wide	(50)
Dicots:	Azalea sp.	Azalea	Gall	Leaf	Exobasidium vaccinii	Fungus	Wide	(24)
	Beta sp.	Sugar beet	Bacterial pocket	Root	Xanthomonas beticola	Bacterium	U.S.A.	(10, 22)
	Beta vulgaris & others	Sugar beet	Gall	Root	Nacobbus batatiformis	Nematode	U.S.A.	(62)
	Brassica	Cabbage	Club root	Root	Plasmodiophora brassiceae	Fungus	Wide	(66)
	Chrysopsis sp.	Golden aster	Wooly bud gall	Bud	Rhopalomyea sp.	Midge	Wide	(23)
	Citrus limonia	Rough lemon	Gall	Root	Hemicycliophora	Nematode	U.S.A.	(64)

Plant (scientific)	Common name	Tumor	Plant part	Causal agent	Type	Distribution	Ref.
Cruciferae	Mustard family	White rust	Flowers, stem	arenaria Albugo candida	Fungus	Wide	(66)
Delphineum sp.	Delphineum	Red leaf gall	Leaf	Synchytrium aureum	Fungus	Wide	(67)
Forsythia sp.	Forsythia	Gall	Stem	Phomopsis sp.	Fungus	Wide	(46)
Frageria sp.	Strawberry	Gall	Leaves, flowers, stem	Ditylenchus dipsaci	Nematode	Wide	(61)
Geranium sp.	Geranium	Pinkish pouch gall	Leaf	Arachnida	Mite	Wide	(23)
Hibiscus sabdariffa	Hibiscus	Gall	Leaf, stem	Rhodochytrium spilanthidis	Red alga	Tropical countries	(44)
Lathyrus sp.	Sweet pea	Fasciation	Stem	Corynebacterium fascians	Bacterium	U. S. A., U.K.	(20, 34)
Lycopersicum esculentum & others	Tomato	Root knot	Roots, leaves, stems, petioles, rhizomes, tubers	Meloidogyne sp.	Nematode	Wide	(35, 61)
Malus sp. and Rosa sp.	Apple, rose	Hairy root	Stem, root	Agrobacterium rhizogenes	Bacterium	U. S. A.	(47)
Medicago sativa	Alfalfa	Galls	Leaves, stem, flowers	Ditylenchus dipsaci	Nematode	Wide	(35, 61)
Medicago sativa	Alfalfa	Crown wart	Stem, root flower	Physoderma alfalfae	Fungus	Wide	(66)
Nerium oleander	Oleander	Gall	Stem, leaf flower	Pseudomonas tonelliana	Bacterium	U. S. A., S & E Africa, Europe	(54, 67)
Nicotiana tabacum	Tobacco	Teratoma	Stem	Agrobacterium tumefaciens	Bacterium	Wide	(55)
Nicotiana sp.	Tobacco	Club root	Root	None	Virus	Wide	(63)
Nicotiana pomiculata	Tobacco	Enations	Leaf	None	Virus	Wide	(36)
Olea sp.	Olive	Olive knot	Stem, leaf, root, fruit	Pseudomonas savastanoi	Bacterium	Europe, Mideast, U. S. A.	(53)
Persicum malum	Peach	Peach wart	Fruit	None	Virus	Wide	(67)
Pisum sativum and other legumes	Pea	Nodule	Root	Rhizobium sp.	Bacterium	Wide	(18)
Populus sp.	Poplar	Vagabond gall	Leaf	Moedevilkoja vagabunda	Aphid	Wide	(23)
Prunus persica	Peach	Leaf curl	Leaf	Taphrina deformans	Fungus	Wide	(13)
Prunus sp.	Cherry	Black knot	Stem	Dibotryon morbosum	Fungus	Wide	(45)
Quercus sp.	Oak	Gouty oak gall	Stem	Plagiotrochus punctatus	Wasp	Wide	(23)
Quercus sp.	Oak	Wool sower gall	Leaf	Callirytis seminator	Wasp	Wide	(45)
Rosa sp.	Rose	Gall	Root	Xiphenema diversicaudatum	Nematode	U. S. A.	(51)
Rosaceae and others	Rose family	Crown gall	Stem, roots	Agrobacterium tumefaciens	Bacterium	Wide	(31)
Rubus sp.	Blackberry, raspberry	Cane gall	Stem	Agrobacterium rubi	Bacterium	U. S. A.	(30)

Table 49.1, Continued

Plant group	Host Common name	Host Scientific name	Type of Neoplasm	Tissue Involved	Incitant Scientific name	Incitant Common name	Distribution	Ref.
	Sorrel	Rumex acetora	Wound tumor	Roots	None	Virus	Wide	(7)
	Potato	Solanum tuberosum	Black wart	Tuber	Synchytrium indobioticum	Fungus	Wide	(66)
	Golden rod	Solidago sp.	Knotty gall	Stem	Lasioptera solidaginis	Midge	Wide	(23)
	Blueberry	Vaccinium macrocarpon	Gall	Root	Hemicycliophora similis	Nematode	U. S. A., Canada	(35)
	Blueberry	Vaccinium macrocarpon	Gall	Stem	Nocardia vaccinii	Actinomycete	U. S. A.	(15, 16)
	Cranberry	Vaccinium oxycoccos	Gall	Root	Hemicycliophora similis	Nematode	U. S. A., Canada	(35)
	Grape	Vitis sp.	Gall	Leaf, root	Phylloxera vitafoliae	Aphid	Wide	(23)

appropriate to suggest here a distinction of different types of tumor growth in plants which may be comparable to animal and human tumors. Beside those types of abnormal growth like repair, hypertrophic growth, and others, plant tumors in general can be divided between those with limited and those with unlimited growth. The first group comprises types of abnormal growth generally known as gall which will cease their growth after the removal of the stimulus. These galls can to a certain degree be compared to benign tumors in animals and man, perhaps on a phylogenetically somewhat lower level. The second group comprises the tumor types with unlimited growth which may be really called neoplasms. They are so unlimited in growth it is appropriate to consider them as malignant. This group of neoplasms comprises the crown gall tumors, the virus-induced tumors such as the wound tumor, the genetic tumors such as of *Nicotiana*-hybrids, and perhaps tumors induced by chemical carcinogens and Whites' spruce tumor of *Picea glauca* and *Piscea sitchensis*.

BACTERIAL GALLS

Representative bacterial galls included in Table 49.1 are induced by organisms in two different parts (8th edition of *Bergey's Manual of Determinative Biology* (6), Part 7, "Gram-Negative Aerobic Rods and Cocci": *Agrobacterium*, *Pseudomonas*, *Rhizobium* and *Xanthomonas*; and Part 17, "Actinomycetes and Related Organisms": *Corynebacterium* and *Nocardia*. *Xanthomonas beticola* and *Pseudomonas savastanoi* are organisms of uncertain affinity at the present time (Ref. 6; see also Lelliot (40), and Schroth and Hildebrand (52). These organisms incite hyperplasia or hypertrophy, or both, on their plant hosts causing abnormal proliferation of tissue on stem, leaf, roots, or flower.

Among the plant galls, the crown gall disease, induced by *Agrobacterium tumefaciens*, because of many similarities to animal tumors, has perhaps been most extensively studied. Smith and Townsend (56) described this disease on Paris Daisy and this was the first evidence that bacteria could induce galls. The crown gall has been the model in plant oncology for more than 70 years. A summary by Lippincott (41), reviews the evidence that an *Agrobacterium* plasmid is the tumor-inducing principle (see also 37). Many details of the etiology of this disease are dis-

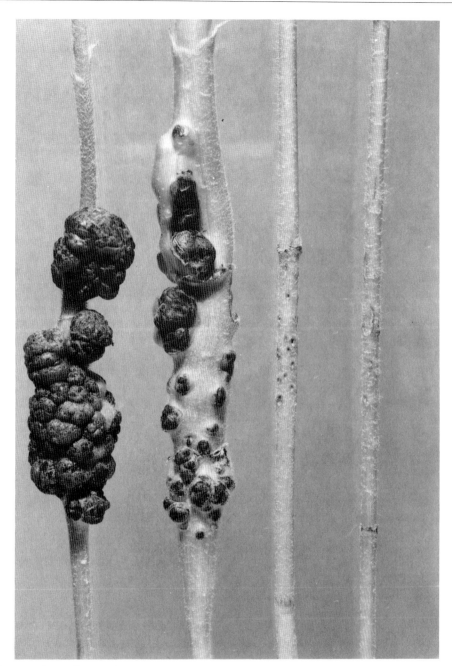

Figure 49.1. Stems of sunflower 6 weeks after inoculation with strains (left to right) A6K1 and A6-6K1 of *Agrobacterium tumefaciens*, strain R1001 of *Agrobacterium radiobacter* and control (*right*).

cussed in another part of this book and will not be further elaborated here (Chapters 50–52).

Two other diseases caused by bacteria in the same genus are the hairy root disease of apples incited by *Agrobacterium rhizogenes* and cane gall of raspberries and related plants incited by *Agrobacterium rubi*. Riker *et al.* (48) distinguished crown gall from hairy root, and showed that the hairy root organism has a much more limited host range than does the crown gall organism. Banfield (3) distinguished crown gall from cane gall and E. M. Hildebrand (30) named the causal organism as a separate species. This

organism is confined to the genus *Rubus*. Hairy root is distinguished from crown gall by the production of an excessive amount of roots from the stem (66) and cane gall by ridges or small swellings on the stem. In cases of severe infection with *A. rubi* the canes may split open and the leaves dry up.

The formation of galls or nodules on the roots of legumes in response to the species of *Rhizobia* is considered a symbiotic relationship with the host. The bacteria take nitrogen from the air and convert it into a form that can be used by the leguminous plants. Graham (27) studied the entire Rhizobiaceae family and concluded that some strains of *Rhizobia* are less closely related to one another than to certain strains of *Agrobacterium*. While there is still some controversy about these conclusions, they have been supported by the work of DeLey (14), and Dixon (18), using the techniques of molecular biology: DNA base ratios of certain species of *Rhizobium* and *Agrobacterium* and DNA homologies between certain species (see also DeLey (14)). Dixon (18) is of the opinion that the modes of action of rhizobia and agrobacteria are probably similar even though there are many differences among root nodules, crown galls, cane galls, or hairy roots.

The leafy gall or fasciation of sweet pea and other plants incited by *Corynebacterium fascians* is a mass of short, thick, fleshy stems with distorted leaves developing at or below soil line. The leafy gall on older plants may resemble a witches broom although it usually is not found more than a few centimeters above the ground.

The bacterial pocket disease of sugar beet incited by *Xanthomonas beticola* was first described by Brown (10). It apparently is limited to the United States. The overgrowths on the beet occur just about at soil level and extend down into the main part of the root. A good portion of the root must therefore be cut off before the sugar beet can be processed (22).

Bacterial knot of olive incited by *Pseudomonas savastanoi* is different from the rest in that it is insect transmitted (11). The olive fly has morphological modifications in the larvae, pupae, and adults to insure survival of the bacteria. The galls, which start as small swellings and may increase to several inches, occur on almost all parts of the plant. A similar gall on ash is apparently caused by a similar species of bacterium (67).

Bacterial gall of oleander incited by *Pseudomonas tonelliana* is not found on the underground parts of the plant. Small swellings may develop on the leaves and an ooze containing quantities of bacteria may be exuded from the veins. The galls are also found on stem and flowers (59, 67).

Hua (33) has reported the presence of DNA plasmids in tumor-inducing *Pseudomonas* strains including *P. savastanoi* and *P. tonelliana*. Hua states they may have important implications in the etiology of the diseases.

Nocardia vaccinii incites the blueberry bud-proliferating galls which are similar to crown gall and are formed at the soil line. Abnormal buds may grow into weak shoots forming a witches broom effect (15, 16, and 67).

Bacteria have also been reported to cause galls on algae and gymnosperms (43).

NEMATODE GALLS

In Table 49.1 we listed some representative galls caused by nematodes on mosses and flowering plants. Nematode galls are also found on algae, fungi, and liverworts (43). The gall-forming nematodes are found in the genera *Anguillulina*, *Anguina*, *Ditylenchus*, *Hemicycliophora*, *Meloidogyne*, and *Xiphenema*. All plant parasitic nematodes can be identified by their stylets which other nematodes lack. Most nematodes parasitize roots and other below-ground parts of plants (rhizomes, tubers, etc.) but some nematodes are also found on stem, leaf, flower, and seed. The gall-forming nematodes may induce hypertrophy or hyperplasia, or both, in host tissues. Possibly the best known galls are the root knots incited by *Meloidogyne* sp. on at least 1865 different species of plants (49). The first specific mention of root knot nematodes was that of Cornu in 1879 who described the causal agent of galls on the roots of *Onobrychis* (61). These nematodes do not always cause good galls and for this reason the extent of the host range was not realized immediately. Staining of root tissues shows, however, that salivary secretions of these nematodes make certain root cells stain more deeply than surrounding cells (Dr. G. Thorne, personal communication). The mechanism of gall formation is not known but is thought to be connected with growth substances within the root (35), particularly auxins.

The classic case of galls on aerial parts of plants is that of the bulb or stem nematode, *Ditylenchus dipsaci*. This nematode incites galls on leaves, flowers, and stems of alfalfa and many other hosts. It rarely occurs in root tissues. The mechanism of gall formation is unknown. *Ditylenchus radiciolus*, a related species, causes galls on roots (35, 61). This nematode can also invade leaf tissue that is touching the ground and galls have been known on leaf petioles of African violet (*Saintpaulia*) after internal migration of second-stage larvae (35).

The cellular responses of plants to nematode infections have been reviewed by Dropkin (21).

GALLS ON ALGAE AND FUNGI

A number of galls are induced on algae by algae, bacteria, fungi, nematodes, rotifers and copepods (43). Red, green, and brown algae induce galls on algae and other plants.

Fungus galls are induced on the alga *Spacelaria* by the fungus *Olpidium spacelarum*.

Galls are also induced on fungi by other fungi; outgrowths appear on mycelia of *Pilobolus crystallinus* induced by the fungus *Pleatrachelus fulgens* (39) and deformations produced on *Boletus* induced by *Sepedonium chrysosperum* (65). *Mycogone rosea* induces galls on fruiting bodies of *Clitocybe* and *Tricholoma*. Galls also have been reported induced by insects on fungus fruiting bodies (60).

The galls on lichens are often induced by Cyanophyceae which develop crusty and warty malformations (43). The lichens are also the only thallophytes on which mites induce galls.

Galls are induced on liverworts by *Nostoc lichinoides* and on ferns by fungi, mites, and insects (43).

INSECT GALLS

Many different types of insect galls may be observed on plants (11, 23). The feeding habits of the insects on plant cells and the resulting irritations to the plant induce plant cells and tissues to develop often in a manner that provides not only food but also shelter and protection for the gall-inciting insect. Thus, the gall is induced to protect the insect in the insect feeding process and is injurious rather than beneficial to the plant. The many insects, especially aphids, gall midges and gall wasps, as well as mites, have used their feeding habits not only to satisfy their food needs, but also to obtain shelter and protection from many unfavorable environments and predators.

The less highly developed gall producers such as the plant mites (mites are not insects but are sufficiently closely related to be considered here) but also many other gall producers, induce the development of single galls or leaf malformations or rolls. Other insects induce complex plant galls, often many-chambered and enlarged structures not typical of the normal plant morphology. The feeding and accompanying irritation are usually controlled to the extent that abnormal growth is induced without excessive injury and death to the plant cells and tissues. Usually, the galls are induced by the immature forms of the insects.

Many gall producers are found among the mites, aphids, midges, and wasps. The various types of galls produced have been given common names for ease of identification. These include one-celled bullet galls, mostly on oak twigs, produced by gall wasps; bud galls that may be small or large swellings and often are induced by midges; leaf galls such as induced on *Populus* sp. leaf blades and petioles by aphids; many-celled galls such as the mossy rose gall; oak apples including the large galls produced on *Quercus* sp. by members of the gall wasp genus *Amphibolips*; pouch or pocket galls consisting of depressions of various sizes and depths and often with hairy openings on the leaf blade produced by mites and aphids; root galls on grape, and stem and leaf galls as seen on *Quercus*; and other genera produced by members of the genus *Phylloxera*.

The plant mites produce many leaf deformations such as pocket or pouch galls, often with excessive development of plant hairs at the pouch opening.

The aphids have well-developed sucking mouth parts. Several genera produce galls. The *Adelges* produces a common cone gall on Norway spruce. Leaf blade and petiole galls are seen on cottonwood poplars induced by *Pemphigus* aphids and on grape leaves by *Phylloxera* aphids.

The gall midges produce galls of many forms on hickory trees and on different parts of many plant species.

The gall wasps (Cynipids) attack principally the various oaks. The maggot forms are present in the closed galls. Members of this group (*Amphibolips*) produce oak apples and oak bullet galls (*Disolcaspis*).

The mechanism of gall induction and development is generally poorly understood. Many galls appear to result from local irritation from one or more stages of the insect. This may start with the injury induced by the laying of the egg on or under the plant surface. Subsequent development may be associated with the young or larvae of the gall maker located within the plant part. The size and shape of many galls may be influenced by the numbers present of the infesting insects. The initiation of the gall may result from the irritation and injury induced by the feeding of the insects. Subsequent proliferation of new cells from the plant surface may be stimulated by the salivary products of the insect especially certain growth-regulating substances including IAA (3 indol acidic acid (heteroauxin)) and nucleic acids. Otherwise, the waste materials dropped by the insect in the gall cavity may also provide irritating, and other cell growth-stimulating, chemicals. Similar conditions are illustrated by the midrib gall of ash. In this case, the larval secretions stimulate the plant cells directly below, and deeper layers of cells subsequently react to the larval secretions. The thickness and size of the gall are proportional to the numbers of larvae present on the leaf. Many galls are initiated when the plant parts are young and tender and developing. Young buds, leaves, and stems respond well to the irritation of feeding injury and insect secretions.

The malignant or nonmalignant condition of the plant cells comprising the gall tissues has been closely studied only in recent years and then on a limited scale. Tissue culture studies of grape *Phylloxera* gall cells and normal grape stem cells in tissue culture have been useful to clarify similarities and differences in gall and normal grape cells (see Hildebrandt (32) and Arya and Hildebrandt (2) and references therein). Results of these tissue culture studies suggested that the cells of the galls are transformed from their normal growth patterns only in the presence of the insect or so long as insect secretions are present. Unlike the irreversible cellular changes produced by crown gall bacteria, the insect gall cells apparently return to normal cellular activities once the insect or its secretions are removed from the gall. Tissue culture studies have indicated that crown gall cells will continue to grow and divide in an unregulated manner if grafted into a normal plant. However, insect gall cells when grafted to a healthy plant stop growth.

Gall midges, gall wasps, aphids, and gall mites are the main gall inducers on plants in many areas of the world.

Felt (23) described over 2000 American insect-induced galls: 805 induced by gall wasps (Cynipidae), and nearly 700 induced by gall midges. The remaining galls are induced by other four-winged flies including 80 aphid galls. The wasps incite galls in 6 botanical families, in about 20 genera, with about 750 on members of the Fagaceae, mainly oaks. Of the 805 Cynipid galls, 41 are on roots, 45 on buds, 175 on twigs, branches and trunks, 275 on leaves, 21 on flowers, and 34 on acorns. There are 62 wasp galls on members of the family Rosaceae. These galls are produced on practically every part of the host plant. There are 700 gall midges in 69 of 78 plant families known to be attacked by gall insects. Aphid galls occur on many plant species. The *Phylloxera* galls on grapes are well-known for their destructiveness. They attack roots, stems and leaves. Mites induce 158 types of galls in 38 plant families. The mite-induced galls are relatively simple and are often characterized by abnormal hairy growths, known as erineums, and they frequently originate in buds. A few gall insects produce galls on either flowers, leaves, or young stems. Some representative galls, the incitants, and their distribution are listed in Table 49.1. Articles in the references will give extensive and additional details.

GENETIC GALLS

Genetic tumors have been reported on certain interspecific hybrids in the genera *Brassica* (roots), *Datura* (ovules), *Lilium* (seedlings), *Nicotiana* (several plant parts), and *Lycopersicum* (leaves). The tumor induction has resulted on the interspecific hybrids and not on the parent species (see Ahuja (1) and Smith (57) and references therein).

ENVIRONMENTAL GALLS

Galls have been reported induced by physical and chemical means.

White spruce (*Picea glauca*) galls on branches, roots, and trunks are widespread in certain areas along the Maine coast near the ocean in the United States. These burllike structures have also been noted on many other species of trees but are often associated with insect, bacterial, or fungus incitants. Each gall is initiated from a single cell (68). Chemically induced gall formation has been observed on *Picea abies* by Kaiser (38).

Wound-induced gall formation has been reported on *Datura* (29) and on kidney bean (26).

References

1. Ahuja, M. R. (1965): Genetic control of tumor formation in higher plants. *Q. Rev. Biol.*, 40:329–340.
2. Arya, A. C., and Hildebrandt, A. C. (1969): Differential sensitivity to gamma radiation of *Phylloxera* gall and normal grape stem cells in tissue culture. *Can. J. Bot.*, 47:1623–1628.

3. Banfield, W. M. (1934): Life history of the crown gall organism in relation to its pathogenesis on the red raspberry. *J. Agr. Res.*, 48:761–87.
4. Barton, E. S. (1891): On the occurrence of galls on *Rhodymenia palmata*. *J. Bot.*, 29:65–68.
5. Beiderbeck, R. (1977): *Pflanzentumoren (Plant Tumors)*. Eugen Ulmer, Stuttgart.
6. Buchanan, R. E., and Gibbons, N. E., (editors), *Bergey's Manual of Determinative Bacteriology* Ed. 8 (1974): Williams and Wilkins Co., Baltimore.
7. Black, L. M. (1952): Plant virus tumors. *Ann. N. Y. Acad. Sci.*, 54:1067–1075.
8. Braun, A. C. (1969): *The Cancer Problem.* Columbia University Press, New York.
9. Braun, A. C. (1969): *Plant Tumor Research.* (*Progress in Experimental Tumor Research*), Vol. 15. S. Karger, New York.
10. Brown, N. A. (1928): Bacterial pocket disease of the sugar beet. *J. Agr. Res.*, 37:155–168.
11. Carter, W. (1973): *Insects in Relation to Plant Disease*, Ed. 2. John Wiley & Sons, New York.
12. Connold, E. T. (1902): *British Vegetable Galls*. E. P. Dutton & Co., New York.
13. Darlington, A. (1968): *The Pocket Encyclopedia of Plant Galls in Color.* Philosophical Library, New York.
14. DeLey, J. (1972): *Agrobacterium*: Intrageneric relationships and evolution, in *Proceedings of the Third International Conference on Plant Pathogenic Bacteria*, Wageningen, 14–21 April 1971, edited by H. P. Geesteranus. University of Toronto Press, Toronto, Canada.
15. Demaree, J. B. (1947): A proliferating gall on blueberry plants caused by an *Actinomyces*. *Phytopathology*, (Abstract) 37:438.
16. Demaree, J. B., and Smith, N. R. (1952): Nocardia vaccinii N. sp. causing galls on blueberry plants. *Phytopathology*, 42:249–252.
17. Dixon, H. N. (1905): Nematode galls on mosses. *J. Bot.*, 43:251–252.
18. Dixon, R. O. D. (1969): Rhizobia (with particular reference to relationships with host plants). *Ann. Rev. Microbiol.*, 23:137–158.
19. Docters Van Leeuwen-Reijnvaan, J., and Docters Van Leeuwen (1926): *The Zoocecidia of the Netherlands East Indies.* Batavia, Drukkerij de Unie.
20. Dowson, W. J. (1957): *Plant Diseases Due to Bacteria.* Cambridge University Press, Cambridge.
21. Dropkin, V. H. (1969): Cellular responses of plants to nematode infections. *Ann. Rev. Phytopathol.*, 7:101–122.
22. Elcock, H. A. (1931): Phytomonas beticola. *Phytopathology*, 21:13–40.
23. Felt, E. P. (1965): *Plant Galls and Gall Makers.* Hafner Publishing Co., New York.
24. Forsberg, J. L. (1963): *Diseases of Ornamental Plants.* University of Illinois Special Publication No. 3. University of Illinois Press, Chicago.
25. Goodey, T. (1945): *Anguillulina brenari*, sp. nov. a nematode causing galls on the moss *Pottia bryoides*. *Mitt. J. Helminthol.*, 21:105–110.
26. Goto, M., Arai, K., and Uchino, M. (1977): Wound induced gall formation on kidney bean plants. *Plant Dis. Rep.*, 61:142–145.
27. Graham, P. H. (1964): The application of computer techniques to the taxonomy of the root-nodule bacteria of legumes. *J. Gen. Microbiol.*, 35:511–517.
28. Gronemann, C. F. (1930): Fifty common plant galls of the Chicago area, in *Botany Leaflet 16.* Field Museum of Natural History, Chicago.
29. Hildebrand, D. C., Thompson, J. P., and Schroth, M. N. (1966): Bacterial enhancement of self-limiting outgrowth formation on *Datura*. *Phytopathology*, 56:365–366.
30. Hildebrand, E. M. (1940): Cane gall of brambles caused by Phytomonas rubi n. sp. *J. Agr. Res.*, 61:685–706.
31. Hildebrandt, A. C. (1950): Some important galls and wilts of plants and the inciting bacteria. *Bacteriol. Rev.*, 14:259–272.
32. Hildebrandt, A. C. (1963): Growth of single cell clones of diseased and normal tissue origins, in *Plant Tissue Culture and Morphogenesis*, pp. 1–22 edited by H. D. Brown. Scholars Library, New York.
33. Hua, S. S. (1977): Plasmids in plant tumor-inducing Pseudomonas strains. *Abstr. Annu. Meet. Am. Soc. Microbiol.*, 77:141.
34. Jacobs, S. G., and Mohanty, U. (1951): Factors influencing infection by Corynebacterium fascians (Tilford) Dowson. *Ann. Appl. Biol.*, 38:237–245.
35. Jenkins, W. R., and Taylor, D. P. (1967): *Plant Nematology.* Reinhold Publishing Co., New York.
36. Jensen, J. H. (1934): Leaf enations resulting from tobacco mosaic infection in certain species of Nicotiana. *Contrib. Boyce Thompson Inst. Plant Res.*, 5:129.
37. Kado, C. I. (1977): Nature of Plasmids in Phytopathogenic Bacteria with Special Reference to Agrobacterium tumefaciens Plasmids, in *Beltsville Symposia in Agricultural Research, I Virology in Agriculture.* Universe Books, New York.
38. Kaiser, H. E. (1974): Reaction of plant tissues to mammalian carcinogens. XIIth International Cancer Congress, Florence, Oct. 20–26.
39. Küster, E. (1911): *Die Gallen der Pflanzen. Ein Lehrbuch des Botanikers und Entomologen*, Hirzel, Leipzig.
40. Lelliot, R. A. (1972): The genus *Xanthomonas*, in *Proceedings of the Third International Conference on Plant Pathogenic Bacteria*, Wageningen, 14–21 April 1971, edited by H. P. Geesteranus. University of Toronto Press, Toronto.
41. Lippincott, J. A. (1977): Molecular basis of plant tumour induction. *Nature*, 269:465–466.
42. Lyon, H. L. (1921): Three major cane diseases. *Hawaiian Sugar Planters Assoc. Expt. Sta. Bull. Bot. Series 3:1.*
43. Mani, J. S. (1964): *Ecology of Plant Galls.* W. Junk Publishers, The Hague.
44. Palm, B. T. (1931): A disease of Hibiscus sabdariffa caused by Rhodochytrium. *Phytopathology*, 21:1201–1202.
45. Pirone, P. P. (1978): *Diseases and Pests of Ornamental Plants.* John Wiley & Sons, New York.
46. Pirone, P. P., Dodge, B. O., and Rickett, A. W. (1960): *Diseases and Pests of Ornamental Plants.* Ronald Press, London.
47. Riker, A. J., and Banfield, W. M. (1930): Studies on infectious hairy root of nursery apple trees. *J. Agr. Res.*, 41:507–540.
48. Riker, A. J., Spoerl, E., and Gutsche, A. E. (1946): Some comparisons of bacterial plant galls and of their causal agents. *Bot. Rev.*, 12:57–82.
49. Sasser, J. N. (1954): Identification and host-parasite relationships of certain root-knot nematodes (Meloidogyne sp.). *Bull. Md. Agric. Expt. Sta. A-77.*
50. Schindler, A. J. (1942): Insect transmission of wallaby ear disease of maize. *J. Aust. Inst. Agr. Sci.*, 8:35–37.
51. Schindler, A., and Braun, A. J. (1957): Pathogenicity of an ectoparasitic nematode Xiphinema diversicaudatum, on strawberries. *Nematologica*, 2:91–93.
52. Schroth, M. N., and Hildebrand, D. C. (1972): Current taxonomic thinking on the genus Pseudomonas, with emphasis on the plant pathogens, in *Proceedings of the Third International Conference on Plant Pathogenic Bacteria*, Wageningen, 14–21 April 1971, edited by H. P. Geesteranus, University of Toronto Press, Toronto.
53. Smith, C. O. (1922): Pathogenicity of the olive knot organism on hosts related to the olive. *Phytopathology*, 12:271–278.
54. Smith, C. O. (1928): Oleander bacteriosis in California. *Phytopathology*, 18:503–518.
55. Smith, E. F. (1917): Embryomas in plants. *Johns Hopkins Med. J.*, 28:1–105.
56. Smith, E. F., and Townsend, C. O. (1907): A plant tumor of bacterial origin. *Science*, 25:671–673.
57. Smith, H. H. (1972): Plant Genetic Tumors, in: *Plant Tumor Research*, (*Progress in Experimental Tumor Research*), Vol. 15, pp. 138–164, edited by A. C. Braun. S. Karger, New York.
58. Swanton, E. W. (1912): *British Plant-Galls.* Methuen & Co., London.
59. Streets, R. B. (1972): *The Diagnosis of Plant Diseases.* The University of Arizona Press, Tucson, Arizona.
60. Thom, C. (1903): A gall upon a mushroom. *Bot. Gaz.*, 36:223–225.
61. Thorne, G. (1961): *Principles of Nematology.* McGraw-Hill Book Co., New York.
62. Thorne, G., and Schuster, J. L. (1956): Nacobbus butatiformis n. sp. (Nematoda: Tylenchidae) producing galls on the roots of sugar beets and other plants. *Proc. Helminthol. Soc. Wash.* we(2):128–134.
63. Valleau, W. D. (1947): Clubroot of tobacco: a wound tumor-like graft-transmitted disease. *Phytopathology*, 37:580.
64. Van Gundy, S. D. (1957): The first report of a species of Hemicycliophora attacking citrus roots. *Plant Dis. Rep.*, 41:1017–1018.
65. Vuillemin, P. (1895): Sur une maladie der agaric prodinte par une association parasitaire. *Bull. Soc. Mycol. Fr.*, 11:16.
66. Walker, J. C. (1969): *Plant Pathology*, Ed. 3. McGraw Hill & Co., New York.
67. Westcott, C. (1971): *Plant Disease Handbook*, Ed. 3. Van Nostrand Reinhold Co., New York.
68. White, P. R. (1958): A tree tumor of unknown origin. *Proc. Natl. Acad. Sci. U. S. A.*, 44:339–344.

50

Cellular Transformation in Crown Gall

Emil Y. Chi and Edward A. Smuckler

INTRODUCTION

Crown gall is an autonomous neoplastic disease of dicotyledonous plants (2). The transformation of plant cells to the cancer-like growth can be induced in wounds infected by specific varieties of *Agrobacterium tumefaciens*. The resultant proliferating cell population forms an irregular, expanding mass that can be propagated in culture and can be successfully grafted onto suitable hosts. Invasion of adjacent structures does not occur, and mobility of these plant cells does not occur in normal structures. This plant model resembles mammalian (human) tumors widely; differences as described by Lippincott (see p. 833) are given through normal variation between plant and animal cells (without and with rigid cell wall), and are due to the variation in body fluids of eumetazoan animals and vascular plants. Plant neoplasms are unable to metastasize.

The usefulness of this induced plant neoplasm for the analysis of structural and functional changes associated with cell transformation is readily apparent. The unique advantages to be obtained utilizing a bacterial inciting agent and plant tissue which can be propagated both *in vivo* and *in vitro* makes this a model suited for direct analysis of both agent-cell interactions and cellular modifications induced in neoplasia (4). In spite of a considerable wealth of information on the biology of crown gall, it has not been established what cells are at risk for transformation into this autonomous plant neoplasm (8). The following study was carried out utilizing both light and electron microscopy, to attempt

to identify those cells transformed in sunflower stems utilizing *A. tumefaciens* as the inducing agent. It would appear that transformation in this model system selects that cell population undergoing replication; that is, the cambium cells of the vascular bundle.

MATERIALS AND METHODS

Young sunflower plants were grown from seeds under greenhouse conditions. Four-week-old young stems, 3–4 mm in diameter, were wounded at internodal areas; control wounds were carried out with sterile toothpicks and test systems were wounded with toothpicks carrying *Agrobacterium tumefaciens*. The plants were sacrificed at different intervals following wounding, with or without inoculation, from 6 hr to 6 weeks. Transverse and longitudinal sections of the wounded area were prepared for both light and electron microscopy. The sites of inoculation were cut from the stems and immediately placed in 4% paraformaldehyde plus 5% glutaraldehyde in 0.1 M cacodylate buffer at pH 6.8. These millimeter-thick discs or sections were permitted to fix for 2 hr at room temperature. After fixation, the tissues were washed three times with buffer and then prepared separately for light and electron microscopy. For light microscopic studies, the tissues were dehydrated in alcohol and embedded in glycol methacrylate (3). Sections of 1 or 2 μm in thickness were cut with a Sorvall JB-4 microtome using a glass knife. Plant tissues were stained with hematoxylin and eosin, or with periodic acid and Schiff reagent. For electron microscopic studies, the tissues were postfixed in 1% osmium tetroxide and dehydrated and embedded in Epon according to the method of Luft (9). Thin sections were stained with uranyl acetate and lead hydroxide and examined in a JEOL-100B electron microscope at 60 kV accelerating voltage.

RESULTS

The morphology of sunflower stems has been previously described. Our material was not different from these studies (5). Figure 50.1 is a micrograph of a vascular bundle, showing the surrounding parenchyma. The latter appears as almost empty cell walls, scant organized cyto-

plasm is apparent. Nuclei, because of their small size in comparison to the cell volume, seem scant. The vascular bundle shows an outer phloem separated from an inner xylem by the vascular cambium. These cells have the most easily identified cytoplasmic and nuclear structures.

Wounding without subsequent infection was associated with repair (Figs. 50.2 and 50.4). Some cells adjacent to the wound collapsed, and extruded their cytoplasmic content. Healing took place into the wound sites by proliferation of the undifferentiated pith (parenchyma) and from the cambium of the vascular bundles (1). The first cell divisions produced cells parallel to existing wound walls and, with continued growth, the wound defect was filled. The contribution of parenchyma seemed to exceed the vascular cambium.

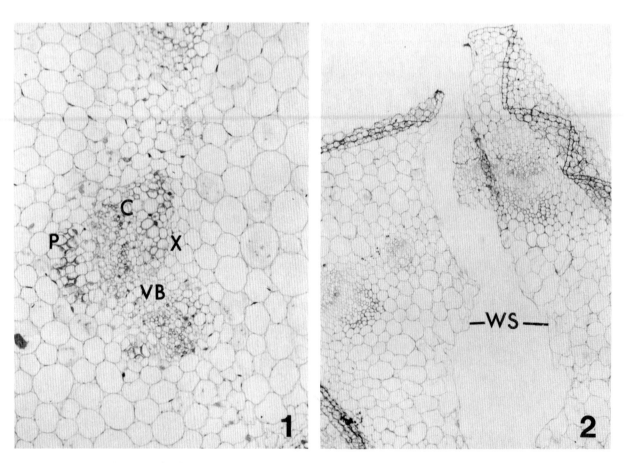

Figure 50.1. This micrograph shows a partial cross section of a young sunflower stem, and one of its vascular bundles (*VB*). Surrounding the bundle are large pith cells with scant organized cytoplasmic structure. The central section of the bundles is the vascular cambium (*C*). The cells in this area are smaller, but have easily identified nuclei and prominent cytoplasm. On the inner aspect, the specialization is to xylem (*X*) while the outer cells form phloem (*P*).

Figure 50.2. This micrograph shows a fresh (4 hr) control wound. The architecture of the stem is not modified; some cells in the surface adjacent to the wound (*WS*) have collapsed (see also Fig. 50.4). Magnification ×540.

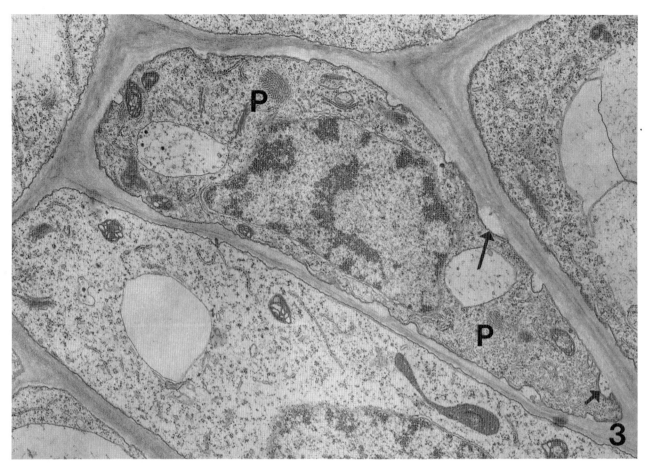

Figure 50.3. Electron micrograph of a 4-day-old wound tissue regenerating shows the cell beginning to differentiate. Note the P-protein (*P*) and cell wall (*arrows*). Magnification ×12,000.

TUMOR FORMATION

Wounding sunflower stems with toothpicks inoculated with *A. tumefaciens* resulted in crown gall formation. The morphology of these wounds was not different from sterile wounds during the first 6 hr. Dead cells were noted that extruded cytoplasm and debris into the wound. By electron microscopy, however, bacteria could be identified and were plentiful in dead cells (Fig. 50.5). In other areas, the bacteria seemed to penetrate between cells and were located several cells distant from the wound margin (Fig. 50.6). After 24 hr the morphology of the wound was not different from controls even at the ultra-structural level. Bacteria could no longer be found even though an extensive search was made for them. The organisms could not be identified by light microscopy using special staining techniques (6, 7).

The earliest tumor nodules were noted by 4 days. Cell masses with a decidedly haphazard structure seemed to arise in or from the vascular bundles (Figs. 50.7–50.9). Some preservation of the vascular architecture remains but the ordered arrays are disturbed by cells varying in size, shape, and a wide zone of vascular cambium of undifferentiated cells accumulates. Within this zone, there are many cells that both lack orientation to one another but also expand in mass into the adjacent parenchyma seemingly forcing it aside. Parenchymal contribution seemed small. By light microscopy, these cells resembled vascular cambium, but they did not appear to differentiate into either xylem or phloem. Electron microscopy shows structures more reminescent of immature meristem cells with abundant cytoplasm, prominent nuclei and nucleoli, and little storage material or transport specializations (Figs. 50.10 and 50.11).

With continued growth, the mass expanded forcing aside adjacent parenchyma and other vascular bundles. The cell pattern became more irregular, the cells were variable in size, shape, and staining reaction (Fig. 50.12). In some areas,

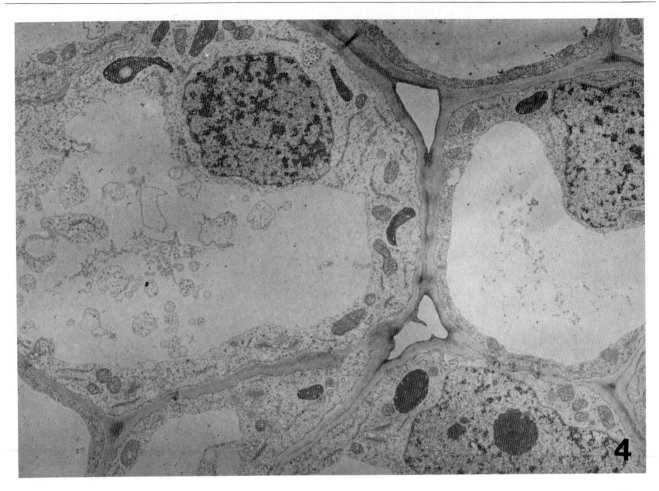

Figure 50.4. This micrograph taken from a 4-day-old wound control tissue shows newly formed cells beginning to vacuolate and thickening cell wall. These cells are larger in size as compared to the tumor cells. Magnification ×8000.

differentiation took place with the formation to sieve cells. On other areas, structure with resemblances to vascular bundles formed (Fig. 50.13). Electron microscopy revealed structural patterns reminescent of immature and very young cells. Occasionally, newly differentiated phloem are observed (Fig. 50.14). No bacteria were seen.

DISCUSSION

There is increasing evidence that neoplastic transformation involves cells in germinal pools (10). This implies that only cells with potential replication capacity can become malignant. In *in vitro* carcinogenesis experiments, there is even evidence to suggest that at least one round of replication is necessary in order to fix the changes associated with cell transformation. A similar suggestion has been made for crown gall induction (4). This notion has the very pragmatic value of providing a ready explanation for the phenotypic expressions seen in malignancy. Transformed cells are capable of further differentiation demonstrated both morphologically and functionally, to more adult tissues.

In crown gall, under our conditions, we have demonstrated that the earliest nodule of tumor formation seemed to be derived from the vascular cambium or meristem. This group of cells represents the replicating germinal pool whose continued growth results in stem enlargement and in the differentiation either to pith (or re-

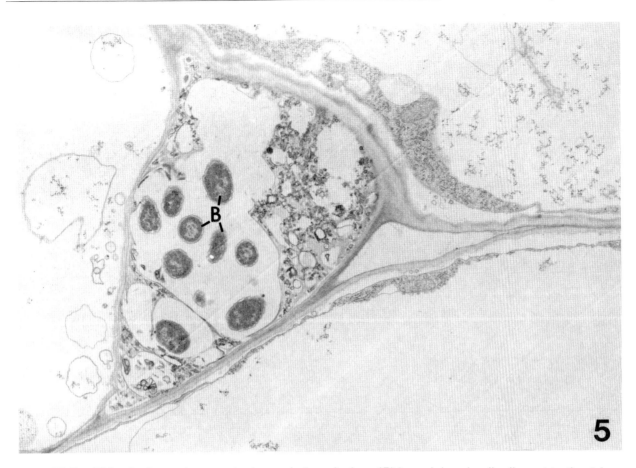

Figure 50.5. This electron micrograph shows *A. tumefaciens* (B) in an injured cell adjacent to the 4-hr wound. The cytoplasmic structures adjacent to the bacterial growth are clumped. Two adjacent cells are not remarkable, there is significant vacuolization of the cytoplasm. Magnification ×14,000.

serve cells) as well as the functioning portion of the vascular bundle (xylem and phloem). The selection of these cells for transformation provides an explanation for the subsequent modification seen in these tumors. Formation of sieve cells (phloem) and teratoma-like structures represents no more than an aberrant form of differentiation in this autonomous growth. It involves no "de-differentiation " in a mature cell population, but, rather, represents a modification of the differentiation in the transformed call population.

A very real and practical issue concerns the mechanism by which this transformation is brought about. The appearance of bacteria early in the wound and their disappearance from the wound before the occurrence of tumor formation suggests their role may be only as carriers of the transforming agency—a concept consistent with other observations made by biochemical means in these tumors (2, 4). It suggests that plasmid transfer must occur within several hours of infection, and provides further evidence for only an indirect role for the intact bacterium. The absence of bacteria at times not synchronous with maximal transforming further points to a peculiarity of bacterial growth and rejection in the cycle of restorative cell population.

The identification of the cell population for transformation as meristem, the growth of the meristem cells in culture, and their transformation under these circumstances points to a commonality of the plant tumor with the mammalian malignant cells and further points to areas for investigation in the mechanisms of transformation.

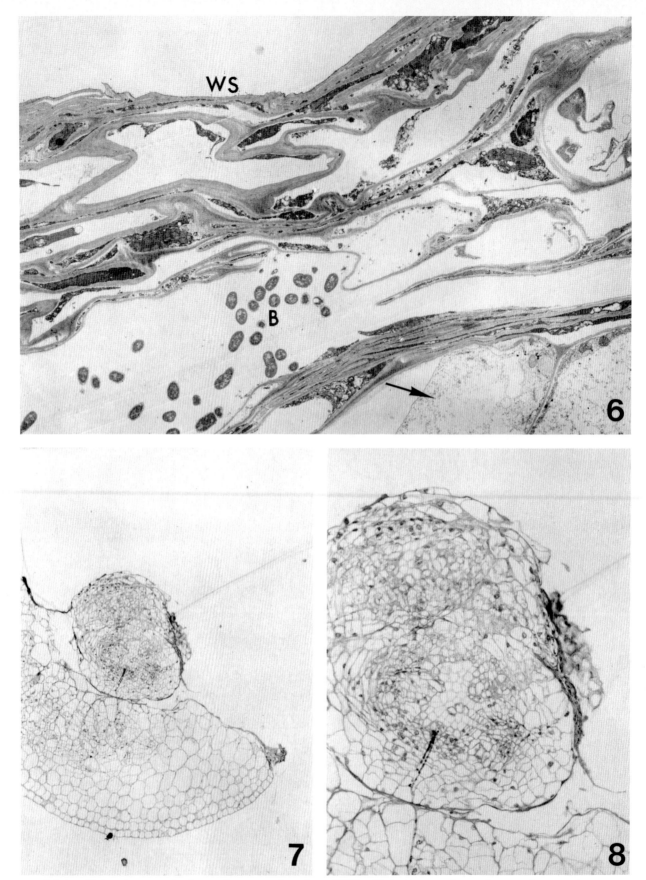

Figure 50.6. This micrograph shows the wound surface (*WS*) with juxtaposed membranes from collapsed cells. The cells adjacent to this zone also exhibit aggregation of cytoplasmic structure. Bacteria (*B*) permeate between cells away from the wound itself, and are located in an area of injured and normal cells (*arrow*). Magnification ×5000.

Figure 50.7. This micrograph shows the morphology of an early gall, formed by 4 days following inoculation. The growth arises from, and resembles, a vascular bundle. Its cells, even at this magnification, show more prominent nuclei. Magnification ×540.

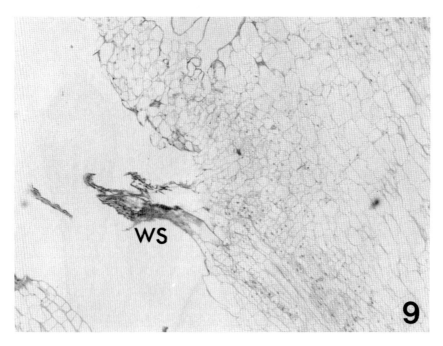

Figure 50.9. The longitudinal section taken also from a 4-day-old wound also shows a disorderly growth of cells protruding into the wound (*WS*). Magnification ×540.

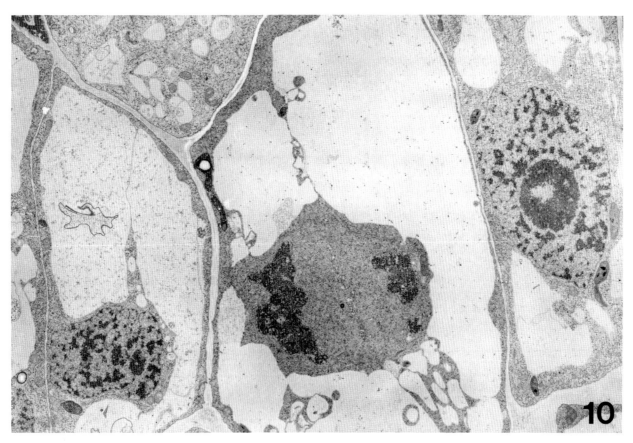

Figure 50.10. This electron micrograph shows tissue from the 4-day-old tumor. The cells have abundant cytoplasm and prominent nuclei, but cytoplasmic specialization are lacking. One cell is dividing (*middle*) a second shows condensed chromatin (*right*). Magnification ×3800.

Figure 50.8. This more detailed picture shows the disorderly growth of cells, resembling in part a vascular bundle. There are dead cells adherent to part of the mass which seems to force aside adjacent structures and bulge into the wound. Magnification ×860.

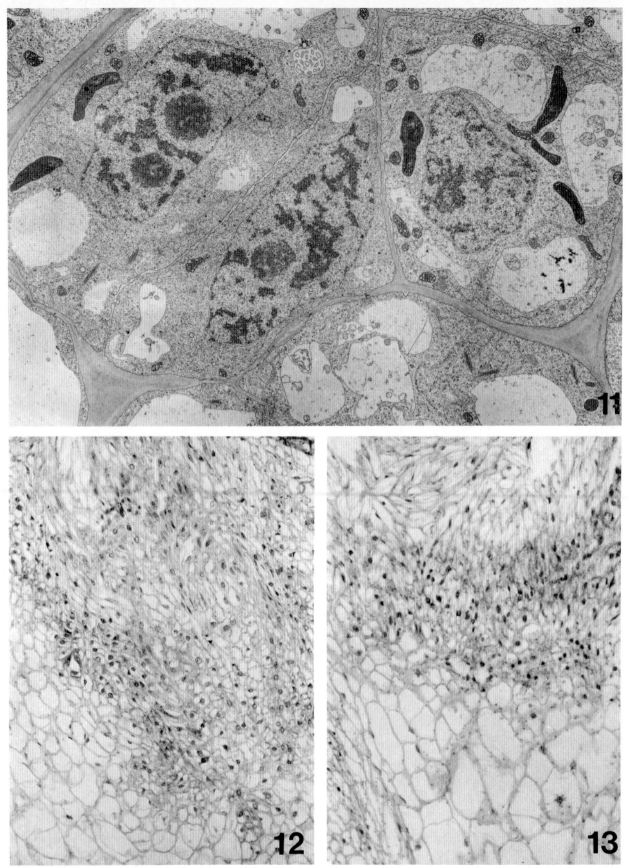

Figure 50.11. This micrograph, taken from tissue of an older tumor (8 days) shows more immature cells. They have abundantly formed cytoplasm with prominent ergastoplasm and Golgi. No histological evidence of differentiation is noted. Magnification ×7200.

Figure 50.12. This micrograph is a 4-week-old tumor, and shows a diffuse, disorganized growth of cells differing in size and shape. The growth pattern lacks specialization and the cells show characteristics of both xylem and phloem. Magnification ×860.

Figure 50.13. This tumor, from a 6-week-old plant shows an undifferentiated mass; vascular structure is poorly defined. Magnification ×860.

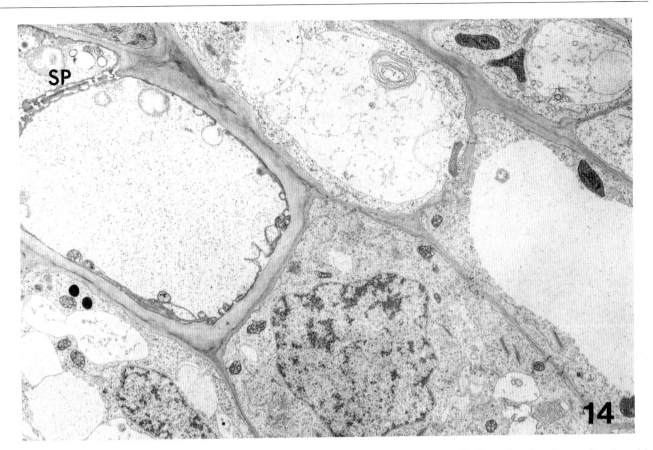

Figure 50.14. This micrograph, taken from the center mass of a gall, reveals the ultrastructure of cells with differentiated structural features. A sieve plate (*SP*) is readily distinguishable. The surrounding cells do not show similar specialization but their cytoplasmic structure includes more well defined vacuoles and less ergastoplasm (compare to Fig. 50.9). Magnification ×7600.

SUMMARY

The cell origin of crown gall was sought by light and electronmicroscopic examination of infected healing wounds. Sunflower stems were injured by toothpicks contaminated with *A. tumefaciens*. Histological and ultrastructural analyses were carried out at intervals in normal healing wounds and in wounds in which crown gall developed. Normal healing took place by cell division in the parenchyma and to a lesser extent in the vascular cambium. Infected wounds resembled normal ones except that bacteria could be identified for the first 6–18 hr, thereafter they were not detectable by morphological techniques. The earliest tumor formation appeared to arise from and resemble the vascular cambium. Further growth was associated with an expansile mass, some of those cells differentiated to vascular elements. We concluded that crown gall involves the transformation of cells from a germinal pool and resembles the animal model of carcinogenesis.

References

1. Barker, W. G. (1954): A contribution to the concept of wound repair in woody stems, *Can. J.Bot.*, 32:486–490.
2. Braun, A. C. (1974): *The Biology of Cancer.* Addison-Wesley, Reading, Mass.
3. Chi, E. Y., and Smuckler, E. A. (1976): A rapid method for processing liver biopsies for two-micron sectioning. *Arch. Pathol. Lab. Med.*, 100: 457–462.
4. Drlica, K. A., and Kado, C. I. (1968): Crown gall tumors: are bacterial nucleic acids involved? *Bacteriol. Rev.*, 39:186–196.
5. Esau, K. (1962): *Anatomy of Seed Plants,* pp. 238–242. John Wiley & Sons, New York.
6. Gee, M. M., Sun, C. N., and Dwyer, J. D. (1966): Subcellular observations on sunflower crown gall induced by *Agrobacterium tumefaciens*. *Am. J. Bot.*, 53:622.
7. Gee, M. M., Sun, C. N., and Dwyer, J. D. (1967): An electron microscope study of sunflower crown gall tumor. *Protoplasma, 64:195.*
8. Kupila-Ahvenniemi, S., and Thurman, E. (1968): Morphogenesis of crown gall. *Adv. Morphog.,* 7:45–78.
9. Luft, J. (1961): Improvements in epoxy resin embedding methods. *J. Biophys. Biochem. Cytol.,* 9:409–414.
10. Pierce, G. B. (1974): Neoplasms, differentiation and mutations. *Am. J. Pathol.,* 77:103.

51

Crown Gall,
a "Malignant Plant Tumor"

James A. Lippincott and Barbara B. Lippincott

INTRODUCTION

Amorphous and organoid hyperplasias are formed by many plants in response to infection by members of the bacterial genus *Agrobacterium* as was first clearly proven by Smith and Townsend (58) in 1907. A recent tabulation indicates that members of minimally 93 different families of dicotyledonous flowering plants and gymnospermous (principally conifer) seed plants are susceptible to transformation by agrobacteria (17) and this host range undoubtedly could be extended by further testing. The autonomous growth characteristics of these tumors was suggested by the results of White and Braun (65) and Braun and White (10) who showed that the tumors continued to grow in tissue culture in the absence of the initiating bacterium and in the absence of growth factors required for the proliferation of normal tissues. Furthermore, bacteria-free tumor tissue proliferated in an unrestricted fashion when grafted onto healthy plants, whereas normal tissues did not. In this respect, therefore, these tumors behave like malignant animal tumor cells. The relatively rigid cell wall which encloses each plant cell and is formed concomitantly with cell division, however, constitutes a formal barrier to any metastatic spread of crown gall cells in the host. Thus, while these tumor cells fulfill all other criteria for true cancer cells, this unique aspect of plants precludes the presence of cancer *in sensu strictu*.

In many ways, the crown gall system offers important advantages as a model system with which to study autonomous neoplastic disease. The tumors are induced at will in a relatively short time by simple inoculation procedures, and the hosts themselves are much less complex in terms of their organization and hormonal regulation than are vertebrates. Plants lack a true immune system, parts can be grafted from one plant to another, haploid plants are readily obtained, both normal and tumor cells are easily grown in tissue culture on simple media relative to that required for animal tissues, and entire plants can be regenerated from tissue-cultured cells growing as amorphous clusters. Also, clones of tissue derived from single cells are readily established. These characteristics have contributed directly to the development of important concepts in crown gall research concerning the nature of the tumorous state which are of increasing relevance to the animal cancer field, e.g. transformation involves the activation of biosynthetic pathways that contribute to metabolic and hormonal independence, and the autonomous state is potentially reversible (6).

CAUSAL AGENT

The agrobacteria are the only bacteria demonstrated to cause formation of autonomous proliferations in any host. They are short, motile, Gram-negative rods closely related to the rhizobia that induce nitrogen-fixing nodules in legumes. The agrobacteria are currently classified into four genera, based primarily on phytopathological considerations: *Agrobacterium tumefaciens*, the agent of the crown gall disease; *Agrobacterium rubi*, the agent of the cane gall disease; *Agrobacterium rhizogenes*, the agent of the hairy root disease; and *Agrobacterium radiobacter*, a nonpathogenic species (1). Pathogenicity, however, is now known to depend on a large DNA plasmid, the Ti-plasmid, carried by the virulent species, but which is absent or defective in the nonpathogenic forms (see following articles). The different *Agrobacterium*-induced diseases, all characterized by abnormal host proliferation, seem to represent evolutionary variations in which the pathogen and/or the Ti-plasmid have adapted to particular hosts rather than being due to different initiation mechanisms (36). Newer taxonomic studies based on physiological characteristics, numerical analysis, and DNA hybridization studies are consistent in indicating that most agrobacteria fall into two major groups, biotypes 1 and 2 (18, 26, 29, 51). Independently, there are two major kinds of Ti-plasmids that confer virulence, the octopine-type and the nopaline-type, which occur with about equal frequency in each biotype (14, 42).

The agrobacteria are a common component of the soil microflora, generally grow best below 30°C and are distributed worldwide in both cultivated and virgin areas. They appear to multiply preferentially near plant roots and show a positive chemotactic response to the growing portion of a root (57). In nature, crown gall tumors are most commonly found at the juncture of the root and stem (crown) at or just below the soil surface and on the upper part of the roots. The susceptibility of this portion of the plant to wounding, a necessary prerequisite for tumor formation, and the proliferation of the bacterium in the surrounding rhizosphere presumably contributes to this relationship. Experimentally, however, all parts of host plants, with the possible exception of embryonic regions, are susceptible to the bacterium.

TRANSFORMATION PROCESS

Virulent strains of *Agrobacterium* in a viable state seem capable of transforming only wound-stimulated plant cells (36). The wound requirement may be essential for three reasons: it provides a medium which supports tumorigenic activities of the bacterium, it exposes sites to which the bacterium can attach, and it stimulates metabolic changes in host cells (termed conditioning) which lead to development of a transformation-susceptible state. Competition studies have demonstrated what is currently the earliest detectable stage in the transformation process,

Agrobacterium attachment or adherence to a site in the wound (33). This adherence shows considerable specificity and seems to involve molecular recognition between the polysaccharides in the outer cell envelope membrane of the bacterium with polygalacturonic acid molecules in the outermost part of host cell walls (35, 38, 39). Both the Ti-plasmid and the main chromosome of virulent agrobacteria can determine adherence (64). On bean leaves, the adherence step is complete within 15 min after inoculation while in other host systems where wound drying is slower, as long as 6 hr may be required for adherence of the maximum number of bacteria.

From adherence to the time when a tumor is first detectable, 2–6 days later depending on the host system, little direct information about the transformation process is available. Attempts to stage the transformation process have been made by temperature transitions (transformation but not tumor or bacterial growth is prevented at 32°C and proceeds at maximum efficiency at 27°C) and antibiotic or antimetabolite application. These results narrow the time required for all transformations to 20–96 hr, depending on the host, after bacterial inoculation. This broad time span seems to represent an asynchrony of transformation rather than the true time requirement; the minimal transformation time is probably a few hours or less once both the host cell and attached bacterium have each reached a "competent" state. A critical stage in the wound-stimulated cell division process is considered to constitute the host competence stage (7, 32). After inoculation, bacterial synthesis of both protein and nucleic acid appear essential for the development of bacterial competence and this is probably true also of potential host cells (24, 36).

All evidence indicates that the bacteria remain external to the cells they transform and are not required beyond the initial 20–96-hr period for tumor progression and subsequent growth. The presence of bacterial plasmid DNA in tumors grown in tissue culture free of the inducing bacterium (13) indicates that part or all of the Ti-plasmid is transferred from the bacterium to the host cell during this process. Other evidence suggests that either bacterial or host-produced growth hormone of the auxin type is essential in the transformation (9). Efforts to induce these tumors with nucleic acid, hormones or both, however, have thus far not succeeded. This suggests that either some unique mechanism or additional components are necessary for transformation.

The enhanced initiation of tumors obtained

when certain avirulent strains of *Agrobacterium* carrying defective Ti-plasmids are inoculated with virulent strains (34, 40) has led to the demonstration that certain pairs of avirulent strains can complement to initiate tumors (41). Analysis of these data suggests that plasmid genes involved in the transfer of the plasmid from bacterium to bacterium also participate in transfer of plasmid DNA to host cells (Lippincott and Lippincott, unpublished data). Thus, these plasmid genes, which appear to be localized outside that part of the plasmid found in stable tumor cells, also seem to be essential for bacterial tumorigenicity. Tempe *et al.* (61) have shown that the conjugative transfer of the Ti-plasmid from bacterium to bacterium is inhibited at temperatures above 30°C. The temperature sensitivity of the plasmid transfer process to plant cells, therefore, may explain the unusual temperature sensitivity of tumor initiation process.

Tumor cells many generations removed from the initial transformation event may contain 20–30 copies of only about a 5% portion of the Ti-plasmid (13, 19, 31). At some stage in either the transformation process or during subsequent tumor development, amplification of certain plasmid DNA sequences must occur whereas the majority of plasmid DNA is either never transferred or is lost during tumor cell divisions. Indirect evidence indicates that a single attached bacterium can transform 30 or more surrounding cells (36). Thus, a very marked synthesis of plasmid DNA must occur either in the bacterium or in the host cell to which it is directly attached to account for the presence of 20 copies in each of 30 cells.

TUMOR DEVELOPMENT

Once the tumor initiation process has passed the stage sensitive to elevated temperature, even less is known about the tumors until they have attained measurable size. By varying the time at permissive and nonpermissive temperatures during the critical initiation period, Braun (3) obtained evidence for progression in the transformation process: the various degrees of progression characterized by increasing ability of the tumors, when cultured, to synthesize their growth requirements on a simple, defined medium with sucrose as carbon source. Progressive quantitative variations in the ability of cultured normal tissue to produce growth substances may be a model for this type of phenomenon (46).

The growth rate of crown gall tumors is initially fast, but with time growth declines to a very low rate unless the tumor is transplanted to a new host or is grown in tissue culture (37). Initial tumor growth is directly correlated with the number of tumor cells in a particular area and appears to depend on tumor production of diffusible products whose level can be rate limiting if optimal levels are not maintained. Levels of certain nonprotein amino acids in particular may be growth limiting, since γ-aminobutyric acid, octopine, and nopaline have been shown to have this effect (37, 53).

With further development, these tumors may remain smooth, erupt into a rough callus mass, or produce abnormal to fully normal appearing plant structures such as roots or shoots (Fig. 51.1) (37). Variables known to influence formation of these latter organs include the infecting bacterial strain, host species, portion of the host inoculated, and the physiological state of the host when inoculated. The ability of these organoid crown galls (teratomas) to produce organ-like outgrowths is frequently maintained when the tissue is grown in culture (5); Braun and Meins (8) suggest that these different kinds of tumors represent different but inherently stable developmental states.

In certain hosts, "secondary" tumors may arise at some distance from the initial wound inoculation without any apparent cellular connection with the primary tumor (37). In many species, however, the bacterium can spread systematically throughout the plant via the vascular tissues and this spread, coupled with natural growth wounding or bacterial hormone-induced growth wounding, may account for the appearance of these tumors (21). The bacteria are known to produce plant growth factors of both the auxin (55, 60) and cytokinin types (12, 25). In many cases, secondary tumors appear to be free of any agrobacteria (10) which has supported considerable speculation that a transmissible agent other than the bacterium might be responsible for these tumors.

Secondary tumors of a potentially different nature have been induced by grafting sterile cultured tumor cells to normal hosts whose cells are cytologically distinguishable from those of the tumor (44). Secondary tumors induced in this manner, however, only arise in the wound-stimulated cells immediately adjacent to the grafted tumor cells. These latter secondary tumors appear equivalent to other crown gall tumors in terms of their nutritional requirements in culture and their growth when grafted into healthy hosts. Further tests are needed, however,

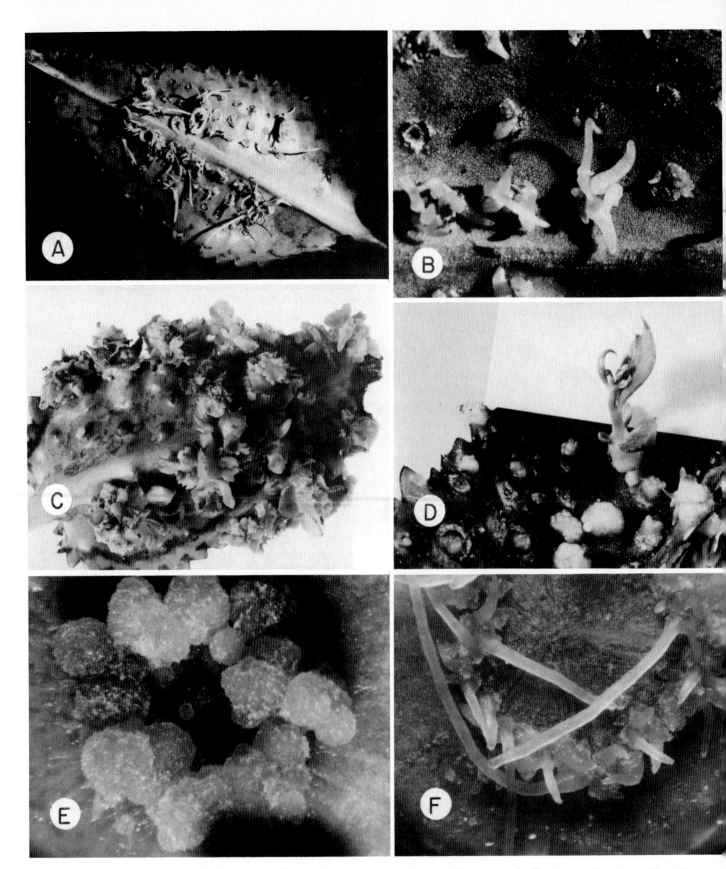

Figure 51.1. Morphological aspects of neoplasms induced by agrobacteria. *A,* Tumor and root proliferation induced by *Agrobacterium rhizogenes* strain 15834 on leaves of *Kalanchoe daigremontiana* (*ca.* ×1), *B,* Detail of leaf similar to that shown in *Part A* (*ca.* ×5); *C,* Teratomas induced by *Argobacterium tumefaciens* strain T37 on *Kalanchoe daigremontiana* leaves (*ca.* ×1.5); *D,* Detail of a leaf inoculated as in *Part C* with normal-appearing shoot and flower primordia (*ca.* ×3); *E,* Rounded amorphous tumors formed by *Agrobacterium tumefaciens* strain B6 on a carrot root slice (*ca.* ×5); and *F,* Tumors and roots induced on a carrot root slice by *Agrobacterium rhizogenes* strain TR7 (*ca.* ×5).

to show whether these tumors are metabolically analogous to the primary tumors used in their initiation or whether they represent a phenomenon called habituation which occurs in varying degree in normal tissues grown in culture.

TUMOR PHYSIOLOGY AND METABOLISM

The demonstration by Braun (4) that crown gall tumors produce a sufficient amount of two classes of growth hormones (auxin-type and cytokinin-type) to grow in tissue culture without these growth factors, whereas most normal tissues require both, suggested that the basic premise that underlies autonomous growth consists of the ability to synthesize compounds that are typically in growth-limiting supply for normal tissues in differentiated portions of the host. This phenomenon, clearly demonstrable in crown gall tumors, establishes a concept which, in possibly less obvious ways, may be the basic explanation of tumor autonomy generally. The nature of these growth regulators, principally β-indoleacetic acid (16, 20, 52) and ribosyl-trans-zeatin (Miller) (47, 49, 54) suggests that the normal plant synthetic pathways, though repressed in differentiated tissues, are responsible for the production of these growth factors. Transformation, therefore, results in the derepression of these biosynthetic pathways that are usually expressed only in embryonic and meristematic (continuously embryonic) portions of the mature plant. Thus, in their ability to produce normal plant growth hormones, the tumors resemble embryonic tissues. Addition of these two growth hormones to plant tissue culture media is sufficient in many plants to allow growth in culture comparable to that shown by the tumor tissues in the absence of the growth factors.

One of the unusual characteristics of most crown gall tumors is their ability to synthesize either the arginine derivative octopine [N^2-(D-1-carboxyethyl)-L-arginine] or nopaline (N^2(?-1,3-dicarboxypropyl)-L-arginine]. Tumors that produce octopine also produce comparable derivatives of lysine, ornithine, and histidine (27, 36, 56). The presence of these compounds in normal tissues has been controversial (e.g., Wendt-Gallitelli and Dobrigkeit (63); Schilperoort and Bomhoff (56); Montoya et al.) (48). Unequivocal evidence that octopine and octopine dehydrogenase occur in embryonic bean tissues has been obtained ((15) and unpublished data) and the enzyme octopine dehydrogenase readily accepts

lysine, histidine, and ornithine to produce the corresponding carboxyethyl derivatives in the presence of pyruvate and reduced NADP (2, 22, 23, 50). Formation of these compounds by the tumors, therefore, seems to be another example of derepression of characteristically embryonic genes in the transformation process.

An additional example of this phenomenon can be found in the cell wall metabolism that characterizes normal and tumor tissues (38, 39). Cell walls isolated from normal tissues have sites to which *Agrobacterium* can adhere whereas cell walls isolated from embryonic tissues and from crown gall tumors do not. In each case, methylation of cell wall polygalacturonic acids can account for the type of response, the lower the degree of methylation the greater the ability of the cell walls to bind *Agrobacterium*. The tumor transformation, therefore, results in an alteration of plant cell wall metabolism to one which is analogous in some respects to that of embryonic tissues.

Additional changes which characterize crown gall tumors generally include changes in metabolism that result in a more highly reduced state and changes generally associated with a more anaerobic type of metabolism (30, 59). The tumors also show an enhanced ability to accumulate potassium and phosphate relative to normal tissues growing at similar rates (66). Phosphate uptake by the tumors is not sensitive to 2,4-dinitrophenol inhibition, whereas that of normal tissue in culture is inhibited (67).

PERMANENCE OF THE TUMOROUS STATE

The dramatic results of Braun (5) showing that shoot-like outgrowths from cultured crown gall tumors could, on grafting to normal hosts, give rise eventually to normal sexually fertile plants have established an important concept in the tumor field. Autonomous tumor growth is potentially reversible. Additional evidence of this potential is gradually building in the animal field (see Braun, Ref. 6). The normal appearing plants derived from these tumors, however, continue to produce one of the unusual arginine derivatives, and when segments of the plant are introduced into tissue culture they quickly revert to tumorous-type growth characterized by auxin and cytokinin independence (11). Seeds obtained from these plants, however, appear fully normal, suggesting there is no carryover of tumor tendencies through the fertilized egg cell (62).

These results, and those showing that many unusual tumor characteristics are representative of normal embryo metabolism, suggest that the tumors represent a stabilized pattern of gene expression similar in part to embryonic tissues which, with certain manipulations, can revert to patterns of gene expression typical of normal differentiated tissues. Meins (45) has shown, using certain tissue culture phenotypes, that elevated or low temperature treatment can promote transitions between apparently stable phenotypes. The nopaline-type tumor culture used in these investigations appears to respond to several products of glutamate metabolism (43). Since α-ketoglutarate and arginine are combined to produce nopaline in nopaline-type tumors, glutamate metabolism may have a key regulatory function in the control of transitions between different phenotypic states.

SUMMARY

Crown gall tumors are the most thoroughly studied of plant tumors. They exhibit numerous characteristics in common with the autonomous neoplasms of vertebrates, including anaerobic-type metabolism and reversion to many embryonic-type features of metabolism. The concepts concerning the physiological basis of tumor autonomy and the potential reversibility of the tumorous phenotype developed through studies in this system are of major relevance to the field of cancer biology. More recently, the demonstration of the presence of a small amount of a unique part of bacterial plasmid DNA in sterile tumors shows that this transformation may have much in common with DNA virus-induced neoplasms. Continued progress in this field should contribute additional concepts and information of potentially leading importance for tumor studies generally.

References

1. Allen, O. N., and Holding, A. J. (1974): Agrobacterium, in: Bergey's Manual of Determinative Bacteriology, Ed. 8, pp. 264–267, edited by R. E. Buchanan and N. E. Gibbons. Williams & Wilkins, Baltimore.
2. Birnberg, P. R., Lippincott, B. B., and Lippincott, J. A. (1977): Two octopine dehydrogenases in crown-gall tumour tissue. Phytochemistry, 16:647–650.
3. Braun, A. C. (1953): Bacterial and host factors concerned in determining tumor morphology in crown-gall. Bot. Gaz., 114:363–371.
4. Braun, A. C. (1958): A physiological basis for autonomous growth of the crown-gall tumor cell. Proc. Natl. Acad. Sci. U. S. A., 44:344–349.
5. Braun, A. C. (1959): A demonstration of the recovery of the crown-gall tumor cell with the use of complex tumors of single cell origin. Proc. Natl. Acad. Sci. U. S. A. 45:932–938.
6. Braun, A. C. (1972): The relevance of plant tumor systems to an understanding of the basic cellular mechanisms underlying tumorigenesis. Prog. Exp. Tumor Res., 15:165–187.
7. Braun, A. C., and Mandle, R. J. (1948): Studies on the inactivation of the tumor inducing principle in crown gall. Growth, 12:255–269.
8. Braun, A. C., and Meins, F., Jr. (1970): The regulation of the expression of cellular phenotypes in crown-gall teratoma tissue of tobacco. Symp. Int. Soc. Cell Biol., 9:193–204.
9. Braun, A. C., and Stonier, T. (1958): Morphology and physiology of plant tumors. Protoplasma., 10(5a):1–93.
10. Braun, A. C., and White, P. R. (1943): Bacteriological sterility of tissues derived from secondary crown-gall tumors. Phytopathology, 33:85–100.
11. Braun, A. C., and Wood, H. N. (1976): Suppression of the neoplastic state with the acquisition of specialized functions in cells, tissues, and organs of crown gall teratomas of tobacco. Proc. Natl. Acad. Sci. U. S. A., 73:496–500.
12. Cherayl, J. D., and Lipsett, M. N. (1977): Zeatin ribonucleosides in the transfer ribonucleic acid of Rhizobium leguminosarum, Agrobacterium tumefaciens, Corynebacterium fascians, and Erwinia amylovora. J. Bacteriol., 131:741–744.
13. Chilton, M. D., Drummond, M. H., Merlo, D. J., Sciaky, D., Montoya, A. L., Gordon, M. P., and Nester, E. W. (1977): Stable incorporation of plasmid DNA into higher plant cells: the molecular basis of crown gall tumorigenesis. Cell, 11:263–271.
14. Chilton, M. -D., Montoya, A. L., Merlo, D. J., Drummond, M. H., Nutter, R., Gordon, M. P., and Nester, E. W. (1978): Restriction endonuclease mapping of a plasmid that confers oncogenicity upon Agrobacterium tumefaciens strain B6-806. Plasmid, 1:254–269.
15. Creaser, V. R. (1977): Establishment of tissue cultures of individual bean leaf crown-gall tumors and examination of their guanidino content. Ph.D. Dissertation. Northwestern University, Evanston, Ill.
16. Davies, F. S., Mau, S. -L. C., and Nooden, L. D. (1975): Auxin synthesis in crown gall tumor tissue: a comparison of three putative precursors. Physiol. Plant., 33:39–41.
17. De Cleene, M., and De Ley, J. (1976): The host range of crown gall. Bot. Rev., 42:389–466.
18. De Ley, J., Tijtgat, R., de Smedt, J., and Michiels, M. (1973): Thermal stability of DNA: DNA hybrids within the genus Agrobacterium. J. Gen. Microbiol., 78:241–252.
19. Drummond, M. H., Gordon, M. P., Nester, E. W., and Chilton, M. -D. (1977): Foreign DNA of bacterial plasmid origin is transcribed in crown gall tumors. Nature, 269:535–536.
20. Dye, M. H., Clarke, G., and Wain, R. L. (1962): Investigations on the auxins in tomato crown-gall tissue. Proc. Roy. Soc. Lond. B, 155:478–492.
21. El Khalifa, M. D., El Nur, E. E., Lippincott, B. B., and Lippincott, J. A. (1973): Crown gall on castor bean leaves. II. Formation of secondary tumours. J. Exp. Bot., 24:1117–1129.
22. Goldmann, A. (1977): Octopine and nopaline dehydrogenases in crown-gall tumors. Plant Sci. Lett. 10:49–58.
23. Hack, E., and Kemp, J. D. (1977): Comparison of octopine, histopine, lysopine, and octopinic acid synthesizing activities in sunflower crown gall tissues. Biochem. Biophys. Res. Commun., 78:785–791.
24. Kado, C. I. (1976): The tumor-inducing substance of Agrobacterium tumefaciens. Annu. Rev. Phytopathol., 14:265–308.
25. Kaiss-Chapman, R. W. and Morris, R. O. (1977): Trans-zeatin in culture filtrates of Agrobacterium tumefaciens. Biochem. Biophys. Res. Commun., 76:453–459.
26. Keane, P. J., Kerr, A., and New, P. B. (1970): Crown gall of stone fruit. II. Identification and nomenclature of Agrobacterium isolates. Aust. J. Biol. Sci., 23:585–595.
27. Kemp, J. D. (1977): A new amino acid derivative present in crown gall tumor tissue. Biochem. Biophys. Res. Commun., 74:862–868.
28. Kerr, A. (1974): Soil microbiological studies on Agrobacterium radiobacter and biological control of crown gall. Soil Sci. 118:168–172.
29. Kersters, K., De Ley, J., Sneath, P. H. A., and Sackin, M. (1973): Numerical taxonomic analysis of Agrobacterium. J. Gen. Microbiol., 78:227–239.
30. Lance, C. (1968): Les oxydases terminales des tumeurs vegetales. in: Les Cultures de Tissus de Plantes, pp. 279–289, edited by R. J. Gautheret and L. Hirth. Colloq. Int. Cent. Nat. Rech. Sci., No. 920.
31. Ledeboer, A. M. (1978): Large plasmids in Rhizobiaceae. I. Studies on the transcription of the tumour inducing plasmid from Agrobacterium tumefaciens in sterile crown gall tumour cells. II. Studies on large plasmids in different Rhizobium species. PhD. thesis. University of Leiden.
32. Lipetz, J. (1966): Crown gall tumorigenesis. II. Relations between wound healing and the tumorigenic response. Cancer Res., 26:1597–1605.
33. Lippincott, B. B., and Lippincott, J. A. (1969): Bacterial attachment to a specific wound site as an essential stage in tumor initiation by Agrobacterium tumefaciens. J. Bacteriol., 97:620–628.
34. Lippincott, B. B., Margot, J. B., and Lippincott, J. A. (1977): Plasmid content and tumor initiation complementation by Agrobacterium tumefaciens strain IIBNV6. J. Bacteriol. 132:824–831.
35. Lippincott, B. B., Whatley, M. H., and Lippincott, J. A. (1977): Tumor induction by Agrobacterium involves attachment of the bacterium to a site on the host plant cell wall. Plant Physiol., 59:388–390.

36. Lippincott, J. A., and Lippincott, B. B. (1975): The genus *Agrobacterium* and plant tumorigenesis. *Annu. Rev. Microbiol., 29:*377–405.

37. Lippincott, J. A., and Lippincott, B. B. (1976): Morphogenic determinants as exemplified by the crown-gall disease. in: *Encyclopedia of Plant Physiology,* New Series, Vol. 4, *Physiological Plant Pathology,* pp. 356–388, edited by R. Heitefuss and P. H. Williams. Springer-Verlag, Berlin.

38. Lippincott, J. A., and Lippincott, B. B. (1977): Nature and specificity of the bacterium-host attachment in *Agrobacterium* infection. in: *Cell Wall Biochemistry Related to Specificity in Host-Plant Pathogen Interactions,* p. 439–451, edited by H. Solheim and J. Raa. Norway Universitetsforlaget, Oslo.

39. Lippincott, J. A., and Lippincott, B. B. (1978): Cell Walls of crown-gall tumors and embryonic plant tissues lack *Agrobacterium* adherence sites. *Science,* 199:1075–1078.

40. Lippincott, J. A., and Lippincott, B. B. (1978): Tumor initiation complementation on bean leaves by mixtures of tumorigenic and non-tumorigenic *Agrobacterium rhizogenes. Phytopathology,* 68:365–370.

41. Lippincott, J. A., and Lippincott, B. B. (1978): Crown-gall initiation by mixtures of two avirulent bacteria. *Plant Physiol.,* 61:S72.

42. Lippincott, J. A., Lippincott, B. B., and Starr, M. P. (1980): The genus *Argobacterium.* in: *The Prokaryotes,* edited by M. P. Starr, H. Stolp. H. G. Truper, A. Balows, and H. G. Schlegel. Springer-Verlag, Berlin.

43. Meins, F., Jr. (1971): Regulation of phenotypic expression in crown-gall teratoma tissues of tobacco. *Dev. Biol.,* 24:287–300.

44. Meins, F., Jr. (1974): Mechanisms underlying tumor transformation and tumor reversal in crown-gall, a neoplastic disease of higher plants. in: *Developmental Aspects of Carcinogenesis and Immunity, 32nd Symposium of the Society for Developmental Biology,* pp. 23–39, edited by T. J. King. Academic Press, New York.

45. Meins, F., Jr. (1975): Temperature-sensitive expression of auxin-autotrophy by crown-gall teratoma cells of tobacco. *Planta,* 122:1–9.

46. Meins, F., Jr. and Binns, A. (1977): Epigenetic variation of cultured somatic cells: evidence for gradual changes in the requirement for factors promoting cell division. *Proc. Natl. Acad. Sci. U. S. A.,* 74:2928–2932.

47. Miller, C. O. (1975): Cell-division factors from *Vinca rosea* L. crown gall tumor tissue. *Proc. Natl. Acad. Sci. U. S. A.,* 72:1883–1886.

48. Montoya, A. L., Chilton, M. -D., Gordon, M. P., Sciaky, D., and Nester, E. W. (1977): Octopine and nopaline metabolism in *Agrobacterium tumefaciens* and crown gall tumor cells: role of plasmid genes. *J. Bacteriol.,* 129:101–107.

49. Morris, R. O. (1977): Mass spectroscopic identification of cytokinins: glucosylzeatin and glucosyl ribosylzeatin from *Vinca rosea* crown gall. *Plant Physiol.,* 59:1029–1033.

50. Otten, L. A. B. M., Vreugdenhil, D., and Schilperoort, R. A. (1977): Properties of D(+)-lysopine dehydrogenase from crown gall tumour tissue. *Biochim. Biophys. Acta,* 485:268–277.

51. Panagopoulos, C. G., and Psallidas, P. G. (1973): Characteristics of Greek isolates of *Agrobacterium tumefaciens* (E. F. Smith & Townsend) Conn. *J. Appl. Bacteriol.,* 36:233–240.

52. Pengelly, W., and Meins, F. Jr. (1977): A specific radioimmunoassay for nanogram quantities of the auxin, indole-3-acetic acid. *Planta, 136:*173–180.

53. Peters, K. E., and Lippincott, J. A. (1976): Induction of a tumour growth factor (GABA) by *Agrobacterium* strains and the effect of GABA on crown-gall tumour initiation and growth. *Physiol. Plant Pathol.,* 9:331–338.

54. Peterson, J. B., and Miller, C. O. (1977): Glucosylzeatin and glucosylribosylzeatin from *Vinca rosea* L. crown gall tumor tissue. *Plant Physiol.,* 59:1026–1028.

55. Rodriguez de Lecea, J., de la Rosa, C., and Beltra, R. (1972): Substancias de crecimiento en *Agrobacterium tumefaciens* y en sus formas L fijas: su influencia en la induccion aseptica de tumores. *Phyton (Horn), 29:* 119–126.

56. Schilperoort, R. A., and Bomhoff, G. H. (1975): Crown gall: a model for tumor research and genetic engineering. in: *Genetic Manipulations with Plant Material,* pp. 141–162, edited by L. Ledoux. Plenum Publishing Corp., New York.

57. Schroth, M. N., Weinhold, A. R., McCain, A. H., Hildebrand, D. C., and Ross, N. (1971): Biology and control of *Agrobacterium tumefaciens. Hilgardia,* 40:537–552.

58. Smith, E. F., and Townsend, C. O. (1907): A plant tumor of bacterial origin. *Science,* 25:671–673.

59. Stonier, T., and Yang, H. -M. (1973): Studies on auxin protectors. XI. Inhibition of peroxidase-catalyzed oxidation of glutathione by auxin protectors and O-dihydroxyphenols. *Plant Physiol.,* 51:391–395.

60. Sukanya, N. K., and Viadyanathan, C. S. (1964): Aminotransferases of *Agrobacterium tumefaciens.* Transamination between tryptophan and phenylpyruvate. *Biochem. J.,* 92:594–598.

61. Tempe, J., Petit, A., Holsters, M., Van Montagu, M., and Schell, J. (1977): Thermosensitive step associated with transfer of the Ti plasmid during conjugation: possible relation to transformation in crown gall. *Proc. Natl. Acad. Sci. U. S. A.,* 74:2848–2849.

62. Turgeon, R., Wood, H. N. and Braun, A. C. (1976): Studies on the recovery of crown gall tumor cells. *Proc. Natl. Acad. Sci. U. S. A.,* 73: 3562–3564.

63. Wendt-Gallitelli, M. F., and Dobrigkeit, I. (1973): Investigations implying the invalidity of octopine as a marker for transformation by *Agrobacterium tumefaciens. Z. Naturforsch.,* 28:768–771.

64. Whatley, M. H., Margot, J. B., Schell, J., Lippincott, B. B., and Lippincott, J. A. (1978): Plasmid or chromosomal determination of *Agrobacterium* adherence specificity. *J. Gen. Microbiol.* 107:395–398.

65. White, P. R., and Braun, A. C. (1942): A cancerous neoplasm of plants. Autonomous, bacteria-free crown-gall tissue. *Cancer Res.,* 2:597–617.

66. Wood, H. N. (1967): Plant carcinogenesis. *Prog. Exp. Tumor Res.,* 9:286–311.

67. Wood, H. N., and Braun, A. (1965): Studies on the net uptake of solutes by normal and crown-gall tumor cells. *Proc. Natl. Acad. Sci. U. S. A.,* 54:1532–1538.

52

Molecular Studies on Crown Gall Tumors: Role of Nucleic Acids, of Agrobacterium Tumefaciens Incorporated Into the Crown Gall Cell

Eugene W. Nester

INTRODUCTION

This section of crown gall tumors concerns the evidence that plasmid DNA of *Agrobacterium tumefaciens* is stably incorporated into the plant tumor and transcribed into RNA. It also considers the evidence that the foreign DNA codes for proteins are unique to the plant tumor. Review articles which deal with some of this same material have recently appeared (21, 22).

DETECTION OF PLASMID GENES IN TUMOR DNA

Because the unique characteristics of crown gall tumors are stably inherited, numerous investigators have attempted to identify bacterial or viral nucleic acid as the tumor-inducing principle. Although many reports have appeared purporting to show the presence of both bacterial and viral genes in DNA isolated from the tumors (26, 28, 29, 31), subsequent studies have indicated that all of these data were interpreted incorrectly (5, 9, 27). However, the possibility that a small fragment of bacterial DNA might be

present in sterile tumor callus was revived when Schell and his colleagues (36) reported that all of the oncogenic but none of the nononcogenic strains of *Agrobacterium* that they examined contained large plasmids. Studies in a number of laboratories have convincingly confirmed their conclusions—that a large plasmid is indeed essential for oncogenicity (4, 32, 35). Several laboratories have shown that the molecular basis of crown gall tumor induction is the incorporation of a portion of the plasmid into the plant cell (7, 8, 18).

The most successful approach for detecting foreign DNA in tumor cells in the crown gall system has been to measure the kinetics of reassociation of small amounts of radioactive single-stranded plasmid DNA (probe) in the presence and absence of large amounts of tumor DNA (driver). If plasmid sequences are present in the tumor DNA, then the concentration of probe DNA is raised in the presence of tumor DNA and it will reassociate more rapidly. The kinetics of reassociation depend both on the number of copies of the plasmid sequences and on the fraction of the plasmid which is present in tumor DNA. The kinetics of reassociation of the total plasmid in the presence and absence of tumor DNA are presented in Fig. 52.1 in the form of a P_0t plot (5). There is a slight but detectable

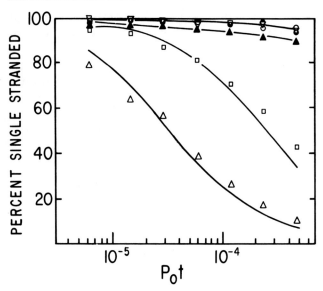

Figure 52.1. Renaturation kinetics of *Agrobacterium tumefaciens* A277 plasmid DNA in the presence of tumor DNA and control DNAs. ^{32}P-labeled plasmid DNA (33×10^6 cpm/μg, 9×10^{-4} μg/ml) was allowed to reassociate in the presence of the following sheared DNA samples: (○) 2.2 mg/ml salmon DNA; (●) 1.9 mg/ml tobacco normal callus DNA; (▲) 2.3 mg/ml crown gall tumor E9 DNA; (▽) DNAase-treated crown gall tumor E9 DNA (originally 2.3 mg/ml); (□) 1.9 mg/ml salmon DNA + 0.038 μg/ml A277 plasmid DNA (0.8 copy model); and (△) 2.3 mg/ml salmon DNA + 0.46 μg/ml A277 plasmid DNA (10 copy model). Ideal second-order reaction curves are drawn for the two reconstruction reactions only. P_0t is in units of moles of nucleotide · liter^{-1} · sec.

increase in the rate of reassociation of single-stranded plasmid DNA in the presence of tumor DNA. This shift is not observed when the probe DNA is incubated with either salmon DNA or DNA isolated from normal callus. Significantly, if the tumor DNA is incubated with DNase prior to incubation with the probe, the rate increase is abolished. These experiments strongly suggest that plasmid DNA is present in the tumor. The most reasonable interpretation for only a slight increase in the rate of reassociation is that only a small fragment (less than 10%) of the total plasmid (120×10^6 daltons) is present in the tumor.

In order to identify the fragment of plasmid DNA present in the tumor, the Seattle investigators cleaved the radioactive plasmid with the restriction endonuclease SMA I and separated the resulting 24 fragments by electrophoresis on agarose gels. Each DNA band was then eluted from the gel, denatured and its kinetics of reassociation followed in the presence and absence of tumor DNA. The rates of reassociation of DNA bands 1 and 2 were not accelerated in the presence of tumor DNA, but the single-stranded DNA of band 3 reassociated significantly more rapidly in the presence of tumor DNA (Fig. 52.2). An analysis of the data suggested that only about 40% of the DNA of band 3 was present, about 4×10^6 daltons of DNA. Further, from the rate of reassociation, these authors concluded that 10–40 copies of this fragment are present. These same investigators presented evidence that DNA from band 10 is also present in the tumor. The amount of DNA from this source was judged to be 2.3×10^6 daltons.

TRANSCRIPTION OF PLASMID DNA SEQUENCES IN TUMOR

The Seattle investigators also reported that they could detect RNA transcripts of at least some of the plasmid DNA in the tumor. To detect these transcripts, ^{32}P-pulse-labeled RNA was isolated from tumor and normal tobacco callus tissues. Plasmid was isolated from the bacteria, fragmented with the restriction enzyme, SMA I and the resulting fragments were separated by electrophoresis on an agarose gel. The DNA bands were then denatured and transferred by "blotting" to a strip of nitrocellulose (30). The position of the bands on the nitrocellulose are identical to their position on the agarose. The ^{32}P-labeled RNA was then incubated with the nitrocellulose strips and autoradiograms prepared. The DNA corresponding to band 3 but not band 10 hybridized indicating that RNA transcripts of this DNA fragment were present in the tumor (10). It is not clear whether the DNA of band 10 is not transcribed at all in the tumor or the transcripts are in too low a concentration to be detected. When similar experiments were done using [^{32}P]RNA isolated from normal callus, none of the DNA bands of the plasmid hybridized to the tumor RNA. These experiments demonstrate in a convincing fashion that at least some of the plasmid DNA in the tumor is transcribed. They also confirm, by an independent approach, that a small fragment of the plasmid is present in the tumor.

POSSIBLE EXPRESSION OF PLASMID DNA SEQUENCES IN TUMOR

Before there was any physical evidence for the presence of bacterial DNA in crown gall tumors, Morel and his associates (12) obtained biological data which they suggested could be most readily interpreted by assuming that tumors contained bacterial DNA. These investigators isolated and identified two unusual amino acids from crown gall tumors that are not present in the uninfected plant (12, 13). These compounds, octopine and nopaline, are formed by the condensation of arginine with pyruvate and arginine with α-ketoglutarate, respectively. (Fig. 52.2) Tumors contain either octopine or nopaline but never both compounds (3, 12, 20, 25). Some tumors contain neither (20, 25). Several additional unusual amino acids, all derivatives of basic amino acids, have been shown to be present in tumor tissue. These include histopine, lysopine, and octopinic acid. (1, 15, 19). Two enzymes appear to be responsible for the synthesis of these compounds; one enzyme, octopine dehydrogenase, has been partially purified and catalyzes the synthesis of octopine, octopinic acid, histopine, and lysopine (15, 23). The other enzyme, nopaline dehydrogenase, catalyzes the synthesis of nopaline (13). This enzyme has also been partially purified from tumor tissue (11). Neither enzyme activity has been demonstrated in the plant prior to infection (2, 11, 14, 16).

Morel's group (12, 13) also demonstrated that *Agrobacterium* has the ability to degrade either octopine or nopaline (rarely both) and, more recently, it was shown that the vast majority of virulent strains degrade either octopine or nopaline (17). This degradation results initially in the formation of arginine and pyruvate, in the case of octopine and arginine, and α-ketoglutaric acid in the case of nopaline. Arginine can be further metabolized through the action of arginase to yield ornithine and urea which, in turn, can be metabolized to provide a source of carbon and nitrogen to the cell. The initial step in the degradation of octopine and nopaline requires a permease specific for octopine or nopaline as well as octopine or nopaline oxidase. Both activities are inducible by either octopine or nopaline, respectively. Nopaline oxidase can degrade octopine, although octopine cannot induce its synthesis (24). Morel and his colleagues (12, 13) were the first to draw attention to a relationship between the degradation of these unusual amino acids by agrobacteria and their synthesis by the tumors induced by these bacteria. Strains of *Agrobacterium* that degrade octopine induce tumors that synthesize octopine and strains that degrade nopaline induce tumors that synthesize nopaline (25). One exception to this correlation is that a few bacterial strains that degrade nopaline induce tumors that synthesize neither octopine nor nopaline. The few strains that degrade neither octopine nor nopaline induce tumors that synthesize neither octopine nor nopaline. Based on this correlation, Morel and colleagues (25) proposed that the gene coding for octopine/nopaline oxidase in the bacteria was transferred to the plant, where it functioned in the opposite direction (octopine/nopaline dehydrogenase). This notion seemed reasonable in view of the fact that the enzyme catalyzing the synthesis and degradation of octopine in the octopus has been highly purified and has been shown to be a single enzyme, having a pH optimum of approximately 6.6 for the biosynthetic reaction and 9.8 for the degradation reaction (33). However, in the crown gall tumor, present evidence suggests that the enzyme responsible for degradation in the bacteria is not the same enzyme that catalyzes the synthesis. Unfortunately, only the biosynthetic enzyme has been purified to a significant extent so a comparison of the properties of the oxidase and dehydrogenase are not totally convincing. However, it appears that the oxidase enzymes are membrane bound and have no cofactor requirement, whereas the dehydrogenase activities are soluble and require NADPH (2). Further, the nopaline oxidase of bacteria can degrade both octopine and nopaline whereas nopaline dehydrogenase does not catalyze the synthesis of octopine (11).

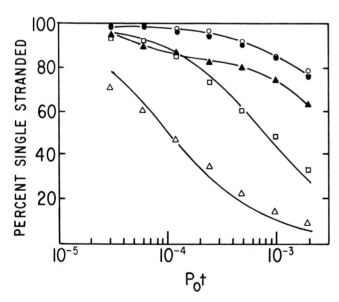

Figure 52.2 Renaturation kinetics of *Agrobacterium tumefaciens* plasmid Sma 1 digest band 3 DNA in the presence of tumor DNA and control DNAs. ^{32}P-labeled DNA (8.2×10^6 cpm/μg, 3.7×10^{-3} μg/ml) was allowed to reassociate in the presence of various sheared DNA samples. Details and symbols are exactly as for Figure 52.1.

Genetic analyses also suggest that the degradative ability of the bacteria and the biosynthetic activity of the tumor do not reside on a single protein. Bacterial mutants which cannot degrade octopine or nopaline still induce tumors which synthesize the same amounts of octopine or nopaline as the parental strains (3, 20 and J. Tempe, personal communication). These latter experiments cannot rule out the possibility that the biosynthetic reaction, which has not been demonstrated in either the bacteria or the uninfected plant, may result from the interaction of protein subunits from the bacterium and the plant. The bacterium may contribute the subunit responsible for the specificity of the amino acid synthesized and the plant may contribute the catalytic subunit.

The mechanism by which the specificity of octopine and nopaline synthesis is determined remains one of the most provocative mysteries in crown gall tumor research. At this time, it is only possible to state with absolute certainty that the specificity is determined by the Ti plasmid. The curing of an oncogenic strain of its virulence-associated plasmid results in the strain not only losing its ability to induce tumors but also its ability to degrade the unusual amino acid (32, 35). The transfer of the virulence-associated plasmid into this cured strain results in its re gaining tumor inducing ability, as well as its ability to both degrade and induce tumors which synthesize the same amino acid as the strain from which the plasmid was derived (6, 35). Another line of evidence that emphasizes the importance of the plasmid has been uncovered by studying strains of *Agrobacterium* which can utilize both octopine and nopaline. Eight such strains induce tumors that synthesize only nopaline. When plasmid from any of these strains is transferred to a plasmidless recipient strain, the latter strains induce tumors that synthesize nopaline but never octopine. From these data, it appears that only the utilization of nopaline is coded by the plasmid and only nopaline is synthesized by the tumor. These observations rule out the possibility that some intermediates in the degradation of octopine activate a plant gene to synthesize octopine. Rather, it emphasizes that the information for synthesis of the unusual amino acid by the plant must be coded by a plasmid gene.

SUMMARY

The information presented in this review makes clear that the stable incorporation of a fragment of a bacterial plasmid is the molecular basis of crown gall tumor induction. There is solid evidence that at least part of this foreign DNA is transcribed into RNA. However, the data are not compelling enough to conclude that some of the transcribed DNA is translated into octopine dehydrogenase or nopaline dehydrogenase. The data reveal just how similar plant and animal tumors actually are when viewed at the molecular level. These observations raise a number of obvious questions which, when answered, will provide considerably more insight into how the foreign DNA functions in transforming plant cells. Where are the plasmid sequences located in the plant cell? Are they covalently integrated into plant DNA? Do all tumors contain the same foreign DNA? What is the basis for the difference between disorganized tumors and teratomas? Is the transformation a result of the site at which the foreign DNA is located, a result of the protein product of the incorporated genes, or a combination of both? Fortunately, the technology of molecular biology has advanced to the stage that these questions are amenable to answeriing.

References

1. Bieman, K., Lioret, C., Asselineau, K., Lederer, E., and Polonski, J. (1960): Sur la structure chimique de la lysopine nouvel acide amine[1] isole de tissue de crown gall. *Bull. Soc. Chim. Biol.*, 42:979.
2. Bomhoff, G. H. (1974): Studies on crown gall—a plant tumor. Ph. D thesis. University of Leyden, Leyden, The Netherlands.
3. Bomhoff, G. H., Klapwijk, P. M., Kester, H. C. M., Schilperoort, R. A., Hernalsteens, J. P., and Schell, J. (1976): Octopine and nopaline synthesis and breakdown genetically controlled by a plasmid of *Agrobacterium tumefaciens*. *Mol. Gen. Genet.*, 145:177-181.
4. Chilton, M.-D., Currier, T. C., Farrand, S. K., Bendich, A. J., Gordon, M. P., and Nester, E. W. (1974): Is there foreign DNA in crown gall tumor DNA? in: *Second Annual John Innes Symposium: Modification of the Information Content of Plant Cells*, pp. 297-311, edited by R. Markham, D. R. Davies, D. A. Hopwood, and P. W. Horne, North-Holland Publishing Co., Amsterdam.
5. Chilton, M.-D., Currier, T. C., Farrand, S. K., Bendich, A. J., Gordon, M. P., and Nester, E. W. (1974): *Agrobacterium tumefaciens* DNA and PS8 bacteriaphage DNA not detected in crown gall tumors. *Proc. Natl. Acad. Sci. U. S. A.*, 71:3672-3676.
6. Chilton, M.-D., Farrand, S. K., Levin, R., and Nester, E. W. (1976): RP4 promotion of transfer of a large *Agrobacterium* plasmid which confers virulence. *Genetics*, 83:609-618.
7. Chilton, M.-D., Drummond, M. H., Merlo, D. H., Sciaky, D., Montoya, A. L., Gordon, M. P., and Nester, E. W. (1977): Stable incorporation of plasmid DNA into higher plant cells: the molecular basis of crown gall tumorigenesis. *Cell*, 11:263-271.
8. Chilton, M.-D., Drummond, M. H., Gordon, M. P., Merlo, D. J., Montoya, A. L., Sciaky, D., Nutter, R., and Nester, E. W. (1978): Foreign genes of plasmid origin detected in crown gall tumor. in: *Microbiology* pp. 136-138, edited by D. Schlesinger American. Society. for Microbiology., Washington, D. C.
9. Drlica, K. A., and Kado, C. I. (1974): Quantitative estimation of *Agrobacterium tumefaciens* DNA in crown gall tumor cells. *Proc. Natl. Acad. Sci. U. S. A.*, 71:3677-3681.
10. Drummond, M. H., Gordon, M. P., Nester, E. W., and Chilton, M.-D. (1977): Foreign DNA of bacterial plasmid origin is transcribed in crown gall tumors. *Nature*, 269:535-536.
11. Goldman, A. (1977): Octopine and Nopaline dehydrogenases in crown gall tumors. *Plant Sci. Lett.*, 10:49-58.
12. Goldman, A., Tempe, J., and Morel, G. (1968): Quelques particularites de diverse souches d'*Agrobacterium tumefaciens*. *C. R. Soc. Biol. (Paris)*, 162:630-631.
13. Goldman, A., Thomas, D. W., and Morel, G. (1969): Sur la structure de la nopaline, metabolite anormale de certaines tumeurs de crown gall. *C. R. Acad. Sci. (D) (Paris)*, 268:852-854.

14. Gordon, M. P., Farrand, S. K., Sciaky, D., Montoya, A. L., Chilton, M.-D., Merlo, D. J., and Nester, E. W. (1979): The crown gall problem. in: *A Symposium on the Molecular Biology of Plants*, pp. 291–331, edited by I. Rubenstein, University of Minneapolis Press, Minneapolis.

15. Hack, E., and Kemp, J. D. (1977): A new amino acid derivative present in crown gall tumor tissue. *Biochem. Biophys. Res. Commun.*, 78:785–791.

16. Kemp, J. D. (1976): Octopine as a marker for the induction of tumorous growth by *Agrobacterium tumefaciens* strain B₆. *Biochem. Biophys. Res. Commun.*, 69:816–822.

17. Lippincott, J. A., Beiderbeck, R., and Lippincott, B. B. (1973): Utilization of octopine and nopaline by Agrobacterium. *J. Bacteriol.*, 116:378–383.

18. Matthysse, A. G. (1977): Variations in plasmid DNA sequences present in crown gall tumour lines. *J. Gen. Microbiol.*, 102:402–430.

19. Menage, A., and Morel, G. (1965): Sur la presence d'octopine dans les tissus de crown gall. *C. R. Acad. Sci. (D) (Paris)*, 261:2001.

20. Montoya, A. L., Chilton, M.-D., Gordon, M. P., Sciaky, D., and Nester, E. E. (1977): Octopine and nopaline metabolism in *Agrobacterium tumefaciens* and crown gall tumor cells: role of plasmid genes. *J. Bacteriol.*, 129:101–107.

21. Nester, E. W., Chilton, M.-D., Drummond, M., Merlo, D., Montoya, A., Sciaky, D., and Gordon, M. P. (1977): Search for bacterial DNA in crown gall tumors, in: *Recombinant Molecules: Impact on Science and Society*, pp. 179–188, edited by R. F. Beers, Jr. and Bassett, E. G. Raven Press, New York.

22. Nester, E. W., Merlo, D. J., Drummond, M. H., Sciaky, D., Montoya, A. L., and Chilton, M.-D. (1977): The incorporation and expression of *Agrobacterium* plasmid in genes in crown gall tumors, in: *Genetic Engineering for Nitrogen Fixation*, pp. 181–196, edited by A. Hollander, R. H. Burris, P. R. Day, R. W. Hardy, D. R. Helinski, M. R. Lamborg, L. Owens, and R. C. Valentine. Plenum Press, New York.

23. Otten, L., Vreugdenhil, A. B. M., and Schilperoort, R. A. (1977): Properties of D(+)-lysopine dehydrogenase from crown gall tumor tissue. *Biochim. Biophys. Acta*, 485:268–277.

24. Petit, A., and Tempe, J. (1976): Étude du metabolisme de l'un de ses analogues par l'*Agrobacterium tumefaciens*. *C. R. Acad. Sci. (D) (Paris)*, 282:69–71.

25. Petit, A., Delhaye, S., Tempe, J., and Morel, G. (1970): Recherches sur les guanidines des tissus de crown gall. Mise en evidence d'une relation biochimique specifique entre les soucles d'*Agrobacterium tumefaciens* et les tumeurs qu'elles induisent. *Physiol. Veg.*, 8:205–213.

26. Quetier, F., Huguet, T., and Guille, E. (1969): Induction of crown gall; partial homology between tumor cell DNA, bacterial DNA and the GC rich DNA of stressed normal cells. *Biochem. Biophys. Res. Commun.*, 34:128–133.

27. Schilperoort, R. A., Dons, J. J. M., and Ras, H. (1975): Characterization of the complex formed between PS8 cRNA and DNA isolated from A6-induced sterile crown gall tissue, in: *Second Annual John Innes Symposium*, pp. 253–286, edited by R. Markham, D. R. Davies, D. A. Hopwood, and R. W. Hoyne, North Holland Publishing Co., Amsterdam.

28. Schilperoort, R. A., Van Sittert, N. J., and Schell, J. (1973): The presence of both phage PS8 and *Agrobacterium tumefaciens* A6 DNA base sequences in A6-induced sterile crown gall tissue cultured in vitro. *Eur. J. Biochem.*, 33:1–7.

29. Schilperoort, R. A., Veldstra, H., Warnaar, S. O., Mulder, G., and Cohen, J. A. (1967): Formation of complexes between DNA isolated from tobacco crown gall tumors and RNA complementary to *Agrobacterium tumefaciens* DNA. *Biochim. Biophys. Acta*, 145:523–525.

30. Southern, E. M. (1975): Detection of specific sequences among DNA fragments separated by gel electrophoresis. *J. Mol. Biol.*, 98:503–517.

31. Srivastava, B. I. S. (1970): DNA-DNA hybridization studies between bacterial DNA, crown gall tumor cell DNA and the normal cell DNA. *Life Sci.*, 9:889–892.

32. Van Larebeke, N., Engler, G., Holsters, M., Van den Elsaker, S., Zaenen, I., Schilperoort, R. A., and Schell, J. (1974): Large plasmid in *Agrobacterium tumefaciens* essential for crown gall-inducing activity. *Nature*, 252:169–170.

33. Van Thoai, N., Hac, C., Pho, D. B., and Olowacki, A. (1969): Octopine dehydrogenase purification et propertietes catalytiques. *Biochim. Biophys. Acta*, 191:46–57.

34. Veldstra, H. (1972): Plant tumors and crown gall, an analysis of autonomous growth, in: *Proceedings of the Third International Conference on Plant Pathogens*, pp. 213–222, edited by H. Geesteranus, University of Toronto Press, Toronto.

35. Watson, B., Currier, T. C., Gordon, M. P., Chilton, M.-D., and Nester, E. W. (1975): Plasmid required for virulence of *Agrobacterium tumefaciens*. *J. Bacteriol.*, 123:255–264.

36. Zaenen, I., Van Larebeke, N., Teuchy, H., Van Montagu, M., and Schell, J. (1974): Supercoiled circular DNA in crown-gall inducing *Agrobacterium* strains. *J. Mol. Biol.*, 86:109–127.

VII

Conclusions

53

Conclusions and Future Progress Concerning Comparative Oncology

Hans E. Kaiser

Abnormal growth is manifested in many different forms such as those with which we are familiar from teratology, from the hypertrophies, the hyperplasias and last, but not least, from the neoplasms, to mention only the most conspicuous examples. The granulation tissues immediately come to mind. In this connection, we should recall the decentralization of fossil organisms that lead to extinction on the one hand and, on the other, anomalies, existing for millions of years, as the nucleic anomalies of the protista, neoplastic cell accumulations, and other similar developments.

Abnormal growth may derive from each state of normal growth. It is, therefore, a biological phenomenon. In its phylogenetic development, the process of abnormal growth evidences a step-by-step acquisition of the characteristics of neoplastic growth.

A number of years ago, the opinion prevailed that the first appearance of neoplasms in the cancerous growth occurred in the fishes. Today, it is accepted that not only abnormal growth but also true neoplasms may develop additionally from the true tissues of invertebrate eumetazoans as well as from the tissues of vascular plants. It is self-evident that the neoplasms of man, vertebrates, invertebrates, and plants exhibit not only characteristics common to all but also those that are species-specific. This holds true of neoplasms of more limited categories, such as the tumors of vertebrates.

The principle of classification of neoplastic growth is derived from a deeper understanding of the development of the normal tissues of the organisms. Given such an understanding, the working principle of histogenesis can be applied to the task of placing neoplasms of similar host tissues but of different species upon a comparable base. It should be borne in mind that the same viewpoint is applicable to comparable groups of tissues in both kingdoms, such as, for example, the covering membranes.

Aside from this finding, each classification of tumor growth should originate from human neoplasms as those composing the best understood, most highly developed, forms of neoplastic growth. Histologically, they are precisely defined. It is thus essential that these human neoplasms be compared to animal and plant neoplasms on the basis of the principle of histogenesis. Common factors already previously indicated are: limited and unlimited growth, infiltrative growth, transplantability, inferiority of the neoplastic tissue in comparison with the parent tissue, and an increased growth rate, among others.

The phylogenetic elements of neoplastic growth have been accomplished along convergent lines in different states. As of today, however, only a parallelism of the following categories involving man, animals, and plants has been demonstrated.

1. Nonhistological anomalies
    a. In ascending development trend
        1) Anomalies of procaryotic cells
        2) Nucleic anomalies of eucaryotic unicellular organisms
        3) Abnormalities of the growth of plant thalli (algae)
    b. As a tissue-like persistence at the cellular condition can be considered
        1) The experimentally produced, pure, cellular ascites tumor
        2) Leukemias of man and animals
        3) Certain neoplasms of highly developed animals,

849

including man, deriving from cells such as the spindle- and round-cell sarcomas.

2. Neoplasms assigned to the tissues of animal, plant and man with a differing degree of differentiation and malignancy: neoplasms in the stricter sense of the word.

The phylogenetic appearance of certain neoplasms can be held to be either possible or impossible in conformation with the given character of the tissue. The rhabdomyomas or chordomas provide examples. Comparison of the parent tissues must be considered as the basis of a theoretical indication of direction of development.

There exists species specific, morphologically ascertainable, differences in the spontaneous or experimental reaction to certain cancer-causing compounds ("carcinogens"). These species-specific variations can be demonstrated through biochemical or biophysical investigations. The different pathways taken by carcinogenic factors, can be recognized in species-specific experiments and later checked in human organ culture.

Contributions of comparative pathology of abnormal growth to the practical control of cancer and other neoplasms are to be found in:

1. Epidemiologic studies and, especially, experimental studies with animals closely associated with man, such as dogs, may point the way toward model experiments.

2. Due to the fact that the reactions toward the seven groups of neoplastic growth (chemicals, radioactive emissions, physical agents, viruses, genes, bacteria, and parasites) can be more easily studied in different species, comparative oncology offers important

Table 53.1
Basic Conclusions

Topics	Fields Where Major Contributions to Cancer Treatment May Arise[a]
Basic aspects	Understanding of chemical pathways of neoplastic metabolism, including histogenesis and whole body metabolism of cancer patient (background for information about principles of metastatic growth and cachexia)
Prevention of neoplastic development	Preservation of a healthy environment
	Comparative epidemiology for environmental evaluation.
	Comparative toxicology.
Treatment of existing neoplasms and prevention of metastatic growth and cachexia	Destruction of primary tumor with gaining increase immunity
	Immunology
	Chronooncology
	Preoperative prevention and postoperative treatment of metastatic growth
	Preoperative prevention and postoperative treatment of cachexia

[a] Personal opinion of H. E. Kaiser.

advantages to an understanding of human neoplasms. In the foreground of interest stand two points of view

a. The variable pathways of chemical carcinogens from the human environment can be checked and, in their variability, understood in different species

b. From the knowledge of these pathways, it should be possible to gain a better understanding of the species-specific immunologic defense

It may be stated with some assurance, that no living organism exists for which the factors of abnormal growth cannot be identified.

The fields of expected special progress are summarized in Table 53.1.

54

Appendix I: Use of Model Microcosmos in Simulating the Role of the Environment in Comparative Experimental Oncology

A. V. Arstila and Hans E. Kaiser

Many carcinogenic hazards in the environment are dependent upon complex chain and metabolic reactions at the various trophy levels. Noncarcinogenic compounds such as pesticides or herbicides may, therefore, via such reactions and interactions, be transformed to carcinogens in various animal species including fish, mammals, and ultimately man. The elucidation of such pathways is extremely difficult since the same carcinogen may not affect in the same way all species due to the pronounced differences in cellular detoxication mechanisms. Such species-specific differences in the carcinogenic effects of many environmental chemicals and residues are well known.

As set forth earlier in this volume in the investigation of the possible carcinogenic effect of a compound on animals, a variety of species should, therefore, be tested. Because of the enormous task of doing such studies, the animal species are, however, limited to one or two laboratory animals such as rat or mouse. In case of very important compounds, these studies may also include tests with larger animals such as a dog or a miniature swine.

In recent years, the need to simulate natural ecosystems has led to a rapid development in the field of model ecosystem and microcosmos studies. To a certain extent, such systems have been used to develop mathematical models to explain dynamics in the biomagnification and biodegradation of foreign compounds. Such model microcosmoses are usually based on terrestrial, aquatic, or combined aquatic-terrestrial aquariums, in which the major trophy levels are represented. For instance, in aquatic models, various species of plankton, water plants, *Daphnia*, molluscs, and one or two types of small fish may be included. The water supply may be closed or based on continuous flow of fresh water into the model.

Since such models are usually based on dynamic equilibrium between the various trophy levels, such models may last for several months and therefore allow testing of the effects of chemical compounds for long periods of time. These models offer also excellent possibilities for subchronic and chronic toxicity tests since the bioavailability of the foreign compounds are much more similar than in typical animal feeding studies and since many species can be studied at the same time. Although such microcosmos models so far have not been studied from the point of chemical carcinogenesis they may, in the future, give much better insight on the possibilities of environmental carcinogenicity of various chemicals than the present systems based on one or two animal species.

55

Appendix II: Cancer Information Sources

Constantine J. Gillespie

Research in the field of cancer[1] is being conducted by many investigators in all parts of the world. Interest in cancer, other neoplasms and abnormal growth is not limited to just research in humans and higher animals, but also to neoplasms in lower animal forms and plants. Data gathered on invertebrate neoplasms, plant tumors, and other forms of abnormal growth may well reveal areas of vital relevance to cancers and neoplastic growth in higher animal life. This research, naturally, is generating vast amounts of literature in the form of journal articles, monographs, conference proceedings, and symposia. Researchers and other investigators must be aware of the sources where this cancer and cancer-related data can be found and they must be especially aware of those sources which are the best to consult for retrieving data in specific areas of oncology.

The first source of cancer data that should be considered is the International Cancer Research Data Bank (ICRDB) of the National Cancer Institute. The ICRDB program was developed in response to a congressinal directive which states that the National Cancer institute shall:

"Collect, analyze, and disseminate all data useful in the prevention, diagnosis, and treatment of cancer, including the establishment of an international cancer research data bank to collect, catalog, store, and disseminate, insofar as feasible, the results of cancer research undertaken in any country for the use of any person involved in cancer research in any country."

In August 1977, the ICRDB released a publication entitled *Directory of Cancer Research Infor-mation Resources* which is an extremely valuable tool for identifying publications and services related to cancer research. The *Directory* has 12 sections listing the following: (a) primary publications which contain original research papers or reviews; (b) secondary publications which contain abstracts, bibliographies, or indexes to the literature; (c) selected classification schemes for cancer and general medicine, and for various biomedical information systems. It also contains sections for the following cancer-related services: (d) libraries which contain books, primary journals and other sources of cancer information; (e) special collections of unique oncological materials; (f) computer-based cancer information services; (g) audio-visual information services; (h) dial-access services which disseminate cancer information via telephone lines to health science professionals; (i) cancer registries; (j) sources of information on cancer research projects undertaken in many countries of the world; (k) organizations that sponsor professional meetings or symposia that relate to cancer or provide funding for research in the form of fellowships, grants, scholarships, assistantships, travel grants, etc.; and (l) listings of national Institutes of Health programs, publications, and services related to cancer.

There are many computerized data bases that contain information on cancer. While some of these data bases deal with cancer exclusively, others cover all areas of biology or biomedicine.

The National Library of Medicine's MEDLINE (for *MEDLARS On-Line*) data bases are the largest single sources of citations that deal with the entire field of cancer. The four MEDLINE files (each covering a 3-year period) are not exclusively cancer, but do contain a total of

---

[1] In the sense of cancer, other neoplasms and related disorders of abnormal growth.

346,831 cancer citations out of a total file size of 3,346,831 citations, as indicated Table 1.

These files are searchable by means of the controlled vocabulary, called *Medical Subject Headings* (MeSH), developed by the National Library of Medicine, or by means of free text searching on significant words in the titles or abstracts of articles that are cited in the files. The controlled vocabulary provides exact and rapid searching of well known concepts while free text searching adds a very useful dimension because any new concept that is desired can be searched easily just as soon as it is used in the published literature. In addition to original journal articles, selected monographs, published proceedings of various congresses and symposia, and multiauthored works are included in the MEDLINE data bases.

The published equivalents of the MEDLINE data bases are the monthly *Index Medicus* and the annual *Cumulated Index Medicus*. The same MeSH vocabulary used in computerized searching is used in finding citations on cancer subjects in these printed indexes. Of course, a large number of citations on cancer topics can be found in the printed indexes without the need to resort to computerized searching; it is when complex and multiple interactions between subject concepts exist that computerized searching is most valuable and timesaving.

Index Medicus and the MEDLINE files deal with cancer subjects mostly in relation to human and experimental medicine. There are some citations that deal with cancers in nonvertebrates, but this is far from comprehensive coverage. Citations on plant tumors will be found very rarely, if at all, in the MEDLINE files since agricultural topics are mostly out of scope for these publications and data bases.

The CANCERLIT file (formerly called CANCERLINE) contains more than 230,000 abstracts from January 1963 through 1980. The file was developed by the ICRDB and is operated and maintained by the National Library of Medicine through its MEDLINE family of on-line data bases. About 75% of the CANCERLIT abstracts appeared in a series of secondary sources: Carcinogenesis Abstracts (from 1963), and Cancer Chemotherapy Abstracts (from 1967) and expanded to Cancer Therapy Abstracts in 1974. Both of these sources were discontinued in 1979. All of these abstracts are directly related to cancer subjects and are searched on-line by a free text vocabulary based on the significant words in the titles and abstracts of the articles. A useful feature of this data base is the presence of abstracts for all entries in the data base and the ability to print them out in full, if desired. The file has been updated with approximately 25,000 abstracts annually, although in the past year more than 42,000 new abstracts were added to the file to bring it up to its present size.

Another file offered by the ICRDB is the CANCERPROJ (for *Cancer Projects*) file, which contains descriptions of ongoing cancer research projects in the United States as well as in other countries. The size of the file varies from about 16,000 to 20,000 reports and will always be limited to just the two most recent years. As of 1980, the file contains about 18,000 reports. The data for this file are provided by the Science Information Exchange of the National Technical Information Service and consists of the following information: supporting agency name and identification number, location where research is being performed, funding period, index terms, type of award, names of investigators, and a description of the project. This file, too, is searchable at any location where MEDLINE service is available.

The publications and services of the Biosciences Information Service of Biological Abstracts (BIOSIS) should be used in finding information on cancers in all animal species, especially nonvertebrates, and in plants. BIOSIS covers the complete range of the biological literature with 245,000 articles indexed or abstracted annually. *Biological Abstracts* provides 140,000 abstracts annually while *BioResearch Index* provides indexes only to an additional 105,000 articles annually. Keyword-in-context (KWIC) indexes based on the significant words in article titles, CROSS Codes (for broad subject concepts), Biosystematic Codes (for broad taxonomic categories), author indexes, and genus-species name indexes are provided for both publications and give multiple means of accessing the specific kinds of information needed.

BIOSIS also provides a computerized data base, called BIOSIS Previews, which is split into two parts: Citations for 1969–1973, and 1974–

Table 1
Cancer Citations in Medline Files[a]

Time Period	Total Citations	Cancer Citations	Percentage
1966–1968	545,463	48,629	8.92
1969–1971	649,346	65,614	10.10
1972–1974	671,116	69,588	10.37
1975–1980	1,495,476	163,000	10.90
TOTALS	3,361,401	346,831	10.32

[a] As of November 1, 1980.

1980. There are no abstracts contained in BIOSIS Previews and the file is searched using the same types of index entries that appear in the published volumes of *Biological Abstracts* and *BioResearch Index*. The BIOSIS Previews file contains cancer citations that cover all areas of biology, including invetebrate cancers and plant tumors. The *BIOSIS Search Guide*, published in 1977, is an extremely useful tool for formulating searches of the BIOSIS Previews file. The Master Index of this *Guide* lists approximately 9,200 words or concepts in the field of biology and displays for each one information regarding how that concept is searchable in BIOSIS Previews. Various cancer terms are listed in the Master Index and it will give an indication of the concepts that should be considered in formulating a search. The Master Index gives approximate total frequency counts or postings counts for each word or stem word based on the BIOSIS Previews file for 1974–1980. The listing below gives the postings counts for various keywords (the asterisk * represents a truncation symbol and the postings count is for any string of characters beginning with those given and for the CROSS Codes covering the topics Neoplasms and Neoplastic Agents.

Cancer Keywords in BIOSIS Previews and Their Postings Counts

Cancer*	22,779
Carcinoma*	24,658
Neoplasia*	1,003
Neoplasm*	2,398
Neoplastic*	14,840
Oncogen*	1,030
Oncology*	616
Tumor*	38,705
Tumorigen*	1

Postings Counts for Entries under CROSS Codes for Neoplasms and Neoplastic Agents

Biochemistry	41,183
Blood and Reticuloendothelial Neoplasms	36,524
Carcinogens and Carinogenesis	53,656
Diagnostic Methods	26,836
General	2,260
Immunology	29,109
Neoplastic Cell Lines	36,776
Pathology; Clinical Aspects; Systemic Effects	27,281
Therapeutic Agents; Therapy	56,144

These postings are given here only to give an indication of the range of cancer topics that can be searched in BIOSIS Previews and to show the extensive number of potential citations. Since BIOSIS Previews is a coordinate searching system, these keywords or CROSS Codes would be ANDED with special animal or plant names or other pertinent concepts to narrow the retrieval down to a reasonable number of citations that would be relevant to the individual's area of exact interest.

The plant literature is covered very extensively by the BIOSIS publications, and services and information on plant tumors can be found in these sources. However, another source for information on plant tumors is the *Bibliography of Agriculture*, published each month by Oryx Press of Phoenix, Ariz. from bibliographic data provided by the National Agricultural Library in Beltsville, Md. The National Agricultural Library also provides this data in a computerized file of over 1 million items, called AGRICOLA, that offers on-line access to the worldwide journal and monographic literature on agriculture and related subjects from 1970 to the present time. AGRICOLA is a natural-language searching system based on keywords in the titles of articles.

Finally, mention should be made of two additional sources of cancer information that should be considered by researchers.

Excerpta Medica abstracts more than 3500 worldwide biomedical journals and publishes these abstracts in some 47 different subject-oriented sections. All of the cancer-related abstracts are brought together and published in a separate cancer section of *Excerpta Medica* comprising 30 issues per year. Indexes to these abstracts are provided in each issue and every 10th issue of the journal provides cumulative indexes which make it easier to locate a large number of pertinent abstracts.

The Oak Ridge National Laboratory in Oak Ridge, Tenn. established the Environmental Mutagen Information Center (EMIC) as a means of gathering the worldwide literature on this subject. Mutagenesis information is an important part of research programs directed toward understanding the mechanisms of carcinogenicity. EMIC has created a computerized file of this data which is one of the component files of the National Library of Medicine's TOXLINE data base. TOXLINE contains two EMIC files: the most recent containing 28,257 records for the time period 1971 through October 1980, and the earlier file containing 5,765 records for the years 1968–1970. These files are searchable using an open-ended free text vocabulary.

A short, very useful summary of basic neoplastic literature, *Neoplasia—A Guide to Sources of Information* by Ione Auston, Reference Section, National Library of Medicine, Bethesda, Maryland, 1980 (27 pp.), lists major sources available at that library.

In summary, the publications, computerized data bases, and specialized information sources reviewed here indicate the many sources that are available for gathering cancer information. There are some other sources beyond those listed here, for example, *Chemical Abstracts* which may be useful in searching for carcinogenic chemicals but, for the most part, those listed here represent the major sources which have been found to provide the greatest value.

GLOSSARY

I. SCOPE OF FIELDS IMPORTANT TO COMPARATIVE ONCOLOGY

Anthropology—Study of the interrelationships of biological, cultural, geographical, and historical aspects of the human race

Bacteriology—Study and science of bacteria; a specialized branch of microbiology

Biochemistry—Study of chemical substances that occur in living organisms, the processes by which these substances enter into or are formed in the organisms and react with each other, and the environment and the methods by which the substances and processes are identified, characterized, and measured

Biophysics—Hybrid science involving the methods and ideas of physics and chemistry to study and explain the structures of living organisms and the mechanics of life processes

Botany—That branch of biological science which embraces the study of plants and plant life; deals with taxonomy, morphology, physiology, and other aspects

Chemistry—the scientific study of the properties, composition, and structure of matter, the changes in structure and composition of matter, and accompanying energy changes

Chronobiology—The study of the effect of time on living systems

Cytology—The branch of biological science which deals with the structure, behavior, growth, and reproduction of cells and the function and chemistry of cells and cell components

Embryology—The study of the development of the organism from the zygote, or fertilized egg

Genetics—The science concerned with biological inheritance, that is, with the causes of the resemblances and differences among related individuals

Geography—The science that deals with the description of land, sea, and air and the distribution of plant and animal life, including humans

Geology—The study or science of earth, its history, and its life as recorded in the rocks; includes the study of the geologic features of an area, such as the geometry of rock formations, weathering, and erosion and sedimentation

Histology—The study of the structure and chemical composition of animal and plant tissues as related to their function

Immunology—The division of biological science concerned with the native or acquired resistance of higher animal forms and humans to infection with microorganisms

Medicine—The study of cause and treatment of human disease, including the healing arts dealing with diseases which are treated by a physician or a surgeon

Organic Chemistry—The study of the composition, reactions and properties of carbon compounds except CO_2, CO, and certain ionic compounds

Pathology—The branch of biological science which deals with the nature of disease, through study of its causes, its processes, and its effects, together with the associated alterations of structure and function; and the laboratory findings of disease, as distinguished from clinical signs and symptoms

Virology—The science that deals with the study of viruses

Zoology—The science that deals with the taxonomy, behavior, and morphology of animal life

II. SELECTED SYNONYMS OF HUMAN NEOPLASMS

Adamantinoma—Ameloblastoma; adamanto-blastoma; multilocular cyst of jaw; epithelial odontome

Adenocystic Carcinoma—Cylindroma

Adenolymphoma—Papillary cystadenoma lymphomatosum; oncocytoma; Warthin's tumor; branchioma; orbital inclusion cyst; branchiogenic adenoma

African Lymphoma—Burkitt's tumor

Ameloblastic Fibroma—Soft odontome

Angioreticuloma—Hemangioblastoma; hemangioendothelioma (Cushing and Bailey)

Angiosarcomas—Angioendotheliomas, angioblastic sarcomas

Basal-Cell Carcinoma—Rodent ulcer; Jacob's ulcer; Basalzellenkrebs of Krompecher

Benign Chondroblastoma—Cartilage-containing giant cell tumor; calcifying giant cell tumor; epiphyseal chondromatous giant cell tumor

Benign Cutaneous Melanoma—Pigmented nevus

Benign Giant Cell Synovioma—Myeloid tumor; xanthoma; villonodular synovitis; tumeur à myeloplaxes

Benign Nodular Hyperplasia—Benign prostatic hypertrophy; chronic lobular prostatitis

Bronchiolar Carcinoma—Alveolar-cell carcinoma; alveolar-cell tumor; pulmonary adenomatosis; bronchio-alveolar carcinoma

Calcifying Epithelial Odontogenic Tumor—Adenoid adamantoblastoma (Thoma and Goldman)

Capillary Haemangioblastoma—von Hippel's disease, von Hippel-Lindau disease

Carotid Body Tumor—Juxtacarotid chemodectoma; nonchromaffin paraganglioma; potato tumor

Carcinoid Tumors gastrointestinal tract)—Enterochromaffinoma, argentaffinoma; karinoide Tumoren (Oberndorfer)

Carcinoma of the Kidney—Hypernephroma, Grawitz tumor; malignant nephroma

Cavernous Angiomas—Cavernoma

Cholangiohepatocarcinoma—Hepatobiliary cancer

"Chondroma" or Chondromatous Hamartoma—Chondroadenoma

Chorion-Epithelioma or Choriocarcinoma—Choriopapillary trophocarcinoma (Friedman and Di Rienzo)

Clear-Cell Hydradenoma—Clear-cell papillary carcinoma; clear-cell myoepithelioma

Clear-Cell Tumor—Adenocarcinoma with clear cells (Hypernephroid) of ovary; mesonephric tumor)

Colloid Cysts of the Third Ventricle—Paraphyseal cysts; neuroepithelial cysts

Craniopharyngioma—Adamantinoma of the pituitary; suprasellar cyst; suprasellar epidermoid cyst; Rathke's pouch tumor, ameloblastoma

Cystic Hyperplasia—Brodie's benign cystic disease; cystophorus desquamative epithelial hyperplasia; Schimmelbusch's disease; fibroadenosis (Atkins); maladie cystique de réclus; Semb's fibroadenomatosis cystica

Desmoid Tumor—Desmoma; desmoid fibromatosis

Diktyoma—Medulloepithelioma

Dysgerminoma—Seminoma; alveolar carcinoma; embryonal carcinoma with lymphoid stroma (Ewing); large cell carcinoma; gonocytoma (Teilum)

Embryonal Carcinoma (Scully and Parham)—Embryoma; teratocarcinoma; trophocarcinoma (Friedman and Di Rienzo)

Embryonic Tumors (of liver)—Embryonal mixed tumor; embryonic hepatoma; hepatoblastoma

Epidermoid Cysts—(Cholesteatoma)

Epithelioma Adenoides Cysticum—Trichoepithelioma

Fibroblastoma (Mallory, Penfield)—Meningioblastoma (Oberling)

Fibroma—Nonosteogenic fibroma; nonossifying fibroma; metaphyseal fibrous defect (Hatcher)

Follicular Adenocarcinoma—Angioinvasive carcinoma or malignant adenoma

Follicular lymphoma—Brill-Symmer disease; lymphoid follicular reticulosis (Robb-Smith); giant follicular lymphadenopathy (Symmer); giant lymph follicle hyperplasia (Brill, Baehr, and Rosenthal)

Ganglioneuroblastomas—Malignant ganglioneuromas

Ganglioneuroma—Ganglioma; sympathicocytoma

Germinoma—Atypical teratoma; pinealoma

Giant-Celled Glioblastomas—Monstrocellular; gigantocellular glioblastoma; spongioblastoma ganglioides

Giant Osteoid Osteoma (Dahlin)—Benign osteoblastoma (Jaffe); osteogenic fibroma (Lichtenstein)

Haemangio-Endothelioma—Angiosarcoma

Hodgkin's Paragranuloma—Early Hodgkin's disease (Jackson); benign Hodgkin's disease (Harrison); indolent Hodgkin's disease (Symmer); reticular lymphoma (Lumb); lymphoreticular medullary reticulosis (Robb-Smith)

Juvenile Aponeurotic Fibroma—Calcifying fibroma

Kaposis Disease—Idiopathic multiple haemorrhagic sarcoma

Keratoacanthoma—Molluscum sebaceum; molluscum pseudocarcinomatosum

Leiomyoma—Myoma; fibroid; fibromyoma

Lipoid-cell Tumor—Adrenocorticoid tumor of ovary; ovarian hypernephroma; luteoma; masculinovoblastoma (Merivale and Forman; Rottino and McGrath)

Liver-Cell Carcinoma—Hepatocellular cancer; malignant hepatoma

Lymphosarcoma—Lymphocytoma; lymphoblastoma; lymphocytic reticulosarcoma; reticulum-cell sarcoma; reticulosarcoma; reticulum-cell lymphosarcoma; stem-cell lymphoma; clasmatocytic lymphoma

Malignant Hydatidiform Mole—Chorioadenoma destruens

Malignant Nonchromaffin Paraganglioma—Alveolar soft-part sarcoma; malignant granular-cell myoblastoma

Malignant Synovioma—Synovioma (Smith); synovialoma; synovial sarcoma; mesothelioma of joints; sarcomesothelioma; malignant angiofibroma

Meningioma—Psammoma (Virchow); dural endothelioma (Golgi, Ribbert); arachnoidal fibroblastoma (Mallory, Penfield); meningioblastoma (Oberling)

"Mesodermal Mixed Tumors" of the Uterus—Malignant mesenchymoma; mesenchymal sarcoma (Ober and Tovell); adenosarcoma (Sophian); dysontogenetic tumor (McFarland); malignant mixed Müllerian neoplasm (Krupp *et al.*)

"Mixed Tumors" of Salivary Glands—Composite tumors; polymorphic adenomas; adenomes metaplastiques polymorphes; enclavomas

Multiple Enchondromatosis—Dyschondroplasia

Multiple-Endocrine-Adenoma Syndrome—Polyendocrine adenomas; pluriglandular adenomatosis; adenomatosis of endocrine glands; familial endocrine adenomatosis

Multiple Myeloma—Mollities ossium (McIntyre, 1850); myelogenous pseudoleukaemia (Zahn, 1885); Köhler's disease (1889); senile osteomalacia (Marchand, 1896); plasma-cell myelosarcoma; myeloma; plasma-cell myeloma; plasmacytoma

Multiple Osteochondromatosis—Diaphysial aclasis (Keith); hereditary deforming dyschondroplasia

Myxoma—Myxosarcoma

Nephroblastoma—Wilms' tumor of kidney, adenosarcoma; embryonal nephroma, "mixed" tumor of kidney; embryonic adenosarcoma

Neurilemoma—Neurolemmoma; Schwann cell tumor, Schwannoma

Neuroblastoma (Wright)—Sympathicoblastoma

Nodular Fasciitis—Subcutaneous pseudosarcomatous fibromatosis; proliferative fasciitis

Osteoclastoma—Giant cell tumor; myeloid sarcoma; tumeur à myeloplaxes

Osteosarcoma—Osteogenic sarcoma; osteoblastic sarcoma

Parosteal Osteosarcoma—Parosteal osteosarcoma; parosteal osteoma (Geschickter and Copeland); juxtacortical osteogenic sarcoma (Jaffe and Selin); parosteal osteogenic sarcoma (Dwinnel *et al.*)

Phaeochromocytoma—Chromaffinoma

Pineoblastoma—Pinealoblastoma

Pineocytoma—Pinealocytoma

Pinealoma—Atypical teratoma of the pineal body

Primary Tumors of Coelomic Surfaces—Mesothelioma

Progressive Recurring Dermatofibroma—Dermatofibrosarcoma protuberans

Reticulum-Cell Sarcoma—Reticulosarcoma; reticulum-cell lymphosarcoma; stem-cell lymphoma; clasmatocytic lymphoma

Retinoblastoma—Neuroblastoma retinae; glioma retinae; neuroepithelioma of the retina; ependymoma retinae

Rhabdoblastic sarcomas—Rhabdosarcomas

Seborrheic Keratosis—Verruca senilis; pigment-forming papilloma; basal-cell papilloma

Seminoma—Spermatocytoma; embryoma; embryonal carcinoma with lymphoid stroma; large cell carcinoma testis; germinoma

Solid Alveolar Carcinoma—Medullary carcinoma; solid carcinoma with amyloid stroma

Solitary Osteochondroma—Solitary osteocartilaginous exostosis

Subependymal Astrocytomas—Subependymal glomerate astrocytoma, subependymoma

Subependymal Giant-Celled astrocytomas—Tuberose sclerosis (syn. Astrocytome sousependymaire à grosses cellules fusiformes, Roussy and Oberling, 1931.)

Subependymomas—Subependymal glomerate astrocytoma (Boykin *et al.*, 1954); subependymal astrocytoma (French and Bucy, 1948)

Syringocystadenoma Papilliferum—Superficial

hidradenoma

Tumors of Specialized Gonadal Stroma (Mostofi)—Androblastoma (Teilum); Sertoli-cell tumor (Collins and Symington); granulosa-theca-cell tumor of testis

III. GENERAL TERMS

Anaplasia (ONCOL)—Reversion of cells to an embryonic, immature, or undifferentiated state; degree usually corresponds to malignancy of a tumor

Carcinogen (ONCOL)—Any agent that incites development of a carcinoma or any other sort of malignancy

Carcinoid (Argentaffinoma) (ONCOL)—A potentially malignant tumor of the argentaffin cells of the stomach and intestine

Carcinoid Syndrome (ONCOL)—A complex of symptoms arising from the metastasis of a carcinoid tumor to the liver

Carcinoma (ONCOL)—A malignant neoplasm arising from epithelial tissue

Carcinoma *in situ* (ONCOL)—A true malignant tumor of squamous or glandular epithelium in which no invasion of underlying or adjacent structures has occurred

Chronobiology—The study of the effect of time on living systems: also: (a) Anachronobiology—the study of the constructive effects (growth, development, and maturation) of time on a living system; (b) Catachronobiology—the study of the deleterious effects of time on a living system

Chronooncology—The new developing discipline studying the influence of biological rhythms on neoplastic growth; the application of these findings for therapeutical use is included

Differentiation (ONCOL)—Specialization of a tissue or organ to perform a particular function; it is accompanied by characteristic morphologic alterations simulating parent tissue

Epigenesis (EMBRYOL)—Development in gradual states of differentiation

Epigenous (BOT)—Developing or growing on a surface, especially of a plant or plant part

Gall (Phytopathology)—A swelling, tumor, or neoplasm of plant tissue

Genome (GEN)—Genetic endowment of a species

Geochronology (GEOL)—The dating of the events in the earth's history

Immunopathology (MED)—The study of various human and animal diseases in which humoral and cellular immune factors seem important in causing pathological damage to cells, tissues, and the host

Immunotherapy (MED)—The treatment of disease by means of human or animal serum containing antibodies; (a) also known as serotherapy; (b) therapy utilizing immunosuppressives (any drugs or agents used to suppress antibody production)

Malignant (ONCOL)—Pertaining to the invasive, neoplastic growth into the surrounding tissues; malignancy of tumors in animals is generally connected with the seeding of neoplastic cells to distant body regions, mainly via the blood and lymph vessels; autonomous plant neoplasms, such as crown gall disease, exhibit characteristics of malignancy without metastasis which does not occur in plants; similarly, not all malignant human or animal neoplasms metastasize; theoretically, benign neoplasms in man or animals may practically behave malignantly (such as certain "benign" inoperable brain tumors, exerting pressure in the skull capsule and being uninfluenced by therapy)

Meristem (BOT)—Formative plant tissue composed of undifferentiated cells capable of dividing and giving rise to other meristematic cells as well as to specialized cell types; meristematic cells typically are small, with dense cytoplasm and a large nucleus; representative meristems occur at the tip of stems and roots, and are responsible for the growth of the plant; new cells produced in these regions enlarge and then mature and differentiate; these are primary meristems of the plant; other meristems are the *cambium* which produces secondary *vascular* tissues and the cork cambium, which produces the *periderm*

Metabolite (BIOCH)—A product of intermediary metabolism

Metastasis (ONCOL)—Transfer of the causal

agent (cell or microorganism) of a disease from a primary focus to a distant one through the blood or lymphatic vessels; in oncology: secondary neoplasm derived from the primary malignant neoplasm by the seeding of neoplastic cells

Morphogenesis (EMBRYOL)—Transformation involved in the growth and differentiation of cells and tissue; also known as topogenesis

Mutagen (GEN)—An agent (chemical carginogens?) that raises the frequency of mutation above the spontaneous rate

Neoplasm (ONCOL)—An actively growing tissue composed of cells which have undergone an abnormal type of irreversible differentiation; a cellular tumor that may either be benign or malignant

Papilloma (ONCOL)—A growth pattern of epithelial tumors in which the proliferating epithelial cells grow outward from a surface accompanied by vascularized cores of connective tissue, to form a branching structure

Papillomatous (ONCOL)—Characterized by or pertaining to a papilloma

Papillary Carcinoma (ONCOL)—A carcinoma characterized by finger-like outgrowths

Parenchyma (HISTOL)—(a) In animals, the essential and characteristic tissue of an organ, or a neoplasm, such as the parenchyma of the liver, composed of the hepatocytes in contrast to the supporting stroma of the organ; the liver parenchyma is a type of glandular epithelium; (b) in plants, the basic, fundamental, or ground tissue with photosynthethic, assimilatory, respiratory, storage, supporting, secretory, and excretory functions; parenchyma occurs in leaves, stems, limbs, roots, fruits, and seeds and is at least theoretically comparable to certain members of the group of connective tissues in animals

Pathogenesis (MED)—The study of the origin and course of the development of disease

Polyp (ONCOL)—A nonspecific term signifying a tissue growth of mucous membrane which may be an inflammatory lesion or a true tumor; there are two kinds: (a) pedunculated polyp—a mass of tissue attached to an organ by a freely movable, narrow stalk or pedicle; (b) sessile polyp—a mass of tissue attached by a broad base

Polyposis (ONCOL)—The presence of multiple polyps, usually occurring in the gastrointestinal tract

Sarcoma—A nonepithelial malignant neoplasm deriving from connective, muscle, or nervous tissues

Totipotence (EMBRYOL)—Capacity of a blastomere to develop into a fully formed embryo; (b) ability to generate or regenerate a whole organism from a part

Tumor (MED, PAL, ZOOL, BOT)—(a) Widely used term for a neoplasm as a new growth of tissue, serving no function; (b) a swollen or distended part of the body, or as used in paleontology of a fossil, such as a skull or bone; (c) sometimes also used for a genus-specific phylogenetic condition of bones and known as pachyostosis; (d) in botany and phytopathology, used for a gall

Tumorigenesis (MED)—The study of the origin and course of the development of tumors

FIELD ABBREVIATIONS

ANTH	Anthropology	GEN	Genetics
BACT	Bacteriology	GEOG	Geography
BIOCH	Biochemistry	GEOL	Geology
BIOPH	Biophysics	HIST	Histology
BOT	Botany	IMMUN	Immunology
CHEM	Chemistry	ONCOL	Oncology
CHRBIOL	Chronobiology	PATH	Pathology
CYTOL	Cytology	VIROL	Virology
EPID	Epidemiology	ZOOL	Zoology

Author Index

Subject Index

Genera and Species Index

The content of the book is set in a broad biological background. Many genera and species of the different kingdoms are mentioned. The attached index facilitates the easy use of the genera and species involved. Each species is given with its Latin name (binary nomenclature).

The species of the first kingdom, Animalia (animals), are coded with the A and the number of the phylum (01, 0, 1–31) to which the species belong. The designation is given on the left. In the cases of the vertebrates the classes are also identified (simplified in the case of fishes).* The species numbers are given at the left. Species of the second kingdom, Plantae (plants), are designated by a P. Species of the third kingdom, Fungi (mushrooms) are characterized by F. Species of the fourth kingdom, Protista (Eukaryotic unicells

and colonies), are designated with Pr. Species of the fifth kingdom, Monera (prokaryotic unicells and colonies), are assigned an M. Units of the sixth kingdom, Virus, Chlamidiae, Bedsoniae, have a V before the species name.

Subspecies, races (e.g. in man), breeds (especially in domesticated animals), and strains (especially of laboratory animals and horticultural and agricultural plants) are included in the index as subheadings.

In the cases of man, dog, cat, rat, and mouse the main entry is the popular name, e.g. dog, followed by the different breeds such as the miniature poodle. This is necessary because the dog generally appears as "dog" in the text and not as *Canis familiaris*.

Coding of Taxonomic Units

A = Kingdom ANIMALIA (animals)
A01 = Phylum Mesozoa, mesozoans
A0 = Phylum Porifera, sponges
A1 = Phylum Cnidaria, coelenterates
A2 = Phylum Ctenophora, comb jellies
A3 = Phylum Platyhelminthes, flatworms
A4 = Phylum Nemertea (Nemertinea, Nemertini. (Rhynchocoela), ribbon worms
A5 = Phylum Gnathostomulida, gnathostome worms
A6 = Phylum Acanthocephala, spiny headed worms
A7 = Phylum Entoprocta, pseudocoelomate polyzoans
A8 = Phylum Rotifera, rotifers, wheel animalcules
A9 = Phylum Gastrotricha, gastrotichs
A10 = Phylum Kinorhyncha, kinorhynch worms

A11 = Phylum Nematoda, roundworms
A12 = Phylum Nematomorpha, hairworms
A13 = Phylum Priapulida, priapulid worms
A14 = Phylum Mollusca, molluscs
A15 = Phylum Sipunculida (Sipuncula), peanut worms
A16 = Phylum Echiurida (Echiura), spoon worms
A17 = Phylum Annelida, segmented or annelid worms
A18 = Phylum Onychophora, onychophorans
A19 = Phylum Pentastomida Pentastoma (Linguatulida), tongue worms
A20 = Phylum Tardigrada, water bears
A21 = Phylum Arthropoda, arthropods
A22 = Phylum Phoronida, lophophorate, phoronid worms
A23 = Phylum Ectoprocta, Bryozoa,

Moss animals
A24 = Phylum Brachiopoda, lamp shells
A25 = Phylum Echinodermata, echinoderms
A26 = Phylum Chaetognatha, arrow worms
A27 = Phylum Pogonophora, Brachiata, beard worms
A28 = Phylum Hemichordata, acorn worms
A29 = Phylum Tunicata (Urochordata), sea squirts
A30 = Phylum Cephalochordata, lancelets
A31 = Vertebrata, vertebrates
A31^f = Fishes
A31^a = Amphibians
A31^r = Reptiles
A31^b = Birds
A31^m = Mammals

(The arrangement of the animal phyla is based on Chapter 3.)

* Identification by coding is omitted or simplified where the taxonomy is apparent from the text.

Footnote: Genera and species cited only on pages 252 and 253 were used in the tabular material and are not mentioned in the text.

P = Kingdom Plantae (plants)
P1 = Phylum (division)
     Rhodophyta, red algae
P2 = Phylum (division)
     Phaeophyta, brown algae

P3 = Phylum (division)
     Chlorophyta, green algae
P4 = Phylum (division)
     Charophyta, stoneworts
P5 = Phylum (division)

Bryophyta, liverworts, hornworts, mosses
P6 = Phylum (division)
     Tracheophyta, vascular plants

F = Kingdom Fungi (mushrooms)
Pr = Kingdom Protista (eukaryotic unicells and colonies)

M = Kingdom Monera (prokaryotic unicells and colonies)

V = Kingdom Virus, Chlamydiae, Bedsoniae

Example of the coding system, as followed through in the index:

A (Kingdom) Animals	31 (Phylum) Vertebrate	m (Subgroup, Class) Mammal	Generic and Species Name *Procavia* *capensis*	Popular Name Hyrax

Remarks

Popular names have been given for the convenience of the reader. Major emphasis has been placed on fish, birds, and mammals, because more information is available about them.

In other cases, e.g., *Leo leo*, the lion, the correct name is *Panthera leo* but *Leo leo* is left in the index because it is used in certain cited papers. The index entry reads: A31 *Leo leo* = *Panthera leo*, the lion (followed by page numbers).

In a case such as *Phalanger cuscus* two species may be involved, either *Phalanger maculatus* or *Phalanger orientalis*. We cannot undertake to correct errors of nomenclature made in the original literature.

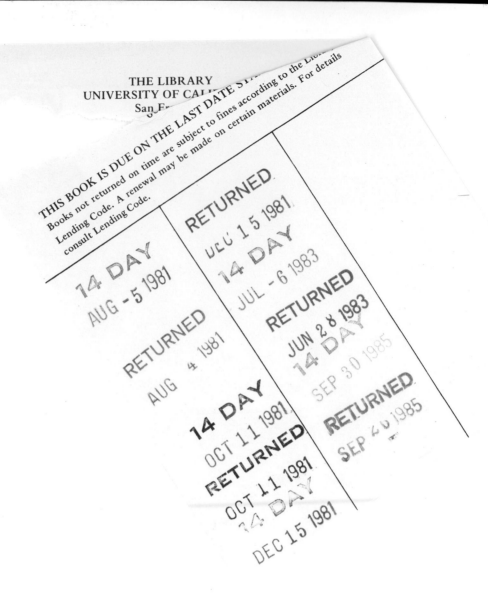